Handbook of BIOLOGICAL PSYCHIATRY

EXPERIMENTAL AND CLINICAL PSYCHIATRY

Series Editor

HERMAN M. VAN PRAAG
Psychiatric University Clinic
Academic Hospital
State University of Utrecht
Utrecht, The Netherlands

Associate Editors

Malcolm H. Lader
Department of Pharmacology
Institute of Psychiatry
University of London
London, England

Samuel Gershon
Department of Psychiatry
New York University Medical Center
New York, New York

Morris Lipton
Department of Psychiatry
Biological Sciences Research Center
University of North Carolina
Chapel Hill, North Carolina

Arthur J. Prange, Jr.
Department of Psychiatry
Biological Sciences Research Center
University of North Carolina
Chapel Hill, North Carolina

Volume 1: HANDBOOK OF BIOLOGICAL PSYCHIATRY, *edited by Herman M. van Praag, Malcolm H. Lader, Ole J. Rafaelsen, and Edward J. Sachar*

Part I: Disciplines Relevant to Biological Psychiatry
Part II: Brain Mechanisms and Abnormal Behavior—Psychophysiology
Part III: Brain Mechanisms and Abnormal Behavior—Genetics and Neuroendocrinology
Part IV: Brain Mechanisms and Abnormal Behavior—Chemistry
Part V: Drug Treatment in Psychiatry—Psychotropic Drugs
Part VI: Practical Application of Psychotropic Drugs and Other Biological Treatments

Volume 2: A PSYCHODYNAMIC APPROACH TO ADOLESCENT PSYCHIATRY: THE MOUNT SINAI EXPERIENCE, *edited by Don R. Heacock*

Volume 3: PSYCHIATRIC CONSULTATION IN THE GENERAL HOSPITAL, *Lewis S. Glickman*

Volume 4: PSYCHOTROPIC DRUGS: PLASMA CONCENTRATION AND CLINICAL RESPONSE, *edited by Graham D. Burrows and Trevor R. Norman*

Volume 5: PSYCHIATRY AROUND THE GLOBE: A TRANSCULTURAL VIEW, *Julian Leff*

Volume 6: PSYCHOPHARMACOLOGY UPDATE: TRENDS FOR THE 1980s, *edited by John J. Schwab*

(other volumes in preparation)

Handbook of BIOLOGICAL PSYCHIATRY

in six parts

PART IV

Brain Mechanisms and Abnormal Behavior—Chemistry

Editor

HERMAN M. VAN PRAAG

Psychiatric University Clinic, Academic Hospital
State University of Utrecht, Utrecht, The Netherlands

Associate Editors

Malcolm H. Lader

Department of Pharmacology, Institute of Psychiatry
University of London, London, England

Ole J. Rafaelsen

Psychochemistry Institute, Rigshospitalet
Copenhagen, Denmark

Edward J. Sachar

New York State Psychiatric Institute and Department of
Psychiatry, College of Physicians and Surgeons, Columbia
University, New York, New York

MARCEL DEKKER, INC. New York and Basel

Library of Congress Cataloging in Publication Data
Main entry under title:

Brain mechanisms and abnormal behavior–chemistry.

(Handbook of biological psychiatry ; pt. 4) (Experimental and clinical psychiatry ; v. 1, pt. 4)
Includes indexes.
1. Brain chemistry. 2. Mental illness. 3. Brain–Diseases. 4. Psychotropic drugs. I. Praag, H. M. van (Herman Meir van), [date]. II. Series. III. Series: Experimental and clinical psychiatry ; v. 1, pt. 4.
[DNLM: 1. Endocrinology–Handbooks. 2. Mental disorders–Handbooks. 3. Neurochemistry–Handbooks. 4. Psychiatry–Handbooks. 5. Psychopharmacology–Handbooks. 6. Psychophysiology–Handbooks. 7. Psychotropic drugs–Handbooks. W1 EX465 v.1 1979 / WM 100 H2336]
RC455.4.B5H35 pt. 4 [QP376] 616.89'071s [616.8'071]
ISBN 0-8247-6966-X 81-5489
AACR2

MARCEL DEKKER, INC.
270 Madison Avenue, New York, New York 10016

Current printing (last digit):
10 9 8 7 6 5 4 3 2 1

PRINTED IN THE UNITED STATES OF AMERICA

Contents

Contributors to Part IV

*David V. M. Ashley, Ph.D.** Research Fellow, Miriam Marks Department of Neurochemistry, Institute of Neurology, The National Hospital, London, England

Jules Angst, M.D. Professor of Psychiatry and Director, Research Department, Psychiatric University Clinic, Burghölzli, Zurich, Switzerland

James C. Ballenger, M.D.† Ward Chief, Section on Psychobiology, Biological Psychiatry Branch, National Institute of Mental Health, Bethesda, Maryland

Guiseppe Bartholini, M.D. Director, Department of Research and Development, Synthélabo-L.E.R.S., Paris, France

Cesario Bellantuono, M.D. Assistant, Department of Psychiatry, University of Bari, Bari, Italy; and Visiting Scientist, Laboratory of Clinical Pharmacology, Mario Negri Pharmacology Research Institute, Milan, Italy

Edward D. Bird, M.D.‡ Clinical Scientist, Medical Research Council Neurochemical Pharmacology Unit, Department of Pharmacology, University of Cambridge Medical School, Addenbrooke's Hospital, Cambridge, England

William E. Bunney, Jr., M.D. Chief, Biological Psychiatry Branch, National Institute of Mental Health, Bethesda, Maryland

Doris H. Clouet, Ph.D. Assistant Director, Research Laboratory, Bureau of Laboratories and Testing, New York State Division of Substance Abuse Services, Brooklyn, New York

Silvana Consolo, Ph.D. Laboratory Chief, Laboratory of Cholinergic Neuropharmacology, Mario Negri Pharmacology Research Institute, Milan, Italy

Present Affiliations:

*Senior Research Scientist, Psychobiology, Nestlé Products Technical Assistance Co., Ltd., La-Tour-de-Peilz, Switzerland

†Director of Research and Inpatient Services, Department of Behavioral Medicine and Psychiatry, University of Virginia Medical School, Charlottesville, Virginia

‡Associate Professor of Neuropathology, McLean Hospital and Harvard Medical School, Belmont, Massachusetts; Clinical Associate in Neuropathology, Massachusetts General Hospital, Boston, Massachusetts; and Director of the Brain Tissue Bank, Ralph Lowell Laboratories, McLean Hospital, Belmont, Massachusetts.

Arthur H. Crisp, M.D., D.Sc., F.R.C.P.(E.), F.R.C.Psych. Professor of Psychiatry, Department of Psychiatry, St. George's Hospital Medical School, London, England

Timothy J. Crow, Ph.D., F.R.C.P., M.R.C.Psych. Head, Division of Psychiatry, Clinical Research Centre, Northwick Park Hospital, Harrow, Middlesex, England

*Glenn Craig Davis, M.D.** Chief, Unit on Drug Abuse, Biological Psychiatry Branch, National Institute of Mental Health, Bethesda, Maryland

Alan N. Davison, Ph.D., D.Sc., F.R.C.Path. Professor of Neurochemistry, Department of Neurochemistry, Institute of Neurology, The National Hospital, London, England.

Daniel X. Freedman, M.D. Professor and Chairman, Department of Psychiatry, The University of Chicago, Chicago, Illinois

Silvio Garattini, M.D. Director, Mario Negri Pharmacology Research Institute, Milan, Italy

C. G. Gottfries, M.D. Professor, Psychiatry Research Center, University of Göteborg, St. Jörgen's Hospital, Göteborg, Sweden

Norbert Herschkowitz, M.D., Ph.D. Department of Pediatrics, University of Berne, Berne, Switzerland

Oleh Hornykiewicz, M.D. Professor and Chairman, Institute of Biochemical Pharmacology, University of Vienna, Vienna, Austria

Leslie L. Iversen, Ph.D. Director, Medical Research Council Neurochemical Pharmacology Unit, Department of Pharmacology, University of Cambridge Medical School, Addenbrooke's Hospital, Cambridge, England

Jerome H. Jaffe, M.D.† Professor of Psychiatry, Department of Psychiatry, College of Physicians and Surgeons of Columbia University, and New York State Psychiatric Institute, New York, New York

Irwin J. Kopin, M.D. Chief, Laboratory of Clinical Science, Division of Clinical and Behavioral Research, National Institute of Mental Health, Bethesda, Maryland

Herbert Ladinsky, Ph.D. Chief, Laboratory of Cholinergic Neuropharmacology, Mario Negri Pharmacology Research Institute, Milan, Italy

John M. Littleton, B.Sc., M.B., B.S., Ph.D. Reader in Pharmacology, Department of Pharmacology, University of London, King's College, London, England

Present Affiliations:

*Director, Psychiatric Clinical Research Unit, and Associate Professor of Psychiatry, Department of Psychiatry, The University of Tennessee Center for the Health Sciences, Memphis, Tennessee

†Professor of Psychiatry, Department of Psychiatry, The University of Connecticut Medical School, Farmington, Connecticut, and Veterans Administration Hospital (Newington), Connecticut

Erling T. Mellerup, M.Sc., M.D. Psychochemistry Institute, Rigshospitalet, Copenhagen, Denmark

J. Mark Ordy, Ph.D. Head, Department of Neurobiology, Delta Regional Primate Research Center, Tulane University, Covington, Louisiana

Carlo Perris, M.D. Professor of Psychiatry and Chairman, Department of Psychiatry, Umeå University, Umeå, Sweden

Agu Pert, Ph.D. Research Psychologist, Biological Psychiatry Branch, National Institute of Mental Health, Bethesda, Maryland

Candace B. Pert, Ph.D. Pharmacologist, Biological Psychiatry Branch, National Institute of Mental Health, Bethesda, Maryland

Robert M. Post, M.D. Chief, Section on Psychobiology, Biological Psychiatry Branch, National Institute of Mental Health, Bethesda, Maryland

Ole J. Rafaelsen, M.D. Professor of Biological Psychiatry, Psychochemistry Institute, Rigshospitalet, Copenhagen, Denmark

Henk Rigter, Ph.D. CNS Pharmacology Department, Organon International B.V., Oss, The Netherlands

*Werner T. Schlapfer, Ph.D.** Research Physiologist, Veterans Administration Medical Center, San Diego, California; and Department of Psychiatry, University of California at San Diego School of Medicine, La Jolla, California

Mogens Schou, M.D., F.R.C.Psych.(Hon.) Professor and Research Director, Psychopharmacology Research Unit, Aarhus University Institute of Psychiatry, The Psychiatric Hospital, Risskov, Denmark

John R. Smythies, M.D. Ireland Professor of Psychiatric Research and Biochemistry, University of Alabama in Birmingham, Birmingham, Alabama

Larry R. Squire, Ph.D. Psychologist, Psychology Service, Veterans Administration Medical Center, San Diego, California; and Associate Professor of Psychiatry, Department of Psychiatry, University of California at San Diego School of Medicine, La Jolla, California

Marie E. Stewart, B.Sc.(Hons) Bedford College, University of London, London, England

Herman M. van Praag, M.D., Ph.D. Professor and Head, Department of Psychiatry, Psychiatric University Clinic, Academic Hospital, State University of Utrecht, Utrecht, The Netherlands

Henk van Riezen, M.D., Ph.D. Methodology Group, Medical Unit, Organon International B.V., Oss, The Netherlands

Willem M. A. Verhoeven, M.D. Psychiatrist and Neurologist, Department of Psychiatry, Academic Hospital, State University of Utrecht, Utrecht, The Netherlands

**Present Affiliation:* Chief, Western Research and Development Office, Veterans Administration Medical Center, Livermore, California

Contents of Other Parts of the Handbook

Part I: Disciplines Relevant to Biological Psychiatry

The History and Scope of Biological Psychiatry, *E. Robins and V. E. Ziegler* Statistics, *B. Andersen* • Research Planning: Studies of Cerebrospinal Fluid Metabolites and Blood Cell Enzymes, *R. M. Post and D. L. Murphy* • Measurement in Psychiatry, *M. Hamilton* • Experimental Psychology, *A. F. Sanders* The Relevance of Epidemiological Methods, Techniques, and Findings for Biological Psychiatry, *R. W. Shapiro and E. Strömgren* • Human Ethology and Psychiatry, *J. Richer* • Child Development, *P. Graham* • Cyclic Processes and Abnormal Behavior, *F. A. Jenner and J. Damas-Mora* • Genetic Concepts for Psychopathology, *D. R. Hanson and I. I. Gottesman* • Animal Models of Relevance to Biological Psychiatry, *S. D. Iversen* • Animal Models of Psychiatric Disorders, *R. Kumar* • The Teaching of Psychopharmacology, *O. J. Rafaelsen* • The Teaching of Research in Biological Psychiatry, *B.-E. Roos* • Classification of Psychiatric Disorders, *N. C. Andreasen and R. L. Spitzer*

Part II: Brain Mechanisms and Abnormal Behavior—Psychophysiology

General Considerations, *L. C. Walrath and J. A. Stern* • Peripheral Measures, *D. A. T. Siddle, G. Turpin, J. A. Spinks, and D. Stephenson* • Peripheral Measures of Schizophrenia, *P. H. Venables* • Central Measures in Schizophrenia, *B. Saletu* • Peripheral Indices of Depressive States, *M. J. Christie, B. C. Little, and A. M. Gordon* • Central Measures of Depression, *C. Perris* The Psychophysiology of Anxiety, *M. H. Lader* • Psychopathy, *R. D. Hare* Alcoholism, *P. Naitoh* • Aggression, *J. W. Hinton* • Brain-Damaged Patients, *F. A. Holloway and O. A. Parsons* • Sleep and the Sleep Disorders, *E. L. Hartmann* • Psychophysiology of Sexual Dysfunction, *J. Bancroft* • Childhood Disorders, *E. Taylor* • Psychological Factors in Physical Disease, *J. P. Henry*

Part III: Brain Mechanisms and Abnormal Behavior—Genetics and Neuroendocrinology

Genetic Aspects of Schizophrenia, *D. Rosenthal* • Genetics of Affective Psychoses, *E. Zerbin-Rüdin* • Genetic Factors in Neurosis, Psychopathy, and Alcoholism, *E. Zerbin-Rüdin* • The Relevance of Psychiatric Genetics to Psychiatric Epidemiology and Nosology, *J. Mendlewica* • Neuroanatomy and Neuropharmacological Regulation of Neuroendocrine Function, *S. Lal and J. B. Martin* • Neuroendocrine Approaches to Psychoneuropharmacologic Research, *E. J. Sachar* • Clinical Application of Neuroendocrine Research in Depression, *B. J. Carroll* • Hormonal Response to Stress in Mental Illness, *M. Ackenheil*

Handbook of
BIOLOGICAL PSYCHIATRY

BIOCHEMICAL DETERMINANTS OF ABNORMAL BEHAVIOR

1

Biochemical Determinants of Schizophrenic and Toxic Psychoses

Timothy J. Crow
Clinical Research Centre, Northwick Park Hospital
Harrow, Middlesex, England

I. NATURE OF SCHIZOPHRENIA

A. Identification of the Syndrome

Studies of the chemical basis of schizophrenia are unlikely to progress unless they take account of disagreements as to the nature of the disease and its differentiation from other psychiatric illnesses. Biological studies have been influenced by increasing interest in standardized systems of diagnosis such as the Present State Examination, and it is possible that such studies will themselves contribute to the identification of core or nuclear syndromes, if such exist, and perhaps to the subdivision of the group of schizophrenias into diseases of fundamentally differing pathogenesis.

The distinction between functional and organic psychoses has traditionally been made on the basis of the presence of intellectual impairment in the latter case. Such a dichotomy carries the implication that the mechanisms of pathogenesis in the two cases are quite different, but the distinction may not be so well founded as has been generally supposed. Some recent studies (e.g., Lilliston, 1973; Depue, 1976) focused on impairments of intellectual function in patients with chronic schizophrenia, and in the past there have been claims that schizophrenic patients with the "severe nuclear" form of the disease (Asano, 1967) or with "mental deterioration" (Haug, 1962) show increased ventricular size on pneumoencephalography. These findings are consistent with those of a recent study with the EMIscan (computerized axial tomography) technique, in which it was demonstrated that a group of chronic institutionalized schizophrenic patients showed increased ventricular size by comparison with an age- and premorbid-occupation-matched control group, and that within the schizophrenic group increased ventricular size was correlated with indices of intellectual impairment (Johnstone et al., 1976, 1978b). Thus, there are some patients with long-standing schizophrenia whose illness resembles an organic psychosis more closely than had been thought. Arguments based upon the distinction between the features of the organic states and acute schizophrenia may therefore be less cogent when applied to the chronic state.

Similar issues arise in relation to the differentiation of schizophrenia from the affective disorders. Kraepelin's criterion of deterioration identifies, at least with hindsight, a group of patients who differ in a fundamental respect from patients with affective disorders, but also from many patients who would be considered to suffer from a schizophrenic illness by other criteria. Unfortunately, the phenomenon of deterioration has attracted relatively little interest as a dimension for chemical research. Yet it may be argued, even on the basis of current findings, that there are basic biological differences between acute and chronic schizophrenic patients, and possibly also between acute and chronic schizophrenic illnesses.

Attempts to avoid the difficulties associated with the retrospective Kraepelinian criterion have focused on the possibility of identifying characteristic psychopathological features in the acute presentation. Bleuler's fundamental symptoms of disturbed association and affectivity, and ambivalence (the altered simple functions) have the substantial shortcoming that they lack an operational definition. Schneider's first rank symptoms are in this respect superior and have been incorporated with some modifications into the standardized diagnostic system of the Present State Examination (Wing et al., 1974).

While diagnostic rules based upon such standard systems can identify a particular group of patients (e.g., those with the nuclear syndrome) with a degree of reliability, it does not necessarily follow either that this group of patients will resemble each other in some fundamental disturbance or that, if such a disturbance exists, it does not also occur in some other nonnuclear schizophrenic patients. Thus the status of patients suffering from schizo-affective psychoses (Kasanin, 1933), schizophreniform psychoses (Langfeldt, 1937), psychogenic psychoses (Faergeman, 1945), and cycloid psychoses (Leonhard, 1959; Perris, 1974) remains ambiguous, at least for the time being. From the point of view of biochemical studies there is no alternative to specifying with whatever precision can be achieved the diagnostic criteria adopted. Where possible, different systems of diagnosis should be applied to the clinical data in an attempt to identify chemical or biological correlates of specific psychopathological features (see, e.g., Rodnight et al., 1976).

B. Meaning of the Characteristic Symptoms

The fact that functional psychoses can be differentiated phenomenologically from organic states may throw some light on pathogenesis. As Bonhoeffer (1909) pointed out, the psychological features of acute psychotic reactions associated with physical disease (the "exogenous psychoses") as various as infection, cachexia, anemia, uremia, jaundice, diabetes, and thyroid disturbance can hardly be distinguished. Although the metabolic disturbance in each of these cases must be quite different, the psychiatric consequences are similar. This suggests that in each case there is a generalized disturbance of cerebral metabolism in cells involved in cognitive activities. Similar arguments apply to the chronic organic states, the dementias, illnesses which share with the acute organic psychoses disturbances of learning capacity and intellect.

Yet the functional psychoses can with certain reservations (see Section I.A) be distinguished phenomenologically from the acute and chronic organic psychoses. Therefore, it may be argued that if the organic psychoses are the indiscriminate end result of a variety of metabolic and structural insults on a significant fraction of the total cerebral cell mass, the functional psychoses must result from a cellular disturbance of a more discrete nature, i.e., which affects only a proportion of these cells. Moreover, if only certain cells or cell systems are affected by these disturbances, these cells presumably must have chemical characteristics which distinguish them from other systems of cells not so affected. The identity of the neurotransmitter is a functionally important feature which distinguishes systems of neurons. It may be suggested, therefore, that the phenomenology of the functional psychoses is consistent with the hypothesis that there is a neurohumoral disturbance but is more difficult to reconcile with any theory which predicts a generalized disturbance of neuronal function.

The case that the underlying disturbance in schizophrenia is of a specific chemical nature would be greatly strengthened by evidence that these psychological changes could be either improved or exacerbated in patients, or induced in normal subjects, by specific drugs. For such evidence to be compelling, however, it is necessary to demonstrate that where such changes are induced in normal subjects they are of a characteristically schizophrenic type and where drug-induced improvements or exacerbations are observed in schizophrenic patients the changes occur in the typically schizophrenic symptoms.

C. Precipitants of Schizophrenic Psychoses

The fact that illnesses similar to schizophrenia occur in association with certain neurological disorders and can be precipitated by various physical and chemical insults may provide a clue to the nature of the disorder. It is sometimes suggested that a diagnosis of schizophrenia should be considered only in the absence of evidence of organic brain disease. Thus defined, schizophrenia is a disease of unknown etiology with an incidence which diminishes with increasing knowledge. It seems a more rational procedure (McClelland et al., 1976) to diagnose the syndrome on the basis of the presenting features. Thus the physical and other causes of schizophrenia-like psychoses may throw some light on the nature of the disturbance.

The best established association of schizophrenia-like psychoses is with temporal lobe epilepsy. Gruhle (1936) reviewed a number of earlier case studies and described eight cases in which epilepsy and a chronic paranoid psychosis had coexisted; in seven of these cases the epilepsy preceded the schizophrenic illness by several years. Pond (1957) described a series of epileptic patients who had paranoid ideas which could be systematized: ideas of influence, auditory hallucinations, and occasional thought disorder with neologisms and condensed words. However, Pond felt that there were differences, at least of a quantitative kind, between these paranoid states and true schizophrenic psychoses in that in his series of cases there was little affective change and no deterioration into a hebephrenic state.

The most systematic study, involving a total of 69 cases, of epilepsy and schizophrenia was carried out by Slater and Beard (1963). They concluded that it was most unlikely that the association was a chance one and that the onset of the psychosis occurred after epilepsy had been present for a mean of 14.1 years. The onset was often insidious, and many patients progressed to a chronic state. Most showed delusion formation and auditory hallucinations of a typically schizophrenic kind. These authors concluded that there was no cardinal feature of schizophrenia, including affective change, which could not be seen in their patients. Nevertheless, catatonic phenomena were unusual and loss of affective response was considered to occur at a later stage and be less severe than in a comparable group of schizophrenic patients. Among these patients there was a great excess (77%) with evidence of a temporal lobe focus. There is thus a strong case for regarding temporal lobe epilepsy as a precipitant of an illness which has typically schizophrenic features.

Other neurological precipitants of schizophrenia are less certain. Slater and Beard (1963) found a small number of cases in which the epileptic focus was centrencephalic. In this case the association with schizophrenia may be a chance one. Feuchtwanger and Mayer-Gross (1938) and Hillbom (1960) both described schizophrenic psychoses apparently following brain injury. Hillbom reported 11 such cases from a total of 415 cases of brain injury. A number had lesions in the temporal lobe, although some were parietal or frontal.

Recently there has been renewed interest in the possibility that there may sometimes be viral precipitants of schizophrenic illnesses (see, e.g., Torrey and Petersen, 1976; Crow, 1978). Catatonic symptoms are occasionally seen in association with diseases of an infective, presumably viral, etiology (Penn et al., 1972; Raskin and Frank, 1974) and schizophrenia-like psychoses have been reported in association with influenza (Menninger, 1926). Schizophrenic symptoms may also be the presenting feature of illnesses which later appear likely to have been acute viral encephalitides (Weinstein et al., 1955; Sobin and Ozer, 1966; Misra and Hay, 1971). The features, if any, by which such illnesses can be differentiated from schizophrenia are unclear, as is the question of whether schizophrenia-like symptoms may be associated with particular viruses. The fact that some experimental viral encephalitides in mice may induce specific changes in catecholamine systems (Lycke and Roos, 1975) suggests that such agents sometimes interact with chemically identified neuronal systems. Moreover, recognition of the existence of slow viral infections of the nervous system with insidious onset and without the characteristic histopathological changes of the more acute encephalitic processes (Johnson and Herndon, 1974) has reopened the question of infection as a possible factor in some functional psychoses.

A virus-like agent has recently been detected in the CSF of a proportion of patients with apparently typical schizophrenic illnesses (Tyrrell et al., 1979; Crow et al., 1979a) with tissue culture techniques. This agent has not been regularly passaged and for this reason knowledge of its characteristics is limited. The same or an apparently similar agent has been detected in patients with other serious or progressive neurological or psychiatric disease, e.g., multiple sclerosis and Huntington's chorea. The relationship between the presence of this agent or agents and the disease process is as yet unclear, but one possibility is that a previously unidentified virus (or group of viruses) is widely distributed in the population but has pathogenic effects only in subgroups of individuals with a genetic predisposition to particular neurological or psychiatric diseases.

By far the most fertile models for schizophrenia, however, have been the drug-induced psychoses. Following the discovery of its hallucinogenic properties (see Hofmann, 1970), much interest centered on lysergic acid diethylamide (LSD). More recently, and principally because the psychotic changes have been thought to resemble acute paranoid schizophrenia more closely, amphetamine has attracted both clinical and experimental attention. The precise features of these psychoses and the extent to which they may provide a model for schizophrenia are discussed in Section III. Less well publicized have been the psychoses induced by alcohol abuse (alcoholic hallucinoses), which can be distinguished from delirium tremens and other manifestations of the withdrawal syndrome. The question as to whether these illnesses if indistinguishable from schizophrenia can be attributed to a direct action of alcohol has yet to be resolved (Section III). Because these conditions may be chronic and even progressive, there is a possibility that they provide a more faithful model of the schizophrenic process of deterioration than other drug-induced conditions.

The fact that in patients with schizophrenia acute psychotic episodes can be precipitated by environmental stress must also be taken into account. Birley and Brown (1970) found that crises and life changes occurred in the 3-week period preceding relapse in 72% of patients with an acute exacerbation of schizophrenia but in only 23% of patients in a control period. Such an excess of life events was not found in patients who had relapsed after discontinuing medication. These findings were confirmed in a later study (Brown et al., 1972), and Vaughn and Leff (1976) analyzed the extent to which drug therapy appears to protect patients against factors, including an adverse family environment, tending to precipitate relapse.

The paranoid psychoses of later life have much in common with schizophrenic illnesses of earlier onset (Kay and Roth, 1961; Post, 1966), including response to drug therapy, but a striking excess of patients suffer from some form of sensory impairment, particularly deafness. It is likely that deafness per se does not predispose to an increased incidence of schizophrenia (Altschuler and Sarlin, 1963), and the overrepresentation of those with hearing difficulties in samples of patients suffering from paranoid psychoses in later life is therefore probably associated with an onset of hearing loss in adult life. The precise mechanisms involved remain obscure (Cooper, 1976).

D. The Genetic Component

An adequate theory of pathogenesis must take account of the extent to which schizophrenic psychoses are predisposed to by genetic influences. The most compelling evidence for genetic determination comes from concordance studies of mono- and dizygotic twin pairs. In a recent review Shields (1976) concluded that the accumulated evidence from 11 studies suggests that the concordance rate for monozygotic twins lies between 45.6% in the most recent and 65.3% in the older and perhaps somewhat less critical studies. Similar rates are observed in those few studies of monozygotic twins reared apart. By contrast, the concordance rate in same sex dizygotic twins is between 12 and 13.7%. A substantial genetic contribution is further supported by studies of the incidence of schizophrenia in adoptive children (Heston, 1966; Kety et al., 1971) in which it was found that rates of schizophrenia in the children resemble more closely those of their biological than their adoptive parents.

Although this evidence for a genetic component is persuasive, the fact that concordance in monozygotic twins is less than 100% indicates that other factors are also relevant. Moreover, in schizophrenia, unlike Huntington's chorea, data on the mode of inheritance within families are not readily compatible with any one simple theory of genetic transmission (Shields, 1976). In these respects schizophrenia resembles chronic diseases such as diabetes mellitus and rheumatoid arthritis. In both cases there is a substantial genetic predisposition but the factors which precipitate the disease at a point in adult life are mostly obscure.

II. NEUROHUMORAL HYPOTHESES

Besides the hypothesis that there is a dysfunction (either an excess or insufficiency) of one or more neurotransmitters in schizophrenia, two other concepts have been advanced: (1) that some abnormal and psychotogenic substance is synthesized within the body and (2) that some normal metabolic process (e.g., methylation) is quantitatively deranged to give rise to psychogenic derivatives of normal body constituents. However, in either case it is necessary to explain how such postulated "toxins" exert their psychotogenic effects. This must presumably occur by an interaction with some normal and functionally important brain component. The disturbance in acute schizophrenia is likely to be limited to certain neuronal systems (Section I.B), and endogenous psychotogens must presumably interact with specific neurohumoral mechanisms to exert their effects. Therefore, if such psychotogens exist it might be more profitable to look for the neurochemical disturbance rather than the unidentified psychotogen. Thus the toxin or abnormal metabolite theories can be reduced in each case to a simpler neurohumoral hypothesis.

Thudichum, the father of neurochemistry, appears to have taken a similar view. While he held that "many forms of insanity are unquestionably the external manifestations of the effects upon the brain substance of poisons fermented in the body," he did not agree with those who wished to avoid attempting to understand the normal chemistry of the brain and proposed "to carry on research by a kind of fishing for supposed disease poisons, of which, according to my view of the subject, the attempt of the boy to catch a whale in his mother's washing tub is an appropriate parabole." The neurohumoral approach is an attempt to understand brain chemistry at the point of interaction between neurons; neurohumoral hypotheses of schizophrenia are based on the premise that the fundamental disturbance in these conditions occurs at this level.

The first such hypothesis was advanced by Gaddum (1954) and Woolley and Shaw (1954). These authors, impressed by the specificity of the blockade by lysergic acid diethylamide of some pharmacological effects of serotonin, proposed that the psychotogenic effects of LSD were due to central serotonin receptor blockade. By analogy the symptoms of schizophrenia might be attributable to lack of serotonin or a failure of serotonergic transmission. Problems for this hypothesis have been the extent to which the features of the LSD psychosis may differ from those of schizophrenia, and the precise mechanism of action of LSD on central serotonergic processes (see Section III.A).

A distinct but analogous approach has developed from observations on the psychoses induced by amphetamine. Randrup and Munkvad (1966) and their colleagues demonstrated that amphetamine-induced behavioral changes in animals are dependent upon dopamine release and are selectively blocked by administration of drugs which exert antipsychotic effects in humans (Randrup and Munkvad, 1965). From these observations has been developed the hypothesis that neuroleptic drugs exert their antipsychotic effects by blocking cerebral dopamine receptors (the dopamine receptor blockade hypothesis of neuroleptic action) and the related but distinct hypothesis that dopaminergic processes are excessively active in schizophrenia (the dopamine overactivity hypothesis of schizophrenia). These have been the most heuristically fertile concepts in the past 10 years.

More recently the hypothesis has been advanced (Stein and Wise, 1971) that a degeneration of central nonradrenaline-containing neurons might account not so much for the acute florid symptoms of the disease but for the affective flattening and progressive deterioration seen in some schizophrenic illnesses. The theory rests upon observations on the behavioral effects of administration of the neurotoxin 6-OH-dopamine to experimental animals but breaks new ground in attributing a behavioral function (the mediation of the effects of rewarding stimuli) to a specific neurochemical system and attempting to relate a disturbance of this function to the symptoms of the disease.

There have been other neurohumoral hypotheses. Before the defects of GABA function in Huntington's chorea had been described, Roberts (1972) elaborated the theory that there is a deficit of GABA systems. A variant of the dopamine hypothesis is that phenylethylamine is released in excess in schizophrenia. This theory (Sandler and Reynolds, 1976) postulates a neurotransmitter role for phenylethylamine and rests on much of the evidence which is also relevant to the dopamine hypothesis. The discovery of pharmacologically active polypeptides in the brain, and the possibility that some of these peptides have a neurohumoral function, has enlarged the field of speculation. In particular, the opiate peptides can induce catatonia-like syndromes when injected intraventricularly in animal experiments, and this has led to suggestions that such peptides may be either in excess (Bloom et al., 1976) or in deficit (Jacquet and Marks, 1976) in schizophrenia. Somewhat similar considerations stimulated the theory that prostaglandin synthesis may be excessive (Feldberg, 1976), although the opposite view has also been held (Horrobin, 1977). A problem here is the obscurity of the relationship between prostaglandins and specific neurotransmitter mechanisms. However, with both the prostaglandin hypothesis and that concerning the opiate peptides there appear to be testable predictions concerning the therapeutic effects of particular drug regimes.

It will be seen that many of these theories have been influenced by observations on the effects of psychotomimetic drugs, or on drug effects thought to mimic some aspect of schizophrenia, and by the therapeutic effects of neuroleptic drugs. It is arguable that such observations have contributed more to our understanding of the neurochemistry of the psychoses than have the large number of experiments designed to detect possible disturbances of metabolism in these conditions. The strategy of attempting to influence psychological function as a dependent variable is more powerful as a means of elucidating mechanisms than the strategy of following changes correlated with the development or remission of the psychosis. The latter may always be secondary phenomena.

III. MODEL PSYCHOSES

Bonhoeffer (1909), who developed the concept of the "exogenous psychotic reaction," psychoses precipitated by physical disease or by intoxication (the deliria or confusional states, and toxic psychoses), emphasized that a psychological disturbance of a basically uniform kind could be provoked by a wide variety of exogenous influences. While it is true that a number of drugs do induce a clinical picture identical to an acute confusional state, it has been increasingly recognized that there are agents which induce psychotic changes without impairment of consciousness, i.e., without disturbances of memory and orientation. Such drug-induced changes therefore challenge Bonhoeffer's generalization and provide a possible model for schizophrenia.

The variety of substances reported to induce psychotic changes is rather wide (for a comprehensive review, see Davison, 1976). Many of these reports are no more than isolated case studies, but for a number of drugs there have been extensive compilations of data from the clinical literature and for some compounds experimental studies on volunteers. Those of particular relevance to schizophrenia are observations on psychoses provoked by LSD and amphetamine and related stimulant drugs. The psychotic changes associated with alcoholism have been neglected as "model" psychoses and also deserve consideration in this context.

A. LSD Psychosis

LSD, the nucleus of the ergot alkaloids, was synthesized in 1938 by Stoll and Hofmann. Its potent hallucinogenic properties were not discovered until 1943 when Hofmann accidentally ingested a very small quantity (Hofmann, 1970). LSD is now the best studied of the psychotomimetic drugs, a group which also includes mescaline (3,4,5-trimethoxyphenylethylamine), DMT (N,N-dimethyltryptamine), and bufotenin (N,N-dimethyl-5-hydroxytryptamine).

A number of at least partly distinguishable psychotic reactions to LSD are described below.

1. Acute Psychotic State

The effects of LSD in normal subjects (Hollister, 1968) usually last for 6–10 hr and include (1) somatic symptoms: dizziness, weakness, tremors, nausea, drowsiness, paresthesia, and blurred vision; (2) perceptual symptoms: alterations of shape and color, difficulty in focusing, increased auditory acuity, synesthesia; and (3) psychic symptoms: alterations in mood, distortions of time sense, depersonalization, and visual hallucinations.

The extent to which these changes resemble or differ from those seen in schizophrenia has been debated. Sandison (1959) using rating scales concluded that there were a number of differences (see Table 1): the predominance of perceptual changes and the presence of visual and olfactory hallucinations, distortions of bodily image, lability of affect, and retention of insight in the LSD psychosis; and the predominance of auditory hallucinations, flattening of affect, and loss of insight in schizophrenia.

However, this comparison ignores the difficulty of the LSD psychosis being transient and occurring in a setting in which psychotic changes are expected. Schizophrenic illnesses are often insidious in onset and inexplicable. These discrepancies might well account for the differences in affect and insight at least.

Recently, Young (1974) compared the taped responses to a questionnaire of 20 subjects who had experienced an LSD psychosis with 20 young schizophrenic patients and 20 normal controls. Visual hallucinations were only modestly less frequent in the schizophrenic group (45%) than the LSD group (60%). There were no significant differences in measures of thought disorder, motor disturbance, or identity loss. However, delusions were found in 25% of the schizophrenic group and in none of those who had had LSD, and the latter subjects usually retained insight. Unfortunately, in these studies,

Table 1 Comparison of Clinical Features of Acute LSD Reaction and Schizophrenia

Clinical feature	Acute LSD reaction	Schizophrenia
Memory and recall	Mild impairment	Normal
Awareness and concentration	Unimpaired	Unimpaired
Existing perceptions	Distorted or elaborated	Unaffected
Visual hallucinations	Frequent	Rare
Olfactory hallucinations	Frequent	Rare
Tactile hallucinations	Frequent	Frequent
Auditory hallucinations	Rare	Frequent
Insight	Retained	Impaired
Thought block	Frequent	Frequent
Thought distintegration	Very frequent	Very frequent
Flight of ideas	Occasional	Very frequent
Compulsive ideas	Occasional, rational	Frequent, irrational
Delusional thought	Occasional, mainly paranoid	Very frequent
Affect	Labile, anxiety agitation	Flat, incongruous
Relationship to reality	Subjective impairment	Failure to relate to external reality
Body image distortion	Frequent	Rare
Impulsive irrational behavior	Frequent	Frequent
Response to chlorpromazine	Affect and behavior improved	Thought disorder and behavior improved

Source: From Sandison, 1959 as reproduced by Davison, 1976.

relatively little attention was paid to those features (i.e., Schneiderian first rank symptoms) which might be considered particularly characteristic of schizophrenia.

Within these limitations it appears that, although there are differences between LSD psychosis and schizophrenia, it is still possible that such differences be attributable to the circumstances of administration and the time course of the LSD effect.

2. *Prolonged Psychotic Reaction*

Occasional prolonged psychoses, lasting from over 48 hr to several weeks or even months, are reported following single doses of LSD. The incidence may be as high as 9 per 1000 LSD administrations (Malleson, 1971) and paranoid delusions, schizophrenia-like auditory hallucinations and thought disorder, and affective changes are reported as common features (Dewhurst and Hatrick, 1972).

3. *Chronic Psychoses*

After repeated LSD abuse some patients are reported (Cohen and Ditman, 1963; Frosch et al., 1965; Glass and Bowers, 1970) to develop states which closely resemble chronic schizophrenia with flattening of affect, paranoid delusions, thought disorder, and volitional loss. The factors which predispose to such changes and the precise circumstances in which they occur are difficult to determine.

4. *Spontaneous Recurrences ("Flashbacks")*

Recurrences of the hallucinatory experience are reported weeks or even months after recovery from the effects of an acute LSD reaction. Although these experiences can be frightening, insight is usually retained.

In each of these psychoses other than the acute reaction (Section III.A.1) the changes appear to be unpredictable and idiosyncratic. Therefore, although in each case (and particularly in the case of chronic psychoses) the mechanism may be of relevance to the pathogenesis of schizophrenic illnesses, the implications of the clinical observations remain obscure. Only the more or less reliable phenomena of the acute psychosis can reasonably be made the basis for speculation on the pharmacological mechanisms of the psychotic change.

The pharmacological actions have been well studied. At low doses LSD inhibits the firing of the serotonin-containing neurons of the raphe nuclei (Aghajanian et al., 1970), and reduces the turnover of serotonin (Andén et al., 1968). These effects have been interpreted as resulting from stimulation of serotonin receptors, on either the pre- or postsynaptic neuron. LSD may also activate dopamine receptors (Pieri et al., 1974; Da Prada et al., 1975) although some other psychotomimetic drugs such as psilocybin may lack this effect (Fuxe et al., 1976).

B. Amphetamine-Induced Psychosis

Although some earlier cases were reported (e.g., Young and Scoville, 1938; Herman and Nagler, 1954), it is only since the publication of a monograph by Connell (1958) that it has been widely recognized that single large or repeated doses of amphetamine can induce a psychosis which closely resembles paranoid schizophrenia. Connell reported 42 cases and described the clinical picture as "primarily a paranoid psychosis with ideas of reference, delusions of persecution, auditory and visual hallucinations, in a setting of clear consciousness." He stated that there were no physical signs diagnostic of amphetamine psychosis and suggested that the mental picture might be indistinguishable from acute or chronic paranoid schizophrenia. Several of his patients described first rank Schneiderian symptoms.

In an attempt to further define the features of the psychosis, Ellinwood (1967) compared the symptoms of amphetamine abusers with and without psychotic reactions in the acute admission ward of the USPHS Narcotic Hospital in Lexington, Kentucky. Symptoms common to both psychotic and nonpsychotic states included hand-face touching and picking, gritting and gnashing of the teeth, an acute sense of novelty and distortion of time sense, as well as physiological changes including insomnia, alertness, lack of appetite, difficulties in micturition, thirst, diaphoresis, and increased energy. Ellinwood notes that most addicts experienced increased talkativeness, a sense of cleverness and "crystal clear thinking," and appeared to have a hyperacute memory during the period of abuse for both relevant and extraneous material. As the psychosis developed, fear, suspiciousness, awareness of being watched, and visual hallucinations in the periphery increased. In psychotic patients delusions of persecution appeared to be an extension of the feeling of suspicion and awareness of being watched. Fear was prominent and sometimes diminished when a delusional explanation was developed. Auditory hallucinations occurred in half the psychotic patients and developed from the perception of simple noises or voices calling the patient's name. Visual hallucinations were as common and appeared to develop from fleeting glimpses of images in the peripheral field. The voices were usually of unknown identity, were perceived as friendly or evil, and were sometimes conversed with. Gross distortions of bodily image were common. Ellinwood describes how some patients felt that others could see their feelings and read their minds, and others felt capable of projecting themselves to distant locales and of controlling by thought people and objects which might in turn control them. There was a preoccupation with faces and eyes, and strangers were often identified and approached as friends. Ideas of reference developed from suspicion and self-consciousness and into the feeling that messages were directed to the patient from the news media. The more severely disturbed patients talked directly to the television or radio, and these were sometimes viewed as instruments of control and manipulation. With increasing curiosity and changes in awareness, the patient regarded neutral objects as having emotional significance. Changes in libido were variable. With increasing severity of psychosis physical activity tended to decrease and patients were found to be withdrawn and passive.

The close similarity between these changes and many seen in schizophrenic illnesses is apparent. Angrist et al. (1974a) considered whether preservation of affective responsivity as suggested by Slater (1959) or absence of thought disorder as suggested by Bell (1965) might be features which distinguished amphetamine psychosis from idiopathic schizophrenia. However, both flattening of affect and thought disorder were seen in Angrist et al.'s subjects, as was anhedonia in the stage of withdrawal and depression which occurred in most subjects before the onset of the psychosis.

It remained possible that the psychotic changes seen in amphetamine abusers were due not to the pharmacological actions of the drug itself but occurred either as an idiosyncratic response, perhaps in a population predisposed to schizophrenic illnesses, or were secondary to some other consequence of drug ingestion, such as sleep deprivation. These possibilities were demonstrated to be remote in the first study of experimentally induced amphetamine psychoses (Griffith et al., 1972). Nine volunteers who had previously abused amphetamines, but of whom four had never experienced a psychotic reaction, were administered small but frequent doses of dextroamphetamine under close observation. Eight developed typical paranoid psychotic changes, and in two cases this occurred within 24 hr, before sleep deprivation could have been a factor. Thus the psychotic changes are almost certainly a consequence of the pharmacological actions of the drug.

Possible pharmacological mechanisms were pursued by Angrist et al. (1971), who in light of previous evidence that the two isomers of amphetamine differ in their relative effects on noradrenergic and dopaminergic mechanisms compared the psychotomimetic potencies of the two isomers.

D-amphetamine was found to be approximately 1.3 times as potent as l-amphetamine in provoking a psychosis. However, interpretation of this finding is made difficult by the fact that there is substantial disagreement in the literature concerning the relative effects of the two isomers on noradrenergic and dopaminergic mechanisms, some part of this disagreement arising from differences in the relative potencies of the two isomers in different systems, e.g., in inhibiting catecholamine uptake or increasing turnover (Matthysse, 1974). However, the view that excess dopamine release occurs in humans following amphetamine administration is supported by a study of homovanillic acid (HVA) concentrations in CSF following prebenecid administration by Angrist et al. (1974a). These authors observed a substantial increase in the rise in the CSF HVA levels following probenecid administration when the subject was pretreated with amphetamine 250 mg over the 21 hr before lumbar puncture. Thus there is evidence that dopamine release is increased following doses of amphetamine which induce psychotic changes.

The effectiveness of drugs in reversing amphetamine-induced psychological changes may also throw light on the mechanisms of these changes. Espelin and Done (1968) described a series of young children with amphetamine intoxication. In these cases, the symptoms, sometimes including hyperactivity, confusion, mania, and self-injury in addition to thermoregulatory and cardiovascular changes, were rapidly reversed by modest doses of chlorpromazine.

Gunne et al. (1972) observed in experimental subjects that amphetamine-induced euphoria could be reduced by the catecholamine synthesis inhibitor α-methyl-p-tyrosine 3 g daily, and was also reversed by chlorpromazine 50 mg 3 times a day for 5 days. The euphoria was not reduced by α- or β-adrenergic receptor blocking drugs but was effectively inhibited by the relatively selective dopamine receptor antagonist pimozide. Angrist et al. (1974b) administered haloperidol 5 mg i.m. to a series of eight patients with symptoms, in several cases including psychotic changes, induced either by self-administered amphetamine or by amphetamine administered in a controlled situation. Approximately 45 to 60 min after haloperidol administration there was a reduction in symptoms with a significant decrease in ratings of suspiciousness and excitement. Thus it appears likely that at least some of the symptoms induced by amphetamine in humans are reduced by drugs which are known to be potent dopamine receptor blockers.

In animal experiments these issues have been explored in detail. A behavioral syndrome of increasingly stereotyped and repetitive behaviors, often including sniffing, licking, and gnawing, following amphetamines and related compounds has been described in rodents by Randrup and his colleagues, and similar behavioral changes have been seen in a variety of other species (for review, see Randrup and Munkvad, 1967). These behaviors are selectively reversed by neuroleptic drugs (Randrup and Munkvad, 1965) and are abolished by α-methyl-p-tyrosine but not by dopamine-β-hydroxylase inhibition (Randrup and Munkvad, 1966). Thus, there is a strong case that these behaviors are dependent upon central dopamine release, and the involvement of dopaminergic mechanisms is supported by observations (Ernst, 1967) that many of the components of the syndrome can be evoked by administration of the dopamine receptor stimulating drug apomorphine. More recently it has been possible to demonstrate that elements of the syndrome can be eliminated by selective destruction with 6-OH-dopamine of certain central dopaminergic pathways (Creese and Iversen, 1975).

From these observations it is apparent that the major components of the behavioral syndrome induced by amphetamine in animals is dependent upon increased neurotransmitter release from the terminals of central dopamine neurons, and in humans there is evidence both that doses of the amphetamines similar to those which induce schizophrenia-like symptoms increase central dopamine turnover and that at least some of the psychological changes induced by amphetamine can be reversed by drugs such as haloperidol and pimozide, which are relatively selective dopamine receptor blocking agents.

C. Psychoses Provoked by Other Stimulant Drugs

Psychoses provoked by stimulant drugs related to amphetamine are of interest particularly insofar as variations in structure and pharmacological action may be associated with differing psychotomimetic properties. Unfortunately, the available evidence is sparse and is dependent upon individual case reports of uneven quality.

Two types of amphetamine-like action upon central catecholamine neurons are described (Scheel-Krüger, 1972). Drugs such as amphetamine, methylamphetamine, and phenmetrazine are believed to act by releasing the reserpine-resistant (or newly synthesized) catecholamine pool. Psychoses are reported with each of these compounds (for references, see Davison, 1976). A second group of compounds (the pipradol group), including pipradol and methylphenidate, is thought to act by releasing the reserpine-sensitive catecholamine pool. The actions are relatively resistant to single doses of α-methyl-p-tyrosine (Scheel-Krüger, 1972). Nevertheless, psychoses are also reported following administration of compounds of the pipradol group (McCormick and McNeel, 1963; Lucas and Weiss, 1971; Spensley and Rockwell, 1972), although they appear to have been noted less frequently than with drugs of the amphetamine group.

These observations suggest that psychoses resembling the amphetamine psychosis may be provoked by any drug which induces excess catecholamine release from nerve endings. However, paranoid psychoses following cocaine are also well recognized (Kraepelin, 1923; Jacobi, 1927; Post, 1975) and the action of cocaine differs from that of both the groups of stimulant drugs described by Scheel-Krüger. In behavioral experiments cocaine does not by itself induce dopamine release but when administered in combination with monoamine oxidase inhibitors provokes typical amphetamine-like effects (Christie and Crow, 1973). These findings are compatible with catecholamine uptake blocking activity (Trendelenburg, 1966). Thus it sppears that paranoid psychoses can be induced by drugs which potentiate central catecholaminergic transmission either by inducing amine release or inhibiting the reuptake process. The fact that such psychoses are not observed following administration of tricyclic antidepressant drugs, many of which are potent inhibitors of the noradrenaline and serotonin uptake processes, once more focuses attention upon dopaminergic transmission.

An interesting case is that of ephedrine. Apparently typical psychoses are reported with this drug (Herridge and A'Brook, 1968). Yet ephedrine is a much less effective releaser of dopamine than the amphetamines (Christie and Crow, 1971) and resembles noradrenaline in possessing a β-hydroxy group on the ethylamine side chain. It is therefore interesting that in one case the psychotic symptoms were resistant to treatment with phenothiazines. There appears to be a possibility that the mechanism of the ephedrine psychosis is not identical with that of the amphetamine-induced syndrome.

D. Alcohol-Induced Psychoses

Of the various psychiatric syndromes associated with alcoholism, the chronic hallucinosis which occurs without clouding of consciousness and can be distinguished from delirium tremens is of particular interest. The relation of the syndrome to withdrawal is not entirely clear, and in some cases a schizophrenia-like picture continues in spite of abstinence (Benedetti, 1952; Victor and Hope, 1958). Some suggest (e.g., Alpert and Silvers, 1970) that there are differences between the phenomenology of alcoholic and schizophrenic hallucinations, e.g., that the hallucinations in the former case are more frequent and continuous, are localized in space rather than in the body, and are often unintelligible and emerge from a background of noise. Others e.g., Victor and Hope, 1958) have maintained that the illnesses are indistinguishable.

Heavy alcohol consumption is associated with admission to hospital with a diagnosis of schizophrenia (Davison, 1976), and a comparison of alcoholics with and without hallucinosis (Schuckit and Winokur, 1971) revealed no excess family or previous history of schizophrenia. Therefore, it seems possible that in some patients alcohol abuse is a direct precipitant of a schizophrenia-like illness. The mechanisms by which this may occur have so far attracted no serious attention.

E. Other Potential Psychotomimetic Drugs

A variety of drugs with modes of action distinct from the amphetamines also induce psychotic reactions, but in most of these cases the form of the psychosis is recognizably different from the typical amphetamine-induced paranoid syndrome. In some cases (e.g., following anticholinergics) the form of the psychosis can be linked to a specific site of action. In others (e.g., following dopamine receptor stimulant agents, such as apormorphine) the failure to observe a paranoid syndrome, or to observe such a syndrome consistently, may throw some light on the possible mechanisms of the amphetamine psychosis.

1. Anticholinergic Drugs

The psychological effects of cholinergic blockade are well described following atropine administration to psychiatric patients (Forrer and Miller, 1958) and after hyocine in normal volunteers (Crowell and Ketchum, 1967). Besides the effects of peripheral cholinergic blockade, the major features are disorientation and confusion with visual hallucinations. Illusions and auditory hallucinations, and abnormal, nonpurposive, and sometimes repetitive behaviors may also occur.

Similar features are noted in parkinsonian patients treated with anticholinergic drugs (Stephens, 1967), although in such patients anxiety and delusions of persecution are also recorded. Symptoms appear to be more common in elderly patients, particularly those with evidence of arterial disease, and in those with previous episodes of confusion induced by drugs.

Anticholinergic drugs therefore induce a typical exogenous psychotic reaction or acute confusional state. Since a central feature which differentiates the organic from the functional psychoses is impairment of learning capacity, it is of particular interest that anticholinergic drugs appear to exert relatively specific effects upon performance on learning tasks (Crow and Grove-White, 1973; Crow et al., 1976a; Drachman and Leavitt, 1974). It appears that a cholinergic link is a necessary component of the mechanism for processing new information into memory, and that interference with this step can provoke all the symptoms of an acute organic reaction. That the role of cholinergic mechanisms in the organic states is not confined to acute psychoses is suggested by recent observations that choline acetyltransferase activity is significantly and relatively selectively diminished in the brains of patients with Alzheimer's disease (Davies and Maloney, 1976) and senile dementia (Bowen et al., 1976; Perry et al., 1977).

2. L-dopa

The effectiveness of L-dopa as replacement therapy in parkinsonism has encouraged the view that this precursor may act as a dopamine receptor agonist. However, this may not be the case. Intact catecholamine uptake processes and mechanisms for egulating amine synthesis may tolerate changes in precursor availability within wide limits without changes in dopamine release taking place. Psychiatric changes following L-dopa are observed in up to 20% of parkinsonian patients (Goodwin, 1972) but are most heterogeneous in type. Affective changes and confusion are common, and paranoid changes also occur but are probably less frequent. A similar range of psychiatric changes was noted when L-dopa was administered to nonpsychotic psychiatric patients in doses up to 8.8 g/day (Sathananthan et al., 1973). It seems unlikely that these rather diverse psychiatric changes can be attributed to a single pharmacological consequence of L-dopa administration.

3. Apomorphine

Any simple theory that increased activation of dopamine receptors underlies the development of paranoid symptoms predicts that drugs such as apomorphine, which appears to act directly upon the dopamine receptor (Ernst, 1967), will provoke such symptoms. However, there is little evidence that this is the case. Before the introduction of neuroleptics apomorphine was quite widely used in the treatment of psychiatric patients (Feldman et al., 1945) yet exacerbations of psychotic symptoms were not noted, nor have they been seen more recently in the treatment of parkinsonism with this drug. In a carefully controlled trial, Lal and de la Vega (1975) examined the effects of apomorphine 1 mg 3 times daily for 14 days in 40 subjects. No schizophrenic symptoms or increase in ratings of symptoms associated with schizophrenia were noted.

4. *ET-495*

ET-495, like apomorphine, appears to activate the dopamine receptor by a direct action (Corrodi et al., 1971). Oral or intravenous administration of ET-495 to schizophrenic patients, some nonschizophrenic psychiatric patients, and one or two normal subjects failed to provoke the psychotic changes or exacerbations which had been expected (Gershon et al., 1977).

5. *Disulfiram*

Disulfiram (tetraethylthiuramdisulfide) inhibits aldehyde dehydrogenase but also inhibits dopamine-β-hydroxylase and depletes brain noradrenaline stores (Goldstein and Nakajima, 1967). Its psychological effects are therefore of interest and there are many reports of psychotic reactions occurring during the course of the drug's use in the treatment of alcoholism. A review of 52 cases in the literature (Liddon and Satran, 1967) concluded that in approximately 80% of cases signs of delirium (disorientation, slurred speech, ataxia, or drowsiness) were present. Affective, paranoid, and delusional changes were often also present, and such changes could occur in the absence of delirium. However, when this was the case affective symptoms were common and in only one patient were the psychiatric symptoms thought to resemble those of paranoid schizophrenia. A more recent survey (Hotson and Langston, 1976) concluded that in those cases which were adequately reported the incidence of disorientation and impairment of memory is even higher (at 90%). Therefore, insofar as the psychiatric symptoms can be attributed to dopamine-β-hydroxylase inhibition the literature provides little evidence that central noradrenaline depletion is associated with a schizophrenia-like picture.

F. Summary

The literature on the model psychoses induced by centrally acting drugs has proved a most productive source of hypotheses concerning the chemical mechanisms of the schizophrenias. It is apparent that many of the features of schizophrenia occur in the LSD psychosis, although at least in the short term delusions are less common and insight is better preserved in this condition than in schizophrenia. Since activation of the serotonin receptor, whether pre- or postsynaptic, appears to underly many of the actions of LSD, disturbances at this site in schizophrenia must be considered. However, by far the least well-understood aspect of the actions of LSD are the mechanisms of the prolonged and, if they are really to be attributed to the drug, chronic psychoses.

Connell's thesis that the amphetamine psychosis very closely resembles acute paranoid schizophrenia is now well established. The psychosis appears to be a direct pharmacological effect of the drug, and there is evidence that dopamine release is increased in man by these doses of amphetamine. The psychosis is seen following drugs such as pipradol and methylphenidate which act upon the reserpine-sensitive catecholamine pool, as well as those like amphetamine which act upon newly synthesized catecholamines. The fact that paranoid psychoses are seen following cocaine but not following drugs such as the tricyclic antidepressants, which inhibit the uptake process into noradrenaline- and serotonin- but not dopamine-containing neurons, again focuses attention on dopaminergic processes. However, the fact that schizophrenia-like psychoses or changes are not commonly reported following drugs which act directly upon dopamine receptors and are seen following ephedrine, which is not a potent dopamine-releasing agent, raises difficulties for the dopamine hypothesis.

The psychosis seen following anticholinergic drugs and disulfiram appear to have the features of an acute confusional state rather than schizophrenia.

IV. DRUG-INDUCED IMPROVEMENTS IN SCHIZOPHRENIA

A. Specificity of Neuroleptics

The effectiveness of neuroleptic drugs in acute schizophrenia is well established (for references, see Klein and Davis, 1969). That the effect is not due to simple sedation was established in trials in which phenothiazine compounds were compared with barbiturates and placebo (Casey et al., 1960a,b). The results of these studies (Fig. 1) suggest that barbiturates are no more effective than placebo and also that there are some phenothiazines (e.g., promazine) which are quantitatively less effective than the prototype compound chlorpromazine. A review of the extensive literature of controlled trials in acute schizophrenia (Klein and Davis, 1969; see their table 1) suggests that many phenothiazines have a therapeutic effectiveness equal but not unequivocally superior to chlorpromazine although one of two compounds (e.g., promazine, mepazine) are less effective. This suggests that there is a pharmacological property shared by many phenothiazines which when present gives maximum therapeutic benefit in schizophrenia but that mepazine and promazine have less of this activity than the standard neuroleptics.

An analysis of the placebo-drug differences over a wide range of symptoms in a 4-week trial reveals something of the nature of the antipsychotic effect (Goldberg et al., 1965). The results (Fig. 2) suggest that the drugs are effective not only in ameliorating the more florid (e.g., ideas of persecution,

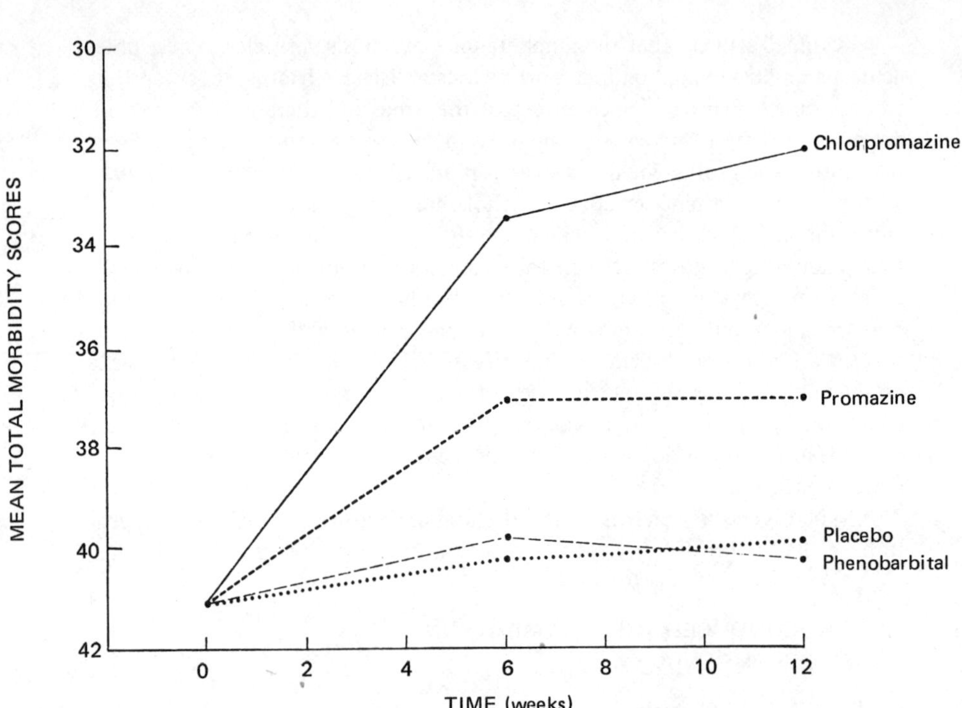

Figure 1 Reductions in total morbidity scores in acute schizophrenia in patients treated with chlorpromazine or promazine compared to placebo or phenobarbital. (From Klein and Davis, 1969; data from Casey et al., 1960a, 1961.)

hallucinations, agitation, and tension) but also some negative or "passive" features (e.g., indifference to the environment, lack of self-care and social participation). It has also been claimed (Klein and Davis, 1969; see their table 7) that the evidence from several studies suggests that drug-control differences are at least as great on Bleuler's fundamental symptoms (thought disorder, blunting of affect, withdrawal, and autism) as on the accessory symptoms (hallucinations, paranoid ideation, grandiosity, hostility, resistiveness), and greater on both of these groups than on nonschizophrenic symptoms.

The findings certainly suggest that neuroleptic drugs can modify a range of typically schizophrenic symptoms and thus may be considered to have antipsychotic rather than antianxiety or other tranquilizing or sedative effects. The question of whether these effects cover the whole range of schizophrenic symptoms is considered below (Section IV.B).

B. Mechanism of the Antipsychotic Effect

It was early recognized that phenothiazines with antipsychotic activity often induce a syndrome with all the features of Parkinson's disease and suggested (e.g., Flügel, 1953; Deniker, 1960) that extrapyramidal effects might be related to the antipsychotic action. This was debated (Cole and Clyde, 1961; Bishop et al., 1965; Chein and di Mascio, 1967) and generally discounted on the grounds that there are some drugs (e.g., thioridazine) which exert antipsychotic effects equal to chlorpromazine but have a lesser incidence of extrapyramidal side effects (NIMH-PSC, 1964).

However, with the introduction of the thiaxanthenes and butyrophenones, many of which have been demonstrated to have antipsychotic effects and also

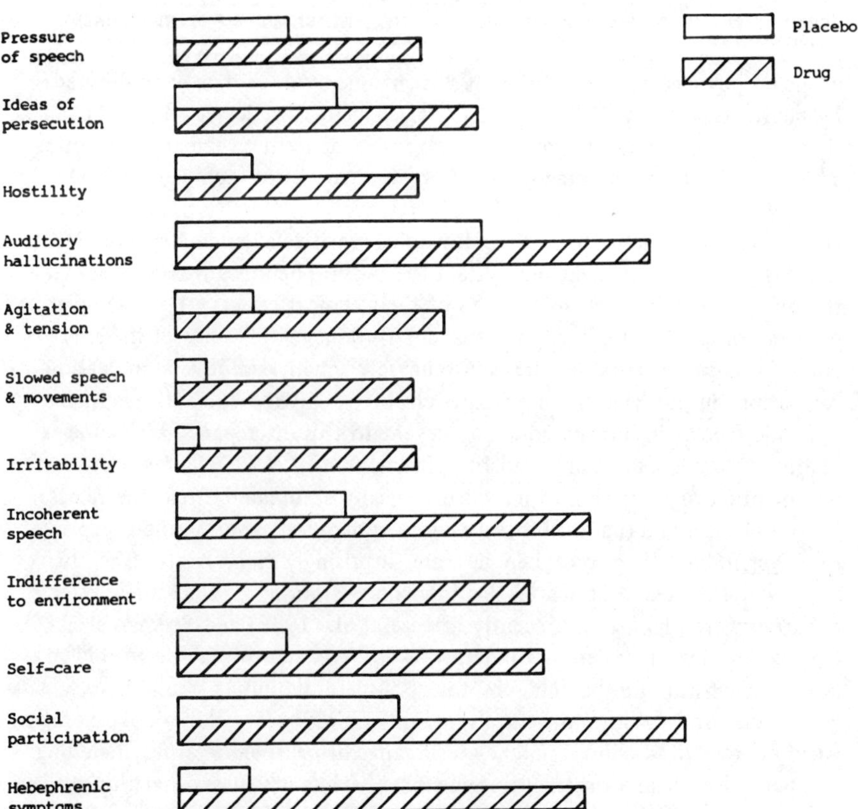

Figure 2 Improvements in individual symptoms on drug and placebo in the NIMH-PSC (1964) trial. (Data taken from Goldberg et al., 1965).

induce extrapyramidal effects, the relationship between the two actions appeared more compelling. Ehringer and Hornykiewicz (1960) demonstrated that the concentration of dopamine is reduced in the corpus striatum in patients dying from Parkinson's disease, and Carlsson and Lindqvist (1963) found that neuroleptic drugs, while they do not deplete brain dopamine, induce increased dopamine turnover as assessed by concentrations of the metabolite HVA. They suggested that this effect might represent a feedback response of the dopamine neuron to blockade of the post synaptic receptor. The concept that neuroleptics block central dopamine receptors is supported by observations that these drugs selectively inhibit dopamine-dependent behaviors induced by amphetamine (Randrup and Mankvad, 1965) and the behavioral changes seen after administration of the dopamine receptor stimulant apomorphine (Andén et al., 1967; Ernst, 1967).

Research on dopaminergic mechanisms has been greatly facilitated by the development of in vitro techniques for investigating receptor mechanisms. Kebabian et al. (1972) described an adenylate cyclase sensitive to dopamine in the corpus stratum. Activation of this enzyme by dopamine was inhibited by neuroleptic drugs (Miller et al., 1974; Clement-Cormier et al., 1974) and there was found to be an approximate correspondence between antipsychotic activity and dopamine antagonism. For example, drugs such as promazine and promethazine, which are probably relatively ineffective antipsychotic agents, were weak inhibitors of the dopamine-sensitive adenylate cyclase (Miller et al., 1974). However, in this system the butyrophenones were less active than might be expected on the basis of their clinical effects. For example, haloperidol is 62.5 times as potent as chlorpromazine in terms of its daily clinical dosage but the drugs are approximately equally effective in molar concentrations in blocking the dopamine-sensitive adenylate cyclase. Pharmacodynamic factors in humans may be relevant to this discrepancy but some alternative explanations are available. Seeman and Lee (1975) reported that neuroleptic drugs are able to inhibit electrically stimulated dopamine release in striatal slices and that in this situation the potencies of various neuroleptic drugs, including the butyrophenones, are surprisingly closely related to their antipsychotic effects. However, the drug concentrations at which these effects occurred were high. More recently, Creese et al. (1976) and Seeman et al. (1976) described haloperidol binding sites in brain which may be related to at least one form of dopamine receptor. Haloperidol binding is inhibited by neuroleptic drugs at low concentrations, and inhibition of haloperidol binding is closely related to clinical potency for a range of neuroleptic drugs, including haloperidol itself and other butyrophenones. Thus it appears that the two in vitro assays of dopamine receptor activity, dopamine-sensitive adenylate cyclase and haloperidol binding, may identify either different dopamine receptors or different states of a single receptor, and that the antipsychotic

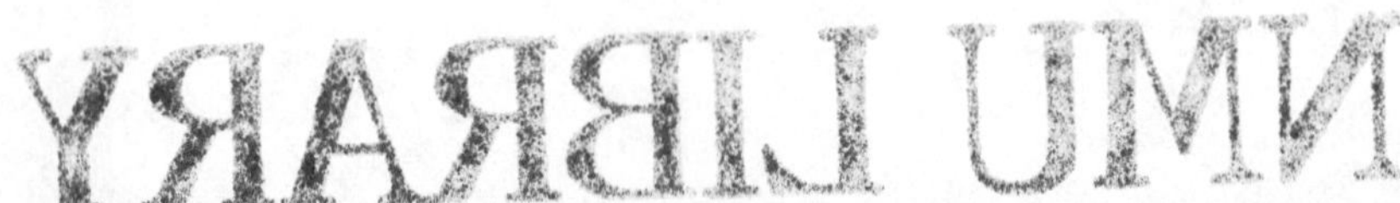

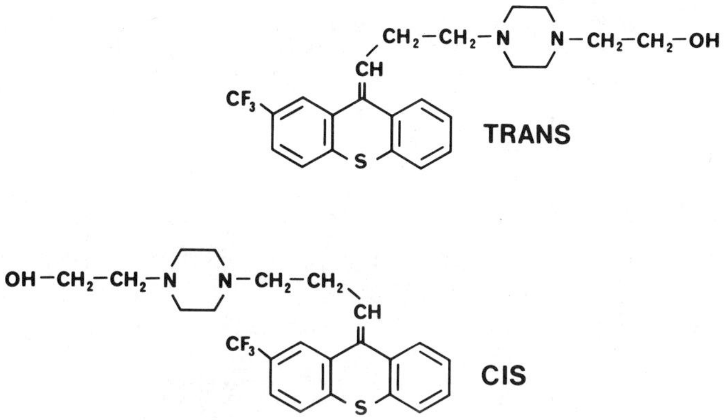

Figure 3 Cis-(α) and trans-(β) isomers of flupenthixol.

activity of neuroleptic drugs is more closely related to actions on the receptor or state identified by the haloperidol binding technique.

A direct clinical test of the dopamine blockade hypothesis of neuroleptic action was made possible by studies on the molecular requirements for antagonist activity in in vitro tests. In the thiaxanthene group of compounds the side chain is linked to the heterocyclic ring system by a carbon-carbon double bond. These drugs exhibit geometric isomerism since the side chain can project either toward (in the cis form) or away from (in the trans form) the halogen substituent in the ring system (Fig. 3). It was demonstrated by Miller et al. (1974) that the two isomers differ in their ability to block the dopamine-sensitive adenylate cyclase, the cis isomer being more active in each case; this is particularly true for flupenthixol, the α (or cis) isomer being highly active but the β (trans) isomer almost devoid of activity (Fig. 4). A similar discrepancy has been demonstrated between the abilities of the two isomers to inhibit haloperidol binding (Enna et al., 1976).

Since the two isomers are included in the standard oral preparation available for clinical use, it was possible to design a trial to determine whether the antipsychotic effect was selectively associated with one or other of the two isomers (Crow and Johnstone, 1977; Johnstone et al., 1978a). The two isomers were separated and administered in a double-blind placebo-controlled trial to recently admitted patients with symptoms of acute schizophrenia as defined by Present State Examination (Wing et al., 1974) criteria. The results established that antipsychotic activity was associated only with the α (cis) isomer of the drug, patients on the β isomer showing slightly but not significantly less improvement than those on placebo (Fig. 5).

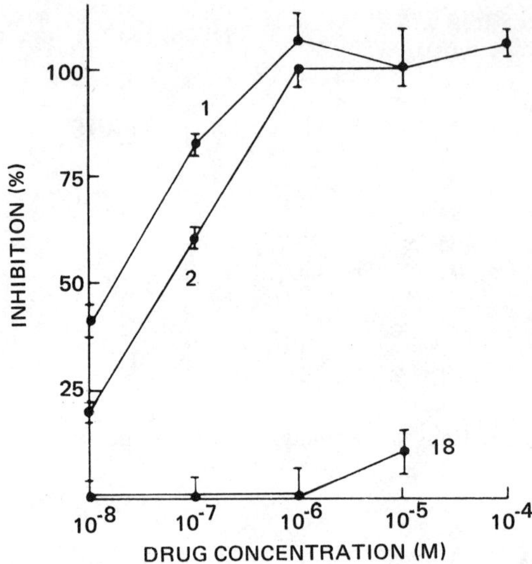

Figure 4 Effects of the α isomer (1) and the β isomer (18), and of the racemate (2), of the two isomers of flupenthixol in inhibiting the dopamine-induced stimulation of adenylate cyclase in the corpus striatum. (Reprinted with permission from Miller et al., 1974.)

The pharmacological interpretation of this result is complicated by the fact that the two isomers differ from each other in their actions on assays of serotonin receptor activity (Enna et al., 1976). However, since both α- and β-flupenthixol have similar potencies in blocking noradrenaline receptors (as assessed by effects on noradrenaline-sensitive adenylate cyclase; Horn and Phillipson, 1975; Miller, 1976) and on acetylcholine and opiate receptors (Enna et al., 1976), actions on these receptors can probably be excluded as the mechanism of the antipsychotic effect. Moreover, since there is no evidence of a significant relationship between serotonin antagonism, as assessed by the LSD binding technique, and neuroleptic activity (Bennett and Snyder, 1975), it seems likely that an action on the serotonin receptor can also be excluded.

The nature of the antipsychotic effect can be further elucidated by an analysis of the clinical data obtained in this trial. Although patients were included on the basis of the presence of nuclear schizophrenic symptoms as defined by Present State Examination criteria, it is possible to further subdivide the population according to the presence or absence of other features. For example, when the total group of 45 patients was divided into a schizo-affective group (where affective symptoms were also present) and a "pure" schizophrenic group, the superiority of α- over β-flupenthixol and placebo was greater in the latter group and virtually absent in the former. Again when patients were subdivided according to the presence or absence of evidence of deterioration over a 6-month period (as defined by the criteria of Feighner et al., 1972) the improvement attributable to α-flupenthixol as compared to the β isomer and placebo was as great in the core group, with evidence of deterioration, as in the remaining patients.

An analysis of symptom change revealed that the effects of α-flupenthxol were most apparent upon positive symptoms (delusions, hallucinations, and thought disorder). On negative symptoms (poverty of speech, retardation, and flattening of affect) and on nonschizophrenic symptoms (anxiety and depression) there were many fewer significant differences between α-flupenthixol and either the β isomer or placebo. This finding appears to conflict with earlier findings (e.g., Goldberg et al., 1965) that significant drug effects are observed over a wide range of manifestations of the disease. The apparent discrepancy may be due to the type of assessment used, since in the trial of the isomers of flupenthixol (Crow et al., 1977b; Johnstone et al., 1978a) this was by intensive clinical interview based on standardized rating scales, and in the earlier study, as in many trials of neuroleptics in schizophrenia, at least partly by ward behavior rating scales. It seems possible that some negative features (e.g., lack of self-care and social withdrawal) as assessed on such scales may be a secondary consequence of positive symptoms (e.g., delusions,

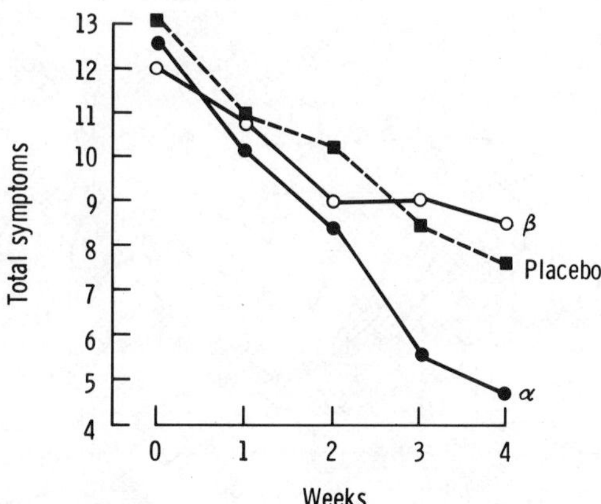

Figure 5 Effects of α- and β-flupenthixol compared to placebo on the symptoms of acute schizophrenia. (From Crow and Johnstone, 1977; Johnstone et al., 1978a.)

hallucinations, and thought disorder). Therefore, while the antipsychotic effect occurs in patients with the most characteristically schizophrenic illnesses and is seen with typically schizophrenic symptoms, the evidence suggests that it is the positive symptoms of delusions, hallucinations, and thought disorder rather than the negative features, including changes in affect, which are the focus of the drug effect.

C. Site of the Antipsychotic Effect

If the antipsychotic effects are, as suggested by these findings, due to antagonism of the dopamine receptor, the possible sites of action within the brain are quite limited. Dopamine-containing neurons have been described in some detail with histochemical techniques (Ungerstedt, 1971; Lindvall and Björklund, 1974). Besides the well-known nigrostriatal pathway, there are dopaminergic innervations of the nucleus accembens, olfactory tubercle and some related nuclei (together constituting the mesolimbic dopamine system), and some areas of frontal cortex (the mesocortical dopamine system). Both these latter innervations appear to arise from cell bodies of the A10 region (the ventral tagmental area) immediately above the interpeduncular nucleus and medial to the pars compacta of the substantia nigra (the A9 area) (Fig. 6).

It is generally assumed that the extrapyramidal effects of neuroleptics are a consequence of dopamine receptor blockade in the corpus striatum. If this is the case, the antipsychotic effects cannot also occur at this site since these two actions are clinically dissociable as demonstrated by a comparison

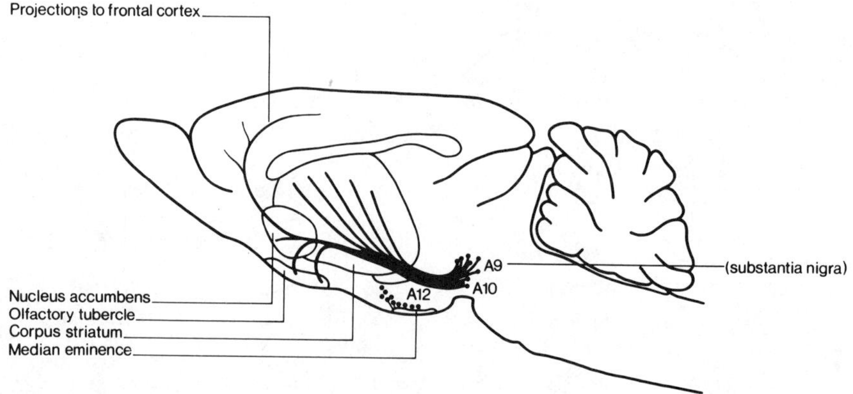

Figure 6 Ascending dopaminergic pathways. (Adapted from Ungerstedt, 1971; Lindvall and Björklund, 1974.)

of thioridazine and chlorpromazine (NIMH-PSC, 1964). Therapeutically equivalent doses of the two drugs differ substantially in their ability to inhibit amphetamine-induced turning in rats with nigrostriatal lesions (an animal model for assessing drug action on nigrostriatal dopaminergic transmission; Crow and Gillbe, 1974).

By exclusion, therefore, one must consider the mesolimbic and mesocortical systems as a possible site of the antipsychotic effect. Although there is no evidence from studies on dopamine uptake or on the dopamine-sensitive adenylate cyclase (Horn et al., 1974) that dopaminergic mechanisms in the two areas are different, it is possible that the effect of drugs on the dopamine receptor is differentially modified by other systems in the two areas. Several authors using assessments of dopamine metabolites (e.g., Andén, 1972; Andén and Stock, 1973; Stawarz et al., 1975) and tyrosine hydroxylase activity (Zivkovic et al., 1975) found that the relative effects of neuroleptic drugs on dopaminergic systems may differ in the two areas. In general, drugs such as thioridazine and clozapine, which have a low incidence of extrapyramidal effects, have a higher relative activity on the mesolimbic system. Nevertheless, it has been suggested (Stawarz et al., 1975) that, although the discrepancy between thioridazine and chlorpromazine is reduced in the mesolimbic system, the residual difference is such as to cast doubt on the dopamine blockade hypothesis. However, in a recent study (Crow et al., 1977b) in which therapeutically equivalent doses of fluphenazine, chlorpromazine, and thioridazine were examined for their effects on dopamine turnover in striatum and nucleus accumbens (dissected out from neighboring mesolimbic structures), the effects in the latter structure were strikingly related to the antipsychotic action.

These findings are consistent with the hypothesis that the antipsychotic effect occurs by dopamine receptor blockade in the nucleus accumbens. An action on mesocortical dopamine receptors is also possible, and studies on dopamine turnover in this region (Scatton et al., 1975a, 1976; Westerink and Korf, 1976) suggest the effects of neuroleptic drugs here resemble those in the mesolimbic system.

The reasons for the differences between the mesolimbic and mesocortical systems on the one hand and the nigrostriatal system on the other are not clear. It has been suggested (Miller and Hiley, 1974; Snyder et al., 1974) that the ability of some neuroleptic drugs to antagonize the muscarinic cholinergic receptor is relevant. These authors have demonstrated an inverse relationship between cholinergic blocking activity and incidence of extrapyramidal effects and suggest that some drugs (e.g., thioridazine) possess their own built-in antiparkinsonian activity. This view is supported by observations (Muller and Seeman, 1974) that the inhibitory effects of chlorpromazine on nigrostriatal transmission (assessed on turning behavior) can be reversed by scopolamine.

D. Time Course of the Antipsychotic Effect

There is evidence from controlled trials (e.g., Casey et al., 1960b) that the therapeutic benefit of neuroleptic drugs is greater after 12 than after 4 weeks of administration (see also Fig. 1). This time course suggests that more complex interactions than reversal of a simple neurohumoral imbalance are taking place.

This delay between dopamine receptor blockade and antipsychotic effect has been documented in the trial of the isomers of flupenthixol (Cotes et al., 1977; Cotes et al., 1978). In patients on α-flupenthixol there was a substantial rise in plasma prolactin concentration, presumably as a result of blockade of the tuberoinfundibular dopamine system (Fuxe et al., 1969) by the end of the 1st week of treatment. However, the clinical improvement which could be attributed to drug therapy (calculated as the difference in scores between patients on α- and those on β-flupenthixol and placebo) was minimal until the end of the 2nd week and showed its greatest increase between the 2nd and 3rd weeks of treatment (Fig. 7). There is thus a delay of at least 2 weeks between the establishment of central dopamine blockade and the emergence of a therapeutic effect which can be attributed to drugs. Therefore, if dopamine receptor blockade is necessary for the antipsychotic effect, this may be because

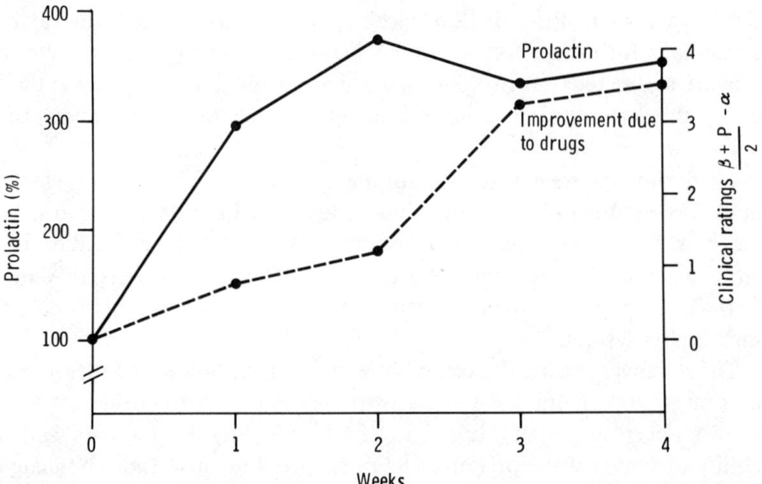

Figure 7 Delay between onset of dopaminergic blockade, as assessed by increases in prolactin secretion, and clinical improvement attributable to neuroleptic medication (calculated as the difference between mean ratings on placebo and β-flupenthixol and ratings on α-flupenthixol). (From Cotes et al., 1977).

such blockade is a condition for some other, rather slow, process to take place (see also Crow et al., 1979b).

Some changes observed after neuroleptics may be relevant to the time course of the antipsychotic effect. Thus Post and Goodwin (1975) reported that patients who had been on neuroleptics for brief periods (15-19 days) showed evidence of increased dopamine turnover as assessed by probenecid induced accumulations of HVA in CSF while patients on extended (25-77 days) treatment had normal levels of HVA. Thus it appears that dopamine turnover returns to normal at about the time at which the antipsychotic effect emerges.

There is evidence from animal studies of adaptation to the effects of neuroleptics. O'Keefe et al. (1970) found that HVA was no longer increased in cat or monkey caudate nucleus following prolonged drug administration. Bowers and Rozitis (1974) found that the effects of neuroleptic drugs on HVA concentrations in the striatum decreased with chronic administration but that effects on the limbic system (including nucleus accumbens, olfactory tubercle, and septum) were largely unchanged. These findings were substantially confirmed for the mesolimbic system and extended to the mesocortical dopamine system in studies in which radioactively labeled tyrosine was used to assess dopamine turnover (Scatton et al., 1976); these authors had previously established (Scatton et al., 1975b) that dopamine turnover is actually decreased in striatum 24 hr after the last of a series of daily neuroleptic injections, but this phenomenon is not seen in the mesolimbic or mesocortical systems. Thus the antipsychotic effect resembles the action on mesolimbic and mesocortical systems in not demonstrating tolerance but may occur at a time when tolerance is emerging in the nigrostriatal system. If one looks only at dopamine systems one might propose the hypothesis that antipsychotic effect is a consequence of a change in the balance between striatal and nonstriatal systems, and occurs when mesocortical and mesolimbic dopaminergic transmission remains inhibited (as shown by the continued increase in dopamine turnover) but when transmission in the striatal system has overcome the initial blockade induced by the drug.

It has been suggested that the phenomenon of receptor supersensitivity may be related to these changes. Following chronic nuroleptic administration increased sensitivity to the dopamine agonist apomorphine is seen in its effects on both dopamine turnover (Gianutsos et al., 1975) and behavior (Christensen et al., 1976), and increased receptor binding activity is reported (Burt et al., 1977). However, some receptor changes are reported to develop rapidly, possibly within hours of a single drug dosage. Thus the time course of some receptor changes is much shorter than that of the antipsychotic effect.

E. Therapeutic Effects Unrelated to Dopamine Receptor Blockade

Since it appears that the antipsychotic effects of standard neuroleptic drugs may be entirely due to their ability to block dopamine receptors, one may ask whether there is evidence that any therapeutic effects are mediated by nondopaminergic mechanisms.

1. L-dopa

Two trials suggest that L-dopa therapy in combination with neuroleptics may have therapeutic effects. Inanaga et al. (1975) reported that patients on L-dopa (200–600 mg daily) and phenothiazines showed significantly greater improvement than patients on placebo and phenothiazines, the effects being greatest in patients ill for less than 5 years and with symptoms of loss of spontaneity, abulia, apathy, and autism. Similar findings were reported by Gerlach and Luhsdorf (1975) in a double-blind crossover trial in 18 young patients with simple schizophrenia (without paranoid delusions or hallucinations in the previous 6 months) of L-dopa and a peripheral decarboxylase inhibitor and placebo. Patients were already established on neuroleptic mediation, and on L-dopa there were significant improvements on an activity-withdrawal scale and on Brief Psychiatric Ratings.

Thus there is a suggestion that in patients on neuroleptic drugs L-dopa may diminish some negative features of the disease. A possible consequence of L-dopa administered in these conditions is a potentiation of noradrenergic mechanisms.

2. Tryptophan, 5-HTP, and Serotonin Antagonists

Attempts to demonstrate beneficial effects of tryptophan (Gillin et al., 1976) or 5-hydroxytryptophan (5-HTP) (Wyatt et al., 1972) have yielded negative or inconsistent results. In the former case L-tryptophan in doses up to 20 g/day with or without pyridoxine induced no significant clinical change in eight male chronic schizophrenic patients (Gillin et al., 1976). In the latter case there were inconsistent changes in a group of young chronic patients following combinations of 5-hydroxytryptophan and a peripheral decarboxylase inhibitor (Wyatt et al., 1972).

Trials of serotonin antagonists have been equally unsuccessful. Cinanserin, a drug with antiserotonin and immunosuppressive effects, was without significant effect in two trials in chronic schizophrenia (Gallant and Bishop, 1968; Holden et al., 1971) in either ameliorating or exacerbating the condition.

3. GABA-Mediated Effects

It has been argued (Fuxe et al., 1975a) that mesencephalic dopamine systems, including the mesolimbic projection, are under inhibitory control from a system of GABA neurons. On this basis it was suggested that GABA agonist drugs might have therapeutic effects on schizophrenia. In spite of claims based on uncontrolled trials of the GABA analogue baclofen (Fredericksen, 1975), this appears unlikely (Gulman et al., 1976; Davis et al., 1976; Simpson, 1976).

An interesting and related question is whether the benzodiazepines, which may possess GABA-mimetic properties (Haefely et al., 1975), have therapeutic effects in schizophrenia. In their effects on unit firing of A10 dopamine cells the benzodiazepines closely resemble antipsychotic drugs (Bunney and Aghajanian, 1976) and this action may be dependent upon intensified GABAergic transmission (Keller et al., 1976). However, few controlled clinical studies have been carried out, although in a carefully balanced multiple crossover study on six patients Kellner et al. (1975) described a response to chlordiazepoxide in two patients which appeared to include schizophrenic symptoms. Thus there is a case for further investigations of the possible role of benzodiazepines and GABA mechanisms in schizophrenia.

F. Summary

The undoubted antipsychotic effects of neuroleptic drugs in acute schizophrenia may be entirely attributable to their ability to block central dopamine receptors, probably at a site or sites within the mesolimbic or mesocortical systems. However, the time course of the antipsychotic effect is such as to suggest that the clinical changes are not a direct consequence of occupation of the receptor site but are the result of a process taking perhaps as long as 2 weeks which is initiated or permitted by receptor blockade. The antipsychotic effect occurs in the most characteristically schizophrenic patients but may be limited to the positive features of the disease: hallucinations, delusions, and thought disorder.

There is no unequivocal evidence that therapeutic effects occur as a consequence of pharmacological actions other than dopamine receptor blockade but the possibility that significant improvments can be observed after L-dopa in combination with neuroleptics and, in some patients, after benzodiazepines deserves to be further investigated.

V. DRUG-INDUCED EXACERBATIONS OF SCHIZOPHRENIC SYMPTOMS

The pharmacological mechanisms by which schizophrenic symptoms may be exacerbated are of as much theoretical interest as those by which they may be diminished. In spite of ethical problems there have been a number of significant observations.

A. Amphetamine and Methylphenidate

The dopamine overactivity hypothesis predicts by analogy with the amphetamine psychosis that the symptoms of schizophrenia will be exacerbated by amphetamine and amphetamine-like drugs.

Concerning this prediction there is a very striking discrepancy in the literature. Janowsky et al. (1973) and Janowsky and Davis (1976) investigated the effects of administering methylphenidate and some amphetamines to a series of young, relatively acutely ill schizophrenic patients. Methylphenidate 0.5 mg/kg i.v. provoked a highly significant increase in psychosis ratings, and similar but less severe exacerbations were seen after equivalent doses of d- and l-amphetamine. It has also been claimed (Janowsky et al., 1977) that the changes observed cannot be attributed to increased verbalization but represent an increase in specifically schizophrenic symptoms. These observations are therefore consistent with the dopamine hypothesis. Directly contrary observations were reported by Kornetsky (1976). In a series of 10 chronic schizophrenic patients doses of 20–40 mg of d-amphetamine caused no exacerbation of the disease process, had little effect on sleep duration, and had little or no effect on performance on a variety of behavioral tests.

Davis (1974) argues that the dose of methylphenidate which exacerbated psychotic symptoms in his schizophrenic patients would produce only mild euphoria in normal subjects; Kornetsky (1976) that the doses of d-amphetamine he used would produce more severe insomnia, and disturbance of test performance, in controls than in his schizophrenic patients. The factor which could account for these discrepancies is the selection of acute or chronic patients. It seems possible, as Kornetsky has argued, that hyporesponsiveness to amphetamine is characteristic of the chronic state. An unequivocal answer to this point appears of particular importance.

B. L-dopa, ET-495, and Apomorphine

In a series of 10 schizophrenic patients L-dopa in doses of 3–6 g/day was reported to induce behavioral worsening (Angrist et al., 1975), although whether this deterioration was to be viewed as a selective activation of the schizophrenic process or nonspecific behavioral stimulation was unclear. In similar nonblind observations on ET-495, a drug with dopamine receptor stimulating activity, some symptomatic exacerbation was observed but this was noted to be less both than that seen after L-dopa and in experiments (Janowsky and Davis, 1976) with methylphenidate. In a carefully controlled study, Smith et al. (1977) observed no exacerbations of psychotic symptoms in four chronic schizophrenic patients after 1.5–6 mg of apomorphine.

C. Monoamine Oxidase Inhibitors

Price and Hopkinson (1968) reviewed a small number of controlled trials in which monoamine oxidase inhibitors appeared to exert no significant effects in chronic schizophrenia. On the other hand, Heinrich (1960) reported exacerbations of symptoms by monoamine oxidase inhibitors in early schizophrenia, and suggested this might be of diagnostic value. Pleasure (1954) described a number of patients in whom schizophrenia-like symptoms occurred during treatment with iproniazid for tuberculosis. There appears therefore to be some evidence that schizophrenic symptoms can be exacerbated or perhaps precipitated by monoamine oxidase inhibitors.

D. Methionine and Other Methyl Donors

Stimulated by the hypothesis (Osmond et al., 1952) that schizophrenia is a disease in which excessive transmethylation occurs, a number of studies have aimed to establish whether or not schizophrenic symptoms are exacerbated by methionine and other methyl donors. A recent review (Cohen et al., 1974) attempted to assess the extent to which the changes observed could be regarded as schizophrenic and whether they could be attributed to methionine administration. Unfortunately, in many of these studies monoamine oxidase inhibitors were also administered, and since these drugs may themselves exacerbate schizophrenic symptoms (see Section V.C) this fact complicates the interpretation of 8 of the 10 studies. Neurological symptoms and symptoms of an organic psychosis were common. Of the 107 patients in these studies, 27% demonstrated one of the features of confusion, disorientation, or delirium without other psychotic changes and 46.7% had these features with or without other psychotic symptoms. Affective changes were also common. Therefore, if methionine provokes schizophrenic symptoms, these are by no means the only psychological changes induced. Nevertheless there were judged to be 35 patients who showed evidence of a worsening of psychosis without confusion or delirium, and on this basis it might be argued that there is evidence for exacerbation of the schizophrenic process itself. However, in view of the high incidence of organic and neurological symptoms and also the difficulties raised by the use of monoamine oxidase inhibitors, it seems doubtful as to whether this point can be regarded as established.

Investigations of abnormalities of methylation in schizophrenia have yielded no very definite conclusions. Price (1972) studied o-methylation by loading with protocatechuic acid, a substance which is extensively methylated in humans, and observed no significant differences between 21 acute schizophrenics and 55 control subjects. Israelstam et al. (1970) found that methionine administration did not greatly increase total body methylation in schizophrenics and did not increase methylation of biogenic amines.

E. Anticholinergics

Some behavioral effects of neuroleptics can be reversed by cholinergic antagonists (e.g., Muller and Seeman, 1974) and the exacerbations of psychosis observed following methylphenidate are reversed by the cholinesterase inhibitor physostigmine (Davis and Janowsky, 1975). Therefore, it is tempting to suppose that schizophrenic symptoms may be modified by changes in cholinergic transmission. However, the widespread use of anticholinergic drugs with neuroleptics is presumably based on a clinical impression that this is not the case. Moreover, in their experiments with physostigmine, Davis and Janowsky (1975) observed no change in the basal ratings of psychosis while observing an interaction with methylphenidate. However, there are some reports (Pfeiffer and Jenney, 1957; Rosenthal and Bigelow, 1973) of therapeutic benefits following cholinomimetic agents in uncontrolled trials. That anticholinergic agents may actually exacerbate schizophrenic symptoms is suggested by the work of Singh and Kay (1975), who examined the effects of various anticholinergic agents on the rates of clinical improvement seen in patients with acute schizophrenia on neuroleptic drugs. However, the type of statistical analysis applied to this date has been criticized in another context (Levy and Weinreb, 1976; Smith, 1976). It appears that the deleterious effects of anticholinergics cannot yet be regarded as established.

F. Summary

Schizophrenic symptoms are exacerbated by methylphenidate and drugs of the amphetamine group, and there is some evidence from psychometric tests that this may be a selective accentuation of the disease process. This effect is reported in acute schizophrenia; the apparent insensitivity of chronic schizophrenics to amphetamine suggests new approaches to the nature of the defect state. Behavioral worsening is also seen in some schizophrenic patients following monoamine oxidase inhibitors and L-dopa, but to a much lesser extent, if at all, after the dopamine receptor stimulants apomorphine and ET-495. It appears that many of the symptoms seen in schizophrenic patients after methionine administration are of an organic type, and the schizophrenic character of the psychotic changes seen after methionine alone has not been established. Whether or not changes in cholinergic transmission exert a direct effect upon schizophrenic symptoms is also not clear.

VI. POSTMORTEM STUDIES

If the neurochemical defect in schizophrenia is either a degeneration of certain neurotransmitter-related pathways or a deficiency or abnormality of enzymatic processes, it is possible that this might be detected in tissue removed at postmortem. The potential of this approach is well attested by studies of parkinsonism (Ehringer and Hornykiewicz, 1960) and Huntington's chorea (Perry et al., 1973; Bird and Iversen, 1974). Many enzymes are well preserved after death, and some neurotransmitters, including polypeptides, are relatively resistant to degradation. A number of postmortem studies in schizophrenia have focused on current monoamine and other hypotheses (Table 2).

A. Monoamine Oxidase

Utena et al. (1968) found no differences in MAO activity in several brain areas between five schizophrenic patients and five controls. Schwarz et al. (1974a) examined MAO activity in four cortical areas, basal ganglia, areas in the limbic system, and brain stem in nine schizophrenic and nine control subjects using [^{14}C] tryptamine as substrate. No significant differences between schizophrenics and controls were observed in mean MAO activity or in activities in specific brain regions. In the same series of specimens Schwarz et al. (1974b) investigated the activities of types A and B MAO with serotonin and β-phenylethylamine as substrates, and with clorgyline and deprenyl as inhibitors of the two enzymes, respectively. The enzymes were found to be rather uniformly distributed in the brain and there were no differences between schizophrenic patients and normal subjects.

Similarly, Domino et al. (1973) found no differences in MAO activity assessed with a [^{14}C] tryptamine technique in 15 brain areas in 6 schizophrenic patients, 4 normal subjects, and 3 patients with an organic brain disease, and Cross et al. (1977a) found no differences in MAO assessed with several substrates in 9 schizophrenic patients and 9 controls. These investigations therefore gave no support to the suggestion arising from studies on platelets (Murphy and Wyatt, 1972) that there might be a deficiency of monoamine oxidase activity in the brain in schizophrenia.

B. Dopamine-β-hydroxylase

Dopamine-β-hydroxylase (DBH) activity is specifically associated with noradrenergic neurons. Interest in this enzyme was stimulated by the hypothesis of Stein and Wise (1971) that degeneration of these neurons might be the defect underlying progressive deterioration. In a series of 18 schizophrenic and 12 control brains, Wise et al. (1975) reported significant reductions in DBH activity in the patients using tyramine as substrate. These authors felt that the reductions (of the order of 30-40%) were not attributable to differences in age, cause of death, time since death, or conditions of storage, and, on the basis of animal experiments, were unlikely to be due to neuroleptic drug treatment. They suggested that it was a relatively specific deficit since, in agreement with the above studies, no differences in MAO activity were found between groups,

Table 2 Neurochemical Studies on Postmortem Brains in Schizophrenia

Assay	Reductions in patients	No significant patient-control differences	Increases in patients
Dopamine-β-hydroxylase	Wise and Stein, 1973; Wise et al., 1974 (18)[a]	Wyatt et al., 1975(9) Cross et al., 1977b(9)	
Monoamine oxidase		Utena et al., 1968(5) Domino et al., 1973(6) Wise et al., 1974(11) Schwarz et al., 1974a,b; Schwarz et al., 1975; Cross et al., 1977a (9)	
Catechol-o-methyltransferase	diencephalon: Wise et al., 1974(18)	pons medulla: Wise et al., 1974(17)	
Acetylcholinesterase	septum: Domino et al., 1973(4)	other areas: Domino et al., 1973(6)	
Pseudocholinesterase			Domino et al., 1973(6)
Choline acetyltransferase	Wise et al., 1974(18) (reductions less in age-matched sample)	Other areas: Domino et al., 1973(6)	medial amygdala: Domino et al., 1973(5)
N-methyltransferase		Domino et al., 1973(6)	
Superoxide dismutase	Wise et al., 1974(8)		
Dopamine-sensitive adenylyl cyclase		Carenzi et al., 1975(7)	

[a] No. in parens = no. in schizophrenic sample.

and there were no differences in the activities of some other enzymes, including lactate dehydrogenase and superoxide dismutase. There were, however, modest reactions in choline acetyltransferase and catechol-O-methyltransferase activity.

These findings were challenged by a report by Wyatt et al. (1975) that in a series of nine schizophrenic and nine control brains DBH activities were not significantly different. It was argued (Wise and Stein, 1975) that the discrepancy might be due to failure to distinguish paranoid from nonparanoid schizophrenic illnesses and that when this was done a deficit in DBH in the nonparanoid patients was observed. In a recent study in nine schizophrenic and nine control brains no differences in DBH activity were observed (Cross et al., 1977b, 1978), although nearly all of these patients would be classified as suffering nonparanoid illnesses. At the present time, therefore, the evidence for deficits in DBH activity is inconsistent.

C. Dopaminergic Mechanisms

In spite of the interest in dopamine blockade in the action of neuroleptics dopaminergic mechanisms until recently have attracted relatively little attention in postmortem studies. Carenzi et al. (1975) investigated receptor mechanisms by assaying dopamine stimulation of adenylyl cyclase in caudate nucleus. Such activity was found to be present in stored brains and was inhibited by haloperidol. In eight normal and seven schizophrenic subjects baseline and stimulated activities were not different. Within the schizophrenic group (but not the controls) there was a significant negative correlation between baseline and stimulated levels which probably could not be attributed to neuroleptic medication. Therefore, there was a possibility that a subgroup of patients with low levels of activity might have an adenylyl cyclase which was particularly sensitive to dopamine, or alternatively that there might be a group with high levels and insensitivity to dopamine.

Owen et al. (1978) attempted a systematic evaluation of the dopamine overactivity hypothesis by assessing dopamine, its metabolites, and dopamine receptors (assessed by spiroperidol binding) in 19 schizophrenic and 19 control brains. There was a modest increase in dopamine concentrations in caudate nucleus ($P < .05$) in schizophrenic patients, but this was not present in putamen or nucleus accumbens, and there was no evidence of an increase in dopamine turnover as assessed by the concentrations of HVA or dihydroxyphenylacetic acid (DOPAC). However, in all three dopaminergically innervated areas there was evidence of an increase in numbers of dopamine receptors. Assessed as maximum spiroperidol binding (a method which avoids the complication introduced by interference with the assay produced by neuroleptic which remains in the brain after death), two-thirds of the patient group fell outside the range of control values, and there was a mean increase of approximately 100%.

Significant increases were found in some patients who apparently had not received neuroleptic medication for the year before death. The findings are consistent with those of a report by Lee et al. (1978) that haloperidol binding is increased in the brains of schizophrenics in comparison to controls.

D. Other Changes

Some changes have been reported in enzyme activity in specific brain areas. For example, Wise et al. (1974) found a 30% reduction in catechol-O-methyl transferase (COMT) activity in samples of tissue from the diencephalon but not from the pons medulla. They also reported reductions in choline acetyltransferase, although these reductions were less marked when age was taken into account. Domino et al. (1973) in a small series found no change in this enzyme in most areas, but an increase in the medial amygdala.

Domino et al. (1973) also found pseudocholinesterase activity to be increased in their schizophrenic sample, but thought that this might well be a secondary consequence of neuroleptic medication.

E. Summary

The few studies so far conducted on postmortem brains (see Table 2) have revealed no evidence of abnormalities of monoamine oxidase activity or of a uniform change in dopamine-sensitive adenylate cyclase in schizophrenia. Reports of deficiencies of DBH activity remain controversial.

Dopamine turnover does not seem to be increased in schizophrenic brain, but two recent studies using butyrophenone binding techniques have demonstrated an increase in numbers of dopamine receptors. This change occurs in some patients who apparently had been untreated with neuroleptic drugs for the year before death.

VII. CSF STUDIES

The utility of studies of CSF concentrations of monoamine metabolites as an index of central monoamine neuron function has been widely debated (Garelis et al., 1974). The technique of administering probenecid, which blocks the egress from CSF of the acid metabolites HVA and 5-HIAA (5-hydroxyindoleacetic acid), and of measuring increases in the concentrations of these metabolites has yielded significant findings in the effective disorders (van Praag and Korf, 1971; Sjöström and Roos, 1972).

In schizophrenia the probenecid technique has been used to investigate the dopamine hypothesis. Bowers (1974) found HVA accumulations following probenecid to be less in 17 patients with acute schizophrenic illnesses than in 11 with affective illnesses, and there is evidence (e.g., van Praag and Korf, 1971;

Sjöström and Roos, 1972) that these latter patients may have low dopamine turnover, as assessed by this technique, in comparison with normal controls. Post et al. (1975) found no differences between schizophrenic patients and affectively disordered and normal controls but within the schizophrenic group they described an inverse relationship between HVA accumulation and severity of illness, assessed by number of Schneiderian first rank symptoms. These findings are therefore in direct conflict with the prediction of increased dopamine turnover in schizophrenia. Within the schizophrenic group Bowers (1974) found those patients with indicators of poor prognosis ("typical" schizophrenics) to have lower HVA levels after probenecid than those of good prognosis ("atypical" schizophrenics). In a later study, Kirstein et al. (1976) found HVA accumulations in a group of 10 acute schizophrenic patients to be higher than those in a group of 10 depressed patients. The results therefore differed somewhat from those of Bowers (1974), in which the control group of patients with affective disorders had included some with mania. Kirstein et al. (1976) found no relationship between HVA accumulation and motor activity; but in a group of patients with psychogenic and schizophrenic psychoses van Praag and Korf (1975) found HVA accumulation to be increased only in a subgroup with marked motor agitation and anxiety.

Post et al. (1975), who studied a group of acute schizophrenics of generally good prognosis, found HVA accumulations to be within the normal range at the time of the illness but to be significantly reduced by comparison with controls when assessed in a phase of recovery.

The effects of neuroleptic drugs on dopamine turnover in animals are well established and analogous findings with the probenecid technique are reported for humans (van Praag and Korf, 1975). Most interesting here, however, is the time course of the effect. Both Post and Goodwin (1975) and van Praag (1977) have reported that the increase in dopamine turnover seen in patients who have recently started on neuroleptic medication disappears after the first few weeks.

In two studies (Bowers, 1974; Post et al., 1975) no significant differences between patients and controls were observed in 5-HIAA accumulation with probenecid. Post et al. (1975) found 5-HIAA accumulations to be less in patients with a greater number of Schneiderian symptoms, and Bowers (1975) found 5-HT turnover, assessed in this way, to be less in acute than in chronic patients. Bowers (1975) suggested that this might reflect a primary decrease in serotonergic neuronal activity in some acute psychotic states. 5-HIAA was negatively correlated with ratings of agitation and a measure of activity. On the basis of evidence that serotonergic systems may inhibit motor activity, Bowers argues that hyporesponsiveness of these systems may be related, either as a primary defect or as a secondary consequence, to pathological overarousal in acute psychotic states.

The noradrenaline metabolite 3-methoxy-4-hydroxyphenylglycol (MHPG) is little changed in CSF following probenecid administration but the levels may provide an index of central noradrenergic function. In a series of eight schizophrenic patients, as in manic patients, mean MHPG levels were found to be modestly but significantly above those of controls but most values in patients fell within the normal range (Shopsin et al., 1973). In a later study (Post et al., 1975) the mean concentration in 17 schizophrenic patients was similar to that in 10 normal controls; but within the schizophrenic group there was an inverse relationship between MHPG and degree of subjective distress.

A. Summary

CSF studies of monoamine metabolites after probenecid have provided little evidence that dopamine turnover is increased in acute or chronic schizophrenia. On the contrary, there is evidence that dopamine turnover may decrease with increasing severity, as assessed by number of Schneiderian symptoms, and with poor prognosis. Similarly, serotonin turnover may decrease with increasing Schneiderian symptoms and with increasing agitation and anxiety. However, there is no evidence from CSF studies of a disturbance of monoamine function which is characteristic of schizophrenia.

VIII. INDICES OF MONOAMINE METABOLISM IN BLOOD AND URINE

The extensive literature on investigations of monoamine metabolites in blood and urine (e.g., as reviewed by Kety, 1959; Brune, 1965; Weil-Malherbe, 1967; Faurbye, 1968; Wyatt et al., 1971) reveals the many difficulties of this type of approach to CNS metabolism. Doubts concerning the validity of measures of monoamine metabolites, or related compounds, in blood or urine as indices of central turnover, their susceptibility to environmental, e.g., dietary, influences, and observed failures of replication of differences between schizophrenics and controls have combined to make such studies less numerous in recent years. However, there have been a number of foci of interest.

A. Platelet MAO

A report (Murphy and Wyatt, 1972) that monoamine oxidase activity in platelets was reduced by 50–60% in patients with schizophrenia provoked considerable interest and was confirmed by other workers (e.g., Meltzer and Stahl, 1974). The possible implication of the finding that there might be a generalized deficit of intracellular monoamine oxidase activity in schizophrenics has not been confirmed in postmortem studies of MAO in brain (see Section VI), and the interest of the original observation was therefore reduced. More recent studies have yielded widely varying results. In acute schizophrenic patients

Friedman et al. (1974) and Carpenter et al. (1975) found no differences in platelet MAO between patients and controls with series of 40 and 26 patients, respectively. Brockington et al. (1976) found no significant differences in platelet MAO between 56 patients with chronic schizophrenia, all of whom had been drug-free for at least 6 months, and age-matched controls; Belmaker et al. (1976) reported similar findings in 18 schizophrenic patients receiving phenothiazines and 19 controls. Drug effects of some neuroleptics are reported on both platelet MAO (Brockington et al., 1976) and other aspects of platelet function (Orr and Boullin, 1976), and it remains a possibility that there are specific and perhaps relatively longlasting effects of certain neuroleptics on platelet MAO levels. It appears unlikely that low platelet MAO can be directly related to the primary disturbance or that it is a genetic marker for the disease.

B. Noradrenaline Metabolites in Urine

The discovery that noradrenaline in brain is metabolized mainly to the alcohol 3-methoxy-4-hydroxyphenylglycol (MHPG) (Mannarino et al., 1963; Rutledge and Jonason, 1967) reopened the possibility of studies of noradrenaline metabolites in urine as indicators of central noradrenaline turnover. Maas and Landis (1968) estimated that as much as 25% of urinary MHPG might derive from the CNS. Moreover, it has been suggested (Bond and Howlett, 1974) that MHPG from the CNS is conjugated as sulfate while a high proportion of MHPG arising from noradrenaline metabolism in the periphery is conjugated as glucuronide. Thus assessments of MHPG sulfate in urine might be a better index of turnover in CNS than either total MHPG or the glucuronide.

In a study of 18 drug-free chronic schizophrenic patients (Joseph et al., 1976), MHPG sulfate, but not glucuronide, was found to show a significant inverse correlation with total symptom score but the mean 24-hr excretion did not differ between patients and controls. This finding is therefore consistent with the suggestion that MHPG sulfate may be a more direct index of CNS changes than is either total MHPG or the glucuronide. If MHPG sulfate is a valid index of central noradrenaline turnover, the failure to find a difference between patients and controls is inconsistent with the hypothesis that in schizophrenia noradrenergic mechanisms are impaired. A possible explanation of the inverse correlation between MHPG sulfate excretion and total symptom score is that a high turnover of noradrenaline in some way protects the individual against a severe form of the disease.

C. Dimethyltryptamine

While few toxic metabolite theories have been seriously pursued in recent years, one hallucinogenic substance, dimethyltryptamine, has continued to attract interest in part because possible mechanisms for its generation in the body have been described. Tryptamine is known to be present in brain

(Saavedra and Axelrod, 1972) and the presence of an enzyme capable of dimethylating tryptamine was reported in human red cells, plasma, and platelets (Wyatt et al., 1973a). However, it now seems doubtful that the product of this reaction is DMT (Boarder and Rodnight, 1976). Nevertheless, levels of 0.5-2.0 ng/ml of DMT were reported in human plasma using a gas-chromatographic mass-spectrometric isotope dilution assay, but there were no significant differences between patients with schizophrenia or depression and controls (Wyatt et al., 1973b). There has been a claim (Narasimhachari et al., 1972) that DMT can be detected in the urine of patients wich schizophrenia but not in that or normal subjects. This claim was subjected to a carefully controlled study (Rodnight et al., 1976) in which 122 recently admitted psychiatric patients were assessed by a series of diagnostic criteria. DMT was more frequently detected in psychiatric patients than in controls and in patients with psychotic rather than neurotic diagnoses. It was concluded, however, that schizophrenic symptoms were not major determinants of DMT excretion. In more recent studies with quantitative techniques (Rodnight, personal communication) increased excretion of DMT in schizophrenic and other psychiatrically disturbed group of patients has been described. However, the significance of these findings remains in doubt since the quantities detected are small in comparison with those seen in the urine of subjects who had received psychotomimetic doses of DMT (Kaplan et al., 1974).

IX. NEUROENDOCRINE APPROACHES TO THE SCHIZOPHRENIC DEFECT

The discovery of a complex pattern of innervation of the endocrine hypothalamus by monoamine-containing nerve terminals (Fuxe and Hökfelt, 1967) initiated a new approach to monoamine neuron function in humans. It may be argued that if there are disturbances of particular neurohumoral mechanisms in the functional psychoses these disturbances will affect monoamine mechanisms in the hypothalamus and median eminence as well as elsewhere in the brain. Thus the underlying disturbance might be detected either in abnormalities of pituitary trophic hormone secretion or in the hormonal response to agents acting on central monoamine mechanisms. In particular the inhibitory influence of the tuberoinfundibular dopamine system on prolactin secretion (Fuxe et al., 1969) is well established and has been the focus of a number of investigations.

A. Acute Schizophrenia

The dopamine overactivity hypothesis of schizophrenia predicts that prolactin secretion will be low in patients untreated by neuroleptic drugs. However, in a series of 22 acutely disturbed patients prolactin concentrations were found to be within the normal range (Meltzer et al., 1974) and this was true for patients with and without paranoid features.

After administration of neuroleptic drugs serum prolactin levels increase. This occurs following chlorpromazine, where a relationship with plasma drug levels has been demonstrated (Kolakowska et al., 1975), and also after administration of thioridazine (Wilson et al., 1975) in spite of the lesser incidence of extrapyramidal side effects induced by this drug. A significant positive relationship has been demonstrated between activity in increasing prolactin release and antipsychotic potency for seven neuroleptic drugs (Langer et al., 1977).

In a trial of the isomers of flupenthixol a rise in serum prolactin was seen in patients on the antipsychotic α isomer but not in those on the β-isomer or placebo (Cotes et al., 1977, 1978). Increased prolactin secretion is therefore closely associated with the antipsychotic effect. There was, however, a clear dissociation in the time course of the two pharmacological actions (see Section IV.D). Whereas the increase in prolactin was well established at the end of the 1st week the therapeutic changes which could be attributed to medication (the difference in ratings between those on α-flupenthixol and on the one hand and β-flupenthixol and placebo on the other) were significantly increased only at the end of the 3rd week (Fig. 7). This finding suggests that dopamine receptor blockade, if as seems likely it is associated with the antipsychotic effect, is necessary only insofar as it permits other, slower changes to take place which themselves become manifest in a change in clinical state.

Although this evidence suggests a temporal dissociation between dopamine receptor blockade, as assessed by prolactin secretion, and the therapeutic effect, there is another respect in which the prolactin response resembles the antipsychotic action. Whereas some actions of neuroleptic drugs on dopaminergic mechanisms show tolerance (Bowers and Rozitis, 1974; Post and Goodwin, 1975) there is no evidence that this occurs with the antipsychotic effect, and prolactin levels remain elevated after administration of neuroleptics over a 3-month period (Meltzer and Fang, 1976). This dissociation has been most clearly demonstrated in a study (van Praag, 1977) in which the probenecid-induced accumulation of HVA in CSF was compared with the serum prolactin level after 2 weeks, 1 month, and at 6 months on chlorpromazine. HVA after probenecid rose to 240% of control values at 2 weeks and fell to approximately 130% at 1 month and to control levels at 6 months. Prolactin rose to approximately 500% at 2 weeks and was at 470% at 1 month and 440% at 6 months (Fig. 8).

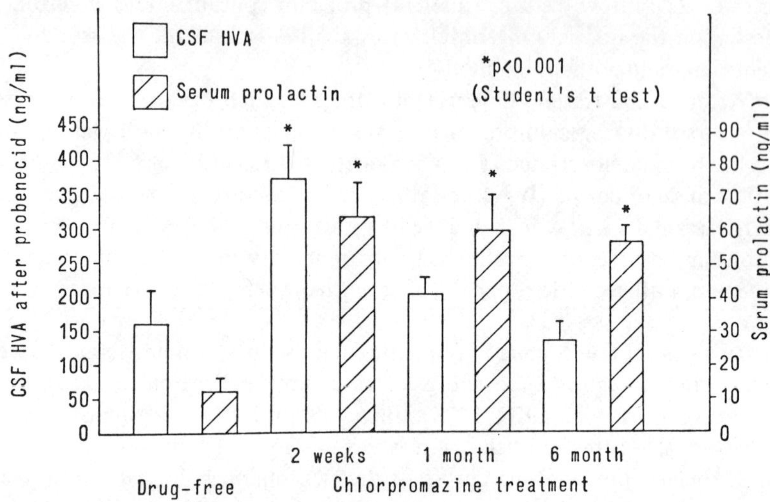

Figure 8 Effects of chlorpromazine on prolactin secretion and probenecid-induced accumulation of homovanillic acid (HVA). (Reprinted with permission from van Praag, 1977.)

B. Chronic Schizophrenia

In a series of 16 unmedicated patients which chronic schizophrenia (Johnstone et al., 1977) prolactin levels were found to be within the normal range or, in a few cases, above this range. When estimated on two occasions, a significant inverse relationship was observed between prolactin secretion and the positive features of the disease (delusions, hallucinations, and thought disorder) suggesting that as symptoms get worse dopamine release from the tuberoinfundibular system may be increasing. Brambilla et al. (1976a) also observed mean prolactin levels to be somewhat increased in a group of 20 mixed sex patients with chronic schizophrenia.

Attempts to use drugs acting on aminergic mechanisms as provocative tests of the integrity of monoamine control of endocrine function have yielded conflicting results. Rotrosen et al. (1976) found growth hormone responses to apomorphine to be significantly more variable in young schizophrenics. They claimed that abnormally high responses were seen only in the three patients who failed to respond to drug therapy. Ettigi et al. (1976) found lower GH responses to apomorphine in chronic schizophrenic patients than in controls, and lower responses in patients with oral dyskinesia than in those without. The increase in prolactin following apomorphine was similar in patients and controls. The data from this study thus provide no evidence of dopamine receptor supersensitivity in chronic schizophrenia, either in unselected patients or in those with oral dyskinesias.

There is some evidence for endocrine changes in schizophrenia less directly related to dopaminergic mechanisms. LH levels are reported to be low in unmedicated chronic schizophrenics (Brambilla et al., 1975; Johnstone et al., 1977) and increase on haloperidol (Brambilla et al., 1975). Although both LH and FSH concentrations in serum were reported lower in a group of 15 chronic schizophrenic patients than in 15 oligophrenic controls the response of both these hormones to gonadotropin-releasing hromone (Gn-RH or LH-RH) was greater and lasted longer in the psychotic patients (Brambilla et al., 1976b). These data suggest that LH-RH secretion may be reduced in chronic schizophrenia but that this reduction can be reversed by neuroleptic medication. There is evidence (Fuxe et al., 1975b) of an inhibitory dopaminergic influence on LH-RH release and an excitatory role for serotonin (Wuttke et al., 1977). The changes observed in schizophrenia are therefore consistent with a relative excess of dopamine with respect to serotonin.

TRH (thyrotropin-releasing hormone) stimulates the release of both thyrotropin and prolactin. In chronic schizophrenic patients it has been reported that the thyrotropin response to TRH is normal (Lindström et al., 1977) but the prolactin response may be enhanced (Brambilla et al., 1976a), although the patients in this latter study had been drug-free for rather short periods. The mechanism of this effect remains obscure.

X. EVALUATION OF THE NEUROHUMORAL HYPOTHESES

An attempt to integrate the diverse findings concerning possible neurotransmitter defects in schizophrenia is bound to fail at the present time. Too many questions concerning, say, the validity of techniques for assessing monoamine turnover or the unitary nature, or otherwise, of acute and chronic, or paranoid and nonparanoid, schizophrenia, remain. Nevertheless, there has been progress in evaluating the various neurotransmitter hypotheses, and this can be summarized in relation to each of the major theories.

A. Dopamine Overactivity

The strengths of the dopamine hypothesis have been its ability to explain the two major pharmacological facts about schizophrenia: symptoms are ameliorated by neuroleptic drugs and mimicked or exacerbated by amphetamines. That the former effect is associated with dopamine receptor blockade now seems highly probable. Some other mechanisms of action can be ruled out, and some earlier contradictions (lack of correlation with extrapyramidal side effects, apparent low potency of butyrophenones as dopamine receptor blockers) resolved. That the psychotogenic effects of the amphetamines and related substances are due to their ability to enhance dopamine release is plausible but not unequivocally established. The psychotomimetic effects of drugs differing from the amphetamines in their actions, such as the ephedrines, require further investigation.

Major weaknesses of the dopamine overactivity hypotheses have been revealed in the search for evidence of increased dopamine release or receptor activation in untreated schizophrenic patients. CSF studies of HVA after probenecid suggest that dopamine turnover is not increased either in acute or chronic schizophrenia; on the contrary, there is evidence that in acute schizophrenia with increasing symptom severity dopamine turnover is decreased. Moreover schizophrenia-like illnesses can occur in patients with preexisting Parkinson's disease and the presence of the features of the one illness does not substantially modify those of the other (Crow et al., 1976c). Since it is now established that dopamine depletion occurs in the mesolimbic as well as the striatal system in Parkinson's disease this finding suggests that increased dopamine release is not necessary for the manifestation of schizophrenic symptoms. The fact that prolactin secretion is not decreased in either acute or chronic schizophrenia suggests that excess dopamine release from the tuberoinfundibular system probably does not occur. On the other hand, there is some evidence in chronic schizophrenia that increasing symptoms are associated with decreasing prolactin secretion (i.e., possibly with increased dopamine release from the tuberoinfundibular system).

The most parsimonious explanation of these findings is that the dopamine blockade hypothesis of neuroleptic action may be correct but the dopamine overactivity hypothesis of schizophrenia mistaken. Thus the primary defect in schizophrenia might be either a relative deficiency of a system which opposes a dopaminergic pathway or supersensitivity of the dopamine receptor (Bowers, 1974; Crow et al., 1976b). Two recent studies (Owen et al., 1978; Lee et al., 1978) presented evidence for a substantial increase in numbers of dopamine receptors in the brains of schizophrenic patients, and this increase occurs in some patients who appear to have been untreated with neuroleptics for the year before death. At the present time this increase in dopamine receptors appears to be the most promising correlate of the primary disturbance in some schizophrenic illnesses.

There are still some problems with the dopamine hypothesis. First, it is uncertain whether neuroleptics are really acting on the entire range of symptoms of the disease. It seems possible that they do not influence the negative symptoms, and therefore that their effectiveness may provide no clues to the nature of the progressive deterioration, where this occurs, or of the defect state. The relative insensitivity of chronic schizophrenic patients to amphetamine may also indicate that dopaminergic mechanisms are not as relevant to the chronic state as to the acute psychosis. Second, the time course of the antipsychotic effect can be clearly dissociated from blockade of dopamine receptors in the tuberoinfundibular system. It appears likely that dopamine receptor blockade, if it is associated with the therapeutic effect, is necessary insofar as it allows some other, and longer term, restitutive process to take place.

B. Noradrenaline Deficiency

The noradrenaline deficiency hypothesis attempted to explain a prominent feature of the defect state (anhedonia) in terms of the postulated functions of a specific neurochemical system (the locus coeruleus system). Although the functions of the locus coeruleus are still obscure the evidence for the suggested degenerative changes in this system is equivocal. The modest reduction originally reported in postmortem brain DBH activity has not been a constant finding and no subgroup of patients has yet been identified with specific noradrenergic defects.

There are, however, some unexplained relationships between schizophrenic symptoms and central noradrenergic activity. There is an inverse relationship between degree of subjective stress and CSF concentration of the noradrenaline metabolite MHPG in acute schizophrenia, and in chronic schizophrenia MHPG sulfate excretion is inversely related to total symptom severity, although mean excretion rates are not significantly different between patients and controls. Whether or not these changes are directly related to the symptoms can probably only be established in experiments in which central noradrenergic activity is manipulated as an independent variable. L-dopa in combination with neuroleptic administration might enhance central noradrenaline release or receptor activation relative to dopaminergic activity, and reports that this combination may have significant therapeutic effects on some negative symptoms in chronic schizophrenia therefore deserve particular attention. If confirmed, this finding is perhaps the only therapeutic change which cannot at the present time be explained in terms of dopamine receptor blockade.

C. Serotonergic Influences

The possible role of serotonin remains the least well-investigated aspect of monoamine function in schizophrenia. The phenomena of the LSD psychosis may differ less from some forms of schizophrenia than has recently been thought, but the pharmacological mechanism, whether by activation of the postsynaptic receptor or inhibition of the presynaptic neuron, or possibly by an action on the dopamine receptor, remains obscure.

From CSF studies on 5-HIAA after probenecid there are suggestions that serotonin turnover is inversely related either to agitation and motor activity, or to number of first rank Schneiderian symptoms. There is as yet little evidence that increasing serotonin release will inhibit these features of the disease although pharmacologically precise therapeutic agents for manipulating serotonin are not available. On the basis of present evidence it seems unlikely that the antipsychotic effects of neuroleptic drugs are related to their ability to interact with the serotonin receptor.

Thus there is little evidence that serotonergic processes are abnormal in schizophrenia or that changes in serotonergic function have therapeutic effects. In a recent postmortem investigation (Joseph et al., 1979) no major changes were found in tryptophan, kynurenin, 5-HIAA, or serotonin in nine brains from chronic schizophrenic patients when compared to nine normal controls.

D. Cholinergic Influences

Both Davis and Janowsky (1975) and Davis et al. (1975) suggested that a relative lack of acetylcholine, perhaps with respect to dopamine, may contribute to the expression of schizophrenic symptoms. It has been claimed that the exacerbation of symptoms induced by methylphenidate (but not the pre-existing symptoms) can be reversed by physostigmine (Davis and Janowsky, 1975) and also that the cholinomimetic agent arecoline can, at least transiently, ameliorate schizophrenic symptoms (Pfeiffer and Jenney, 1957). However, the exacerbation of symptoms by anticholinergic drugs has not yet been unequivocally established, and the hypothesis that acetylcholine lack plays a major part in the pathogenesis of schizophrenia has to be reconciled with the fact that anticholinergic agents induce an acute confusional state rather than a schizophrenia-like psychosis. However, an examination of cholinergic mechanisms in those types of chronic defect state in which intellectual changes are prominent (Stevens et al., 1978) appears to be of considerable interest.

E. Other Neurohumoral Hypotheses

With the possible exception of the changes in the dopamine receptor which have yet to be extensively evaluated no one neurohumoral hypothesis can be confidently advanced. In each case there are deficiencies, and it is plausible that the primary defect (or defects) lies elsewhere. Yet other neurotransmitter theories have been less well investigated. The theory that GABA mechanisms are deficient (Roberts, 1972) is consistent with observations that paranoid changes are often seen early in Huntington's chorea (Panse, 1942) in which loss of GABA-containing cells is prominent (Bird and Iversen, 1974) but this theory does not explain why schizophrenic illnesses do not progress to

Huntington's chorea. It has been proposed, largely on the basis of the same observations, that central opiate-like transmitters are either in excess (Bloom et al., 1976) or deficient (Jacquet and Marks, 1976) in schizophrenia but little evidence has yet been collected from patients with the disease which would be relevant to this hypothesis. Likewise the hypotheses that prostaglandins are in excess (Feldberg, 1976) or deficit (Horrobin, 1977) have yet to be evaluated. (See Table 3.)

XI. CONCLUSIONS

The most significant advances toward understanding the chemical basis of schizophrenic illnesses have come from an understanding of the pharmacological mechanisms by which schizophrenic symptoms can be ameliorated or exacerbated. The dopamine receptor blockade hypothesis of neuroleptic action has been notably successful in explaining the efficacy of a range of drugs, and some earlier difficulties for this hypothesis have been satisfactorily resolved. It seems possible that blockade of dopamine receptors, probably at a site within the mesolimbic or mesocortical systems, is the sole mechanism of the antipsychotic effect. However, it has not yet been satisfactorily established that neuroleptic drugs do more than reverse some of the positive features (delusions, hallucinations, and thought disorder) of the disease, and the mechanism of the antipsychotic effect may not be relevant to an understanding of the progressive deterioration which sometimes occurs or the features of the defect state. The rather slow time course of the antipsychotic effect also remains to be explained since clear dissociation has been established between this course and the onset of dopamine receptor blockade as assessed by actions on the tuberoinfundibular system.

The hypothesis that there is overactivity of dopamine neurons in schizophrenia has met with increasing difficulties. Evidence from CSF studies of HVA and now from postmortem brains reveals no increase of dopamine turnover. By contrast there is evidence from two studies with ligand binding techniques that dopamine receptors are increased in perhaps two-thirds of patients, and there is some evidence that this increase occurs in patients who have been free of neuroleptic drugs. It seems possible that in some cases the increase in dopamine receptor numbers is associated with the disease process.

Outstanding questions, concerning which little neurochemical information is available, are the possible heterogeneity of the group of schizophrenias (e.g., the paranoid-nonparanoid dichotomy) and the nature of the acute-chronic dimension. There is a notable lack of evidence that neuroleptics are effective in reversing or arresting any of the features of progressive deterioration, when this occurs, and some evidence that with the change from the acute to the chronic state there is a quantitative change in the response to amphetamine. In

Table 3 Evaluation of Some Neurohumoral Hypothesis of Schizophrenia

Hypotheses	Model psychoses (Section III)	Antipsychotic effects (Section IV)	Drug-induced exacerbations (Section V)
Dopamine overactivity:			
For	Amphetamine (and related) psychoses (Section III.B)	Neuroleptic effects probably due to DA blockade	Methylphenidate (could act by increased DA release) (Section V.A)
Against	Failure of apomorphine, ET-495 to induce psychotic changes (Section III.E)		Failure of apomorphine to exacerbate schizophrenia,[a] relative insensitivity of chronic schizophrenics to amphetamine[b]
Dopamine receptor supersensitivity:			
For	As above	As above	As above
Against	As above		As Above

[a]Smith et al., 1977.
[b]Kornetsky, 1976.
[c]Owen et al., 1978.

Postmortem studies (Section VI)	CSF studies (Section VII)	Urine metabolites (Section VIII)	Endocrine changes (Section X)	Other
No increase in DA however in postmortem brain[a]	HVA accumulation after probenecid not increased		Prolactin not decreased in acute or chronic schizophrenia	Parkinsonism and schizophrenia can coexist[d]
Increased DA receptors[c,e]	HVA accumulation after probenecid decreases with increasing severity[f]			
No increase in adenylyl cyclase[g]			No consistent increase in GH response to apomorphine	

[d]Crow et al., 1976.
[e]Lee et al., 1978.
[f]Post et al., 1975.
[g]Carenzi et al., 1975.

Table 3 (Continued)

Hypotheses	Model psychoses (Section III)	Antipsychotic effects (Section IV)	Drug-induced exacerbations (Section V)
Noradrenaline deficiency:			
For		L-dopa plus neuroleptics may have therapeutic effects in some chronic patients	
Against	Disulfiram psychosis does not resemble schizophrenia		
Serotonin deficiency:			
For	?LSD (and related) psychoses		
Against		5-HTP and tryptophan not effective	
Serotonin excess:			
For	?LSD (and related) psychoses		
Against		Serotonin antagonists probably ineffective	

Postmortem studies (Section VI)	CSF studies (Section VII)	Urine metabolites (Section VIII)	Endocrine changes (Section X)	Other
	MHPG inversely related to subjective distress[f]	MHPG inversely related to symptom severity in chronic schizophrenia		
DBH not consistently reduced[f]	MPHG not reduced[f]	MPHG not reduced[h]		
	5-HIAA accumulation after probenecid inversely related to agitation[i]			
5-HT and 5-HIAA not reduced[j]				
	5-HIAA after probenecid not increased			

[h] Joseph et al., 1976.
[i] Bowers, 1975.
[j] Joseph et al., 1979 (unpublished).

Table 3 (Continued)

Hypotheses	Model psychoses (Section III)	Antipsychotic effects (Section IV)	Drug-induced exacerbations (Section V)
ACh deficit:			
For		?Cholinomimetic drugs have therapeutic effects	?Anticholinergic drugs exacerbate symptoms
Against	Anticholinergic drugs induce a toxic confusional state, not schizophrenia		
GABA deficit:			
For			
Against		Baclofen does not exert therapeutic effects	
Opiate excess:			
For	Intraventricular opiates induce a "catatonia-like" state	?Naloxone has antipsychotic effects[k]	
Against	Opiate agonists do not induce schizophrenic symptoms in humans	Neuroleptic effects are unrelated to opiate receptor blockade	

[k] Gunne et al., 1976.
[l] Feldberg, 1976.
[m] Falloon et al., 1978.

Postmortem studies (Section VI)	CSF studies (Section VII)	Urine metabolites (Section VIII)	Endocrine changes (Section X)	Other
No consistent change in choline acetyl transferase				
				Huntington's chorea is associated with paranoid psychotic changes[n]
	?Increased opiate-like activity in CSF[o]			Some chronic schizophrenics may be insensitive to pain[p]

[n] Panse, 1942.
[o] Terenius et al., 1976.
[p] For references see Horrobin, 1977.

Table 3 (Continued)

Hypotheses	Model psychoses (Section III)	Antipsychotic effects (Section IV)	Drug-induced exacerbations (Section V)
Prostaglandin excess:			
For	Intraventricular prostaglandin E induces "catatonia-like" changes[l]		
Against		Paracetamol does not exert therapeutic effects[m]	
Prostaglandin deficit:			
For		Neuroleptics stimulate prolactin secretion and prolactin stimulates prostaglandin synthesis[q]	
Against	Prostaglandin antagonists (e.g., antimalarials) induce a toxic confusional state rather than schizophrenia		

[q]Horrobin, 1977.

Postmortem studies (Section VI)	CSF studies (Section VII)	Urine metabolites (Section VIII)	Endocrine changes (Section X)	Other
				Occasional febrile changes in acute schizophrenia[l]
				Some chronic schizophrenics may be insensitive to pain; rheumatoid arthritis and schizophrenia occur together less frequently than would be expected[q]

the chronic defect state very little attention has so far been devoted to neurochemical, pharmacological, or endocrine characteristics which may distinguish between patients with and without evidence of neurological or intellectual deterioration.

REFERENCES

Aghajanian, G. K., Foote, W. E., and Sheard, M. H. (1970). Action of psychotogenic drugs on single midbrain raphe neurons. *J. Pharmacol. Exp. Ther. 171*, 178–187.

Alpert, M., and Silvers, K. N. (1970). Perceptual characteristics distinguishing auditory hallucinations in schizophrenia and acute alcoholic psychoses. *Am. J. Psychiatry 127*, 298.

Altschuler, K. Z., and Sarlin, M. B. (1963). Deafness and schizophrenia: a family study. In *Family and Mental Health Problems in a Deaf Population*, J. D. Rainer, K. Z. Altschuler, F. J. Kallman, and W. E. Denning (Eds.). Columbia University, New York.

Andén, N-E. (1972). Dopamine turnover in the corpus striatum and the limbic system after treatment with neuroleptic and anti-acetylcholine drugs. *J. Pharm. Pharmacol. 24*, 905–906.

Andén, N-E., and Stock, G. (1973). Effect of clozapine on the turnover of dopamine in the corpus striatum and the limbic system. *J. Pharm. Pharmacol. 26*, 738–740.

Andén, N-E., Rubenson, A., Fuxe, K., and Hökfelt, T. (1967). Evidence of dopamine receptor stimulation by apomorphine. *J. Pharm. Pharmacol. 19*, 627–629.

Andén, N-E., Corrodi, H., Fuxe, K., and Hökfelt, T. (1968). Evidence for a central 5-hydroxytryptamine receptor stimulation by lysergic acid diethylamide. *Br. J. Pharmacol. 34*, 1–7.

Angrist, B. M., Shopsin, B., and Gershon, S. (1971). Comparative psychotomimetic effects of stereoisomers of amphetamine. *Nature 234*, 152–153.

Angrist, B., Sathananthan, G., Wilk, S., and Gershon, S. (1974a). Amphetamine psychosis: behavioural and biochemical aspects. *J. Psychiatr. Res. 11*, 13–23.

Angrist, B., Lee, H. K., and Gershon, S. (1974b). The antagonism of amphetamine-induced symptomatology by a neuroleptic. *Am. J. Psychiatry 131*, 817–819.

Angrist, B., Thompson, H., Shopsin, B., and Gershon, S. (1975). Clinical studies with dopamine-receptor stimulants. *Psychopharmacologia 44*, 273–280.

Asano, N. (1967). Pneumoencephalographic study of schizophrenia. In *Clinical Genetics in Psychiatry*, H. Mitsuda (Ed.). Igaku-Shoin, Tokyo, pp. 209–219.

Bell, D. S. (1965). Comparison of amphetamine psychosis and schizophrenia. *Br. J. Psychiatry 111*, 701–707.

Belmaker, R. H., Ebbesen, K., Ebstein, R., and Rimon, R. (1976). Platelet monoamine oxidase in schizophrenia and manic depressive illness. *Br. J. Psychiatry 129*, 227–232.

Benedetti, G. (1952). *The Alcohol Hallucinoses.* Thieme, Stuttgart.

Bennett, J. P., and Snyder, S. H. (1975). Stereospecific binding of D-lysergic acid diethylamide (LSD) to brain membranes: relationship to serotonin receptors. *Brain Res. 94*, 523–544.

Bird, E. D., and Iversen, L. L. (1974). Huntington's chorea: postmortem measurement of glutamic-acid-decarboxylase, choline acetyltransferase and dopamine in basal ganglia. *Brain 97*, 457–472.

Birley, J. L. T., and Brown, G. W. (1970). Crises and life changes preceding the onset or relapse of acute schizophrenia: clinical aspects. *Br. J. Psychiatry 116*, 327–333.

Bishop, M. P., Gallant, D. M., and Sykes, T. F. (1965). Extrapyramidal side effects and therapeutic response. *Arch. Gen. Psychiatry 13*, 155–162.

Bloom, F. E., Segal, D., Ling, N., and Guillemin, R. (1976). Endorphins: profound behavioural effects in rats suggest new etiological factors in mental illness. *Science 194*, 630–632.

Boarder, M. R., and Rodnight, R. (1976). Tryptamine-N-methyltransferase activity in brain tissue: a re-examination. *Brain Res. 114*, 359–364.

Bond, P. A., and Howlett, D. R. (1974). Measurements of the two conjugates of 3-methoxy-4-hydroxyphenyl-glycol in urine. *Biochemical. Med. 10*, 219–228.

Bonheoffer, K. (1909). Zur Frage der exogenen Psychosen. *Zentbl. Nervenheilk 32*, 499–505 [Translated and reprinted in *Themes and Variations in European Psychiatry*, 1974, S. R. Hirsch and M. Shepherd (Eds.). John Wright, Bristol, 1974].

Bowen, D. M., Smith, C. B., White, P., and Davison, A. N. (1976). Neurotransmitter-related enzymes and indices of hypoxia in senile dementia and other abiotrophies. *Brain 99*, 459–496.

Bowers, M. B. (1974). Central dopamine turnover in schizophrenic syndromes. *Arch. Gen. Psychiatry 31*, 50–54.

Bowers, M. B. (1975). Serotonin (5HT) systems in psychotic states. *Psychopharmacol. Comm. 1*, 655–662.

Bowers, M. B., and Rozitis, A. (1974). Regional differences in homovanillic acid concentrations after acute and chronic administration of antipsychotic drugs. *J. Pharm. Pharmacol. 26*, 743–745.

Brambilla, F., Guerrini, A., Guastalla, A., Rovere, C., and Riggi, F. (1975). Neuroendocrine effects of haloperidol therapy in chronic schizophrenia. *Psychopharmacologia 44*, 17–22.

Brambilla, F., Guastalla, A., Guerrini, A., Rovere, C., Legnani, G., Sarno, M., and Riggi, F. (1976a). Prolactin secretion in chronic schizophrenia. *Acta Psychiatr. Scand. 54*, 275–286.

Brambilla, F., Rovere, C., Guastalla, A., Guerrini, A., and Riggi, F. (1976b). Gonadotropin response to synthetic gonadotropin hormone-releasing hormone (GnRH) in chronic schizophrenia. *Acta Psychiatr. Scand. 54*, 131–145.

Brockington, I., Crow, T. J., Johnstone, E. C., and Owen, F. (1976). An investigation of platelet monoamine oxidase activity in schizophrenia and schizoaffective psychosis. In *Monoamine Oxidase and its Inhibition*. K. F. Tipton and M. B. H. Youdim (Eds.), CIBA Foundation, Elsevier, Amsterdam, pp. 353–362.

Brown, G. W., Birley, J. L. T., and Wing, J. K. (1972). Influence of family life on the course of schizophrenic disorders: a replication. *Br. J. Psychiatry 121*, 241–258.

Brune, G. G. (1965). Biogenic amines in mental illness. *Int. Rev. Neurobiol. 8*, 197–220.

Bunney, B. S., and Aghajanian, G. K. (1976). The effect of antipsychotic drugs on the firing of dopaminergic neurons: a reappraisal. In *Antipsychotic Drugs: Pharmacodynamics and Pharmacokinetics*, G. Sedvall (Ed.), Pergamon, Oxford, pp. 305–318.

Burt, D. R., Creese, I., and Snyder, S. H. (1977). Antischizophrenic drugs: chronic treatment elevates dopamine receptor binding in brain. *Science 196*, 326–328.

Carenzi, A., Gillin, J. C., Guidotti, A., Schwartz, M. A., Trabucchi, M., and Wyatt, R. J. (1975). Dopamine-sensitive adenylyl cyclase in human caudate nucleus. A study in control subjects and schizophrenic patients. *Arch. Gen. Psychiatry 32*, 1055–1059.

Carlsson, A., and Lindqvist, M. (1963). Effect of chlorpromazine or haloperidol on formation of 3-methoxytryamine and normetanephrine in mouse brain. *Acta Pharmacol. Toxicol. 20*, 140–144.

Carpenter, W. T., Murphy, D. L., and Wyatt, R. J. (1975). Platelet monoamine oxidase activity in acute schizophrenia. *Am. J. Psychiatry 132*, 438–441.

Casey, J. F., Bennett, I. F., Lindley, C. J., Hollister, L. E., Gordon, M. H., and Springer, N. N. (1960a). Drug therapy in schizophrenia. A controlled study of the relative effectiveness of chlorpromazine, promazine, phenobarbital and placebo. *Arch. Gen. Psychiatry 2*, 210–220.

Casey, J. F., Lasky, J. J., Klett, C. J., and Hollister, L. E. (1960b). Treatment of schizophrenic reactions with phenothiazine derivatives. A comparative study of chlorpormazine, triflupromazine, mepazine, prochlorperazine, perphenazine and phenobarbital. *Am. J. Psychiatry 117*, 97–105.

Casey, J. F., Hollister, L. E., Klett, C. J., Lasky, J. J., and Caffey, E. M. (1961). Combined drug therapy of chronic schizophrenics. Controlled evaluation of placebo, dextro-amphetamine, imipramine, isocarboxazid, and trifluoperazine added to maintenance doses of chlorpromazine. *Am. J. Psychiatry 117*, 997–1003.

Chien, C. P., and Di Mascio, A. (1967). Drug-induced extrapyramidal symptoms and their relations to clinical efficacy. *Am. J. Psychiatry 123*, 1490–1498.

Christensen, A. V., Fjalland, B., and Mϕller-Nielsen, I. (1976). On the supersensitivity of dopamine receptors, induced by neuroleptics. *Psychopharmacology 48*, 1–6.

Christie, J. E., and Crow, T. J. (1971). Turning behaviour as an index of the action of amphetamines and ephedrines on central dopamine-containing neurones. *Br. J. Pharmacol. 43*, 658–667.

Christie, J. E., and Crow, T. J. (1973). Behavioural studies of the actions of cocaine, monoamine oxidase inhibitors and iminodibenzyl compounds on central dopamine neurones. *Br. J. Pharmacol. 47*, 39–47.

Clement-Cormier, Y. C., Kebabian, J. W., Petzold, G. L., and Greengard, P. (1974). Dopamine-sensitive adenylate cyclase in mammalian brain: a possible site of action of antipsychotic drugs. *Proc. Nat. Acad. Sci. USA 71*, 1113–1117.

Cohen, S., and Ditman, K. S. (1963). Prolonged adverse reactions to LSD. *Arch. Gen. Psychiatry 8*, 475–480.

Cohen, S. M., Nichols, A., Wyatt, R., and Pollin, W. (1974). The administration of methionine to chronic schizophrenic patients. *Biol. Psychiatry 8*, 209–225.

Cole, J. O., and Clyde, O. (1961). Extrapyramidal side effects and clinical response to the phenothiazines. *Rev. Can. Biol. 20*, 565–574.

Connell, P. H. (1958). Amphetamine psychosis. Oxford University Press, London.

Cooper, A. F. (1976). Deafness and psychiatric illness. *Br. J. Psychiatry 129*, 216–226.

Corrodi, H., Fuxe, K., and Ungerstedt, U. (1971). Evidence for a new type of dopamine receptor stimulating agent. *J. Pharm. Pharmacol. 23*, 989–991.

Cotes, P. M., Crow, T. J., and Johnstone, E. C. (1977). Serum prolactin as an index of dopamine receptor blockade in acute schizophrenia. *Br. J. Clin. Pharmacol. 4*, 651P.

Cotes, P. M., Crow, T. J., Johnstone, E. C., Bartlett, W., and Bourne, R. C. (1978). Neuroendocrine changes in acute schizophrenia as a function of clinical state and neuroleptic medication. *Psychol. Med. 8*, 657–665.

Creese, I., and Iversen, S. D. (1975). The pharmacological and anatomical substrates of the amphetamine response in the rat. *Brain Res. 83*, 419–436.

Creese, I., Burt, D. R., and Snyder, S. H. (1976). Dopamine receptor binding predicts clinical and pharmacological potencies of antischizophrenic drugs. *Science 192*, 481–483.

Cross, A. J., Crow, T. J., Glover, V., Lofthouse, R., Owen, F., and Riley, G. J. (1977a). Monoamine oxidase activity in postmortem brains of schizophrenics and controls. *Br. J. Clin. Pharmacol. 4*, 719P.

Cross, A. J., Crow, T. J., Kilpack, W. S., Longden, A., Owen, F., and Riley, G. J. (1977b). A comparison of dopamine-β-hydroxylase activity in postmortem brains in schizophrenics and controls. *Br. J. Clin. Pharmacol. 4*, 720P.

Cross, A. J., Crow, T. J., Killpack, W. S., Longden, A., Owen, F., and Riley, G. J. (1978). The activities of brain dopamine-β-hydroxylase and catechol-o-methyl transferase in schizophrenics and controls. *Psychopharmacology 59*, 117–121.

Crow, T. J. (1978). Viral causes of psychiatric disease. *Postgrad. Med. J. 54*, 763–767.

Crow, T. J., and Grove-White, I. G. (1973). An analysis of the learning deficit following hyoscine administration to man. *Br. J. Pharmacol. 49*, 322–327.

Crow, T. J., and Gillbe, C. (1974). Brain dopamine and behaviour. A critical analysis of the relationship between dopamine antagonism and therapeutic efficacy of neuroleptic drugs. *J. Psychiatr. Res. 11*, 163–172.

Crow, T. J., and Johnstone, E. C. (1977). Stereochemical specificity in the antipsychotic effects of flupenthixol in man. *Br. J. Pharmacol. 59*, 466P.

Crow, T. J., Grove-White, I. G., and Ross, D. G. (1976a). The specificity of the action of hyoscine on human learning. *Br. J. Clin. Pharmacol. 2*, 367–368P.

Crow, T. J., Deakin, J. F. W., Johnstone, E. C., and Longden, A. (1976b). Dopamine and schizophrenia. *Lancet 2*, 563–566.

Crow, T. J., Johnstone, E. C., and McClelland, H. A. (1976c). The coincidence of schizophrenia and Parkinsonism: some neurochemical implications. *Psychol. Med. 6*, 227–233.

Crow, T. J., Frith, C., and Johnstone, E. C. (1977a). The clinical effects of the isomers of flupenthixol: the consequences of dopamine receptor blockade in acute schizophrenia. *Br. J. Clin. Pharmacol. 4*, 648P.

Crow, T. J., Deakin, J. F. W., and Longden, A. (1977b). The nucleus accumbens: possible site of antipsychotic action of neuroleptic drugs? *Psychol. Med. 7*, 213–221.

Crow, T. J., Ferrier, I. N., Johnstone, E. C., Macmillan, J. F., Owens, D. G. C., Parry, R. P., and Tyrrell, D. A. J. (1979a). Characteristics of patients with schizophrenia or neurological disease and virus-like agent in cerebrospinal fluid. *Lancet 1*, 842–844.

Crow, T. J., Johnstone, E. C., Londgen, A., Owen, F., and Ridley, R. M.

(1979b). The time course of the antipsychotic effect in schizophrenia and some changes in post-mortem brain and their relation to neuroleptic medication. Advances in Biochemical Psychopharmacology (in press).

Crowell, E. B., and Ketchum, J. S. (1967). The treatment of scopolamine-induced delirium with physostigimine. *Clin. Pharmacol. Ther. 8*, 409–414.

da Prada, M., Saner, A., Burkard, W. P., Bartholini, G., and Pletscher, A. (1975). Lysergic acid diethylamide: Evidence for stimulation of cerebral dopamine receptors. *Brain Res. 94*, 67-73.

Davies, P., and Maloney, A. J. F. (1976). Selective loss of central cholinergic neurons in Alzheimer's disease. *Lancet 2*, 1403.

Davis, J. M. (1974). A two-factor theory of schizophrenia. *J. Psychiatr. Res. 11*, 25–29.

Davis, K. L., Hollister, L. E., and Berger, P. A. (1976). Baclofen in schizophrenia. *Lancet 4*, 1245.

Davis, J. M., and Janowsky, D. (1975). Cholinergic and adrenergic balance in mania and schizophrenia. In *Neurotransmitter Balances Regulating Behaviour*, E. F. Domino and J. M. Davis (Eds.), NPP Books, Ann Arbor,. pp. 135–148.

Davis, K. L., Hollister, L. E., Berger, P. A., and Barchas, J. D. (1975). Cholinergic imbalance hypotheses of psychoses and movement disorders: strategies for evaluation. *Psychopharmacol. Comm. 1*, 533–543.

Davison, K. (1976). Drug-induced psychoses and their relationship to schizophrenia. In *Schizophrenia Today*, D. Kemali, G. Bartholini, and D. Richter (Eds.), Pergamon, Oxford, pp. 105–133.

Deniker, P. (1960). Experimental neurological syndromes and the new drug therapies in psychiatry. *Comprehens. Psychiatry 1*, 92–102.

Depue, R. A. (1976). An activity withdrawal distinction in schizophrenia: behavioural, clinical, brain damage and neurophysiological correlates. *J. Abnorm. Psychol. 85*, 174–185.

Dewhurst, K., and Hatrick, J. A. (1972). Differential diagnosis and treatment of LSD induced psychosis. *Practitioner 209*, 327.

Domino, E. F., Krause, R. R., and Bowers, J. (1973). Various enzymes involved with putative neurotransmitters. Regional distribution in the brain of deceased mentally normal, chronic schizophrenics or organic brain syndrome patients. *Arch. Gen. Psychiatry 29*, 195–201.

Drachman, D. A., and Leavitt, J. (1974). Human memory and the cholinergic system. A relationship to ageing? *Arch. Neurol. 30*, 113–121.

Ehringer, H., and Hornykiewicz, O. (1960). Verteilung von Noradrenalin und Dopamin (3-Hydroxytyramin) im Gehirn des Menschen und ihr Verhalten bei Erkrankungen des Extrapyramidalen-Systems. *Klin. Wochenschr. 38*, 1236–1239.

Ellinwood, E. H. (1967). Amphetamine psychosis. I. Description of the individuals and process. *J. Nerv. Ment. Dis. 144*, 274-283.

Enna, S. J., Bennett, J. P., Burt, D. R., Creese, I., and Snyder, S. H. (1976). Stereospecificity of interaction of neuroleptic drugs with neurotransmitters and correlation with clinical potency. *Nature* (London) *263*, 338–347.

Ernst, A. M. (1967). Mode of action of apomorphine and d-amphetamine for gnawing compulsion in rats. *Psychopharmacologia 10*, 316–323.

Espelin, D. E., and Done, A. K. (1968). Amphetamine poisoning: effectiveness of chlorpormazine. *N. Engl. J. Med. 278*, 1361–1365.

Ettigi, P., Nair, N. P. V., Lal, S., Cervantes, P., and Guyda, H. (1976). Effect of apomorphine on growth hormone and prolactin secretion in schizophrenic patients, with or without oral dyskinesia, withdrawn from chronic neuroleptic therapy. *J. Neurol. Neurosurg. Psychiatry 39*, 870–876.

Faergeman, P. M. (1945). *Psychogenic Psychoses* (translated 1963). Butterworth, London.

Falloon, I., Watt, D. C., Lubbe, K., MacDonald, A., and Shepherd, M. (1978). N-Acetyl-p-amino-phenol (paracetamol, acetaminophen) in the treatment of acute schizophrenia. *Psychol. Med. 8*, 495–499.

Faurbye, A. (1968). The role of amines in the aetiology of schizophrenia. *Comprehens. Psychiatry 9*, 155–177.

Feighner, J. P., Robins, E., Guze, S. B., Woodruff, R. A., Winokur, G., and Munoz, R. (1972). Diagnostic criteria for use in psychiatric research. *Arch. Gen. Psychiatry 26*, 57–63.

Feldberg, W. (1976). Possible association of schizophrenia with a disturbance in prostaglandin metabolism: a physiological hypothesis. *Psychol. Med. 6*, 359–369.

Feldman, F., Susselman, S., and Barrera, S. E. (1945). A note on apomorphine as a sedative. *Am. J. Psychiatry 102*, 403–405.

Feuchtwanger, E., and Mayer-Gross, W. (1938). Hirnverletzung und Epilepsie. *Schwiez. Arch. Neurol. Psychiatr. 41*, 17.

Flügel, F. (1953). Thérapeutique par médication neuroléptique obtenue en réalisant systématiquement des états Parkinsoniformes. *L'Encephale 45*, 1090–1092.

Forrer, G. R., and Miller, J. J. (1958). Atropine coma: a somatic therapy in psychiatry. *Am. J. Psychiatry 115*, 455–458.

Frederiksen, P. K. (1975). Preliminary note on Lioresal (Baclofen) on treatment of schizophrenia. *Läkartidningen 72*, 456–458.

Friedman, E., Shopsin, B., Sathananthan, G., and Gershon, S. (1974). Blood platelet monoamine oxidase activity in psychiatric patients. *Am. J. Psychiatry 131*, 1392–1394.

Frosch, W. A., Robins, E. S., and Stern, M. (1965). Untoward reactions to LSD resulting in hospitalisation. *N. Engl. J. Med. 273*, 1235–1239.

Fuxe, K., and Hökfelt, T. (1967). The influence of central catecholamine neurons on the hormone secretion from the anterior and posterior pituitary. In *Neurosecretion*, F. Stutinsky (Ed.), IVth International Symposium on Neurosecretion. Springer-Verlag, Berlin, pp. 166–177.

Fuxe, K., Hökfelt, T., and Nilsson, P. (1969). Factors involved in the control of the activity of the tubero-infundibular dopamine neurons during pregnancy and lactation. *Neuroendocrinology 5*, 257–270.

Fuxe, K., Hökfelt, T., Ljungdahl, A., Agnati, L., Johansson, O., and Perez de la Mora, M. (1975a). Evidence for an inhibitory gabergic control of the mesolimbic dopamine neurons: possibility of improving treatment of schizophrenia by combined treatment with neuroleptics and gabergic drugs. *Med. Biol. 53*, 177–183.

Fuxe, K., Löfström, A., Agnati, L. F., Everitt, B. J., Hökfelt, T., Jonsson, G., and Wiesel, F-A. (1975b). On the role of central catecholamine and 5-hydroxytryptamine neurons in neuroendocrine regulation. In *Anatomical Neuroendocrinology*, W. E. Stumpf and L. D. Grant (Eds.), Karger, Basel, pp. 420–432.

Fuxe, K., Everitt, B. J., Agnati, L., Fredholm, B., and Jonsson, G. (1976). On the biochemistry and pharmacology of hallucinogens. In *Schizophrenia Today*, D. Kemali, G. Bartholini, and P. Richter (Eds.), Pergamon, Oxford, pp. 125–157.

Gaddum, J. H. (1954). Drugs antagonistic to 5-hydroxytryptamine. In *Ciba Foundation Symposium on Hypertension*, G. W. Wolstenholme (Ed.), Little Brown, Boston, pp. 75–77.

Gallant, D. M., and Bishop, M. P. (1968). Cinanserin (SQ. 10,643): a preliminary evaluation in chronic schizophrenic patients. *Curr. Ther. Res. 10*, 461–463.

Garelis, E., Young, S. N., Lal, S., and Sourkes, T. L. (1974). Monoamine metabolites in lumbar csf: the question of their origin in relation to clinical studies. *Brain Res. 79*, 1–8.

Gerlach, J., and Luhdorf, K. (1975). The effect of L-dopa on young patients with simple schizophrenia, treated with neuroleptic drugs. *Psychopharmacologia 44*, 105–110.

Gershon, S., Angrist, B., and Shopsin, B. (1977). Pharmacological agents as tools in psychiatric research. In *The Impact of Biology on Modern Psychiatry*, E. S. Gershon, R. H. Belmaker, S. S. Kety, and M. Rosenbaum (Eds.), Plenum, New York, pp. 65–93.

Gianutsos, G., Hynes, M. D., and Lal, H. (1975). Enhancement of apomorphine-induced inhibition of striatal dopamine-turnover following chronic haloperidol. *Biochem. Pharmacol. 24*, 581–582.

Gillin, J. C., Kaplan, J. A., and Wyatt, R. J. (1976). Clinical effects of tryptophan in chronic schizophrenic patients. *Biol. Psychiatry 11*, 635–639.

Glass, G. S., and Bowers, M. B. (1970). Chronic psychosis associated with long-term psychotomimetic drug abuse. *Arch. Gen. Psychiatry 23*, 97–103.

Goldberg, S. C., Klerman, G. L., and Cole, J. O. (1965). Changes in schizophrenic psychopathology and ward behaviour as a function of phenothiazine treatment. *Br. J. Psychiatry 111*, 120–133.

Goldstein, M., and Nakajima, K. (1967). The effect of dilsulfiram on catecholamine levels in the brain. *J. Pharmacol. Exp. Ther. 157*, 96–102.

Goodwin, F. K. (1972). Behavioural effects of L-dopa in man. In *Psychiatric Complications of Medical Drugs*, R. I. Shader (Ed.), Raven, New York, pp. 149–174.

Griffith, J. D., Cavanaugh, J., Held, J., and Oates, J. A. (1972). Dextroamphetamine: evaluation of psychotomimetic properties in man. *Arch. Gen. Psychiatry 26*, 97–100.

Gruhle, H. W. (1936). Ueber den Wahn bei Epilepsie. *Z. ges. Neurol. Psychiat. 154*, 395.

Gulmann, N. C., Bahr, B., Andersen, B., and Eliassen, H. M. M. (1976). A double-blind trial of baclofen against placebo in the treatment of schizophrenia. *Acta Psychiatr. Scand. 54*, 287–293.

Gunne, L. M., Anggard, E., and Jönsson, L. E. (1972). Clinical trials with amphetamine blocking drugs. *Psychiatr. Neurol. Neurochir. 75*, 225–226.

Gunne, L. M., Lindström, L., and Terenius, L. (1976). *J. Neurol. Transmission 40*, 13–18.

Haefely, W., Kulcsar, A., Möhler, H., Pieri, L., Pelc, P., and Schaffner, R. (1975). Possible involvement of GABA in the central actions of benzodiazepines. In *Mechanism of Action of Benzodiazepines*, E. Costa and P. Greengard (Eds.), Raven, New York, pp. 131–151.

Haug, J. O. (1962). Pneumoencephalographic studies in mental disease. *Acta Psychiatr. Scand. 38*, supplement 165.

Heinrich, K. (1962). Die gezielte symptomprovokation mit monoaminoxydasehemmenden substanzen in diagnostik und therapie schizophrenen psychosen. *Nervenarzt 31*, 507.

Herman, M., and Nagler, S. H. (1954). Psychoses due to amphetamine. *J. Nerv. Ment. Dis. 120*, 268.

Herridge, C. F., and A'Brook, M. F. (1968). Ephedrine psychosis. *Br. Med. J. 1*, 160.

Heston, L. L. (1966). Psychiatric disorders in foster home reared children of schizophrenic mothers. *Br. J. Psychiatry 112*, 819–825.

Hillbom, E. (1960). After effects of brain injuries. *Acta Psychiatr. Neurol. Scand.* supplement 142.

Hofmann, A. (1970). The discovery of LSD and subsequent investigations on naturally occurring hallucinogens. In *Discoveries in Biological Psychiatry*, F. J. Ayd and B. Blackwell (Eds.), Lippincott, Philadelphia, pp. 91-106.

Holden, J. M. C., Itil, T., Keskiner, A., and Gannon, P. (1971). A clinical trial of an antiserotonin compound, cinanserin, in chronic schizophrenia. *J. Clin. Pharmacol. 11*, 220-226.

Hollister, L. E. (1968). *Chemical Psychoses*, Thomas, Springfield, Ill.

Horn, A. S., and Phillipson, O. T. (1975). Noradrenaline-sensitive adenylate cyclase in rat limbic forebrain homogenates: effects of agonists and antagonists. *Br. J. Pharmacol. 55*, 299-300P.

Horn, A. S., Cuello, A. C., and Miller, R. J. (1974). Dopamine in the mesolimbic system of the rat brain: endogenous levels and effects of drugs on the uptake mechanism and stimulation of adenylate cyclase activity. *J. Neurochem. 22*, 265-270.

Horrobin, D. F. (1977). Schizophrenia as a prostaglandin deficiency disease. *Lancet 1*, 936-937.

Hotson, J. R., and Langston, J. W. (1976). Disulfiram-induced encephalopathy. *Arch. Neurol. 33*, 141-142.

Inanaga, K., Nakazawa, Y., Inoue, K., Tachibana, H., Oshima, M., Kotorii, J., Tanaka, M., and Ogawa, N. (1975). Double-blind controlled study of L-dopa therapy in schizophrenia. *Folia Psychiatr. Neurol. Jap. (Niigata) 29*, 123-142.

Israelstam, D. M., Sargent, T., Finley, N., Winchell, H. S., Fish, M. B., Motto, J., Pollycore, M., and Johnson, A. (1970). Abnormal methionine metabolism in schizophrenic and depressive states: a preliminary report. *J. Psychiatr. Res. 7*, 187.

Jacobi, A. (1927). Die psychische Wirkung des cokains in ihrer Bedeutung fur die psychopathologie. *Arch. Psychiatr. 79*, 383.

Jacquet, Y. F., and Marks, N. (1976). The C-fragment of β-lipotropin: an endogenous neuroleptic or antipsychotogen. *Science 194*, 632-635.

Janowsky, D., and Davis, J. (1976). Methylphenidate, dextroamphetamine and levamphetamine: effects on schizophrenic symptoms. *Arch. Gen. Psychiatry 33*, 304-308.

Janowsky, D. S., El-Yousef, M. K., Davis, J. M., and Sekerke, H. J. (1973). Provocation of schizophrenic symptoms by intravenous administration of methylphenidate. *Arch. Gen. Psychiatry 28*, 185-191.

Janowsky, D. S., Huey, L., Storms, L. H., and Judd, L. L. (1977). Methylphenidate hydrochloride effects on psychological tests in acute schizophrenic and nonpsychotic patients. *Arch. Gen. Psychiatry 34*, 189-194.

Johnson, R. T., and Herndon, R. M. (1974). Virologic studies of multiple sclerosis and other chronic and relapsing neurological disease. *Progr. Med. Virol. 18*, 214-228.

Johnstone, E. C., Crow, T. J., Frith, C. D., Husband, J., and Kreel, L. (1976). Cerebral ventricular size and cognitive impairment in chronic schizophrenia. *Lancet 2*, 924-926.

Johnstone, E. C., Crow, T. J., and Mashiter, K. (1977). Anterior pituitary hormone secretion in chronic schizophrenia: an approach to neurohumoural mechanisms. *Psychol. Med. 7*, 223–228.

Johnstone, E. C., Crow, T. J., Frith, C. D., Carney, M. W. P., and Price, J. S. (1978a). Mechanism of the antipsychotic effect in the treatment of acute schizophrenia. *Lancet 1*, 848–851.

Johnstone, E. C., Crow, T. J., Frith, C. D., Stevens, M., Kreel, L., and Husband, J. (1978b). The dementia of dementia praecox. *Acta Psychiatr. Scand. 57*, 305–324.

Joseph, M. H., Baker, H. F., Johnstone, E. C., and Crow, T. J. (1976). Determination of 3-methoxy-4-hydroxy-phenyl-glycol conjugates in urine. Application to the study of central noradrenaline metabolism in unmedicated chronic schizophrenic patients. *Psychopharmacology 51*, 47–51.

Joseph, M. H., Baker, H. F., Crow, T. J., Riley, G. J., and Risby, D. (1979). Brain tryptophan metabolism in schizophrenia: a post-mortem study of metabolites on the serotonin and kynurenine pathways in schizophrenic and control subjects. *Psychopharmacology 62*, 279–285.

Kaplan, J., Mandel, L. R., Stillman, R., Walker, R. W., van den Heuvel, W. J. A., Gillin, J. C., and Wyatt, R. J. (1974). Blood and urine levels of N,N-dimethyl tryptamine following administration of psychoactive dosages to human subjects. *Psychopharmacologia 38*, 239–245.

Kasanin, J. (1933). The acute schizoaffective psychoses. *Am. J. Psychiatry 13*, 97–126.

Kay, D. W. K., and Roth, M. (1961). Environmental and hereditary factors in the schizophrenias of old age. *J. Ment. Sci. 107*, 649–686.

Kebabian, J. W., Petzold, G. L., and Greengard, P. (1972). Dopamine-sensitive adenylate cyclase in caudate nucleus of rat brain, and its similarity to the "dopamine receptor." *Proc. Nat. Acad. Sci. USA 69*, 2145–2149.

Keller, H. H., Schaffner, R., and Haefely, W. (1976). Interaction of benzodiazepines with neuroleptics at central dopamine neurons. *Naunyn-Schmiedeberg's Arch. Pharmacol. 294*, 1–7.

Kellner, R., Wilson, R. M., Muldawer, M. D., and Pathak, D. (1975). Anxiety in schizophrenia. The responses to chlordiazepoxide in an intensive design study. *Arch. Gen. Psychiatry 32*, 1246–1254.

Kety, S. S. (1959). Biochemical theories of schizophrenia. *Science 129*, 1528–1532 and 1590–1596.

Kety, S. S., Rosenthal, D., Wender, P., and Schulsinger, F. (1971). Mental illness in the biological and adoptive families of adopted schizophrenics. *Am. J. Psychiatry 128*, 87–94.

Kirstein, L., Bowers, M. B., and Heninger, G. (1976). CSF amine metabolites, clinical symptoms, and body movements in psychiatric patients. *Biol. Psychiatry 11*, 421–434.

Klein, D. F., and Davis, J. M. (1969). *Diagnosis and Drug Treatment of Psychiatric Disorders*, Williams & Wilkins, Baltimore.

Kolakowska, T., Wiles, D. H., McNeilly, A. S., and Gelder, M. G. (1975). Correlation between plasma levels of prolactin and chlorpromazine in psychiatric patients. *Psychol. Med. 5*, 214–216.

Kornetsky, C. (1976). Hyporesponsivity of chronic schizophrenic patients to dexamphetamine. *Arch. Gen. Psychiatry 33*, 1425–1428.

Kraepelin, E. (1923). Delirium, hallucinose and dauervirgiftung. *Monatschr. Psychiatr. 54*, 43.

Lal, S., and de la Vega, C. E. (1975). Apomorphine and psychopathology. *J. Neurol. Neurosurg. Psychiatry 38*, 722–726.

Langer, G., Sachar, E. J., Gruen, P. H., and Halpern, F. S. (1977). Human prolactin responses to neuroleptic drugs correlate with antischizophrenic potency. *Nature 266*, 639–640.

Langfeldt, F. (1937). *The Prognosis in Schizophrenia and the Factors Influencing the Course of the Disease*, Humphrey Melford, London.

Lee, T., Seeman, P., Tourtellotte, W. W., Farley, I. J., and Hornykiewicz, O. (1978). Binding of ^{3}H-neuroleptics and ^{3}H-apomorphine in schizophrenic brain. *Nature 274*, 897–900.

Leonhard, K. (1959). *Aufteilung der Endogenen Psychosen*, 2nd ed., Akademie-Verlag, Berlin.

Levy, D. B., and Weinreb, H. J. (1976). Wheat gluten-schizophrenia findings. *Science 194*, 448.

Liddon, S. C., and Satran, R. (1967). Disulfiram (Antabuse) psychosis. *Am. J. Psychiatry 123*, 1284–1289.

Lilliston, L. (1973). Schizophrenic symptomatology as a function of probability of cerebral damage. *J. Abnorm. Psychol. 82*, 377–381.

Lindström, L. H., Gunne, L. M., Ost, L-G., and Persson, E. (1977). Thyrotropin-releasing hormone (TRH) in chronic schizophrenia. *Acta Psychiatr. Scand. 55*, 74, 80.

Lindvall, O., and Björklund, A. (1974). The organisation of the ascending catecholamine neuron system in the rat brain. *Acta Physiol. Scand 92*, supplement 412.

Lucas, A. R., and Weiss, M. (1971). Methylphenidate hallucinosis. *J. Am. Med. Ass. 217*, 1079–1081.

Lycke, E., and Roos, B-E. (1975). Virus infections in infant mice causing persistent impairment of turnover of brain catecholamines. *J. Neurol. Sci. 26*, 49–60.

McClelland, H. A., Roth, M., Neubauer, H., and Garside, R. (1968). Some observations on a case-material based on patients with certain common schizophrenic symptoms. In *Proc. IVth World Congr. Psychiatry*, Excerpta Medica Foundation, Amsterdam, pp. 2955–2957.

McCormick, T. O., and McNeel, T. W. (1963). Acute psychosis and ritalin abuse. *Tex. State J. Med. 59*, 99–100.

Maas, J. W., and Landis, D. H. (1968). In vivo studies of the metabolism of norepinephrine in the central nervous system. *J. Pharmacol. Exp. Ther. 163*, 147–162.

Malleson, N. (1971). Acute adverse reactions to LSD in clinical and experimental use in the United Kingdom. *Br. J. Psychiatry 118*, 229–230.

Mannarino, E., Kirschner, N., and Nashold, B. S. (1963). The metabolism of (^{14}C)noradrenaline by cat brain in vivo. *J. Neurochem. 10*, 373–379.

Matthysse, S. (1974). Dopamine and the pharmacology of schizophrenia: the state of the evidence. *J. Psychiatr. Res. 11*, 107–113.

Meltzer, H. Y., and Fang, V. S. (1976). The effect of neuroleptics on serum prolactin in schizophrenic patients. *Arch. Gen. Psychiatry 33*, 279–286.

Meltzer, H. Y., and Stahl, S. M. (1974). Platelet monoamine oxidase activity and substrate preferences in schizophrenic patients. *Res. Comm. Chem. Pathol. Pharmacol. 7*, 419–431.

Meltzer, H. Y., Sachar, E. J., and Frantz, A. G. (1974). Serum prolactin levels in unmedicated schizophrenic patients. *Arch. Gen. Psychiatry 31*, 564–569.

Menninger, K. A. (1926). Influenza and schizophrenia. *Am. J. Psychiatry 82*, 469–529.

Miller, R. J. (1976). Comparison of the inhibitory effects of neuroleptic drugs on adenylate cyclase in rat tissues stimulated by dopamine, noradrenaline and glucagon. *Biochem. Pharmacol. 25*, 537–541.

Miller, R. J., and Hiley, C. R. (1974). Antimuscarinic properties of neuroleptics and drug-induced Parkinsonism. *Nature* (London) *248*, 596–597.

Miller, R. J., Horn, A. S., and Iversen, L. L. (1974). The action of neuroleptic drugs on dopamine-stimulated adenosine cyclic 3',5'-monophosphate production in neostriatum and limbic forebrain. *Molec. Pharmacol. 10*, 759–766.

Misra, P. G., and Hay, G. G. (1971). Encephalitis presenting as acute schizophrenia. *Br. Med. J. 1*, 532–533.

Muller, P., and Seeman, P. (1974). Neuroleptics: relation between cataleptic and anti-turning actions, and role of the cholinergic system. *J. Pharm. Pharmacol. 26*, 981–984.

Murphy, D. L., and Wyatt, R. J. (1972). Reduced MAO activity in blood platelets from schizophrenic patients. *Nature 238*, 225–226.

Narasimhachari, N., Avalos, J., Fujimori, M., and Himwich, H. E. (1972). Studies of drug-free schizophrenics and controls. *Biol. Psychiatry 5*, 311–318.

NIMH-Psychopharmacology Service Center Collaborative Study Group (1964). Phenothiazine treatment in acute schizophrenia. *Arch. Gen. Psychiatry 10*, 246–261.

O'Keefe, R., Sharman, D. F., and Vogt, M. (1970). Effect of drugs used in psychoses on cerebral dopamine metabolism. *Br. J. Pharmacol. 38*, 287–304.

Orr, M. W., and Boullin, D. J. (1976). The relationship between changes in 5-HT induced platelet aggregation and clinical state in patients treated with fluphenazine. *Br. J. Clin. Pharmacol. 3*, 925–928.

Osmond, H., Smythies, J. R., and Harley-Mason, J. (1952). Schizophrenia: new approach. *J. Ment. Sci. 98*, 309–315.

Owen, F., Cross, A. J., Crow, T. J., Longden, A., Poulter, M., and Riley, G. J. (1978). Increased dopamine-receptor sensitivity in schizophrenia. *Lancet 2*, 223–226.

Panse, F. (1942). *Die Erbchorea*, Leipzig.

Penn, H., Racy, J., Lapham, L., Mandel, M., and Sandt, J. (1972). Catatonic behavior, viral encephalopathy, and death. *Arch. Gen. Psychiatry 27*, 758–761.

Perris, C. (1974). A study of cycloid psychoses. *Acta Psychiatr. Scand., supplement 253.*

Perry, T. L., Hansen, S., and Kloster, M. (1973). Huntington's chorea, deficiency of gamma-aminobutyric acid in brain. *N. Engl. J. Med. 288*, 337–342.

Perry, E. K., Perry, R. H., Blessed, G., and Tomlinson, B. E. (1977). Necropsy evidence of central cholinergic deficits in senile dementia. *Lancet 1*, 189.

Pfeiffer, C. C., and Jenney, E. H. (1957). The inhibition of the conditioned response and the counteraction of schizophrenia by muscarinic stimulation of the brain. *Ann. N.Y. Acad. Sci. 66*, 753–764.

Pieri, L., Pieri, M., and Haefely, W. (1974). LSD as an agonist of dopamine receptors in the striatum. *Nature 252*, 586–588.

Pleasure, H. (1954). Psychiatric and neurological side effects of isoniazid and iproniazid. *Arch. Neurol. Psychiatry 72*, 313.

Pond, D. A. (1957). Psychiatric aspects of epilepsy. *J. Ind. Med. Prof. 3*, 1441.

Post, F. (1966). *Persistent Persecutory States of the Elderly*, Pergamon, London.

Post, R. M. (1975). Cocaine psychoses: a continuum model. *Am. J. Psychiatry 132*, 225–231.

Post, R. M., and Goodwin, F. K. (1975). Time-dependent effects of phenothiazines on dopamine turnover in psychiatric patients. *Science 190*, 488–489.

Post, R. M., Fink, E., Carpenter, W. T., and Goodwin, F. K. (1975). Cerebrospinal fluid amine metabolites in acute schizophrenia. *Arch. Gen. Psychiatry 32*, 1063–1069.

Price, J. (1972). Methylation in schizophrenics: a pharmacogenetic study. *J. Psychiatr. Res. 9*, 345–351.

Price, J., and Hopkinson, G. (1968). Monoamine oxidase inhibitors and schizophrenia. *Psychiatr. Clin.* (Basel) *1*, 65–84.

Randrup, A., and Munkvad, I. (1965). Special antagonism of amphetamine-induced abnormal behaviour. Inhibition of stereotyped activity with increase of some normal activities. *Psychopharmacologia 7*, 416–422.

Randrup, A., and Munkvad, I. (1966). On the role of catecholamines in the amphetamine excitatory response. *Nature* (London) *211*, 540.

Randrup, A., and Munkvad, I. (1967). Stereotyped activities produced by amphetamine in several animal species and man. *Psychopharmacologia 11*, 300–310.

Raskin, D. E., and Frank, S. W. (1974). Herpes encephalitis with catatonic stupor. *Arch. Gen. Psychiatry 31*, 544–546.

Roberts, E. (1972). An hypothesis suggesting that there is a defect in the GABA system in schizophrenia. *Neurosci. Res. Prog. Bull. 10*, 468–482.

Rodnight, R., Murray, R. M., Oon, M. C. H., Brockington, I. F., Nicholls, P., and Birley, J. L. T. (1976). Urinary dimethyltryptamine and psychiatric symptomatology and classification. *Psychol. Med. 6*, 649–657.

Rosenthal, R., and Bigelow, L. B. (1973). The effects of physostigmine in phenothiazine resistant chronic schizophrenic patients: preliminary observations. *Comprehens. Psychiatry 14*, 489–494.

Rotrosen, J., Angrist, B. M., Gershon, S., Sachar, E. J., and Halpern, F. S. (1976). Dopamine receptor alteration in schizophrenia: neuroendocrine evidence. *Psychopharmacology 51*, 1–7.

Rutledge, C. O., and Jonason, J. (1967). Metabolic pathways of dopamine and norepinephrine in rabbit brain in vitro. *J. Pharmacol. Exp. Ther. 157*, 493–502.

Saavedra, J. M., and Axelrod, J. (1972). Psychotomimetic N-methylated tryptamines: formation in brain in vivo and in vitro. *Science 172*, 1365–1366.

Sandison, R. A. (1959). Comparison of drug-induced and endogenous psychoses in man. In *Proceedings of the First International Congress in Neuropharmacology*, Elsevier, London.

Sandler, M., and Reynolds, G. P. (1976). Does phenylethylamine cause schizophrenia? *Lancet 1*, 70–71

Sathananthan, G., Angrist, B. M., and Gershon, S. (1973). Response threshold to L-dopa in psychiatric patients. *Biol. Psychiatry 7*, 139–149.

Scatton, B., Thierry, A. M., Glowinski, J., and Julou, L. (1975a). Effects of thioproperazine and apomorphine on dopamine synthesis in the mesocortical dopaminergic systems. *Brain Res. 88*, 389–393.

Scatton, B., Glowinski, J., and Julou, L. (1975b). Neuroleptics: effects on dopamine synthesis in the nigro-neostriatal, mesolimbic and mesocortical dopaminergic systems. In *Antipsychotic Drugs: Pharmacodynamics and Pharmacokinetics*, G. Sedvall (Ed.), Pergamon, Oxford, pp. 243–255.

Scatton, B., Glowinski, J., and Julou, L. (1976). Dopamine metabolism in the mesolimbic and mesocortical dopaminergic systems after single or repeated administration of neuroleptics. *Brain Res. 109*, 184–189.

Scheel-Krüger, J. (1972). Some aspects of the mechanism of action of various stimulant amphetamine analogues. *Psychiatr. Neurol., Neurochir. 75*, 179–192.

Schuckit, M. A., and Winokur, G. (1971). Alcoholic hallucinosis and schizophrenia: a negative study. *Br. J. Psychiatry 119*, 549–550.

Schwarz, M. A., Aikens, A. M., and Wyatt, R. J. (1974a). Monoamine oxidase activity in brains from schizophrenic and mentally normal individuals. *Psychopharmacologia 38*, 319–328.

Schwarz, M. A., Wyatt, R. J., Yang, H.Y-T., and Neff, N. H. (1974b). Multiple forms of brain monoamine oxidase in schizophrenia and normal individuals. *Arch. Gen. Psychiatry 31*, 557–560.

Seeman, P., and Lee, T. (1975). Antipsychotic drugs: direct correlation between clinical potency and presynaptic action on dopamine neurons. *Science 188*, 1217–1219.

Seeman, P., Lee, T., Chau-Wong, M., and Wong, K. (1976). Antipsychotic drug doses and neuroleptic/dopamine receptors. *Nature* (London) *261*, 717–719.

Shields, J. (1976). Genetics in schizophrenia. In *Schizophrenia Today*, D. Kermali, G. Bartholini, and D. Richter (Eds.), Pergamon, Oxford, pp. 57–70.

Shopsin, B., Wilk, S., Gershon, S., Davis, K., and Suhl, M. (1973). Cerebrospinal fluid MHPG: an assessment of norepinephrine metabolism in affective disorders. *Arch. Gen. Psychiatry 28*, 230–233.

Simpson, G. (1976). Baclofen in schizophrenia. *Lancet 1*, 702.

Singh, M. M., and Kay, S. R. (1975). Therapeutic reversal with benzotropine in schizophrenics. *J. Nerv. Ment. Dis. 160*, 258–266.

Sjöström, R., and Roos, B-E., (1972). 5-hydroxyindoleacetic acid and homovanillic acid in cerebrospinal fluid in manic-depressive psychoses. *Eur. J. Clin. Pharmacol. 4*, 170–176.

Slater, E. (1959). Book review: *Amphetamine Psychosis* by P. H. Connell. *Br. Med. J. 1*, 488.

Slater, E., and Beard, A. W. (1963). The schizophrenia-like psychoses of epilepsy: psychiatric aspects. *Br. J. Psychiatry 109*, 95–150.

Smith, J. M. (1976). Wheat gluten-schizophrenia findings. *Science 194*, 448.

Smith, R. C., Tamminga, C., and Davis, J. M. (1977). Effect of apomorphine on schizophrenic symptoms. *J. Neural Transm. 40*, 171–176.

Snyder, S. H., Greenberg, D., and Yamamura, M. I. (1974). Antischizophrenic drugs and brain cholinergic receptors. *Arch. Gen. Psychiatry 31*, 58–61.

Sobin, A., and Ozer, M. N. (1966). Mental disorders in acute encephalitis. *J. Mt. Sinai Hosp. 33*, 73–82.

Spensley, J., and Rockwell, D. A. (1972). Psychosis during methylphenidate abuse. *N. Engl. J. Med. 16*, 880–881.

Stawarz, R. J., Hill, H., Robinson, S. E., Setler, P., Dingell, J. V., and Sulser, F. (1975). On the significance of the increase in homovanillic acid (HVA) caused by antipsychotic drugs in corpus striatum and limbic forebrain. *Psychopharmacologia 43*, 125–130.

Stein, L., and Wise, C. D. (1971). Possible aetiology of schizophrenia: progressive damage to the noradrenergic reward system by 6-hydroxydopamine. *Science 171*, 1032–1036.

Stephens, D. A. (1967). Psychotoxic effects of benzhexol hydrochloride (Artane). *Br. J. Psychiatry 113*, 213–218.

Stevens, M., Crow, T. J., Bowman, M., and Coles, E. C. (1978). Age disorientation in chronic schizophrenia: a constant prevalence of 25% in a mental hospital population? *Br. J. Psychiatry 133*, 130–136.

Stoll, A., and Hofmann, A. (1943). Partial synthesis of alkaloids of the ergonovine type (6th communication on ergot alkaloids). *Helv. Chim. Acta 26*, 844–965.

Terenius, L., Wahlström, A., Lindström, L., and Widerlov, E. (1976). Increased CSF levels of endorphines in chronic psychosis. *Neurosci. Lett. 3*, 157-162.

Torrey, E. F., and Peterson, M. R. (1976). The viral hypothesis of schizophrenia. *Schizophrenia Bull. 2*, 136–146.

Trendelenburg, U. (1966). Mechanisms of supersensitivity and subsensitivity to sympathomimetic amines. *Pharmacol. Rev. 18*, 629–640.

Tyrrell, D. A. J., Parry, R. P., Crow, T. J., Ferrier, I. N., and Johnstone, E. C. (1979). Detection of a virus-like agent in cerebrospinal fluid in schizophrenia and some neurological conditions. *Lancet 1*, 839–841.

Ungerstedt, U. (1971). Stereotaxic mapping of the monoamine pathways in the rat brain. *Acta Physiol. Scand. supplement 367*, 1–48.

Utena, H., Kanamura, H., Suda, S., Nakamura, R., Machiyama, Y., and Takahashi, R. (1968). Studies of the regional distribution of monoamine oxidase activity in the brains of schizophrenic patients. *Proc. Jap. Acad. 44*, 1078–1083.

van Praag, H. M. (1977). The significance of dopamine for the mode of action of neuroleptics and the pathogenesis of schizophrenia. *Br. J. Psychiatry 130*, 463–474.

van Praag, H. M., and Korf, J. (1971). Retarded depression and the dopamine metabolism. *Psychopharmacologia 19*, 199–203.

van Praag, H. M., and Korf, J. (1975). Neuroleptics, catecholamines and psychoses: a study of their inter-relations. *Am. J. Psychiatry 132*, 593–597.

Vaughn, C. E., and Leff, J. P. (1976). The influence of family and social factors on the course of psychiatric illness. *Br. J. Psychiatry 129*, 125–137.

Victor, M., and Hope, J. M. (1958). The phenomenon of auditory hallucinations in chronic alcoholism. *J. Nerv. Ment. Dis. 126*, 451–481.

Weil-Malherbe, H. (1967). The biochemicstry of the functional psychoses. *Adv. Enzym. 29*, 479–553.

Weinstein, E. A., Linn, L., and Kahn, R. L. (1955). Encephalitis with the clinical picture of schizophrenia. *J. Mt. Sinai Hosp. 21*, 341–354.

Westerink, B. H. H., and Korf, J. (1976). Acidic dopamine metabolites in cortical areas of the rat brain: localisation and effects of drugs. *Brain Res. 113*, 429–434.

Wilson, R. G., Hamilton, J. R., Boyd, W. D., Forrest, A. P. M., Cole, E. N., Boyns, A. R., and Griffiths, K. (1975). The effect of longterm phenothiazine therapy on plasma prolactin. *Br. J. Psychiatry 127*, 71–74.

Wing, J. K., Cooper, J. E., and Sartorious, N. (1974). *Measurement and Classification of Psychiatric Symptoms*, Cambridge University Press.

Wise, C. D., Baden, M. M., and Stein, L. (1974). Postmortem measurement of enzymes in human brain: evidence of a central noradrenergic deficit in schizophrenia. *J. Psychiatr. Res. 11*, 185–198.

Wise, C. D., and Stein, L. (1975). Dopamine-β-hydroxylase activity in brains of chronic schizophrenic patients. *Science 187*, 370.

Woolley, D. W., and Shaw, E. (1954). A biochemical and pharmacological suggestion about certain mental disorders. *Proc. Nat. Acad. Sci. USA 40*, 228–231.

Wuttke, W., Bjørklund, A., Baumgarten, H. G., Lachenmayer, L., Fenske, M., and Klemm, H. P. (1977). De- and regeneration of brain serotonin neurons following 5,7-dihydroxytryptamine treatment: effects on serum LH, FSH and prolactin levels in male rats. *Brain Res. 134*, 317–331.

Wyatt, R. J., Termini, B. A., and Davis, J. (1971). Biochemical and sleep studies of schizophrenia: a review of the literature 1960–1970. *Schizophrenia Bull. NIMH 4*, 8–66.

Wyatt, R. J., Vaughan, T., Galanter, M., Kaplan, J., and Green, R. (1972). Behavioural changes of chronic schizophrenic patients given L-5-hydroxytryptophan. *Science 177*, 1124–1126.

Wyatt, R. J., Saavedra, J. M., and Axelrod, J. (1973a). A dimethyltryptamine-forming enzyme in human blood. *Am. J. Psychiatry 130*, 754–760.

Wyatt, R. J., Mandel, L. R., Ahn, H. S., Walker, R. W., and van den Heuvel, W. J. (1973b). Gas-chromatographic mass spectrometric isotope dilution determination of N,N-dimethyltryptamine concentrations in normals and psychiatric patients. *Psychopharmacologia 31*, 265–270.

Wyatt, R. J., Schwartz, M. A., Erdelyi, E., and Barchas, J. P. (1975). Dopamine-β-hydroxylase activity in brains of chronic schizophrenic patients. *Science 187*, 368–369.

Young, B. G. (1974). A phenomenological comparison of LSD and schizophrenic states. *Br. J. Psychiatry 124*, 64–74.

Young, D., and Scoville, W. B. (1938). Paranoid psychosis in narcolepsy and possible dangers of benzedrine treatment. *Med. Clin. North Am. 22*, 637–643.

Zivkovic, B., Guidotti, A., Revuelta, A., and Costa, E. (1975). Effect of thioridazine, clozapine and other antipsychotics on the kinetic state of tyrosine hydroxylase and on the turnover rate of dopamine in striatum and nucleus accumbens. *J. Pharmacol. Exp. Ther. 194*, 37–46.

2

Course of Schizophrenia and Some Organic Psychoses

Carlo Perris
Umeå University
Umeå, Sweden

I. COURSE OF SCHIZOPHRENIA

A. Introduction

Both Kraepelin (1896), who introduced the concept of dementia praecox, and E. Bleuler (1908), who introduced the concept of schizophrenia, maintained that their grouping together under the same heading of different morbid conditions should be regarded as provisional. Three-quarters of a century later the label "dementia praecox" belongs to the history of psychiatry whereas the more comprehensive label "schizophrenia" is still used provisionally. A unanimous agreement about the boundaries of the disorder to which the label is supposed to refer has yet to be reached. Stephens (1970) points out that the diagnosis of schizophrenia depends almost entirely upon the psychiatrist's conception of it. Notwithstanding, schizophrenia is still treated in textbooks and articles as if it were a unitary nosological entity, or at best a badly defined syndrome or type of reaction. At the same time other authors regard it as an "impossible concept" (van Praag, 1976), a "mystification" (Laing, 1960), or a "myth" (Szasz, 1960). Under such circumstances to write a review of the literature about the course of a condition which is not yet defined and might not exist at all might seem a dubious task. There are many other factors which contribute to making the task difficult. First of all, there is no possibility whatsoever of describing the natural course of the hypothetical conditions labeled schizophrenia since the diagnosis depends upon the psychiatrist's conception of it and because the disorder can last a lifetime. No research worker would be able to collect during his lifetime a series of patients large enough to allow generalizations. Even if this were possible, the problem would remain that the observation in itself could be suspected of influencing the course in an unpredictable way. Furthermore, the course of any disease in general, and of any mental disorder in particular, is always dependent upon the social context within which they occur and must be evaluated against a background of continuous change within the society where they are observed. The course of schizophrenia as it has been described in hundreds of articles and monographs refers to a fragment of the course of a disorder (or group of disorders) observed and described under certain circumstances and in a certain historical epoch. Whatever the case it never refers to the natural course, but to the course as it has been determined by selection, attitudes, expectations, treatments, resources, etc. Since all these variables are seldom explicitly acknowledged, the information obtainable from all these writings taken per se reflects only what has occurred to certain patients who have been classified as schizophrenics and treated in a certain way. If we look at the problem from this angle, then a review of the literature could be useful in that it allows identification of features which recur independently of who observed them, and when and where. It will also be possible to identify features which belonged to certain historical epochs and which are no longer relevant.

In the following, relevant variables about the course of the conditions labeled schizophrenia will be reviewed and analyzed and an attempt made to evidentiate the evolution of opinions over time. No attempt will be made to analyze the different authors' conception of schizophrenia. The data reported in the literature will be summarized as they were originally presented and some sources of error regarding their collection or interpretation will be pointed out. It is the author's belief that from such an impartial survey it is possible that some general conclusions may emerge which can form the basis for further research.

The author does not believe that the label schizophrenia as it is most commonly used today is still meaningful. However, it can be retained for the sake of simplicity in this chapter, and schizophrenia is referred to by such terms as *psychosis, disorder, illness,* and *disease,* exclusively for linguistic reasons. For the same reasons the term *schizophrenia* will be used throughout the chapter in its singular form.

B. Age at Onset

The age limits within which a disorder with a supposed genetic component in its causation can manifest itself for the first time is of importance especially for studies of morbidity rates among the relatives of the proband. In fact, among his criteria in favor of a genetic component in the causation of a certain disorder, Hanna (1965) lists the onset at a certain well-delimited age. Schizophrenic disorders, however, do not fulfill this criterion since a wide range in the distribution of age at onset has been documented by several authors.

The different authors' individual conceptions of schizophrenia are important for the ascertainment of the age limits for the onset of the disorder. Depending upon whether late paraphrenia or paronoic syndromes arising in the senium and early childhood psychosis are regarded as belonging to the group of schizophrenias or not, the percentage distribution of onset in different age groups varies greatly in the literature. Furthermore, it is not easy to trace back the age at onset of a disorder which develops insidiously. Especially if one takes into account that personality disturbances of a certain severity have been regarded in themselves as the earliest manifestation of the disorder. Several authors give an account of the age at onset concerning the cases they have studied (Table 1). However, the definition of *onset* is not consistent and usually is not given at all. Some of the definitions are as follows: "patient's age at the time when his family members or other people in his environment observed his psychotic symptoms" (Achté, 1961, 1967) or "the age at which the patient first displayed psychotic symptoms or marked personality changes indicative of mental illness" (Kay and Lindelius, 1970). However, there are others who feel it impossible to establish the age at the first manifestation of the disorder and prefer instead to use age at first admission as the starting point of a condition for

Table 1 Percent Distribution of Patients with Onset Before Age 20 or After Age 40

Reference	No. of patients	Age limits (yr)		Remarks
		Before 20	After 40	
Kraepelin, 1913	1054	33.9	5.8	Quoted in Mayer-Gross, 1932
Wolfsohn, 1907	618	22.0	13.0	Quoted by Bleuler, 1911
Schneider, 1942	889	20.4	15.4	Quoted in Mayer-Gross, 1932
Schulz, 1933	660	20.2	5.6	
Fromenty, 1937	81	13.6	2.5	
Gerloff, 1937	348	33.3	6.3	
Strömgren, 1938	174	19.5	13.8	
Bleuler, 1941	459	19.8	14.8	
Rennie, 1941	500	21.0	8.0	
Tangerman, 1942	418	13.9	14.6	
Böök, 1953	85	14.1	10.6	
Polonio, 1954	511	16.7	32.6	
Holmboe & Astrup, 1957	255	9.4	18.4	
Johanson, 1958	100	34.0	16.0	
Welner & Strömgren, 1958	72	13.9	19.4	Benign schizophreniform
Hallgren & Sjögren, 1959	246	12.1	17.5	
Marinow, 1959	425	4.9	1.6	Refers to < 15 and > 50 yr
Achté, 1961–1967	100	7.0	27.0	Admitted 1950
	100	8.0	37.0	Admitted 1960

Frøshaug & Ytrehus, 1963	95	2.1	20.0	Admitted 1933-1935	all
	103	6.8	39.8	Admitted 1953-1959	female
Retterstøl, 1966	84	8.1	30.4		
Noreik & Ödegaard, 1967[a]	not given	(9.2)	(13.6)	Male patients 1951-1955	
		10.4	15.2		
		(6.6)	(26.7)	Female patients 1951-1955	
		8.1	30.4		
Hartmann, 1969	861	18.9	19.3		
Kay & Lindelius, 1970	237	16.9	18.1		
Larsson & Nyman, 1970	153	9.2	32.0	All male	
Bleuler, 1972	271	12.0	23.0		
Achté & Niskanen, 1973	100	10.0	24.0	Admitted 1965	
Gross & Huber, 1973	449	20.7	14.7		
Huber et al., 1975a,b	502	24.5	13.9		
Total[b]	9453	16.6	18.3		
		range 2.1-34.0	range 2.5-39.8		

[a]Figures by Noreik & Ödegaard do not appear in the average values.
[b]The series by Welner and Strömgren and by Marinow are not included in the total.

which they want to investigate the further course (Hoch et al., 1962; von Trostorff, 1975). It is evident that both taking into account the occurrence of manifest psychotic symptoms or age at first admission are very crude estimates which might conceal sources of error.

According to Kraepelin's original figures, the age at onset was between 20 and 40 years in 87% of 296 cases and only about 7.6% at an age of 40 or more. Kraepelin maintained, however, that in most instances the origin of dementia praecox could be traced in the very early childhood.

Table 1 shows the percent distribution of patients with onset before age 20 or after age 40. According to the data in the table, which cover about 9500 patients, there are about 16.6% of the patients with onset before the age of 20 and about 18.3% with onset after the age of 40. However, these are average figures. In reality the range is very wide: 2.1-34.0% for the early onset and from 2.5-39.8 for the late onset. These differences cannot but express differences in the conception of what kind of disorders have to be included under the heading schizophrenia. An interesting question is whether or not the age for the first appearance of the respective conditions has changed over the years. M. Bleuler (1972) in comparing his early (1941) and late investigations suggests that the percentage of early onset cases has diminished and that the percentage of late onset cases has increased during the 30 years which elapsed between his two investigations. Figure 1 shows the proportion of early and late onset cases in studies published before 1940 and after 1960. The general picture so obtained seems to support the view maintained by Bleuler. To be noted is the fact that the proportion of the cases who become ill in the age range 20-40 years has not changed in the two periods taken into account and has remained fairly constant at about 67%. Of interest in this context are the studies by those authors who compared series of patients collected in different periods (Bleuler, 1941, 1972;

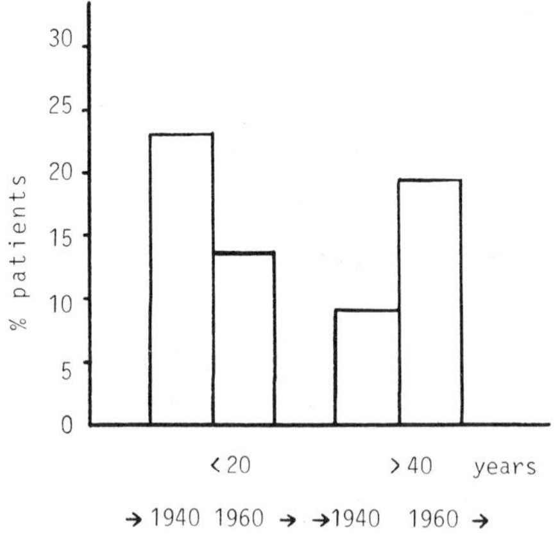

Figure 1 Percentage of patients with age at onset < 20 or > 40 year years in early (before 1940) and late (after 1960) studies. Observe that the percentage of patients with onset between 20 and 40 years has not changed (67.8% vs. 67.1%).

Achté, 1961, 1967; Achté and Apo, 1967; Achté and Niskanen, 1973; Frøshaug and Ytrehus, 1963; Noreik and Ødegaard, 1967) since it can be assumed that the same criteria for defining age at onset have been applied in the comparisons. All these authors clearly point out an increase of late onset cases over the years. However, one wonders what kind of selection has been operating when figures for the late onset as those presented by Frøshaug and Ytrehus (39.8%) or by Achté (37.0% for patients admitted in 1960) have to be evaluated. It has been investigated whether there is any difference between sexes as concerns age at onset. Judging from the data reported in the literature (Helgason, 1964; Noreik and Ødegaard, 1967; Janzarik, 1968; Kay and Lindelius, 1970; Bleuler, 1972) it seems that the mean age at onset is somewhat higher in female than in male patients especially as concerns paranoid forms (Agnst et al., 1973). Tangerman (1942) suggests the occurrence of two different peaks in females: one at about 25 years and one at about 45. As it will be described later females are over-represented in series of patients with late onset, the proportion being about 2.5:1. Such an overrepresentation of females among late onset cases had been found already by Schröder in his study of late catatonia (quoted by Kraepelin, 1913).

Although a differentiation in subtypes of schizophrenic syndromes is less frequently taken into account in the most recent studies, possible differences in age at onset have been reported by several authors. Table 2 gives the figures reported in some studies. In line with classical concepts, hebephrenic and catatonic forms have been found to occur at an earlier age than paranoic ones. Early authors, e.g., Gerloff (1937), maintained that no instance of hebephrenic schizophrenia occurred after the age of 25.

A differentiation as concerns age at onset has also been made as concerns patients with a favorable course and patients with a poor prognosis. Some of the results referring to this issue are summarized in Table 2. On the whole, the same wide range as concerns age distribution at onset has been found in both groups. Perris (1974) reviewed the literature concerning age at onset for those conditions which following Leonhard's (1957) classification are labeled as cycloid psychoses and found that clear-cut recurrent psychotic conditions of this kind very seldom begin after the age of 50. The occurrence of schizo-affective disorders in the elderly, however, has been pointed out by Post (1971).

Kraepelin had been aware that the onset of dementia praecox could be traced back to early childhood and gave a figure of about 6% with onset before the age of 15. Marinow (1959) found a proportion which is quite similar to that by Kraepelin (4.9%) whereas Bradley (1941) and Kallman and Roth (1956) maintain that no more than 1.0-1.9% of all schizophrenic patients become ill before the age of 15. Table 3 shows the percent distribution of patients with onset before 15 according to different authors. Judging from the results summarized in the table, it seems that there have been less variations over time in

Table 2 Mean Age (yr) at Onset or Percent of Patients at a Certain Age of Onset in Subtypes of Schizophrenia

Reference	Simplex	Hebephrenic	Catatonic	Paranoic	Dementia praecox
Kraepelin, 1913				40% < 25 yr	60% < 25 yr
Mayer-Gross, 1932		21.5	25.7	35.0	
Johanson, 1958	21.6	21.6	21.6	34.4	
Leonhard, 1966		23.1	24.2	4.3	
Angst et al., 1973			65% < 30	33% < 30	
Langfeldt, 1937		19.0	23.1	26.9	
Gerloff, 1937			75% < 30		
Achté, 1967		80% < 30	68% < 30	26% < 30	
Tangerman, 1942		95% < 30	72% < 30	38% < 30	
Aghté, 1961		23.5			

Table 3 Percent Distribution of Patients with Onset at an Age Below 15 Years According to Different Authors[a]

Reference	Distribution (%)
Kraepelin	6
Wolfsohn, 1907	4
Fromenty, 1937	3.7
Bradley, 1941	1.0
Böök, 1953	1.2
Kallman & Roth, 1956	1.9
Johanson, 1958	3.0
Marinow, 1959	4.9
Noreik & Ødegaard, 1967	4.6-5.1 male patients 3.3-3.9 female patients
Hartman, 1969	2.2

[a]None of the patients comprised by Bleuler in his 1972 monograph had become ill before age 15.

this special age group than in others. However, the question is still unsettled as to what extent early childhood psychosis or early childhood autism has to be regarded as belonging to the group of schizophrenias or not. It seems fair to assume that the inclusion or exclusion of these conditions under the heading schizophrenia might influence not only opinions about age at onset but also opinions about course. For these reasons a separate survey of the main findings regarding the course of psychotic conditions in childhood will be presented in this chapter.

Contrary to his concept of dementia praecox, Kraepelin admitted the occurrence of cases with onset late in life (after the age of 40). However, paraphrenic and paranoic conditions arising in the senium have for a long time been kept apart from schizophrenia. The concept of late schizophrenia seems to have been introduced by Halberstadt (1925). More recently, schizophrenic conditions arising after the age of 40 have attracted the attention of several authors (Bleuler 1943; Knoll, 1952; Polonio, 1954; Janzarik, 1957; Klages, 1961; Failla et al., 1963; Schimmelpenning, 1965; Berner, 1969; Berner and Gabriel, 1973a,b; Berner et al., 1973; Gabriel, 1974a,b; 1975a,b; Sternberg, 1972; Rostovtseva, 1973; Huber et al., 1975a,b). Late schizophrenia is usually defined according to the criteria set out by Bleuler (1943), i.e., "a psychotic condition arising for the first time after the age of 40 which: 1) on the basis of its symptomatology cannot be distinguished from the schizophrenia arising in earlier age, and b) is not explained by the organic damage of the brain." An onset as late as after the age of 60 was reported in 3.1% out of 644 cases studied by Huber et al. (1975a,b) and 10.2% out of 153 cases studied by Larson and Nyman (1970). Of the cases labeled by Berner et al. (1973a,b) as late schizophrenia 81.6% (out of 110) had had their onset after the age of 40 whereas in the remainder the debute of the condition could be traced to a time before that age. Table 4 shows the age distribution in a series of patients with late onset. In almost all these series female patients predominate.

1. *Comments*

Studies concerned with the age of onset of schizophrenic conditions are loaded with uncertainty and conceal many sources of error. This is reflected in the wide range of the percentage distribution in the different age groups. One major source of inconsistency is to be found in how broad or narrow the conception of schizophrenia is taken to be by the authors who have attempted to sort out this age variable. Another source of inconsistency is the opportunity of obtaining reliable information. However, the inclusion of paraphrenic and late paranoic conditions in the realm of the schizophrenic syndromes has very likely been one main reason for the increase of late forms registered in more recent studies. As in early periods, the most part of the patients (about 67%) seem to become ill for the first time in the age range 20-40 years, the peak being 24-34 years. Taking the results published in the literature at their face value, it would seem that instances of early onset (before age 20) have diminished, whereas instances of late onset (i.e., above age 40) have increased since the early descriptions by Kraepelin and E. Bleuler. In particular a shift toward more frequent late onset seems to have occurred after World War II. No satisfactory explanation of why this change in risk period has occurred has been given. Noreik and Ødegaard tried to relate age at onset with socioeconomic factors as for example periods of economic crisis and unemployment but their results were not clear-cut, and

Table 4 Age Distribution in Series of Patients with Late Onset (> 40)

		Age distribution (%)				
Reference	*n*	40-44	45-49	50-54	55-59	> 61
Bleuler, 1943	94	35.0	33.0	16.0	12.0	–
Knoll, 1952	83	29.0	38.5	26.0	5.0	–
Klages, 1961	53	30.2	32.1	24.5	13.2	–
Failla et al., 1963	50	60.0	26.0	10.0	4.0	–
Schimmelpenning, 1965	117	37.6	29.1	16.2	9.4	7.7
Huber et al., 1975	110	36.3	36.3	24.3		3.1
Larson & Nyman, 1970	49	57.1		32.6		10.2

the authors were unable to explain differences in different periods or differences between sexes. One possible explanation of the increase in late-onset instances has been given above. As concerns a possible decrease of cases with an early onset, it seems fair to assume that the successive development of child psychiatric care in the Western World might have contributed to a more appropriate definition of psychopathological conditions in childhood which in earlier periods might have been regarded as schizophrenic in nature. Almost all the studies in the literature report a somewhat higher age at onset in females than in males, but in most instances the difference hardly reaches statistical significance. If such a difference really exists and if it depends upon sociocultural or biological factors it is still unsettled.

Almost all the studies concerned with age at onset have been carried out in development countries, where no marked differences have emerged. A comparison of age at onset of schizophrenia in patients hospitalized in India and in the USA has been made by Walker (1961), who was unable to find significant differences. Comprehensive studies of different cultural settings, however, are still lacking. Also uncertain is whether studies carried out in the community will give results which are different from those based on hospitalized patients.

The definition of the risk period during which a disorder can manifest itself for the first time is of great importance in family studies for a calculation of the morbidity risk among relatives of probands. For most of the family studies in the literature the period at risk was taken as terminated at 40 years. The figures shown in the present review suggest that such a narrow risk period might have been a source of error which could lead to an overestimation of the expectancy rats among relatives of schizophrenic patients.

C. Type of Onset, Premorbid Characteristics, and Prodroma

Major obstacles to an accurate ascertainment of the age at onset of schizophrenic conditions have been the insidious progressive debut in most instances and the fact that under the heading schizophrenia are listed conditions such as the pseudoneurotic and pseudopsychopathic forms described by Hoch and coworkers (1949, 1962) and more recently by Nyman et al. (1976), as well as the coenesthetic form described by Huber (1957). These forms, schizophrenia classified as latens according to the ICD system, manifest themselves less frequently with clear-cut psychotic episodes. In particular, Hoch et al. (1962) stated that the actual age at onset of illness in their psychoneurotic cases was difficult to determine and that they had gained the impression that many of the patients had had some disability most of their lives.

Also, problems related to the possible identification of a particular personality makeup preceding manifest schizophrenia and its relationship with the disease have contributed to making the issue controversial. Furthermore, a difference in type of onset, i.e., insidious versus acute, has been taken into account in attempts at differentiating between true or nuclear schizophrenic disorders with a poor prognosis and schizophreniform or reactive schizophrenic syndromes which generally have a more favorable outcome. Such a separation might have influenced the selection of patients comprised in follow-up studies of schizophrenics also as concerns age and type of onset.

Kraepelin maintained that the onset of hebephrenia was consistently insidious and protracted over several years, and that for this reason it was very difficult to establish the actual onset of the illness. On the other hand he maintained that the onset was most often subacute in catatonic and acute in paranoid subtypes of dementia praecox. Bleuler considered the possibility of a very acute onset and quoted in this respect an observation by Kahlbaum. However, he maintained that a careful anamnesis very often uncovers early minor manifestations of the disease. This opinion also seems to be valid for more recent authors, such as Bemporad and Pinsker (1974). In particular, Bleuler did not like the concept of prodroma since he believed, as Kraepelin did, that when these prodromal manifestations occurred they were nothing but the first manifestations of the disease which had not been recognized.

In a discussion of the course of schizophrenia the issue of possible premorbid personality characteristics must be taken into account. Kraepelin described peculiar characterological characteristics in about 20% of his patients. He maintained, however, that these characteristics resulted from early episodes of the disease passing unnoticed. Berze (1910) described a personality pattern characterized by shyness and eccentricity not only in the patients but also in their parents and regarded these eccentrics as latent schizophrenics. The linkage of schizophrenia with a particular personality makeup is, however, from a later period.

In 1946 Bellak and Parcell wrote that "one of the more time-honored hypotheses concerning dementia praecox contends that there is a typical prepsychotic personality associated with this disorder." The typical personality pattern they were referring to was that characterized by introversion as conceived by Jung. Bellak and Parcell pointed out that Bleuler, Kretschmer, and Jung himself were responsible for linking introversion with schizophrenia and were the supporters of the hypothesis that schizoid personalities were related to and frequently the forerunners of full-blown schizophrenic pictures. Most of the studies in the early forties showed a very high frequency of schizoid personality traits in schizophrenics (Wittman and Steinberg, 1944), also of the paranoid type (Miller, 1941). In successive years the view that a schizoid personality is a frequent forerunner of schizophrenia has been accepted as part of established psychiatric knowledge in major textbooks (Mayer-Gross et al., 1960, 1969; Noyes and Kolb, 1963; Freedman and Kaplan, 1967), whereas in others a more cautious position is maintained (Ey et al. 1963).

Several authors and most textbooks maintain that a schizoid personality makeup occurs in at least 50% of schizophrenic patients. In particular, the presence of a schizoid personality has been associated with a poor prognosis (Langfeldt, 1937; Kant 1941a,b,c; Polonio, 1954; Vaillant, 1964b; Noreik, 1970). However, Johanson (1958) and Rennie (1941) found no clear-cut correlation between schizoid personality and prognosis. Bleuler (1972) found that patients with a premorbid schizopathic personality were less represented among those who later showed a periodic course but he was unable to find statistical relationships between premorbid personality and further course of the disease. Bellak and Parcell (1946), however, found in their most careful investigation that no more than 28% of their patients had distinct introvert prepsychotic personalities, the remainder being distinctly extravert or "ambivalent." Similar figures are given by Holmboe and Astrup (1957) (24%), Johanson (185) (21%), Retterstøl (1966) (26%). Bleuler (1972) makes a distinction between a premorbid personality "pronounced schizoid but with the norm" and "morbid schizoid"; 28% of his patients were regarded as schizoid within the norm, and 24% as morbid schizoid in their premorbid personality makeup. Although the figures are somewhat smaller than those found in an earlier study (1941) and despite division of the schizoid personality into two subtypes, the results by Bleuler do not deviate from the 50% mentioned in most textbooks.

Studies of the premorbid personality characteristics of schizophrenic patients have been criticized mainly because they have been based upon retrospective recollection of unsystematic information when the patients had already become schizophrenics. However, other approaches have been followed which have contributed considerably to the clarification of this issue. Among them of special interest are the longitudinal studies carried out by Morris et al. (1954), Michael et al. (1957), O'Neal and Robins (1958), Pritchard and Graham (1966), and Mellsop (1973). In these studies both adolescents characterized as schizoid have been followed up into adult age and schizophrenic patients have been identified retrospectively on the basis of school or hospital records at the time they were still children. In all instances the studies failed to support the hypothesis that introversion is forerunner to schizophrenia or that a schizoid personality is the most common among schizophrenics. In particular, only one out of 54 shy, withdrawn children investigated 16-27 years later by Morris et al. developed schizophrenia. On the other hand, out of 606 patients who had been childhood attenders 10 males developed schizophrenia and of these only one had a personality of the introverted type (Michael et al., 1957). Finally, none of the 64 patients studied by Pritchard and Graham who had been hospitalized at the Maudsley both as children and as adults was schizoid. From the report by O'Neil and Robins, on the other hand, it emerged that children referred to a psychiatrist for antisocial behavior were very likely to develop schizophrenia in adulthood.

The occurrence of neurotic manifestations in the history of individuals who later become schizophrenic is mentioned in many textbooks (Tanzi and Lugaro, 1923; Baruk, 1950; Henderson and Gillespie, 1969; Noyes and Kolbe, 1963) and has been the concern of several investigators (Heuyer et al., 1929; Lucena, 1938; Caldwell, 1941a,b; Rubino and Piro, 1954; Gilberti and Gregoretti, 1958; Carletti, 1958; Pritchard and Graham, 1966; Gardner, 1967; Mellsop, 1973). The possible occurrence of neurasthenic and hysterical manifestations was first pointed out by E. Bleuler and later confirmed by Heuyer et al., Lucena, Rubino and Piro, Giberti and Gregoretti, Lambert, and Midenet (1972). However, the most frequent neurotic characteristics seem to be those of anxiety and obsession (Morlaas, 1938; Caldwell, 1941a,b; Müller, 1953; Shneshnevski, 1966, 1970). Stoianov et al. (1969) found that the occurrence of neurotic manifestations prior to manifest schizophrenia decreases with increasing age at onset. In retrospective studies of the type mentioned above, the occurrence of neurotic traits in childhood could be established in 3 of the 64 patients studied by Pritchard and Graham. A high frequency of neurotic manifestations was also found by Gardner and by Mellsop. The latter found that 40% of his adult schizophrenics had been characterized as neurotic during childhood. However, as pointed out by Vallejo-Nagera (1954), none of these preschizophrenic neurotic manifestations is characteristic of schizophrenia, nor is it possible to predict from these manifestations which patients will later develop manifest schizophrenia.

A more peculiar prodromal phase of schizophrenia has been described by Conrad (1958), who in 1941-1942 carefully investigated 107 soldiers during their first hospitalization for schizophrenia. Conrad labeled this prodromal phase as *trema* (which is a German slang for stagefright) and maintained that he had been able to establish its occurrence in all of his patients. The main feature of trema is a lack of volition accompanied by dysphoric affects and impaired flow of thought. According to Conrad the phase of trema varied in duration from a very brief period to several years. A similar variation in duration has been reported recently by Varsamis and Adamson (1971). Other authors who carefully studied early schizophrenia were on the whole able to confirm Conrad's findings (Meares, 1959; Chapman, 1966; Varsamis and Adamson, 1971). However, the occurrence of trema does not seem to be so constant as suggested by Conrad, and Varsamis and Adamson. Premonitory symptoms were also described by Cameron (1938) in 83% of his patients and by Bowers (1968).

The Bonn group takes into account partly the occurrence of prodroma and partly the occurrence of outpost syndromes (Vorposten syndrome) (Gross, 1969; Gross et al. 1973a,b; Huber et al. 1974, 1975a,b, 1977). Prodromal manifestations were found in 44% of the patients. At variance from other authors (Failla et al., 1963), who maintained the absence of prodromal manifestations in cases of late schizophrenia, the Bonn group found prodroma in 31.4% outpost syndromes in 21.4% of their schizophrenic patients with a late onset. In 27.1% of these patients prodromal manifestations among those with late onset was also found by Sternberg (1972), who stressed that these manifestations can last for years. The further course of these prodromal and/or outpost syndromes is different in different patients. These manifestations can remain for a long time as isolated episodes of short duration—from a few weeks to a few months (outpost syndromes)—or develop toward manifest psychosis (prodroma). According to the Bonn group, the longer the prodromal phase the worse the prognosis (Gross et al., 1973a,b). Prodromal manifestations were found to occur in 30.4% of these cases by Giberti and Gregoretti (1958). Abortive episodes of different duration prior to manifest attacks of schizophrenia were found in 22 of 216 patients by Kutsenok (1971). They occurred more frequently in patients with a subsequent remittent course of the disease.

The reported incidence of acute versus insidious onset varies considerably between the different studies. This variation probably depends upon the subtypes of patients taken into account. Table 5 shows the percentage of cases with an insidious (chronic or progressive) onset in different studies. Noteworthy is the difference between the results of Klages (1961) and Schimmelpenning (1965). An acute onset, irrelevant of precipitating factors, has been regarded as a factor related to a favorable prognosis for a long time (Hunt and Appel, 1936; Gerloff, 1937; Langfeldt, 1973; Kant, 1941b,c; Holmboe and Astrup, 1957; Polonio, 1957; Kay and Lindelius, 1970; Noreik, 1970). Patients labeled as cycloid psychotics, schizoaffective psychotics, or reactive psychotics are mainly characterized by an acute onset (Retterstøl, 1966; Perris, 1974). These labels are regarded by some authors as interchangeable with those of periodic, recurrent, or good-prognosis schizophrenia. Furthermore, the conditions so labeled also often have an acute debut (Bleuler, 1941, 1972; Kant, 1941; Rennie, 1941; Polonio, 1954, 1957; Hallgren and Sjögren, 1959, Murtalibov, 1976). Thus it is evident that the different values for acute onset obtained by different authors are to a large degree dependent upon whether or not disorders of this type are included in follow-up studies. Instances of acute onset have not increased lately, according to the results by Bleuler (1972). However, Bleuler points out that instances of acute relapse have increased among the patients comprising his most recent series as compared with the previous ones (1941). According to the results of the international pilot study of schizophrenia (WHO, 1973) a sudden onset of the episode occurred on average in 12% of the cases in all centers participating in the study. The range, however, varied from 1% in Washington and Moscow to 49% in Agra. In a study of Chinese patients from Hong Kong the percentage of acute onset was 34% (Lo and Lo, 1977). According to Bleuler (1973), an acute onset occurs very frequently in Africa.

Table 5 Percent Distribution of Patients with Insidious ("Chronic" or "Progressive") Onset of Disorder in Different Series

References	Insidious onset (%)	Type of patients
Langfeldt, 1937	62.3	
Gerloff, 1937	100.0	Hebephrenic
	52.4	Catatonic
Polonio, 1954, 1957	70.0	Continuous course
	32.0	Periodic course
Freyhan, 1955	76.0	1920 series
	51.0	1940 series
Giberti & Gregoretti, 1958	30.4	
Hallgren & Sjögren, 1959	71.2	Continuous course
	47.0	Periodic course
Marinow, 1959	24.7	
Klages, 1961	33.7	Late schizophrenia
Schimmelpenning, 1965	93.4	Late paranoic syndromes
Retterstøl, 1966	35.0	Paranoic schizophrenia
	10.0	Reactive paranoia
Pritchard, 1967	40.0	1952/53 series
	36.0	1956/57 series
Inghe et al., 1970	56.8	
Kay & Lindelius, 1970	38.0	
Noreik, 1970	50.0	Schizophrenic
	26.0	Schizophrenic?
Bleuler, 1972	38.0	
Huber, 1968b, Huber et al., 1975a,b	22.0	
Lo & Lo, 1977	65.8	Chinese pat. popul. from Hong Kong

1. Comments

The studies reviewed in this section reveal how difficult it is to give conclusive answers to questions concerning relevant variables of the course of schizophrenic syndromes. Cultural changes have greatly influenced current opinions about a particular personality makeup of schizophrenic patients. Unsystematically collected information of dubious reliability has over certain periods been the basis for assuming specific relationships between a peculiar kind of personality structure and a successive schizophrenic development. On the other hand, more recent studies tend to support such a strong relationship. At present, the most reasonable conclusion should be that no particular personality pattern is to be expected in the background of schizophrenic disorders. Only when subgroups are consistently identified and described will studies of a particular personality structure predisposing to the outbreak of the disorder become meaningful. No statistically significant relationships have been found between particular personality types and further course of the disease. However, some consensus seems to exist for a more favorable prognosis in patients with less pronounced deviations in their premorbid personality structure.

About one-third of the patients who manifest overt psychotic schizophrenic syndromes have in their past history psychopathological manifestations of various intensity and duration either in the form of disturbances labeled as neurotic or in the form of outpost syndromes or finally in the form of prodromal manifestations. These previous manifestations can remain isolated for many years or develop further into manifest psychotic conditions.

Formerly insidious onset was regarded as the rule in the hebephrenic and pseudoneurotic forms of schizophrenia. More recent statistics show that a chronic insidious onset characterizes about one-third of the patients labeled as schizophrenics. However, great variations still occur—most of the cases with a favorable outcome have an acute onset whereas particular syndromes with a late onset still show an insidious debut. Any increase over the last few decades of the number of cases with an acute onset seems to not have occurred. On the other hand, it is probable that there is an increase in the number of acute relapse. The nosological position of syndromes labeled as cycloid, schizo-affective, reactive psychosis or recurrent, periodic, remitting, good-prognosis schizophrenia is still uncertain. Since the conditions referred to by these labels might differ from other subtypes of schizophrenic syndromes as concerns both premorbid personality characteristics and type of onset, they should be identified separately in studies concerning the course of schizophrenia.

D. Seasonal Distribution at Onset; Interval Between Onset and Hospital Admission

Contrary to what is generally accepted concering affective disorders, no clear-cut seasonal variations have been maintained as concerns the onset of schizophrenic syndromes. Information in the literature as concerns this course variable is very scanty, and most often the possibility of seasonal variations is not mentioned at all. Mayer-Gross et al. (1960) in their textbook quote Kollibay-Uter, who found that like most acute psychoses, acute schizophrenic attacks occur more frequently in spring or early summer than in other periods of the year. On the contrary, Mentzos (1967) quotes an investigation by Supprion (1964), who found an even distribution of the onset in 500 patients.

In an unpublished study of more than 1000 admissions for a schizophrenic syndrome to a mental hospital where both first admissions and readmissions were taken into account, a summer peak was noted. However, it is uncertain as to what degree factors proper to the schizophrenic disorder or social factors are responsible for the distribution which has been found. Furthermore, the seasonal distribution of hospital admission does not necessarily correspond to the distribution of the onset of the episodes. In view of the insidious onset described in the previous section, studies relating to seasonal distribution are dubious. It is more feasible to map out the seasonal distribution of those disorders with an acute onset. In a study of 182 episodes with an acute onset in a group of patients labeled as cycloid psychotics (Perris, 1974), an even distribution of onset during the whole year was found without any statistically significant deviation for any particular month (Fig. 2). Kirow (1972a), who studied the distribution of 459 episodes in an apparently similar group of patients, found a clear prevalence in early spring and early autumn. However, it is uncertain as to what extent the series by Kirow and Perris are diagnostically comparable. In fact, 46 of the episodes studies by Kirow proved to be self-limiting and the patients recovered in a few days without any treatment. Mentzos (1969) found a higher occurrence in autumn and winter.

The course variable which refers to the interval between the onset of the first psychotic symptoms and the first admission to the hospital is very likely much more indicative of the availability of psychiatric services in a certain community and of the attitudes toward psychiatric care at a certain time than of the real course of the disorder. On the other hand, it could be assumed that the severity of the disorder is reflected in the length of delay before hospital admission, thus giving indirect information about the course of the milder forms of the illness.

The delay between the onset of the psychosis and the first admission to hospital is taken into account in several studies; the main findings are summarized in Table 6. It can be seen that most of the patients experienced a delay of several years from the beginning of the disorder to the time they received psychiatric care. What should be noted in particular is the fact that in some studies a very high percentage of patients had not been admitted to a hospital before more than 5 years had elapsed from the onset of the disorder. Moreover, population studies, as for example those by Böök (1953) and Hallgren and Sjögren (1959), show that a large number of patients are admitted first after decades of illness or not admitted at all. It seems fair to assume that patients with an acute onset are more likely to be admitted to hospital earlier than patients with an insidious onset. Johanson (1958), however, found than an acute onset did not necessarily lead to an acute admission. Niskanen and Achté (1972) found in a comparison of patient series from 1950, 1960, and 1965 that the delay in admission had become significantly longer in the most recent series.

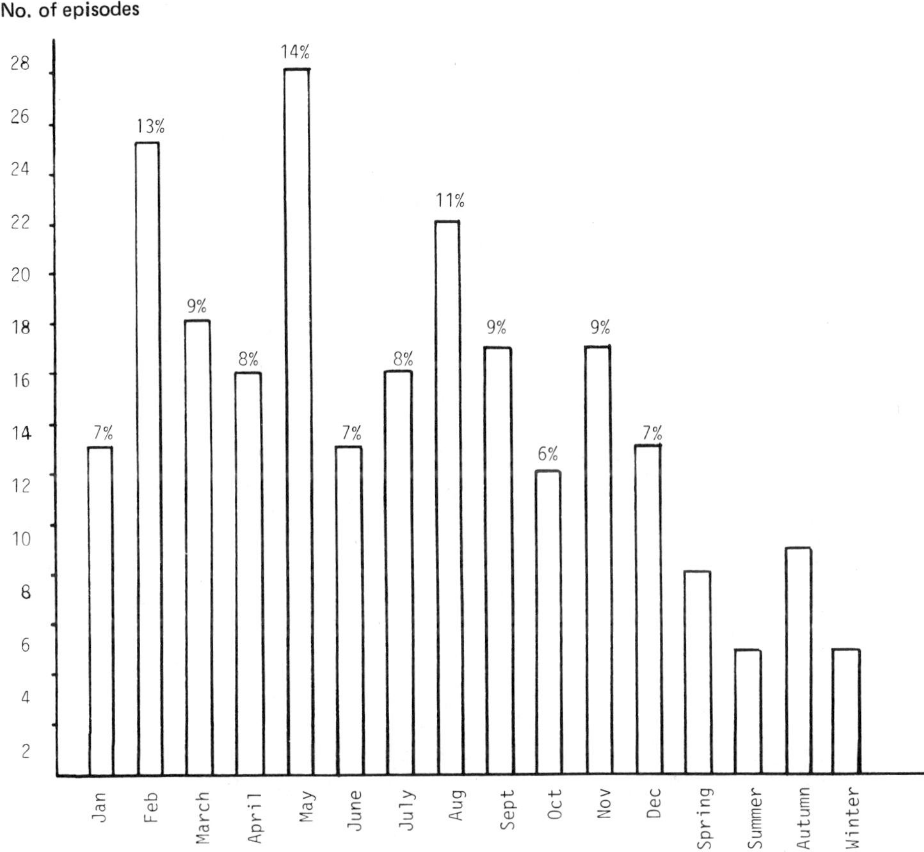

Figure 2 Monthly distribution of acute onset episodes (n = 182), and seasonal distribution of the episodes with an insidious onset (n = 27).

However, the authors do not make any attempt to explain this increase in delay between onset of the disorder and admission. It can be supposed that increased outpatient facilities might have contributed to the increased delay.

1. Comments

It seems that the question as to whether the onset of schizophrenic syndromes shows any particular seasonal distribution comparable to that of affective disorders is still unsettled. The occurrence of an insidious onset makes the mapping out of this course variable uncertain. Patients with an acute onset, which could be regarded as belonging to subgroups of schizophrenia, have been studied in

Table 6 Percent Distribution of Delay Between Onset of Psychosis and First Admission to Hospital

Reference	6 months or less	2 years or more
Gelperin, 1939	< 6 months 43.8%	> 2 years 22.1%
Böök, 1953	< 6 months 17.5%	> 2 years 49.5%
Johanson, 1958	< 6 months 13%	> 3 years 44% only male
Achté, 1961, 1965; Niskanen & Achté, 1972	< 2 months 46% (1935)	> 3 years 9%
	< 1 month 32% (1950)	> 3 years 7%
	< 1 month 36% (1960)	> 3 years 18%
	< 1 month 29% (1965)	> 3 years 25%
Frøshaug & Ytrehus, 1963	< 1 month 7.4% (1933-35)	> 5 years 12.6% only
	< 1 month 12.6% (1953-59)	> 5 years 22.3% female
Retterstøl, 1966	< 1 month 12%	> 2 years 13% schizophr.
	< 1 month 22%	> 2 years 10.2% reactive
Kay & Lindelius, 1970	< 3 months 40%	> 2 years 39%
Noreik, 1970	– –	> 5 years 26%

this respect but the results remain inconsistent, probably due to differences in sampling. Seasonal variations in admission rates very probably depend more upon social factors than factors bound to the illness itself.

A large number of patients are admitted to a hospital after a very long delay from the first onset of the psychotic symptoms. This delay also very likely depends to a large extent upon sociocultural factors. It is, however, still unclear whether and to what extent a long delay in receiving psychiatric care influences the further course of the disorder. Judging from the small amount of data available in the literature, it seems that individuals with a lifelong illness may never be admitted to a hospital and thus not be comprised in statistical evaluations of the course of schizophrenia. Since the fact that these patients remain in the community is very probably dependent upon the degree of tolerance for deviant behavior in the society and/or the availability of psychiatric services, it is difficult to decide whether the disorder these patients suffer from represents a mild subgroup of schizophrenic syndromes or not.

E. Types of Course and Outcome

The Kraepelinian conception of dementia praecox was that of a progressive disorder with a continuous course, but for the catatonic subgroup. As concerns the catatonic form, Kraepelin described the possible occurrence of long-lasting remission in about 20% of his cases. He pointed out that such periods of remission could last as long as up to 20 years but he maintained that most often a relapse occurred within 5 years from the first episode. According to Kraepelin, an acute onset was related to a more favorable prognosis. Since catatonic episodes often have an acute onset, Kraepelin assumed that the catatonic subgroup of dementia praecox had a better prognosis as compared with the other forms of the disease. As regards outcome Kraepelin admitted that in a small number of cases (about 15%) a complete recovery could occur. However, it seems that he was uncertain as to whether or not the morbid process in the cases who recovered was of the same nature as in the others who never recovered. This opinion has dominated for a long time and psychiatrists have insisted on reconsidering the diagnosis when patients recovered from a morbid episode previously diagnosed as schizophrenic. The most common outcome, according to Kraepelin, was a condition of marked clinical improvement with some degree of defect. Finally he described different types of terminal states characterized not only by a defectual impairment of intellectual functions, but also by the persistence and chronicization of different symptoms—hallucinations, delusions, verbal incoherence (schizophasia), apathy, and so on.

E. Bleuler paid very much attention to the concept of "recovery," which he regarded as almost impossible to use. He maintained that some patients could appear as recovered after a morbid episode, and also "better than before" the episode, but he preferred to use the concept "pronounced improvement" instead of "recovery." In fact, he asserted that a "full *restitutio ad integrum*" never occurred. Actually, it seems that what he meant was that the experience of having gone through a psychotic episode cannot be completely cancelled from the sum of experiences which characterize an individual, even when the outcome is the most favorable.

According to Bleuler's statistical data, about 60% of the patients showed marked improvement after the first episode, whereas about 22% showed a severe deterioration. As for terminal states, Bleuler agreed on the whole with the descriptions given earlier by Kraepelin. As is shown in the following, successive authors have not deviated much from those classical conceptions with the exception of the proportion of recoveries. However, there are considerable differences from study to study regarding the sampling of the series, the diagnostic creiteria, the setting where the observations were made, and the time of observation. Thus, any definite agreement as concerns outcome is far from reached.

M. Bleuler has given very careful descriptions of the different types of course. He takes into account two main types—a simple ("einfache") and a wave form ("wellenformig"), which he divides into four subgroups each in relation to the possible outcome. A graphic representation of the different types of course is given in Figure 3. In a comparison of two series of patients studied in two different periods (Bleuler, 1941, 1972), the most significant finding was the complete disappearance of a course characterized by an acute onset followed by a very rapid severe deterioration (5-18% in the 1941 series). Severe deterioration previously found in other types of course also decreased, whereas the types of course tended toward less severe deterioration, and also the "wave form toward recovery" increased slightly in the most recent series. Another important observation by Bleuler was that further dramatic changes toward impairment as well as toward improvement can still occur in patients more than 30 years after the onset of the psychosis.

Russian psychiatrists (Nadsharow and Sternberg, 1965; Shneshnevski, 1966, 1968, 1970; Rumyantseva, 1970; Sternberg, 1972, 1973; Uspenskaia, 1972; Volkova, 1974; Khramelashvili and Liberman, 1976; Molchanova, 1976) consider three main types of course: a progressive, continuous type; a shiftlike ("schübe") type; and a recurrent or periodic form. As to the last form, Russian psychiatrists specify that it corresponds to what other authors label "schizo-affective" or "cycloid" psychosis. According to Russian authors, the outcome of the different forms can be very different in different patient samples.

Rumyantseva describes a shiftlike form with marked and very stable improvement, Volkova a shiftlike form with progressive deterioration and residual hallucinosis, and Molchanova a shiftlike form with periods of remission lasting up to more than 20 years. According to Uspenskaia, a shiftlike followed by a chronic deteriorating course is more frequent in males than in females.

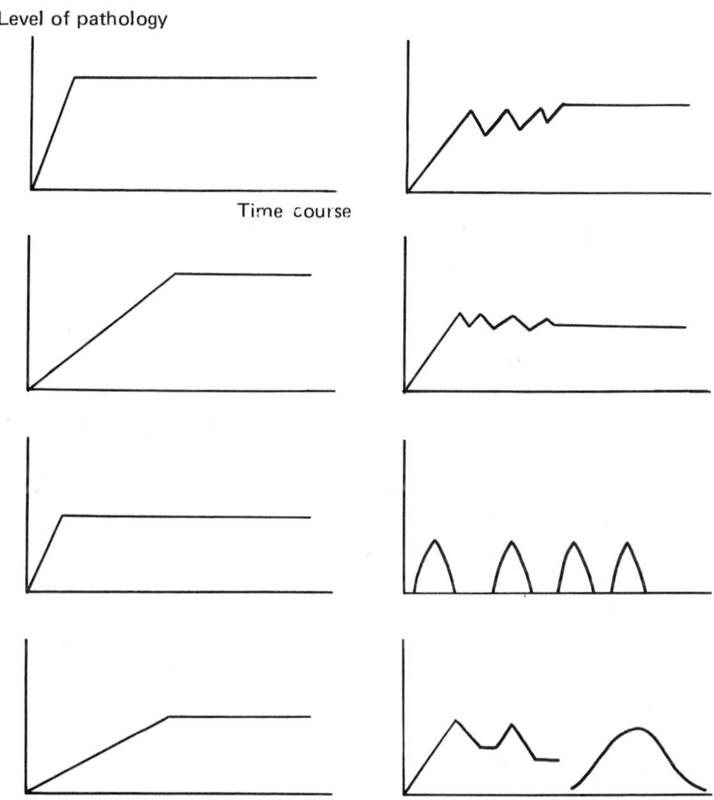

Figure 3 Left, simple course; right, course in attacks ("schub") or episodes.

Favorina (1963a,b) distinguishes two main types of terminal states: one "iterative or hypekinetic," and one "adynamic or akinetic."

Among French authors, Fromenty (1937), referring to the personal observation of 271 patients followed up for several years, maintained that the most frequent feature was that of a continuous progressive course toward a pronounced defect (70%). The remaining 30% were equally divided into those who evolved toward defect through periods of exacerbations and of remissions, and those who showed a complete remission after a series of relapses. Ey et al. (1963) in their textbook describe two main types of course, one toward recovery and one toward defect, each of them divided into two subgroups. According to these authors, about 25% of the patients recover after the first episode and another 22% after periods of exacerbation and remission. About 20% show a continuous development toward chronicity at the first episode whereas the remaining 33% deteriorate after periods of acutization and remission. Lambert and Midenet (1972) distinguish a form characterized by periodic relapsing (of the same symptomatology) with successive stabilization, a form characterized by a periodic course with successive impairment, a form with an evolution toward recovery, a form with a very malignant evolution toward marked deterioration ("schizocaries"), and finally a chronic form either stable or with a continuously deteriorating course.

From the British textbooks, Mayer-Gross et al. (1960) admitted that an illness that may start at any time from puberty to late middle age must necessarily show great variety in course. However, they seemed to be of the opinion that "every condition grouped under the term schizophrenia is associated with a general tendency toward disintegration of the personality." Mayer-Gross et al. admit the occurrence of a course characterized by exacerbations and remissions (especially among catatonics) but maintain that as a rule the prospect of recovery after a third attack is very small. Remissions, however, can according to Mayer-Gross et al., last for a very long time. As an example the authors describe their own observation of a case in which 45 years elapsed between the first and second episodes of illness. The prospects of a longlasting spontaneous remission are, according to Mayer-Gross et al., greatest during the first 2 years of illness to become negligible after 5 years of continuous illness. A series of patients with a very long interval between the first and second attacks of schizophrenia was reported in Switzerland by Wyrsch (1941). Of his 57 patients, 5 had an interval of 40-50 years and 1 more than 50 years. Henderson and Gillespie (rev. 1969) do not take the "course" directly into account; however, it seems that they have been of the opinion that schizophrenia has a chronic course toward a more or less severe deterioration. Paranoid psychoses, according to these authors, should be kept separate from the other forms since they "rarely exhibit the gross intellectual and emotional deterioration which is so characteristic of schizophrenia." Forrest (1973) seemed to accept the possibility of recovery but maintained that "if patients do recover from the psychosis their personality may remain damaged." As concerns outcome he refers to the follow-up study by Wing et al. (1964) according to which 49% of 113 patients followed up for 5 years after discharge from mental hospital were well and able to support themselves whereas 11% had returned to a hospital quite soon and spent the whole period there.

The course of schizophrenia is hardly considered under a particular heading in American textbooks and handbooks. Noyes and Kolb (1963) take into account an intermittent and a progressive course, and point out that a symptom-free remission does not preclude the diagnosis of schizophrenia. Concerning outcome, they maintain that a permanent disorganization of the personality does not invariably follow. It seems, however, that they attribute a particular importantce to etiology in the sense that they regard the forms which lead to recovery as having psychogenic origin. They describe further "episodes of mild fleeting nature with no subsequent recurrence." It is unclear, however, as to whether the authors mean that some degree of defect remains after these episodes. According to their experience, about one-third of hospitalized patients make a fairly complete recovery during their first year of illness, whereas another one-third require indefinite periods of hospital care.

Arieti (1959) divides the evolution of schizophrenia into four stages. The first, comprising three substages, stretches from the beginning of the psychopathology to the formation of psychotic symptoms and is characterized by the following substages: panic; psychotic insight, when experiences are interpreted in a psychotic way; and multiplication of symptoms. The second stage (advanced) is that of apparent acceptance of illness. The third (preterminal) occurs between 5 and 15 years after the onset and is characterized by the fact that many symptoms have burned out and that the subtypes resemble each other. The fourth, finally, is the terminal stage characterized by impulsive and reflex-like behavior. In the second edition of the American handbook, Bemporad and Pinsker (1974) maintain that the course most commonly seen is a series of recurrences and remissions occuring against a background of chronic disability. Redlich and Freedman (1966) divide the course into three main phases: the early, initial; the phase of disintegration; and the phase of deterioration. Concerning evolution they agree with the opinion by other authors distinguishing forms which progress very rapidly, slowly, or remain almost static. An arrest in evolution can occur at any stage, and the course can be characterized by remissions and relapses or be progressive to the "bitter end." A similar view is maintained by Bulgarian authors (Schipkowensky, 1956; Marinow, 1959, 1971). Marinow identifies four types of terminal stages: one apathetic-hypobulic (the most frequent), one hallucinatory-paranoid, one catatonic, and one paranoid.

In Germany different tendencies are expressed in different textbooks: from a strict adherence to Kraepelinian concepts (Mayer-Gross, 1932; Bumke, 1948), to a view more consistent with that of Bleuler (Weitbrecht, 1963). Older authors, and also Kleist and his school, Rümke (1958) in the Netherlands, Brzezicki (1972) in Poland, and Langfeldt (1937, 1965) in Norway, regard "true," or "nuclear," or "process" schizophrenia as a psychotic condition with a continuous progressive course toward defect or deterioration, whereas they considered forms with a more favorable prognosis as schizophreniform or "pseudoschizophrenic." Kleist (1928) and Leonhard (1935-1969) occupy a special position as regards a division of endogenous psychoses in different subgroups with a different course and a different outcome. Leonhard, in particular, distinguishes between cycloid psychoses characterized by a periodic course and complete remission between episodes; nonsystematic schizophrenias (affect-laden paraphrenia, periodical catatonia, and cataphasia) with a course characterized by attacks followed by remissions or sometimes with a periodicity comparable with that of the cycloid psychoses; and the systematic schizophrenias characterized by a continuous course with progressive impairment. The terminal state is also quite different in the three subgroups. Patients suffering from cycloid psychoses almost regularly recover after each episode. In a minority of patients, however, a slight defect can be recognized according to Leonhard after several episodes. The systematic forms, on the contrary, always proceed toward a terminal state which is different in all the subgroups, simple or combined, which Leonhard takes into account. As for the nonsystematic forms, less than one-third of the cases of affect-laden paraphrenia and cataphasia show a progressive course (and of course, none of the cases of periodical catatonia). In about 83% of the cases of periodic catatonia and in about 40% of the other nonsystematic forms the course is characterized by the occurrence of acutizations and remissions. According to Leonhard, remissions may occur also in patients suffering from systematic forms—most frequently in the catatonic (about 20%), least frequently in the hebephrenic subgroup (about 7%). The classification by Leonhard has been used in investigations by Astrup (1957), Fish (1958, 1962), Stephens and Astrup (1963, 1967), and van Epen (1969).

In recent years, important contributions to the study of the course of schizophrenia have been published by Huber and his co-workers in Bonn (Huber, 1964,1966,1968a,b; Huber et al., 1974,1975a,b; Gross et al., 1971a,b,c,1973a,b) (here referred to as the Bonn group). According to the Bonn group the diagnosis of schizophrenia is compatible with a complete remission. Such a complete remission occurred in about 20% out of 449 schizophrenics followed up for more than 20 years; its occurrence was more frequent in patients with a shorter duration of illness [9-14 years, $n = 94$, complete remission 25.5% (Huber et al., 1974)] than in patients with a duration of illness of 25 years or more ($n = 97$), complete remission 13.4%). In an early series (Huber, 1964), two-thirds of the patients showed a simple progressive course and one-third a course characterized by attacks and remissions before reaching a condition of defect. In a later series (Gross et al., 1971a,b,c) the percentage of patients with a simple, progressive course was only 14.5%, whereas that of those with a course in the form of attacks ("schubförmig") had increased to about 42%. As to outcome, a mild to moderate residuum or defect was found in about 39% and a pronounced residuum or defect in another 42% of cases. Moreover, the Bonn group describes the occurrence in the course of schizophrenia of a "2nd positive break" ("sweiter positiver knick") (Huber, 1964; Gross et al., 1973a,b; Huber et al., 1974). This break occurs, according to the authors, spontaneously and not as an effect of pharmacological treatment. It is characterized by complete remission and can occur at any time in chronic patients who have been ill for decades and last for months or years. The age of the patient does not seem to play any role. In fact, this second break was observed in patients in their 20s as well as in patients aged 70 or more. However, it seems to occur most often in patients in the 40s (Gross et al., 1973a,b).

A comparison between the findings obtained by the Bonn group and those obtained by Bleuler in a recent follow-up (Bleuler, 1972; Huber et al., 1974) showed a very high degree of consistency. The most important findings can be summarized as follows: a remission of such a duration that it may be regarded as recovery occurs in about 25% of patients. The favorable courses, i.e., those with a mild residual impairment, occur with about the same frequency as those toward recovery. About three-quarters of the cases reach a stable condition; however, dramatic changes can still occur after decades of stability. Both studies show that a catastrophic course rapidly progressing toward deterioration has become very rare (in 4% of the cases in Bonn, 1% in Zurich).

A thorough review of follow-up studies has been made on two occasions by Stephens (1970, 1978). Judging from his table referring to studies with a follow-up of at least 10 years, the percentage complete recovery in schizophrenia is of about the same as found by Bleuler and by the Bonn group.

1. Comments

From the data reviewed in this section it becomes evident that different types of course have been found in patients classified as schizophrenics. In older studies the opinion prevailed that schizophrenia had a continuous course toward deterioration. However, Kraepelin admitted the possible occurrence of longlasting remissions of such a duration to be considered equivalent to recovery. It is evident that the different authors' conception of schizophrenia largely influences opinions about course and outcome. The percentage of patients who make a complete recovery seems to be about 25% according to the most recent and comprehensive follow up studies carried out in Zurich and Bonn. Results from other countries are consistent with these findings. It seems also that the percentage of cases with a catastrophic course progressing rapidly toward deterioration has clearly diminished in recent years. Most authors defend the opinion that a progressive course toward a chronic terminal stage should not be regarded as a necessary characteristic for the diagnosis of schizophrenia. This change in opinion makes comparisons between old and recent follow-up studies quite impossible. Since the introduction of active methods of treatment the major concern has been to identify, among the schizophrenic patients, those with more favorable prognosis. These efforts have lead to attempts at identifying subgroups with particular characteristics. Beyond these attempts there must be a conviction that at least one form of the disorder has a chronic course and a poor outcome. A clear-cut definition of forms with a good and forms with a poor prognosis is not yet available despite the efforts of several research workers. An important finding in long-term studies is that after decades an apparently stable illness can be susceptible to sudden improvement. It is very likely that the course of schizophrenia is influenced by several factors and that change in it over time are dependent upon factors external to the disease. However, despite changes in attitudes, an increase in treatment facilities, and an increased awareness of the factors which may negatively influence the course of the disease, the percentage of patients who do not completely recover is still about 70-75% and of these 25-30% do not improve at all.

From the comprehensive follow-up studies carried out over several years by the Bonn group evidence is presented that spontaneous longlasting remissions, the s.c. "2nd positive break," can occur at any time in chronic patients who have been ill for decades independent of pharmacological treatment. Moreover, both the studies by the Bonn group and those carried out by Blueler show that dramatic changes toward improvement as well as impairment also can occur in patients who have apparently been stable for years. Both these findings are important for the planning and the evaluation of treatment programs. Furthermore, the possible occurrence of these changes in the condition of the patients, also very old ones, make the concept of terminal stage commonly used by many authors rather dubious.

F. Mortality and Suicide

An overmortality among psychiatric patients has been observed since ancient times when the conditions of care of the mentally ill were very poor. Conditions have obviously changed in the course of the centuries and mortality has drastically diminished, but an excess mortality among psychiatric patients still remains in comparison with mortality rates in the general population.

Kraepelin pointed out that tuberculosis was four to five times more frequent among patients suffering from dementia praecox than in the general population and that this fact lead to a higher mortality rate among patients.

Bleuler (1911) could not find an excess of tuberculosis among his patients as compared with the general population. He quoted a study carried out by Kerner at the Rheinau Hospital in which a mortality rate about twice as high as in the general population has been found in schizophrenic patients. Most of the studies published since that time (Lempp, 1921; Essen-Möller, 1935; Malzberg, 1934, 1943, 1953; Holt and Holt, 1952; Ødegaard, 1952; Böök, 1953; Larsson and Sjögren, 1954) have confirmed an overmortality among schizophrenic patients with ratios of 2-4:1 as compared with the general population. Almost consistently female patients have shown a higher mortality than male patients. One of the early, more comprehensive investigations was that of Alström (1938, 1942), who stressed the importance of tuberculosis as a cause of death among hospitalized patients. According to his figures referring to patients followed during the years 1924-1936, the mortality rate was about twice as high among patients in comparison with the general population and somewhat higher in females than in males.

Successive studies (Freyhan, 1955; Shepherd, 1957; Johanson, 1958; Achté, 1961, 1967; Niswander et al., 1963a,b,c; Retterstøl, 1966, 1970; Hoenig, 1967; Babigian nd Odorff, 1969; Kay and Lindelius, 1970, 1973; Bleuler,

1972; Niskanen and Achté, 1972; Guggenheim and Babigian, 1974; Bland et al., 1976; Ciompi and Medvecka, 1976; Tsuang and Woolson, 1977) have shown a clear-cut decrease in mortality due to tuberculosis, and also a decrease in deaths in general as compared with the older figures. The findings in this respect are, however, less consistent in the different studies. So, for example, whereas Kay and Lindelius, and Tsuang and Woolson did not find an overmortality in their later series of patients as compared with the general population, Helgason (1964), Leyberg (1975), Hartelius (1972), Bland et al. (1976), and Ciompi and Medvecka (1976) still found a highly significant difference between observed and expected deaths among their patient series. It is very likely that the inconsistency depends mainly upon differences of period in which the series were collected, differences in the methods used to calculate excess mortality, and accessibility to adequate figures from the general population. When separate calculations have been made according to subforms of schizophrenia or in relation to the fact whether the patients were in hospital or discharged, some differences emerged: Niswander et al. (1963a) found that an overmortality occurred more in hospitalized than discharged patients, and that it was higher among catatonic patients than patients suffering from other forms. Guggenheim and Babigian found that the relative risk of death was not higher for the catatonic than for the other types of the disease. Ciompi and Medvecka instead found again a maximal overmortality among catatonics (2.6:1 as compared with the general population) whereas the findings in the paranoid subgroup were almost the same as in the general population. One finding reported by Niswander et al. (1963a) refers to the fact that among patients, females die at a younger age than males, which is the contrary of what happens in the general population. Besides tuberculosis no other causes of death (except suicide; see below) have been found to occur consistently more often in patients. Bleuler (1972) points out that malignant tumors occurred less often than expected among the causes of death in his series. The possible occurrence of "sudden death" of unknown cause in single patients has been pointed out by Holt and Holt (1952) and by Bleuler (1972). Within the catatonic forms, a particularly severe type with an acute onset and lethal outcome has been considered [*tödliche Katatonie* by Stauder (1934)]. This particular form is also known as *délire aigu, catatonie pernicieuse,* acute lethal catatonia, or hypertoxic schizophrenia. The question as to whether this form should be considered within the realm of schiozphrenia or as a pseudoschizophrenic syndrome caused by an atypical encephalitic process (Huber, 1954a,b; 1964) is still unsettled. A recent review of the literature has been published by Glatzel (1970). Laskowska et al. (1965) published a follow-up study of a series of 55 patients (12 male and 43 female) collected between 1951 and 1960 and followed up for 2-12 years. Of the patients, 20 (36.4%) died during the acute stage of the illness. Of the surviving 32 patients, 27 (84.4%) became chronic schizophrenics and 5 remained symptom-free during the follow-up.

The problem of suicide is of particular importance because in recent years it has been discussed in relation to modern kinds of treatment, mainly the use of depot neuroleptics. There are many studies concerned with the frequency of suicide among schizophrenic patients or the occurrence of schizophrenia in series of suicides (Dahlgren, 1945; Ettlinger and Flordh, 1955; Rizzo, 1957; Johansson 1958; Achté, 1961, 1967; Dalgård, 1966; Retterstøl, 1966; Babigian and Odoroff, 1969; Kay and Lindelius, 1970, 1973; Bland et al., 1976). The occurrence of suicide has been calculated in different ways in different studies. This makes comparisons between different investigations somewhat uncertain. The frequency of suicide depends largely upon the accuracy of registration of this cause of death and upon the length of the follow-up period. With these limitations in mind, it is fair to assume that the reported data represent minimal estimates and the figures as concerns suicide might in fact be higher. The percentage of deaths due to suicide seems to be of the order of 2-4% when the follow-up has lasted at least several years. A somewhat smaller figure is reported by Dalgård (1966) (1%) and Leyberg (1965) (1.2%). In the "Enquête of Lausanne" carried out by Ciompi (1976) and comprising 5661 former patients followed up for 30-40 years, 4227 had died, among them 1891 in the period 1942-1962 when the patients were 57-77 years old. In this group schizophrenia and allied psychoses (paranoia, unspecified delusional states) showed the lowest suicide rates (3.1% in males, 3.3% in females) as compared with other patients' categories. The suicide rate in the series by Bland and Parker (province of Alberta, Canada) was 28 times higher than the corresponding in the general population. In investigations of suicides and suicide attempts (Dahlgren, 1945; Ettlinger and Flordh, 1955) schizophrenic patients represented 8.7-2.9%. In the series by Bleuler (1972) comprising 208 patients followed up for more than 20 years, 70 patients had died, 9 of them by suicide. This means 4.3% of the patients with suicide representing 12.9% of the causes of death. From the comparison with the Bonn series (Bleuler et al., 1976) it emerged that the corresponding figure in Bonn was about 20%. Eleven percent of the 757 patients of the Bonn series committed suicide during the follow-up period (Gross et al., 1973a,b).

Kay and Lindelius, Lindelius and Kay (1973) have been particularly concerned with changes in the pattern of mortality in schizophrenia in Sweden. From their studies covering different series of patients collected in 1900-1910 and followed up till 1960, 1947-1958 to 1970, and 1961-1965 to 1972 a pronounced increase in suicide emerged clearly. The ratio between observed and expected, in fact, was 0.7 in the first series, 8.6 in the second, and 40.0 in the third. According to the authors, several factors contribute to this pronounced rise in suicide. Among them, the change in treatment policy was an increased tendency toward extramural care plays an important role.

In older studies it had been maintained that the occurrence of suicide was most pronounced in the initial phase of illness. More recent studies by Bleuler (1972), Kay and Lindelius (1973), and the Bonn group (Bleuler et al., 1976) clearly show that the risk of suicide also remains high many years after the onset of the illness. A particular characteristic of suicide among schizophrenic patients is that it occurs in equal proportion among males and females, whereas in the general population male individuals clearly predominate.

1. Comments

Follow-up studies on schizophrenic patients often neglect to take into account mortality. This might introduce a source of error in the long-term evaluation of the course of schizophrenia, especially when comparisons are made with earlier studies. An overmortality among schizophrenics had been consistently documented in several investigations. Recent studies by Kay and Lindelius (1970) have shown that the mean expectation of life was 25-30% lower for males and 35-40% lower for females among patients collected in the periods 1901-1910 and 1941-1950. More recently a decrease in mortality has been reported by Bleuler (1972) and Kay and Lindelius (1973). In earlier periods tuberculosis was one of the causes leading to excess mortality, especially among hospitalized patients. The importance of tuberculosis has now clearly diminished whereas the importance of suicide clearly increased. No special causes of death besides tubercolosis and suicide have been found to occur more frequently among schizophrenics than the general population. To the contrary, malignant tumors, according to findings by Bleuler (1972), might occur less frequently among patients. In early studies it has been maintained that suicides occurred predominantly in the early phases of the illness. More recent investigations show instead that they occur at any time during the course of the disorder as well as several decades after the onset. At variance from what is usually found in the general population, suicides occur to the same extent among males and females in a schizophrenic population. No clear-cut explanation of the increase in suicide rate has yet been proposed. Among the possible explanations, changes in care policy with a decrease in chronic hospitalization has been pointed out. Numerous schizophrenic patients now live socially isolated in the community. This might greatly increase the risk of suicide (Sainsbury, 1955). Instances of sudden death of unknown causes have occasionally been reported in patients prior to the use of neuroleptic drugs.

G. Results of Some Follow-Up Studies

Besides the studies already mentioned in the previous sections, numerous other articles have been published on the subject of the follow-up of schizophrenic patients. These articles deal almost exclusively with a study of hospitalized patients. They are mostly concerned with duration of hospital care at first admission, percentage of patients who have been discharged or who have chronically remained in the hospital, percentage of relapses during the follow-up period, and condition of the patients at the end of the study. Almost all of the above-mentioned variables are dependent upon factors which might not necessarily reflect the true course of schizophrenia. Instead they might be closely related to the social context in which the observations were made and how the different variables were defined. Furthermore, the span of time covered by many follow-up studies is too short to give any valuable information about the long-term course of schizophrenic disorders. The patients involved in these studies have been treated with diverse methods under very different circumstances, and details about treatment are often lacking. Also omitted is a mention of relevant social and psychological factors which might have influenced on onc sidc admission and discharge policy and on the other side the re-entry of the discharged patient into society.

Bearing this criticism in mind, it seems enough within the scope of the present chapter to discuss only the main trends which emerge from these studies. One of them concerns a successive shortening of hospital stay, which has been even more prominent in recent years. At present there are relatively few patients who remain hospitalized for the rest of their life after the first hospital admission. Tangerman (1942) found in patients admitted in 1925-1934 that 43% had never been discharged and another 15% had died in the hospital. Beck (1968) in a study of patients admitted in the periods 1930-1932 and 1940-1942 found 25-35 years later that 64% had been continuously hospitalized. In a 3-year follow-up carried out by Mandelbrote and Trick (1970), only 13.8% remained in the hospital during the whole period. McWalter et al. (1961-1962) found that of patients admitted in 1949-1953, 66% of the males and 68% of the females had been discharged within a year; the percentage for patients admitted in the period 1954-1957 had remained almost unchanged for the male but has risen to 82% for the female patients. In a study by Israel and Johnson (1956) referring to patients admitted to a hospital in the periods 1913-1922 and 1943-1952, the rate of discharge within less than 6 months rose from 21.9% in the first to 40.4% in the second period, whereas the rate of discharge within less than 1 year rose from 35.1% to 59.9% (n = 630 and 1784 patients in the two series). Similar observations have been made by Wing et al. (1964), Brown et al. (1961), Fröshaug and Ytrehus (1963), Apo and Achté (1966), Achté and Apo (1967) and Niskanen et al. (1973), who compared series of patients collected in different periods. Seventy-one percent of the 139 patients studied by Spern et al. (1965) who had been admitted in 1956-1959 were discharged within 1 year. In the follow-up by Leyberg (1965) 75% of the patients admitted in 1963 had been discharged within 3 months.

Another main trend, depending partly upon the first, is a pronounced increase in readmission rates in more recent series. Thus, for example, whereas only 3% of the patients followed up by Gelperin (1939) (admitted 1933-1937) were readmitted within a year after discharge, the percentage of readmission in the series by Schooler et al. (1967) was 41.1%. The percentage of readmission within the 1st year in the series by Israel and Johnson (1913-1952) was on average 11.4% with a peak of 19.2% for the patients (n = 313) first admitted in the period 1923-1932 covering the years of economic depression. Of the patients studied by Leyberg (1965) 21% were readmitted within 1 year and 44% within 3 years. The percentage of patients readmitted within 2 years was 47% in a series of patients first admitted in 1970 and studied by Niskanen et al. (1973). From these two sets of data the question can be raised as to whether or not the total duration of hospitalization has markedly changed if an adequate observation period is taken into account. The question can be answered in the affirmative if the comparison is made with series of patients collected before World War II. On the other hand, the findings are more uncertain if more recent periods are taken into account. In a careful investigation carried out at two Swedish hospitals (Lassenius et al. 1973), strictly defined, first admission schizophrenic patients treated over three different periods (1944-1946, 1955-1956, and 1959-1960) were followed up for 10 years and the duration (in years) of time spent in hospital or any kinds of institution during the follow-up period was calculated. The results of the study are presented in Table 7.

The table shows that there is a gradual increase in the number of admissions from the first to the third period simultaneously as the total period of care decreases. However, the decrease in total period of care is more pronounced from the first to the successive periods and for the male patients. As for the females, no appreciable difference has been found between periods 2 and 3.

Table 7 Time (yr) Spent in Hospital or Any Institution for Patients from Two Mental Hospitals in the North of Sweden During Three Different Periods (10 yr Follow-Up)[a]

		Hospital S			Hospital U		
	Patients	I	II	III	I	II	III
	Male	5.8	3.1	3.4	5.4	3.2	3.6
	Female	6.4	2.6	1.3	5.2	2.6	2.5
Mean no. of admissions to mental hospital	Male	2.0	3.1	3.6	2.8	3.1	3.8
	Female	1.9	3.8	4.1	2.6	3.6	4.2

[a]Refers to patients first admitted 1944-1946 (I), 1955-1956 (II), and 1959-1960 (III).
Source: Adapted from Lassenius et al., 1973.

A different kind of follow-up study is concerned with the percent distribution of patients who have made a recovery, improved, or who are unimproved at the end of the study. Studies of this kind also contain sources of uncertainty, due mainly to selection procedures, length of follow-up, total duration of illness at the time of the last discharge, form of treatment, and kind of support in the community. A very difficult variable in the definition of "recovery" because it seems that it sometimes refers to absence of psychopathology, sometimes to social adjustment ("social remission"), sometimes to an admixture of both. Two very careful and comprehensive reviews of studies of this kind have recently been published by Stephens (1970,1978) whereas a review of main studies has been compiled by Angst (1977). Since both these reviews are easily accessible, only some major studies with the longest follow-up (for each patient) are summarized in Table 8. In line with the data presented in previous sections, the table shows that the percentage of patients who recover or improve is higher and that of those who are severely disabled is lower in more recent than earlier studies.

Recently, a 2-year follow-up of the patients included in the WHO International Pilot Study of Schizophrenia was reported (Sartorius et al., 1977). The results suggest very marked variations of course and outcome over a 2-year period. In particular, schizophrenic patients identified in developing countries had markedly better course and outcome than those in developed countries.

1. Comments

The pattern of admission and of discharge primarily reflects the cultural climate of the period under scrutiny and also the availability of treatment facilities both at hospital and after discharge. Over the years marked changes have occurred as concerns the duration of time in hospital care at the first admission and the number of readmission after discharge from hospital. Significantly fewer patients remain chronically hospitalized from the very beginning. The most pronounced change has occurred when psychothropic drugs have been introduced and more attention has been paid to counteract the negative influence of institutionalization. Increased milieutherapeutic and sociotherapeutic efforts (Hogarty and Goldberg, 1973; Hogarthy et al., 1974) have greatly improved the possibility of schizophrenic patients living in the community. Although the studies reviewed in this section principally illustrate the radical changes in the philosophy of care of schizophrenic patients. However, the findings concerning a decrease in the longlasting severely disturbed states suggests that factors external to the disorder have in the past contributed greatly to the chronicity of the attacks.

On the other hand, the patients who have in recent years remained chronically hospitalized very likely represent a special selection of severely disabled patients, very often without any remaining social connections outside the hospital, who are in need of continuous supervision (see for example, Todd et al., 1976).

H. Course of Childhood Schizophrenia

Impossible as it may seem, a close definition of childhood schizophrenia is even more controversial than the delimitation of schizophrenia in the adult. The occurrence of severe psychopathological disorders, resembling Kraepelin's description of dementia praecox and characterized by a similar catastrophic course, prompted the introduction of the concept of *dementia praecocissima* (De Sanctis, 1906; Costantini, 1911) at the beginning of this century. Since that time the question as to whether childhood schizophrenia did exist and, if so, whether it has any relation with adult schizophrenia has been a matter of much controversy. Homburger presented an extensive discussion of this subject as early as 1926. Since then, many conditions which earlier had been placed under the comprehensive heading *dementia infantilis* have been reclassified when their physio- and anatomopathological bases became better understood and their nature as progressive brian diseases became clarified. A major impulse in the study of childhood schizophrenia occurred in the thirties and early forties with the work by Potter (1933), Grebelskaja-Albatz (1934-1935), Lutz (1937-1938), Despert (1938), Bender (1940), Bradley (1941). In 1943 Kanner introduced the concept of "early infantile autism," and in 1949 Rank described the "atypical child," and in 1952 Mahler published her comprehensive description of "autistic and symbiotic infantile psychoses." Another more generic label, frequently used in the literature, is "infantile psychosis" or "juvenile psychosis" (Anthony, 1958; Esman, 1960; Creak, 1962, 1963a,b; Rutter, 1965; Kolvin, 1971; Dahl, 1976). Although attempts aimed to define and classify all these conditions have been repeatedly made, it seems that these labels are used somewhat inconsistently and as if they were interchangeable. In fact, in most follow-up studies, childhood schizophrenia, early infantile autism, and childhood psychosis are lumped together. However, consensus is growing that the term "childhood schizophrenia" should be reserved for a late-onset disorder in previously healthy children and that "early infantile autism" should be restricted to children who show abnormalities before the age of 2 years, whereas the term "symbiotic childhood psychosis" should refer to a type which develops later than childhood autism in the age group 3-5 years (Rutter, 1967; Knobloch and Pasamanick, 1975).

From the possible distinctions mentioned above it is evident that the onset of childhood schizophrenia is not limited to a certain age. To the contrary, the hypothesis has been proposed that the disorder can be present at birth (cf. the s.c. "no-onset" type described by Despert, 1938). Officially, age at onset of early infantile autism has been established in the WHO classification (Rutter et al., 1969) to be within the first 30 months. There is some agreement that

Table 8 Main Results of Some Follow-Up Studies, Distribution in Percent

Reference	No. of patients	Follow-up (yr)	Outcome (%)			Remarks
			Recovered[a]	Improved	Unimproved	
Bleuler, 1911	515	3-10?	60		40	Follow-up by Zablocka, 1908[b]
Langfeldt, 1937	100	6-10	17	17	66	Unclear form
Langfeldt, 1939	100	6-12	32	25	43	Schizophreniform
Hayashi & Akimoto, 1939	88	12-16	33	25	42	
Rennie, 1939	222	15-26	27	13	60	
Bleuler, 1941	216	10-15	25	25	50	
Holmboe & Astrup, 1957	225	6-18	29	29	42	
Eitinger et al., 1958	110	5-15	5	13	84	Unclear schizophrenia
Eitinger et al., 1958	44	5-15	32	45	23	Schizophreniform
Johanson, 1958	98	10-18	2	35	63	Only males
Shepherd, 1958	123	5	30	31	39	
Marinow, 1959	242	15-18	10	30	40	20% dead at follow-up
Achté, 1961	100	25-27	21	5	29	45% dead at follow-up

Astrup et al., 1962	435	5-22	15	17	68	
Frøshaug & Ytrehus, 1963	84	6-8	19	19	62	Only females
Astrup & Noreik, 1966	271	5-12	6	10	84	Unclear form
Astrup & Noreik, 1966	89	5-12	22	3		"Schizophrenia"?
Astrup & Noreik, 1966	304	5-12	26	46	28	"Reactive psychosis"
Retterstøl, 1966	33	15-18	15	3	82	Paranoid schizophrenia
Retterstøl, 1966	39	15-18	36	18	46	"Paranoid schizophrenia"?
Retterstøl, 1966	54	15-18	59	24	17	Reactive paranoid psychosis
Achté, 1967	200	5	35	25	32	4.5% deat at follow-up
Stephens, 1970	62	10-16	6	39	55	Process schizophrenia
Stephens, 1970	81	10-16	38	51	11	Nonprocess schizophrenia
Uglešić et al., 1970	51	10	24	51	17	7.3% dead at follow-up
Bleuler, 1972	208	23	20	57	24	
Hinterhuber, 1973	157	30	29	53	13	
Huber et al., 1975a	501	20	22	62	16	
Tsuang & Winokur, 1975	139	30-40	19	35	47	

[a]Patients defined as recovered and as very much improved with social recovery have been grouped together.
[b]No duration of follow-up is given. The patients were collected in 1898-1905.

psychotic symptoms of the type as observed in adults, e.g., hallucinations, do not occur before the age of 7 or 8 years (Rutter, 1972; Kolvin, 1972; Eggers, 1973). Age at onset seems to be one of the critical variables as concerns the further course of the psychosis in that the outcome is clearly worse the earlier the onset (Creak, 1951; Eggers, 1973; Harper and Williams, 1975). Other factors related to outcome are level of measured intelligence (Rutter, 1965, 1966; Bender, 1970), severity of behavioral abnormalities (Brown, 1960; Rutter, 1966), and—very important—degree of speech disorder (Eisenberg, 1957; Bender, 1970; Lotter, 1974). Differences in frequency among the sexes have been reported (Eggers, 1973; Dahl, 1976), but these seem to be due to selection effects.

As in the adult, psychotic disorders in children can have an acute or an insidious onset. Acording to Kolvin (1972), an insidious onset is the most common pattern (two-thirds of the cases). Out of the 107 cases studied by Ssuchareva (1932) only 20 had shown an insidious onset. In the series by Eggers (1973) patients with an acute onset (n = 42) outnumbered those with an insidious debut (n = 15). The further course was different in the two groups—the former showing a remitting, the latter a chronic course. An acute-remitting course was found to occur significantly more often in patients in the prepubertal phase (i.e., between 10 and 14 years) than in younger patients. The reverse was true for the chronic forms.

The occurrence of prodromal manifestations in childhood schizophrenia has been pointed out by several authors (Villinger, 1957; Spiel, 1961; Uschakov, 1965; Eggers, 1973). Others maintain that they never occur (Wieck, 1965). An earlier description of their characteristics had been given by Schneider in 1942, who pointed out they consisted most often of lack of initiative, shallow affects, and attention disturbances. Related to the prodromal manifestations are the prepsychotic states described by French authors (Lebovici and Diatkine, 1963). Also the type of course, especially in patients in whom the disorder has its onset in late childhood, can show the same variation as in adults. Eggers describes both simple and attack-like courses quite similar to those described by Bleuler in adults. Uschakov (1965) observed a progressive course in 52% and a periodical in 30% of 225 patients. Kozlova (1967) found a slowly progressive course in 21, an acute recurrent in 12, and a catastrophic course in 24 patients. As mentioned previously, patients with an attack-like course very seldom terminate in a condition of severe deterioration.

Some results obtained in follow-up studies are presented in Table 9. Also in the case of childhood schizophrenia, the evaluation of complete recovery presents severe difficulties and must be taken cautiously. As in follow-up studies of schizophrenia in adults, comparisons between results obtained in different studies of childhood schizophrenia are very dubious since the different series are hardly homogeneous. Taken as a whole the percentage distribution

Table 9 Survey of Some Follow-Up Studies of Childhood Psychotic Conditions

Reference	No. of patients	Follow-up (yr)	Outcome in percent: Good to normal	Improved	Severely disturbed	Remarks
Bender, 1953	330	5-15	33	33	33	Mixed group. Age at onset 1-13 yr
Kanner & Eisenberg, 1955	42	4-19	2	31	67	Early infantile autism
Annesby, 1961	78		19	23	58	
Annell, 1963	115	1-15	14	44	42	Mixed group. 19 childhood schizophr.
Creak, 1963	100	Several years	17	40	43	Mixed group. Age at onset 1-13 yr
Havelkova, 1968	71	4-12		45	41	Preschool age
Rutter and Lockyer, 1969	63	5-15	14	25	61	Age at onset 2-10 yr
Bender, 1970	100	18-35	37		63	
Eggers, 1973	57	5-40	26	16	58	Age at onset 3-14 yr

regarding different types of outcome is not too different from what has been found in adults (cf. Table 8). On the other hand, several authors not represented in the table (Ssuchareva, 1932; Despert and Sherwin, 1958; Alanen et al., 1964; Uschakov, 1965) reported much worse results in the series they investigated. Also, the percentage of patients who in long-term follow-ups showed a passage from childhood to adult schizophrenia is quite different in the literature (Annell, 1963; Uschakov, 1965; Dahl, 1976). Difference in the composition of the series, mainly as concerning the age at the onset of the disorder, and differences in the length of follow-up might be responsible for the inconsistent results. In judging the results of follow-up studies of psychotic disorders in children it must be remembered that different proportions of children included in the studies have shown pronounced neurological manifestations during the follow-up. These neurological disturbances suggest an organic background to the psychotic condition. The occurrence of suicidal thoughts, suicide attempts, and suicide in childhood schizophrenia have been dealt with in particular by Eggers (1974). Out of his 57 patients mentioned above, 11 had attempted suicide and 3 committed it. However, the patients who committed suicide had reached the age of 19, 21, and 22 years.

1. Comments

Childhood schizophrenia is a condition even more heterogeneous than schizophrenia in the adult. Behind this label are concealed a great variety of morbid processes. Many of them are very probably of organic nature and are characterized by the occurrence of neurological manifestations in their further course. Others are of a clear-cut psychogenic nature and susceptible to complete recovery. The question whether very early schizophrenic manifestations accompanied by a poor prognosis should be included within the realm of schizophrenia proper or in that of mental deficiency is still unsettled. Very likely there is a distinction between the forms classified as early infantile autism occurring in early infancy and those closely resembling schizophrenia and occurring in the prepubertal phase. It is quite understandable that cases characterized by a very early severe deterioration can hardly develop into adult forms of the illness. There seems to be sufficient evidence to maintain that most cases of late psychosis in childhood will trespass into adult forms of schizophrenia. Type of onset and types of course and outcome show the same degree of variety as adult schizophrenia.

I. Course of Schizophrenia in the Elderly and the Process of Aging in Schizophrenia

In previous sections it was mentioned that schizophrenia can occur for the first time in the elderly. It has also been mentioned that schizophrenics who reach an advanced age and seem stabilized can show dramatic changes in their condition as well as the s.c. 2nd positive break described by the Bonn group. Besides the papers quoted in the previous sections, there are studies which have been particularly devoted to the aging process of schizophrenic patients and to the possible changes in psychopathology which may occur with increasing age (Riemer, 1950; Barucci, 1955; Janzarik, 1957; Wenger, 1958; Müller, 1959; Berner, 1969; Berner et al., 1973; Gabriel, 1974a,b; 1975a,b; Berner and Gabriel, 1973a,b; Ciompi and Müller, 1976). Early authors, Weygandt (1904) and Cortesi (1909) (both quoted by Barucci) maintained that schizophrenic patients who had been ill for more than 50 years and had reached an advanced age did not show any sign of senility. Since that time the question as to whether schizophrenic patients are more or less pone to age-related psychoorganic syndromes than nonpatients is still unanswered despite the fact that very old chronic patients represent a very high precentage of the chronically hospitalized (see, for example, Hartmann and Meyer, 1974).

Most authors maintain that the symptomatology of those patients who become ill when elderly does not differ markedly from that of younger patients. A delusional-hallucinatoric patterns seems, however, to be the most common (Janzarik, 1957; Klages, 1963). All types of course have been described in the elderly, i.e., both one characterized by an acute onset followed by complete recovery or by a remission with some degree of defect and one characterized by an insidious onset and a chronic course. According to Gabriel (1974), recovery after an acute episode occurs rarely. The occurrence of arteriosclerotic or other brain organic manifestations strongly influences the course toward chronicity (Barucci; Berner and Gabriel; Ciompi and Müller; Gabriel; Klages; Post, 1971). Besides, a destructuration of the delusions often occurs with increasing age (Gabriel). Riemer (1950) in a study of 100 schizophrenic patients who had remained in hospital for more than 25 years found that the incidence of senile psychoses was almost negligible. Wenger (1958) compared 25 hospitalized schizophrenic veterans aged 65-85 years with a similar number of hospitalized veterans who were classified as mentally well, although they were more or less afflicted with physical disabilities. From this comparison no clear-cut intergroup differences could be evidentiated either in the clinical examination or with psychological tests. Organic brain deterioration was disclosed by psychological tests only in the very old late-schizophrenic patients. Barucci (1955) carried a comprehensive investigation of 80 patients aged 70-84 years who were selected according to year of birth among 2000 patients admitted to the psychiatric hospitals in Florence, Italy. Of these 80 patients, 25 (31.2%) were never discharged after first admission and showed a progressive course, whereas the remaining 55 showed a successive course characterized by exacerbations and remission, 5 of them with more than 6 attacks. A careful clinical and psychological investigation showed that arteriosclerotic signs were present in about one-third of the cases. It was also found that neurological signs of focal vascular brain lesion were present in 11% of patients and that about 28% showed severe disorientation. In a further anatomopathological study of 200 patients who died, Barucci could show pronounced arteriosclerotic and senile brain damage in most cases. As for the patients who were still alive, Barucci maintained, contrary to the opinion expressed by other authors, that the schizophrenic substratum was recognizable in most patients and was not completely masked by the senile process. Ciompi and Müller (1976), who published one of the most comprehensive studies, found instead that schizophrenic patients on reaching old age became less unlike nonpsychotic elderly individuals. When the general problems of the aged occupied the foreground, the role of being aged suppressed the role of being a schizophrenic and it became more and more difficult to differentiate the former patients from the rest of the population. The difference between the results of the two studies very probably depends upon the selection of the patients since severely demented patients were scarcely represented in the series by Barucci. Post (1966, 1971), who studied series of patients classified as schizo-affective or late paraphrenics, found that cerebral pathology is not infrequently encountered in elderly patients with persistent paranoid symptoms. Its impact upon the further course cannot always be predicted correctly; some patients show sign of amelioration after treatment whereas others develop rapidly progressing brain deterioration (dementia).

J. Course of Cycloid Psychoses

As mentioned previously, the label cycloid psychosis refers to such psychotic conditions which in other nomenclatures are listed as recurrent or periodic schizophrenia, schizo-affective psychosis, atypical psychosis, etc. This uncertainty in classification and labeling means that the course of these conditions is considered most often under the more comprehensive heading "schizophrenia." In fact, it can be assumed that a great number of patients constituting follow-up studies of schizophrenia who have shown acute onset, a periodic course without any pronounced defect after each phase, and a more favorable long-term prognosis would be referred to as cycloid psychotics if this diagnosis had been taken into account. In particular, Russian psychiatrists, as mentioned previously, regard the diagnoses recurrent schizophrenia and cycloid psychosis as equivalent. Recent reviews of the literature concerning the different eponyms used to denominate quite similar psychotic disorders and their historic development are available (Fish, 1962; Vaillant, 1964a,b; Cerrolaza and Cleghorn, 1971; Perris, 1973, 1974).

One of the main characterisitcs of these psychotic disorders is that they present a mixture of symptomatological features belonging to the affective disorders and of symptoms commonly seen in the course of schizophrenic syndromes either at the same time or during different episodes. For this reason they have also been labeled "mixed psychoses" or, in the German literature, "Legierungspsychoses" (Arnold et al. 1964).

From a more general point of view different possibilities must be taken into account as concerns the long-term course of mixed psychoses and division into subgroups must be considered. The most usual subgrouping is as follows:

1. Disorders which begin with a syptomatology more proper of the affective disorders (depressive or atypical manic syndromes) and which switch in the later course to a more clear-cut schizophrenic symptomatology. Very often the course of this form becomes chronic-progressive and indistinguishable from the course by other schizophrenic patients who did not show any pronounced "affective" symptomatology at the beginning of their illness.

2. Disorders which begin with a schizophrenia-like symptomatology and which after one or more phases show a further course of clear-cut affective type without any admixture of symptoms. In these cases, the further course, as a rule, follows the same pattern as for depressive or manic-depressive psychoses.

3. Cases that for the most part of their course show a clear-cut schizophrenic symptomatology followed by occasional switch toward a depressive symptomatology of a severe degree. The possible occurrence of a depressive symptomatology in the course of schizophrenia has been recognized for a long time and was first described by Kraepelin. The significance of these depressive manifestations, however, has been interpreted differently by different authors (Bleuler, 1911; Eissler, 1951; Mayer-Gross et al., 1960; Sachar et al., 1963; Fadda and Müller, 1957). More recently, they have been interpreted as a possible side effect of a prolonged neuroleptic treatment, which has also been held responsible for the occurrence of suicide. Therefore, it is important to remember that the occurrence of both depression and suicide were well known for a long time before the introduction of neuroleptic drugs. In particular, the authors with a psychodynamic training have consistently regarded these post-psychotic depressive phases as the most important in the whole course of schizophrenia. Both Cohen et al. (1964) and Steinberg et al. (1967) were unable to demonstrate a greater incidence of suicide in patients treated with phenothiazine as compared with untreated.

4. Cases that should be properly labeled as cycloid psychotics. This refers to disorders which from the very beginning, and for almost the entire course, manifest themselves with a polymorphic symptomatology of a mixed type. Additional details about the long-term course of this particular subgroup are given in the following sections. Here it is sufficient to say that these disorders are most frequently characterized by acute psychotic episodes of short duration followed by recovery.

5. Cases in which a schizo-affective symptomatology characterizes the acute onset of an organic disorder in the aged (Post, 1971). In these cases, the further course is that of the underlying organic disorder.

From the description so far it can be assumed that much of the confusion concerning correct classification of mixed psychoses is very probably due to the fact that the diagnosis "schizo-affective psychosis" is improperly used to refer to all of the five subgroups mentioned above.

1. Age at Onset of Cycloid Psychoses

The results in the literature concerning the age at onset of cycloid psychoses are remarkably consistent. In fact, in all main studies (Leonhard, 1957-1969; Angst, 1966; Mentzos, 1967; Kirow, 1972a,b; Perris, 1973,1974) and also in articles which include small series (Sahli, 1959; Kurosawa, 1961; Krüger, 1968) the age at onset was 15 and 50 years with only exceptional instances below or above these age limits. In this respect, cycloid psychoses seem to differ from both schizophrenia and manic-depressive psychosis. No significant difference related to the sex of the patients have been reported as concerns the age at onset.

2. Type of Onset

The most common type of onset is acute. From a state of good health patients become psychotic within a few days or a few hours. The possible occurrence of less definite prodromal disturbances has, however, also been discussed, e.g., by Boeters (1971). On this point agreement seems to exist independently of the label given to the disorder (Vaillant, 1964a,b). In the series by Perris (1974), 45 patients had shown an acute onset at their first episode and 15 an insidious onset. Age, sex, and the occurrence of precipitating factors did not show any relationship to type of onset. The possible occurrence of unspecific prodromal disturbances could not be assessed in detail; in a few cases, however, there was a previous history of mild psychic disturbances, mainly of an anxiety-depressive variety, which had not implied the need for medical care. In the following course of illness there were in all 209 episodes–among these 182 were with an acute and 27 with an insidious onset. The type of onset at the first episode did not have any influence upon the type of onset at successive episodes.

3. Duration of an Episode

Leonard reports in the fourth edition of his textbook (1969) a calculation of the duration of the episodes in his probands made by Laszlo. According to these figures the mean duration was 3.9 months for 101 patients with an anxiety-happiness psychosis, 3.1 months for 88 patients with a confusion psychosis, and 2.8 months for 44 patients with a motility psychosis. Leonhard admits, however, that his figures are merely orientative because all patients were treated. Angst (1966) compared the episode duration in bipolar patients had the longest (average 8.8 months) duration; those with mixed conditions the shortest (average 5.5 months) duration; and periodically depressive patients somewhere in-between (6.1 months). However, since patients with involutional melancholy were considered separately, and since those patients had a longer duration than bipolars (14.1 months), it might be concluded that patients suffering only from depressive episodes have the longest and patients with mixed conditions the shortest duration, with bipolar patients falling in-between. Kirow (1972a) found an episode duration of less than 2 months in 61% and longer than 4 months in only 12% of his 98 cases. Neither Angst nor Kirow discuss their findings in relation to treatment, hospitalization, or changes in philosophical attitudes toward psychiatric care.

Perris (1976) was unable to calculate the duration of illness in each episode satisfactorily. This is mainly due to the fact that the duration of an episode as calculated on the basis of hospital records appeared to be correlated more to particular policies than to the real condition of the patient as described in the notes. First, it seems that the diagnostic label given on admission was of importance, e.g., a diagnosis of schizophrenia on several occasions implied a prolonged insulin coma treatment, the total duration of which seems to relate more to standards concerning this particular therapy than to the actual symptomatology. Such a treatment was seldom used if the diagnostic label given to a symptomatologically similar condition was psychosis per trauma mentale instead. Second, accessibility to new therapeutic methods seems to have played a role: Perris refers to the introduction of neuroleptics and to the policy of putting patients onto long-term treatment with these drugs on their discharge from hospital, once again independent of whether they had recovered of not. Third, many patients have in different episodes been treated by means of electroconvulsive therapy (ECT) with a fairly rapid positive therapeutic response whereas the same patient during other episodes or different patients have received other kinds of treatment.

4. Recurrency

There is a general agreement among authors that psychotic episodes of this kind have a strong tendency to recidivate. However, no definite results have hitherto been published which answer the question: how great is the risk of experiencing successive episodes after having suffered the first one? Some of the patients reported in Leonhard's textbook had suffered from only one episode, but it is not possible from the data available to calculate exactly how long these patients were observed or to draw general conclusions about the recidive risk after the first episode. In Perris' series, the longest observation of patients with ony one episode is 12 years.

The mean number of episodes has been calculated by different authors. According to Leonhard's latest findings, the mean number of episodes is almost the same as in bipolar manic-depressive psychosis, except for anxiety-happiness psychosis which seems to have a lower tendency to recidivate. Male patients have a slightly higher number of recidives than females. The length of the observation period is not given in detail, but it should be about 15 years. Angst

(1966) found a slightly higher number of episodes in his probands (5.5 episodes on average) who were observed for about 10 years. The 98 patients observed by Kirow (1972a) had suffered from 454 episodes, which means an average of 4.6 per patient. The observation period was in this case very long–between 10 and 43 years–for the most part between 15 and 30 years. Angst et al. (1969) in a later paper present some theoretical calculations about recidive frequency in bipolar and in schizo-affective psychotics. According to this calculation a patient suffering from one of these disorders would suffer on average upward of 18 episodes within a 15-year period.

As concerns variations in duration in successive episodes Angst et al. (1969) maintain that, while there is no shortening of the episodes, there is a shortening of the symptom-free intervals. According to Kirow, however, late episodes tend to be shorter than early ones. In this case also the differential effects of treatment must be taken into account before more positive affirmations can be made.

5. *Length of the Intervals*

Angst (1966) calculated that the interval between successive episodes is on average 42.1 months with a pronounced tendency to become shorter after many episodes. In a later paper, Angst et al. (1969) estimated the duration of a "cycle" (i.e., the span of time from the beginning of one episode to the beginning of a successive one) in patients who had suffered from bipolar manic-depressive psychosis and schizo-affective patients and found that the duration of the cycles decreases constantly in these patients by about 10%, the first cycle lasting 2 years. There is no doubt that because of the difficulties about a correct estimation of the duration of single episodes a calculation based on cycles is to be preferred. Such a calculation is relatively easy in patients with cycloid psychosis in which an acute onset is the most frequent, but it might be quite difficult in patients with affective disorders in which an insidious onset is more common.

A calculation of the duration of the cycles in Perris' probands is presented in Tables 10 and 11. As can be seen from the tables, the duration of the cycles is on average 2 years, the duration between the first and the second episodes being twice as long as the average. It seems, moreover, that any pronounced shortening of the cycles does not occur in Perris' series, a fact which is in contrast with the calculations of Angst et al. (1969). A source of error to be taken into account when calculating the duration of intervals or cycles according to Slater (1938b) is that patients with several episodes are more likely to be included in studies of this kind than patients with fewer recidives and that patients of the first type might have from the very beginning shorter intervals than patients with fewer relapses. A comparison of the length of the first cycle in patients with only two and in patients with nine or more episodes is presented

Table 10 Length of Cycle Between Successive Episodes (yr)[a]

Episodes	0.5	1	1.5	2	2.5	3	3.5	4	4.5	5	5.5	6	7	7.5	8	9	10	11	12	13	14	15 yr	n	x (yr)
1-2	9	7	3	8		2		1	1	2		2	2	1	3	2	6	1	1	1		1	53	4.5
2-3	10	8	3	5	2	5	2	2		4		1						1					43	2.3
3-4	10	13		4	4	2	2		1		1												37	1.5
4-5	6	6	2	1	2		2					1			1								24	2.0
5-6	7	8	2	1	2																		19	1.1
6-7	6	5	2			1				1													15	1.2
7-8	5		1	2						1													9	1.4
8-9	2	1	1					1															5	1.5
9-10			1				1																2	2.5
10-11		1		1																			2	1.5
Total	55	49	15	22	10	10	7	4	4	8	1	4	2	1	4	2	6	2	1	1	–	1	209	

[a] Seven patients only one episode. (168) 80.4% < 4 yr.

Table 11 Length of Cycle Between Successive Episodes (mo)[a]

Interval between episodes	No. of intervals	Mean length	Range
1- 2	53	54.9	6-180
2- 3	43	27.7	6-132
3- 4	37	19.1	6- 66
4- 5	24	24.5	6- 76
5- 6	19	13.6	6- 30
6- 7	15	15.2	6- 60
7- 8	9	17.3	6- 60
8- 9	5	18.0	6- 48
9-10	2	30.0	18- 42
10-11	2	18.0	12- 24
Total	209	23.8	6-180

[a]Seven patients only one episode.

Table 12 Mean Length of First Cycle (mo) in Patients with Only Two Episodes as Compared with Patients with Nine or More Episodes[a]

Patients	n	Mean duration
2 episodes	13	49.1 ± 13.5
9 or more episodes	9	48.6 ± 16.2

[a]$t = 0.18$; p = n.s.

in Table 12. No significant difference has been found in this small group, but different results might be obtained in larger series. According to the calculations presented in the tables, about 80% of the cycles were shorter than 4 years.

II. SYMPTOMATIC SCHIZOPHRENIA AND ORGANIC PSYCHOSES

A. Organic Psychoses with a Schizophrenia-Like Symptomatology

There are several psychotic conditions with an organic basis which at a certain phase of their development can manifest themselves with a symptomatology indistinguishable from that occurring in schizophrenic syndromes with a cryptogenic etiology. The most known among these schizophrenia-like psychoses is that related to epilepsy, which is treated in some detail in the following. A schizophrenia-like symptomatology, however, can occur against a vast variety of organic backgrounds including traumatic, tumoral, heredodegenerative, chromotoxic, or infective conditions. The course of such schizophrenia-like psychoses is poorly investigated and information about it must be deduced from studies of single cases or from reports concerning very small series. However, the recognition of such psychoses is of fundamental importance for the planning of treatment and for prognosis. Of these conditions, one major exception refers to the schizophrenia-like psychoses of epilepsy, which have been a matter of much concern and controversy for a long time.

B. Schizophrenia and Epilepsy: Clinical Types and Course

The possible occurrence of epileptic fits in catatonic patients was ascertained by Kahlbaum (1874) before Kraepelin's description of dementia praecox. Later Kraepelin confirmed that epileptic manifestations could occur in about 18% of catatonic patients. He also admitted that the differential diagnosis could sometimes be very difficult, especially in the initial phase of the psychosis. Since then, the most divergent opinions about a possible combination of epilepsy and schizophrenia have been maintained in the literature.

E. Bleuler admitted that epileptic manifestations could be very frequent, but he wrote that he himself had never seen any case with such a "complication." However, he quotes the thesis by Morawitz (1900), which contains one of the earliest and most thorough description of catatonic patients with epileptic manifestations. Tanzi and Lugaro (1916) also describe the occurrence of epileptic fits in the initial stage of dementia praecox and maintain that the epileptic manifestations disappear in the later course of the psychosis. Early studies are characterized by speculations as to whether or not schizophrenia could cause epilepsy or vice versa. Most of the early studies give different figures as to the frequency of epileptic manifestations in schizophrenics or of schizophrenic manifestations in epileptics. Vorkastner (1918) found only 10 cases with epileptic manifestations among 218 schizophrenics. On the basis of these findings he criticized the hypothesis of a possible schizophrenic nature of epilepsy. Hoch (1934) observed the occurrence of a schizophrenia-like development in about 10% of a series of 100 epileptics and the occurrence of epilepsy in only 2 out of 500 schizophrenics. Urstein (quoted by Motta, 1953) in a series of 2700 patients found that epileptic convulsions had occurred in 3.5%. Yde et al. (1941) found epileptic manifestations in 20 of 715 schizophrenic patients. Garland and Sumner (1964) reported a 5% incidence of psychosis "indistinguishable from schizophrenia" in a series of 54 epileptics. Asuni and Pillutla (1976) found 11 cases with schizophrenia-like psychosis among 42 epileptics in Nigeria. The introduction of electroencephalography in clinical routine has also contributed to the discussions about the occurrence of epilepsy in schizophrenia. However, most of the early investigations conceal different sources of error, partly due to the treatment that the schizophrenic patients had received, partly due to an overevaluation of the epileptic nature of certain EEG abnormalities. Later on the widespread use of psychosurgery in schizophrenics, and more recently the widespread use of drugs capable of lowering the convulsive threshold, once again contributed to making the problem controversial. As concerns schizophrenia and epilepsy, two types of course were recognized at a very early stage, one characterized by the development of a schozphrenia-like symptomatology in former epileptics. This symptomatology is sometimes followed and sometimes not by a successive disappearance of the epileptic manifestations [Vorkastner; Notkin, 1929; Langenhorn (quoted by Vitello, 1958); Senise, 1931; Marchand and Ajuriaguerra, 1948; Perris and Stancati, 1954; Bonetti and Perris, 1959; Perris and d'Elia, 1960]. The other course type is instead characterized by the disappearance of the schizophrenic symptomatology following the occurrence of epileptic manifestations (Müller, 1930). Although the coexistence of epilepsy and schizophrenia had been recognized by several authors, the observation by Müller helped to lay the ground for the hypothesis by von Meduna (1935) of a biological antagonism between epilepsy and schizophrenia upon which the introduction of convulsive therapy with cardiazol was based.

C. Types of Succession of the Epileptic and Schizophrenic Manifestations

Thus, the following types of succession have been recognized:

1. Epileptic manifestations precede, sometimes by several years, the occurrence of a schizophrenia-like symptomatology. Afterward:
   a. Epileptic and schizophrenic manifestations coexist in the future course.
   b. The epileptic manifestations disappear, whereas the schizophrenia-like symptomatology becomes most prominent. Occasional seizures, however, can occur in latee periods of the course.
2. Schizophrenic manifestations precede, sometimes by several years, the occurrence of epileptic seizures. Afterward:
   a. The schizophrenic symptomatology disappears, whereas the occurrence of convulsions becomes more pronounced.
   b. The occurrence of epileptic convulsions remains an isolate feature or, more often, there is a recurrence after very long intervals.
3. Both epilepsy and schizophrenic manifestations coexist and there is a progress toward severe demential states.

All these different features have been described in the literature, but there is no possibility of deciding which of them is the most frequent. No special predominance of any sex has emerged from the cases described in the literature. Nor does there seem to be any type of schizophrenic symptomatology which does not occur in combination with epilepsy. To the contrary, it has been pointed out that hebephrenic, catatonic, and paranoid manifestations can be found in the course of schizophrenia-like psychoses of epilepsy (Vorkastner, 1918; Vitello, 1958; Perris and d'Elia, 1960). Paranoid manifestations, however, seem to have been reported more frequently among the single-case reports or in surveys (Golodetz and Ravkin, 1968).

In one of the most thorough studies of these conditions, Slater et al. (1963) maintained that the symptomatology in their patients was clinically indistinguishable from that of clear-cut schizophrenic patients without any history of epilepsy. The study by these authors is very important because it shows in an elegant, scientific way that the schizophrenia-like symptomatology diagnosticized in their patients is epileptic in origin. Apart from the results of calculations aimed at ruling out the possibility of an association by chance of the two disorders, an important finding by Slater and his co-workers was the occurrence of a significant correlation between the ages of onset of epilepsy and psychosis, suggesting that duration of epilepsy plays an etiological role in determining the psychosis. In a later study, however, Slater and Moran (1969) suggested that the age factor might have more importance in female than male patients. Taylor (1975) contrasted a group of patients with "alien tissue" in their resected temporal lobe with a group of patients with mesial temporal sclerosis and suggested that in the alien tissue group females were the most likely to have developed a schizophrenia-like psychosis.

D. Follow-Up and Outcomes

The only comprehensive follow-up study comprising detailed information about outcome is that published by Slater et al. (1963). The authors were able to follow up their 64 patients for an average of 7-8 years after the onset of the schizophrenia-like symptomatology (range 2-25 years). Four of the patients had died, but information about these patients could also be obtained. At the follow-up 30 of the patients were at home, 16 living mainly at home, whereas the remainders had been mainly or permanently in hospital. Forty-five patients no longer had fits. Epilepsy, on the other hand was moderately troublesome in 12 and constituted a severe problem in another 3 cases. As for the schizophrenia-like symptomatology, about one-third of the patients had made a good recovery, one-third were much improved, and one-third were unchanged. Organic personality changes independent of the schizophrenic symptomatology were present in 29 and absent in 31 patients. It must be mentioned, however, that 11 patients has been subjected to a temporal lobectomy.

E. Schizophrenia-Like Psychoses of Huntington's Chorea

When manifest neurological symptoms are present the diagnosis of Huntington's chorea seldom presents difficulties for the experienced clinician. What is often overlooked is that the disease often begins with mental disturbances and that psychopathological manifestations can for a long time assume a schizophrenia-like nature.

The possible occurrence of schizophrenia-like manifestations is acknowledged in psychiatric textbooks (Mayer-Gross et al. 1960; Weitbrecht, 1963), where it is also pointed out that these manifestations often characterize the initial phase of the illness. However, McHugh and Folstein (1975) point out that most often little enthusiasm is kindled for the drawing of subtle psychiatric manifestations in the course of a rare, hereditary disorder in which other clinical characteristics very soon become much more prominent. On the other hand, it is not exceptional to find that several cases of Huntington's chorea have been diagnosed for a long time as schizophrenic or paranoid psychoses (and treated accordingly) before the diagnosis of Huntington's chorea was finally made. Many authors have been concerned with the occurrence of a schizophrenia-like symptomatology in the course of Huntington's chorea (Brothers and Meadows, 1955; Streletzki, 1961; Myrianthopoulous, 1966; Garron, 1973) and the possible occurrence of wrong diagnoses before the appearance of motor disability has been recognized (McHugh and Folstein, 1975). However, follow-up studies of large series of patients are almost nonexistent. In a recent study carried out at Umeå, Mattsson (1974) was able to collect 162 patients and to map the course of their disease. In 48% of the patients the initial phase was characterized by posychiatric manifestations alone, and in another 30% by a combination of neurological and psychiatric symptoms, whereas in only 22% the disease initiated with neurological manifestations. Among the patients with an initial psychiatric symptomatology, 20 (12% of all patients, 25.6% of those with initial psychiatric symptoms) showed a schizophrenia-like or paranoid picture. The time lapse before the appearance of neurological symptoms was, on average, 5.1 s.d. 3.4 years. However, the time lapse from the onset of the psychiatric manifestations to the point when a correct diagnosis was made was 8.8 s.d. 6.5 years. One of the reasons for the delay in correct diagnosis is that choreatic movements appearing in a patient treated for a long time for an assumed schizophrenia may be erroneously regarded as extrapyramidal side effects due to neuroleptic treatment, or in older patients as arteriosclerotic dyskinesis. In Mattsson's patients, the time from the first onset of Huntington's chorea to dementia was about 9 years independent of the type of initial symptomatology.

F. Other Symptomatic Schizophrenic Syndromes

As pointed out at the beginning of this section, schizophrenia-like manifestations may occur in the course of several organic conditions. In particular, the syndromes may occur in patients with previous encephalitic processes, arteriosclerosis, brain tumors, trauma of the brain, intoxications, chromosomal abnormalities, lupus erythematosus, etc. (Hillbom, 1950; Lemke, 1950; Perris and d'Elia, 1960; Alsen, 1961, 1967, 1969; Guze, 1967; Thompson, 1970; Owen, 1972; Penn et al., 1972; Baker, 1973; Nikonova, 1974; Toshcheva, 1974; Foerster et al., 1976; Dorus et al., 1977; Sørensen and Nielsen, 1977). Several case reports have been published concerning these different morbid conditions, but no thorough follow-up studies or detailed information about the long-term course of these schizophrenia-like manifestations have been published. Also in the case of systemic lupus erythematosus a schizophrenia-like symptomatology can occur prior to the somatic manifestations (Baker, 1973; Foerster et al., 1976). On the other hand, a schizophrenia-like symptomatology seems to be a rare feature in the course of this disease whereas anxious-depressive manifestations have been described more frequently. Hillbom (1960), who published a comprehensive investigation of the after-effects of brain injuries, maintained that the occurrence of a schizophrenia-like symptomatology was almost invariably related to a lesion in the temporal lobes. Nikinova (1974) described the course of schizophrenia-like psychoses in 84 patients who had suffered from brain injury. According to her findings, the psychotic manifestation was characterized in the initial phase by an exogenous type of reaction and later on by a slow development with a relatively mild progressiveness.

III. PSYCHOSES IN THE AGED

The course of late schizophrenia and the process of aging in schizophrenic patients has been dealt with in some detail in Section I.I. At this point a short account of the course of the psychoses in the aged is given. However, a comprehensive analysis of the organic psychoses in presenium and senium is beyond the scope of this chapter.

Until the comprehensive work by British psychiatrists in the middle of the fifties—mostly by Roth and his group (Post, 1951; Roth and Morrissey, 1951; Roth, 1955; Kay et al., 1956; Kay 1962)—psychoses arising in old age had been regarded as organic in nature and their course as chronic toward dementia. The lack of therapeutic facilities contributed greatly to a pessimistic view concerning the prognosis of these conditions and most patients were chronically hospitalized. Later, however, the spread of improved electroconvulsive therapy (ECT) under anesthesia and muscular relaxation and, more recently, the introduction of psychotropic drugs have greatly enhance the possibilities of treating psychotic conditions in the elderly. This improvement of treatment facilities led to a revision of classificatory and prognostic concepts. One major advance was the recognition of a pseudodemntial symptomatology in the course of an affective disorder in the aged and the experience that patients showing such a syndrome could still recover if treated appropriately (a recent comprehensive review on this subject was published by Isaacs and Post (1978). Another important finding is that of a psychotic condition with a schizophrenic coloring which presents for the first time late in life (Post, 1966; see also the previous section on late schizophrenia).

Among the series of patients investigated by Roth and his co-workers a separation could be made into subroups on the basis of a careful clinical investigation, and the natural history of these subgroups could be investigated (Roth and Morrissey, 1952; Roth, 1955). The groups taken into account were affective psychoses in the senium, senile psychosis, "late" paraphrenia, acute confusion, and arteriosclerotic psychosis. In making this subdivision, the authors pointed out that many patients with paranoid psychosis in old age had been regarded as paranoid types of senile psychosis on the assumption that the eventual outcome was one of gross disintegration of the intellect and personality. A closer identification of this subgroup seemed particularly important since transient "ever-changing" paranoid ideas are also seen in the organic psychoses (Roth, 1955).

Roth and his group studied 450 patients who were admitted to hospital in two different periods:—1934, 1936 and 1948, 1949—and who were followed up for 2 years. The age of these patients ranged from 60 to 80 years or above at the time of admission to hospital. A first follow-up was made with respect to outcome 6 months after the admission for the patients suffering from affective psychosis. The number "discharged' at the end of the 6 months was almost double for patients admitted in the later years (58%) as compared with those admitted in 1934, 1936. As for the other subgroups, no comparisons were made between the two periods since the treatment given had not altered during the period of observation. However, a comparison was made for all 4 years' material among the diagnostic subgroups. Among the patients with late paraphrenia only about 15% had been discharged within 6 months; 76% were still inpatients and the remainder had died. Of the patients with acute confusion, 50% had been discharged and 40% had died. The highest mortality (58%) occurred among the patients with senile psychosis, who also had the least number of discharges. In the arteriosclerotic psychosis group the difference in proportion between discharged, inpatients, and deaths was more even than in the other four groups.

Patients admitted in 1948, 1949 were followed up for 2 years (318 patients in all). At this second follow-up the percentage of patients with affective psychosis who had been discharged was still the highest (about 60%) and also the percentage of patients who had died was lowest. On the other hand, most of the patients suffering from late paraphrenia were still in hospital (about 60%) and of the remainder one-half had been discharged and the other died. During the 2-year follow-up as many as 80% of the patients with senile psychosis and about 70% of those suffering from arteriosclerotic psychosis had died, whereas very few had been discharged. From the study it became evident also that mortality, especially in the group of senile psychosis, was lower among the women than the men.

A long-term follow-up of functional and organic psychoses in old age with special reference to mortality has been published by Kay (1962). The patients had been admitted to a Swedish hosptial during the period 1931-1937 and the period of follow-up was 16-25 years. This very careful investigation showed that the mortality rate in the late paraphrenic group (53 cases) was not significantly higher than in the general population. In the group of patients with dementia, however, the mortality rate was at least five times as high as in the general population and the length of survival about 25% of the normal or less. The proportion of cases of late paraphrenia in which cerebral arteriosclerosis was associated with the onset of illness was about 5%. Sjögren has for a long time been concerned with the geriatric population at a mental hospital in Sweden. In one of his most comprehensive papers (1964) he furnished data about the average age at onset and about the average duration of the disease in large series of patients. According to his results, the age at onset of presenile psychoses (m. Alzheimer, m. Pick) was 57-63 years and the duration 7-10 years (longest being m. Pick). The age at onset of senile psychosis was on average 77 years and the duration 6-7 years. In a cerebrovascular group the average age at onset was about 69 years and the duration about 4 years. As for late paraphrenia, Sjögren found that the average age at onset was about 61 years and the average age at death about 78 years.

Attempts have been made to identify predictors of short-term outcome and survival in psychogeriatric populations (Kay et al. 1956; McAdam and Robinson, 1957; Epstein et al. 1971; Libow, 1973; Müller et al., 1975; Neiditch and White, 1976). Many of these studies, however, have been concerned with very different categories of patients and with healthy elderly (Libow, 1973) investigated in different settings; therefore, it is difficult to draw general conclusions. However, it seems that some agreement does exist about the prognostic value of EEG. In fact, a generalized EEG slowing and an impaired EEG reactivity have been repeatedly reported as of central importance for the lessening of survival chances (Pampiglione and Post, 1954; McAdam and Robinson, 1957; Obrist and Busse, 1965; Müller et al., 1975).

A. Occurrence of Schizophrenia-Like Symptoms in the Course of Organic Psychoses of the Aged

The course of organic psychoses of the aged is characterized by a more or less rapid decline of intellectual functioning toward a demential disintegration of intellect and personality. The course is almost continuous in the presenile and senile degenerative disorders of the nervous system, whereas it is more fluctuating in psychotic disorders due to cerebral arteriosclerosis. Although memory disturbances, impaired orientation, decreases in efficiency, and personality changes of various degree are ass a rule the most prominent features of the initial stages of all these disorders, transient schizophrenia-like symptoms can also occur. The only exception seems to be m. Pick, wherein a pronounced decay of intellectual functions appears evident from the early stage of the disease and paranoid ideas or hallucinatory episodes are rare (Bolzani, 1959; Mayer-Gross et al., 1960). Sjögren et al. (1952) found a paranoid reaction in only 1 among 18 histopathologically verified cases. They quote, however, an observation by Eiden and Lechner (1950, quoted by Sjögren et al.), who found paranoid psychotic elements in 10 out of 30 cases of m. Pick.

In Alzheimer's disease, auditory and visual hallucinations and paranoid ideas are occasionally present during the initial phase of the disease (Mayer-Gross et al., 1960; Ey et al., 1963). Hallucinations were found in 4 and paranoid ideas in 5 of 18 cases of histopathologically verified m. Alzheimer studied by Sjögren et al. In a series of 10 cases studied by Eiden and Lechner (see above), 4 showed psychotic components in the initial stage. Lauter (1968) found paranoid ideas as initial symptoms in 25 of 177 patients with m. Alzheimer. Taking into account the whole course, paranoid symptoms occurred in 39 patients in all at some stage of the disease.

As for senile psychosis, acute delirious episodes can occur in the early phase of the disease, often precipitated by an acute infection, a fracture, or a sudden change in circumstances (Mayer-Gross et al., 1960; Ey et al., 1963; Weitbrecht, 1963). These episodes of acute delirium are characterized by restlessness, auditory and visual hallucinations, and paranoid suspicion. They are as a rule of short duration and leave behind a more pronounced dementia than was present before their occurrence. Waldton (1973) found transient paranoid symptoms in about one-half of 60 cases of senile dementia.

Greger (1971) paid attention to the course of mental disorders in the aged. Among the diagnostic groups taken into account he described a subgroup comprised of 14 patients with brain organic psychoses (senile psychosis?). These patients were characterized by a paranoid symptomatology. Nine of them showed a very rapid progressive demential disintegration, and all of them died within 2 years after discharge from the hospital. In two other patients the brain organic symptomatology became dominant in the further course and masked the paranoid symptons. In the last three patients, however, the paranoid symtomatology paralleled the course of organic disintegration.

Of 50 patients with arteriosclerotic psychosis studied by Greger (1971), 29 showed a course characterized by marked remissions and 21 a chronic progressive course. In 8 of these patients transient paranoid syndromes were occasionally observed.

B. Comments

The most important finding of the last decades as concerns psychotic conditions in the senium is the recognition that both affective and paranoid disorders can occur for the first time in very old people. In most instances these conditions simulate a demential state and lead to therapeutic nihilism. Experience has proved that a large part of the patients show in such a complex syndrome can be treated successfully. Further details about the course of schizophrenia arising in the senium are discussed in Section I.I. Here it can be mentioned that out of 42 patients with a paranoid-hallucinatoric syndrome investigated by Greger and followed up for 3-17 years, more than one-half showed a periodic or remitting course whereas only 6 showed a chronic progressive course.

ACKNOWLEDGMENTS

Mrs. Doris Cedergren has skillfully contributed in the collection of references and in the preparation of the manuscript.

REFERENCES

Achté, K. A. (1961). Der Verlauf der Schizophrenien und der Schizophreni ormen Psychosen. *Acta Psychiatr. Neurol. Scand., Supplement 155.*

Achté, K. A. (1967). On prognosis and rehabilitation in schizophrenic and paranoid psychoses. *Acta Psychiatr. Scand., Supplement 196.*

Achté, K. A., and Apo, M. (1967). Schizophrenic patients in 1950-1952 and 1957-1959. A comparative study. *Psychiatr. Quart. 42,* 411-422.

Achté, K. A., and Niskanen, P. (1973). Prognosis in schizophrenia and community psychiatry. *Psychiatr. Fennica,* 115-122.

Alanen, Y. O., Arajärvi, T., and Viitamäki, R. O. (1964). Psychoses in childhood. *Acta Psychiatr. Scand., Supplement 174.*

Alsen, V. (1961). Zur Psychopathologie der cerebralen Durchblutungsstörungen. *Acta Neurochir.* (Wien), *Supplement 7,* 118-126.

Alsen, V. (1967). Eine chronische paranoid-hallucinatorische Psychose bei hirntraumatischem Anfallsleiden. *Acta Psychiatr. Scand. 43,* 52-67.

Alsen, V. (1969). Schizophreniforme Psychosen mit belangenvollen körperlichem Befunden. *Fortschr. Neurol. Psychiatr. 37,* 448-457.

Alström, C. H. (1938). Schizophrenie und Tuberkulose. *Z. Ges. Neurol. Psychiatr. 162,* 25-30.

Alström, C. H. (1942). Mortality in mental hospitals with especial regard to tuberculosis. *Acta Psychiatr. Neurol. Scand., Supplement 24.*

Angst, J. (1966). *Zur Ätiologie und Nosologie endogener depressiver Psychosen,* Springer, Berlin.

Angst, J. (1977). Verlauf endogener Psychosen. mimeo. to be published.

Angst, J., Ditrich, A., and Grof, P. (1969). Course of endogenous affective psychoses and its modification by prophylactic administration of imipramine and lithium. *Int. Pharmacopsychiatr. 2,* 1-11.

Angst, J., Baastrup, P. Grof, P., Hippius H., Pöldinger, W., Varga, E., Weis, P., and Wyss, F. (1973). Statistische Aspekte des Beginns und Verlaufs schizophrener Psychosen. In *Verlauf und Ausgang schizophrener Erkrankungen,* G. Huber (Ed.), Schattauer, Stuttgart, New York.

Annell, L. A. (1963). The prognosis of psychotic syndromes in childhood. *Acta Psychiatr. Scand. 39,* 235-297.

Annesby, A. T. (1961). Psychiatric illness in adolescence: presentation and prognosis. *J. Ment. Sci. 107,* 268-277.

Anthony, E. J. (1958). An aetiological approach to the diagnosis of psychosis in childhood. *Res. Psychiatr. Inf. 25,* 89-96.

Apo, M., and Achté, K. A. (1966). Schizofreniundersökning 1950-1952 och 1957-1959. *Nord. Psykiatr. Tidskr. 20,* 125-140.

Arieti, S. (1959). Schizophrenia. In *American Handbook of Psychiatry,* S. Arieti (Ed.), Basic Books, New York, 1st ed.

Arnold, O. H., Gastager, H., and Hofman, G. (1964). Klinische, psychopathologische und biochemische Untersuchungen an Legierungspsychosen. *Wien Zschr. Nervenhelik. 22,* 301-361.

Astrup, C. (1957). Experimentelle Untersuchungen über die Störungen der höheren Nerventätigkeit bei Defekt schizophrenen. *Psychiatr. Neurol. Med. Psychol. 9,* 9-14, 33-38.

Astrup, C. and Noreik, K. (1966). Functional psychoses. *Diagnostic and Prognostic Models,* Thomas, Springfield, Ill.

Astrup, C., Fossum, A., and Holmboe, R. (1962). *Prognosis in Functional Psychoses,* Thomas, Springfield, Ill.

Asuni, T., and Pillutla, V. S. (1967). Schizophrenia-like psychoses in Nigerian epileptics. *Br. J. Psychiatr. 113,* 1375-1379.

Babigian, H. M., and Odoroff, C. L. (1969). The mortality experiences of a population with psychiatric illness. *Am. J. Psychiatr. 126,* 470-480.

Babigian, H. M., Gardner, E. A., Miles, H. C., and Romano, J. (1964). Diagnostic consistency and change in a follow-up study of 1215 patients. *Am. J. Psychiatr. 121,* 895-901.

Baker, M. (1973). Psychopathology in systematic lupus erythematosus. 1. Psychiatric observations. *Sem. Arthr. Rheum. 3,* 95-110.

Barucci, M. (1955). La vecchiaia degli schizofrenici: studio di un gruppo di 80 schizofrenici giunti all'età de oltre 70 ami. *Riv. Pat. Nerv. Ment. 76,* 257-284.

Baruk, E. (1950). *Precis de Psychiatrie,* Masson, Paris.

Beck, M. N. (1968). Twenty-five and thirty-five year follow-up of first admissions to mental hospital. *Can. Psychiatr. Assoc. J. 13,* 219-229.

Bellak, L., and Parcell, M. S. (1946). The pre-psychotic personality in dementia praecox. *Psychiatr. Quart. 20,* 627-637.

Bemporad, J. R., and Pinsker, H. (1974). Schizophrenia: the manifest symptomatology. In *American Handbook of Psychiatry,* S. Arieti (Ed.), Basic Books, New York, 2nd ed., Vol. III, Chap. 23, 524-525.

Bender, L. (1940). Childhood schizophrenia. *Nerv. Child. 1,* 138-153.

Bender, L. (1953). Childhood schizophrenia. *Psychiatr. Quart. 27,* 663-671.

Bender, L. (1970). The life course of schizophrenic children. *Biol. Psychiatr. 2,* 165-170.

Berner, P. (1969). Der Lebensabend der Paranoiker. *Wien Z. Nervenheilkunde 27,* 115-161.

Berner, P., and Gabriel, E. (1973a). Beziehungen zwischen Psychopathologie und Genetik sogenannter "spätschizophrenien." *Wien Z. Nervenheilkunde 31,* 1-11.

Berner, P., and Gabriel, E. (1973b). Sogenannte "spätschizophrenie" in hohen Alter. *Actuelle Gerontologie 3,* 351-357.

Berner, P., Gabriel, E., and Naske, R. (1973). Verlaufstypologie und Prognose bei sogenannten spätschizophrenien. In *Verlauf und Ausgang schizophrener Erkrankungen,* G. Huber (Ed.), Shattauer, Stuttgart.

Berze, J. (1910). *Heredity or Dementia Praecox,* Deuticke, Vienna.

Bland, R. C., Parker, J. H., and Orn, H. (1976). Prognosis in schizophrenia. *Arch. Gen. Psychiatr. 33,* 949-954.

Bleuler, E. (1908). Die Prognose der Dementia praecox (Schizophreniegruppe). *Allg. Z. Psychiatr. 65,* 436-442.

Bleuler, E. (1911). Dementia praecox oder die Gruppe der Schizophrenien. In *Handbuch der Psychiatrie,* G. Aschaffenburg (Ed.), Deuticke, Leipzig.

Bleuler, M. (1941). *Krankheitsverlauf, Persönlichkeit und Verwandschafe Schizophrener und ihre gegenseitigen Beziehungen,* Thieme, Leipzig.

Bleuler, M. (1943). Die spätschizophrenen Krankheitsbilder. *Fortschr. Neurol. 15,* 259-290.

Bleuler, M. (1972). Die Schizophrenen Geistesstörungen im Lichte langjähriger Kranken- und Familiengeschichten, Thieme, Stuttgart.

Bleuler, M. (1973). Die Schizophrenien: die langen Verläufe und ihre Formbarkeit. In *Verlauf und Ausgang schizophrener Erkrankungen,* G. Huber (Ed.), Schattauer, Stuttgart.

Bleuler, M., Huber, G., Gross, G., and Schüttler, R. (1976). Die langfristige Verlauf schizophrener Psychosen. *Nervenarzt 47,* 477-481.

Boeters, V. (1971). Die oneiroiden Emotionspsychosen. *Bibl. Psychiatr. No. 148,* Karger, Basel.

Bolzani, L. (1959). L'atrofia cerebrale circoseritta o morbo di Pick. *Riv. Sper. Freniat. 83,* fs. 2, 1-21.

Bonetti, U., and Perris, C. (1959). Ulteriori considerazioni sui rapporti tra epilessia e schizofrenia. *Rass. Neuropsichiat. 13,* 349-357.

Bowers, M. B. (1968). Pathogenesis of acute schizophrenic psychosis. *Arch. Gen. Psychiatr. 19,* 348-355.

Bradley, C. (1941). *Schizophrenia in childhood.* MacMillan, New York.

Brothers, C. R. D., and Meadows, A. W. (1955). An investigation of Huntington's chrea in Victoria. *J. Ment. Sci. 101,* 548-563.

Brown, G. W. (1960). Length of hospital stay and schizophrenia: a review of statistical studies. *Acta Psychiatr. Scand. 35,* 414-430.

Brown, G. W., Murray Parkes, C., and Wing, J. K. (1961). Admissions and readmissions to three London mental hospitals. *J. Ment. Sci. 107,* 1070-1077.

Brown, G. W., Monch, E. M., Carstairs, G. M., and Wing, J. K. (1962). Influence of family life on the course of schizophrenic illness. *Br. J. Prev. Soc. Med. 16,* 55-68.

Brzezicki, E. (1972). Follow-up observations (catamnesis) and prognosis in acute juvenile psychosis. *Pol. Med. J. 11,* 437-446.

Bumke, O. (1948). *Lehrbuch die Geisteskrankheiten.* 7 Aufl. Bergmann, München.

Böök, J. A. (1953). A genetic and neuropsychiatric investigation of a North-Swedish population. *Acta Genet. 4,* 1-100.

Caldwell, J. (1941a). Neurotic components in psychopathic behaviour. *J. Nerv. Ment. Dis. 99,* 134-136.

Caldwell, J. (1941b). Schizophrenic psychoses: 100 cases in U.S. Army. *Am. J. Psychiatr. 97,* 1061-1072.

Cameron, D. E. (1938). Early schizophrenia. *Am. J. Psychiatr. 95,* 567-578.

Carletti, G. (1958). Esordi nevrotiformi della schizofrenia. *Note Riv. Psichiat. fs. 1* (estratto), 1-13.

Cerrolaza, M., and Cleghorn, R. A. (1971). Atypical psychoses. *Can. Psychiatr. Assoc. J. 16,* 507-514.

Chapman, J. (1966). The early symptoms of schizophrenia. *Br. J. Psychiatr. 112,* 225-251.

Ciompi, L. (1976). Late suicide in former mental patients. *Psychiatr. Clin. 9,* 59-63.

Ciompi, L., and Medvecka, J. (1976). Etude comparative de la mortalité à long terme dans les maladies mentales. *Arch. Suiss Neurol. Neurochir. Psychiatr. 118,* 111-135.

Ciompi, L., and Müller, C. (1976). *Lebensweg und Alter der Schizophrenen. Eine katamnestische Langzeitstudie bis ins Senium,* Springer, Berlin.

Cohen, S., Leonard, C. V., Farberow, N. L., and Shneidman, E. S. (1964). Tranquilizers and suicide in the schizophrenic patient. *Arch. Gen. Psychiatr. 11,* 312-321.

Conrad, K. (1958). *Die beginnende Schizophrenie,* Thieme, Stuttgart.

Costantini, F. (1911). Nuovo contributo allo studio clinico della dementia precocissima. *Riv. Sper. Freniat. 37,* 305-321.

Creak, E. M. (1951). Psychoses in childhood. *J. Ment. Sci. 97,* 545-554.

Creak, E. M. (1962). Juvenile psychosis and mental deficiency. Quoted by Rutter (1967).

Creak, E. M. (1963a). Childhood psychosis. *Br. J. Psychiatr. 109,* 84-89.

Creak, E. M. (1963b). Schizophrenia in early childhood. *Acta Paedopsychiatr. 30,* 42-47.

Dahl, V. (1976). A follow-up study of a child psychiatric clientele with special regard to the diagnosis of psychosis. *Acta Psychiatr. Scand. 54,* 106-112.

Dahlgren, K. G. (1945). *On Suicide and Attempted Suicide,* Lindstedt, Lund.

Dalgård, O. S. (1966). Mortalitet ved funksjonelle psykoser. *Nord. Med. 75,* 680-684.

De Sanctis, S. (1906). Sopra alcune varietà della demenza precoce. *Riv. Sper. Freniat. 32,* 141-180.

Despert, J. L. (1938). Schizophrenia in children. *Psychiatr. Quart. 12,* 366-371.

Despert, J. L., and Sherwin, A. C. (1958). Further examination of diagnostic criteria in schizophrenic illness and psychoses of infancy and early childhood. *Am. J. Psychiatr. 114,* 748-790.

Dorus, E., Dorus, W., and Telfer, M. A. (1977). Paranoid schizophrenia in a 47,XYY male. *Am. J. Psychiatr. 134,* 687-689.

Eggers, C. (1973). *Verlaufsweisen kindlicher und präpuberaler Schizophrenien,* Springer, Berlin.

Eggers, C. (1974). Todesgedanken, Suicide und Suicidversuche in Verlauf kindlicher Schizophrenien. *Nervenarzt 45,* 36-42.

Eisenberg, L. (1957). The course of childhood schizophrenia. *Arch. Neurol. Psychiatr. 78,* 69-77.

Eissler, R. K. (1951). Remarks on the psychoanalysis of schizophrenia. *Int. J. Psychoanal. 32,* 139-156.

Eitinger, L., Laane, C., and Langfeldt, G. (1958). Prognostic value of clinical picture and therapeutic value of physical treatment in schizophrenia and schizophreniform states. *Acta Psychiatr. Scand. 33,* 33-53.

Epen van, J. H. (1969). Defect schizophrenic states (residual schizophrenia). *Psychiatr. Neurol. Neurochir. 72,* 371-394.

Epstein, L. J., Robinson, B. C., and Simon, A. (1971). Predictors of survival in geriatric mental illness during the eleven years after initial hosptial admission. *J. Am. Geriatr. Soc. 19,* 913-921.

Esman, A. H. (1960). Childhood psychosis and childhood schizophrenia. *Am. J. Orthopsychiatr. 30,* 391-396.

Essen-Möller, E. (1935). Untersuchungen über die fruchtbarkeit gewisser

Gruppen von Beisteskranken. *Acta Psychiatr. Neurol. Scand., supplement 8.*

Ettlinger, R. W., and Flordh, P. (1955). Attempted suicides. *Acta Psychiatr. Neurol. Scand., supplement 103.*

Ey, H., and Bonnafous-Serieux, M. (1938). Etudes cliniques et considérations nosographigues sur la D.P. *Ann. Méd. Psychol. 96,* 151-181, 360-394.

Ey, H., Bernard, P., and Brisset, C. (1963). *Manuel de Psychiatrie,* Masson and Cie, Paris.

Fadda, S., and Müller, C. (1975). La depression post-schizophrenique. *Ann. Méd. Psychol. 133,* 65-71.

Failla, E., Grassi, B., and Pisapia, A. (1963). In tema di schizofrenia tardiva. Contributo clinico e nosografico. *Rass. Neuropsichiatr. 17,* 339-360.

Favorina, V. N. (1963a). About the question of the terminal state in schizophrenia (in Russian). *Z. Nevropat. Psihiatr. Korsakoff 63,* 412-420.

Favorina, V. N. (1963b). Idem. communic. III. *Z. Nevropat. Psihiatr. Korsakoff 63,* 1703-1715.

Fish, F. (1958). Leonard's classification of schizophrenia. *J. Ment. Sci. 104,* 943-971.

Fish, F. (1962). *Schizophrenia,* Wright, Bristol.

Foerster, K., Foerster, G., and Glatzel, J. (1976). Symptomatische Schizophrenie bei Lupus erythematodes disseminatus. *Nervenarzt 47,* 265-267.

Forrest, A. (ed.) (1973). *Companion to Psychiatric Studies.* Vol. 3, Churchill Livingstone, Edinburgh.

Freedman, A. M., and Kaplan, H. I. (Eds.) (1967). *Comprehensive Textbook of Psychiatry,* Williams and Wilkins, Baltimore, 1st ed.

Freyhan, F. A. (1955). Course and outcome of schizophrenia. *Am. J. Psychiatr. 112,* 161-169.

Fromenty, L. (1937). Les rémissions dans la schizophrénie. Statistique sur leur fréquence et leur durée avant l'insulinothérapie. *Encéphale 32,* 275-286.

Frøshaug, H., and Ytrehus, A. (1963). The problem of prognosis in schizophrenia. *Acta Psychiatr. Scand., supplement 169.*

Gabriel, E. (1974a). Der langfristige Verlauf schizophrener späterkrankungen im Vergleich mit Schizophrenien aller Lebensalter. *Psychiatr. Clin. 7,* 172-180.

Gabriel, E. (1974b). Über den Einfluss psychoorganischer Beeinträchtigung im alter auf den Verlauf sogenannter Spätschizophrenien. *Psychiatr. Clin. 7,* 358-364.

Gabriel E. (1975a). Das Schicksal katathymer Wahnbildungen im Licht langfristiger Katamnesen. *Psychiatr. Clin. 8,* 81-87.

Gabriel, E. (1975b). Délire chronique et sociolgénèse. *Ann. Méd. Psychol. T2,* 128-135.

Gardner, G. G. (1967). The relationship between childhood neurotic symptomatology and later schizophrenia in males and females. *J. Nerv. Ment. Dis. 144*, 97-100.

Garland, H. G., and Sumner, D. W. (1964). Sulthiame in treatment of epilepsy. *Br. Med. J. 1*, 475-476.

Garron, D. C. (1973). Huntington's chorea and schizophrenia. In *Advances in Neurology*. 1. Huntington's Chorea, A. Bareau, T. N. Chase and G. W. Paulson (Eds.), Raven, New York.

Gelperin, J. (1939). Spontaneous remissions in schizophrenia. *J.A.M.A. 112*, 2393-2395.

Gerloff, W. (1937). Über Verlauf und Prognose der Schizophrenie. *Arch. Psychiatr. Nervenkr. 106*, 585-598.

Giberti, F., and Gregoretti, L. (1958). Modalità di esordio e earatteristiche premorbose nelle sindromi schizofreniche dell'età giovanile. *Riv. Patol. Nerv. Ment. 79*, 1-21.

Glatzel, J. (1970). Die akute Katatonie unter besonderer Berücksichtigung der akuten tödlichen Katatonie. *Acta. Psychiatr. Scand. 46*, 151-179.

Golodetz, R. G., and Ravkin, I. G. (1968). The clinical characteristics of prolonged epileptic psychoses (in Russian). *Z. Nevropat. Psikhiatr. 68*, 1651-1655.

Grebelskaja-Albatz, Z. (1934/35). Zur Klinik der Schizophrenie des frühen Kindesalters. *Schweiz. Arch. Neurol. Psychiatr. 34*, 244; *35*, 30.

Greger, J. (1971). Über Verlaufstendenzen und Prognose psychischer Erkrankungen des höheren Lebansalters. *Psychiatr. Clin. 4*, 281-307.

Gross, G. (1969). Prodrome und Vorpostensyndrome schizophrener Erkrankungen. In *Schizophrenie und Zyklothymie. Erbegnisse und Probleme*, G. Huber (Ed.), Thieme, Stuttgart, pp. 177-187.

Gross, G., and Huber, G. (1973). Zur Prognose der Schizophrenien. *Psychiatr. Clin. 6*, 1-16.

Gross, G., Huber, G., and Schüttler, R. (1971a). Peristatische Faktoren im Beginn und Verlauf schizophrener Erkankungen. *Arch. Psychiatr. Nervenkr. 215*, 1-7.

Gross, G., Huber, G., and Schüttler, R. (1971b). Verlaufs- und Sozialpsychiatrische Erhebungen bei Schizophrenen. *Nervenarzt 42*, 393-396.

Gross, G., Huber, G., Schüttler, R., and Hasse-Sauder, I. (1971c). Uncharakteristische Remissionstypen im Verlauf schizophrener Erkrankungen. In *Ätiologie der Schizophrenien*, G. Huber (Ed.), Schattauer, Stuttgart, pp. 201-214.

Gross, G., Huber, G., and Schüttler, R. (1973a). Probleme der Chroniczität schizophrenerb Erkankungen. In *Chronische endogene Psychosen*, H. Kranz, and K. Heinrich (Eds.), Thieme, Stuttgart, pp. 90-96.

Gross, G., Huber, G., and Schüttler, R. (1973b). Verlaufuntersuchungen bei

Schizophrenen. In *Verlauf und Ausgang schizophrener Erkrankungen,* G. Huber (Ed.), Schattauer, Stuttgart, pp. 101-133.

Guggenheim, F. G., and Babigian, H. M. (1974). Catatonie schizophrenia: epidemiology and clinical course. *J. Nerv. Ment. Dis. 158,* 291-305.

Guze, S. B. (1967). The occurrence of psychiatrie illness in systemic lupus erythematosus. *Am. J. Psychiatr. 123,* 1562-1571.

Halberstadt, G. (1925). La schizophrénie tardive. *L'Encéphale 20,* 655-679.

Hallgren, B., and Sjögren, T. (1959). A clinical and geneticostatistical study of schizophrenia and low-grade mental deficiency in a large Swedish rural population. *Acta Psychiatr. Scand., supplement 140.*

Hanna, B. L. (1965). Genetic studies of family units. In *Genetics and the Epidemiology of Chronic Diseases,* J. O. Neil et al. (Eds.), U.S. Dept. H.E.W., Washington, D.C.

Harper, J., and Williams, S. (1975). Age and type of onset as critical variables in early infantile autism. *J. Autism Child. Schizophrenia 5,* 25-36.

Hartelius, H. (1972). An investigation of mental morbidity in a rural county in the south of Sweden. *Acta Psychiatr. Scand., supplement 228.*

Hartmann, W. (1969). Statistische Untersuchungen an langjährig hospitalisierten Schizophrenen. *Soc. Psychiatr. 4,* 101-114.

Hartmann, W., and Meyer, J. E. (1974). Zur stationären Behandlung chronisch Schizophrener in der Bundesrepublik. *Nervenarzt. 45,* 1-8.

Havelkova, M. (1968). Follow-up study of 71 children diagnosed as psychotic in preschool age. *Am. J. Orthopsychiatr. 38,* 846-859.

Hayashi, S., and Akimoto, H. (1939). Prognosis and therapy of schizophrenia. *Psychiatr. Neurol. Jap. 43,* 705-742.

Helgason, T. (1964). Epidemiology of mental disorders in Iceland. *Acta Psychiatr. Scand., supplement 173.*

Henderson, D., and Gillespie, R. D. (1956, 1969). *Henderson and Gillespie's Textbook of Psychiatry.* Revised by I. R. C. Batchelor, 10th ed., Oxford Univ. Press, London.

Heuyer, G., Badonnel, M., and Bouysson, P. (1929). Les voies d'entrée dan la démence précoce. *Ann. Méd. Psychol. t1,* 30, 117, 199.

Hillbom, E. (1950). Schizophrenia-like psychoses after brain trauma. *Acta Psychiatr. Neurol. Scand., supplement 60,* 36-47.

Hillbom, E. (1960). After-effects of brain-injuries. *Acta Psychiatr. Neurol. Scand., supplement 142.*

Hinterhuber, H. (1973). Zur Katamnese der Schizophrenien. *Fortschr. Neurol. Psychiatr. 41,* 527-558.

Hoch, P. (1934). Quoted by Vitello, 1958.

Hoch, P., and Polatin, P. (1949). Pseudoneurotic form of schizophrenia. *Psychiatr. Quart. 23,* 248-276.

Hoch, P., Cattell, J. P., Strahl, M. O., and Pennes, H. H. (1962). The course and outcome of pseudoneurotic schizophrenia. *Am. J. Psychiatr. 119*, 106-115.

Hoenig, J. (1967). The prognosis of schizophrenia. *Br. J. Psychiatr. Spec. Publ. 1*, 115-132.

Hogarty, G. E., and Goldberg, S. L. (1973). Collaborative study group: Drug and sociotherapy in the after care of schizophrenic patients: one year relapse rate. *Arch. Gen. Psychiatr. 28*, 54-64.

Hogarty, G. E., Goldberg, S., Schooler, N., and Ulrich, R. (1974). Drug and sociotherapy in the aftercare of schizophrenic patients: Two year relapse rates. *Arch. Gen. Psychiatr. 31*, 603-608.

Holmboe, R., and Astrup, A. (1957). A follow-up study of 255 patients with acute schizophrenia and schizophreniform psychoses. *Acta Psychiatr. Scand., supplement, 115.*

Holmboe, R., Noreik, K., and Astrup, C. (1968). Follow-up of functional psychoses at two Norwegian mental hospitals. *Acta Psychiatr. Scand. 44*, 298-310.

Holt, W. L., and Holt, W. M. (1952). Long-term prognosis in mental illness. *Am. J. Psychiatr. 108*, 735-739.

Homburger, A. (1926). *Psychopathologie des Kindesalters,* Springer, Berlin.

Huber, G. (1954a). Zur nosologischen Differenzierung lebenbedrohlicher katatoner Psychosen. *Schweiz. Arch. Neurol. Neurochir. Psychiatr. 74*, 216.

Huber, G. (1954b). Schizophrene Katatonie und atypische Encephalitis. *Zbl. Ges. Neurol. Psychiatr. 130*, 191-217.

Huber, G. (1957). Die coenästhetische Schizophrenie. *Fortschr. Neurol. Psychiatr. 25*, 491-520.

Huber, G. (1964). Schizophrene Verläufe. *Dtsch. Med. Wschr. 89*, 212-216.

Huber, G. (1966). Reine Defektsyndrome und Basisstadien endogener Psychosen. *Fortschr. Neurol. Psychiatr. 34*, 409-426.

Huber, G. (1968a). Zur Frage der Reversibilität im Verlauf von Psychosen. In *Situation und Persönlichkeit in Diagnostik und Terapie*, B. Pauleikhoff (Ed.), Karger, Basel, pp. 43-61.

Huber, G. (1968b). Verlaufsprobleme schizophrener Erkrankungen. *Schweiz. Arch. Neurol. Psychiatr. 101*, 346-368.

Huber, G. (1976). Zur Problematik quantitativer Verlaufsbeobachtungen bei Schizophrenen. *Psychopathometrie 2*, 61-69.

Huber, G., Gross, G., and Schüttler, R. (1974). Course and long-term prognosis of schizophrenic illnesses. In *Schizophrenia and Schizophrenia-like Psychoses*, Igaku Shoin, Tokyo, pp. 139-145.

Huber, G., Gross, G., and Schüttler, R. (1975a). A long-term follow-up study of schizophrenia: psychiatric course of illness and prognosis. *Acta Psychiatr. Scand. 52*, 49-57.

Huber, G., Gross, G., and Schüttler, R. (1975b). Spätschizophrenie. *Arch. Psychiatr Nervenkr. 221*, 53-66.

Huber, G., Gross, G., and Schüttler, R. (1977). Schizophrene Psychosen der 2 Lebenshälfte. *Med. Welt 28(NF)*, 166-168.

Hunt, R. C., and Appel, K. E. (1936). Prognosis in the psychoses lying midway between schizophrenia and manic-depressive psychoses. *Am. J. Psychiatr. 93*, 313-339.

Inghe, G., Inghe, M. B., and Jersild, P. C. (1969). Recovery in schizophrenia. A clinical and sociopsychiatric study. *Acta Soc. Med. Scand., supplement 2.*

Isaacs, A. D., and Post, F. (1978). *Studies in Geriatric Psychiatry.* Wiley, New York.

Israel, R. H., and Johnson, N. A. (1956). Discharge and readmission rates in 4254 consecutive first admissions of schizophrenia. *Am. J. Psychiatr. 112*, 903-909.

Janzarik, W. (1957). Zur Problematik schizophrener Psychosen im höheren Lebensalter. *Nervenarzt. 28*, 535-542.

Janzarik, W. (1968). *Schizophrene Verläufe*, Springer, Berlin.

Johanson, E. (1958). A study of schizophrenia in the male. *Acta Psychiatr. Neurol. Scand., supplement 125.*

Kahlbaum (1874). Quoted by Bleuler, E. (1911).

Kallman, F. J., and Roth, B. (1956). Genetic aspects of preadolescent schizophrenia. *Am. J. Psychiatr. 112*, 599-606.

Kanner, L. (1943). Autistic disturbances of affective contact. *Nerv. Child. 2*, 217-250.

Kanner, L., and Eisenberg, L. (1955). Notes on the follow-up studies of autistic children. In *Psychopathology of Childhood*, P. H. Hoch and J. Zubin (Eds.), Grune and Stratton, New York.

Kant, O. (1941a). A comparative study of recovered and deteriorated schizophrenic patients. *J. Nerv. Ment. Dis. 93*, 616-624.

Kant, O. (1941b). Study of a group of recovered schizophrenic patients. *Psychiatr. Quart. 15*, 262-283.

Kant, O. (1941c). The relation of a group of highly improved schizophrenic patients to one group of completely recovered and another group of deteriorated patients. *Psychiatr. Quart. 15*, 779-789.

Kay, D. W. K. (1962). Outcome and cause of death in mental disorders of old age: a long-term follow-up of functional and organic psychoses. *Acta Psychiatr. Neurol. Scand. 38*, 249-276.

Kay, D. W. K., and Lindelius, R. (1970). Course and prognosis. In *A Study of Schizophrenia*, R. Lindelius (Ed.), *Acta Psychiatr. Scand., supplement 216*, 46-63.

Kay, D. W. K., and Lindelius, R. (1973). Der Wandel in der Prognose der Schizophrenie mit besonderer Berucksichtigung der Mortalität. In *Verlauf und Ausgang schizophrener Erkrankungen*, G. Huber (Ed.), Schattauer, Stuttgart, pp. 149-155.

Kay, D. W. K., Norris, V., and Post, F. (1956). Prognosis in psychiatric disorders of the elderly. *J. Ment. Sci. 102,* 129-140.

Khramelashvili, V. V., and Liberman, I. U. I. (1976). Prognosis of the frequency of attacks of schizophrenia (according to findings from an epidemiologic study). In Russian. *Zh. Nevropatol. Psikhiatr. 76,* No. 5, 747-754.

Kirow, K. (1972a). Untersuchungen über den Verlauf zykloider Psychosen. *Psychiatr. Neurol. Med. Psychol. (Leipzig) 24,* 726-732.

Kirow, K. (1972b). Untersuchung über die Behandlung atypischer phasischer Psychosen. *Psychiatr. Neurol. Med. Psychol. 24,* 160-165.

Klages, W. (1961). *Die Spätschizophrenie,* Enke, Stuttgart.

Klages, W. (1963). Spätmanifestationen schizophrener Psychosen. *Medizin. Klin. 58,* 1289-1294.

Kleist, K. (1928). Über cycloide, paranoide und epileptoide Psychosen und über die Frage der Degenerationspsychosen. *Schweiz. Arch. Neurol. Psychiatr. 23,* 3-37.

Knobloch, H., and Pasamanick, B. (1975). Some etiologic and prognostic factors in early infantile autism and psychosis. *Pediatrics 55,* 182-191.

Knoll, H. (1952). Wahnbildende Psychosen der Zeit des Klimakteriums und der Involution in klinischer und genealogischer Betrachtung. *Arch. Psychiatr. Nervenkr. 189,* 59-92.

Kolvin, I. (1971). Studies in the childhood psychoses. *Br. J. Psychiatr. 118,* 381, 196, 403, 407.

Kolvin, I. (1972). Late onset psychosis. *Br. Med. J. (Sept. 1972),* 816-817.

Kozlova, I. A. (1967). Sur l'évolution de la schizophrénie chez les enfants de bas âge. *J. Nevropat. Psikhiat. 67,* 1516-1531.

Kraepelin, E. (1896). *Dementia praecox and paraphrenia* (Engl. transl.), Livingstone, Edinburgh (1919).

Kraepelin, E. (1913). *Psychiatrie.* Ein Lehrbuch für Studierende und Ärzte. 8th ed., vol. 3, Leipzig.

Krüger, H. (1968). Nachuntersuchungen bei Psychosen, die im Sinne Kraepelin-Bleulerschen Psychiatrie als Schizophrenien aufgefasst wurden. *Psychiatr. Neurol. Med. Psychol. 20,* 135-144.

Kurosawa, R. (1961). Untersuchung der atypischen endogenen Psychosen (periodische Psychosen). *Psychiatr. Neurol. Med. Psychol. 13,* 364-370.

Kutsenok, B. M. (1971). The clinical picture of abortive psychotic episodes preceding the manifest onset of schizophrenia. (In Russian.) *Zh. Nevropatol. Psikhiatr. 71,* No. 5, 720-725.

Laing, R. D. (1960). *The Divided Self,* Tavistock, London.

Lambert, P. A., and Midenet, M. (1972). Evolution actuelle de la schizophrenie. *Ann. Méd. Psychol. T2 133,* 873-891.

Langfeldt, G. (1937). The prognosis in schizophrenia and the factors influencing the course of the disease. *Acta Psychiatr. Neurol. Scand., supplement 13.*

Langfeldt, G. (1965). *Lärebok i klinisk psykiatri.* Aschehoug & Co., Oslo, 3rd ed.

Larsson, C. A., and Nyman, G. E. (1970). Age of onset in schizophrenia. *Human Hered. 20,* 241-247.

Larsson, T., and Sjögren, T. (1954). A methodological psychiatric and statistical study of a large Swedish rural population. *Acta Psychiatr. Neurol. Scand., supplement 89.*

Laskowska, D., Urbaniak, K., and Jus. A. (1965). The relationship between catatonic-delirious states and schizophrenia, in the light of a follow-up study (Stauder's lethal catatonia). *Br. J. Psychiatr. 111,* 254-257.

Lassenius, B., Ottosson, J-O., and Rapp, W. (1973). Prognosis in schizophrenia. The need for institutionalized care. *Acta Psychiatr. Scand. 49,* 295-305.

Lauter, H. (1968). Zur Klinik und Psychopathologie der Alzheimerschen Krankheit. *Psychiatr. Clin. 1,* 85-108.

Lebovici, S., and Diatkine, R. (1963). Essai d'approche de la notion de prépsychose en psychiatrie infantile. *Bull. Psychol. 17,* 20-37.

Lemke, R. (1950). Über die symptomatische Schizophrenie. *Arch. Psychiatr. Z. Neurol. 185,* 756-772.

Lempp, G. (1921). Die Lebens- und Krankheitsdauer bei Geisteskrankheiten. *Arch. Psychiatr. Nervenkr. 63,* 272-310.

Leonhard, K. (1935). Exogene Schizophrenien und die symptomatischen Bestandteile bei den genuinen (idopathischen) Schizophrenien. *Mschr. Psychiatr. Neurol. 91,* 249-269.

Leonhard, K. (1952). Formen und Verläufe der Schizophrenien. *Mschr. Psychiatr. Neurol. 124,* 169-192.

Leonhard, K. (1954). Die zykloiden meist als Schizophrenien verkannten Psychosen. *Psychiatr. Neurol. Med. Psychol. 9,* 359-373.

Leonhard, K. (1957-69). *Aufteilung der endogenen Psychosen,* 1st-4th ed., Akademie Verlag, Jena.

Leonard, K. (1969). Diagnose der Schizophrenie in verschiedenen Verlaufsformen. *Lebenversich. Med. 21,* 73-78.

Leyberg, J. T. (1965). A follow-up study on some schizophrenic patients. *Br. J. Psychiatr. 111,* 617-624.

Libow, L. S. (1973). Pseudo-senility: Acute and reversible organic brain syndromes. *J. Am. Geriatr. Soc. 21,* 112-120.

Lindelius, R., and Kay, D. W. K. (1973). Some changes in the pattern of mortality in schizophrenia in Sweden. *Acta Psychiatr. Scand. 49,* 315-323.

Lo, W. H., and Lo, T. (1977). A ten-year follow-up of Chinese schizophrenics in Hong Kong. *Br. J. Psychiatr. 131*, 63-66.

Lotter, V. (1974). Factors related to outcome in autistic children. *J. Autism Child. Schizophr. 4*, 263-277.

Lucena, J. (1935). Contribuçao ao estudio de algunas manifestaçoes iniciais das esquizofrenias. *Neurobiology 1*, 147-164.

Lutz, J. (1937/38). Über die Schizophrenie im Kindesalter. *Schweiz. Arch. Neurol. Psychiatr. 39*, 355; *40*, 141.

Mahler, M. S. (1952). On child psychosis and schizophrenia: autistic and symbiotic infantile psychosis. *Psychoanalytic Study Child 7*, 286-305.

Malzberg, B. (1934). *Mortality among Patients with Mental Disease.* State Hosp. Press, Utica, New York.

Malzberg, B. (1943). The increase in mental disease. *Psychiatr. Quart. 17*, 488-507.

Malzberg, B. (1953). Further studies of mortality among patients with mental disease. *Acta Med. Scand., supplement 277*, 215-230.

Mandelbrote, B. M., and Trick, K. L. K. (1970). Social and clinical factors in the outcome of schizophrenia. *Acta Psychiatr. Scand. 46*, 24-34.

Marchand, L., and Ajuriaguerra, J. (1948). *Epilepsies,* Desclée de Brouwer, Paris.

Marinow, A. (1959). Über den Verlauf und Endzustand bei der Schizophrenie. *Psychiatr. Neurol. Med. Psychol. 11*, 368-378.

Marinow, A. (1971). Schizophrene Endstadien. *Arch. Psychiatr. Nervenkr. 215*, 46-61.

Mattsson, B. (1974). Huntington's chorea in Sweden: social and clinical data. *Acta Psychiatr. Scand., supplement 255*, 221-236.

Mayer-Gross, W. (1932). Die Schizophrenie. In *Handbuch des Geisteskrankheiten,* O. Bumke (Ed.), Bd IX, Vol. V, Springer, Berlin.

Mayer-Gross, W., Slater, E., and Roth, M. (1960). *Clinical Psychiatry,* 2nd ed., Cassell and Company Ltd., London.

Mayer-Gross, W., Slater, E., and Roth, M. (1969). *Clinical Psychiatry,* 3rd ed., Balliere, Tindall Cassell, London.

McAdam, W., and Robinson, R. A. (1957). Prognosis in senile deterioration. *J. Ment. Sci. 103*, 821-823.

McHugh, P. R., and Folstein, M. F. (1975). Psychiatric syndromes of Huntington's chorea: a clinical and phenomenologic study. In *Psychiatric Aspects of Neurologic Disease,* D. F. Benson, and D. Blumer (Eds.), Grune and Stratton, New York, pp. 267-286.

McWalter, H. S., Mereer, R., Sutherland, M., and Watta, A. (1961/62). Outcomes of treatment of schizophrenia in a North-East Scottish mental hospital. *Am. J. Psychiatr. 118*, 529-533.

Meares, A. (1959). The diagnosis of prepsychotic schizophrenia. *Lancet 1,* 55-58.

Meduna von, L. (1935). Versuche über die biologische Beinflussung des Ablaufes der Schizophrenie. *Z. Neurol. Psychiatr. 152,* 235-262.

Mellsop, G. (1973). Antecedents of schizophrenia: the "schizoid" myth? *Austr. New Zeal. J. Psychiatr. 7,* 208-211.

Mentzos, S. (1967). *Mischzustände und mischbildhafte phasische Psychosen,* Enke, Stuttgart.

Michael, C. M., Morris, D. P., and Soroker, E. (1957). Follow-up studies of shy, withdrawn children. II. Relative incidence of schizophrenia. *Am. J. Orthopsychiatr. 27,* 331-342.

Miller, C. W. (1941). The paranoid syndrome. *Arch. Neurol. Psychiatr. (Chicago), 45,* 953.

Molchanova, E. K. (1976). Attack-like schizophrenia with a "progressive" course and profound long-term remissions in old age. (In Russian.) *Zh. Nevropatol. Psikhiatr. 76,* No. 5, 736-741.

Morlass, J. (1938). La phase préclinique des maladies mentales. *Marseille Méd. 2223,* 177-179.

Morris, D. P., Soroker, E., and Burrus, G. (1954). Follow-up studies of shy, withdrawn children: evaluation of later adjustment. *Am. J. Orthopsychiatr. 24,* 743-751.

Motta, E. (1953). Sull'antagonismo epilessia schizofrenia. *Giorn. Psichiat. Neuropat. 81,* 787-818.

Murtalibov, S. (1976). A catamnestic study of shift-like schizophrenia with long-term remissions. (In Russian.) *Zh. Nevropatol. Psikhiatr. 76,* No. 4, 568-572.

Müller, G. (1930). Anfälle bie schizophrenen Erkrankungen. *Allg. Zeitschr. Psychiatr. 93,* 235-250.

Müller, C. (1953). Der Ubergang von Zwangsneurose in Schizophrenie im Lichte der Katamnese. *Schweiz. Arch. Neurol. Neurochir. Psychiatr. 72,* 218-225.

Müller, C. (1959). Uber das Senium der Schizophrenen, zugleich ein Beitrag zum Problem schizophrener Endzustände. *Bibl. Psychiatr. Neurol. (Basel), 106.*

Müller, H. F., Grad, B., and Engelsmann, F. (1975). Biological and psychological predictors of survival in a psychogeriatric population. *J. Gerontol. 30,* 47-52.

Myrianthopoulous, M. C. (1966). Huntington's chorea. *J. Ment. Genet. 3,* 298-314.

Nadsharow, R., and Sternberg, E. (1965). Uber klinische Untersuchungen auf dem Gegiet der endogenen Psychosen. *Psychiatr. Neurol. Med. Psychol. 70,* 59-66.

Neiditch, J. A., and White, L. (1976). Prediction of short-term outcome in newly admitted psychogeriatric patients. *J. Am. Geriatr. Soc. 24,* 72-78.

Nikonova, T. B. (1974). Data from a comparative study of traumatic, hallucinatory-delusional psychoses and of hallucinatory-delusional schizophrenia in persons who have experienced skull injury. (In Russian.) *Zh. Nevropatol. Psikhiatr. 74,* No. 3, 416-422.

Niskanen, P., and Achté, K. A. (1972). *The Course and Prognosis of Schizophrenic Psychoses in Helsinki,* Monogr. Psychiatr. Dept., Helsinki Univ. Hosp. no. 4.

Niskanen, P., Lönnqvist, J., and Achté, K. A. (1973). Schizophrenic and paranoid psychotic patients first admitted in 1970 with a two-year follow-up. *Psychiatr. Fennica.* 103-112.

Niswander, G. D., Haslerud, G. M., and Mitchell, G. (1963a). Difference in longevity of released and retained schizophrenic patients. *Dis. Nerv. Syst. 24,* 348-352.

Niswander, G. D., Haslerud, G. M., and Mitchell, G. D. (1963b). Changes in cause of death of schizophrenic patients. *Arch. Gen. Psychiatr. 9,* 229-234.

Niswander, G. D., Haselrud, G. M., and Mitchell, G. D. (1963c). Effect of catatonia on schizophrenic mortality. *Arch. Gen. Psychiatr. 9,* 548-551.

Noreik, K. (1970). *Follow-up and Classification of Functional Psychoses with Special Reference to Reactive Psychoses,* Universitetsförlaget, Oslo.

Noreik, K., and Ødegaard, O. (1967). Age at onset of schizophrenia in relation to socio-economic factors. *Br. J. Soc. Psychiatr. 1,* 242-249.

Notkin, Y. (1929). Epileptic manifestations in the group of schizophrenic and manic depressive psychoses. *J. Nerv. Ment. Dis. 69,* 494-508.

Noyes, A. P., and Kolb, L. C. (1963). *Modern Clinical Psychiatry,* 6th ed., Saunders, Philadelphia.

Nyman, G. E., Nyman, A. K., and Nylander, B. I. (1976). *Non-regressive schizophrenia.* Dept. of Psychiat. Res., St. Lars Hosp., Lund, mimeographed.

Obrist, W. D., and Busse, E. W. (1965). The electroencephalogram in old age. In *Application of Electroencephalography in Psychiatry,* W. P. Wilson (Ed.), Duke Univ. Press, Durham, N.C.

Ödegaard, Ö. (1952). The excess mortality of the insane. *Acta Psychiatr. Neurol. Scand. 27,* 358-367.

O'Neal, P., and Robins, L. N. (1958). The relation of childhood behavior problems to adult psychiatric status: a thirty year follow-up study of 150 subjects. *Am. J. Psychiatr. 114,* 961-983.

Owen, D. R. (1972). The XYY male: a review. *Psychol. Bull. 78,* 209-233.

Pampiglione, G., and Post, F. (1958). Value of EEG examination in psychiatric disorders of old age. *Geriatrics 13,* 725-732.

Penn, H., Racy, J., Lapham, L., Mandel, M., and Sandt, J. (1972). Catatonic behavior, viral encephalopathy and death. *Arch. Gen. Psychiatr. 27,* 758-761.

Perris, C. (1973). Cycloid psychosis: historical background and nosology. *Nord. Psykiatr. Tidsrk. 27,* 369-378.

Perris, C. (1974). A study of cycloid psychoses. *Acta Psychiatr. Scand., supplement 253.*

Perris, C., and Stancati, G. (1954). Contributo clinico ed elettroencefalografico allo studio dei rapporti tra epilessia e schizofrenia. *Il Cervello 30,* 515-521.

Perris, C., and d'Elia, G. (1960). Disturbi parossistici dello schema corporeo, ipersessulità ed altri feuomeni psichici oli tipo paranoide in associazone con lesione fronto-pareito-temporale destra. Rass. *Neuropsichiat. 14,* 299-303.

Polonio, P. (1954). Periodic schizophrenia. *Mschr. Psychitr. Neurol. 128,* 265-272.

Polonio, P. (1957). A structural analysis of schizophrenia. *Psychiatr. Neurol. 133,* 351-379.

Post, F. (1951). The outcome of mental breakdown in old age. *Br. Med. J. 1,* 436-440.

Post, F. (1966). *Persistent Persecutory States of the Elderly,* Pergamon, Oxford.

Post, F. (1971). Schizo-affective symptomatology in late life. *Br. J. Psychiatr. 118,* 437-445.

Potter, H. W. (1933). Schizophrenia in children. *Am. J. Psychiatr. 89,* 1253-1261.

Praag van, H. M. (1976). About the impossible concept of schizophrenia. *Comprehens. Psychiatr. 17,* 481-497.

Pritchard, M. (1967). Prognosis of schizophrenia before and after pharmacotherapy. *Br. J. Psychiatr. 113,* 1345-1359.

Pritchard, M., and Graham, P. (1966). An investigation of a group of patients who have attended both the child and adult departments of the same psychiatric hospital. *Br. J. Psychiatr. 112,* 603-612.

Rank, B. (1949). Adaptation of the psychoanalytic technique for the treatment of young children with atypical development. *Am. J. Orthopsychiatr. 19,* 130-139.

Redlich, F. C., and Freedman, D. X. (1966). *The Theory and Practice of Psychiatry,* Basic Books, New York.

Rennie, T. A. C. (1939). Follow-up study of five hundred patients with schizophrenia admitted to the hospital from 1913 to 1923. *Arch. Neurol. Psychiatr. 42,* 877.

Rennie, T. A. C. (1941). Analysis of one hundred cases of schizophrenia with recovery. *Arch. Neurol. Psychiatr. 46,* 197-229.

Retterstøl, N. (1966). *Paranoid and Paranoiac Psychoses,* Scandinavian Univ. Books, Oslo.

Retterstøl, N. (1970). *Prognosis in Paranoid Psychoses,* Scandinavian Univ. Books, Oslo.

Riemer, M. D. (1950). A study of the mental status of schizophrenics hospitalized for over 25 years into their senium. *Psychiatr. Quart. 24,* 309-313.

Rizzo, E. M. (1957). Il tentativo di suicidio degli schizofrenici. *Riv. Patol. Nerv. Ment. 78,* 105-120.

Rostovtseva, T. I. (1973). The clinical picture and course of the so-called senile schizophrenia. (In Russian.) *Zh. Nevropatol. Psikhiatr. 73,* No. 3, 424-430.

Roth, M. (1955). The natural history of mental disorder in old age. *J. Ment. Sci. 101,* 281-301.

Roth, M., and Morrissey, J. O. (1952). Problems in the diagnosis and classification of mental disorder in old age. *J. Ment. Sci. 98,* 66-80.

Rubino, A., and Piro, S. (1954). Psicopatologia delle forme marginali fra nevrosi e schizofrenia. *Acta Neurol. (Napoli), Quad. 7.*

Rumyantseva, G. M. (1970). Concerning one of the favorable varieties of shift-like schizophrenia. (In Russian.) *Zh. Nevropatol. Psikhiatr. 70,* 1235-1242.

Rutter, M. (1965). Classification and categorization in child psychiatry. *J. Child. Psychol. Psychiatr. 6,* 71-83.

Rutter, M. (1966). Prognosis: psychotic children in adolescence and early adult life. In *Childhood Autism: Clinical, Educational and Social Aspects,* J. K. Wing (Ed.), Pergamon, London.

Rutter, M. (1967). Psychotic disorders in early childhood. In *Recent Development in Schizophrenia,* A. Coppen and A. Walk (Eds.), *Br. J. Psychiatr. Spec. Publ. 1,* 133-158.

Rutter, M. (1972). Relationships between child and adult psychiatric disorders. *Acta Psychiatr. Scand. 48,* 3-21.

Rutter, M., and Lockyer, L. (1969). A five to fifteen year follow-up study of infantile psychosis. *Br. J. Psychiatr. 155,* 865 (see also *113,* 1169, 1967).

Rutter, M., Lebovici, S., Eisenberg, L., Shneshnevski, A., Sadou, R., Brooke, E., and Lin, T-Y. (1969). A tri-axial classification of mental disorders in childhood. *J. Child. Psychol. Psychiatr. 10,* 41-61.

Rümke, H. C. (1958). Die klinische differenzierung innerhalb der Gruppe der Schizophrenien. *Nervenarzt. 29,* 49-63.

Sachar, E. J., Mason, J. W., Kolmer, H. S., and Artiss, K. L. (1963). Psychoendocrine aspects of acute schizophrenic reactions. *Psychosom. Med. 25,* 510-537.

Sahli, H. R. (1959). Ubergänge manisch-depressiver und schizophrener Verläufe. *Psychiatr. Neurol. (Basel) 138,* 98-125.

Sainsbury, P. (1965). *Suicide in London. An Ecological Study,* Chapman and Hall, London.

Sartorius, N., Jablenski, A., and Shapiro, R. (1977). Two year follow-up of the patients included in the WHO international pilot study of schizophrenia. *Psychol. Med. 7,* 529-541.

Schimmelpenning, G. W. (1965). *Die paranoiden Psychosen der zweiten Lebenshälfte,* Karger, Basel.

Schipkowensky, N. (1956). *Clinical Psychiatry.* (In Bulgarian.) Sofia.

Schneider, C. (1942). *Die schizophrenen Symptomverbände,* Springer, Berlin.

Schooler, N. R., Goldberg, S. C., Boothe, H., and Cole, J. O. (1967). One year after discharge: Community adjustment of schizophrenic patients. *Am. J. Psychiatr. 123,* 986-995.

Senise, T. (1931). Epilessia e demenza precoce. *Il Cervello 10,* 39-57.

Shepherd, M. (1957). *A Study of the Major Psychoses in an English County,* Maudsley Monogr., London.

Shepherd, M. (1959). Social outcome of early schizophrenia. *Psychiatr. Neurol. 137,* 224-229.

Sherman, L. J., Moseley, E. C., Ging, R., and Bookbinder, L. J. (1964). Prognosis in schizophrenia: a follow-up study of 588 patients. *Arch. Gen. Psychiatr. 10,* 123-130.

Sjögren, H. (1964). Paraphrenic, melancholic and psychoneurotic states in the presenile-senile period of life. *Acta Psychiatr. Scand., supplement 176.*

Sjögren, T., Sjögren, H., and Lindgren, Å, G. H. (1952). Morbus Alzheimer and morbus Pic. *Acta Psychiatr. Neurol. Scand., supplement 82.*

Schneider, K. (1942). Quoted in Mayer-Gross (1932).

Slater, E. (1938a). Zur Erbpathologie der manisch-depressiven Irreseins. *Zschr. ges. Neurol. Psychiatr. 162,* 794-801.

Slater, E. (1938b). Zur Periodik der manisch-depressiven Irreseins. *Zschr. ges. Neurol. Psychiatr. 162,* 794-801.

Slater, E., and Moran, P. A. P. (1969). The schizophrenia-like psychoses of epilepsy: relation between ages of onset. *Br. J. Psychiatr., 115,* 599-600.

Slater, E., Beard, A. W., and Glithero, E. (1963). The schizophrenia-like psychoses of epilepsy. *Br. J. Psychiatr. 109,* 95-150.

Shneshnevski, A. V. (1966). The prognosis of schizophrenia. *Int. J. Psychiatr. 2,* 635-638.

Shneshnevski, A. V. (1968). Evolucao e unidade nosologica da esquizofrenia. *Anais Portug. Psiquiatr. 20,* 71-80.

Shneshnevski, A. V. (1970). Sintomatologia, formas clinicas y nosologia de la esquizofrenia. *Rev. Colombiana Psiquiatr. 2,* 355-371.

Spern, R. A., Morrow, W. R., and Peterson, D. P. (1965). Follow-up of schizophrenic, geriatric and alcoholic first admissions. *Arch. Gen. Psychiatr. 12,* 427.

Spiel, W. (1961). *Die endogenen Psychosen des Kindes- und Jugendalters,* Karger, Basel.

Ssuchareva, G. (1932). Uber den Verlauf der Schizophrenien im Kindesalter. *Z. ges. Neurol. Psychiatr. 142,* 309.

Stauder, K. H. (1934). Die tödliche Katatonie. *Arch. Psychiatr. 121,* 271-285.

Steinberg, H. R., Green, R., and Durell, J. (1967). Depression occurring during the course of recovery from schizophrenic symptoms. *Am. J. Psychiatr. 124,* 699-702.

Stephens, J. H. (1970). Long-term course and prognosis in schizophrenia. *Seminars in Psychiatry 2,* 464-485.

Stephens, J. H. (1978). Long-term prognosis and follow-up in schizophrenia. *Schizophrenia Bull. 4,* 25-47.

Stephens, J. H., and Astrup, C. (1963). Prognosis in "process" and "non-process" schizophrenia. *Am. J. Psychiatr. 119,* 945-953.

Stephens, J. H., Astrup, C., and Mangrum, J. C. (1967). Prognosis in schizophrenia. *Arch. Gen. Psychiatr. 16,* 693-698.

Sternberg, E. (1972). Neuere Forschungsergebnisse bei spätschizophrenen Psychosen. *Fortschr. Neurol. Psychiatr. 40,* 631-643.

Sternberg, E. (1973). Uber den gegenwärtigen Stand der Schizophrenieforschung und einige ihrer aktuellen Aufgaben. *Forschr. Neurol. Psychiatr. 41,* 123-140.

Stoianov, S., Liberman, I., and Goncharova, T. A. (1969). Clinicostatistical characteristics of the pathokinesis of the uninterrupted form of schizophrenia reaching the paraphrenia stage in its development (findings from a continuous study of a patient population). (In Russian.) *Zh. Nevropatol. Psikhiatr. 69,* No. 12, 1852-1859.

Streletzki, F. (1961). Psychosen in Verlauf der Huntingtonschen Chorea unter besonderer Berücksichtigung der Wahnbildungen. *Arch. Psychiatr. Nervenkrankh. 202,* 202-214.

Strömgren, E. (1938). Beiträge zur psychiatrischen Erblehre. *Acta Psychiatr. Neurol. Scand., supplement 19.*

Szasz, T. S. (1960). The myth of mental illness. *Am. Psychol. 15,* 113-127.

Sørensen, K., and Nielsen, J. (1977). Reactive paranoid psychosis in a 47, XYY male. *Acta Psychiatr. Scand. 55,* 233-236.

Tangerman, R. (1942). Spontanremissionen bei Schizophrenie. *Allg. Z. Psychiatr. 121,* 36-57.

Tanzi, E., and Lugaro, E. (1923). *Trattato delle Malattie mentali,* Vol. 2. Soc. Ed. Libraria, Milan.

Taylor, D. C. (1975). Factors influencing the occurrence of schizophrenia-like psychosis in patients with temporal lobe epilepsy. *Psychol. Med. 5,* 249-254.

Thompson, G. N. (1970). Cerebral lesions simulating schizophrenia. *Biol. Psychiatr. 2,* 59-64.

Todd, N. A., Bennie, E. H., and Carlisle, J. M. (1976). Some features of "new long-stay" male schizophrenics. *Br. J. Psychiatr. 129,* 424-427.

Toshcheva, T. E. (1974). Atypical forms of psychoses in the late period after burcellous encephalitis. (In Russian.) *Zh. Nevropatol. Psikhiatr. 74,* No. 2, 236-240.

Tsuang, M. T., and Winokur, G. (1975). The Iowa 500: fieldwork in a 35 year follow-up of depression, mania and schizophrenia. *Can. Psychiatr. J. 20,* 359-365.

Tsuang, M. T., and Woolson, R. F. (1977). Mortality in patients with schizophrenia, mania depression and surgical conditions. *Br. J. Psychiatr. 130,* 162-166.

Uglešić, B., Bahun, Z., and Bokun, P. (1970). Razvojni tok shizofrenije (Evolutional courseof schizophrenia). (In Yugoslavian.) *Neuropsihijatrija 18,* 237-244.

Uschakov, G. K. (1965). Quoted by Eggers, 1973.

Uspenskaia, L. I. (1972). Characteristics of the atypical course of attack-like progressive schizophrenia. *Zh. Nevropatol. Psihiatr. 72,* No. 8, 121--1224.

Vaillant, G. E. (1964a). An historical review of the remitting schizophrenia. *J. Nerv. Ment. Dis. 138,* 48-56.

Vaillant, G. E. (1964b). Prospective prediction of schizophrenic remission. *Arch. Gen. Psychiatr. 11,* 509-518.

Vallejo-Nagera, A. (1954). *Tratado de Psiquiatria,* Salvat, Madrid.

Varsamis, J., and Adamson, J. D. (1971). Early schizophrenia. *Can. Psychiatr. Assoc. J. 16,* 487-495.

Villinger, W. (1957). *Symptomatologie der kindlich-jugendlichen Schizophrenien.* 2nd World Congr. Psychiatr, Zürich. [Proceed, Vol. I, p. 345 (1959)].

Vitello, A. (1958). Ancora in tema di rapporti della schizofrenai con l'epilessia. *Il Pisani 73,* 521-620.

Volkova, R. P. (1974). Hallucinatory remissions in schizophrenia with a favorable course. (In Russian.) *Zh. Nevropatol. Psikhiatr. 74,* No. 5, 716-722.

von Trostorff, S. (1975). Verlauf und Psychose in der Verwandschaft bei den systematischen und unsystematischen Schizophrenien und den zykloiden Psychosen. *Psychiatr. Neurol. Med. Psychol. 27,* 80-100.

Vorkastner, W. (1981). *Epilepsie und Dementia Praecox,* Karger, Berlin.

Waldton, S. (1973). Dementia senilis. Sjukdomsbild och förlopp hos 66 kvinnliga patienter. Thesis, Stockholm.

Walker, R. G. (1961). Comparison of age of onset of schizophrenia among patients hospitalized in Rauchi, India and in Brockton, USA. *J. Neuropsychiatr. 2,* 183-185.

Weitbrecht, H. J. (1963). *Psychiatrie in Grundriss,* Springer, Berlin.

Welner, J., and Strömgren, E. (1958). Clinical and genetic studies on benign schizophreniform psychoses based on a follow-up. *Acta Psychiatr. Neurol. Scand. 33,* 377-399.

Wenger, P. (1958). A comparative study of the aging process in groups of schizophrenic and mentally well veterans. *Geriatrics (June),* 367-370.

WHO (The World Health Organization). (1973). *The International Pilot Study of Schizophrenia,* Vol. 1, Geneva.

Wieck, C. (1965). *Schizophrenie im Kindesalter,* Hirzel, Leipzig.

Wing, J. K. (1963). Rehabilitation of psychiatric patients. *Br. J. Psychiatr. 109,* 635-641.

Wing, J. K., Monck, E., Brown, G. W., and Carstairs, G. M. (1964). Morbidity in the community of schizophrenic patients discharged from London mental hospitals in 1959. *Br. J. Psychiatr. 110,* 10-21.

Wittman, M. P., and Steinberg, D. L. (1944). Prodromal factors in schizophrenia. *Am. J. Psychiatr. 100,* 811-816.

Wolfsohn. (1907). Quoted by Bleuler, E. (1911).

Wyrsch, J. (1941). Beitrag zur Kenntnis schizophrener Verläufe. *Z. Neurol. Psychiatr. 172,* 797-811.

Yde, A., Lohse, E., and Faurbye, A. (1941). On the relation between schizophrenia epilepsy and induced convulsions. *Acta Psychiatr. Neurol. Scand. 16,* 325-338.

3

Central Monoamines and the Pathogenesis of Depression

Herman M. van Praag
Academic Hospital
State University of Utrecht
Utrecht, The Netherlands

I. DESIGN OF THIS CHAPTER

This paper does not present an exhaustive discussion of the question of the possible correlation between central monoamine (MA) metabolism and depressive behavior. Its design is as follows. To begin with it summarizes the observations which have led to the formulation of the MA hypotheses. Next it discusses the research done in order to evaluate these hypotheses. It does not present a comprehensive review, which can be found elsewhere (van Praag, 1977a, 1978a; Post and Goodwin, 1978). Finally, it discusses various recent developments in this field, namely,

1. The neuroendocrinological strategy to study the central MA metabolism
2. The possible significance of disorders of the central MA metabolism as a factor predisposing to the occurrence of depressions
3. The development of MA-specific antidepressants, i.e., compounds which more or less selectively influence one of the central MA
4. Modifications in the substance of the MA hypotheses

It is assumed that the elementary principles of MA metabolism and central MAergic transmission are known. The list of references does not claim comprehensiveness, and whenever possible, review articles are cited.

II. DATA ON THE BASIS OF WHICH THE MONOAMINE HYPOTHESES WERE FORMULATED

A. Antidepressants

Toward the end of the 1950s, two groups of compounds were discovered which could claim the qualification "antidepressant": monoamine oxidase (MAO) inhibitors (prototype: iproniazid; Marsilid) (Pletscher, 1968) and the tricyclic antidepressants (prototype: imipramine; Tofranil) (Sigg, 1968).

Although unrelated in chemical structure, the two groups proved similar on two levels. First of all, on the *psychopathological level,* they exert a beneficial influence on depressions and more particularly on a given *syndromal* depression type known as vital depression. This syndrome is discussed elsewhere (van Praag, 1978b). It corresponds roughly to the *syndrome* described in Anglo-American and German literature as endogenous depression.

Second, the two types of antidepressant proved to be similar on the *biochemical level* in that both increase the amount of 5-hydroxytryptamine (5-HT; serotonin) and noradrenaline (NA) available at the central postsynaptic recepor sites, albeit via different mechanisms: MAO inhibitors by inhibiting degradation, and tricyclic compounds by inhibiting the (re)uptake of 5-HT and NA in the nerve terminals. It is assumed that this (re)uptake pump is the principal mechanism by which the transmitter substance is removed from the synaptic cleft once the postsynaptic receptor has been "hit."

To summarize: Two chemically unrelated groups of compounds both produce an antidepressant effect and potentiate certain MA in the brain. These data directly lead to the hypothesis of a possible relationship between the psychopathological and the neurochemical effects. A derivative hypothesis holds that depressions which show a favorable response to these compounds may involve a central MA deficiency. Both hypotheses are known as "MA hypothesis." In this context we confine ourselves to the latter. This has two components: the *5-HT hypothesis,* which relates depression to central 5-HT deficiency (van Praag, 1962; Coppen, 1967; Lapin and Oxenkrug, 1969), and the *NA hypothesis,* which relates depression to central NA deficiency (Bunney and Davis, 1965; Schildkraut, 1965). Dopamine (DA) plays no role in the original MA hypotheses because the influence of tricyclic antidepressants on DA uptake was found to be slight to absent. (It is to be noted that MAO inhibitors do inhibit DA degradation.)

B. Reserpine

An additional argument in favor of the MA hypotheses was supplied by reserpine research. Reserpine inhibits the uptake of the three MAs already mentioned in the synaptic vesicles (Sulser and Bass, 1968). In the cytoplasm, these MAs are degraded by MAO before they can reach the synaptic cleft. The amount of transmitter substance available for transmission consequently diminishes. In clinical use (as an antihypertensive), reserpine was found to induce depressions of the vital type in a by no means inconsiderable number of patients (Goodwin et al., 1972). In psychopathological and biochemical terms, therefore, reserpine mirrors the antidepressants.

C. A Misunderstanding

A possible relationship between the therapeutic effects of the conventional antidepressants and their MA-potentiating capacity does not imply that antidepressant action depends exclusively on inhibition of MAO and inhibition of MA uptake. To begin with, there are other mechanisms which result in MA potentiation. Moreover, it is quite conceivable that antidepressant effects can also develop without a (direct) influence on MAergic systems. Yet this misunderstanding crops up repeatedly in the literature. The fact that antidepressants have been discovered which are neither MAO inhibitor nor uptake inhibitor (e.g., mianserine) is then used as an argument against involvement of MAergic systems in mood regulation (Berger, 1978). This argument impresses this author as lacking validity.

III. THE FOUNDATION ON WHICH THE MONOAMINE HYPOTHESES REST

In the past few years, several strategies have been used to test the MA hypotheses. The following subsections briefly discuss these strategies and summarize the results obtained by them.

A. Research at the Periphery

1. MA Metabolites in Peripheral Body Fluids

MA metabolites have been determined in blood and urine—not a very efficient strategy for obtaining information on central MA metabolism. 5-HT and NA are known to be relatively abundant at the periphery. Their metabolism at the periphery is influenced by a variety of factors, such as nutrition, physical activity, and renal function. These are all factors which probably do not influence cerebral MA, or do so only slightly or not in the same sense. In other words, it is unlikely that changes in central MA are reliably reflected in peripheral metabolite levels. The peripheral "noise level" is too high for this.

There are two possible exceptions to this general rule. The principal NA metabolite in the brain is not vanillylmandelic acid (VMA) but 3-methoxy-4-hydroxyphenylglycol (MHPG). At the periphery, the reverse is true (Erwin, 1973). There are indications that renal MHPG excretion correlates fairly well with central NA degradation (Ebert and Kopin, 1975) and that motor activity exerts little or no influence on it (Goodwin et al., 1978a). Diminished renal MHPG excretion has been repeatedly found in primary depressions (Goodwin et al., 1978b), suggesting that central NA degradation can indeed be diminished in depressive patients.

A second exception might be the renal excretion of homovanillic acid (HVA) and dihydroxyphenylacetic acid (DOPAC), the principal metabolites of DA. So far, only minute amounts of DA have been found at the periphery. It is quite possible, therefore, that the renal excretion of its metabolites is of value as an indication of DA degradation in the brain. Surprisingly, no research has so far focused on this question.

2. *5-HT Uptake in Blood Platelets*

Blood platelets are considered to be a useful model of nerve terminals of central serotonergic neurons (Stahl, 1977), although their validity as such has been repudiated (Smith et al., 1978). According to Tuomisto and Tuhiainen (1976). 5-HT uptake in blood platelets from depressive patients is diminished. Oxenkrug et al. (1978) confirmed this observation. If this disorder should also apply to central serotonergic neurons it would of course be inconsistent with the 5-HT hypothesis, unless we assume that the diminished uptake is secondary to a functional 5-HT deficiency and meant to increase the concentration of transmitter substance at the postsynaptic receptors.

3. *Enzyme Determinations*

A third peripheral strategy is determination of the activity of enzymes involved in MA metabolism in plasma and blood platelets. Of course, such determinations make sense only if the peripheral activity is representative of the situation in the brain. We have no information on this question, but it seems justifiable for the time being to accept this postulate at least for chronic deviations from normal. After all, it is not very plausible that such a disorder could be localized and become manifest only at the periphery. A more serious handicap of this strategy is that, in most cases, we do not know when an abnormal enzyme concentration starts to have functional implications. Some enzyme systems have very ample safety margins. For example, MAO inhibition may exceed 80% without any deficiency of MA metabolism (Pletscher et al., 1960; Robinson et al., 1978).

MAO, an enzyme involved in the degradation of all MAs, and catechol-O-methyltransferase (COMT), an enzyme involved in DA and NA degradation, have been studied most intensively. The results, however, cannot be unequivocally interpreted. Several investigators (not all: see, for example, Nies et al., 1974) found decreased MAO concentrations in the blood platelets in depressive patients, and more particularly in those with bipolar depressions (Murphy and Weiss, 1972; Landowski et al., 1975). Diminished MAO activity has been found in other diagnostic categories as well, e.g., schizophrenia (Murphy and Wyatt,

1972). This disorder is therefore not specific to depressions. Moreover, it is syndrome-independent, which is to say that it persists even after psychopathological symptoms disappear. In a group of normal test subjects, Buchsbaum et al. (1976) observed that those with the lowest MAO concentrations showed more psychological disorders of various kinds than those with the highest MAO levels. It was therefore suggested that diminished MAO activity might possibly be a biological marker indicating increased psychological vulnerability.

Decreased MAO activity, if present in the brain, seems hardly consistent with central MA deficiency unless the enzyme defect is secondary to the MA deficiency and represents an attempt to "save" MA.

The COMT activity in erythrocytes was likewise found to be decreased in depressions, particularly in women with unipolar depressions (Cohn et al., 1970; Dunner et al., 1971). Shulman et al. (1978) maintain that COMT activity is correlated with motor activity: agitated patients showed increased values, whereas values in patients with motor retardation were decreased. It us uncertain as to whether the enzyme disorders contribute to the development of motor activity or result from it.

4. *Conclusions*

Studies of possible peripheral indices of central MA metabolism in depressive patients have revealed some deviations from the normal but no convincing evidence in support of the MA hypotheses. The only possible exception is the decreased MHPG excretion in some categories of depressive patients, which might be indicative of a diminished NA metabolism in the brain.

B. Postmortem Studies of the Brain

The question as to whether the central MA metabolism can be diminished in depressive patients has been approached directly by postmortem determination of the concentrations of MA, MA metabolites, and enzymes involved in MA metabolism in the brain of suicide victims. This strategy involves two essential difficulties, methodological problems to begin with. The results of postmortem studies are influenced by numerous factors which can hardly be controlled, if at all, e.g., duration of the interval between death and postmortem examination, duration of the death agony, use of pharmaceuticals, nutrition prior to death, and so on. The second essential problem lies in the fact that one has of course no "choice" of test subjects. As a rule, one must resort to suicide victims. Suicide is not a diagnosis but an act which concludes one of several possible patterns of behavior. Sometimes this pattern of behavior can be defined as depressive in the psychiatric sense, but this is by no means always the case. Moreover, it is often difficult to obtain reliable information on the psychological condition of these individuals prior to death. This implies uncertainty as to whether the material studied originates from patients who in terms of psychopathology tend to form a homogeneous group.

This makes it all the more striking that the results of postmortem studies so far done tend to warrant the same conclusion, i.e., that the concentration of 5-HT and/or its principal metabolite 5-hydroxyindoleacetic acid (5-HIAA) tends to be decreased, even though this tendency is not always significant (review: Murphy et al., 1978). According to Lloyd et al. (1974), the decrease in 5-hydroxyindoles is not generalized but confined to certain raphe nuclei (the site of predilection of 5-HT in the brain), i.e., the inferior central nucleus and the dorsal nucleus (Table 1).

Since the various postmortem studies were not coordinated it can hardly be assumed that they concerned patients or individuals of the same type. The fact that the results were nevertheless more or less comparable might indicate that a decrease in central 5-HT metabolism corresponds not so much with the nosological psychiatric concept "depression" as with a given psychological functional disorder, probably disturbed mood regulation or an increased level of anxiety, independent of the nosological context in which this disorder occurs. We revert to this possibility in Section V. Gottfries et al. (1975) reported a 20-40% decrease of the cerebral MAO level in a group of suicide victims, and particularly in those with a history of chronic alcohol abuse. It seems doubtful whether a decrease of this order would have functional implications in vivo.

C. CSF Baseline Studies

1. Imperfections

There are sound reasons for the assumption that the concentration of a MA metabolite in the CSF gives an indication of the amount of mother substance degraded in a given part of the CNS (Moir et al, 1970). This is why concentrations of MA metabolites in the CSF were determined in depressive patients. One imperfection of this method lies in the fact that some MA metabolites are transported directly to the bloodstream instead of via the CSF (Meek and Neff, 1973). The ratio direct/indirect transport is not exactly known; nor is it known whether this ratio is constant. Another imperfection lies in the fact that there is a gradient for MA metabolites, and particularly for 5-HIAA and HVA. The concentrations are highest at the ventricular level and diminish caudadly. This means that CSF flow and CSF pressure (coughing, straining, sneezing) must influence the concentrations measured at the lumbar level (Davson, 1967). These imperfections have in part been overcome with the aid of the probenecid method (Section III.D).

2. 5-HIAA

The results of CSF studies are (therefore?) not unequivocal (review: van Praag, 1977a). Decreased 5-HIAA baseline values have repeatedly been found in depressive patients—an observation consistent with diminished central 5-HT metabolism. However, the decrease found was not always significant; and some

Table 1 Concentrations of 5-HIAA and 5-HT in the Raphe Nuclei of Controls and Suicides

	5-HIAA (μg/g)				5-HT (μg/g)			
	Controls		Suicides		Controls		Suicides	
Raphe nuclei	Mean ± SEM	*n*	Mean ± SEM	*n*	Mean ± SEM	*n*	Mean ± SEM	*n*
Centralis superior	12.37 ± 0.65 (11.25 –14.53)	5	12.39 ± 0.91 (9.19 –14.61)	5	2.25 ± 0.19 (1.88 – 2.97)	5	1.86 ± 0.16 (1.41 – 2.26)	5
Dorsalis	7.04 ± 0.59 (5.85 – 8.63)	5	6.14 ± 0.52 (5.00 – 7.79)	5	2.22 ± 0.13 (1.92 – 2.56)	5	1.55 ± 0.12[a] (1.23 – 1.90)	5
Pontis	7.66 ± 0.57 (6.21 – 8.92)	5	7.12 ± 0.68 (5.42 – 9.55)	5	1.34 ± 0.21 (0.80 – 1.89)	5	1.04 ± 0.13 (0.65 – 1.38)	5
Centralis inferior	4.49 ± 0.43 (3.63 – 5.77)	5	4.01 ± 0.32 (3.14 – 4.67)	5	1.32 ± 0.12 (0.94 – 1.47)	5	0.95 ± 0.07[b] (0.69 – 1.09)	5
Obscurus	2.86 ± 0.24 (2.00 – 3.46)	5	3.36 ± 0.31 (2.46 – 4.24)	5	1.07 ± 0.14 (0.62 – 1.39)	5	1.02 ± 0.14 (0.75 – 1.56)	5
Pallidus	2.28 ± 0.16 (1.85 – 2.67)	5	2.25 ± 0.20 (1.90 – 2.74)	4	0.61 ± 0.09 (0.44 - 0.91)	5	0.42 ± 0.12 (0.28 – 0.76)	4

[a]Significantly different from controls: $P < .01$.
[b]$P < .05$.
Source: From Lloyd et al., 1974.

authors found no decrease at all. A conclusion can therefore not be drawn. This statement stands even in light of one particular study, that of Åsberg et al. (1976), which is the most valid. It is the only baseline study so far which fulfills three important criteria: (1) the number of patients examined was large: 68; (2) the group tended toward psychopathological homogeneity in that all test subjects had a primary depression; (3) 5-HIAA concentrations were determined by gas choromatography/mass spectrometry. This method is more sensitive and more specific than the customary fluorometric procedure. The principal conclusion from this study was that the baseline 5-HIAA concentration in the CSF *can* be decreased in patients with primary depressions. The concentrations proved to show a dichotomous distribution. In other words, the primary depression group included one subgroup with low and one with normal 5-HIAA concentrations. The overlap between the two subgroups was small (Fig. 1). The authors concluded that a 5-HT-deficient subgroup of depressions exists, thereby confirming the observations of van Praag and Korf (1971a) with the probenecid procedure (Fig. 2) (cf. Section III.D).

3. *HVA*

To the DA metabolite HVA, the same applies as to the CSF 5-HIAA concentration: varying results (review: van Praag, 1977a). Although the majority of

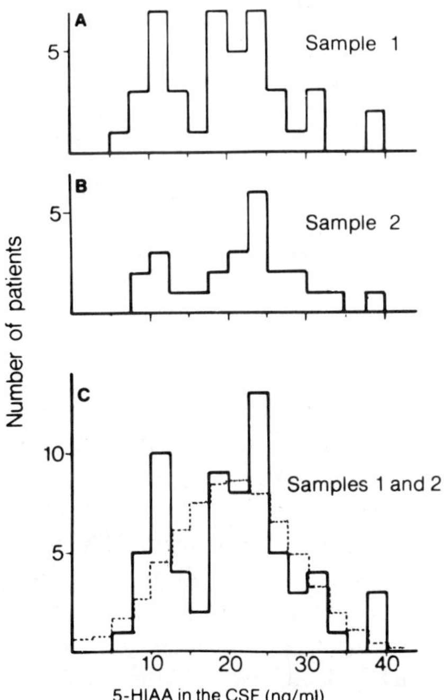

Figure 1 Distribution of 5-HIAA in depressed patients: (A) sample 1, $n = 43$; (B) sample 2, $n = 25$; (C) samples 1 and 2 combined. The dashed line represents the expected normal distribution (mean ± standard deviation = 20.36 ± 7.77). The deviation from normality is significant ($x^2 = 19.76$, 9 d.f., $P = .01$) [Reprinted with permission M. Åsberg, P. Thoren, L. Trashman, L. Bertilsson and V. Ringberger (1976). *Science 191,* 478-480 (6 February). Copyright 1976 by the American Association for the Advancement of Science.]

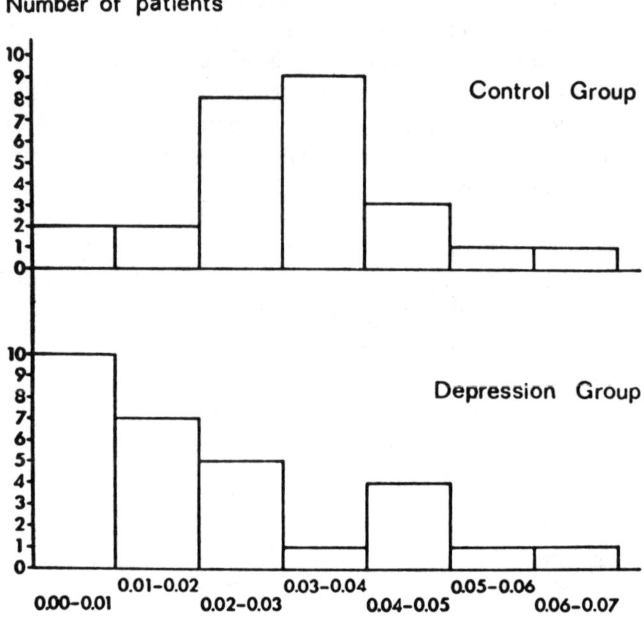

Figure 2 Increase in the 5-HIAA concentration in the CSF following probenecid in the depression group and in the control group. The groups of the oral and the intravenous probenecid test were combined. The columns indicate the number of patients showing the increase in concentration given at the bottom of the column (From van Praag and Korf, 1971a).

authors report a decrease (significant or not) of the CSF HVA concentration in depressive patients, normal values are also mentioned repeatedly. As will be demonstrated, the postprobenecid values are more consistent.

4. MHPG

Before we consider the MHPG levels as reflection of central NA metabolism, two points should be made. First, MHPG studies have been much less numerous than 5-HIAA and HVA studies. This is probably explained by the technical difficulties of MHPG determination. Second, the MHPG concentration shows only a slight craniocaudad gradient (Chase et al., 1973). This means that MHPG in lumbar CSF is probably chiefly a reflection of spinal NA metabolism. Of course, this does not as such disqualify the determination because it is possible that a disorder of NA metabolism, if present, becomes manifest throughout the CNS. However, HVA in lumbar CSF originates largely from the cerebrum, and

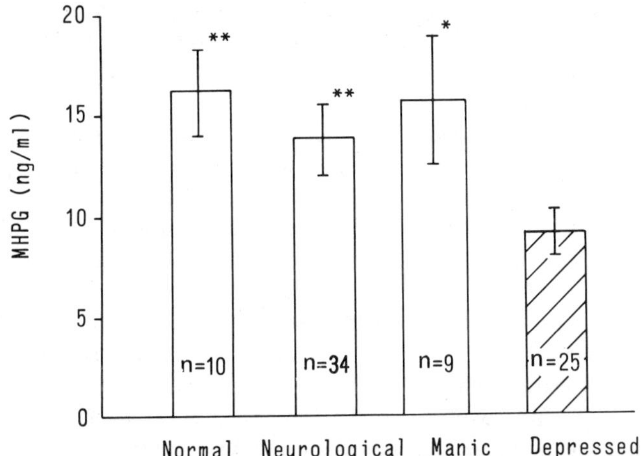

Figure 3 Low MHPG concentration in CSF in depressed patients. Levels of MHPG in depressed patients were significantly lower than those in other groups (* $P < .05$; ** $P < .01$; Student's t test, two-tailed). (From Post et al., 1973.)

5-HIAA for 50%. Consequently, their determination in lumbar CSF is more instructive than that of MHPG.

The group of Goodwin et al. (Post and Goodwin, 1978) established that both MHPG (Fig. 3) and VMA (a subordinate NA metabolite in the CNS) are found in decreased concentrations in the CSF in patients with primary depressions. This dual finding might indicate a reduced NA turnover in the brain. It is to be noted that the concentration of NA itself was not decreased. However, decreased MHPG levels have not been observed by all authors (Shaw et al., 1973).

Simultaneous determination of urinary and CSF MHPG levels in depression patients has so far not been carried out. There are indications, however, that renal and CSF MHPG levels are not correlated (Goodwin et al., 1978b). This fact certainly raises doubt as to the validity of the assumption that renal MHPG levels are indicative of the extent of the central NA metabolism.

D. CSF Probenecid Studies

1. Possibilities and Limitations

About 10 years ago the probenecid technique was introduced in an effort to enhance the instructive value of determination of MA metabolites in human CSF (Roos and Sjöström, 1969; van Praag et al., 1970; Tamarkin et al., 1970). Probenecid blocks the transport of the acid MA metabolites 5-HIAA and HVA from the CNS to the blood stream. Consequently, these metabolites accumulate throughout the CNS, including the CSF. By measuring their accumulation, an impression can be gained of the 5-HT and DA turnover in the entire CNS. Low accumulation indicates a low production of the metabolites and, therefore, low degradation of the mother substance. High accumulation indicates high degradation of the mother substance. The background and application of the probenecid technique have been discussed in detail elsewhere (van Praag 1977a, 1978a).

This method, too, has its disadvantages. It is uncertain, for example, whether probenecid in doses tolerable to the human organism does in fact totally block 5-HIAA and HVA transport. If not, then it incompletely reflects the amine degradation. Moreover, probenecid influences 5-HT metabolism in more ways than solely by blocking 5-HIAA transport. It releases tryptophan in plasma from its protein complex and thus increases the supply of free tryptophan to the CNS. In view of this, one might expect 5-HT synthesis to increase. In actual practice, however, this increase is only very moderate.

Even though the probenecid technique is far from flawless, it can nevertheless be regarded as a (crude) indicator of 5-HT and DA turnover throughout the CNS. In this respect it is more instructive than baseline measurements.

2. *Results*

The probenecid-induced accumulation of 5-HIAA and HVA in lumbar CSF has been studied by five groups. Three found decreased values both for 5-HIAA and for HVA (van Praag et al., 1970; van Praag and Korf 1971a; Sjöström and Roos, 1972; van Praag et al., 1975; Post and Goodwin, 1978). Bowers reported normal values in 1972 but later (1974) found decreased accumulation in bipolar depressions. Jori et al. (1975) were the only investigators to find normal 5-HIAA and HVA accumulation in depressive patients.

3. *Selectivity of Findings*

The Achilles' heel of biological depression research still lies in psychiatric classification. Exact definition of the syndromes studied calls for three-dimensional classification encompassing symptomatology, etiology, and course. In actual practice this is rarely done, but investigators eagerly use one-dimensional concepts such as primary/secondary depression, endogenous/neurotic depression, unipolar/bipolar depression (an evil certainly not confined to the group of depressions, but pervading almost the entire field of psychiatry). It is therefore difficult to compare the results obtained by the various investigators. According to van Praag et al. (1973), decreased postprobenecid 5-HIAA accumulation occurs mainly in the group of vital depressions regardless of their etiology or course (unipolar or bipolar). Moreover, it is not a universal phenomenon within this group, but confined to about 40% of patients. It has so far been impossible to differentiate vital depressive patients with from those without disorders in central 5-HT metabolism on the basis of psychopathological criteria.

According to the van Praag group (van Praag and Korf, 1971b; van Praag et al., 1973; van Praag, 1974), decreased postprobenecid HVA accumulation is chiefly found in depressions with pronounced motor retardation (Table 2). Since the latter occurs mostly in vital depressions, it is chiefly in depressions of this category that this biochemical phenomenon is observed. Banki (1977) confirmed the relationship between decreased HVA accumulation and motor retardation.

MHPG transport is probenecid-insensitive, and consequently the method is not suitable for more exact detection of central NA degradation.

E. Conclusions from the Attempts to Measure Central MA Metabolism Directly

Postmortem and CSF studies have supplied arguments in favor of a disorder of central 5-HT metabolism in a certain category of (vital) depressions. In fact these arguments can be described as fairly strong if one considers the fact that these signals are received in spite of the strong "noise" caused by inadequate depression classification. It is uncertain as to which features of the depressive syndrome the suspected 5-HT defect is related. CSF studies have shown the plausibility of a disorder of central DA metabolism as well, and there are indications that this phenomenon is related to motor retardation.

The changes found are suggestive of diminished 5-HT and DA turnover in the brain but need not necessarily have implications for the functional activity in serotonergic and dopaminergic systems, respectively. A decreased turnover can be a primary phenomenon, in which case it probably leads to reduced neuronal activity in the systems concerned. But it may also be secondary to increased activity in these systems (e.g., as a result of hypersensitivity of postsynaptic receptors). The decrease in turnover in that case probably leads to reduction of hyperactivity or to normalization of neuronal activity in the systems involved. In view of the data discussed in Section VII, we regard the former hypothesis as more plausible than the latter.

The data so far collected on the NA metabolism indicate a draw: The number of studies reporting disorders more or less equals the number of those reporting negative findings. We therefore refrain from formulating any conclusion.

F. Pharmacological Strategies

1. *Expectations Based on MA Hypotheses*

If depressions can involve a central 5-HT and/or NA deficiency, and if this deficiency is of etiological importance, then two expectations seem justified. The *first expectation* is that an increase in the amount of transmitter substance at the central receptor sites should result in alleviation of (certain) depressive

Table 2 Concentration of HVA in CSF in Depressive Patients and Controls Before and After i.v. Probenecid Administration (in μg/ml)[a]

Patients	No. of test subjects	Before probenecid	After probenecid	Difference
Depression (retarded and nonretarded)	20	0.039 ± 0.016 (0.014 – 0.067)	0.082 ± 0.043 (0.027 – 0.185)	0.044 ± 0.038 (0.000 – 0.130)
Retarded depression	8	0.032 ± 0.008 (0.020 – 0.046)	0.053 ± 0.032 (0.027 – 0.114)	0.020 ± 0.028 (0.000 – 0.074)
Nonretarded depression	12	0.043 ± 0.017 (0.014 – 0.067)	0.106 ± 0.036 (0.040 – 0.185)	0.063 ± 0.037 (0.010 – 0.130)
Control	12	0.042 ± 0.016 (0.021 – 0.073)	0.091 ± 0.026 (0.059 – 0.151)	0.050 ± 0.033 (0.023 – 0.122)

[a]Results are given as means ± s.d. (with range).
Source: From van Praag and Korf, 1971b.

symptoms, particularly in patients in whom a deficiency of one or several MA has been demonstrated to be plausible. The second clause of this expectation is ignored in the literature. Most precursor studies, for example, have been based on the assumption that, on the basis of the MA hypotheses, MA precursors can be expected to be universal antidepressants. This is begging for negative results. By way of a crude analogy, in the case of vitamin B_{12} deficiency one should not expect the anemic symptoms to disappear in response to iron repletion.

The *second expectation* mirrors the first: On the basis of the MA hypotheses, decreased central 5-HT and/or NA levels should induce or aggravate depressive symptoms.

2. Studies with 5-HT Agonists

Generally speaking, the first expectation is supported by the empirical data. *Tryptophan studies* are the weak spot in the argumentation (review: Mendels et al., 1975). Some authors ascribe an antidepressant effect to this 5-HT precursor, but virtually as many others refute this. We postulated in 1970 (van Praag and Korf) that this discrepancy might be based on biochemical heterogeneity of the (vital) depressions and advocated a biochemical typology of the depressions in precursor studies. So far as tryptophan is concerned, this design was still absent in 1978; that is to say, it was still unknown whether a (5-HT-deficient) subtype of depression exists which is tryptophan-sensitive. The tryptophan problem, therefore, seems still moot. On the other hand, there are strong indications that the therapeutic effect of MAO inhibitors (e.g., Coppen et al., 1963) and of clomipramine, a tricyclic antidepressant with a marked inhibitory effect on 5-HT reuptake (Walinder et al., 1966), is potentiated by l-tryptophan.

Few studies have been made with the second 5-HT precursor, *5-hydroxytryptophan* (5-HTP), but their results are unequivocal. Several open studies (Sano, 1972; Takahashi et al., 1975; van Hiele, 1980) and three controlled studies (van Praag et al., 1972; Angst et al., 1977; van Praag, 1978b, 1979) led to the conclusion that 5-HTP has antidepressant properties which compare with those of clomipramine (van Praag, 1978b) and imipramine (Angst et al., 1977) (Figs. 4 and 5). Moreover, it was established that the therapeutic efficacy of 5-HTP is maximal in patients with subnormal 5-HIAA accumulation, i.e., those who show indications of central 5-HT deficiency (Fig. 6).

In normal test subjects, 5-HTP was found to have a euphorizing effect (Trimble et al., 1975; Pühringe et al., 1976). In myoclonic patients treated with this compound, (hypo)manic disinhibition was reported as a side effect (van Woert et al., 1977).

A few studies with more or less *selective tricyclic antidepressants* point in the same direction. Clomipramine, a 5-HT reuptake inhibitor, is the most effective agent in the group of 5-HT-deficient depressions. The majority of clomipramine-resistant patients respond favorably to nortriptyline, a selective

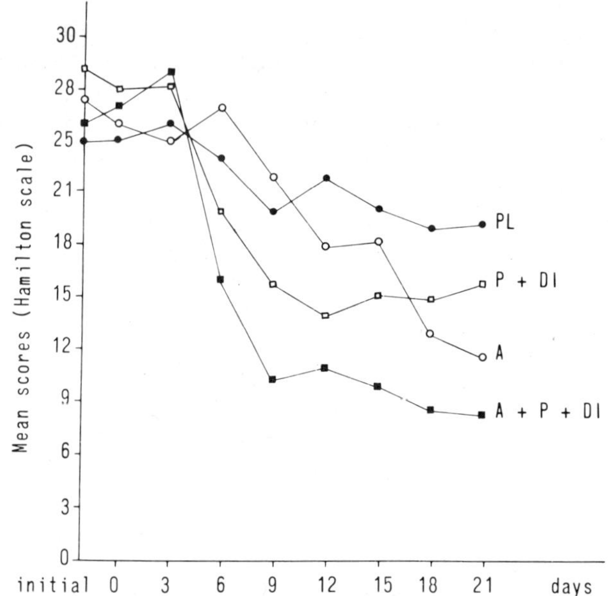

Figure 4 Hamilton scores in four groups of patients suffering from vital depression with uni- and bipolar course before and during a 3-week treatment period with serontonin-potentiating compounds. The groups consisted of 10 patients each, treated respectively with clomipramine alone (225 mg/day; A), 5-HTP alone (P; 200 mg/day, in combination with 150 mg MK 486, a peripheral decarboxylase inhibitor; DI), the combination of clomipramine with 5-HTP and placebo (P1). The design was double blind. 5-HTP ($P = < .05$), clomipramine ($P = < .05$) and the combination treatment ($P = < .01$) are superior to placebo treatment (Wilcoxon test, Mann-Whitney test). (From van Praag, 1978b.)

NA reuptake inhibitor, but in the nortriptyline responders no indications of NA deficiency were found in the CSF (van Praag, 1977b). Moreover, patients with low CSF 5-HIAA values showed a less favorable response to nortriptyline than patients with normal 5-HIAA values (Åsberg et al., 1972).

3. Selectivity of 5-HT Agonists

These results should be interpreted with caution. The selectivity of the compounds used is only relative. Typptophan is a precursor, not only of 5-HT but also of other compounds such as tryptamine and the B-vitamin nicotinic acid. 5-HTP is converted to 5-HT not only in serotonergic but also in catecholaminergic neurons because 5-HTP and DOPA decarboxylase are identical enzymes (Yuwiler et al., 1959). The principle clomipramine metabolite—demethylclomipramine (Westenberg et al., 1977)—is a NA reuptake inhibitor.

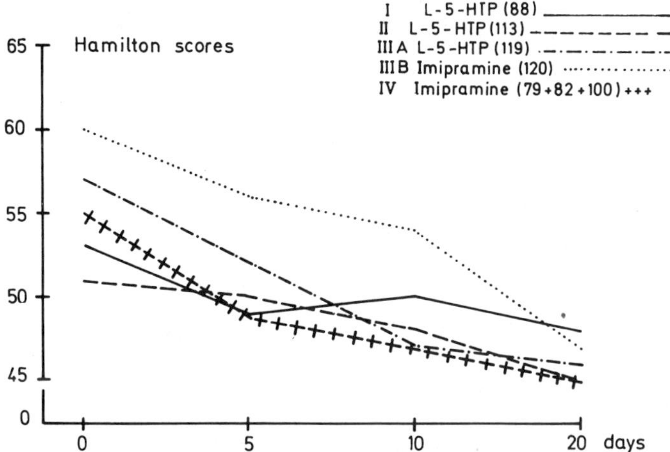

Figure 5 Hamilton scale items 1-17 (unadjusted means) during treatment with 1-5-HTP or imipramine in depression. Studies III and IV were double-blind-controlled. The other two studies were open. (From Angst et al., 1977.)

5-HT agonists which really tend toward selectivity are now being evolved. An example is the selective 5-HT reuptake inhibitor zimilidin. Clinical results obtained with it have so far been promising (Siwers et al., 1977; Cox et al., 1978), but studies correlating these results with CSF 5-HIAA values have yet to be carried out.

4. Studies with DA Agonists

The catecholamine precursor *L-dopa,* which if given systematically is largely converted to DA, has also been tested in depressions. The therapeutic results have not been spectacular but they are nevertheless important from a scientific point of view. In the case of motor retardation, L-dopa activates (Goodwin et al., 1970; van Praag, 1974) and normalizes the HVA response to probenecid, which is usually decreased in these patients (van Praag and Korf, 1975) (Table 3). It exerts little influence on the mood. This is an argument in favor of the hypothesis that DAergic systems are involved in particular in the motor pathology of depression but less in the pathogenesis of mood disturbance (van Praag et al., 1975; van Praag, 1977c).

A similar correlation between pretherapeutic HVA response to probenecid and therapeutic response has been established for two other DA agonists: *nomifensine* and *piribedil.* The former (Van Scheyen et al., 1978) was initially believed to be mostly a DA reuptake inhibitor. Its therapeutic range proved to

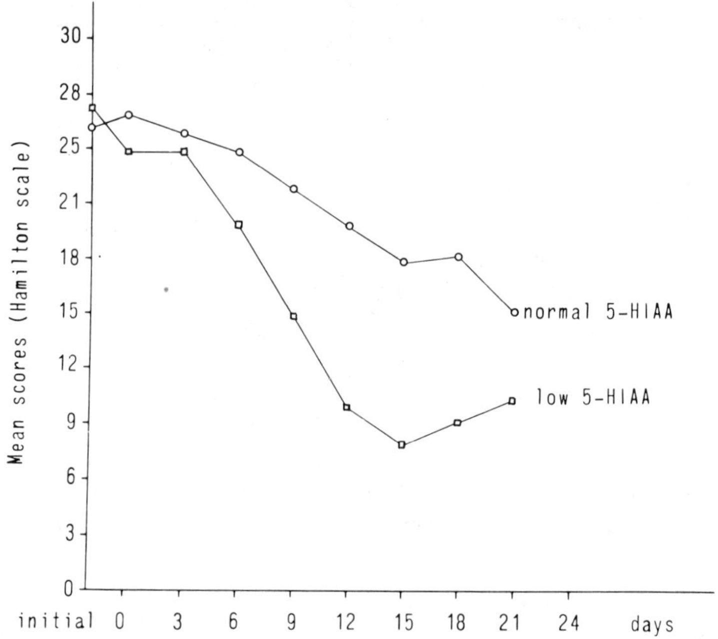

Figure 6 Hamilton scores of 30 patients suffering from vital depression with uni- and bipolar course before and during a 3-week treatment period with serotonin-potentiating compounds, i.e., clomipramine alone, 5-HTP (together with a peripheral decarboxylase inhibitor) alone, and those drugs in combination. The lower curve depicts treatment results in patients with subnormal pretreatment 5-HIAA response to probenecid (n = 13), the upper curve those in patients with normal pretreatment 5-HIAA responses (n = 17). The difference is statistically significant ($P = < .05$, Wilcoxon test; Man-Whitney test). (From van Praag, 1978b.)

differ from that of L-dopa. Not only does it activate, but it behaves like a true antidepressant. This is not necessarily at odds with the above hypothesis that DAergic systems correlate more with motor activity than with mood regulation, for nomifensine was later found to be an inhibitor, not only of DA reuptake but also of NA reuptake. This might explain its behavior like a true antidepressant. The second compound, piribedil, is a stimulator of postsynaptic receptors. Like L-dopa, this compound shows the behavior of a motor activator; but unlike L-dopa, it also produces a feeble antidepressant effect (Post et al., 1978).

Table 3 DA Metabolism Before Treatment and Treatment Response to L-Dopa in Depression

Patients	*n*	HVA accumulation (ng/ml)[a]	Motor retardation[a]	
			Before treatment	After treatment
DA-deficient	5	74 (65-90)	6.8 (4-8)	2.7 (0-3)
Non-DA-deficient	5	121 (107-143)	2.1 (0-3)	2.4 (0-3)

[a]Group mean and range.
Source: Reprinted with permission from H. M. van Praag and J. Korf (1975) *Pharmakopsych. 8,* 322-326. Georg Thieme Verlag, Stuttgart.

5. *Studies with NA Agonists*

After exogenous administration, L-dopa is largely converted to DA and is therefore unsuitable. Clonidine, a stimulator of NA receptors, has so far been tested in depressions only on a very limited scale. No definite conclusion can yet be formulated (Post and Goodwin, 1978). The tetracyclic antidepressant amprotiline (Ludiomil) and the tricyclic antidepressant nortriptyline (Aventyl) are pure NA reuptake inhibitors. They are among the conventional antidepressants, but it is unknown whether depressive patients with a suspected central NA deficiency provide their indication of choice. Such research has been done with the mixed reuptake inhibitor imipramine, which inhibits NA reuptake more strongly than 5-HT reuptake. In the NA-deficient subgroup (with low renal MHPG excretion), this compound was indeed found to be most effective (Beckman and Goodwin, 1975).

6. *Conclusions from the Studies with 5-HT and NA Agonists*

The above observations indicate the plausibility of a correlation between pretherapeutic central MA metabolism and the therapeutic efficacy of compounds which exert a more or less selective influence on central MA metabolism. This is an argument in favor of the MA hypotheses. It is also an argument in support of the primary nature of the biochemical disorders mentioned. That is to say, an argument indicating that these disorders are of importance in the pathogenesis of the depression rather than being a consequence of it.

7. *Monoaminergic Suppression*

We must now consider the complementary hypothesis: A pharmacologically induced MA deficiency leads to depressive symptoms. In fact it can. The best known example is the reserpine-induced vital depression (Goodwin et al., 1972).

Reserpine lowers the levels of catecholamines as well as of 5-HT. Depressions have also been observed as a complication of the use of a few other antihypertensives: α-methyldopa and propranolol (Whitlock and Evans, 1978), which both suppress noradrenergic transmission. Phenothiazine-type neuroleptics block central DA and NA receptors. There are indications that they may induce depression, but this has not been established with certainty (Van Putten and May, 1978). Depressions in response to these compounds are relatively sporadic. This does not necessarily argue against the MA hypotheses. It may well be that additional factors have to be involved (in central MA metabolism or elsewhere) before the depressogenic activity of these compounds can become manifest.

Parachlorophenylalanine (PCPA), an inhibitor of tryptophan hydroxylase and therefore of 5-HT synthesis, has no indication in the treatment of human individuals, with the possible exception of certain instances of carcinoid—an intestinal tumor which produces large amounts of 5-hydroxyindoles. Depressions have not been described, but then the compound's clinical use has been very limited in view of its toxic side effects. An observation of importance in this context was reported by Shopsin et al. (1974), who found that PCPA arrests the therapeutic effect of imipramine within a few days. This would seem to indicate that 5-HT plays a role at least in the antidepressant action of imipramine.

Inhibition of catecholamine synthesis has also been tried, with the aid of α-methyl-p-tyrosine (inhibition of tyrosine hydroxylase) and fusaric acid (inhibition of DA β-hydroxylase) (Sack and Goodwin, 1974; Schildkraut, 1975). The results are uncertain: no distinct depressogenic effect has been observed, but the number of test subjects is too small to warrant any definite conclusion.

8. *Conclusions from the Results Obtained by the Pharmacological Strategy*

In conclusion, I would say that the results of pharmacological research do not repudiate the MA hypotheses but in several ways in fact support them. This applies in particular to the 5-HT hypothesis. It is to be borne in mind, however, that the selectivity of the compounds used for one particular MAergic system is limited. Biological depression research should benefit greatly from more selective compounds. It is therefore fortunate that developments in this direction are in progress. It is no less fortunate that these developments have been greatly stimulated by clinical studies in the field of depressions.

IV. STUDY OF THE CENTRAL MONOAMINES VIA THE NEUROENDOCRINE STRATEGY

A. Strategy

A new strategy to approach human central MAergic system has outlined itself in the past few years: determination of plasma hormone concentratins, and more specifically of the concentrations of hormones originating from the anterior lobe of the hypophysis (review: van Praag, 1978c). These compounds are formed exclusively in the hypophysis. Their release is controlled by the so-called inhibiting and releasing factors (hormones) from the hypothalamus, which in turn are controlled by central MAergic systems. It may therefore be assumed that disorders in central (hypothalamic) MAergic activity are bound to be reflected in the release of anterior hypophyseal hormones. The following subsections discuss the psychoendocrine findings in depressions so far as they are relevant to the MA hypotheses. (See also Volume III of this Handbook.)

B. Growth Hormone

The response of plasma growth hormone (GH) to insulin is decreased in postmenopausal women suffering from unipolar depressions (Gruen et al., 1975). This mechanism has not yet been studied in males, nor in depressive syndromes of a different type. Nor is it known whether the baseline 24-hr profile of GH may be disturbed in depressions.

There are indications that NAergic systems are involved in the release of GH in response to insulin-induced hypoglycemia (Brown et al., 1978). The decreased GH response to insulin might therefore be related to a deficient NAergic system. This interpretation is corroborated by several other observations. To begin with, the GH response to amphetamine and clonidine is also diminished in vital depressive patients (Langer et al., 1973; Matussek et al., 1977). Clonidine is a direct NA agonist. Amphetamine enhances both NAergic and DAergic activity in the brain via several mechanisms. The increase in GH response, however, is probably not based on a DAergic mechanism: The effect persists when amphetamine is combined with pimozide, a substance which blocks DAergic transmission but exerts little influence on NAergic transmission (Sachar et al., 1976).

A second argument lies in the fact that a correlation has been demonstrated between human GH response to insulin and renal MHPG excretion (Garver et al., 1975). MHPG is the principal NA metabolite in the CNS, and its urinary concentration is regarded as a (crude) indicator of NA degradation in the CNS. The correlation is therefore an indication that the GH response to insulin diminishes as central NA turnover diminishes.

If it is true that the GH response to insulin-induced hypoglycemia is effected NAergically, then the above observations are consistent with the hypothesis that a central NA deficiency can play a role in the pathogenesis of vital depressions.

C. Luteinizing Hormone

In depressive patients, another hypothalamic/hypophyseal hormonal system has been studied which is probably controlled by NAergic nuerons: the secretion of luteinizing hormone (LH). This process is activated by a hypothalamic factor:

luteinizing-hormone-releasing factor (LHRF), the production of which is in turn activated by a NAergic system. This can be deduced from observations of the following type.

In rats, gonadectomy causes increased LH secretion because it eliminates the inhibitory influence of gonadal estrogens, particularly estradiol. The estradiol effect is probably produced via a NAergic system (Ojeda and McCann, 1974). The increased plasma LH concentration after gonadectomy is not observed in rats premedicated with a compound which inhibits the conversion of DA to NA, but the increase commences again when the animals are given dihydroxyphenylserine, an amino acid converted to NA directly, without intermediary DA synthesis.

In postmenopausal women the production of estrogens (particularly estradiol) is low, and consequently the plasma LH level rises substantially. In this phase of life the estrogen antagonist clomifene causes no further rise of the LH level (Sachar, 1975) and this implies that in this respect the menopause can be regarded as a state of functional gonadectomy.

Presuming that (1) a central NA deficiency does exist in certain types of vital depression and (2) the LH effect is produced NAergically during the menopause, it is justifiable to expect the plasma LH level in (vital) depressive postmenopausal women to be lower than that in nondepressive postmenopausal women.

Only one adequately controlled study has so far focused on this hypothesis (Altman et al., 1976). It led to the conclusion that the plasma LH level averaged 33% lower in postmenopausal women with unipolar vital depressions than in the control group ($P < 0.05$). This finding is consistent with expectation based on the presumption that central NAergic activity is diminished. In this context I may point out that the facts can also be differently interpreted: by presuming that estrogen production is larger in depressive than in nondepressive postmenopausal women. This possibility can be verified by determining the plasma estradiol concentration. So far, no studies have been carried out to establish whether this phenomenon is specific of the group of vital depressions.

D. Prolactin

Prolactin secretion is regulated by the prolactin-inhibiting factor (PIF) produced in the hypothalamus. There is also a prolactin-releasing factor, but its nature is uncertain (Boyd and Reichlin, 1978). The PIF production is vigorously activated by a DAergic system. Consequently, L-dopa (a DA agonist) lowers the prolactin levels in CSF and blood, whereas neuroleptics (DA antagonists) raise these prolactin levels (review: van Praag, 1977c). Serotonergic systems are claimed to produce the opposite effect, i.e., inhibition of PIF production (Kato et al., 1974), but this is not certain (van Praag et al., 1976).

If disregulation of central DAergic systems should play a role in the pathogenesis of depressive symptoms, then it would be sensible to determine blood (or CSF) prolactin levels as a measure of central DAergic activity. DA research has so far been neglected in depressive patients, virtually all attention having been focused on 5-HT and NA. There are nevertheless some indications which would justify such research. For example, it has been demonstrated that motor disorders in retarded vital depression are probably related to central DA deficiency. Activation of the central DAergic system, whether with the aid of L-dopa or with piribedil (a relatively specific DA agonist), has a therapeutic effect in these cases via improvement of the motor symptoms (Goodwin et al., 1970; van Praag and Korf, 1971b, 1975; Post et al., 1978). Systematic studies of the prolactin secretion in depression are therefore certainly justified. The first study (to the author's knowledge) of the 24-hr prolactin profile in depressive patients and normal volunteers supports the hypothesis that the DAergic system can be hypoactive in certain types of depression (Halbreich et al., 1979).

E. Cortisol

Cortisol is not a hypohyseal but an adrenocortical hormone. It is nevertheless mentioned in this section because (1) if the adrenals are intact, cortisol secretion is virtually parallel with ACTH secretion and (2) there seems to be a relation between peripheral cortisol secretion and central NAergic activity. The cortisol secretion is hormonally regulated by hypophyseal ACTH and hypothalamic corticotropin-releasing factor (CRF). The neuronal regulation of ACTH and CRF secretion is complicated, and involves serotonergic and NAergic as well as cholinergic systems. Moreover, different systems are probably involved in the regulation of the baseline secretion, the 24-hr profile, and the response to stress. Nevertheless, there are strong indications in favor of the existence of a NAergic system with a tonic inhibitory effect on CRF production (van Loon, 1973; Sachar, 1975).

If central NAergic systems should function deficiently in certain types of depression, then hypersecretion of cortisol could be expected. This phenomenon has in fact been repeatedly observed, particularly in vital depressions with a unipolar and bipolar course (Fig. 7) (Sachar et al., 1973; Carroll et al., 1976). Normally, cortisol secretion takes place in bursts, and the strongest of these bursts occur between 0500 and 0900 hr. Cortisol secretion virtually ceases between 2000 and 0200 hr, when the plasma cortisol concentration approaches zero.

In the above-mentioned depressive patients the number of bursts was increased, the cortisol peaks were higher, and cortisol production continued during normally "silent" periods. The abnormalities were much more marked as the depression was more severe and disappeared as the depression abated.

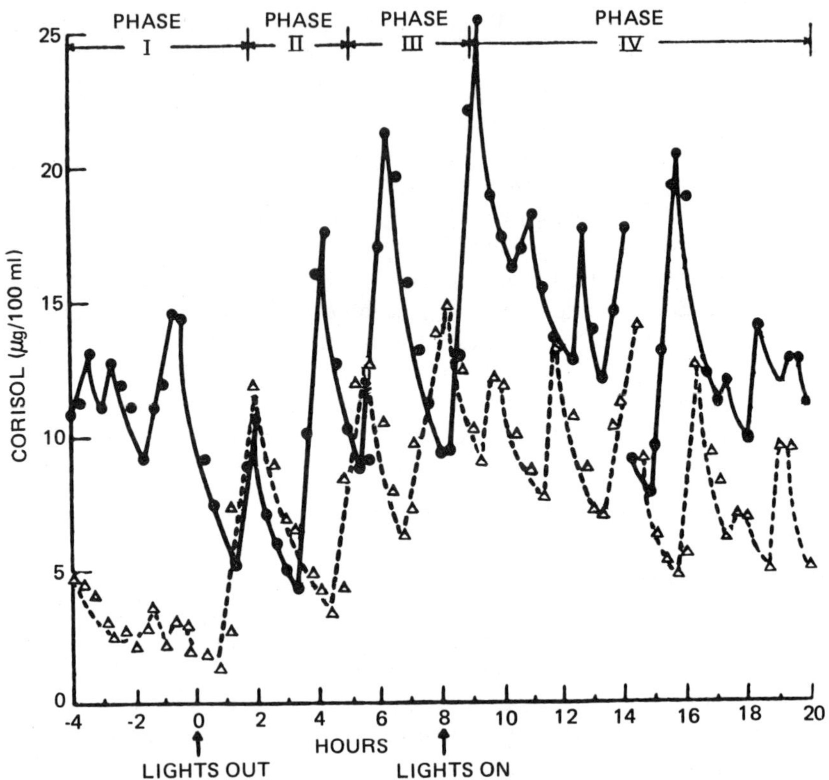

Figure 7 Plasma cortisol pattern (24-hr) in a 52-year-old woman with unipolar vital depression, during the depression (●) and after recovery (Δ). Time 0 is the time at which lights went out for sleep. [Reprinted by permission from E. J. Sachar (1975). Neuroendocrine abnormalities in depressive illness. In *Topics in Psychoendocrinology,* E. J. Sachar (Ed.). Grune & Stratton, New York.]

According to Carroll et al. (1976), these phenomena are highly specific. They are rarely observed in depressions with symptoms other than those known as vital and in conditions not included in the group of affective disorders. For this reason, too, it is unlikely that the cortisol hypersecretion could be a nonspecific stress reaction. There are more arguments against this possibility, e.g., that the phenomenon is observed in agitated as well as in retarded vital depressions, and that it persists even when the patient receives sedative medication (Sachar, 1975).

There is another argument indicating that vital depressions may involve a "failure of the normal inhibitory influence of the brain on the release of ACTH

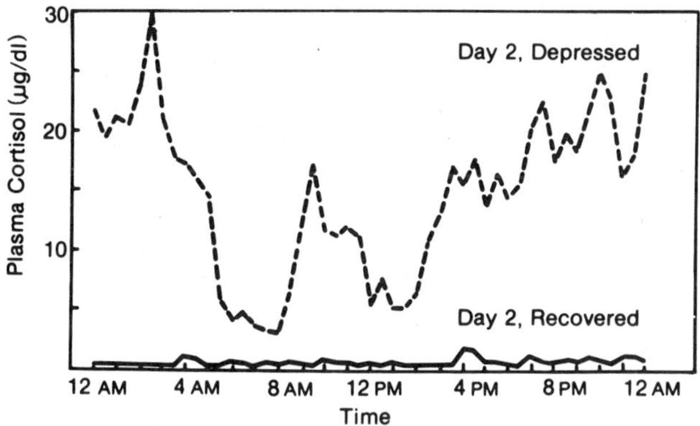

Figure 8 Plasma cortisol concentration after oral administration of 2 mg dexamethasone at midnight in a 58-year-old man with retarded depression of the bipolar type, during the depression (– – –) and after recovery (———). (After Carroll et al., 1976.)

and cortisol" (Carroll et al., 1976): Some 50% of (vital) depressive patients show a subnormal decrease in plasma cortisol in response to dexamethasone (Fig. 8). Normally, this synthetic corticosteroid so suppresses ACTH production that the plasma cortisol level falls to practically zero. Patients with vital depressions, however, are much more resistant to this dexamethasone effect.

F. Thyroid-Stimulating Hormone

In this context we arrive at the observation that vital depressive patients may show a subnormal thyroid-stimulating hormone (TSH) response to thyrotropin-releasing hormone (TRH) (Fig. 9) (Prange et al., 1972; Hollister et al., 1976; van den Burg et al, 1975, 1976). A decreased TSH response to TRH is generally indicative of an increased production of thyroid hormones, for the latter reduce the sensitivity of the hypophysis to TRH. In the depressive patients in question, however, thyroid function was normal.

A possible explanation of this phenomenon lies in an increased production of GH-inhibiting factor. This peptide inhibits not only the release of GH but also that of TSH after administration of TRH (Prange et al., 1978). The hypothesis is attractive because it also affords an explanation of the fact that the GH response to insulin-induced hypoglycemia in depressions can be decreased (Section IV.B).

Another, likewise speculative explanation is that the autochthonous TRH production in these patients is subnormal, causing the hypophysis to "unlearn" its response to TRH excess by vigorous TSH secretion. This explanation is con-

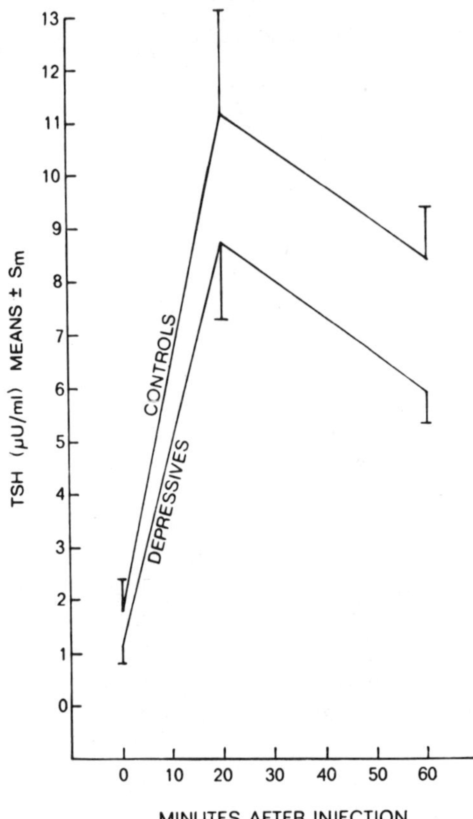

Figure 9 TSH response curves after administration of 500 μg TRH intravenously, showing mean increment in plasma TSH after 20 and 60 min for a sample of depressive patients ($n = 10$) and for a matched control group ($n = 23$). (Reprinted with permission from W. van den Burg et al., 1975. Cambridge University Press, publishers.)

sistent with the fact that the TSH response is restored when TRH administration is relatively prolonged, i.e., by continuous drip for a few hours (Fig. 10) (van den Burg et al., 1976).

G. Conclusions

The hormonal findings in vital depressions—particularly those concerning GH, LH, and cortisol—are consistent with the presence of a functional NA deficiency as postulated in the context of the MA hypotheses. The suggested relation is speculative, but this speculation is justifiable because it can be tested in a clinical setting. After all, the plausibility of such a relation would greatly increase if the disorders in central NA metabolism and those in the secretion of the abovementioned hormones were found to occur in patients of the same type.

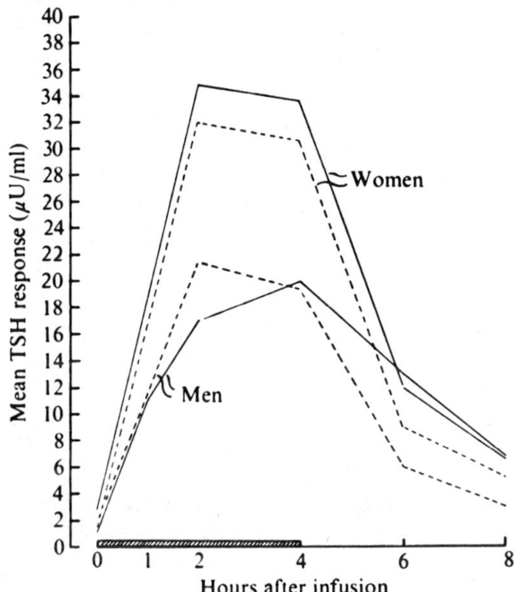

Figure 10 TSH response after a 4 hr infusion of 1000 μg TRH (striped bar on abscissa) in depressive patients (———) and in normal subjects (– – –); men and women separately plotted; the −½- and 0-hr values of the depressive patients were averaged, no 1-hr value was assessed in the normal group; standard deviations, omitted for the sake of clarity, were rather high. (Reprinted with permission from W. van den Burg, 1976. Cambridge University Press, publishers.)

V. IMPORTANCE OF DISORDERS OF MONOAMINE METABOLISM IN THE PATHOGENESIS OF DEPRESSIONS

A. MA Deficiency: Causative or Predisposing Factor?

The above findings warrant the following conclusions (which of course are still merely working hypotheses).

1. The group of vital depressions includes a subgroup with signs of central 5-HT deficiency. Precursor studies indicate the likelihood that this defect plays a role in the pathogenesis of depressions rather than being a consequence of them.
2. In depressions with marked motor retardation, central DA metabolism is diminished. In view of the results of precursor studies, this phenomenon seems to be causally related to the motor pathology.

3. Disorders of central NA metabolism also occur within the group of vital depressions, but it is uncertain whether they indicate a separate subgroup. Nor has it been established whether these disorders are causative or secondary phenomena.

Let us assume that at least the disorders of central 5-HT and DA metabolism are of importance in the pathogenesis of depressions. This assumption raises the following question: Do they play a role in manifestation of the depression, or do they represent a presidsposing factor? In the latter case the metabolic disorders would be an expression in biological terms, as it were, of the increased tendency of some individuals to respond to menacing internal or external (psychological or material) stimuli by developing a (vital) depression.

B. Longitudinal MA Studies

The only available strategy to gain some insight into the above-mentioned problem lies in longitudinal studies, i.e., studies of biochemical variables which are repeated when the patient has been free from symptoms and without medication for some time. Absence of the metabolic disorder on the second occasion argues in favor of its direct causative importance. Persistence indicates that it is more likely a predisposing factor. Pertinent data are available on the probenecid-induced accumulation of 5-HIAA and HVA in CSF (Table 4). The data show that the HVA response is normalized as retardation abates. The decreased 5-HIAA response, however, persists in the majority of patients. This prompted our hypothesis that central 5-HT deficiency is a factor presidposing to the development of the depression (van Praag, 1977d, 1979). This hypothesis was tested via two strategies:

1. Precursor studies. If the predisposition hypothesis is correct, then normalization of central 5-HT metabolism, e.g., with the aid of 5-HT precursors, could be expected to exert a stabilizing influence on the mood.

Table 4 Number of Depressive Patients After Probenecid Loading with Low or Normal Response of CSF 5-HIAA and CSF HVA Before Treatment and After Clinical Recovery

	Before treatment		After recovery	
Response	5-HIAA	HVA[a]	5-HIAA	HVA[a]
Low	19	15	10	1
Normal	31	35	40	49

[a]HVA is the main degradation product of DA.
Source: van Praag, 1977d.

2. Studies of the depression frequency in patients with and without demonstrable disorders of central 5-HT metabolism and in their respective relatives. The finding of an increased depression frequency in the 5-HT-deficient subgroup and their relatives would support the predisposition hypothesis.

C. 5-HTP Prophylaxis

The question as to whether chronic administration of 5-HTP reduces the frequency of vital depressions was studied in 20 patients, 5-HTP (200 mg/day) was always combined with a peripheral decarboxylase inhibitor (150 mg carbidopa/day); 5-HTP was given in tablets with a coating that does not dissolve until pH = 8.6 (in order to avoid gastrointestinal side effects).

The patients studied fulfilled the following criteria:

1. They were suffering from recurrent vital depressions.
2. The relapse rate was high: three or more depressive episodes in the preceding 4 years.
3. The probenecid-induced 5-HIAA accumulation was either persistently subnormal (i.e., demonstrable in depressive phases and in symptom-free intervals) or persistently normal; values below the lower limit of the range of variation in a control group were considered subnormal (van Praag et al., 1973).

Ten patients were given 5-HTP one year, and a placebo the next; in the other ten the order was reversed. At least once every 4 weeks the patients were seen for evaluation of the mental condition, scored on a 4-point overall rating scale and on the Hamilton scale for depressions. A relapse of depression was considered to have occurred if the overall score was 2 or 3, or if the Hamilton score exceeded 21. In that case clomipramine was prescribed (150-225 mg/day), in principle in an outpatient setting unless suicidal tendencies necessitated hospitalization.

The results of this study can be summarized as follows:

1. In both groups the depression frequency was significantly higher during the placebo than during the 5-HTP periods. This applies to the number of patients who showed a relapse as well as to the total number of relapses (Table 5).
2. Comparison of mean depression scores over the entire year reveals not only that the relapse rate differed but that the depressive morbidity over the entire 5-HTP period was lower than that in the placebo period (Fig. 11).

Table 5 Number of Patients Who Developed Relapses, and Number of Relapses, During Placebo and 5-HTP Medication[a]

Group	Number of test subjects	Number of patients who developed relapses		Number of relapses	
		Placebo period	5-HTP period	Placebo period	5-HTP period
A[b]	10	9	3	14	3
B[c]	10	8	3	10	4

[a]The difference in relapse rate is statistically significant both in group A ($P < .005$ sign test; $P < .05$ McNemar test) and in group B ($P < .05$ sign test; $P < .05$ McNemar test).
[b]One year of 5-HTP medication, followed by one year of placebo medication.
[c]One year of placebo medication, followed by one year of 5-HTP medication.

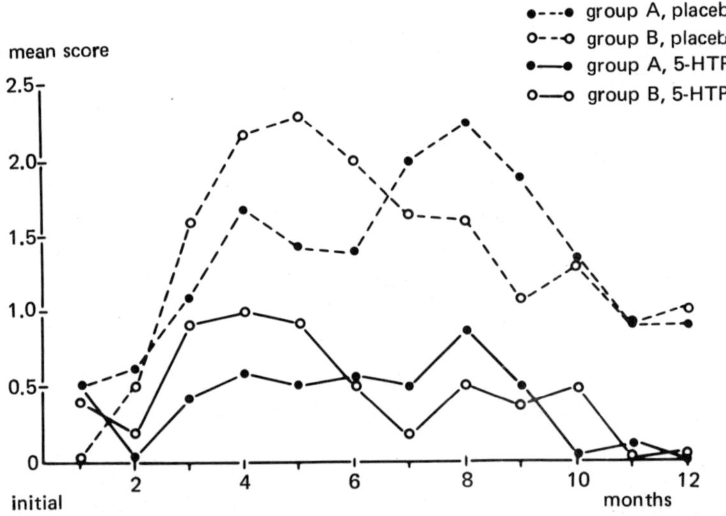

Figure 11 Mean depression score during 5-HTP and placebo medication on a 4-point depression scale in group A (1 year of 5-HTP follwed by 1 year of placebo medication) and group B (reversed sequence). The mean depression score over the placebo year significantly exceeds that over the 5-HTP year both in group A ($P = .001$, sign test) and in group B ($P = .001$, sign test). (From van Praag, 1979.)

Table 6 Number of Relapses During 5-HTP Periods in Patients with Normal and Subnormal Postprobenecid CSF 5-HIAA Concentrations[a]

Patients	Number of patients	Relapse during 5-HTP	No relapse during 5-HTP
Persistent normal postprobenecid CSF 5-HIAA	7	5	2
Persistent subnormal postprobenecid CSF 5-HIAA	13	1	12

[a] The relapse rate in the 5-HT deficient subgroup is significantly lower than that in the normoserotonergic subgroup ($P < .02$, Fisher's exact probability test, two-tailed). "Persistent" means: during depressive episodes *and* in symptom-free intervals.

3. The prophylactic effect of 5-HTP was significantly more pronounced in the group with persistently subnormal postprobenecid CSF 5-HIAA levels than in that without this metabolic disorder (Table 6).

We concluded that 5-HTP has a prophylactic effect on rapidly recurrent vital depressions, and that this effect seems most marked in the 5-HT-deficient subtype. Should these findings be corroborated, then 5-HTP prophylaxis is the first form of prophylaxis in psychiatry which is target-oriented, i.e., deliberately aimed at elimination of a suspected biological vulnerability factor.

D. Depression Frequency and 5-HT Deficiency

Patients in whom a possible relation between central 5-HT metabolism and depression frequency was studied, were selected as follows. In the past 10 years we examined 54 patients hospitalized with vital depressions characterized by subnormal postprobenecid CSF 5-HIAA values. This finding was persistent (demonstrable during depressive phases and symptom-free intervals) in 33. They constitute the low 5-HIAA group. During the same period we examined 69 other patients hospitalized with vital depressions characterized by a persistently normal 5-HIAA level. The 33 patients with the highest 5-HIAA values in this group constitute the normal 5-HIAA group (Table 7).

In these two groups, the number of psychiatric hospitalizations was established in interviews with the patient and a relative. The hospitalization data were verified by contacting the hospitals in question. Similar data were collected on these patients' closest relatives, i.e., their parents, grandparents, brothers, and sisters.

Table 7 Some Biographical and Diagnostic Data on Patients in the Subnormal and Normal 5-HIAA Groups

Data	Subnormal 5-HIAA group	Normal 5-HIAA group
Males	12	14
Females	21	19
Age	52 (37-62)	49 (34-64)
First depressive phase	5	9
Unipolar vital depression	18	19
Bipolar vital depression	10	5
Postprobenecid CSF 5-HIAA ± s.d.	39 ± 10.3	139 ± 36.7

In the patients themselves, the depression frequency proved to be significantly higher in the low 5-HIAA group than in the normal 5-HIAA group (Tables 8 and 9). A similar tendency was observed in their relatives: an increased depression frequency in the low 5-HIAA group (Table 10). It is still a moot question whether the relatives likewise show a disorder of 5-HT metabolism in the CNS. Investigation of this question encounters ethical problems with regard to (1) lumbar puncture; (2) the question of whether one may focus the attention of a group of individuals on the possibility of a familial increased depression vulnerability. Rates of hospitalization with other psychiatric syndromes did not significantly differ in the two groups.

A few years ago, Buchsbaum et al. (1976) carried out a similar study with regard to MAO activity in blood platelets. They studied normal test subjects and found that (1) this variable showed a marked range of variation and (2) low

Table 8 Psychiatric Morbidity in Subnormal (n = 33) and Normal (n = 33) 5-HIAA Groups

Number of admissions	Subnormal 5-HIAA group	Normal 5-HIAA group	Probability
For depression	89	61	$P < .002$
For mania	19	10	n.s.
For other psychiatric conditions	7	6	n.s.

Table 9 Frequency of Admission for Depression of Patients in the Subnormal and Normal 5-HIAA Groups[a]

Group	Number of admissions per patient for depression					Total number of admissions
	1	2	3	4	5	
Subnormal 5-HIAA	5	9	12	5	2	89
Normal 5-HIAA	9	20	4	–	–	61

[a]The number of hospitalizations for depression in the subnormal 5-HIAA group significantly exceeds that in the normal 5-HIAA group ($P < .002$, Mann-Whitney U test, two-tailed).

MAO activity was associated with increased psychiatric morbidity, not confined to depressions but involving psychiatric disorders in general (Table 11). Assuming that a MAO deficiency exists in the brain also, two hypotheses on a relation between our findings and those reported by Buchsbaum et al. are conceivable:

1. The 5-HT deficiency is a primary, and the diminished MAO activity a secondary phenomenon: an attempt to "save" 5-HT.
2. The diminished MAO activity is a primary, and the 5-HT deficiency a secondary phenomenon: an attempt to prevent "overproduction" of 5-HT.

Table 10 Psychiatric Morbidity in Relatives of Subnormal and Normal 5-HIAA Probands[a]

Reason for admission	Number of relatives admitted to psychiatric institution: Subnormal 5-HIAA group	Normal 5-HIAA group	Probability
Depression	138	67	$P < .001$
Mania	37	42	n.s.
Alcoholism	26	18	n.s.
Other psychiatric conditions	24	16	n.s.

[a]Relatives of low 5-HIAA probands has significantly more admissions for depression than relatives of normal 5-HIAA probands ($P < .001$, Mann-Whitney U test, two-tailed).

Table 11 Occurrence of Psychosocial Problems in Male Subjects and Their Familes in Relation to Platelet MAO

Psychosocial problems[a]	Low-MAO probands	High-MAO probands	Probability
In self	(n = 19)	(n = 17)	
Psychiatric contact	7	2	n.s.
Psychiatric hospitalization	2	0	n.s.
Convicted of offenses	7	0	.006
In jail	7	3	n.s.
Suicide attempts	2	0	n.s.
Any of above	12	5	.045
Psychiatric hospitalization, suicide attempt, conviction, or jail	10	3	.032
In family	(n = 17)	(n = 17)	
Psychiatric contact	7	9	n.s.
Psychiatric hospitalization	6	2	n.s.
Problems with the law	3	1	n.s.
Suicide or suicide attempts	6	1	.043
Any of above	11	10	n.s.
Psychiatric hospitalization, suicides or attempts, problems with the law	10	3	.016

[a]Subjects were questioned about sibs, parents, parents' sibs, and grandparents; information on a total of 203 relatives of low-MAO probands and 214 relatives of high-MAO probands was obtained. The table reports the number of probands with one or more family members exhibiting psychosocial problems; actual rates of occurrence in the family populations were higher. Two low-MAO individuals were adopted and therefore excluded as probands in tabulations of family problems. Probabilities for the Fisher exact probability test are given when $P < .05$, one-tailed.

Source: Reprinted with permission from M. S. Buchsbaum, R. D. Coursey, and D. L. Murphy (1976). *Science 199,* 339-341 (15 October). Copyright 1976 by the American Association for the Advancement of Science.

E. Conclusions

The influence of 5-HTP on central 5-HT is not "punctiform." It is also taken up in catecholaminergic nerve terminals, where dopa (= 5-HTP) decarboxylase converts it to 5-HT, which may function locally as a false transmitter. The combination of findings described—a prophylactic effect of 5-HTP in depressions and a correlation between a low (persistent) postprobenecid CSF 5-HIAA value and depression frequency–suggests, however, that the prophylactic effect of 5-HTP is related to the influence of this compound on the central 5-HT system.

Bearing this in mind, the findings discussed in this section warrant two conclusions:

1. Persistent disorders of central 5-HT metabolism increase the risk of development of vital depressions, i.e., they are a factor predisposing to depression;
2. The vulnerability to this type of depression can be reduced by increasing the amount of 5-HT available in the brain.

VI. MONOAMINE-SELECTIVE ANTIDEPRESSANTS

A. Developments

The classical antidepressants–tricyclic compounds and MAO inhibitors–exert a pronounced influence on central MA metabolism. They prompted studies of central MA metabolism in patients with depressions. As pointed out, this research has provided us with indications that, particularly in the group of vital depressions, disorders of central MA metabolism can play a pathogenetic role. These results in turn stimulated the development of pharmaceuticals with a selective effect on the central MA. In other words, pharmaceutical which exert their influence on one MAergic system in particular, leaving other systems more or less unaffected. Exponents of this development are the selective 5-HT reuptake inhibitors recently evolved by several pharmaceutical companies. Zimilidine is an example (Åberg and Holmberg, 1979). These compounds greatly inhibit the (re)uptake of 5-HT in synaptosomes, but exert little or no influence on the (re)uptake of catecholamines. This also applies to their metabolites. With the classical tricyclic antidepressant clomipramine (Anafranil) this is different. This compound likewise selectively inhibits 5-HT (re)uptake, but the desmethyl derivative which is its principal metabolite (Westenberg et al., 1977) is a pronounced NA reuptake inhibitor. The selective 5-HT reuptake inhibitors are still in an experimental stage, but preliminary experience with them has been promising (Siwers et al., 1977; Cox et al., 1978).

Substances with a similar selective effect on NA (re)uptake are also being developed (Saletu et al., 1977), but data on their clinical efficacy are not yet available. On the basis of the NA hypothesis, depressions have also been treated with β-adrenergic stimulants, particularly salbutamol. Successes of this strategy have been reported (Lecrubier et al., 1977).

The interest in selective DA agonists derives more from Parkinson research than from depression research. Nevertheless, these compounds have also been used in depressions; an example is piribedil (Post et al., 1978). The results correspond with those obtained with the DA precursor L-dopa (Section III.F).

Motor activity, if affected, is restored; but the influence of the mood level is inconsiderable.

B. Significance

For several reasons the development of MA-selective compounds is of great importance:

1. In practical terms, they will probably extend the possibilities of pharmacotherapy in depressions.
2. These agents can be expected to be most effective in patients with disorders of that MAergic system that is more or less selectively influenced by them. Their use, therefore, calls for a biochemical classification of depressive patients. This implies the operationalization of a fourth diagnostic dimension in psychiatry: pathogenesis, or the cerebral substrate that creates the instrumental conditions for the development of certain types of disturbed behavior. This can only enhance the conventional three-dimensional diagnosis based on the criteria symptomatology, etiology, and course.
3. Attempts to develop MA-selective compounds would probably never have been made without the results of biological depression research. They represent a promising example of a productive interaction between pharmacological and clinical research. Pharmaceuticals stimulate research into biological determinants of depressive behavior. And this research in turn stimulates the development of pharmaceuticals with a selective influence on certain systems of the cerebral apparatus which, it is suspected, make depressive behavior instrumentally possible.
4. All the conventional antidepressants have been chance findings, but the above-mentioned compounds are the products of purposeful research. Research based on a knowledge of the central substrates of depressive behavior (however fragmentary this knowledge may as yet be). This implies an essentially new course taken in psychopharmacology, a course which seems very promising.

VII. MODIFICATIONS OF THE MONOAMINE HYPOTHESES

A. Classical and Alternative MA Hypotheses

The classical MA hypothesis comprises two components:

1. A postulate on the mechanism of action of conventional antidepressants. Their therapeutic effect is claimed to be related to their ability to increase the amount of MA available at the central postsynaptic receptors. The decrease in MA synthesis observed after (chronic) administration of these compounds is regarded as a side effect secondary to the increased availability of transmitter substance.

2. A postulate on the pathogenesis of (certain types of) vital depressions. The signs indicative of MA deficiency are regarded as primary. That is to say, the subnormal neuronal activity of MAergic systems is considered to be the biological substrate of certain depressive symptoms (or syndromes).

Two observations cannot be readily reconciled with this hypothesis:

1. Reuptake inhibition and MAO inhibition in response to tricyclic antidepressants and MAO inhibitors, respectively, develop much earlier than the therapeutic effects, if any, which usually do not become apparent until 10-20 days later.
2. Chronic administration of tricyclic antidepressants and MAO inhibitors reduces the sensitivity of adenylcyclase in central NAergic systems (Sulser et al., 1978), a phenomenon which might indicate diminished NAergic receptor function.

In view of these facts, an alternative MA hypothesis was formulated (Bunney et al., 1977; Sulser et al., 1978; Aprison et al., 1978). This, too, has two components. The first postulates that the primary disorder in (certain types of) vital depression lies in hypersensitivity of postsynaptic 5-HT and/or NA receptors. The central MA deficiency suggested in these patients is secondary: an attempt to neutralize the hypersensitivity of the receptors. The second component postulates that the therapeutic efficacy of the conventional antidepressants is based on their ability to suppress MA synthesis. Thus they support the mechanism of neutralization already activated autochthonously. Diminished MA synthesis is interpreted, not as an accessory phenomenon but as reponsible for the therapeutic efficacy of these antidepressants.

B. Arguments in Favor of the Alternative MA Hypothesis

The two observations which could not be readily reconciled with classical MA hypotheses are in fact quite consistent with the alternative. Suppression of MA synthesis takes time, and this could explain the long latency of these compounds. The decreased NAergic receptor function after chronic administration of antidepressants is likewise consistent with the alternative hypothesis.

C. Observations at Odds with the Alternative and in Favor of the Classical MA Hypotheses

Observations at odds with the alternative and in favor of the classical MA hypotheses can be listed in concise form because most of them already have been discussed in the above.

1. According to the alternative hypothesis, antidepressants should initially cause aggravation of the depression, namely, when reuptake inhibition has occurred but MA synthesis inhibition has not. There are no indications of this.
2. Although little is known about the action of α-methyl-p-tyrosine and p-chlorophenylalanine (inhibitors of catecholamine and 5-HT synthesis, respectively), there is no indication that they might have an antidepressant effect.
3. The stimulant effect of L-dopa on motor activity and the antidepressant effect of 5-HTP argue strongly in favor of the classical hypotheses.
4. Studies of the function of the anterior lobe of the hypophysis also fail to support the alternative hypothesis (Section IV).

The long latency, moreover, is not inconsistent per se with the classical hypotheses. It should be borne in mind that a latent phase occurs not only with traditional antidepressants but also with 5-HTP. It is therefore conceivable that the capacity to synthesize 5-HT and NA is so reduced that after reuptake inhibition, inhibition of degradation, or precursor administration some time elapses before a sufficient amount of transmitter substance has accumulated at the postsynaptic receptor sites.

That receptor sensitivity might gradually diminish during antidepressant medication is not inconsistent per se with the classical hypotheses either. Increased availability of transmitter substance should induce compensatory mechanisms. One such mechanism we know: diminished synthesis of transmitter substance. If overstimulation is nevertheless imminent, then receptor sensitivity (synthesis) conceivably diminishes. Perhaps the ultimate balance between transmitter availability, transmitter synthesis, and receptor sensitivity is in fact individually variable.

D. Conclusions

The disorders of central MA metabolism found in (vital) depressions are for the time being best placed in the context of the classical MA hypothesis in which MAergic hypoactivity is the central postulate. An additional advantage of the "classical" theory is that, at least hypothetically, it affords an explanatory model for the fact that vital depression and (hypo)mania are relatively often observed in the same patients. As a result of transmitter deficiency, one may reason, the postsynaptic MAergic receptors become hypersensitive. If the production of transmitter substance increases at a given moment, for whatever reason, then the system enters a state of hyperactivity. This neuronal hyperactivity might induce the manic syndrome (Bunney, personal communication).

VIII. SUMMARY AND CONCLUSIONS

In view of all the findings obtained by the various research strategies (peripheral studies, postmortem studies of the brain, CSF studies with and without probenecid loading, hormonal studies, and pharmacological manipulation of central MA), one conclusion is inevitable: Disorders of central MA metabolism can be present in depressions and, more particularly, in the vital depressive syndrome.

This conclusion raises several questions. The first is whether these metabolic disorders play a role in the pathogenesis of the depression or represent a secondary phenomenon. With regard to the disorders in central 5-HT and DA metabolism, it seems justifiable at this time to conclude that they are causative. This conclusion is based on the observation that pharmacological interventions aimed at alleviation of the metabolic disorder lead to alleviation of the depressive symptoms. The DA disorders seem to be unmistakably related to motor pathology, whereas the 5-HT disorders may be more (or also) related to the disturbed mood regulation.

With regard to NA disorders there are no data either in favor of or against the plausibility of their playing a causative role in depressions.

Assuming that at least the 5-HT and DA disorders play a primary (i.e., causative) role, the question of the nature of this causality arises. Are they directly responsible for the development of the (or of certain) depressive symptoms, or is their signficance more that of a predisposing factor?

With regard to the DA disorders a direct causative role seems probable in view of the fact that they disappear as the depressive symptoms (particularly the motor symptoms) disappear.

With regard to 5-HT disorders, a predisposing role seems more plausible because in a majority of patients these disorders persist after abatement of the depression. Moreover, chronic 5-HTP medication reduces the relapse rate in these patients. Finally, it has been demonstrated that the risk of (vital) depression is increased in individuals with persistent 5-HT disorders. Whether the 5-HT disorders are related to instability of mood regulation or to other personality characteristics remains obscure.

MA research in depressions has given great impetus to purposeful efforts to develop MA-specific pharmaceuticals. It has thus introduced a new phase in psychopharmacology, which hitherto has been largely dependent on chance findings. In its turn, the development of MA-specific pharmaceuticals has led to intensification of the efforts to test the MA hypotheses on the pathogenesis of depressions in a clinical setting.

If anywhere, it is in the field of the depressions that the productiveness of the interaction between biological psychiatry and psychopharmacology can be demonstrated.

REFERENCES

Åberg, A., and Holmberg, J. (1979). Preliminary clinical test of Dimildine, a new 5-HT reuptake inhibitor. *Acta Psychiatr. Scand. 59,* 45-58.

Altman, N. E., Sachar, E. J., Gruen, P. H., Halpern, F. S., and Eto, S. (1976). Reduced plasma LH concentration in postmenopausal depressed women. *Psychosom. Med. 37,* 274-276.

Angst, J., Waggon, B., and Schoepf, J. (1977). The treatment of depression with 1-5-hydroxytryptophan versus imipramine. *Arch. Psychiatr. Nervenk. 224,* 175-186.

Aprison, M. H., Tahahashi, R., and Tachiki, K. (1978). Hypersensitive serotonergic receptors involved in clinical depression. A theory. In *Neuropharmacology and Behavior,* B. Haber and M. H. Aprison (Eds.), Plenum, New York, pp. 76-99.

Åsberg, M., Bertilsson, L., Tuck, D., Cronholm, B., and Sjöqvist, F. (1972). Indoleamine metabolites in the cerebrospinal fluid of depressed patients before and during treatment with nortriptyline. *Clin. Pharmacol. Ther. 14,* 227-286.

Åsberg, M., Thoren, P., Trashman, L., Bertilsson, L., and Ringberger, V. (1976). "Serotonin depression": a biochemical subgroup within the affective disorders? *Science 191,* 478-480.

Banki, C. M. (1977). Correlation between cerebrospinal fluid amine metabolites and psychomotor activity in affective disorders. *J. Neurochem. 28,* 255-257.

Beckman, H., and Goodwin, F. K. (1975). Antidepressant response to tricyclics and urinary MHPG in unipolar patients. *Arch. Gen. Psychiatry 32,* 17-21.

Berger, Ph.A. (1978). Medical treatment of mental illness. *Science 200,* 974-981.

Bowers, M. B., Jr. (1972). Cerebrospinal fluid 5-hydroxyindoleacetic acid (5-HIAA) and homovanillic acid (HVA) following probenecid in unipolar depressives treated with amitriptyline. *Psychopharmacologia 23,* 26-33.

Bowers, M. B., Jr. (1974). Amitriptyline in man: decreased formation of central 5-hydroxyindoleacetic acid. *Clin. Pharmacol. Ther. 15,* 167-170.

Boyd, A. E., and Reichlin, S. (1978). Neural control of prolactin secretion in man. *Psychoneuroendocrinology 3,* 113-130.

Brown, G. M., Seggie, J. A., Chambers, J. W., and Ettigi, P. G. (1978). Psychoendocrinology and growth hormone: a review. *Psychoneuroendocrinology 3,* 131-153.

Buchsbaum, M. S., Coursey, R. D., and Murphy, D. L. (1976). The biochemical high-risk paradigm: behavioral and familial correlates of low platelet monoamine oxidase activity. *Science 199,* 339-341.

Bunney, W. E., Jr., and Davis, J. M. (1965). Norepinephrine in depressive reactions: a review. *Arch. Gen. Psychiatry 13,* 483-494.

Bunney, W. E., Post, R. M., Andersen, A. E., and Kopanda, R. T. (1977). A hypothesised neuronal receptor sensitivity mechanism in affective illness. *Psychopharmacol. Comm. 1*, 393-406.

Carroll, B. J., Curtis, G. C., and Mendels, J. (1976). Neuroendocrine regulation in depression. I. Limbic system-adrenocortical dysfunction. I. Discrimination of depressed from nondepressed patients. *Arch. Gen. Psychiatry 33*, 1039-1044; *33*, 1051-1058.

Chase, T. N., Gordon, E. K., and Ng, L. K. Y. (1973). Norepinephrine metabolism in the central nervous system of man: studies using 3-methoxy-4-hydroxyphenylethylene glycol levels in cerebrospinal fluid. *J. Neurochem. 21*, 581-587.

Cohn, C. K., Dunner, D. L., and Axelrod, J. (1970). Reduced catechol-O-methyltransferase activity in red blood cells of women with primary affective disorder. *Science 170*, 1323-1324.

Coppen, A., Shaw, D. M., and Farrell, J. P. (1963). Potentiation of the antidepressive effects of a monoamine oxidase inhibitor by tryptophan. *Lancet 1*, 79-81.

Coppen, A. (1967). Biochemistry of affective disorders. *Br. J. Psychiatry 113*, 1237-1264.

Cox, J., Moore, G., and Evans, L. (1978). Zimildine: a new antidepressant. *Prog. Neuro-Psychopharmacol. 2*, 379-384.

Davson, H. (1967). *Physiology of the Cerebrospinal Fluid*, Churchill, London.

Dunner, D. L., Cohn, C. K., Gershon, E. S., and Goodwin, F. K. (1971). Differential catechol-O-methyltransferase activity in unipolar and bipolar affective illness. *Arch. Gen. Psychiatry 25*, 348-353.

Ebert, M., and Kopin, T. J. (1975). Differential labeling of origins of urinary catecholamine metabolites by dopamine C^{14}. *Trans. Assoc. Am. Phys. 28*, 256-264.

Ervin, G. V. (1973). Oxidative-reductive pathways for metabolism of aldehydes. In *Frontiers of Catecholamine Research*, E. Usdin and S. Snijder (Eds.), Pergamon, New York, pp. 161-166.

Garver, D. L., Pandey, G. N., Dekirmenjian, H., and Deleon-Jones, F. (1975). Growth hormone and catecholamines in affective disease. *Am. J. Psychiatry 132*, 1149-1154.

Goodwin, F. K., Brodie, H. K. H., Murphy, D. L., and Bunney, W. E., Jr. (1970). L-Dopa, catecholamines and behavior: a clinical and biochemical study in depressed patients. *Biol. Psychiatry 2*, 341-366.

Goodwin, F. K., Ebert, M. H., and Bunney, W. E., Jr. (1972). Mental effects of reserpine in man: a review. In *Psychiatric Complications of Medical Drugs*, R. I. Shader (Ed.), Raven, New York, pp. 73-101.

Goodwin, F. K., Cowdry, R., Gold, P. W., and Wehr, F. (1978a). Central monoamine metabolism in depression and mania. In *Neurotransmission and*

Disturbed Behavior. H. M. van Praag and J. Bruinvels (Eds.), Spectrum Publications, New York, pp. 34-60.

Goodwin, F. K., Muscettola, J., Gold, P. W., and Wehr, F. (1978b). Biochemical and pahrmacological differentiation of affective disorder: an overview. In *Psychiatric Diagnosis*, H. S. Akishal and W. C. Webb (Eds.), Spectrum Publications, New York, pp. 313-336.

Gottfries, C. G., Orland, L., Wiberg, A., and Winblad, B. (1975). Lowered monoamine oxidase activity in brains from alcoholic suicides. *J. Neurochem. 25*, 667-673.

Gruen, P. H., Sachar, E. J., Altman, N., and Sassin, J. (1975). Growth hormone response to hypoglycemia in postmenopausal depressed women. *Arch. Gen. Psychiatry 32*, 31-33.

Halbreich, H., Grunhaus, L., and Ben-David, M. (1979). Twenty-four-hour rhythm of prolactin in depressive patients. *Arch. Gen. Psychiatry 36*, 1183-1186.

Hollister, L. E., Kenneth, L. D., and Berger, P. A. (1976). Pituitary response to thyrotropin-releasing hormone in depression. *Arch. Gen. Psychiatry 33*, 1393-1396.

Jori, A., Dolfini, E., Casati, C., and Argenta, G. (1975). Effect of E.C.T. and imipramine treatment on the concentration of 5-HIAA and HVA in the cerebrospinal fluid of depressed patients. *Psychopharmacologia 44*, 87-90.

Kato, Y., Manakai, Y., Imura, H., Chihara, K., and Ohgo, S. (1974). Effect of 5-hydroxytryptophan (5-HTP) on plasma prolactin levels in man. *J. Clin. Endocrin. Metab. 38*, 695-697.

Landowski, J., Lysiak, W., and Angielski, S. (1975). Monoamine oxidase activity in blood platelets from patients with cyclophrenic depressive syndromes. *Biochem. Med. 14*, 347-354.

Langer, G., Heinze, G., Reim, B., and Matussek, N. (1976). Reduced growth hormone responses to amphetamine in "endogenous" depressive patients. *Arch. Gen. Psychiatry 33*, 1471-1475.

Lapin, I. P., and Oxenkrug, G. F. (1969). Intensification of the central serotonergic process as a possible determinant of the thymoleptic effect. *Lancet 1*, 132-136.

Lecrubier, Y., Jouvent, R., Puech, A. J., Simon, P., and Wildlöcher, D. (1977). Effect anti-depresseur d'un stimulant bêta-adrenergique. *Nouvelle presse medical 6*, 2786.

Lloyd, K. J., Farley, I. J., Deck, J. H. N., and Hornykiewicz, O. (1974). Serotonin and 5-hydroxyindoleacetic acid in discrete areas of the brainstem of suicide victims and control patients. *Ad. Biochem. Psychopharmacol. 11*, 387-397.

Matussek, N., Ackenheil, M., Hippius, H., Schröder, H.Th., Schults, H., and Wasilewski, B. (1977). *Effect of Clonidine on HGH Release in Psychiatry Patients and Controls.* L. Martini and F. W. Ganony (Eds.), VI. World Congress of Psychiatry, Hawaii.

Meek, J. L., and Neff, N. H. (1973). Is cerebrospinal fluid the major avenue for the removal of 5-hydroxyindoleacetic acid from the brain? *Neuropharmacology 12,* 497-499.

Mendels, J., Stinnet, J. L., Burns, D., and Frazer, A. (1975). Amine precursors and depression. *Arch. Gen. Psychiatry 32,* 22-30.

Moir, A. T. B., Ashcroft, G. W., Crawford, T. B. B., Eccleston, D., and Guildberg, H. C. (1970). Cerebral metabolites in cerebrospinal fluid as a biochemical approach to the brain. *Brain 93,* 357-368.

Murphy, D. L., and Weiss, R. (1972). Reduced monoamine oxidase activity in blood platelets from bipolar depressed patients. *Am. J. Psychiatry 128,* 1351-1357.

Murphy, D. L., and Wyatt, R. J. (1972). Reduced monoamine oxidase activity in blood platelets from schizophrenic patients. *Nature 238,* 225-226.

Murphy, D. L., Campbell, I. C., and Costa, J. L. (1978). The brain serotonergic system in the affective disorders. *Prog. Neuro-psychopharmacol. 2,* 1-31.

Nies, A., Robinson, D. S., Harris, L. S., and Lamborn, K. R. (1974). Comparison of MAO substrate activities in twins, schizophrenics, depressives and controls. *Psychopharmacol. Bull. 10,* 10-11.

Ojeda, S. R., and McCann, S. M. (1974). Evidence for participation of a catecholaminergic mechanism in the post-castration rise in plasma gonadotrophins. *Neuroendocrinology 12,* 295-315.

Oxenkrug, G. F., Prakhje, I., and Mikhalenko, I. N. (1978). Disturbed circadian rhythm of 5-HT uptake by blood platelets in depressive psychoses. *Activitas Nervosa Superior (Praha) 20,* 66-67.

Pletscher, A., Gey, K. F., and Zeller, P. (1960). Monoamin oxydase-hemmer. biochemie, chemie, pharmakologie, *Klin. Fortschr. Arzneimittelforsch. 2,* 417-590.

Pletscher, A. (1968). Monoamine oxidase inhibitors: effects related to psychostimulation. In *Psychopharmacology: A Review of Progress 1957-1967,* D. H. Eon (Ed.), Public Health Service Publications no. 1836, Washington, D.C., 649-655.

Post, R. M., and Goodwin, F. K. (1978). Approaches to brain amines in psychiatric patients: a reevaluation of cerebrospinal fluid studies. *Handbook Psychopharmacol. 13,* 147-185.

Post, R. M., Gerner, R. H., Carman, J. L., Gillin, Ch., Jimmerson, D. C., Goodwin, F. K., and Bunney, W. F. (1978). Effects of a dopamine agonist piribedil in depressed patients. *Arch. Gen. Psychiatry 35,* 609-615.

Prange, A. J., Jr., Wilson, I. C., Lara, P. P., Alltop, L. B., and Breese, G. R. (1972). Effects of thyrotropin releasing hormone in depression. *Lancet 11,* 999-1022.

Prange, A. J., Jr., Nemberoff, Ch. B., Lipton, M., Breese, G. R., and Wilson, I. C. (1978). Peptides and the central nervous system. *Handbook Psychopharmacol. 13,* 1-108.

Pühringe, W., Wirz-Justice, A., Graw, P., Lacoste, V., and Gastpar, M. (1976). Intravenous 1-5-hydroxytryptophan in normal subjects: an interdisciplinary precursor loading study. Part I. Implication of reproducible mood elevation. *Pharmakopsychiatrie Neuropsychopharmacol. 9,* 260-268.

Robinson, D. S., Nies, A., Ravaris, C. L., Ives, J. O., and Barlett, D. (1978). Clinical pharmacology of phenelzine. *Arch. Gen. Psychiatry, 35,* 629-638.

Roos, B. E., and Sjoström, R. (1969). 5-Hydroxyindoleacetic acid and homovanillic acid levels in the cerebrospinal fluid after probenecid application in patients with manic-depressive psychosis. *J. Clin. Pharmacol. 1,* 153-155.

Sachar, E. J. (1975). Neuroendocrine abnormalities in depressive illness. In *Topics in Psychoendocrinology,* E. J. Sachar (Ed.), Grune & Stratton, New York, p. 135.

Sachar, E. J., Hellman, L., Roffwarg, H. P., Halpern, F. S., Fukushima, D. K., Gallagher, R. F., and Bronx N.Y. (1973). Disrupted 24 hour patterns of cortisol secretion in psychotic depression. *Arch. Gen. Psychiatry 28,* 19-24.

Sachar, E. J., Gruen, P. H., Altman, N., and Sassin, J. (1976). Use of neuroendocrine techniques in psychopharmacological research. In *Hormones, Behavior and Psychopathology.* E. J. Sachar (Ed.), Raven, New York, p. 161.

Sack, R. L., and Goodwin, F. K. (1974). Inhibition of dopamine-β-hydroxylase in manic patients. *Arch. Gen. Psychiatry 31,* 649-654.

Saletu, B., Krieger, P., Grünberger, J., Schanda, H., and Sletten, I. (1977). Tandamine, a new norepinephrine reuptake inhibitor. *Pharmacopsychiatry 12,* 137-152.

Sano, I. (1972). L-5-hydroxytryptophan (1-5-HTO)-therapie bei endogener Depression. *Münchener Med. Wochenschr. 144,* 1713-1716.

Schildkraut, J. J. (1965). The catecholamine hypothesis of affective disorders: a review of supporting evidence. *Am. J. Psychiatry 122,* 509-522.

Schildkraut, J. J. (1975). Depressions and biogenic amines. In *American Handbook of Psychiatry.* VI. D. Hamburg (Ed.), Basic Books, New York.

Shaw, D. M., O'Keefe, R., and McSweeney, D. A. (1973). 3-Methoxy-4-hydroxyphenylglycol in depression. *Psychol. Med. 3,* 333-336.

Shopsin, B., Gershon, S., Goldstein, M., Friedman, E., and Wilk, S. (1974). Use of synthesis inhibitors in defining a role for biogenic amines during imipramine treatment in depressed patients. *Psychopharmacol. Bull. 10,* 52-55.

Shulman, R., Griffiths, J., and Diewold, P. (1978). Catechol-O-methyl transferase activity in patients with depressive illness and anxiety states. *Br. J. Psychiatry 132,* 133-138.

Sigg, E. B. (1968). Tricyclic thymoleptic agents and some newer antidepressants. In *Psychopharmacology. A Review of Progress 1957-1967.* D. H. Efron (Ed.), Public Health Service Publication no. 1836. Washington, D.C., pp. 655-671.

Siwers, B., Ringberger, V., Tuck, J. R., and Sjoqvist, F. (1977). Initial clinical trial based on biochemical methodology of zimildine (a serotonin uptake inhibitor in depressed patients). *Clin. Pharmacol. Ther. 21,* 194-200.

Sjöström, R., and Roos, B. E. (1972). 5-Hydroxyindoleacetic acid and homovanillic acid in cerebrospinal fluid in manic-depressive psychosis. *Eur. J. Clin. Pharmacol. 4,* 170-176.

Smith, L. T., Hanson, D. R., and Omenn, G. S. (1978). Comparison of serotonin uptake by blood platelets and brain synaptosomes. *Brain Res. 146,* 400-403.

Stahl, S. M. (1977). The human platelet: a diagnostic and research book for the study of biogenic amines in psychiatric and neurologic disorders. *Arch. Gen. Psychiatry 34,* 509-516.

Sulser, F., and Bass, A. D. (1968). Pharmacodynamic and biochemical considerations of the mode of action of reserpine-like drugs. In *Psychopharmacology: A Review of Progress 1957-1967,* D. H. Efron (Ed.), Public Health Service Publication no. 1836, Washington, D.C., pp. 1065-1077.

Sulser, F., Vetulani, J., and Mobley, Ph. L. (1978). Mode of action of antidepressant drugs. *Biochem. Pharmacol. 27,* 257-261.

Takahashi, S., Kondo, H., and Kato, N. (1975). Effect of 1-5-hydroxytryptophan on brain monoamine metabolism and evaluation of its clinical effects in depressed patients. *J. Psychiatr. Res. 12,* 177-187.

Tamarkin, N. R., Goodwin, F. K., and Axelrod, J. (1970). Rapid elevation of biogenic amine metabolites in human CSF following probenecid. *Life Sci. 9,* 1397-1408.

Trimble, M., Chadwick, D., Reynolds, E., and Marsden, C. D. (1975). L-5-hydroxytryptophan and mood. *Lancet 1,* 583.

Tuomisto, J., and Tuhiainen, E. (1976). Decreased uptake of 5-hydroxytriptamine in blood platelets from depressed patients. *Nature 262,* 596-598.

van den Burg, W., van Praag, H. M., Bos, E. R. H., Piers, D. A., van Zanten, A. K., and Doorenbos, H. (1976). TRH by slow continuous infusion: an antidepressant. *Psychol. Med. 6,* 393-397.

van den Burg, W., van Praag, H. M., Bos, E. R. H., van Zanten, A. K., Piers, D. A., and Doorenbos, H. (1975). TRH as a possible quick-acting but short-lasting antidepressant. *Psychol. Med. 5,* 404-412.

van Hiele, L. J. (1980). 5-hydroxytryptophan in depression. The first substitution therapy in psychiatry? *Neuropsychobiology 6,* 230-240.

van Loon, G. R. (1973). Brain catecholamines and ACTH secretion. In *Frontiers in Neuroendocrinology,* L. Martini and F W. Ganong (Eds.), Oxford University Press, New York, pp. 209-231.

van Praag, H. M. (1962). A critical investigation of the significance of MAO inhibition as a therapeutic principle in the treatment of depressions. Utrecht, Ph.D. thesis.

van Praag, H. M. (1974). Towards a biochemical typology of depressions? *Pharmacopsychiatry 7,* 281-292.

van Praag, H. M. (1977a). *Depression and Schizophrenia. A Contribution on Their Chemical Pathologies,* Spectrum Publications, New York.

van Praag, H. M. (1977b). Evidence of serotonin-deficient depression. *Neuropsychobiology 3,* 56-63.

van Praag, H. M. (1977c). The significance of dopamine for the mode of action of neuroleptics and the pathogenesis of schizophrenia. *Br. J. Psychiatry 130,* 463-474.

van Praag, H. M. (1977d). Significance of biochemical parameters in the diagnosis, treatment and prevention of depressive disorders. *Biol. Psychiatry 12,* 101-131.

van Praag, H. M. (1978a). Amine hypotheses of affective disorders. In *Handbook of Psychopharmacology, Vol. 13. Biology of Mood and Antianxiety Drugs,* L. L. Iversen, S. D. Iverson and S. H. Snijder (Eds.), Plenum, New York, Amsterdam, London.

van Praag, H. M. (1978b). *Psychotropic Drugs. A Guide for the Practitioner,* Brunner/Mazel, New York.

van Praag, H. M. (1978c). Neuroendocrine disorders in depression and their significance for the monamine hypothesis of depression. *Acta Psychiatr. Scand. 57,* 389-404.

van Praag, H. M. (1979). Central serotonin. Its relation to depression vulnerability and depression prophylaxis. In *Biological Psychiatry Today,* J. Obiols (Ed.). Elsevier/North Holland Biomedical Press, Amsterdam, pp. 1185-1198.

van Praag, H. M., and Korf, J. (1970). L-Tryptophan in depression. *Lancet 2,* 612.

van Praag, H. M., and Korf, J. (1971a). Endogenous depressions with and without disturbances in the 5-hydroxytryptamine metabolism: a biochemical classification? *Psychopharmacologia 19,* 148-152.

van Praag, H. M., and Korf, J. (1971b). Retarded depression and the dopamine metabolism. *Psychopharmacologia 19,* 199-203.

van Praag, H. M., and Korf, J. (1975). Central monoamine deficiency in depression: causative or secondary phenomenon? *Pharmakopsychiatria 8,* 321-326.

van Praag, H. M., Korf, J., and Puite, J. (1970). 5-Hydroxyindoleacetic acid levels in the cerebrospinal fluid of depressive patients treated with probenecid. *Nature 225,* 1259-1260.

van Praag, H. M., Korf, J., Dols, L. C. W., and Schut, T. (1972). A pilot study of the predictive value of the probenecid test in application of 5-hydroxytryptophan as antidepressant. *Psychopharmacologia 25,* 14-21.

van Praag, H. M., Korf, J., and Schut, T. (1973). Cerebral monoamines and depression. An investigation with the probenecid technique. *Arch. Gen. Psychiatry 28,* 827-831.

van Praag, H. M., Korf, J., Lakke, J. P. W. F., and Schut, T. (1975). Dopamine metabolism in depressions, psychoses and Parkinson's disease: the problem of the specificity of biological variables in behaviour disorders. *Psychol. Med. 5,* 138-146.

van Praag, H. M., Korf, J., and Lequin, R. M. (1976). An unexpected effect of 1-5-hydroxytryptophan-ethylester combined with a peripheral decarboxylase inhibitor on human serum prolactin. *Psychopharmacol. Comm. 2,* 369-378.

van Putten, T., May, P. R. A. (1978). Akinetic depression in schizophrenia. *Arch. Gen. Psychiatry 35,* 1101-1107.

van Scheyen, J. D., van Praag, H. M., and Korf, J. (1977). A controlled study comparing nomifensine and clomipramine in unipolar depression, using the probenecid technique. *Br. J. Clin. Pharmacol. 4,* 179S-184S.

van Woert, M. H., Rosenbaum, D., Howieson, J., and Bowers, M. B. (1977). Long term therapy of myoclonus and other neurological disorders with 1-5-hydroxytryptophan and carbidopa. *N. Engl. J. Med. 296,* 70-75.

Walinder, J., Skott, A., Carlsson, A., Nagy, A., and Roos, B. E. (1976). Potentiation of the antidepressant action of clomipramine by tryptophan. *Arch. Gen. Psychiatry 33,* 1384-1387.

Westenberg, H. G. M., de Zeeuw, R. A., de Cuyper, H. J. A., van Praag, H. M., and Korf, J. (1977). Bioanalysis and pharmacokinetics of clomipramine and desmethylclomipramine in man by means of liquid chromatography. *Postgrad. Med. J. 53 suppl. 4,* 124-130.

Whitlock, F. A., and Evans, L. E. J. (1978). Drugs and depression. *Drugs 15,* 53-71.

Yuwiler, A., Geller, E., and Eidulson, S. (1959). Studies on 5-hydroxytryptophan decarboxylase. I. In vitro inhibition and substrate interaction. *Arch. Biochem. 80,* 162-173.

4

Electrolyte Metabolism and Manic-Melancholic Disorder

Erling T. Mellerup and Ole J. Rafaelsen
Psychochemistry Institute, Rigshospitalet
Copenhagen, Denmark

I. INTRODUCTION

The biological basis of mental disease, including manic-melancholic disorder, is not fully understood. Theories, ideas, and concepts change following advances in the fields of neurochemistry, neuroendocrinology, and neurophysiology. For more than 10 years monamines have been the focus of research in biological psychiatry; now receptors, neuropeptides, and hypothalamic hormones are also entering the scene, and membranes, pumps, and specific brain proteins are waiting behind. However, among the first biological variables studied in mental disease were the electrolytes, mainly sodium, potassium, and calcium; anions and trace elements have also been investigated. Despite the interest in other variables, research in electrolyte metabolism of psychiatric patients has continued and is still carried out.

There are several reasons for studying electrolyte metabolism in connection with mental disease. First is the profound knowledge of the role of cations in nearly all aspects of nerve cell function. Second, it is also known that disturbances in peripheral electrolyte metabolism very often are accompanied by mental symptoms. Third, the use of lithium salts in the treatment of manic-melancholic disorders has emphasized the possible role of other cations. Finally, the results up till now of the studies of electrolyte metabolism in manic-melancholic patients are such that it is still impossible to decide whether electrolytes are involved or not involved in the biology of affective illness.

II. ROLE OF CATIONS IN NERVOUS FUNCTION

The two properties which are the basis for the integrated functions of neurons are nerve cell excitability and synaptic transmission. Both of these phenomena depend on a very precise regulation of extracellular and intracellular concentrations as well as transmembranal movements of sodium, potassium, magnesium, and calcium.

The excitability of a nerve cell is due to the high concentration of potassium inside the cell and the high concentration of sodium outside the cell. This uneven distribution is caused by the Na^+-K^+-ATPase sodium pump located in the membrane which transports sodium out of cell and potassium into the cell against concentration gradients. In a resting nerve cell the permeability of potassium is higher than that of sodium. This means that the resting electrical potential of the cell is due mainly to uneven potassium distribution. When the cell is stimulated chemically or electrically changes occur in the cell membrane, making the membrane much more permeable to sodium. As a consequence, the electrical potential changes from the resting (potassium) potential of about −60 mV to the action (sodium) potential of about +20 mV. The magnitudes of these potentials obviously depend on the concentration gradients of potassium and sodium. Thus, when potassium is increased extracellularly, the resting potential is diminished (tends to depolarize, approaches zero). When intracellular sodium, on the other hand, is increased, the positive peak of the action potential decreases or may even disappear. It is seen that both these changes could be brought about by inhibition of the sodium pump in the cell membrane; but other factors may also influence the distribution and permeability of sodium and potassium. Studies of brain slices have thus shown that both sodium and potassium content of the brain tissue strongly depend on the calcium concentration in the surrounding fluid (Lolley and McIlwain, 1964). In addition, the excitability is influenced by calcium and magnesium; low extracellular concentrations of these divalent cations cause hyperexcitability, which may go as far as constant spontaneous firing of the nerve cell (Lorente de Nó, 1947), and the resting conductance to potassium as well as the increased flow of potassium during depolarization is dependent on the concentration of intracellular calcium (Meech, 1974; Eckert and Tillotson, 1978).

The synaptic transmission is the transmission of a signal, the nerve impulse, across the synaptic cleft. Presynaptically, the electrical impulse causes the release of a neurotransmitter into the synaptic cleft, and this substance by diffusion reaches the postsynaptic membrane, where it is bound to a specific receptor, which in turn initiates an action potential. The whole mechanism of this phenomenon, and particularly the coupling between the depolarization and the release of neurotransmitters, is strongly infuenced by cations.

The most investigated cation in this respect is calcium. In the last century it was observed that calcium was necessary in the bathing fluid for neuromuscular impulse transmission to occur (Locke, 1894). In recent years it has been found that calcium has to cross the presynaptic membrane, or more correctly that intracellular calcium has to increase before neurotransmitter release takes place (Katz and Miledi, 1967; Miledi, 1973; Llinás and Nicholson, 1975).

Intracellular calcium concentration is very low compared with extracellular concentration, and as depolarization of a nerve terminal leads to an increased calcium permeability, calcium will enter the nerve terminal after an action potential as the result of the electrochemical gradient across the membrane. Accordingly, the amount of neurotransmitter released is related to the extracellular calcium concentrations (Dodge and Rahaminoff, 1967). However, neurotransmitter secretion may also be triggered alone by calcium ions released from intracellular stores (Katz and Edwards, 1973). The storage system for calcium in the cell consists of a sarcoplasmic reticulum-like system (Kendrick et al., 1977), calcium-binding macromolecules, including membrane components (Oschman et al., 1974; Baker and Schlaepfer, 1975), synaptic vesicles (Politoff et al., 1974), and mitochondria (Scarpa, 1976). All these mechanisms are responsible for the immediate return to low calcium concentrations after a transient increase, whereas the permanent steady-state concentration gradient is due to the calcium efflux across the nerve membrane (Blaustein and Oborn, 1975; Mullins and Brinley, 1975). In relation to the biogenic amine hypotheses for manic-melancholic disorders, all these neurochemical findings may be of potential interest because disturbances in any of the mechanisms regulating intra- as well as extracellular calcium concentrations may lead to changes in neurotransmitter secretion of a kind postulated to be important for affective disorders. The fact that reserpine is one of the many metabolic inhibitors or drugs which affect the storage of calcium is of particular interest. This drug has been found to decrease brain calcium, probably by releasing calcium from a cellular storage before the well-known reserpine induced decrease in noradrenaline, dopamine, and serotinin was seen. Furthermore, injection of calcium before reserpine administration prevented not only the decrease of brain calcium but also the depletion of cerebral monamines (Boyaner and Radouco-Thomas, 1971; Radouco-Thomas et al., 1971).

It should be emphasized that calcium is important not only in the presynaptic part of the synaptosomal complex but also at the postsynaptic membrane. It has been suggested that calcium may serve to couple hormone-receptor interaction to the following intracellular or membrane-located effects (Douglas, 1968; Rasmussen, 1970), and other studies have indicated that calcium ions are essential for the inhibitory effects of biogenic amines on cortical neurones (Yarbrough et al., 1974).

The function of the other cations in synaptic transmission does not seem to be of the same importance as that of calcium, and often their influence may be seen as secondary to their effect on calcium. Thus, with respect to the release of neurotransmitters, magnesium seems to be antagonistic to calcium (Hutter and Kostial, 1954), and the same may be true for sodium because it has been found that calcium releases more neurotransmitter when the incubation medium has a low sodium concentration (Rahaminoff and Colomo, 1967). The rate of calcium entry into synaptosomes increases with increasing extracellular potassium concentrations (Blaustein, 1975), whereas calcium efflux is coupled to sodium influx (Blaustein and Russell, 1975).

It should also be mentioned that oubain, which inhibits the sodium pump, also inhibits the uptake of biogenic amines into nerve endings, and that sodium and potassium are necessary for the uptake and storage of noradrenaline and serotonin (Hughes and Brodie, 1959; Bogdanski et al., 1968).

III. MENTAL SYMPTOMS IN DISORDERS OF PERIPHERAL ELECTROLYTE METABOLISM

Considering the importance of cations for nervous function, one would anticipate that disturbances in electrolyte metabolism generally are accompanied by mental symptoms. However, this seems not to be true in contrast to neurological symptoms commonly found. Mental abnormalities are often seen in both Cushing's disease and Addison's disease, but in these conditions many other parts of the overall metabolism are changed, and thus the mental disturbances may be caused by several other factors than changes in electrolyte metabolism. Reduction in serum sodium is seen in a number of conditions such as diarrhea, vomiting, profuse sweating, excessive diuresis, low salt intake, and psychogenic diabetes insipidus. The symptoms in these cases are mostly somatic but may include drowsiness, apathy, confusion, coma, and convulsions. Mental symptoms are, rare, however. Similarly, disorders with excess of sodium in the body are known in several conditions, e.g., diarrhea without corresponding loss of sodium and renal disorders. Also in such cases a number of neurological symptoms are found without obvious mental changes (Ford, 1973). Hypokalemia and hyperkalemia, where the changes in potassium are of a magnitude that can lead to cardiac failure, may alter the electroencephalogram but have not been clearly associated with changes in mood or behavior (Baer, 1973). High doses of magnesium may have narcotic and antiepileptic activity whereas magnesium deficiency is accompanied by a large number of neurological symptoms, but psychotic behavior has also been described in this condition (Wallach et al., 1962).

Again with respect to disorders of calcium metabolism, neurological signs and symptoms are usual, but in these patients psychiatric manifestation are commonly found. All kinds of mental symptoms have been described, including cyclic manic-depressive states. In one study of patients with secondary hypoparathyroidism after surgical removal of the parathyroids, the decrease in serum calcium was correlated with the increase in depression measured on a rating scale (Christie-Brown, 1968). In hyperparathyroidism emotional disturbances are among the mental changes found in this condition, and the affective disturbances may often be the first psychic symptoms. The severity of the mental changes was proportional to the level of serum calcium and independent of the cause of the hypercalcemia (Smith et al., 1972).

IV. LITHIUM AND OTHER CATIONS

Although sodium, potassium, magnesium, and calcium not are the only metal cations occurring in biological systems, they are the only ones occurring in relatively high concentrations because all the other biologically important cations are found only as trace elements. Furthermore, these other cations are often strongly bound to transport proteins or enzymes, which means that the concentrations of the free ions are extremely low. However, due to the use of lithium in the treatment of manic-melancholic disorders, many patients now have a fifth "major" cation in their body. Despite the fact that lithium normally does not occur in biological systems, except for trace amounts, and that no known biochemical or physiological role exists for this ion, lithium is tolerated in the body year after year in concentrations around 1 mmol/liter, a concentration as high as serum magnesium and serum ionized calcium.

Lithium is the third element in the periodic system and the first of the alkali metals; accordingly, it is similar in many respects to sodium and potassium, and also (due to the so-called diagonal realtionship) to magnesium and calcium. The lithium ion has one positive charge like sodium and potassium, a radius similar to that of the magnesium ion, and a charge density close to that of the calcium ion (Mellerup and Jørgensen, 1975). Theoretically, the lithium ion might thus be handled in the organism by the same mechanisms as the other cations. This is also true for some systems, e.g., it is well known that lithium is the only other metal cation able to replace sodium in the fluid surrounding an isolated neuron, without changing the resting or the action potential. Another example is that lithium in the kidney is handled like sodium in the proximal tubules (Thomsen et al., 1969). In certain experimental settings lithium, like calcium and magnesium, may increase the stimulation threshold for nerve excitability (Ichiokia, 1955). Also, like calcium and magnesium, lithium may be found in higher concentrations in bone than in any other tissue (Birch and Hullin, 1972). Such examples emphasize the possibility that lithium may to varying degrees replace or compete with sodium, potassium, magnesium, and calcium at any place these cations are bound or transported, thereby explaining all lithium effects, including the psychotrophic effects, as secondary to a primary change in the function of a cation at some pertinent site. The actual changes in cation metabolism during lithium treatment are mentioned in connection with the following review of the single cations.

V. ELECTROLYTE METABOLISM IN MANIC-MELANCHOLIC PATIENTS

A. Sodium

Sodium is probably the most studied cation, apart from lithium, in manic-melancholic patients. Several studies have found serum sodium values to be in the normal range (Altschule, 1953; Bjørum, 1972; Bech et al., 1978), and CSF values have been reported normal (Bech et al., 1978) as well as slightly decreased (Ueno et al., 1961) and slightly increased (Bjørum et al., 1972a). Urinary studies have in some cases shown that sodium is retained in the organism during a depressed phase (Klein and Nunn, 1945; Ström-Olsen and Weil-Malherbe, 1958). However, in a balance study of 15 depressed patients who were in a metabolic ward from 14 to 35 days, recovery from depression did not induce any significant change in the balance of sodium (Russell, 1960).

Sodium metabolism in manic-melancholic patients has also been studied by techniques more elaborate than blood, urine, and CSF concentration analyses. Coppen (1960) analyzed the transfer of sodium from serum to CSF in depressed patients. Radioactive sodium was injected intravenously, lumbar puncture was performed 60 min later, and from the radioactivity measurements the rate of entry of sodium into CSF could be calculated. The procedure was repeated when the patients had recovered, and it was found that sodium in depressed patients entered the CSF at a rate which was about half of the values after recovery and half that of control patients. The results were not due merely to a general decreased fluid transfer because control studies with tritiated water revealed no differences between the transfer in depressed and neutral phases. This study has been partially repeated by other groups. In one of the studies the patients were compared with a control group of schizophrenic patients, and no significant difference in transfer rate was obtained; however, a small group of severely depressed patients showed lower values than the whole group of depressed patients (Fotherby et al., 1963). In a study of 11 patients, 7 showed an increase in transfer rate after recovery, while 4 were unchanged or decreased; the statistical analysis showed no significant change (Carroll et al., 1969). The study of Baker (1971) showed that manic as well as depressed patients had significantly lower transfer rates than a group of control patients. Carroll (1972) not only retested his own patients, but also pooled the results from all the studies, and from this he concluded that both manic and depressed patients had a significantly lower transfer rate for sodium than recovered patients and controls.

Radioactive sodium has also been used in order to determine the amount of exchangeable body sodium and in three studies the results indicated that exchangeable sodium decreased upon recovery from depression (Gibbons, 1960; Shaw and Coppen, 1966; Baer et al., 1969). When in addition to exchangeable sodium extracellular volume and therefore extracellular sodium were estimated, it was possible to calculate the difference between exchangeable sodium and extracellular sodium. This difference, called residual sodium, supposedly consisted of all intracellular sodium and some of the bone sodium. Using these methods, Coppen and his co-workers (Coppen et al., 1966; Shaw and Coppen, 1966) reported that residual sodium decreased upon recovery from both depression and mania. Provided that exchangeable bone sodium is independent of changes in mood, the results indicated that intracellular sodium was higher during the depressed phase and decreased following recovery. This finding was even more pronounced in manic patients. In relation to these studies it has also been observed that depressed patients had a relatively increased intracellular waterspace and a decreased extracellular space (Hullin et al., 1967) and that a shift of fluid from intracellular to extracellular spaces took place during improvement (Brown et al., 1963). The results of such studies are difficult to interpret, first because the procedure includes the difference between two large indirect measurements, body sodium and extracellular volume, giving rise to high statistical uncertainty, and second because bone sodium may not necessarily be independent of mood changes.

Direct analysis of the sodium content in the brains of deceased patients showed that sodium concentrations were lower in the brains of depressed suicides (Shaw et al., 1969) but the changes were small.

In addition, red blood cells have been used in the study of sodium metabolism in manic-melancholic patients. Sodium content of red blood cells was higher in depression than after recovery (Naylor et al., 1971); in mania, on the other hand, sodium content was reduced (Glen and Reading, 1973). The Na^+, K^+-dependent ATPase activity in red blood cells was found to be correlated with the degree of depression in endogenous depression but not in neurotic depression (Dick et al., 1972). In manic patients the red blood cell sodium pump activity was low during maina as well as during remission (Hokin-Neaverson et al., 1974).

Among the large number of studies of sodium metabolism in manic-melancholic patients, a few seem to have shown consistent changes. The low transfer rate of sodium from blood to CSF, may reflect a low rate of turnover of sodium by the nervous system, thus being consistent with the postulated increase in intracellular sodium and therefore also with an increased retention of sodium during depression. The explanations for such findings may be changes in the sodium pump activity, in the aldosterone secretion (Murphy et al., Burney, 1969; Alsoop et al., 1972) in kidney function, in acid base metabolism, or in the calcium content of the cell membranes (Triggle, 1972).

Regardless of the mechanism behind the possible changes in sodium metabolism, another question is what influence these changes may have on the course of the illness. Even if they are secondary to some basic mechanism directly involved in the etiology of the mental disturbance, changes in sodium metabolism may inevitably influence all excitable cell membranes including nerve cells.

B. Potassium

Serum potassium in manic-melancholic patients has been reported as normal (Altschule, 1953; Bech et al., 1978), increased (Jacobi, 1925; Klemperer, 1925; Sharma et al., 1970), and decreased (Bjϕrum, 1972). In a more elaborate study in which total extracellular and intracellular potassium were stimated, no changes in any of the variables were found when the patients were examined in depressed phase and after recovery (Coppen and Shaw, 1963). In a balance study in which patients were studied during a depressive phase from a treatment period to recovery, no changes in potassium metabolism were found (Russell, 1960). Urinary studies of depressed patients and a control group of neurotic patients showed no difference between the two groups, either in total output of potassium or in diurnal fluctation (Lobban et al., 1963). In a longitudinal study of two patients on a fixed diet with regular changes between depression and mania, it was found that excretion of potassium decreased in mania and increased in depression (Cookson et al., 1969). In CSF one study showed a slight increase in potassium concentration in depressed patients compared with control persons (Bjϕrum et al., 1972a), whereas another study found no differences (Bech et al., 1978).

In three patients with alternating periods of mania and depression, sweat potassium was found to be about 10 times as high during mania as during depression (Paschalis et al., 1977).

Lithium treatment seems not to alter potassium metabolism very much; plasma levels are unchanged and, except for an initial small increase, urine excretion of potassium is unchanged (Hullin, 1975; Saran and Russell, 1976). Sleep deprivation and tricyclic antidepressants did not change serum potassium but the ratio between erythrocytes and serum potassium decreased with both treatments (Bojanovsky et al., 1974).

Whole-body counting has been used to estimate total body potassium (Platman et al., 1970), and total brain potassium concentration has been measured in the brain of suicide patients (Shaw et al., 1969); however, neither of the methods uncovered significant changes between depressed patients and controls.

C. Magnesium

The role of magnesium in manic-melancholic disorders has not been very intensively investigated, and the few studies have not been in agreement, i.e., serum magnesium has been reported as unchanged (Naylor et al., 1972), elevated (Cade 1964; Bjørum, 1972), or decreased (Frizel et al., 1969). In one study serum magnesium in depressed females was lower than in depressed males, although such a difference was not observed in controls (Herzberg and Herzberg, 1977).

Magnesium concentrations in CSF in depressed patients were not different from those of controls and did not change upon recovery (Dreyer and Quadbeck, 1965; Bjørum et al., 1972a; Bech et al., 1978).

In one study it was found that urinary magnesium increased during recovery from depression (Bjørum et al., 1972b). With respect to treatment it is noteworthy that lithium in most studies increases serum magnesium (Nielsen, 1964; Aronoff et al., 1971; Christiansen et al., 1975; Mellerup et al., 1976). This seems to be a very specific lithium effect because no other treatment or condition (except for renal failure) is known to increase serum magnesium.

D. Calcium

Despite the role of calcium in both nerve cell excitability and synaptic transmission, and despite the reports of mental disturbances in hypo- and hypercalcemic states, calcium metabolism has not been thoroughly studied in manic-melancholic patients. One reason for this might be that the studies that have been done generally do not support the hypothesis that calcium metabolism should be changed in these patients.

Most studies of serum calcium in manic-melancholic patients have not shown any consistent changes when the patients were compared before and after recovery or were compared with various control groups (Weston and Howard, 1922; Jacobi, 1925; Klemperer, 1925; Frizel et al., 1969; Faragalla and Flach, 1970; Naylor et al., 1972; Bojanovsky et al., 1974; Bech et al., 1978). Two studies found a statistically significant decrease of serum calcium after recovery from depression (Bjørum, 1972; Carman et al., 1977). However, none of these studies measured ionized calcium or corrected the serum calcium for possible changes in protein concentration. Serum calcium shows a distinct diurnal variation, which, however, is due solely to changes in serum protein concentrations and thereby to the changes in the protein-bound fraction of calcium. When corrections are made for the changes in protein concentration, serum calcium is almost constant throughout the 24-hr period (Mellerup et al., 1976). In a study of ECT-treated manic-melancholic patients, a decrease in serum calcium was found very shortly after the ECT treatment, but also this decrease could be accounted for by changes in serum protein concentrations (Mellerup et al., 1979). Sleep deprivation therapy is followed by an increase in serum calcium at the first day after the sleep deprivation (Bojanovsky et al., 1974), and lithium therapy is also accompanied by slight increases in serum calcium (Christiansen et al., 1975; Mellerup et al., 1976).

CSF calcium has been analyzed in a few studies with manic-melancholic patients; no differences were found when calcium concentrations before and after recovery were compared, or when the patients were compared with control groups (Scholberg and Goodall, 1926; Katzenelbogen, 1935; Bjørum et al., 1972a; Bech et al., 1978). In a group of patients treated with ECT, CSF calcium was decreased in all patients 1 hr after the last ECT compared with pretreatment values. In patients who had a third determination of CSF calcium 2 weeks later, the reduction in calcium concentration persisted (Carman et al., 1977). When patients treated with tricyclic antidepressants and those treated with ECT were compared both before and 1 week after recovery from depression, no changes in CSF calcium could be demonstrated (Mellerup et al., 1979).

Urinary calcium excretion has been found to be within normal range in manci-melancholic patients (Malleson et al., 1968; Bjørum et al., 1972b). However, some investigators observed that during recovery from depression urinary calcium excretion decreased (Flach, 1964; Flach and Faragalla, 1970; Fischbach, 1971; Ferrari, 1973). When balance techniques and isotopes were used to study calcium metabolism in depressed patients, it was found that recovery was associated with increased calcium absorption from the gut, or decreased urinary excretion, or both (Faragalla and Flach, 1970). In this connection it is of interest that lithium treatment is followed by an immediate reduction in urinary calcium excretion (Crammer, 1975; Bjørum et al., 1975), which persists during several years of lithium treatment (Mellerup et al., 1976). In balance studies lithium treatment induces not only a decrease in urinary calcium but also an increased absorption of calcium from the gut (Plenge and Rafaelsen, 1981).

Paradoxically, this increase in the body content of calcium seems to be associated with a decrease in bone mineral content in manic-melancholic patients treated with lithium (Christiansen et al.,1975; Baastrup et al.,1978). In connection with the latter results it should be noted that a high incidence of osteoporosis has been observed among depressed female patients (Varga et al.,1968; Faragalla and Flach, 1970).

The old observation that a large proportion of manic-melancholic patients have a body build of the pycnic type has not lead to further investigations into bone physiology or bone metabolism of the patients and of the pycnic group in general.

VI. CONCLUSION AND SUMMARY

The strongest evidence for the hypothesis that electrolytes, and particularly cations, should be of etiological importance for affective disorders is probably our knowledge of the importance of these cations for nearly all aspects of nerve function. With respect to a multifaceted function calcium is by far the most interesting cation in the nervous system and, accordingly, the one which should be involved in the biology of mental disturbances.

Generally, however, disturbances in peripheral electrolyte metabolism are not accompanied by mental symptoms. Neurological symptoms may be much more common, and even in cases of hyper- and hypoparathyroidism where psychiatric symptoms have been described such symptoms are not seen in all patients. One explanation for this situation is that electrolyte metabolism in the brain to a certain degree may be regulated independent of peripheral electrolyte metabolism, first because the permeability of the blood-brain barrier is very low for cations and second because active mechanisms, in, e.g., the choroid plexus or the glia cells may regulate the ionic composition of the extracellular milieu of the central nervous system. The fact that changes in serum calcium concentrations in some cases can give rise to mental symptoms may perhaps be an indication of a higher permeability of the blood-brain barrier in smaller parts of the brain, e.g., the hypothalamic area.

The effect of lithium in the treatment of manic-melancholic disorders is another bit of evidence favoring the electrolyte hypothesis. The suggestion that the effects of lithium are primarily brought about by lithium-induced changes in function and metabolism of the other cations may eventually be tested if similar changes, e.g., an increase in serum magnesium, could be produced by some other kind of treatment.

Finally, the changes in electrolyte metabolism in manic-melancholic patients are small and normal conditions seem to be the general rule. Although many kinds of findings have been reported, a single finding which everybody can agree upon does not exist at this time.

Two kinds of changes have been repeatedly reported by independent workers. One is based on different findings in sodium metabolism which all suggest that sodium may be retained in the body during depression, eventually due to an increase in intracellular concentration. The other is the observation that calcium excretion is decreased upon recovery from depression. Both findings may be secondary to increased secretion of cortical steroids. And for both findings it is unknown as to whether they have any influence on the brain.

There are several explanations as to why the many studies of electrolyte metabolism have failed to demonstrate more consistent changes in manic-melancholic patients. The first is that such changes are not in any way related to affective disturbances. However, this possibility cannot be proven by the existing data. Another explanation is that manic-melancholic patients are heterogenous from a biological point of view, and thus electrolyte disturbances may only be of etiological importance in a subgroup. A third possibility is that the pertinent variables have not yet been studied. It is obvious that the function of a cation in a biological system always depends on the enzyme, the binding site, the transport mechanism, the membrane protein, etc., with which the cation reacts. Such cation-binding molecules are well known, and it might be fruitful to study this field in relation to affective disorders. It is also known that the balance of cations and the ratio between them might be more important than their individual concentrations (Burton, 1972). This point of view may prove useful in the study of electrolyte metabolism in manic-melancholic patients.

REFERENCES

Alsopp, M. N. E., Levell, M. J., Stitch, S. R., and Hullin, R. P. (1972). Aldosterone production rates in manic-depressive psychosis. *Br. J. Psychiatry 120,* 399-404.

Altschule, M. D. (1953). *Bodily Physiology in Mental and Emotional Disorders,* Grune & Stratton, New York.

Aranoff, M. S., Evens, R. G., and Durell, J. (1971). Effect of lithium salts on electrolyte metabolism. *J. Psychiatr. Res. 8,* 139-159.

Baastrup, P. C., Christiansen, C., and Transbøl, I. (1978). Calcium metabolism in lithium-treated patients. *Acta Psychiatr. Scand. 57,* 124-128.

Baer, L. (1973). Electrolyte metabolism in psychiatric disorders. In *Biological Psychiatry,* J. Mendels (Ed.), Wiley, New York, pp. 199-234.

Baer, L., Durrell, J., Bunney, W. E., Levy, B. S., and Cardon, P. V. (1969). Sodium-22 retention and 17-hydroxycorticosteroid excretion in affective disorders: a preliminary report. *J. Psychiatr. Res. 6,* 289-297.

Baker, E. F. W. (1971). Sodium transfer to cerebrospinal fluid in functional psychiatric illness. *Can. Psychiatr. Assoc. J. 16,* 167-170.

Baker, P. F., and Schlaepfer, W. (1975). Calcium uptake by axoplasm extruded from giant axons of *Loligo*. *J. Physiol. 249,* 37P-38P.

Bech, P., Kirkegaard, C., Bock, E., Johannesen, M., and Rafaelsen, O. J. (1978). Hormones, electrolytes, and cerebrospinal fluid proteins in manic-melancholic patients. *Neuropsychobiology 4,* 99-112.

Birch, N. J., and Hullin, R. P. (1972). Distribution and binding of lithium following its long-term administration. *Life Sci. 11,* 1095-1099.

Bjφrum, N. (1972). Electrolytes in blood in endogenous depression. *Acta Psychiatr. Scand. 48,* 59-68.

Bjφrum, N., Plenge, P., and Rafaelsen, O. J. (1972a). Electrolytes in cerebrospinal fluid in endogenous depression. *Acta Psychiatr. Scand. 48,* 533-539.

Bjφrum, N., Mellerup, E. T., and Rafaelsen, O. J. (1972b). Electrolytes in urine in endogenous depression. *Acta Psychiatr. Scand. 48,* 337-349.

Bjφrum, N., Hornum, I., Mellerup, E. T., Plenge, P. K., and Rafaelsen, O. J. (1975). Lithium, calcium, and phosphate. *Lancet 1,* 1243.

Blaustein, M. P. (1975). Effects of potassium, veratridine, and scorpion venom on calcium accumulation and transmitter release by nerve terminals *in vitro*. *J. Physiol. 247,* 617-655.

Blaustein, M. P., and Oborn, C. J. (1975). The influence of sodium on calcium fluxes in pinched-off nerve terminals *in vitro*. *J. Physiol., 247,* 657-686.

Blaustein, M. P., and Russell, J. M. (1975). Sodium-calcium exchange in interally dialyzed squid giant axons. *J. Membr. Biol., 22,* 285-312.

Bogdanski, D. F., Tissani, A., and Brodie, B. B. (1968). The effects of inorganic ions on uptake, storage, and metabolism of biogenic amines in nerve endings. In *Psychopharmacology: A Review of Progress 1957-1967,* D. H. Efron (Ed.), Public Health Service, Washington, D.C., pp. 17-26.

Bojanovsky, J., Koch, W., and Tölle, R. (1974). Elektrolytveränderungen unter antidepressiver Therapie. *Arch. Psychiatr. Nervenkr. 218,* 379-386.

Boyaner, H. G., and Radouco-Thomas, S. (1971). Effect of calcium on reserpine-induced catalepsy. *J. Pharm. Pharmacol. 23,* 974-975.

Brown, D. G., Hullin, R. P., and Roberts, J. M. (1963). Fluid distribution and the response of depression to E.C.T. and imipramine. *Br. J. Psychiatry 109,* 395-398.

Burton, R. F. (1973). The balance of cations in the plasma of vertebrates and its significance in relation to the properties of cell membranes. *Comp. Biochem. Physiol. 44A,* 781-792.

Cade, J. F. J. (1964). A significant elevation of plasma magnesium levels in schizophrenia and depressive states. *Med. J. Aust. 1,* 195-196.

Carman, J. S., Post, R. M., Goodwin, F. K., and Bunney, W. E. (1977). Calcium and electroconvulsive therapy of severe depressed patients. *Biol. Psychiatry 12,* 5-17.

Carroll, B. J. (1972). Sodium and potassium transfer to cerebrospinal fluid in severe depression. In *Depressive Illness. Some research studies,* B. Davies, B. J. Carroll, and R. M. Mowbray (Eds.), Thomas, Springfield, Ill. pp. 247-257.

Carroll, B. J., Steven, L., Pope, R. A., and Davies, B. (1969). Sodium transfer from plasma to CSF in severe depressive illness. *Arch. Gen. Psychiatry 21,* 77-81.

Christiansen, C., Baastrup, P. C., and Transbøl, I. (1975). Osteopenia and dysregulation of divalent cations in lithium treated patients. *Neuropsychobiology 1,* 344-354.

Christie-Brown, J. R. W. (1968). The psychiatric aspects of disturbed calcium metabolism. *Proc. Roy. Soc. Med. 61,* 1121-1123.

Cookson, B. A., Huszka, L., Quarrington, B., and Stancer, H. (1969). Longitudinal studies of diurnal excretion patterns in two cases of cyclical affective disorder. *J. Psychiatr. Res. 7,* 63-81.

Coppen, A. J. (1960). Abnormality of the blood-cerebrospinal fluid barrier of patients suffering from a depressive illness. *J. Neurol. Neurosurg. Psychiatry 23,* 156-161.

Coppen, A., and Shaw, D. M. (1963). Mineral metabolism in melancholia. *Br. Med. J. 2,* 1439-1444.

Coppen, A., Shaw, D. M., Malleson, A., and Costain, R. (1966). Mineral metabolism in mania. *Br. Med. J. 1,* 71-75.

Crammer, J. (1975). Lithium, calcium, and mental illness. *Lancet 1,* 215-216.

Dick, D. A. T., Dick, E. G., le Poidevin, D., and Naylor, G. J. (1972). Sodium and potassium transport in depressive illness. *J Physiol. 227,* 30-31P.

Dodge, F. A., Jr., and Rahamimoff, R. (1967). Cooperative action of calcium ions in transmitter release at the neuromuscular junction. *J. Physiol. 193,* 419-432.

Douglas, W. W. (1968). Stimulus-secretion coupling: the concept and clues from chromaffin and other cells. *Br. J. Pharmacol. 34,* 451-474.

Dreyer, U., and Quadbeck, G. (1965). Der Gehalt der Liquor cerebrospinalis an Magnesium und andere Kationen bei zentralnervösen Erkrankungen. *Dtsch. Z. Nervenheilk. 187,* 595-607.

Eckert, R., and Tillotson, D. (1978). Potassium activation associated with intraneuronal free calcium. *Science 200,* 437-439.

Faragalla, F. F., and Flach, F. F. (1970). Studies of mineral metabolism in mental depression. *J. Nerv. Ment. Dis. 151,* 120-129.

Ferrari, G. (1973). On some biochemical aspects of affective disorders. *Riv. Sper. Freniat. 97,* 1167-1175.

Fischbach, R. (1971). Veränderungen des Calcium-Stoffwechsels bei Depressionen während der Verabreichung von Thymoleptica. *Arzneimittel-Forsch. 21,* 27-28.

Flach, F. F. (1964). Calcium metabolism in states of depression. *Br. J. Psychiatry 110,* 588-593.

Flach, F. F., and Faragalla, F. F. (1970). The effects of imipramine and electric convulsive therapy on the excretion of various minerals in depressed patients. *Br. J. Psychiatry 116,* 437-438.

Ford, F. R. (1973). *Disease of the Nervous System,* 6th ed., Thomas, Springfield, Ill.

Fotherby, K., Ashcroft, G. W., Affleck, J. W., and Forrest, A. D. (1963). Studies on sodium transfer and 5-hydroxyindoles in depressive illness. *J. Neurol. Neurosurg. Psychiatry 26,* 71-73.

Frizel, D., Coppen, A., and Marks, V. (1969). Plasma magnesium and calcium in depression. *Br. J. Psychiatry 115,* 1375-1377.

Gibbons, J. L. (1960). Total body sodium and potassium in depressive patients. *Clin. Sci. 19,* 133-138.

Glen, A. I. M., and Reading, H. W. (1973). Regulatory action of lithium in manic-depressive illness. *Lancet 2,* 1239-1241.

Herzberg, L., and Herzberg, B. (1977). Mood change and magnesium. *J. Nerv. Ment. Dis. 165,* 423-426.

Holin-Neaverson, M., Spiegel, D. A., and Lewis, W. C. (1974). Deficiency of erythrocyte sodium pump activity in bipolar manic-depressive psychosis. *Life Sci. 15,* 1739-1748.

Hughes, F. B., and Brodie, B. B. (1959). The mechanism of serotonin and catacholamine uptake by platelets. *J. Pharmacol. Exp. Ther. 127,* 96-102.

Hullin, R. P. (1975). The effects of lithium on electrolyte balance and body fluids. In *Lithium Research and Therapy,* F. N. Johnson (Ed.), Academic, London, pp. 359-379.

Hullin, R. P., Bailey, A. D., McDonald, R., Dransfield, G. A., and Milne, H. B. (1967). Body water variations in manic-depressive psychosis. *Br. J. Psychiatry 113,* 584-592.

Hutter, O. F., and Kostial, K. (1954). Effect of magnesium and calcium ions on the release of acetylcholine. *J. Physiol. (London) 124,* 234-241.

Ichioka, M. (1955-56). The effects of Na, K, Ca and Li upon threshold and 'latency' at a node of Ranvier. *Jap. J. Physiol. 5,* 222-230.

Jacobi, W. (1925). Ueber den Calcium und Kalium-Blutserumspiegel bei katatonen Erregungszuständen, chronischen Schizophrenien und Melancholien im Klimakterium. *Mschr. Psychiatr. Neurol. 59,* 130-139.

Katz, N. L., and Edwards, C. (1973). Effects of metabolic inhibitors on spontaneous and neurally evoked transmitter release from frog motor nerve terminals. *J. Gen. Physiol. 61,* 259.

Katz, B., and Miledi, R. (1967). A study of synaptic transmission in the absence of nerve impulses. *J. Physiol. 192,* 407-436.

Katzenelbogen, S. (1935). *The Cerebrospinal Fluid and Its Relation to the Blood,* Johns Hopkins Press, Baltimore.

Kendrick, N. C., Blaustein, M. P., Fried, R. C., and Ratzlaff, R. W. (1977). ATP-dependent calcium storage in presynaptic nerve terminals. *Nature 265,* 246-248.

Klein, R., and Nunn, R. F. (1945). Clinical and biochemical analysis of a case of manic-depressive psychosis showing regular weekly cycles. *J. Ment. Sci. 91,* 79-88.

Klemperer, E. (1925). Untersuchungen über den Stoffwechsel bei manishen und depressiven Zustandsbildern. Veränderungen des Kalzium- und Kaliumspiegels des Gesamtblutes. *Jb. Psychiatr. Neurol. 45,* 32-62.

Llinás, R., and Nicholson, C. (1975). Calcium role in depolarization-secretion coupling: an aequorin study in squid giant synapse. *Proc. Nat. Acad. Sci. USA 72,* 187-190.

Lobban, M., Tredre, B., Elithorn, A., and Bridges, P. (1963). Diurnal rhythms of electrolyte excretion in depressive illness. *Nature 199,* 667-669.

Locke, F. S. (1894). Notiz über den Einfluss physiologischer Kochsalzlösung auf die elektrische Erregbarkeit von Muskel und Nerv. *Zantralbl. Physiol. 8,* 166-167.

Lolley, R. N., and McIlwain, H. (1964). Effects of calcium on sodium and potassium of mammalian cerebral tissue. *Biochem. J. 93,* 12P-13P.

Lorento de Nó, R. (1947). A study of nerve physiology. *Stud. Rockefeller Inst. Med. Res. 132.*

Malleson, A., Frizel, D., and Marks, V. (1968). Ionized and total plasma calcium and magnesium before and after modified E.C.T. *Br. J. Psychiatry 114,* 631-633.

Meech, R. W. (1974). Prolonged potentials in aplysia neurons injected with EGTA. *Comp. Biochem. Physiol. A48,* 397-402.

Mellerup, E. T., and Jørgensen, O. S. (1975). Basic chemistry and biological effects of lithium. In *Lithium Research and Therapy,* F. N. Johnson (Ed.), Academic, New York, pp. 353-358.

Mellerup, E. T., Lauritsen, B., Dam, H., and Rafaelsen, O. J. (1976). Lithium effects on diurnal rhythm of calcium, magnesium and phosphate metabolism in manic-melancholic disorder. *Acta Psychiatr. Scand. 53,* 360-370.

Mellerup, E. T., Bech, P., Sørensen, T., Fuglsang-Frederiksen, A., and Rafaelsen, O. J. (1979). Calcium and electroconvulsive therapy of depressed patients. *Biol. Psychiatry 14,* 711-714.

Miledi, R. (1973). Transmitter release induced by injection of calcium ions into nerve terminals. *Proc. R. Soc. B183,* 421-425.

Mullins, L. J., and Brinley, F. J., Jr. (1975). Sensitivity of calcium efflux from squid axons to changes in membrane potential. *J. Gen. Physiol. 65,* 135-152.

Murphy, D. L., Goodwin, F. K., and Bunney, W. E., Jr. (1969). Aldosterone and sodium response to lithium administration in man. *Lancet 2,* 458-460.

Naylor, G. J., McNamee, H. B., and Moody, J. P. (1971). Changes in erythrocyte sodium and potassium on recovery from a depressive illness. *Br. J. Psychiatry 118,* 219-223.

Naylor, J., Fleming, L. W., Stewart, W. K., McNamee, H. B., and le Poideven, D. (1972). Plasma magnesium and calcium levels in depressive psychosis. *Br. J. Psychiatry 120,* 683-684.

Nielsen, J. (1964). Magnesium-Lithium Studies 1. *Acta Psychiatr. Scand. 40,* 190-196.

Oschman, J. L., Hall, T. A., Peters, P. D., and Wall, B. J. (1974). Association of calcium with membranes of squid giant axnon: ultrastructure and microprobe analysis. *J. Cell. Biol. 61,* 156-165.

Paschalis, C., Jenner, F. A., Lee, C. R., Hill, S. E., Jennings, G., and Triccas, G. (1977). Sweat electrolytes in manic-depressive illness. *Lancet 2,* 502.

Platman, S. R., Fieve, R. R., and Pierson, R. N. (1970). Effects of mood and lithium carbonate on ttal body potassium. *Arch. Gen. Psychiatry 22,* 297-300.

Plenge, P., and Rafaelsen, O. J. (1981). Lithium effects on calcium, magnesium and phosphate balance in man. To be publsihed.

Politoff, A. L., Rose, S., and Pappas, G. D. (1974). The calcium binding sites of synaptic vesicles of the frog sartorius neuromuscular junction. *J. Cell. Biol. 61,* 818-823.

Radouco-Thomas, S., Tessier, L., Lajeunesse, N., and Garcin, F. (1971). Role of calcium in the reserpine-induced cerebral monamines depletion. *Int. J. Clin. Pharmacol. 5,* 5-11.

Rahamimoff, R., and Colomo, F. (1967). Inhibitory action of sodium ions on transmitter release at the motor end-plate. *Nature 215,* 1174-1176.

Rasmussen, H. (1970). Cell communication, calcium ion, and cyclic adenosine monophosphate. *Science 170,* 404-412.

Russell, G. F. M. (1960). Body weight and balance of water, sodium and potassium in depressed patients given electroconvulsive therapy. *Clin. Sci. 19,* 327-336.

Saran, B. M., and Russell, G. F. M. (1976). The effects of administering lithium carbonate on the balance of Na, K, and water in manic-depressive patients. *Psychol. Med. 6,* 381-392.

Scarpa, A. (1976). Kinetic and thermodynamic aspects of mitochondrial calcium transport. In *Mitochondria Bioenergetics, Biogenesis and Membrane Structure,* L. Packer and A. Gómez-Puyou (Eds.), Academic, New York, pp. 31-45.

Sharma, S. D., Shah, P. B., and Acharya, P. T. (1970). Urinary 17-hydroxycorticosteroids levels and urine electrolytes in depression. *Dis. Nerv. Syst. 31*, 343-347.

Shaw, D. M., and Coppen, A. (1966). Potassium and water distribution in depression. *Br. J. Psychiatry 112*, 269-276.

Shaw, D. M., Frizel, D., Camps, F. E., and White, S. (1969). Brain electrolytes in depressive and alcoholic suicides. *Br. J. Psychiatry 115*, 69-77.

Smith, C. K., Barish, J., Correa, J., and Williams, R. H. (1972). Psychiatric disturbance in endocrinologic disease. *Psychosom. Med. 34*, 69-86.

Ström-Olsen, R., and Weil-Malherbe, H. (1958). Humoral changes in manic-depressive psychosis with particular reference to the excretion of catechol amines in urine. *J. Ment. Sci. 104*, 696-704.

Thomsen, K., Schou, M., Steiness, I., and Hansen, H. E. (1969). Lithium as an indicator of proximal sodium reabsorption. Pflügers Arch. Europ. *J. Physiol. 308*, 180-184.

Triggle, D. J. (1972). Effects of calcium on excitable membranes and neurotransmitter action. *Progress in Surface and Membrane Science 5*, 267-331.

Ueno, Y., Aoki, N., Yabuki, T., and Kuraishi, F. (1961). Electrolyte metabolism in blood and cerebrospinal fluid in psychoses. *Folia Psychiatr. Neurol. Jap. 15*, 304-326.

Varga, E., Csaba, C., Holló, and Koref, O. (1968). Androgen deficit and osteoporosis in depressed female patients. *Activ. Nerv. Sup. 10*, 12-14.

Wallach, S., Cahill, L. N., Rogan, F. H., and Jones, H. L. (1962). Plasma and erythrocyte magnesium in health and disease. *J. Lab. Clin. 59*, 195-210.

Weston, P. G., and Howard, M. Q. (1922). The determination of Na, Ca, and Mg in the blood and spinal fluid of patients suffering from manic-depressive insanity. *Arch. Neurol. Psychiatry 8*, 179-183.

Yarbrough, G. G., Lake, N., and Phillis, J. W. (1974). Calcium antagonism and its effect on the inhibitory actions of biogenic amines on cerebral cortical neurones. *Brain Res. 67*, 77-88.

5

Course of Affective Disorders

Jules Angst
Psychiatric University Clinic
Zurich, Switzerland

I. INTRODUCTION

Interest in the course of psychiatric disorders is historically old. Kraepelin had already based his dichotomy of schizophrenia and affective disorders on the course and outcome of the two groups; since then many studies have been devoted to the problem. Since the introduction of modern drug treatments of affective disorders, mainly the long-term lithium or antidepressant treatment, there is a new and increasing interest in the natural or spontaneous course in the evaluation of treatments. Another significant question concerns the variables (sex, age, personality, etc.) that could influence the prognosis of affective disorders. Finally, it is of great interest to develop mathematical models for the prognosis.

Research on the course of affective disorders is full of pitfalls:

1. The natural or spontaneous course cannot be studied separately from the treated course. All over the world patients suffering from depression or mania are treated and we do not know to what extent the course is modified by this type of treatment. There do not exist any studies of representative samples of patients that give reliable prospective data.

2. All studies on the course of affective disorders are either retrospective or both retrospective and prospective. The ideal of a purely prospective study cannot be realized. In many instances the patient had already suffered from several episodes before consulting a medical doctor. An affective disorder, especially a bipolar manic-depressive disorder, can last for decades and therefore a prospective study would be a work of several generations of research workers. There is a loss of information in retrospective data and we may miss a lot of milder episodes or hypomanic syndromes. Figures on morbidity of affective disorders are therefore minimal figures.

3. The patient samples studied up to now are not at all representative of the population of the patients. Epidemiological studies have shown that not more than 10% of the patients are likely to be hospitalized or seen by a psychiatrist. Most of the patients with depression are treated by general practitioners or are not treated at all. Therefore the studies that are usually carried out, which are based on hospitalized patients, cannot be completely representative. Future research in that field is needed.

4. A substantial error in studies on the course of affective disorders is created by the change of diagnosis (Angst et al., 1978). Unipolar depressions may change prospectively into bipolar affective illness or schizoaffective psychoses; the latter is also true for bipolar manic-depressive disorders. Furthermore, an original diagnosis of reactive or neurotic depression may have to be changed in the future to "affective psychosis."

The aim of this chapter is to describe the results of a new follow-up study of originally hospitalized patients with affective disorders based on the dichotomy of the diagnoses of unipolar depressions (ICD 296.2 + 296.0) and bipolar psychoses (ICD 296.1 + 296.3).

II. PATIENT SAMPLE AND METHODOLOGY

The patient sample consists of all hospital admissions to the Psychiatric University Clinic Burghölzli in Zurich during the years 1959-1963. All patients with a diagnosis of ICD 296 (affective psychosis) were selected ($n = 254$). First admissions and readmissions were included. The patients were originally examined between 1959 and 1963 during their stay in the hospital and some of the findings for a part of the sample were published in a monograph in 1966. The original sample described in the monograph comprised only patients who were admitted with a depressive syndrome. Since then this sample has been complemented by another group of bipolar patients admitted with a manic syndrome.

The study consists of a retrospective period until 1959 and a prospective period since 1959. Follow-up examinations were carried out every fifth year in 1965, 1970, and 1975. Furthermore, many patients were seen in between because they had to be treated again. The follow-up was usually done by a telephone interview with the patient and at least one of his next relatives, and by letter to the doctors who were in charge of the patients. Furthermore, all available records were studied. At each follow-up a standardized set of questions was asked about necessity of treatment, capacity to work, and manifestations of secondary cases in the families. A last investigation was carried out by two co-workers (Frey and Felder) in 1975.

Eleven patients dropped out of the study; eight were excluded because they were foreigners and no further information on them could be obtained; another three had to be dropped for other reasons (one with a wrong diagnosis, and two were excluded erroneously). Two patients with a chronic course of depression were excluded because they would have disturbed most of the analyses of the remaining 159 unipolar depressed patients.

Table 1 gives some descriptive information about the patient sample: There are some marked differences between bipolar affective disorder ($n = 95$) and unipolar depression ($n = 159$). Thus we found 37% of the total sample to be bipolar. The sex ratio in both samples favors the females especially in unipolar depression. This sex difference results not only from social factors determining the hospital admission; in unipolar depression especially, a true difference is also to be found in epidemiological investigations of a normal population. The two diagnostic groups are also described in terms of "early onset" and "late onset" cases, dichotomized at the age of 50. It shows that 15% of the bipolar and 45% of the unipolar patients have a late onset of the disorder. The latter were usually called late or involutional depression. But from a genetic point of view they belong to unipolar depression (Angst, 1966).

Thirty-seven percent of the bipolar versus fifty-nine percent of the unipolar patients were first admissions when they entered the study in the period 1959-1963. The lower first admission rate of bipolar patients is explained by the higher frequency of ambulatory episodes before their first hospitalization, mainly due to hypomanic syndromes.

The average age at the final follow-up shows a difference between the two groups: 61 years in the bipolar and 64 years in the unipolar sample. The former

Table 1 Patient Sample

Diagnosis	Bipolar affective Illness, ICD 296.3 + 296.1		Unipolar depression, ICD 296.2 + 296.0		*P*
	n	%	*n*	%	
Number of patients	95	37	159	63	
Sex: males	37	39	39	25	.05
females	58	61	120	75	
Early onset (<50 years)	81	85	88	55	.001
Late onset (⩾50 years)	14	15	71	45	
First admissions (when entering the study)	35	37	94	59	.001
Readmission (when entering the study)	60	63	65	41	
Patients who died	26	27	66	42	n.s.
(dead by suicide)	3	3	16	10	
In years	$\bar{x}$	s	$\bar{x}$	s	
Age at first onset	34.7	13.9	45.3	16.6	.001
Age at final follow-up	61.0	13.2	64.3	13.9	.001
Average duration of observation	26.4	11.9	19.0	11.4	.001
Duration of illness	23.8	12.5	13.9	11.7	.001

has been observed on the average during 26 and the latter during 19 years. The difference is explained by the earlier onset of the bipolar group (34.7 versus 45.3 years). The death rate is higher in the unipolar (42%) than in the bipolar (27%) depressed group. It can be explained to some extent by the age difference but is also influenced by the marked difference of the suicide rate (3% versus 10%).

III. RESULTS

In this section the course of bipolar and monopolar depressive affective illness is described comparatively in terms of the following characteristics: age at first onset, total number of episodes, length of episodes, length of cycles, outcome, couse of syndromes in bipolar affective illness, and typology of bipolar affective disorder.

A. Age at First Onset

As mentioned in Table 1, the age of first onset of bipolar patients is significantly lower than that of monopolar depressive patients (34.7 ± 13.9 versus 45.3 ± 16.6). This difference is well known (Angst, 1966; Perris, 1966). A more interesting question is the distribution of the age of first onset shown in histograms. Kraepelin's original data based on 903 cases showed a unimodal distribution with a peak at the age of 20, but Slater's data (1938) based on 2532 cases showed a bimodal distribution also confirmed by Kielholz (1959), who found a first peak between 26 and 30 years and a second between 41 and 45 years (n = 232).

In an international cooperative study (Angst et al., 1973) of 1027 patients with affective disorders we found again a bimodal distribution and explained it first by the difference in age of onset between patients with bipolar and unipolar disorders. This explanation cannot be maintained any more because we now have the same trend in a more homogeneous group of bipolar affective illness as shown in Figure 1.

In bipolar illness we find a first peak of the manifestation between 20 and 29 years and a second between 40 and 49, especially between 45 and 49. There is a trend to a difference between males and females, the latter being more prone to have a late manifestation perhaps connected with the menopause. However, a similar trend for males cannot yet be excluded because the figures available are too few. The question as to whether the age of onset of bipolar patients shows a bimodal distribution is of great importance because it may point to a heterogeneity of that group. The distribution may be discussed again for subtypes of bipolar patients (see Section III.G).

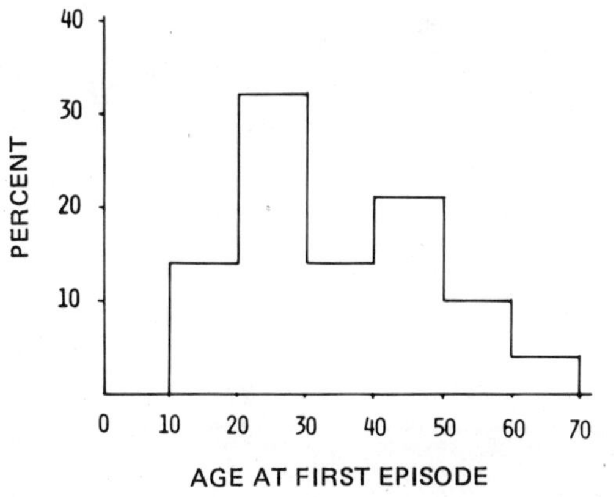

Figure 1 Hererogeneity of bipolar illness. Bipolar psychoses (n = 95) and age at first episode.

There may be a bimodal distribution of age of onset in unipolar depression as well. The mode in our sample lies between 50 and 59 with a shift of the curve to the right. The relatively high frequency of manifestations in the age period of 20 to 29 may be explained by the heterogeneity of the sample and may be due to some not recognized bipolar cases.

B. Total Number of Episodes

Of course, the total number of episodes depends on the time of observation, a fact neglected in many publications. The total number of episodes is far higher in bipolar than in unipolar psychoses (Table 2). The median in the first is 9, in the latter 4 episodes. It is remarkable that 58% of the bipolar patients suffered from 10 or more episodes. We may actually have missed some milder episodes; the true figure may be even higher. In any case, the results confirm the well-known fact that bipolar psychoses show a higher recurrence than unipolar (Perris, 1966; Angst, 1966).

Only two patients had suffered two episodes and none were single-episode patients. On the other hand, unipolar depression was frequently observed only once (16%) or twice (22%). If we should exclude depressed patients with one or two episodes, we would eliminate 37% of the material and the remaining 63%

Table 2 Total Number of Episodes

Total number of episodes	Bipolar disorder (n = 95)		Unipolar depression (n = 159)	
	n	% (cum.)	n	% (cum.)
1	—	—	24	16
2	2	2	35	37
3	6	8	*19*	*49*
4	7	16	*21*	62
5	10	26	9	68
6	4	30	13	76
7	11	42	10	82
8	3	45	4	85
9	5	51	2	86
10	7	58	6	90
>10	40	100	16	100
Median	9		9	
Length of observation (years)	*26.4*		*19.0*	

would no longer be representative. Of course, patients with few episodes are more frequent in the group with a late onset of the disorder and also more frequent in first admission selected in the years 1959-1963. If we base the calculation on first admissions only, we find 94 unipolar depressives and a total number of episodes as shown in Table 3. The table describes the frequency of episodes splitted by patients followed up after first admission on the one hand and after readmission on the other. The table shows that in bipolar patients this selection criterion is of no importance. The unipolar depressives have been splitted into early onset cases (age of onset beyond 50 years) and late-onset cases. Single-episode patients are found in 19% of early-onset and in 26% of late-onset patients. Patients with two episodes are found in 19% in the early and in 29% in the late group.

It is interesting to compare first admitted and readmitted patients (Table 3). Therefore, "unipolar patients" in the definition of Perris (1966) with three or more episodes are found in 62% of first admitted, early-onset patients and 45% of first admitted, late-onset patients. As expected, the readmitted patients show a much higher frequency of episodes as a consequence of their selection. On the whole, 22 of 94 (23%) of first admitted unipolar patients suffered from one episode only and another 24 (26%) from two episodes.

Table 3 Total Number of Episodes, First Admitted Versus Readmitted Patients

Patients	Total number of episodes	First admitted		Readmitted		
		n	%	*n*	%	*P*
Bipolar patients	1	—	—	—	—	
	2	1	3	1	2	n.s.
	⩾3	34	97	59	98	
Unipolar patients onset < 50 years	1	8	18	1	2	
	2	10	23	6	14	.01
	⩾3	26	59	37	84	
Unipolar patients onset ⩾ 50 years	1	14	28	1	5	
	2	14	28	5	24	.05
	⩾3	22	44	15	71	

Unipolar <50 years versus ⩾50 years n.s.

C. Length of Episodes

The length of episodes in affective illness shows a more or less log normal distribution, short episodes being much more frequent than long ones. The distributions were described earlier (Angst and Weis, 1967). Therefore the arithmetic mean of the duration of an episode is not a suitable description. It makes more sense to give the logarithmic mean or the median with the quartiles (Table 4).

The figures show that the length of episode in bipolar patients is on the average shorter than that in unipolar depression. An earlier analysis (Angst et al., 1973) did not find a great difference in length of episodes between cohorts of patients with few or many episodes. The length of episode has intraindividually a certain trend to be constant but shows a high variance. Multiple-regression analyses using length of episodes as the dependent variable reflect a certain influence of the following independent variables: the number of episode, the age at first episode, or age. The influence of these variables is the following: The trend of episodes to become shorter and shorter is 8% from one episode to the subsequent episode in unipolar depression and 4.3% in bipolar disorders. These figures basically mean that patients with many episodes show a relatively shorter length of episodes than those with few episodes. Age lengthens the duration of episodes by a factor of 1% (unipolar) to 2.6% (bipolar) disorders for each year of age. In unipolar depression the female patients show considerably longer episodes than the males.

An interesting question is whether in bipolar illness depressive, manic, and manic-depressive episodes vary in length. The figures in Table 4 show a greater length for manic episodes (median 4.0 months) than depressive episodes (2.5 months). This finding could be an artefact of an underreporting of hypomania or the expression of a more severe pathophysiological change than in manic-depressive and in depressive episodes. The data contradict the hypothesis that manic-depressive episodes are in their length the sum of a manic and a depressed episode. These data support the hypothesis that manic syndromes are manifestations of a more severe biochemical dysfunction than depressed episodes. The data give a hint to the assumption that a bipolar manic-depressive episode has about the same duration as a depressed episode or may be slightly longer.

D. Length of Cycles

In contrast to the earlier studies that analyzed the distance from one episode to the the other by the length of the free interval (see Angst, 1966) we decided to base the calculations on the length of cycles. A cycle is defined as the time from the onset of an episode to the time of the onset of the subsequent episode. This measurement is more recommended because it has become extremely difficult

Table 4 Length of Episodes in Months

Type of episode	No. of episodes	Arithmetic		log n		Median	Quartiles	
		$\bar{x}$	s	$\bar{x}$	s		1	3
Bipolar illness	1030	4.6	8.4	.991	.993	3.0	1.5	5.0
Unipolar depression	649	7.7	14.4	1.305	1.131	3.5	2.0	7.0
Bipolar illness								
manic episodes	241	5.1	9.8	1.232	.797	4.0	2.0	6.0
manic and depressive episodes	289	5.5	9.5	1.102	1.020	3.0	1.5	6.0
depressive episodes	500	4.0	7.3	.816	1.038	2.5	1.0	4.1

to determine the end of an episode and consequently the beginning of a free interval because the therapeutic changes of an episode frequently hide their total length.

The length of cycles shows a log normal distribution (Angst and Weiss, 1967). Tables 5 and 6 give mean values for the length of cycles separately for

Table 5 Length of Cycles in Unipolar Depression in Months

Cycle no.	n	Median	Quartile 1	Quartile 3	ln $\bar{x}$	s
1	159	65.0	20.0	144.0	3.989	1.168
2	133	28.0	11.0	86.0	3.359	1.237
3	100	22.5	9.0	62.0	3.091	1.260
4	80	20.0	9.5	50.0	3.032	1.099
5	60	12.5	8.0	48.0	2.939	1.108
6	48	12.5	6.5	43.0	2.774	1.211
7	37	12.0	7.0	20.0	2.480	1.113
8	28	7.5	5.0	12.5	2.143	.920
9	24	9.0	6.0	13.5	2.399	1.064
10	22	10.0	5.0	17.0	2.301	1.609
⩾11	81	8.0	5.0	15.0	2.263	.976

Table 6 Length of Cycles in Bipolar Disorder in Months

Cycle no.	n	Median	Quartile 1	Quartile 3	ln $\bar{x}$	s
1	95	48	12	89	3.518	1.232
2	95	22	11	49	3.120	1.044
3	93	24	12	71	3.314	1.076
4	87	14	10	35	2.941	.987
5	80	12	8	30.5	2.750	1.045
6	70	12	7	24	2.619	.977
7	66	12	6	24	2.522	1.041
8	55	12	7	31	2.681	.982
9	52	9.5	6	15	2.355	.869
10	47	12	6	24	2.492	1.033
11	431	7	5	12	2.045	.863

cycles 1, 2, and so on. The results show the trend for progressive shortening of the cycles in agreement with other authors (Kraepelin, Lange, Kinkelin, Kielholz; see Kielholz, 1959). To interpret these data one must consider that in unipolar depression especially there are a lot of patients who do not have a higher recurrent type of disorder but may show, after a certain time, an interruption of the process. Therefore the figures themselves may be misleading if they are not interpreted together with the total number of expected episodes and with the final outcome.

A multiple-regression analysis shows that the length of each cycle is shortened by 10% in unipolar and 5% in bipolar disorder by each episode and 1% by each year of age.

E. Outcome

Outcome is defined as the state of the patient at the time of the last follow-up. Then, 9 of 95 bipolar patients (10%) and 25 of 159 depressed patients (16%) were dead. A trend shows that fewer bipolar than unipolar patients commit suicide (3 versus 10.1%) (Table 7).

Table 7 Outcome at Time of Last Follow-Up

	Bipolar patients		Unipolar depressed patients		
Outcome	*n*	%	*n*	%	*P*
Patient actually suffers an episode	12	13	7	4.4	.05
Died in an episode from suicide	3	3	16	10.1	.10
Died for other reasons	7	7	9	5.7	n.s.
Full remission for					
⩾5 years	11	12	50	31.4	.001
<5 years	23	24	16	10.1	
Partial remission	26	25	33	20.8	n.s.
Organic brain syndrome					
mild	2	2	12	7.5	n.s.
severe	11	12	14	8.8	
Unknown	0	0	2	1.2	n.s.
Total	95	100	159[a]	100.0	

[a]Of 161 patients with a chronic course of the disorders, 2 were excluded.

Of the bipolar 13% and of the unipolar 4.4% suffered a new episode at the time of the last follow-up. We have to add to the figure of the unipolar patients the two chronically depressed patients who have been excluded from the whole study. These two cases would raise the percentage from 4.4 to 5.6%. The trend that more bipolar patients suffered actually from an episode confirms the finding that bipolar psychoses are active during decades and that the relapse rate is very high.

It is amazing that full and partial remissions are found in both groups about equally frequently, 36% of bipolar and 41.5% of unipolar patients showed full remission at the time of the follow-up. The proportion of full remission versus partial remission is more favorable in the unipolar group ($P < .001$). An organic brain syndrome is equally frequent in both groups but severe organic brain syndromes are relatively more frequent (not significant) in the bipolar group despite of the fact that the average age is lower.

These data on outcome at time of last follow-up have to be interpreted together with the dimension of time. An important criterion for the outcome is whether the patient has remained relapse-free during the last 5 years of the follow-up period. Relapse-free means that he or she did not suffer a new affective episode. In this sense only 11 of 95 (12%) of bipolar and 50 of 159 (31.4%) of unipolar patients were "cured."

These figures show that unipolar psychoses have a much better prognosis than bipolar disorders and they show also that in many unipolar cases one should consider seriously stopping a prophylactic lithium treatment when the patient does not suffer from residual symptoms for 3 or more years. In this connection it has to be mentioned that only 16 of 95 bipolar and 6 of 159 unipolar patients were treated with lithium for at least 12 months.

F. Course of Syndromes in Bipolar Affective Illness

The course of syndromes can be analyzed from different points of view:

Is there a sex difference in the ratio of depression to mania?

How frequent are monosyndromal versus bisyndromal episodes, i.e. how many episodes are either depressed or manic and how many consist of both syndromes?

How frequent is a switch from an initial mild depression or hypomania to a severe bipolar mood swing?

How frequently do hospitalized depressive patients switch to hypomania?

Does the ratio between depression and mania change with increasing recurrency of the disorder?

How high is the risk that a diagnosis of unipolar depression has to be changed in the future?

These questions can be answered very briefly (for details see Angst, 1978). The conclusions are based on the analysis of the course of 95 manic-depressive patients with 1162 episodes.

Figure 2 shows an amazing stability over time of the ratio between depressive and manic syndromes for both sexes. During the first five episodes the proportion of depressive syndromes is a bit higher than later but this may be an artefact resulting from underreporting of hypomanic episodes at the onset of the disorder.

Table 8 shows the patterns of syndromes observed in all (1176) episodes split by sex From this table it is evident that monosyndromal episodes are twice as fequent as bipolar (cyclic) episodes consisting of mania and depression.

Females suffer much more frequently (60%) than males (35.5%) from depressive episodes. The contrary is true for manic syndromes: females suffer in 13.6% and males in 35.3% from purely manic syndromes. We do not think this difference is due to a difference in self-observation and reporting.

In males the distribution of frequency of depression and mania is equal. Therefore a random process may be underlying. In females we have a strong shift in favor of depression that may be explained by an additional factor (i.e., endocrine changes).

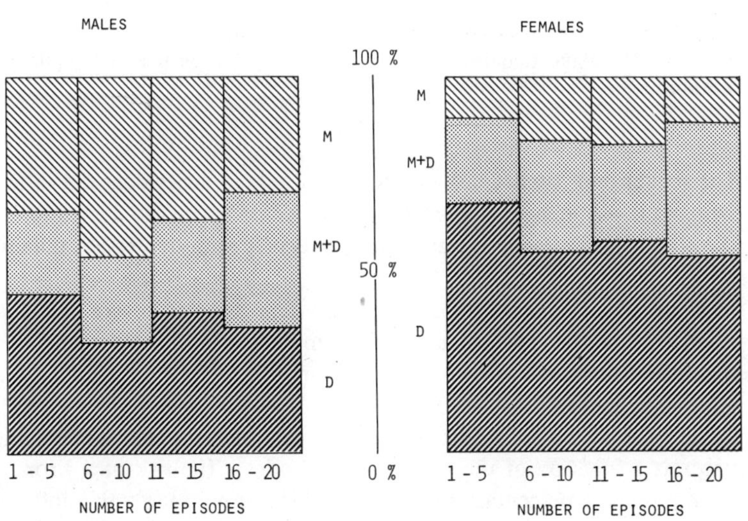

Figure 2 Cross-sectional proportion of depressive (D), manic (M), and manic-depressive (M + D) syndromes during the first 20 episodes.

Table 8 Frequency of Syndrome Patterns in Bipolar Psychoses and Sex (95 Patients, 1176 Episodes)

Pattern of syndromes[a]	Males		Females		Males (%)	Females (%)
	n	%	*n*	%		
D	80	18.3	194	26.3	35.5	60.0
d	75	17.2	246	33.7		
M	127	29.1	75	10.1	35.3	13.6
m	27	6.2	26	3.5		
DM	5	1.1	15	2.0		
Dm	23	5.3	66	8.9	15.3	16.6
dM	7	1.6	4	0.5		
dm	32	7.3	39	5.2		
MD	2	0.5	11	1.5		
Md	19	4.3	18	2.4	12.6	9.2
mD	3	0.7	11	1.5		
md	31	7.1	28	3.8		
Questionable, unknown	6	1.4	6	0.8		

[a]D = Severe depression (requiring hospitalization). d = Mild depression (not requiring hospitalization). M = Mania (requiring hospitalization). m = Hypomania (not requiring hospitalization).

The sequence of syndromes within one episode in males does not differ if we compare the sequence "depression to mania" or "mania to depression." In females the episodes seem to start more frequently with depression than with mania.

In hospitalized patients the switch from depression to severe mania is observed in 1-2% of the cases and a switch from depression to hypomania in 5% (males) and 9% (females). This may be of importance for comparisons with drug-induced switches.

Table 9 shows the probability of originally depressed patients becoming manic later as a function of the number of episodes. The risk of a wrong diagnosis is given as a percentage figure for the bipolar group ($n = 95$) and for a total sample of hospital admissions with affective disorders ($n = 254$) including all unipolar depressive patients. The table shows that after three depressive episodes 29 of 95 bipolar patients (31%) could not yet have been diagnosed

Table 9 How Frequently are Bipolar Patients Diagnosed as Depressed?

Number of Episodes	ICD 296	Diagnosed as ICD 296.3	Remaining ICD "296.2"	Not yet Diagnosed ICD 296.3	Not yet Diagnosed % ICD 296.3
1	254	32	222	63	28
2	230	15	215	48	22
3	193	19	174	29	17
4	168	5	163	24	15
5	140	4	136	20	15
6	121	4	117	16	14
7	104	5	99	11	11
8	83	1	82	10	12
9	76	2	68	8	12
10	69	2	63	6	10
>10	56	6	50	–	–

because they switched in a later episode to mania. The risk for this diagnostic error is about 16% calculated for the total group of affective disorders. The last column in the table shows that this error cannot be reduced substantially by selecting patients with more and more episodes. This may be due to the fact that patients with many episodes have a higher chance of belonging to the bipolar group than patients with few episodes.

G. Typology of Bipolar Affective Disorders

An attempt was made to classify bipolar patients in three groups:

Type Md — During his life the patient has suffered once or several times from a mania requiring hospitalization, but he has shown only mild or no depression. This type is called prevailingly manic type and corresponds with the bipolar I group of Dunner et al., (1976).

Type MD — The patient has shown both mania and depression requiring hospitalization (nuclear type of bipolar illness). This type corresponds with bipolar I patients.

Type Dm — The patient has required hospitalization for depression but has shown only hypomania (prevailingly depressed type). This type corresponds with bipolar II patients (Dunner et al., 1976).

Of course it makes sense to classify patients by such a typology only if we have observed the course of the illness for a long time because the total information of all episodes has to be included.

Figure 3 shows the frequency of the three types split by sex. Again the findings of Section III.F are confirmed with an amazing accuracy: male patients belong preponderantly to the nuclear type (MD) with both severe mania and severe depression. The other two types (Md, Dm) are less frequent. Assuming a continuum between the three subtypes, this may represent a normal distribution in male patients.

To the contrary, in female patients there is a high preponderance of the depressed subtype in 59%, and we find a marked underrepresentation of type Md. Further studies will be necessary to confirm this marked difference between the sexes and to find the reasons for it.

If we stick to the hypothesis of a normal distribution of the subtypes of affective disorders in general, the extrapolation gives an expectation rate of about three times more depressive than bipolar patients suffering from the same disorder. This expectation is widely confirmed by the genetic studies, which show that the first degree relatives of bipolar patients suffer much less frequently from mania or bipolar manic-depressive disorders than from unipolar depression or neurotic depression, or they die from suicide without other diagnosis (Angst et al. 1980). Therefore we have to assume that the biological disorder "bipolar manic-depressive illness" shows depression as its phenotype much more frequently than mania or bipolar illness. This assumption is not yet a conclusive

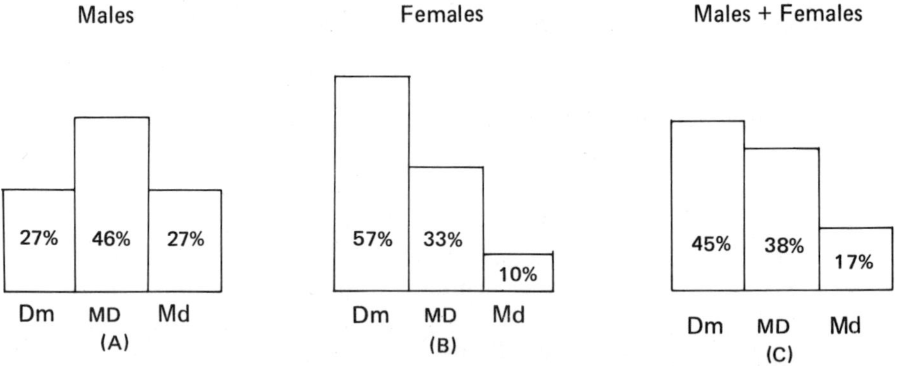

Figure 3 Typology of bipolar patients. Males, $n = 37$; females, $n = 58$; males and females, $n = 95$. (A) Type MD: patient suffered at least once from a severe manic and a severe depressive syndrome, = bipolar type. (B) Type Md: patient suffered at least once from a severe manic syndrome, but showed only mild depressive symptomatology, = prevailingly manic type. (C) Type Dm: patient suffered at least once from a severe depressive syndrome but showed only hypomanic symptoms, = prevailingly depressed type.

argument in favor of a complete continuum between bipolar and unipolar illness, but it strongly supports the hypothesis that the group of unipolar patients is very heterogeneous and consists in general of a remarkable proportion of patients who must suffer from a basic bipolar disorder.

IV. SYNTHESIS OF RESULTS

A. Bipolar Manic-Depressive Versus Unipolar Depressive Disorders

The course of the two disorders can be distinguished by different characteristics. The bipolar psychosis shows a more malignant course illustrated by earlier age of onset, higher frequency and total number of episodes during life, lower rate of spontaneous remissions (defined by a relapse-free period of 5 years), shorter length of cycles, and attentuated chance for a full remission in favor of the partial remission only; furthermore, there is a higher risk of developing severe organic brain syndrome. Finally, bipolar psychoses last much longer than unipolar depressive disorders. Some of the differences may be explained by the earlier age of onset of the bipolar group, but the differences are still valid even if we compare early onset unipolar with early-onset bipolar patients. It is remarkable, however, that the suicide rate up to now seems to be lower in the bipolar than in the unipolar group.

Unipolar depression has a distinctly better prognosis illustrated by later age of onset, lower number of episodes, shorter length of the duration of the illness, and longer distances between the episodes. The final outcome is better, showing fuller remissions. On the other hand, the episodes in unipolar depression last longer; the suicide rate seems to be higher. A relapse-free remission during the last 5 years was found in 31.4% of unipolar patients and in 37% of unipolar patients who were selected as first admissions.

B. Syndrome Patterns of Bipolar Illness

In addition to the classification of bipolar patients into bipolar I and bipolar II proposed by Dunner et al. (1976), we propose a classification into three groups of bipolar patients: the prevailingly manic, the nuclear bipolar, and the prevailingly depressed type of bipolar patients. The most important finding of this analysis points to a striking sex difference in the frequencies of these subtypes. Male patients are mainly being found to belong to the nuclear type, female patients mainly to the prevailingly depressed type of the disorder. An extrapolation from these findings and from the distribution of secondary cases in the first degree relatives of bipolar patients suggests the existence of a spectrum of phenotypes of the disorder bipolar manic-depressive illness: recurrent mania, subtypes of bipolar psychoses, recurrent depression, suicide, neurotic depression, and cycloid personality. It is suggested to assume that the phenotype is more frequently a depressed than a bipolar or manic disorder and that therefore the diagnoses "unipolar depression" and "neurotic depression" are unreliable and this material heterogeneous.

REFERENCES

Angst, J. (1966). *Zur Aetiologie und Nosologie endogener depressiver Psychosen,* Monogr. Gesamtgebiet Neurol. Psychiat., Heft 112, Springer, Berlin, Heidelberg, Stuttgart.

Angst, J. (1978). The course of affective disorders. II. Typology of bipolar manic-depressive illness. *Arch. Psychiatr. Nervenkr. 226,* 65-73.

Angst, J., and Weis, P. (1967). Periodicity of depressive psychoses. *Proc. Int. Except. Med. Found. Int. Congr. Series, No. 129,* Elsevier Amsterdam, pp. 703-710.

Angst, J., Baastrup, P., Grof, P., Hippius, H., Pöldinger, W. and Weis, P. (1973). The course of monopolar depression and bipolar psychoses. *Psychiatr. Neurol. Neurochir.* (Amst.) *76,* 489-500.

Angst, J., Felder, W., Frey, R., and Stassen, H. H. (1978). The course of affective disorders. I. Change of diagnosis of monopolar, unipolar, and bipolar illness. *Arch. Psychiatr. Nervenkr. 226,* 54-64.

Angst, J., Frey, R., Lohmeyer, B., and Zerbin-Rüdin, E. (1980). Bipolar manic-depressive psychoses: Results of a genetic investigation. *Human Genet.* In press.

Dunner, D. L., Fleiss, J. L., and Fieve, R. R. (1976). The course of development of mania in patients with recurrent depression. *Am. J. Psychiatry 133,* 905-908.

Kielholz, P. (1959). Klinik, Differentialdiagnostik und Therapie der depressiven Zustandsbilder. Documenta Geigy. *Acta Psychosom. 2,* Basel.

Kraepelin, E. (1896). *Compendium der Psychiatrie,* 5th ed. Barth, Leipzig.

Perris, C. (1966). A study of bipolar (manic-depressive) and unipolar recurrent depressive psychoses. *Acta Psychiatry Scand. supplement 194.*

Slater, E. (1938). Zur Periodik des manisch-depressiven Irreseins. *Z. ges. Neurol. Psychiat. 162,* 794-801.

6

Biochemical Aspects of Alcohol Tolerance and Dependence

John M. Littleton
University of London, King's College
London, England

I. INTRODUCTION

Alcohols can be classed pharmacologically with other drugs which produce a general depression of the central nervous system. Alcohol tolerance and dependence inevitably share many characteristics with tolerance and dependence on other central depressant drugs. The uniqueness of alcohols, and particularly ethanol, is their importance, socially and medically, as constituents of alcoholic drinks. The use of ethanol in this way has become an integral part of some civilizations. Consumption of ethanol in moderation may have beneficial properties, but there is little doubt that the pathological consequences of excessive consumption affect millions. Despite the realization that alcoholism is a crippling condition, and despite efforts to elucidate the mechanisms by which ethanol produces its harmful effects, our understanding is still vague. Partly the problem has been that alcoholism defines a condition which seems uniquely human. It is only recently that some aspects of alcoholism, namely, tolerance and physical dependence, have been produced in laboratory animals (for review, see Friedman and Lester, 1977) and this achievement has provided the stimulus for an explosion of research on the biochemical basis of alcohol tolerance and dependence during the last 5 years.

The term alcoholism simply indicates that an individual suffers harmful effects—be they physical, psychological, or social—from habitual ingestion of alcohol. The relation between alcoholism and tolerance and dependence on alcohol is quite complex. Thus it is clearly possible that an individual can be an alcoholic (i.e., suffer harmful effects) without being dependent on the drug. Equally, it is theoretically possible that an individual can be dependent on alcohol without suffering harmful effects. However, in reality, it seems likely that all alcoholics demonstrate signs of alcohol tolerance and dependence and that the presence of dependence on the drug should itself be regarded as harmful. Discussion of patients in terms of their alcohol tolerance or dependence rather than their alcoholism does have advantages in that the former terms are more objectively definable (for discussion, see Edwards and Gross, 1976).

An attempt is made in Figure 1 to show the relationship between alcohol consumption, tolerance, dependence, and pathological effects. The consumption of alcohol produces effects fairly typical of a central depressant drug (see Section II). Repeated consumption leads to tolerance, in which higher doses of the drug are required to produce the same degree of central depression. This tolerance may be cellular (in which neurons appear capable of functioning normally at concentrations of ethanol higher than those tolerated in a naive individual), metabolic (in which the rate of elimination of ethanol from the body is increased), or behavioral (implying a learned adaptation to the behavioral effects of ethanol). These different mechanisms of tolerance are discussed in Section III.

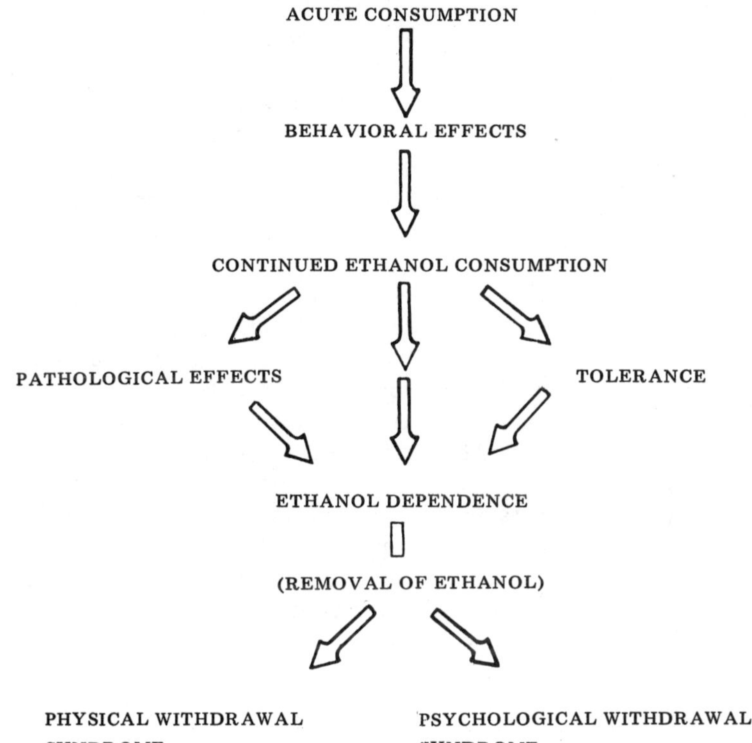

Figure 1 Relationship between effects produced by acute and chronic consumption of ethanol.

During the repeated consumption of ethanol, pathological changes may appear in several organs. The organ most frequently affected is the liver, but pathological effects on heart, brain, peripheral nerves, and pancreas are all recognized. It is not known whether any of these changes influence the induction of tolerance or dependence on alcohol. Dependence on ethanol, like that on other central nervous system depressants, may be described as physical or psychological. It is likely that these coexist in most clinical alcoholics. The paradox of dependence is that it can only be demonstrated to exist by removal of the drug in question, thus destroying the state of dependence.

Removal of ethanol from a human subject, or animal, in a state of ethanol dependence results in a withdrawal syndrome. If this syndrome is primarily physical (e.g., major convulsions, tremors, autonomic disturbances), the dependence is characterized as physical dependence. If the syndrome is primarily psychological (e.g., craving for the drug, anxiety, sleep disturbances), the dependence is classified as psychological dependence. These syndromes often coexist in ethanol withdrawal and seem to be merely at opposite ends of a spectrum of severity of changes induced by ethanol withdrawal. There seems little justification in considering them as separate and thus little merit in attempting to rigidly distinguish psychological dependence on alcohol from physical dependence on alcohol. When the biochemical bases of both are better understood, they may be shown to possess a common mechanism. However, in this chapter the terms are retained because they are understood and are often useful descriptively.

The only alcohol discussed here will be ethanol because it is clear that this compound accounts for the great majority of the pharmacological effects of alcoholic drinks. Also, no attempt will be made to cover the possibility that pharmacological effects of ethanol are due to its metabolite, acetaldehyde (see Truitt and Walsh, 1971), although there is evidence that ethanol physical dependence may be reproduced by acetaldehyde (e.g.,Ortiz et al., 1974). Each section has been divided into a discussion of the effects of alcohol at either the level of neuronal membranes or the level of neurotransmitter metabolism. Protein synthesis has been considered under the first heading and cyclic nucleotide metabolism under the second. Although this kind of division may seem arbitrary, it does represent a division of approach between the molecular biologist and the traditional neuropharmacologist. It should become clear in this chapter that these different levels of organization cannot really be considered as separate in any way.

II. EFFECTS OF ACUTE ADMINISTRATION OF ETHANOL

A. Introduction

The results of acute self-administration of ethanol will be known to most readers of this volume. They include initial excitability, volubility, and euphoria, followed, at increasing concentrations of ethanol in blood, by incoordination, sometimes aggression, and eventually unconsciousness and death. This spectrum of effects is fairly typical of those produced by a general depressant of the central nervous system. Other effects of alcohol, such as respiratory depression and hypothermia, are also commonly associated with a general depression of activity in the brain. There are, however, some effects of ethanol which may have a more specific basis (see Section II.C).

There is good evidence that central depressant drugs, including the anesthetics and higher alcohols, interact with cell membranes in a physical way to produce their effects. Ethanol, too, may act in this way (Section II.B). The acute effects of ethanol are to some extent determined by the rate of absorption of the drug (dependent on the form in which the ethanol was consumed, presence of food in the stomach, etc.) and are limited by the rate of elimination of ethanol from the body. This factor is mainly controlled by the rate at which the liver metabolizes ethanol (Section II.D).

B. Actions of Ethanol at Level of Neuronal Membranes

The simple nature of the chemical structure of ethanol and the characteristics it shares with other central depressant drugs, which also have simple, but dissimilar, chemical structures, suggest that ethanol may act nonspecifically on cell membranes, as anesthetic agents are thought to do, rather than through any receptor mechanism. Anesthetic agents expand membranes (Seeman, 1972) and can be shown to increase the fluid nature of both biological and model mebranes (e.g., Metcalfe et al., 1968). Recently it was shown (Chin and Goldstein, 1977a) that ethanol, in concentrations associated with intoxication rather than anesthesia, can induce an increased fluidity in cell membranes obtained from mice. The addition of ethanol in low concentrations in vitro increased the physical fluidity of membranes from brain synaptosomes, brain mitochondria, and erythrocytes. This increase in fluidity of neuronal membranes produced by ethanol would be expected to produce widespread changes in synaptic transmission. One would predict that the activity of many membrane-associated enzymes in brain would also be affected (see Farias et al., 1975). This biophysical effect of ethanol on synaptic membranes may represent the basic mechanism for its central depressant action.

Another property of ethanol which may play an important part in its functional effects is its ability to interfere with calcium binding to cell membranes. Calcium is critically involved in many basic functions at the level of the synapse, probably playing some part in release of transmitter (e.g., Douglas, 1968), neurotransmitter-receptor interactions (see Triggle, 1971), and coupling of receptor activation and neuronal response (e.g., Rasmussen, 1970; Phillis, 1974). Calcium also has important effects on the control of neurotransmitter biosynthesis (e.g., Knapp et al. 1975). Some of the relationships between calcium and synaptic function are shown in Figure 2. It is thus clear that effects on neuronal calcium metabolism can produce widespread alterations in brain function. Ethanol is thought to act as a calcium antagonist (e.g., Hurwitz et al., 1962; Late et al., 1973) and the acute administration of low doses of ethanol in vivo depletes calcium in various brain regions (Ross et al., 1974). Exactly what these effects mean at the level of neuronal membrane binding or release of calcium is not yet clear. Seeman et al. (1971) suggested that volatile anesthetics, including alcohol, increase the binding of calcium to cell membranes. This, together with the results mentioned above, suggests that the overall effect of ethanol on calcium metabolism may be to reduce its release from cell membranes, preventing its access to some intracellular site of action. However, it has recently been shown (Tyler and Erickson, 1977) that intracerebral

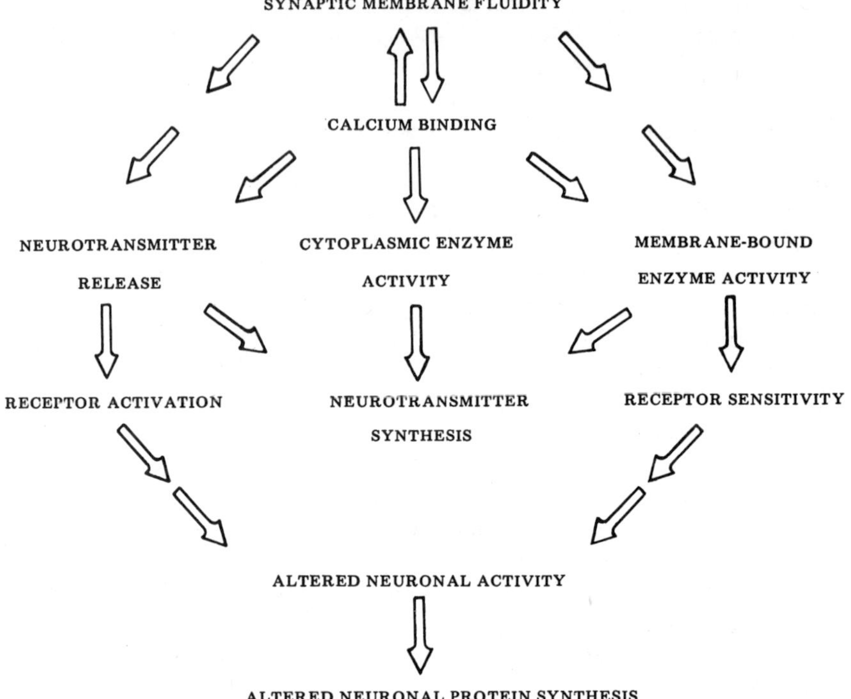

Figure 2 It is only necessary to postulate some effect by ethanol on a basic property of the synaptic membrane, such as its physical fluidity or ability to bind calcium, to explain the many reported effects of ethanol on neuronal chemistry and function. An alteration in either of these variables can produce changes in all the aspects of synaptic function shown here.

administration of calcium potentiates ethanol-induced central depression. Similarly, the administration of calcium-chelating agents antagonizes ethanol. These results suggest that it is potentiation of calcium at some intracerebral site that is important in the depressant effects of ethanol. At present it is not certain how these differences can be resolved.

It is possible that the effects of ethanol on calcium binding by membranes may not be the primary action but may be secondary to the physical effects of ethanol on the membrane. The increase in membrane fluidity referred to previously is probably mediated by an effect on the phospholipid structural components of the membrane; membrane phospholipids are also important calcium binding sites (see Triggle, 1971). The relationships between membrane fluidity, calcium binding, and basic functions of the synapse are shown in Figure 2.

Other functions of the neuron which may play important roles in membrane excitability are also altered by ethanol. Thus, the acute administration of ethanol has often been reported to reduce the incorporation of amino acids into protein in the brain (e.g., Kuriyama et al., 1971). A reduced capacity for synthesis of proteins, including proteins incorporated into neuronal membranes, could play some part in the acute or chronic effects of ethanol. Ethanol is reported to inhibit the activity of the membrane-bound enzyme [Na^+, K^+]-dependent ATPase in synaptosomes of humans and animals (Sun and Samorajski, 1975) and this, or some more direct effect on activation of the Na^+ channel (for review, see Noble and Tewari, 1977), may explain some of the acute effects of ethanol on neuronal excitability. Here again it seems likely that these changes are secondary to some fundamental alteration of physical properties of membranes rather than being the event of primary importance.

C. Actions of Ethanol at Level of Neurotransmitter Metabolism

In the intact animal the effect of ethanol on neurotransmitter metabolism is complicated by the "stressing" effect of acute administration of large doses of the drug. This may be the reason for the initial increase in central catecholamine synthesis often reported (e.g.,Hunt and Majchrowicz, 1974a) but some direct effect on catecholamine neurons may also be involved. After this initial increase in catecholamine biosynthesis this variable falls to below normal levels (e.g., Hunt and Majchrowicz, 1974a; Pohorecky, 1974). The initial increase in catecholamine synthesis may play some part in ethanol-induced excitation in animals (Carlsson et al., 1972) and euphoria in humans (Ahlenius et al. 1973). The excitation in animals seems predominantly to result from increase in noradrenaline rather than dopamine, functional activity (see Carlsson et al.,1974).

The later central depressent effects of ethanol in vivo may also be related to some effect on monoamine metabolism (e.g., Blum et al., 1973; Smith et al., 1976). Indirect evidence favors amino acids as also playing a part (e.g., Blum et al., 1972; Iida and Hikichi, 1976; Hakkinen and Kulonen, 1976). The acute administration of ethanol is reported to cause an increase in brain γ-amino butyric acid (GABA) concentrations (e.g. Sutton, 1973) but the extent of this increase does not correlate with genetic differences in the central depression produced (Chan, 1976). Acetylcholine release from the cerebral cortex is decreased by the in vivo administration of ethanol (Phillis and Jhamandas, 1971) but drugs which modify cholinergic transmission seem not to affect ethanol-induced central depression (Graham and Erickson, 1974).

When experiments are carried out in vitro most reports show that ethanol inhibits many aspects of neurotransmitter function. Thus, release of several neurotransmitters from cortical slices is inhibited by ethanol (Carmichael and Israel, 1975) and the reuptake of neurotransmitters is also inhibited, although not to a great extent (Roach et al., 1973). It should be emphasized that, although these effects are qualitatively the same for several transmitters, there are differences in the extent to which different systems are affected. If as seems likely these actions can be ascribed to some direct effect on neuronal membranes, than ethanol must show selectivity for some membranes rather than others. This might depend, for example, on differing membrane structure or compositions at different synapses.

In conclusion, the effects of acute administration of ethanol on neurotransmitter metabolism probably involve mainly a depression of neuronal functional activity. There may be exceptions to this rule, particularly catecholaminergic nerves, and some neuronal systems may be affected to a greater extent than others. As a result, some physiological or behavioral effects of ethanol may relate to specific effects on neurotransmitter systems, but the overall picture is of generalized depression of central neuronal function.

D. Metabolism of Ethanol After Acute Administration

The rate of elimination of ethanol from the body may determine the peak alcohol concentration attained in the bloodstream and partly determines the duration of the pharmacological effects of the drug. It is therefore an important consideration in discussing the effects of acute administration of ethanol. By far the most important factor determining the rate of elimination is the metabolism of ethanol by the liver. Other routes of ethanol elimination, such as in the breath and urine, although of medicolegal importance, have little significance in the total clearance of ethanol from the body. Other organs, apart from the liver, metabolize ethanol but, once again, these sites are not important in the overall removal of ethanol.

The metabolism of ethanol has been one of the most exhaustively studied topics in biochemistry. There is still controversy over its exact nature. Probably the main pathway for the metabolism of ethanol by the liver is oxidation by alcohol dehydrogenase (for review, see Thurman and McKenna, 1975; for recent experimental results, see Havre et al., 1977). However, at high concentrations of ethanol in the bloodstream, other pathways of ethanol metabolism may become important. A major controversy exists here as to whether it is catalase, present in hepatic peroxisomes, which is responsible (see Thurman and McKenna, 1975) or whether an alternative, microsomal, pathway, the microsomal ethanol-oxidizing system, is important (e.g., Lieber and De Carli, 1970). The weight of evidence at present favors catalase as the more important, but the question is still not settled.

Alcohol dehydrogenase

$$CH_3CH_2OH + NAD^+ \rightarrow CH_3CHO + NADH + H^+$$

Catalase

$$CH_3CH_2OH + H_2O_2 \rightarrow CH_3CHO + 2H_2O$$

Microsomal ethanol oxidizing system

$$CH_3CH_2OH + NADPH + H^+ + O_2 \rightarrow CH_3CHO + NADP + 2H_2O$$

Figure 3 These pathways probably contribute to the metabolism of ethanol although their relative importance is controversial (see text). Alcohol dehydrogenase is located in the cytoplasm, catalase mainly in the hepatic peroxisomes, and the microsomal ethanol-oxidizing system is thought to be associated with the membranes of the endoplasmic reticulum. In all cases the major metabolite of ethanol is acetaldehyde which may itself have important pharmacological properties.

The pathways of ethanol metabolism are shown in Figure 3. In the normal individual the rate of elimination of ethanol from the body is between about 100 and 200 mg/kg per hr, but in laboratory animals elimination rates may be much higher (see Kalant, 1971). As stated previously, elimination is due largely to metabolism of ethanol by the liver; adaptive alterations in ethanol elimination rate are similarly related to changes in metabolism by liver (see Section III.D).

III. DEVELOPMENT OF TOLERANCE TO ETHANOL

A. Introduction

Tolerance to ethanol implies that after repeated administration of the drug a subject is able to function relatively normally after doses of ethanol which would previously have produced a behavioral deficit. Conversely, after repeated doses of ethanol, higher doses of the drug are required to produce the same behavioral deficit. There are several aspects to tolerance; the individual may eliminate ethanol more rapidly from the body, so that the peak concentration of ethanol achieved in the bloodstream is lower and the duration of maintenance of concentrations of ethanol at pharmacologically active levels is reduced. This form of tolerance is known as metabolic tolerance. Alternatively, the individual may become capable of functioning at higher concentrations of ethanol than hitherto. This sort of tolerance can be viewed in two ways. At the level of the intact animal, or human subject, there may be some kind of learned response involved, so that the individual becomes able to disguise the behavioral deficit produced by alcohol. This kind of tolerance, sometimes described as behavioral tolerance, has recently been discussed by Leblanc and Cappell (1977). Tolerance, to maintain function in the presence of higher concentrations of ethanol than those normally tolerated, can also be considered at the level of the neuron. Here, it is assumed that some fundamental adaptive process causes ethanol to be less effective in disrupting neuronal function. This is called cellular, or alternatively, physiological, tolerance.

There are studies on the development of tolerance to ethanol in the intact animal that indicate that it may develop within minutes or hours (e.g., after a single dose of ethanol, Leblanc et al., 1975). However, the extent of ethanol tolerance is probably relatively small compared to that of some other drugs, e.g., morphine. Animals made tolerant to ethanol seem to be able to function at ethanol concentrations only about double those which had previously produced a behavioral deficit (e.g., Majchrowicz and Hunt, 1976).

B. Tolerance to Ethanol at Level of Neuronal Membranes

Since many of the acute central depressant effects of ethanol may be explained by some biophysical action of the drug on neuronal membranes (see Section II), it seems logical to look at the level of the membrane for the mechanism of cellular tolerance to ethanol. Hill and Bangham (1975) proposed that since alcohols increased membrane fluidity by some physical interaction with the lipid part of the membrane, then an intrinsic reduction of fluidity by the lipids of the membrane may account for tolerance. This suggestion may prove to be correct. Tolerance to ethanol at the level of the synaptic membrane has now been shown to exist (Chin and Goldstein, 1977b). These workers obtained synaptic and erythrocyte membranes from ethanol-tolerant and dependent mice and exposed them to moderate concentrations of ethanol in vitro. The fluidization of membranes from these animals produced by ethanol (measured by incorporation of an electron spin resonance label into membranes) was significantly less than that produced in membranes from naive animals. The membranes themselves had therefore become tolerant to this physical effect of ethanol. Interestingly, Chin and Goldstein were unable to find any differences in the intrinsic fluidity of tolerant and naive membranes, but this may reflect methodological difficulties. Intrinsic fluidity may here be defined as the physical nature of the membranes in the absence of drug.

As tolerance does exist at the level of the synaptic membrane it is necessary to consider the mechanisms which account for its development. Hill and Bangham (1975) suggested that some alteration in the lipid composition of the membrane may be involved. Evidence in favor of this suggestion was provided by Ingram (1976), who investigated the fatty acid composition of membrane phospholipids from bacteria grown in different media. On addition of ethanol to the medium, bacterial growth rate slowed, then returned to normal with a time course similar to an alteration in the incorporation of different fatty acids into phospholipids. Paradoxically, Ingram observed an increase in incorporation of polyunsaturated fatty acids into bacterial phospholipids in the presence of ethanol. This change would be expected to further increase membrane fluidity (presumably already increased by the physical effect of ethanol on cell membranes). It is difficult to see how this could account for cellular tolerance. Clearly, differences may exist between mammalian synaptic membranes and bacterial cell membranes, and between complex synaptic functions and a gross parameter such as bacterial cell division. The position at mammalian synapses may now have been resolved. Littleton and John (1977) recently reported that in ethanol-tolerant and dependent mice, reduced proportions of polyunsaturated fatty acids are found in phospholipids of the synaptosomal fraction of brain. Of course, this change would reduce the intrinsic fluidity of the synaptosomal membranes, rendering them less affected by the fluidization produced by the continuous presence of ethanol.

The change in phospholipid composition described above may therefore form the basis for the cellular adaptation to ethanol at the level of the synaptic membrane. There are still many questions unresolved. As already stated, Chin and Goldstein (1977b) were unable to find any difference in the intrinsic fluidity of ethanol-tolerant membranes. Such a difference is, however, predicted by the results of Littleton and John (1977). The variation in membrane fluidity inevitably encountered in the experiments of Chin and Goldstein may have obscured differences in intrinsic fluidity, but the situation may be even more complex, since genetic differences may also contribute to differences in lipid adaptation (Littleton and John, 1977; Griffiths et al., 1977). A possible answer to these difficulties may come from the work of Garrett and Ross (1977) where, using fluorescent probe binding to synaptic membranes as an index of biochemical change, it was suggested that the initial alteration induced by ethanol was in the lipid portion of the membrane whereas long-term exposure to ethanol resulted in adaptation of both lipid and protein regions. Taken together, all the observations made on synaptic membranes suggest that more than one adaptive mechanism is at work. These may be first a rapid mechanism involving a change in membrane lipids and perhaps leading to a reduction in the intrinsic fluidity of the membrane; second, a slower mechanism, supplanting or supplementing the lipid change as the basis for cellular tolerance and probably based on altered membrane protein synthesis (see below). Such a change need not necessarily cause any change in intrinsic membrane fluidity. Perhaps genetic differences in development of ethanol tolerance and dependence simply reflect differences in the relative importance of these mechanisms in an individual.

This is a simplified view of the changes in the membrane lipid and protein interactions which may be responsible for tolerance to ethanol. It must be remembered that the membrane composition is in a dynamic state, particularly with regard to the fatty acids incorporated into phospholipids. Not only the overall composition may be altered at any one point in time, but the rate of turnover of individual components of the membrane may also be altered. There is recent evidence that the turnover of arachidonic acid in synaptosomes is increased by chronic administration of ethanol to rats (Sun et al., 1977). This evidence comes from the observation of increased activity in the enzyme system responsible for specific acylation of phosphoglycerides. It seems likely, therefore, that both membrane composition and turnover of membrane constituents should be considered as contributory factors in determining the chronic effects of ethanol at the level of the synapse.

With respect to the ability of membranes to bind calcium, some adaptive mechanism to repeat administration of ethanol may also exist here. Ross et al. (1977) recently reported that tolerance to the reduction in brain calcium concentration produced by ethanol occurs after its repeated administration. Reduced calcium binding in brain may also occur after chronic ethanol administration. This altered calcium binding might be a function of altered protein binding sites, or of alterations in phospholipids. In the scheme discussed above both could be important, but with a differing time course.

Chronic administration of ethanol has been reported to induce some changes in brain protein synthesis, but it does not seem likely that the changes can be involved in the development of tolerance to ethanol. Although Kuriyama et al. (1971) found that chronic ethanol intake caused a stimulation of ribosomal protein synthesis (an effect which might be considered a possible basis for tolerance), several subsequent papers (for review, see Noble and Tewari, 1977) indicate that significant inhibition of brain protein synthesis occurs in animals maintained chronically on ethanol. The inhibition of protein synthesis seems likely to be related to some defect in the ribosomes from ethanol-treated animals (see Noble and Tewari, 1977). Such a defect may flow from alterations in ribosomal membranes, but this has not yet been established.

Alterations of [Na^+, K^+]-dependent ATPase activity after chronic administration of ethanol seems a possible mechanism for tolerance. Most workers report that the acute depression of [Na^+, K^+]-ATPase by ethanol is followed by an increase in activity after chronic administration of ethanol (e.g., Israel et al., 1970). Other ATPases may also be affected (see Noble and Tewari, 1977). Alterations in ion flux which may follow such changes in membrane-bound enzyme activity could play a part in overcoming the neuronal depressant properties of ethanol. However, it should be emphasized once again that effects of ethanol on membrane composition and fluidity may influence the activity of membrane-bound enzymes including [Na^+, K^+]-ATPase (see Farias et al., 1975).

This section has been speculative. This is inevitable in the light of our present knowledge, but it seems important to attempt a discussion of the way in which ethanol affects the fundamental processes of neurotransmission. Changes in neurotransmitter metabolism and receptor sensitivy (see Section III.C) can be discussed only against the background realization that they may not be the event of primary significance, but may reflect alterations in neuronal function at a very much more basic level.

C. Tolerance to Ethanol at Level of Neurotransmitter Metabolism

The chronic administration of ethanol to laboratory animals, presumably producing tolerance in many instances, has been reported to produce a bewildering variety of changes in neurotransmitter metabolism. Unfortunately, only rarely has any attempt been made to establish whether any similarities exist between the time course of the neurotransmitter change and the development of tolerance, or whether prevention of the neurotransmitter change influences ethanol tolerance. There is, however, some evidence for causal relationships between specific alterations in neurotransmitter metabolism induced by ethanol, and development of ethanol tolerance. Most evidence favors the monoamine neurotransmitters.

Chronic administration of ethanol produces increases in endogenous catecholamine levels (Griffiths et al., 1973, 1974a; Post and Sun, 1973) and in catecholamine synthesis (Pohorecky, 1974; Hunt and Majchrowicz, 1974a). Concentrations of catecholamine metabolites in brain are also increased (Karoum et al., 1976), arguing increased release of these transmitters. In contrast to all these changes, which suggest increase in catecholaminergic functional activity in brain, the receptors for catecholamines are reported to show decreased sensitivity (e.g., Israel et al., 1972; French et al., 1974; Hoffman and Tabakoff, 1977). The administration of a drug which destroys catecholaminergic nerve terminals (6-hydroxydopamine) has been reported by Ritzmann and Tabakoff (1976) to inhibit the development of tolerance to ethanol with respect to its hypothermic effects. It is not certain as to whether this effect can be ascribed to interference with noradrenergic (Tabakoff et al, 1977a) or dopaminergic systems (Hoffman and Tabakoff, 1977). The alteration in dopamine receptor sensitivity reported by Hoffman and Tabakoff seems the most likely candidate for a change specifically related to ethanol tolerance.

The situation with respect to 5-hydroxytryptamine (5-HT) involvement in ethanol tolerance is even less clear. Several authors (e.g., Griffiths et al., 1973, 1974b; Pohorecky et al., 1974b; Gothoni and Ahtee, 1977) have reported a small increase in 5-HT concentration in brain produced by chronic ethanol administration but reports of changes in rate of synthesis are contradictory (e.g., Pohorecky et al., 1974b; Hunt and Majchrowicz, 1974b). Information on sensitivity of 5-HT receptors during the induction of tolerance to ethanol seems to be lacking. Despite the absence of any clear indication as to how 5-HT metabolism is altered by chronic ethanol administration, tryptaminergic mechanisms do seem to be involved in the development of some apsects of tolerance to ethanol. Frankel et al. (1975) showed that administration of p-chlorophenylalanine, an inhibitor of 5-HT biosynthesis, inhibits the development of behavioral tolerance to ethanol and pentobarbital.

This evidence suggests that monoamine pathways are involved in the development of tolerance to ethanol or at least are involved in the expression of some aspects of tolerance to ethanol. The fact that similar pathways play important roles in the learning process has been advanced as evidence for a connection between acquisition of tolerance and learned behavior (e.g., Leblanc and Cappell, 1977; Tabakoff et al., 1977a). At present such a connection can be regarded as only speculative.

If changes in transmitter receptor sensitivity play a part in the development of tolerance to ethanol (see this section), then the fundamental change may be at the level of cyclic nucleotide metabolism. Volicer and Hurter (1977) reported that tolerance develops to the reduction in brain cAMP which results from acute administration of ethanol, but that the similar change in cGMP does not demonstrate tolerance. However, Hunt et al. (1977) presented evidence which suggests that the reduction in cGMP produced by acute administration of ethanol is less, at similar blood ethanol concentrations, after chronic administration of the drug. The results suggest that tolerance to the effects of ethanol on metabolism of both cyclic nucleotides develops. It may be that neuronal adaptation involves some alteration in adenyl or guanyl cyclase or in the intracellular concentration of cyclic nucleotides. This could be the basis for tolerance to ethanol at the level of neurotransmitter release or receptor activation.

Neurotransmitters other than monoamines are affected by the chronic administration of ethanol and so may play some part in the development of tolerance. Acetylcholine release, which is decreased in vivo by the acute administration of ethanol (see Section II), is also reduced when ethanol is added in vitro to cortical slices (Kalant and Grose, 1967). The chronic administration of ethanol to animals abolishes the subsequent ability of ethanol to reduce acetylcholine release in vitro (Kalant and Grose, 1967). The cholinergic terminals seem therefore to have become tolerant to this effect of ethanol. Concentrations of acetylcholine in brain are usually reported to be decreased by chronic administration of ethanol (e.g., Hunt and Dalton, 1976) and the enzymes of acetylcholine metabolism may also be affected (see Feldstein, 1971). There seems to be no evidence of alterations in acetylcholine receptor sensitivity induced by ethanol or of alteration in development of ethanol tolerance by drugs affecting cholinergic nerves.

Changes in γ-aminobutyric acid (GABA) concentration have been reported in mammalian brain during the chronic administration of ethanol, but the results seem contradictory. For example, Sutton (1973) and Rawat (1974) have reported increases in GABA concentration, whereas Sytinsky et al. (1975) and Griffiths and Littleton (1977a) have reported decreases. Different concentrations of ethanol achieved in vivo may explain these differences. There is at present no evidence to link brain GABA, or alterations in other amino acids induced by ethanol (Griffiths and Littleton, 1977a), with the development of tolerance to ethanol. It must be acknowledged that other putative neurotransmitters or neuromodulators (e.g., peptides, prostaglandins) may have a role in the development of ethanol tolerance, but at present there is no direct evidence for this.

D. Development of Metabolic Tolerance to Ethanol

There seems to be no doubt that the elimination rate of ethanol increases after its chronic administration, and it is also certain that this increase is due to increased metabolism of ethanol by the liver. At this stage agreement ends; the adaptive change in hepatic metabolism of ethanol remains controversial.

The extent of the development of metabolic tolerance by animals and humans is probably not great. Most workers report an increase in the rate of metabolism of ethanol by experimental animals to about double the normal rate (see Thurman and McKenna, 1975). The situation in human studies is complicated by liver dysfunction found in chronic alcoholics. Healthy volunteers and alcoholics certainly seem able to increase metabolism of ethanol after its chronic administration (e.g., Mendelson et al., 1966) but there appears to be no significant difference between alcoholics and normal subjects after a period of abstinence (Mendelson, 1968).

The reason for the increased rate of ethanol metabolism after its chronic administration is not understood. There are many conflicting reports as to whether the activity of hepatic alcohol dehydrogenase is increased (see Thurman and McKenna, 1975), but this is probably irrelevant anyway since the rate-limiting step in this pathway is the dissociation rate of reduced cofactor from the enzyme (Theorell and Chance, 1951). There is some evidence (Thurman and McKenna, 1975) that an adaptive increase in the rate of NADH reoxidation can occur, thereby activating the alcohol dehydrogenase pathway at this step. Evidence for altered activities of catalase and the mitochondrial ethanol-oxidizing system after the chronic adminsitration of ethanol is also conflicting. Once again the problem may be that the enzyme activities themselves are not rate limiting. Change in rate of ethanol metabolism through any of these putative pathways may depend on availability of other factors.

Regardless of the reason for the increase in hepatic metabolism of ethanol resulting from its chronic administration, there is little doubt that such a change does make a significant contribution to ethanol tolerance. There is also the possibility that ethanol tolerance may be due partly to induction of alcohol dehydrogenase in the brain. Although such a change was reported by Raskin and Sokoloff (1972), this does not appear to have been observed by other workers. It seems likely that such metabolic tolerance as exists to ethanol is seated primarily in the liver.

IV. RELATIONSHIP BETWEEN TOLERANCE AND DEPENDENCE

A. Introduction

In one sense there is an obvious relationship between tolerance and dependence. The development of tolerance makes it necessary for the individual to increase intake to produce the same behavioral effect. This increased intake may then predispose toward the development of dependence. However, this section is concerned not with any indirect relationship of this sort but with the possibility that tolerance and dependence share the same mechanism and can be regarded as different aspects of the same process. Several authors have considered this possibility in the past (e.g., Jaffe and Sharpless, 1968; Mendelson, 1971).

B. Basic Unitary Hypothesis for Tolerance and Dependence

The hypothesis relies on the empirical observation that the withdrawal syndrome always represents a change opposite to that produced by the acute administration of the drug. This can be explained most simply by supposing that during the chronic administration of the drug the neuronal pathways affected adapt to its presence to reach a relatively normal level of function. This adaptation, or cellular tolerance, may relate to a number of mechanisms (e.g., receptor synthesis, Collier, 1965; enzyme expansion, Goldstein and Goldstein, 1968; alteration in synaptic membranes, Hill and Bangham, 1975). When this adaptation has been achieved, removal of the drug leaves the neuronal pathway exposed at its "new" level of functional activity, and the withdrawal syndrome results. A diagrammatic representation of the way in which this scheme may apply to the central depression produced by ethanol is shown in Figure 4. It should be noted that rapid removal of the drug, accentuated by the development of metabolic tolerance, may make the withdrawal syndrome more precipitate, but is not necessary for the production of the syndrome (e.g., Littleton et al., 1974).

This hypothesis is attractive because of its simplicity. It does explain the almost invariable association between cellular tolerance and physical dependence,

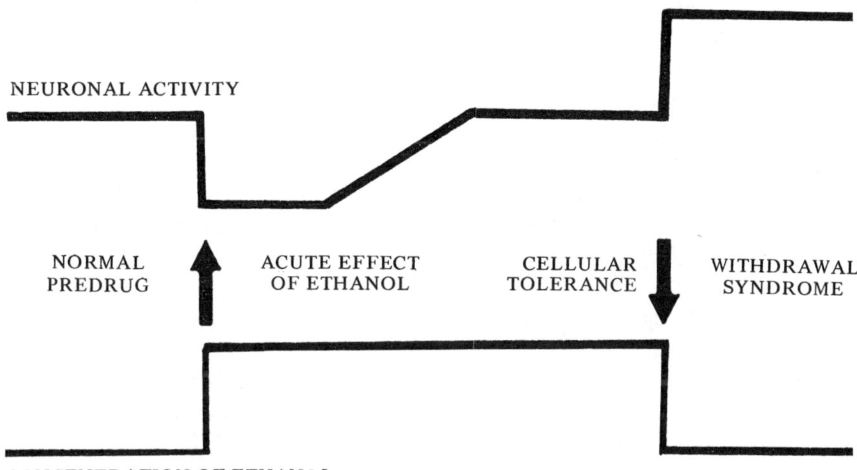

Figure 4 Simplified view of the unitary hypothesis of drug dependence. The concentration of ethanol in the vicinity of the neuron is assumed to be either zero or effective in causing neuronal depression. In vivo, of course, this is not the case. Concentrations of ethanol in the brain may rise relatively quickly after its peripheral administration, but tend to decay slowly as ethanol is metabolized by the liver. Metabolic tolerance to ethanol may cause concentrations of ethanol in brain to fall more rapidly and thus precipitate a withdrawal syndrome more quickly (see text and Fig. 5).

and also the relation between the acute effects of a drug and the withdrawal syndrome. There seems certain to be much truth in the hypothesis, but there are some disturbing discrepancies between predictions based on the hypothesis and experimental observations.

C. Arguments Against Unitary Hypothesis

Even on a brief consideration it is unlikely that the unitary hypothesis of tolerance and dependence can be strictly true. Chronic administration of many drugs acting on the central nervous system, e.g.,antidepressants and neuroleptics, can be shown to produce aspects of cellular tolerance (e.g. Asper et al., 1973) but these drugs are not considered to produce dependence since their removal does not lead to an overt withdrawal syndrome. Of course, the critical point here is to establish what is meant by an "overt withdrawal syndrome." It may be that removal of these drugs from a tolerant individual does produce a functional change in the central nervous system but that current methods of objective investigation are not sufficiently sensitive to observe this.

We can propose a similar argument based on observations of the relationship between cellular tolerance and dependence on ethanol. The time course of development of cellular tolerance may be extremely short—hours, or even minutes (e.g., Leblanc et al., 1975)—but the induction of dependence usually requires several days of continuous administration of ethanol (see Freund, 1969; Goldstein and Pal, 1971; Griffiths et al., 1973; Majchrowicz and Hunt, 1976). There is no overt evidence of ethanol dependence within hours of a single dose of ethanol, yet tolerance can be seen at that time (see above), suggesting that there is no direct connection between the two. Even this statement may be untrue. If "evidence of dependence" is simply some functional change on removal of the drug, then ethanol-induced "hangover" can be taken as evidence of dependence after a single dose of the drug. Also, although overt signs of a withdrawal syndrome cannot be seen, McQuarrie and Fingl (1958) showed that mice have a lower seizure threshold for a short period following a single dose of ethanol. The best counter to this argument is that at least the time course of hangover and the decrease in seizure threshold is less than that of the withdrawal syndrome, but this merely implies a quantitative rather than a qualitative difference.

Majchrowicz and Hunt (1976) presented evidence based on the time courses of development of maximal ethanol tolerance and dependence which suggests that their mechanisms are different. Also, Ritzmann and Tabakoff (1976) demonstrated that tolerance to the hypothermic effects of ethanol can be separated from physical dependence by administration of other drugs. Evidence of the kind presented here does not disprove a relationship between cellular tolerance and physical dependence, but it does suggest that the simple, direct relationship of the unitary hypothesis requires modification.

D. A Concept of Dependence Based on Time Course of Neuronal Adaptation

Figure 4 shows that removal of ethanol from an animal in the drug-tolerant state should produce a functional change in the central nervous system causing the withdrawal syndrome. This functional change will continue until the neurons return to their original, predrug, state, i.e., until they adapt to the absence of the drug. Since this should involve merely the reversal of the change which induced drug tolerance, it is difficult to see why it should have a very different time course. As stated previously, tolerance to ethanol in the rat can be observed after a single dose of the drug, i.e., within 1 hr. The functional change on withdrawal should therefore be very brief (see Fig. 5). In fact, the withdrawal syndrome in the rat lasts about 72 hr, (see Walker and Zornetzer, 1974). Clearly, if the above arguments are true, the long duration of the withdrawal

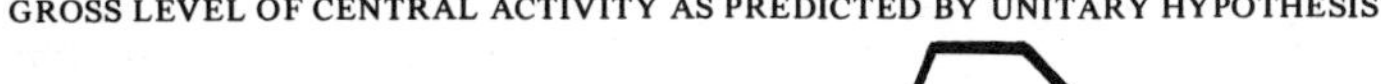

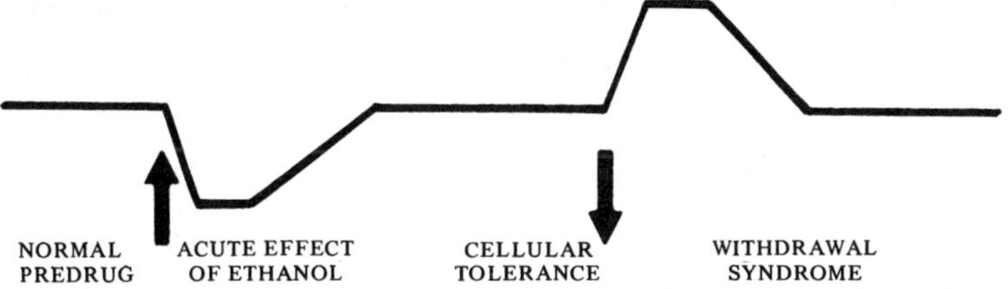

GROSS LEVEL OF CENTRAL ACTIVITY SUGGESTED BY EXPERIMENTAL RESULTS

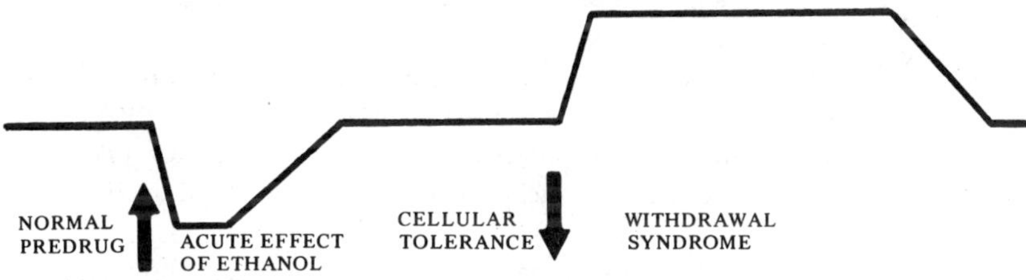

Figure 5 Highly diagrammatic attempt to show relationships between the development of tolerance and the withdrawal syndrome.

syndrome, and perhaps its very existence, represents a failure of the rapid adaptive mechanism of neurons. Evidence is presented in Section III which suggested that the initial adaptation of neuronal membranes to the presence of ethanol is by an alteration in membrane phospholipid composition. Some aspects of this change seem to occur within 2 hr of the continuous administration of ethanol to mice (Littleton and John, 1977). Cellular tolearance may therefore become dependence only when this mechanism of membrane lipid adaptation fails for some reason. Failure of other neuronal adaptive mechanisms could equally account for the discrepancy between the time courses of tolerance development and the withdrawal syndrome.

The modification of the unitary hypothesis of tolerance and dependence which is proposed here is, therefore, that cellular tolerance on ethanol develops into physical dependence when the rapid adaptational mechanism of neuronal membranes is inhibited in some way. The reasons for supposing some alteration of lipid metabolism associated with dependence are discussed in the next section.

V. DEVELOPMENT OF DEPENDENCE ON ETHANOL

A. Introduction

Dependence on ethanol can be considered as of the physical and psychological type, as can that of most central depressant drugs. The use of these terms has already been considered (see Section I). Psychological dependence on ethanol is obviously very difficult to study in laboratory animals and presents problems of definition even in humans. There is some evidence that catecholaminergic nerves are involved in pathological ethanol consumption (e.g., Sprince et al., 1972) whereas recent evidence (e.g., Myers and Melchior, 1977) suggests that this may be mediated by alkaloids of the tetrahydropapaveroline type (see also Davis and Walsh, 1970).

Physical dependence represents a much easier field of study in that objective criteria for the condition can be established. These are based on the observation of a physical syndrome of withdrawal on removal of ethanol. This syndrome in animals and in humans includes signs of anxiety and excitation (which may be followed by prostration), tremor, and convulsions. Hallucinations occur in humans and behavior suggestive of hallucinations is observed in animals (e.g., see Victor, 1970; Goldstein and Pal, 1971; Hammond and Schneider, 1973; Walker and Zornetzer, 1974). Increased voluntary alcohol consumption by animals during the physical withdrawal syndrome has also been described (e.g., Hunter et al., 1974). The time required to produce physical dependence in animals is of the order of days (see review by Friedman and Lester, 1977). Probably longer is required in humans, but it seems unlikely under optimum conditions that the time required would be more than a few weeks (e.g., Isbell et al., 1955). An important consideration is that administration of ethanol should be continuous (e.g., see Goldstein, 1974). The withdrawal syndrome itself lasts for some 10-12 hr in mice (e.g., Griffiths et al., 1974a) and several days in humans (see Victor, 1970). Other laboratory animals probably show syndromes intermediate in duration.

The criterion of physical dependence is the presence of a withdrawal syndrome. The only way to demonstrate dependence, therefore, is by removal of the drug in question. This itself removes the state of dependence. An additional problem is that no quantitative measure of physical dependence exists. One can measure the severity of the withdrawal syndrome (e.g., Goldstein and Pal, 1971) but in comparison between treatment groups (e.g., Goldstein, 1971; Griffiths et al., 1974a,b) or between different strains (e.g., Goldstein and Kakihana, 1974; Griffiths and Littleton, 1977b) this cannot be taken as an indication of the extent of preexisting dependence. Individuals may be equally physically dependent, but the expression of the withdrawal syndrome may differ. Until every aspect of dependence and the withdrawal syndrome can be measured this problem cannot be overcome.

B. Dependence on Ethanol at Level of Neuronal Membranes

Hill and Bangham (1975) formulated a hypothesis of central depressant tolerance and dependence which attempted to explain these phenomena at the level of the neuronal membrane. Their hypothesis does not distinguish between cellular tolerance and dependence, and therefore suffers from the same drawbacks as other unitary hypotheses (see Section IV). However, the results of Chin and Goldstein (1977b) and Littleton and John (1977) suggest that some alteration of synaptosomal membranes does occur in ethanol-dependent animals. It seems that this alternation can more easily explain cellular tolerance than dependence.

In Section IV it is argued that cellular tolerance may become physical dependence when the neuronal mechanism of rapid adaptation becomes inhibited. Rapid adaptaton of neuronal membranes may be by alteration of phospholipid fatty acid composition. There is indirect evidence (Abu Murad et al., 1977; Griffiths et al., 1977) suggesting that some general disorder of fatty acid metabolism accompanies the development of ethanol physical dependence. This disorder of fatty acid metabolism may also contribute to some of the pathological effects of ethanol, including the accumulation of triglyceride in different organs. Thus, the accumulation of triglyceride in liver which is induced by chronic administration of ethanol seems to be genetically linked to the severity of the ethanol physical withdrawal syndrome (Griffiths et al., 1977). Also the administration of (±)-carnitine to animals during the induction of physical dependence on ethanol prevents some aspects of the change in lipid metabolism normally associated with dependence and reduces the severity of the subsequent withdrawal syndrome (Abu Murad et al., 1977). These results and those which suggest synaptic membrane alteration are suggestive of an important role for membrane lipids in the development of dependence, but a great deal more work is required.

It seems unlikely that the lipid fraction only of the membrane is involved in the induction of dependence. In Section IV it is suggested that adaptation in membrane proteins played a role in the later development of cellular tolerance and that protein adaptation may eventually supplant lipid adaptation as the mechanism for tolerance. If so, then it will be this alteration in membrane proteins which will eventually be responsible for the expression of the withdrawal syndrome. Information is lacking on the rate of synthesis of specific neuronal proteins in ethanol dependence and withdrawal, but, in general terms, brain protein synthesis is depressed in ethanol-tolerant animals (see Section IV) and in ethanol-dependent animals, and may become further depressed during the withdrawal syndrome (see Tewari and Noble, 1977). With regard to membrane proteins specifically related to neuronal excitability, it seems unlikely that alterations in activity of [Na^+, K^+]-ATPase can be important in ethanol dependence or in the withdrawal syndrome (Goldstein and Iraael, 1972) but this is not yet certain. There are numerous other possibilities not yet fully investigated, including altered proportions of calcium binding proteins, altered numbers of ion channels through the membrane, and alterations in neurotransmitter receptor proteins (see Section V.C).

C. Dependence on Ethanol at Level of Neurotransmitter Metabolism

In general, the changes in neurotransmitter metabolism associated with the dependent state are similar to those discussed in Section III under tolerance. Thus there is a tendency for increased catecholamine concentrations, synthesis and metabolites, reduction in acetylcholine concentration and release, and changes in metabolism of several amino acid putative neurotransmitters (for references, see Section III). Decreased concentrations of cyclic nucleotides in brain are also found in the ethanol-dependent state, and reduced sensitivity of adenyl cyclase to neurotransmitters probably also exists (see Section III). All these changes may represent a complex pattern of adaptation to one primary alteration in neurotransmitter metabolism or, alternatively, may simply reflect a change induced by ethanol at the level of the neuronal membrane. It is not possible to be certain whether these changes in neurotransmitter metabolism play an important role in the genesis of dependence. All that can be said is that many seem to be important in the expression of dependence, i.e., they play some part in the genesis of the withdrawal syndrome.

During withdrawal of ethanol from dependent animals several changes in neurotransmitter metabolism occur. There is a rapid increase in concentration and synthesis of noradrenaline in brain but some doubt as to whether similar changes occur in brain dopamine (Griffiths et al., 1973, 1974a; Hunt and Majchrowicz, 1974a). Noradrenaline metabolites are increased (Karoum et al., 1976). Urinary excretion of catecholamines and their metabolites increases during withdrawal of alcohol from alcoholics (see Feldstein, 1971). There seems to be some correlation between severity of the ethanol withdrawal syndrome and excretion of catecholamines.

This increase in central (and probably also in peripheral) catecholamine synthesis and release may be simply a response to the stress of alcohol withdrawal. However, there is evidence from the administration of inhibitors of noradrenaline biosynthesis that this neurochemical change may mediate the excitation observed in animals at the beginning of the withdrawal syndrome (Griffiths et al., 1974a).

Following the increase in catecholamine synthesis there is an increase in sensitivity of adenyl cyclase to catecholamines (e.g., French and Palmer, 1973; French et al., 1975; Smith et al., 1977). Once again the evidence for increased noradrenaline receptor sensitivity is more convincing than that for dopamine.

These changes reflect a tendency for increased functional activity in catecholaminergic nerves during the physical syndrome of withdrawal from ethanol. Several workers have attempted to modify the withdrawal syndrome by administration of drugs which interfere with catecholamine synthesis or receptor activation. In general, the results indicate that the increase in functional activity in catecholaminergic nerves is a protective mechanism, acting to reduce the severity of ethanol withdrawal convulsions and tremor (e.g., Goldstein, 1973; Griffiths et al., 1973,1974a; Blum and Wallace, 1974; Blum et al., 1976a; Littleton et al., 1976). These changes in catecholamine neurotransmitter metabolism seem, therefore, unlikely to play any direct role in the production of the major signs of the physical withdrawal syndrome. They may, of course, be important in other signs, such as anxiety, autonomic changes, and sleep disturbances.

Changes in 5-HT metabolism, generally suggesting increased functional activity, have also been reported during the ethanol withdrawal syndrome (e.g., Griffiths et al., 1974a; Pohorecky et al., 1974b; Gothoni and Ahtee, 1977) but these do not seem to be as marked as the changes observed in catecholamine metabolism. Sensitivity of 5-HT-stimulated adenyl cyclase is also reported to increase (French et al., 1975). Recently Tabakoff et al. (1977b) reported that serotonergic neurons in brain show reduced synthesis of 5-HT from labeled tryptophan during the withdrawal syndrome. It cannot therefore be stated with any certainty whether increased or decreased 5-HT functional activity is associated with ethanol withdrawal. There is also controversy over whether 5-HT-containing neurons play any role in withdrawal, since suppression of 5-HT synthesis seems to have no obvious effect on the withdrawal syndrome (e.g., Goldstein, 1973; Griffiths et al., 1974b), but antagonism of 5-HT receptors potentiates withdrawal convulsions (Blum et al., 1976b). A role for 5-HT-containing neurons in ethanol withdrawal head twitches has also been proposed (Collier et al., 1974, 1976). In this case it may be the balance between 5-HT and catecholamine systems which is important.

There is little information on dynamic aspects of acetycholine metabolism during the ethanol withdrawal syndrome. Hunt and Dalton (1976) report that the decrease in acetylcholine concentrations observed in brains of ethanol-dependent rats does not persist into the withdrawal syndrome. In testing drugs which interfere with cholinergic transmission, Goldstein (1972) was unable to demonstrate any alteration in the ethanol withdrawal syndrome. Although it cannot be stated with certainty, it seems unlikely, on present evidence, that central cholinergic nerves play an important part in the ethanol withdrawal syndrome.

In 1973, Patel and Lal reported that brain GABA concentrations were reduced in mice undergoing the physical syndrome of ethanol withdrawal. Goldstein (1973) had previously suggested, on the basis of drug-induced alteration of ethanol withdrawal convulsions, that a functional reduction in brain GABA may be involved in the withdrawal syndrome. Griffiths and Littleton (1977a) showed that GABA concentrations were reduced in the brains of ethanol-dependent mice and that concentrations reverted to normal during the withdrawal syndrome with a time course similar to that of the behavioral change. The reduction in brain GABA concentration has also been shown to be strain-dependent (Griffiths and Littleton, 1977b), strains showing the most severe withdrawal syndromes exhibiting the greatest reduction in brain GABA concentration. In addition, it has been reported (Cooper et al., 1977) that intracerebral GABA can inhibit the development of seizures during ethanol withdrawal. Clearly there is now good evidence for supposing that GABA-containing neurons have reduced functional activity during the ethanol withdrawal syndrome and that this plays some part in the genesis of withdrawal convulsions. Evidence for involvement of other amino acids in ethanol withdrawal is slight, but proline and aspartic acid may prove interesting candidates (see Griffiths and Littleton, 1977a,b).

Many of the changes in functional neurotransmitter metabolism which occur during the withdrawal syndrome may be related to alterations in intracellular cyclic nucleotide concentrations or to changes in sensitivity of membrane-bound adenyl or guanyl cyclase. The work of Volicer and Hurter (1977) shows that levels of cyclic nucleotides, although reduced in the dependent state, may increase to supranormal concentrations during the ethanol withdrawal syndrome. Paralleling this increase in cyclic nucleotide concentation, French et al. (1975) reported that sensitivity of adenyl cyclase to several neurotransmitters is increased during the ethanol withdrawal syndrome. A relationship between GABA and these changes in adenyl cyclase may also exist (e.g., French et al., 1975). The changes in cyclic nucleotides, and in adenyl cyclase reported here, seem to fulfill many of the requirements of a fundamental basis for tolerance and dependence. However, the changes may reflect an even more fundamental alteration at the neuronal membrane level. Functions and composition of synaptic membranes and activity of membrane-bound enzymes are certain to be closely interrelated. More basic research is required before the cellular basis of ethanol dependence can be ascribed to any one of these changes.

VI. CONCLUSIONS

Ethanol tolerance and dependence are important aspects of the pathological effects of alcohol consumption, and as such they have great medical and social significance. It is necessary to reach an understanding of the mechanisms underlying tolerance and dependence on ethanol for these practical reasons. The development of tolerance and dependence is also of tremendous theoretical interest because it throws light on the fundamental processes by which neurons adapt to prolonged stimulation or depression.

From the evidence presented in this chapter, it seems likely that many of the effects of acute administration of ethanol may be accounted for by some biophysical effect of ethanol on neuronal cell membranes. The development of tolerance to ethanol, although it may occur rapidly, does not seem to reach the extent shown by tolerance to morphine. Tolerance to ethanol appears to take place at several levels of organization of the central nervous system. At the level of the synaptic membrane, tolerance develops to the biophysical effects of ethanol, and this may be due to an adaptive change in the lipid or protein composition of the membrane. Changes in neurotransmitter metabolism may also be important; probably the best evidence favors alteration in neurotransmitter receptor sensitivity as a basis for tolerance. The monamine neurotransmitters appears to be particularly closely involved. At the level of the intact animal the development of tolerance seems to have characteristics in common with learned behavior. In addition to these aspects of tolerance, a change in the metabolism of ethanol contributes to the process. Increased metabolism of ethanol by the liver, perhaps by increased oxidation of ethanol by alcohol dehydrogenase, leads to more rapid elimination of the drug in the tolerant subject.

There seems to be a strong connection between tolerance at the cellular level and the development of physical dependence on ethanol. It has been suggested here that physical dependence cannot be simply a facet of cellular tolerance, as has been proposed by others, but that it represents a "fixing" of the state of cellular tolerance by failure of some adaptive mechanism within the neuron. The result is that when ethanol is withdrawn from a dependent subject, readaptation to the absence of the drug cannot occur and a functional change, the withdrawal syndrome, results. The withdrawal syndrome from ethanol seems to be expressed, at least partly, through pathways utilizing amine and amino acid neurotransmitters. The increased level of central excitation associated with withdrawal may be closely related to changes in cyclic nucleotide metabolism which occur at this time.

Research on alcohol tolerance and dependence now seems to be approaching an understanding of the fundamental basis of these conditions. It is not certain as to whether this approach will necessarily lead to any rapid improvement in clinical treatment of alcoholics. This is partly because the complexity of the social, psychiatric, and medical problems associated with alcoholism preclude direct comparisons with animal experimentation. However, the information gained in such studies should be of value in early diagnosis of the ethanol-dependent state and should facilitate consideration of some logical therapeutic possibilities. In this connection, study of dependence at the level of neurotransmitter metabolism may initially be of greater benefit because current neuropharmacological and psychiatric thinking concentrates on manipulation of neurotransmitter function as a means of producing a therapeutic effect. In the long run, study of dependence at the level of composition and function of the synaptic membrane may prove to be most valuable. Precise manipulation of neuronal excitability, in terms of the response to different drugs or neurotransmitters, may become possible, providing a whole new armory for neuropharmacologists and psychiatrists.

In conclusion, although we cannot yet be said to understand alcohol tolerance and dependence at any level of organization, it is important that we continue to try. Approaches based on the single neuron, neurotransmitter pathways, and complex behavior are all valuable and provide information of great theoretical and practical importance. The uneasy balance between pleasurable and harmful effects of alcohol may be tipped in our favor by such information. Few would argue that this would not be of great benefit to our society.

REFERENCES

Abu Murad, C., Begg, S. J., Griffiths, P. J., and Littleton, J. M. (1977). Hepatic triglyceride accumulation and the ethanol physical withdrawal syndrome in mice. *Br. J. Exp. Path. 58,* 606-615.

Ahlenius, S., Carlsson, A., Engel, J., Svensson, T. H., and Sodersten, P. (1973). Antagonism by alpha methyltyrosine of the ethanol-induced stimulation and euphoria in man. *Clin. Pharmacol. Ther. 14,* 586-591.

Asper, H., Baggiolini, M., Burki, H. R., Lanenr, H., Ruch, W., and Stille, G. (1973). Tolerance phenomena with neuroleptics catalepsy apomorphine stereotypes and striatal dopamine metabolism in the rat after single and repeated administration of loxapine and haloperidol. *Eur. J. Pharmacol. 22,* 287-294.

Blum, K., and Wallace, J. E. (1974). Effects of catecholamine synthesis inhibition on ethanol-induced withdrawal symptoms in mice. *Br. J. Pharmacol. 51,* 109-111.

Blum, K., Wallace, J. E., and Geller, I. (1972). Synergy of ethanol and putative neurotransmitters: glycine and serine. *Science 176,* 292-294.

Blum, K., Calhoun, W., Merritt, J., and Wallace, J. E. (1973). L-DOPA: effect on ethanol narcosis and brain biogenic amines in mice. *Nature 242,* 406-409.

Blum, K., Eubanks, J. D., Wallace, J. E., and Schwertner, H. A. (1976a). Suppression of ethanol withdrawal by dopamine. *Experientia 32,* 493-495.

Blum, K., Wallace, J. E., Schwertner, H. A., and Eubanks, J. D. (1976b). Enhancement of ethanol-induced withdrawal convulsion by blockade of 5-hydroxytryptamine receptors. *J. Pharm. Pharmacol. 28,* 832-835.

Carlsson, A., Engel, J. H., and Svensson, T. H. (1972). Inhibition of ethanol-induced excitation in mice and rats by alpha-methyl-p-tyrosine. *Psychopharmacologia 26,* 307-312.

Carlsson, A., Engel, J., Strombom, U., Svensson, T. H., and Waldeck, B. (1974). Suppression by dopamine agonists of the ethanol-induced stimulation of locomotor activity and brain dopamine synthesis. *Naunyn Schmiedeberg's Arch. Pharmacol. 283,* 117-128.

Carmichael, F. J., and Israel, Y. (1975). Effects of ethanol on neurotransmitter release by rat brain cortical slices. *J. Pharmacol. Exp. Ther. 193,* 824-834.

Chan, A. W. K. (1976). Gamma aminobutyric acid in different strains of mice. Effect of ethanol. *Life Sci. 19,* 596-604.

Chin, J. H., and Goldstein, D. B. (1977a). Effects of low concentrations of ethanol on the fluidity of spin-labelled erythrocyte and brain membranes. *Mol. Pharmacol. 13,* 435-442.

Chin, J. H., and Goldstein, D. B. (1977b). Drug tolerance in biomembranes: a spin label study of the effects of ethanol. *Science 196,* 684-685.

Collier, H. O. J. (1965). A general theory of the genesis of drug dependence by induction of receptors. *Nature 205,* 181-182.

Collier, H. O. J., Hammond, M. D., and Schneider, C. (1974). Biogenic amines and head twitches in mice during ethanol withdrawal. *Br. J. Pharmacol. 51,* 310-311.

Collier, H. O. J., Hammond, M. D., and Schneider, C. (1976). Effects of drugs affecting endogenous amines or cyclic nucleotides on ethanol withdrawal head twitches in mice. *Br. J. Pharmacol. 58,* 9-16.

Cooper, B. R., Viik, K., Sato, T., and White, H. L. (1977). GABA and susceptibility to audiogenic seizures during alcohol withdrawal in the rat. *Fed. Proc. 36* (3), 286 No. 83.

Davis, V. E., and Walsh, M. J. (1970). Alcohol, amines and alkaloids: a possible basis for alcohol addiction. *Science 167,* 1005-1007.

Douglas, W. W. (1968). Stimulus-secretion coupling: the concept and clues from chromaffin and other cells. *Br. J. Pharmacol. 34,* 451-474.

Edwards, G.,and Gross, M. M. (1976). Alcohol dependence: provisional description of a clinical syndrome. *Br. Med. J. 1* (6017), 1058-1061.

Farias, R. N., Bloj, B., Morero, R. D., Sineriz, F., and Trucco, R. E. (1975). Regulation of allosteric membrane-bound enzymes through changes in membrane lipid composition. *Biochim. Biophys. Acta 415,* 231-251.

Feldstein, A. (1971). In *The Biology of Alcoholism.* Vol. 1. *Biochemistry,* B. Kissin and H. Begleiter (Eds.), Plenum, New York, pp. 127-160.

Frankel, D., Khanna, J. M., Leblanc, A. E., and Kalant, H. (1975). Effect of para-chlorophenylalanine on the acquisition of tolerance to ethanol and pentobarbital. *Psychopharmacologia 44,* 247-252.

French, S. W., and Palmer, D. S. (1973). Adrenergic supersensitivity during ethanol withdrawal in the rat. *Res. Commun. Chem. Pathol. 6,* 651-662.

French, S. W., Reid, P. E., Palmer, D. S., Narold, M. E., and Ramey, C. W. (1974). Adrenergic subsensitivity of the rat brain during chronic ethanol ingestion. *Res. Commun. Chem. Path. Pharmacol. 9,* 575-578.

French, S. W., Palmer, D. S., and Narold, M. E. (1975). Effect of withdrawal from chronic ethanol ingestion on the cAMP response of creebral cortical slices using the agonists histamine, serotonin and other neurotransmitters. *Can. J. Physiol. Pharmacol. 53,* 248-255.

Freund, G. (1969). Alcohol withdrawal syndrome in mice. *Arch. Neurol. 21,* 315-320.

Friedman, H. J. and Lester, D. (1977). In *Alcohol and Opiates,* K. Blum (Ed.), Academic, New York, London, San Francisco, pp. 1-20.

Garrett, K. M., and Ross, D. H. (1977). Fluorescent probe binding to synaptic membranes after acute and chronic ethanol exposure. *Fed. Proc. 36* (3), 314, No. 229.

Goldstein, D. B. (1973). Alcohol withdrawal reactions in mice: effects of drugs that modify neurotransmission. *J. Pharmacol. Exp. Ther. 186,* 1-9.

Goldstein, D. B. (1974). Rates of onset and decay of alcohol physical dependence in mice. *J. Pharmacol. Exp. Ther. 190,* 377-383.

Goldstein, A., and Goldstein, D. B. (1968). In *The Addictive States,* A. Wikler (Ed.), Williams and Wilkins, Baltimore, pp. 265-267.

Goldstein, D. B., and Israel, Y. (1972). Effects of ethanol on mouse brain [$Na^+ + K^+$]-activated adenosine tryphosphatase. *Life Sci. 11.II,* 957-963.

Goldstein, D. B., and Kakihana, R. (1974). Alcohol withdrawal reactions and reserpine effects in inbred strains in mice. *Life Sci. 15,* 415-425.

Goldstein, D. B., and Pal, N. (1971). Alcohol dependence produced in mice by inhalation of ethanol: grading the withdrawal reaction. *Science 172,* 288-290.

Gothóni, P., and Ahtee, L. (1977). 5-Hydroxytryptamine and 5-hydroxyindoleacetic acid concentrations in brains of rats during ethanol intoxication and withdrawal. *Acta Pharmacol. Toxicol. 41, suppl. IV,* 49.

Graham, D. T., and Erickson, C. K. (1974). Alteration of ethanol-induced CNS depression: ineffectiveness of drugs that modify cholinergic transmission. *Psychopharmacologia 34,* 173-180.

Griffiths, P. J., and Littleton, J. M. (1977a). Concentrations of free amino acids in brains of mice during the induction of physical dependence on ethanol and during the ethanol withdrawal syndrome. *Br. J. Exp. Path. 58,* 19-27.

Griffiths, P. J., and Littleton, J. M. (1977b). Concentrations of free amino acids in brains of mice of different strains during the physical syndrome of withdrawal from ethanol. *Br. J. Exp. Path. 58,* 391-399.

Griffiths, P. J., Littleton, J. M., and Ortiz, A. (1973). Evidence for a role for brain monamines in ethanol dependence. *Br. J. Pharmacol. 48,* 354P.

Griffiths, P. J., Littleton, J. M., and Ortiz, A. (1974a). Changes in monamine concentrations in mouse brain associated with ethanol dependence and withdrawal. *Br. J. Pharmacol. 50,* 489-498.

Griffiths, P. J., Littleton, J. M., and Ortiz, A. (1974b). Effect of p-chlorophenylalanine on brain monamines and behaviour during ethanol withdrawal in mice. *Br. J. Pharmacol. 51,* 307-309.

Griffiths, P. J., Abu Murad, C., and Littleton, J. M. (1977). Ethanol-induced heptatic triglyceride accumulation in mice and genetic differences in the ethanol physical withdrawal syndrome. *Br. J. Addict. 74,* 37-42.

Hakkinen, H. M., and Kulonen, E. (1976). Ethanol intoxication and gamma-aminobutyric acid. *J. Neurochem. 27,* 631-633.

Hammond, M. D., and Schneider, C. (1973). Behavioural changes induced in mice following termination of ethanol administration. *Br. J. Pharmacol. 47,* 667P.

Havre, P., Abrams, M. A., Corrall, R. J. M., Yu, L. C., Szcepanik, P. A., Feldman, H. B., Klein, P., Kong, M. S., Margolis, J. M., and Landau, B. R. (1977). Quantitation of pathways of ethanol metabolism. *Arch. Biochem. Biophys. 182,* 14-23.

Hill, M. W., and Bangham, A. D. (1975). General depressant drug dependency: a biophysical hypothesis. *Adv. Exp. Med. Biol. 59,* 1-9.

Hoffman, P. L., and Tabakoff, B. (1977). Alterations in dopamine receptor sensitivity by chronic ethanol treatment. *Nature 268,* 551-553.

Hunt, W. A., and Dalton, T. K. (1976). Regional brain acetylcholine levels in rats acutely treated with ethanol or rendered ethanol dependent. *Brain Res. 109,* 628-631.

Hunt, W. A., and Majchrowicz, E. (1974a). Alterations in the turnover of brain norepinephrine and dopamine in alcohol dependent rats. *J. Neurochem. 23,* 549-552.

Hunt, W. A., and Majchrowicz, E. (1974b). Turnover rates and steady state levels of brain serotonin in alcohol dependent rats. *Brain Res. 72,* 184-184.

Hunt, W. A., Redos, J. D., Dalton, T. K., and Catravos, G. N. (1977). Alterations in brain cyclic guanosine 3′:5′-monophosphate levels after acute and chronic treatment with ethanol. *J. Pharmacol. Exp. Ther. 201,* 103-109.

Hunter, B. E., Walker, D. W., and Riley, J. N. (1974). Dissociation between physical dependence and volitional ethanol consumption: role of multiple withdrawal episodes. *Pharmacol. Biochem. Behav. 2,* 523-529.

Hurwitz, L., Battle, F., and Weiss, G. B. (1962). Action of the calcium antagonists cocaine and ethanol on contraction and potassium efflux of smooth muscle. *J. Gen. Physiol. 46,* 315-332.

Iida, S., and Hikichi, M. (1976). Effect of taurine on ethanol-induced sleeping time in mice. *J. Stud. Alcohol 37,* 19-26.

Ingram, L. O. (1976). Adaptation of membrane lipids to alcohols. *J. Bacteriol. 126,* 670-678.

Isbell, H., Fraser, H. F., Wikler, A., Belleville, R. E., and Eisenman, A. J. (1955). An experimental study of the etiology of "rum fits" and delirium tremens. *Quart. J. Stud. Alc. 16,* 1-33.

Israel, Y., Kalant, H., Leblanc, A. E., Bernstein, J. C., and Salazar, I. (1970). Changes in cation transport and [$Na^+ + K^+$]-activated adenosine triphosphatase produced by chronic administration of ethanol. *J. Pharmacol. Exp. Ther. 174,* 330-336.

Israel, Y., Kimura, H., and Kuriyama, K. (1972). Changes in activity and hormonal sensitivity of brain adenyl cyclase following chronic ethanol administration. *Experientia 28,* 1322-1323.

Jaffe, J. H., and Sharpless, S. K. (1968). In *The Addictive States,* A. Wikler (Ed.), Williams and Wilkins, Baltimore, pp. 226-243.

Kalant, H. (1971). In *The Biology of Alcoholism, Vol. I. Biochemistry,* B. Kissin andH. Begleiter (Eds.), Plenum, New York, pp. 1-62.

Kalant, H., and Grose, W. (1967). Effects of ethanol and pentobarbital on release of acetylcholine from cerebral cortex slices. *J. Pharmacol. Exp. Ther. 158,* 386-393.

Karoum, F., Wyatt, R. J., and Majchrowicz, E. (1976). Brain concentrations of biogenic amine metabolites in acutely treated and ethanol dependent rats. *Br. J. Pharmacol. 56,* 403-411.

Knapp, S., Mandell, A. J., and Bullard, W. P. (1975). Calcium activation of brain tryptophan hydroxylase. *Life Sci. 16,* 1583-1594.

Kuriyama, K., Sze, P. Y., and Rauscher, G. E. (1971). Effects of acute and chronic ethanol administration on ribosomal protein synthesis in mouse brain and liver. *Life Sci. 10.II,* 181-189.

Lake, N., Yarbrough, G. G., and Phillis, J. W. (1973). Effects of ethanol on cerebral cortical neurons: interaction with some putative transmitters. *J. Pharm. Pharmacol. 25,* 582-584.

Leblanc, A. E., and Cappell, A. E. (1977). In *Alcohol and Opiates: Neurochemical and Behavioural Mechanisms,* K. Blum (Ed.), Academic, New York, pp. 65-77.

Leblanc, A. E., Kalant, H., and Gibbins, R. J. (1975). Acute tolerance to ethanol in the rat. *Psychopharamacologia 41,* 43-46.

Lieber, C. S., and De Carli, L. M. (1970). Hepatic microsomal ethanol oxidising system. *J. Biol. Chem. 245,* 2505-2512.

Littleton, J. M., and John, G. (1977). Synaptosomal membrane lipids of mice during continuous exposure to ethanol. *J. Pharm. Pharmacol. 29,* 579-580.

Littleton, J. M., Griffiths, P. J., and Ortiz, A. (1974). The induction of ethanol dependence and the ethanol withdrawal syndrome: the effects of pyrazole. *J. Pharm. Pharmacol. 26,* 81-91.

Littleton, J. M., Griffiths, P. J., and Abu Murad, C. (1976). The significance of biochemical changes in mouse brain and liver during the induction of physical dependence on ethanol in mice. *Anglo-French symposium on Alcoholism. INSERM Proceedings 54,* 141-150.

Majchrowicz, E., and Hunt, W. A. (1976). Temporal relationship of the induction of tolerance and physical dependence after continuous intoxication with maximum tolerable doses of ethanol in rats. *Psychopharmacology 50,* 107-112.

McQuarrie, D. G., and Fingl, E. (1958). Effects of single doses and chronic administration of ethanol on experimental seizures in mice. *J. Pharmacol. Exp. Ther. 124,* 264-271.

Mendelson, J. H. (1968). Ethanol-1-C^{14} metabolism in alcoholics and non-alcoholics. *Science 159,* 319-321.

Mendelson, J. H. (1971). In *The Biology of Alcoholism, Vol. 1, Biochemistry,* B. Kissin and H. Begleiter (Eds.), Plenum, New York, pp. 513-544.

Mendelson, J. H., Stein, S., and McGuire, M. T. (1966). Comparative psychophysiological studies of alcoholic and non-alcoholic subjects undergoing experimentally induced ethanol intoxication. *Psychosom. Med. 28,* 1-12.

Metcalfe, J. C., Seeman, P., and Burgen, A. S. V. (1968). The proton relaxation of benzyl alcohol in erythrocyte membranes. *Mol. Pharmacol. 4,* 87-95.

Myers, R. D., and Melchior, C. L. (1977). Alcohol drinking: abnormal intake caused by tetrahydropapaveroline in brain. *Science 196,* 554-556.

Noble, E. P., and Tewari, S. (1977). In *Metabolic Aspects of Alcoholism,* C. S. Lieber (ed.), M.T.P. Press, Lancaster, Eng., pp. 149-185.

Ortiz, A., Griffiths, P. J., and Littleton, J. M. (1974). A comparison of the effects of chronic administration of ethanol and acetaldehyde to mice: evidence for a role of acetaldehyde in ethanol dependence. *J. Pharm. Pharmacol. 26,* 249-260.

Patel, G. J., and Lal, H. (1973). Reduction in brain gamma-aminobutyric acid and in barbital narcosis during ethanol withdrawal. *J. Pharmacol. Exp. Ther. 186,* 625-629.

Phillis, J. W. (1974). The role of calcium in the central effects of biogenic amines. *Life Sci. 14,* 1189-2101.

Phillis, J. W., and Jhamandas, K. (1971). The effects of chlopromazine and ethanol on *in vivo* release of acetylcholine from the cerebral cortex. *Comp. Gen. Pharmacol. 2,* 306-310.

Pohorecky, L. A. (1974). Effects of ethanol on central and peripheral noradrenergic neurons. *J. Pharmacol. Exp. Ther. 189,* 380-391.

Pohorecky, L. A., Jaffe, L. S., and Berkeley, H. A. (1974a). Ethanol withdrawal in the rat: involvement of noradrenergic neurons. *Life Sci. 15,* 427-437.

Pohorecky, L. A., Jaffe, L. S., and Berkeley, H. A. (1974b). Effects of ethanol on serotonergic neurons in the rat brain. *Res. Commun. Chem. Path. Pharmacol. 8,* 1-11.

Post. M. E., and Sun, A. Y. (1973). The effect of chronic ethanol administration on the levels of catecholamines in different regions of rat brain. *Res. Commun. Chem. Path. Pharmacol. 6,* 887-894.

Raskin, N. H., and Sokoloff, L. (1972). Ethanol-induced adaptation of alcohol dehydrogenase activity in rat brain. *Nature 236,* 138-140.

Rasmussen, H. (1970). Cell communication, calcium ion and cyclic adenosine monophosphate. *Science 170,* 404-412.

Rawat, A. K. (1974). Brain levels and turnover rates of presumptive neurotransmitters as influenced by administration and withdrawal of ethanol in mice. *J. Neurochem. 22,* 915-922.

Ritzmann, R. F., and Tabakoff, B. (1976). Dissociation of alcohol tolerance and dependence. *Nature 263,* 418-420.

Roach, M. K., Davis, D. L., Pennington, W., and Nordyke, E. (1973). Effect of ethanol on the uptake by rat brain synaptosomes of (^{3}H)DL-norepeinephrine, (^{3}H)5-hydroxytryptamine, (^{3}H)-GABA and (^{3}H)glutamate. *Life Sci. 12,* 433-441.

Ross, D. H., Kibler, B. C., and Cardenas, H. L. (1977). Modification of glycoprotein residues as Ca^{2+} receptor sites after chronic ethanol exposure. *Drug and Alcohol Dependence 2,* 305-316.

Ross, D. H., Medina, M. A., and Cardenas, H. L. (1974). Morphine and ethanol: selective depletion of regional brain calcium. *Science 186,* 63-65.

Seeman, P. (1972). The membrane actions of anaesthetics and tranquillisers. *Pharamcol. Rev. 24,* 583-655.

Seeman, P., Chan, M., Goldberg, M., Sanko, T., and Sax, L. (1971). The binding of calcium to the cell membrane increased by volatile anaesthetics (alcohol, acetone, ether) which induce sensitisation of nerve and muscle. *Biochim. Biophys. Acta 225,* 185-193.

Smith, A. A., Engelsher, C., and Croftord, M. (1976). Respiratory or analgesic actions of ethanol and other narcotics: modulation by biogenic amines. *Ann. N.Y. Acad. Sci. 273,* 256-262.

Smith, T., Shen, A., Jacobyansky, A., and Thurman, R. G. (1977). Rapid adaptation of norepinephrine-stimulated adenylate cyclase of rat brain cerebral cortex during ethanol withdrawal reaction. *Fed. Proc. 36* (3), 331, No. 325.

Sprince, H., Parker, C. M., Smith, G. G., and Gonzales, L. J. (1972). Alcoholism: biochemical and nutritional aspects of brain amines aldehydes and amino acids. *Nut. Rep. Int. 5,* 185-200.

Sun, A. Y., and Samorakjski, T. (1975). The effects of age and alcohol on [Na^+, K^+] ATPase activity of whole homogenate and synaptosomes prepared from mouse and human brain. *J. Neurochem. 24,* 161-164.

Sun, G. Y., Creech, D. M., Corbin, D. R., and Sun, A. Y. (1977). The effect of chronic ethanol administration on arachidonyl CoA: 1-acyl-glycerophosphorylcholine acyl CoA transferase activity in rat brain synaptosomal-rich fraction. *Fed. Proc. 36* (3), 334, No. 342.

Sutton, I. (1973). Effects of acute and chronic ethanol on the GABA system in rat brain. *Biochem. Pharmacol. 22,* 1685-1692.

Sytinsky, I. A., Guzikov, B. M., Gomanko, M. V., Eremin, V. P., and Konovalova, N. N. (1975). The gamma-aminobutyric acid system in brain during acute and chronic ethanol ingestion. *J. Neurochem. 25,* 43-48.

Tabakoff, B., Ritzmann, R. F., and Yanai, J. (1977a). Tolerance to sedative hypnotics, memory and noradrenergic systems. *Fed. Proc. 36* (3), 315, No. 234.

Tabakoff, B., Hoffman, P., and Moses, E. (1977b). Neurochemical correlates of ethanol withdrawal: alterations in serotonergic function. *J. Pharm. Pharmacol. 29,* 471-476.

Theorell, H., and Chance, B. (1951). Studies on liver alcohol dehydrogenases. II. The kinetics of the compound of horse liver alcohol dehydrogenase and reduced diphosphopyridine nucleotide. *Acta Chem. Scand. 5,* 1127-1144.

Thurman, R. G., and McKenna, W. R. (1975). In *Biochemical Pharmacology of Ethanol,* E. Majchrowicz (Ed.), Plenum, New York, pp. 57-76.

Triggle, D. J. (1971). *Neurotransmitter-Receptor Interactions.* Academic, New York, London.

Truitt, E. B., Jr., and Walsh, M. J. (1971). In *The Biology of Alcoholism,* B. Kissin and H. Begleiter (Eds.), Plenum, New York, pp. 161-196.

Tyler, T. D., and Erickson, C. K. (1977). Identification of a calcium pool within mouse brain involved in ethanol-induced narcosis. *Fed. Proc. 36* (3), 331, No. 327.

Victor, M. (1970). The alcohol withdrawal syndrome; theory and practice. *Postgrad. Med. 4,* 68-72.

Volicer, L., and Hurter, B. P. (1977). Effects of acute and chronic ethanol administration and withdrawal on adenosine 3′:5′-monophosphate and guanosine 3′:5′-monophosphate in the rat brain. *J. Pharmacol. Exp. Ther. 200,* 298-305.

Walker, D. W., and Zornetzer, S. F. (1974). Alcohol withdrawal in mice: electroencephalographic and behavioural correlates. *Electroenceph. Clin. Neurophys. 36,* 233-243.

7

Opioid Dependence: Links Between Biochemistry and Behavior

Jerome H. Jaffe*
College of Physicians and Surgeons, Columbia University, and
New York State Psychiatric Institute
New York, New York

Doris H. Clouet
New York State Division of Substance Abuse Services
Brooklyn, New York

*Present Affiliation: The University of Connecticut Medical School, Farmington, Connecticut and Veterans Administration Hospital (Newington), Connecticut.

I. INTRODUCTION

The past decade has witnessed an explosive increase in our knowledge of the mechanisms of action of opioid drugs (reviewed in Martin and Sloan, 1978; Snyder, 1978; Simon and Hiller, 1978; Beaumont and Hughes, 1979; Snyder and Childers, 1979), the behavioral effects of opioid drugs in laboratory settings (reviewed in O'Brien, 1975; Schuster, 1978; Mello and Mendelson, 1978), and the treatment and natural history of opioid dependence (Vaillant, 1973; Robins, 1974; Stimson et al., 1978; and reviewed in Platt and Labate, 1976). Despite these advances, we are still uncertain as to the relationship between events at the biochemical level and the various behavioral patterns associated with the opioids: episodic self-administration, drug-seeking behavior of varying degrees of intensity (including the pattern called "addiction" or "dependence"), and the phenomenon of relapse.

Interdisciplinary barriers have made it difficult to translate discoveries at one level of experimentation into intelligible and useful information at another level. This chapter considers some of the biological factors that may contribute to opioid use, dependence, and relapse, and points to some ways in which recent findings at the biochemical and behavioral levels might help us to understand the complex and perplexing issues that challenge the clinician. It is not intended to be an exhaustive review of either the pharmacology of the opioids, the behavioral pharmacology of the opioids, or the clinical aspects of opioid dependence. Other recent reviews that cross disciplines are those of Platt and Labate, 1976; Jaffe, 1977; and Martin, 1978.

II. OPIOID-USING BEHAVIORS

There is little argument that in any given society the major factors affecting the initial use of opioids are availability and general cultural attitudes toward their use for medical and recreational purposes. But, given any set of societal attitudes, some individuals deviate from the norm. Even where opioid use is considered highly deviant, some people obtain such drugs from illicit channels, use them recreationally, and having experienced the effects continue to use opioids until, at some point, they seem to place the use of the drug above other values. These individuals seem to have a reduced capacity to control their use of opioids; they have lost plasticity, they are "dependent" or "addicted." Precise definitions for these terms, whether they are used to refer to drug-taking behavior or to the altered biochemical state that is also called opioid physical dependence, will probably never be available—for good reasons. At the physiological and biochemical level, the changes that opioids induce which eventually become obvious as withdrawal phenomena when the drugs are stopped seem to begin with the first dose. At the behavioral level, the difficulty with definitions is not that dependence begins with the first dose, but that there is no sharp line that separates the casual opioid user from the individual who exhibits a pattern of compulsive use. Agreement among observers is easy only at the extremes. Nevertheless, it is important to ask what psychological, biological, and pharmacological factors play a role in determining which users will continue beyond casual use, which will become dependent, and which will relapse repeatedly after periods of detoxification.

III. OPIOIDS AS REINFORCERS

Animals will self-administer opioids as well as a number of other classes of pharmacological agents (reviewed by Thompson and Young, 1978; Schuster, 1978; Spealman and Goldberg, 1978). Self-administration of opioids can be demonstrated in a number of species and by several routes of administration (oral, intravenous, intragastric); analogous models can be established with human volunteers. In both animals and humans, if an inert drug is substituted, behavior is not maintained. In short, the opioids can be positive reinforcers of the antecedent drug self-administration. One major avenue of research has been the effort to understand which of the multiple actions of opioid drugs are responsible for its reinforcing properties. Former heroin addicts given acute doses of opioids such as morphine, heroin, or methadone experience a reduction in anxiety, a rise in self-esteem, less concern about boredom, and an increase in the ability to "cope" with everyday events (Martin et al., 1978). In addition, when opioids are given intravenously the user reports a sudden, brief sensation, a "rush" or "flash" that is exceedingly pleasurable and is likened to an orgastic sensation experienced in the abdomen (Jaffe and Martin, 1975).

Heroin addicts self-administering heroin in a research ward appear to develop tolerance to the anxiety-relieving and mood-elevating effects of opioids, so that over a period of several weeks they report feelings of anxiety and dysphoria and a return of somatic concerns. However, even when there is considerable tolerance, single injections continue to produce brief periods (30-60 min) of positive mood (Mirin et al., 1976). The loss of mood-elevating effects and appearance of "hypophoria" and hypochondriasis has also been observed with other opioids (e.g., methadone) administered to addicts in a research setting (Martin et al., 1973a). Similarly, increasing dysphoria soon replaces the initial euphoria in hospitalized alcoholics who are permitted to drink alcohol in large amounts (Mendelson and Mello, 1978).

It has been postulated that when opioid self-administering humans become tolerant and experience dysphoria (or hypophoria), they continue to self-administer the opioids primarily to prevent unpleasant withdrawal phenomena. But it is unlikely that such an interpretation accounts for all the phenomena. In animals with electrodes implanted in selected brain regions (medial forebrain bundle, ventral tegmentum, mesencephalic gray, and tip of locus coeruleus), low doses of opioids seem to lower the threshold for electrical self-stimulation, suggesting that exogenous opioids somehow lower the threshold or increase the intensity of the hedonic effect. Tolerance does not appear to develop to this facilitation of self-stimulation with electrical current (Esposito and Kornetsky, 1977). In addition, interviews with heroin users who were tolerant and physically dependent indicated that despite such tolerance they continued to experience a brief euphoric effect immediately following the injection of an opioid (McAuliffe and Gordon, 1974).

Attempts to clarify the mechanism of the acute reinforcing properties of opioids have involved measurement of altered reinforcing effects after discrete brain lesions and after pharmacological manipulation of various neurotransmitters and other cellular mechanisms. Some general findings include the following. In animals that are not physically dependent, lesions of the caudate nucleus, as well as lesions of the substantia nigra (the origin of dopaminergic input to the caudate), decrease opioid self-administration (Glick et al., 1975). Such lesions also lower the threshold for detecting rewarding properties. These observations were interpreted to indicate that destruction in these areas increased the sensitivity to morphine's rewarding effects. In animals self-administering opioids, dorsal raphe and locus coeruleus lesions had no effect (Glick et al., 1975) and lesions in ventral-noradrenergic bundle, medial forebrain bundle, ventrolateral hypothalamus, and cingulate gyrus appear to decrease opioid consumption, but it is unclear whether the above lesions alter the rewarding effects of opioid or decrease the aversiveness of withdrawal (Pert, 1978).

The electrode placement sites for self-stimulation with electrical current are found in monoaminergic projection areas such as the noradrenergic dorsal tegmental bundle from the locus coeruleus to the hippocampus (Segal and Bloom, 1976); in periventricular areas in the hypothalamus (Stein et al., 1976); in dopaminergic neurons in the substantia nigra, entorhinal and anterior cingulate cortex (Wise, 1978); and in serotonergic pathways in the medial raphe (Liebeskind et al., 1973). Drugs that alter catecholamine function tend to disrupt self-stimulation (Wise, 1978). While some of these drugs also cause decreases in general activity and other reward behavior, effects on self-stimulation can be distinguished from these general effects in some cases, usually by using lower doses of the drugs (Rolls et al., 1974). In a critical review of the evidence implicating catecholamines in electrical self-stimulation, Fibiger has concluded that the evidence for the noradrenergic system as the exclusive mediator of central reinforcement processes must be rejected, although it probably participates in a nonessential manner, and that the evidence supports a major role for dopamine in the striatum and a modulating role in other areas such as the hypothalamus (Fibiger, 1978).

Electrical stimulation of certain brain areas produces profound analgesia. Tolerance develops to stimulation-produced analgesia (SPA) and the analgesia is partially antagonized by naloxone, suggesting involvement of endorphins (see Sandberg and Segal, 1978; Cannon et al., 1978). When electrodes were implanted in periaqueductal gray, analgesia was produced in opioid-naive animals but not in opioid-tolerant ones (Mayer and Hayes, 1975). Since stimulation-tolerant animals were not opioid tolerant, it was proposed that stimulation produces a focal tolerance, while opioids administered chronically act at multiple sites to produce tolerance. Although the sites for stimulation-produced analgesia overlapped to some extent those of self-stimulation reward (periaqueductal gray and substantia nigra), the two phenomena can be separated. There are self-stimulation sites in which analgesia is not produced (hippocampus and cortical areas) while some sites that yield analgesia seem to produce aversive effects (Cannon et al., 1978). Stein and Belluzzi (1978) postulated that endogenous opioids play a role in normal regulation of mood and function as "natural euphorigens." They noted that many of the brain sites that support self-stimulation are rich in enkephalins as well as catecholamines, and that when the electrodes are in these areas naloxone suppresses self-stimulation. It is highly unlikely, however, that the endogenous opioids are the sole mediators of "euphoria," or of the reinforcing effects of self-stimulation or other environmental stimuli that produce "pleasure" or positive reinforcements. Former heroin addicts maintained on large doses of the opioid antagonist naltrexone continue to experience pleasurable effects from food, sex, cigarettes, and a variety of nonopioid drugs.

The self-administration of powerful reinforcers such as amphetamine or cocaine may be related to catecholaminergic mechanisms because both drugs act on catecholamine systems in vitro. The administration of drugs that disrupt catecholamine synthesis or block receptors attenuate the reinforcing properties of cocaine and amphetamines (Pickens et al., 1968). Opioid self-administration has been related to dopaminergic and serotonergic pathways in the central nervous system (CNS). On the basis of lesioning studies in rats, the reinforcing power of morphine was related to ascending monoaminergic pathways projecting to the frontal cortex and hippocampus (Glick and Cox, 1978), areas that are also associated with electrical self-stimulation. As was pointed out by Wise (1978), the anatomical data are at best correlational. That is, when the activation of a specific catecholaminergic pathway coincides with reward stimulation, the activation may be either an important mediator of the response or an unimportant consequence of stimulation. In addition, the monoaminergic pathways may delineate the route through which internal stimuli act, but say nothing about the formation and consolidation of the internal stimuli.

At a recent interdisciplinary conference on drug dependence, it was emphasized that the "reinforcing" property did not reside solely in the drug or the stimulus. Depending on the previous history of the organism and the temporal arrangements (the schedule), animals will continue to press a level to self-administer electrical shocks of the same intensity that they previously worked hard to avoid. In such a model the high-level shock is a reinforcer in that it maintains the behavior that leads to the shock. The behaviorists concluded that a reinforcer, whether a drug or a nonpharmacological event, can only be defined as a behavioral consequence that maintains the behavior which produced it (Kalant, 1978).

IV. OPIOIDS: A CHANGING DEFINITION

The term "opioid" was coined more than 20 years ago to eliminate the awkward phrase "morphine, semisynthetic morphine-like drugs, and synthetic analgesics." It was intended to refer to all substances that produced morphine-like effects, regardless of their source or chemical structure. With the advent of drugs which had both agonist (morphine-like) effects and antagonist (naloxone-like) effects, this simple definition began to break down. A number of synthetic opioids, when given acutely, produced typical morphine-like subjective effects: analgesia, sedation, euphoria, and decreased anxiety, as well as typical morphine-like physiological effects, such as decreased respiratory rate, decreased intestinal motility, and pupillary constriction. These drugs also prevented the appearance of the morphine withdrawal syndrome when substituted for morphine in dependent humans or animals and exhibited cross-tolerance with morphine. These easily fit the definition. Other drugs created problems. Pentazocine, a weak antagonist, produced largely morphine-like subjective and physiological effects at low to moderate doses, but it did not substitute for morphine in physically dependent subjects, and at higher doses induced hallucinogenic effects similar to those seen with the antagonists nalorphine and cyclazocine. Still another drug, SKF-10, 047, N-allylnormetazocine, had almost no morphine-like activity, but it did antagonize the effects of morphine and was a potent hallucinogen. These observations prompted Martin to suggest that there are probably several distinct opioid receptors in the nervous system: a μ receptor at which morphine produced its typical effects, a κ receptor which when activated by a model drug such as ketocyclazocine produces analgesia and certain sedative effects, and σ receptor which is responsible for hallucinogenic activity (Martin et al., 1976).

The actions of mixed agonist-antagonist drugs such as nalorphine, pentazocine, and cyclazocine are explained by postulating that they are agonists at the κ and σ receptors and are competitive antagonists at the μ receptor. A drug like naloxone would be viewed as a relatively pure competitive antagonist which has greater affinity for the μ receptor than the κ or σ receptor. This view would explain why it requires so much more naloxone to antagonize the subjective effects of cyclazocine than the effects of morphine and related μ agonists. Despite the differences in activity, all of the drugs described interact with opiate receptors and those with agonistic activity are viewed as opioids.

V. ENDORPHINS AND ENKEPHALINS

The discovery of stereospecific, saturable opioid receptors that are distributed unequally throughout the central nervous system and in peripheral nerves (see reviews by Simon and Hiller, 1978; Beaumont and Hughes, 1979; Snyder and Childers, 1979) helped to explain the many earlier studies showing that opioids exert actions at many sites in the body (Table 1). It also paved the way for the even more exciting discovery of naturally occurring ligands for these receptors—endogenous opioid-like substances. The first of these, isolated from pig brain, were a pair of pentapeptides designated leucine enkephalin (leu-enkephalin) (H-tyrosine-glycine-glycine-phenylalanine-leucine-OH) and methionine enkephalin (met-enkephalin) (H-tyrosine-glycine-glycine-phenylalanine-methionine-OH) (Hughes et al., 1975). The latter was noted to be the amino acid sequence 61-65 contained within the 91 amino acid pituitary hormone β-lipotropin (β-LPH), which had been isolated by C. H. Li (1964).

Several larger peptide segments of β-lipotropin also have opioid-like activity. The most potent of these is the terminal or C fragment (β-LPH 61-91), which was designated β-endorphin (Li and Chung, 1976; Guillemin, 1978); the others, which are probably produced during extraction, were designated α-endorphin (β-LPH-61-76) and λ-endorphin (β-LPH-61-77) (Bradbury et al., 1976). A comparison of the activities of β-endorphin, met- and leu-enkaphalin with those of morphine, ketocyclazocine, and etorphine was made in three in vitro model systems: action on guinea pig ileum (GPI) and mouse vas deferens (MVD) preparations and inhibition of specific binding of leu-enkephalin in brain homogenates. Three sets of responses were found: The enkephalins were more active on MVD, β-endorphin and morphine were about equally active on MVD and GPI, and ketocyclazocine was much more active on GPI (Kosterlitz and Hughes, 1978). From the MVD/GPI potency ratios of these compounds, it was concluded that the MVD and the GPI are populated by different types of receptors. The data indicating different types of receptors mean that theoretical models for opioid action will not have to accommodate all of the actions of opioids at a single receptor and, also, open the possibility that drugs can be synthesized for therapeutic use that are specific for a single receptor type. In any event, the term opioid now covers both exogenous and endogenous substances with rather diverse actions.

Table 1 Localization of Opiate Receptors in the Nervous System[a]

Location	Functions influenced by opiates
Spinal cord	
Laminae I and II	Pain perception in body
Brainstem	
Substantia gelatinosa of spinal tract of caudal trigeminal	Pain perception in head
Nucleus of solitary tract, nucleus commissuralis, nucleus ambiguus	Vagal reflexes, respiratory depression, cough suppression, orthostatic hypotension, inhibition of gastric secretion
Area postrema	Nausea and vomiting
Locus coeruleus	Euphoria
Habenula-interpeduncular nucleus-fasciculus retroflexus	Limbic, emotional effects, euphoria
Pretectal area (medial and lateral optic nuclei)	Meiosis
Superior colliculus	Meiosis
Ventral nucleus of lateral geniculate	Meiosis
Dorsal, lateral, medial terminal nuclei of accessory optic pathway	Endocrine effects through light modulation
Dorsal cochlear nucleus	Unknown
Parabrachial nucleus	Euphoria in a link to locus coeruleus
Diencephalon	
Infundibulum	ADH secretion
Lateral part of medial thalamic nucleus, internal and external thalamic laminae, intralaminar (centromedian) nuclei, periventricular nucleus of thalamus	Pain perception
Telencephalon	
Amygdala	Emotional effects
Caudate, putamen, globus pallidus, nucleus accumbens	Motor rigidity
Subfornical organ	Hormonal effects
Interstitial nucleus of stria terminalis	Emotional effects

[a]The localization of opiate receptors is shown in the left hand panel, with possible functions associated with the area shown in the right hand panel. *Source:* From Snyder, 1978. (Copyright by the American Psychiatric Association, 1978. Reprinted by permission.)

VI. ROLE OF THE ENDOGENOUS OPIOID SUBSTANCES

The role of endogenous opioids in normal and abnormal behavior is unclear (see reviews by Verebey et al., 1978; Beaumont and Hughes, 1979). The enkephalins are distributed widely in the nervous system, and their distribution tends to correlate with that of the opioid receptors. They are present in brain areas that are presumed to be related to pain (laminae I and II of the spinal cord, spinal trigeminal nucleus, periaqueductal gray, and medullary raphe nuclei); to movement and behavior (globus pallidus, stria terminalis); to neuroendocrine effects (median eminence); and to self-stimulation and reward (substantia nigra, caudate nucleus, medial forebrain bundle) (Simantov et al., 1977; Hökfelt et al., 1977; Stein and Belluzzi, 1978). In contrast, β-endorphin is found primarily in a few fibers in the hypothalamus and midbrain, but is present in high concentration in the pituitary where little or no enkephalin is present (Bloom et al., 1978). Although the amino acid sequences for β-endorphin and met-enkephalin are found in the pituitary hormone β-LPH, there is no evidence that pituitary β-LPH hydrolysis is the source of brain met-enkephalin. Furthermore, the levels of endorphin and enkephalin in the hypothalamus are not reduced by hypophysectomy.

The very short half-life of the enkephalins, their proximity to opioid receptors, their calcium-dependent release following depolarization of brain or intestinal tissues, and their location in synaptosomes, as well as other evidence, makes it likely that the enkephalins act as neurotransmitters or neuromodulators of synaptic function (Snyder, 1978).

Both β-endorphin and the enkephalins produce opioid-like responses when administered acutely if the term opioid is used in its broadest sense. These responses are blocked by narcotic antagonists and tolerance and physical dependence develop upon chronic exposure to the endorphins (Tseng et al., 1976). Similarly, β-endorphin and enkephalin and other analogs produce biochemical changes also produced by exogenous opioids (Biggio et al., 1978).

Like the exogenous opioids, the enkephalins interact with a number of other transmitter substances: dopamine, acetylcholine, GABA, substance P, and neurotensin. The role of β-endorphin is less clear; its longer half-life and its presence in the pituitary suggest that it may act as a neurohormone.

Of particular interest are the effects of endogenous opioid peptides, as well as exogenous opioids on the release of hormones from the pituitary gland. The acute administration of morphine and other opioids produces an inhibition of release of luteinizing hormone (LH), follicle stimulating hormone (FSH), and thyroid stimulating hormone (TSH) and a stimulation of release of growth stimulating hormone (GH), adrenocorticotropic hormone (ACTH), vasopressin, and prolactin (Pang and Zimmerman, 1975; Lotti et al., 1969). The effects are blocked by opioid antagonists and some degree of tolerance develops with chronic drug use (George and Kokka, 1976). This action of opioids appears to involve polypeptide-releasing factors synthesized in and released from hypothalamic nuclei. Endogenous opioids seem to have similar effects. Leu-enkephalin administered intraventricularly stimulated the release of GH and prolactin (Shaar et al., 1977), and β-endorphin stimulated the release of the same two trophic hormones (Dupont et al., 1977; Rivier et al., 1977). The action of endogenous opioids on pituitary hormones also appears to be exerted on the hypothalamic nuclei. In turn, some of these hormones, their fragments, and target tissue hormones have subtle but important effects on behavior and this may be important for an understanding of the reinforcing effects of opioids and the conditions that predispose to the development of behavioral dependence and relapse.

Studies exploring the actions of endogenous opioids in brain have been based on two general techniques: (1) treatment of animals or humans with narcotic antagonists to block the action of endogenous opioids on the assumption that antagonists will displace endogenous opioids from their receptors with consequent alterations in any function for which these substances are needed; and (2) assay of levels of endogenous opioids in brain, pituitary gland, blood, urine, or cerebrospinal fluid (CSF) in normal or abnormal subjects, or after procedures designed to activate endogenous opioid processes.

The narcotic antagonists naloxone and naltrexone have been tested on various parameters in humans and animals. In opioid-naive human subjects naltrexone produces effects that are much more subtle and difficult to detect than the analgesic and subjective effects usually observed with more potent opioid agonists. Dose-dependent changes in mood and behavior (Jones, 1978) and sleepiness and dysphoria (Gorodetsky, 1974), as well as autonomic changes in respiratory rate and body temperature (Martin et al., 1973b) have been described. The effects of narcotic antagonists on pain seem to depend to some extent on the sensitivity of the individual to pain. In pain-insensitive humans, naloxone produced a hyperalgesia (increased sensitivity to pain) (Buchsbaum et al., 1977). However, using tourniquet-induced ischemia as the pain stimulus, Grevert and Goldstein (1978) did not find naloxone-induced mood changes or hyperalgesia in healthy subjects. In rodents, naloxone also produced a hyperalgesic response: a decrease in latency time to escape a hot-plate (McMillan and Morse, 1967). Since this response to naloxone was not obtained in hypophysectomized animals, the pituitary gland seems to be required for the response. In humans, naloxone also antagonizes the analgesia produced by acupuncture, suggesting a role for endogenous opioids in this situation (Pomeranz and Chiu, 1976).

In humans, levels of endogenous opioids have been measured in CSF, blood, and urine. The major difficulty with such measurements is that the number of molecular species of endogenous opioids in each of these fluids is not known, so that measurements of total opioid-like activity do not describe the species measured and measurements specific for a single species may not measure total activity. There are several molecular species in the CSF with opioid activity. One species with an approximate weight of 1200, termed fraction I by the Swedish group of researchers, is present in lower quantities in patients with chronic pain than in healthy individuals or in patients with psychogenic pain (Terenius, 1978). The Swedish group has characterized individuals with low fraction I levels as not depressed and not tolerant to pain and individuals with high levels as pain-insensitive and depressed. The levels of substances with opioid-like activity increased 20-fold in lumbar CSF in human subjects undergoing electrical stimulation analgesia. In both blood and urine endogenous opioid activity has been found without chemical or immunological correspondence to known endorphins or enkephalins (Wüster et al, 1978). Since a nonpeptide substance with opioid activity has been found in brain and CSF (Schorr et al., 1978), it is possible that other molecular species exist in brain and body fluids.

VII. TOLERANCE AND PHYSICAL DEPENDENCE

It has become an accepted view that one motive for continued use of opioids is the avoidance of the opioid withdrawal syndrome. However, this general view leaves many questions unanswered. How soon in the course of opioid use does the physical dependence develop? Is the withdrawal syndrome equally distressing to all people? Do some people develop physical dependence more easily than others? And how long does physical dependence last?

In humans the withdrawal syndrome after chronic morphine withdrawal consists of a number of discrete signs and symptoms which for the most part are opposite in direction to the acute effects of the opoioid drug. They include hyperalgesia, anxiety, dysphoria, hyperactive spinal polysynaptic reflexes, dilated pupils, increased respiratory sensitivity to CO_2, nausea, vomiting, increased bowel motility, increased blood pressure, and increased body temperature. Since different techniques are used to elicit and to measure these signs and symptoms, it is not certain that they all develop and decay at the same rate. In humans, the administration of the opioid antagonist naloxone can produce nausea and dilated pupils after only a day or two of therapeutic doses of opioid drugs. In former addicts on a prison ward naloxone can unmask some symptoms of opioid withdrawal 1 week after a single 40-mg dose of methadone (reviewed in Jaffe and Martin, 1980).

Clinically, opioid withdrawal syndromes appear to follow a general rule: If an opioid leaves the receptor gradually (because it is slowly metabolized or excreted), the withdrawal syndrome is slower to appear and is more protracted with the acute phase lasting a number of days. If the opioid is rapidly metabolized, the syndrome is more rapid in onset—within hours after the last dose—

and the acute phase is briefer and more intense. The administration of an antagonist which displaces the opioid from the receptor produces a rapid onset of symptoms (reviewed in Jaffe and Martin, 1980).

As noted above, tolerance develops unevenly to the various actions of opioid drugs. Some acute effects which may be related to their reinforcing properties may still occur at a time when there is rather marked tolerance to other effects. But much depends on the sensitivity of the measures used to detect tolerance.

Not long ago it could be said that opioids exhibit cross-dependence, i.e., physical dependence induced by one opioid can be suppressed by giving another. This statement must now be modified as a result of increased recognition of receptor heterogeneity. There may be several varieties of opioid tolerance and physical dependence which vary with the receptor type involved. Thus, morphine, believed to act primarily at the μ receptor, and ketocyclazocine, thought to act primarily at the κ receptor, both produce tolerance and physical dependence in monkeys upon repeated exposure. There is, however, limited cross-tolerance or cross-dependence between the two drugs; ketocyclazocine will not suppress morphine withdrawal (Martin et al., 1976). Thus, it is possible that tolerance and dependence may be specific to a single receptor type if it is produced by an opioid with actions that occur predominantly at one type of receptor.

Both β-endorphin and met-enkephalin also produce tolerance when infused into cerebral ventricles in rodents (Wei and Loh, 1976) or injected intravenously in a human (Catlin et al., 1978). Cross-tolerance and cross-dependence between morphine and endogenous opioids has been demonstrated in rodents. It is proposed that enkephalins and β-endorphin are normally sequestered so that an endogenously produced tolerance and physical dependence does not occur.

In some experimental models tolerance and physical dependence have been separated. In spinal dogs, nalorphine evokes abstinence before signs of tolerance are discernible during chronic morphine treatment. In rodents, many factors have been shown to affect the development of tolerance and physical dependence differently (Way and Bhargava, 1976). When the narcotic effects of morphine are blocked by the concurrent administration of an antagonist, tolerance does not develop, although abstinence can be induced (Mushlin and Cochin, 1976). One problem affecting the validity of the interpretation of such findings is that the sensitivity of the assays for tolerance and dependence may not have been equal.

The general view that in humans opioid physical dependence is readily reversible and the withdrawal syndrome is relatively short-lived (a matter of days of weeks) must be modified in the light of findings that in experimental subjects, after the acute withdrawal phenomena subside, deviations from baseline on selected physiological and psychological parameters persist for up to 24 weeks following withdrawal from chronically administered methadone (Martin et al., 1973a). The role that this "protracted" or "secondary" abstinence syndrome plays in relapse is a matter of considerable practical and theoretical significance.

The processes involved in the development of opioid tolerance and physical dependence can be separated from those involved in the acute effects of opioids. As noted previously in the description of reinforcers, the acute reinforcing effects may be sufficient to maintain drug-seeking behavior, but undoubtedly the capacity of opioids to alleviate the regularly recurring dysphoria that is part of the withdrawal syndrome sets up a distinct and powerful mechanism for reinforcing opioid-using behavior (Wikler, 1965, 1973). Recent efforts to understand the role of physical dependence in opioid-related behavior has moved along two distinct lines: studies which attempt to elucidate the relationship between withdrawal phenomena and drug-seeking behavior, and those which focus on the biochemical and neurophysiological substrates of physical dependence and withdrawal phenomena per se.

VIII. MECHANISMS OF TOLERANCE AND PHYSICAL DEPENDENCE: SOME RECENT FINDINGS

There are several theories of opioid physical dependence which attempt to account for the general observation that withdrawal phenomena tend to be opposite in direction to the acute effects produced by the drugs. To a considerable degree these theories are all variations on Himmelsbach's homeostatic concept, which postulates that the acute effects of opioids elicit homeostatic (counteradaptive) responses which build up if the drug administration is continued. When the drug is withdrawn or displaced from its receptor by an antagonist, the counteradaptive mechanisms are unopposed, producing the withdrawal phenomena. The theories differ in the level of explanation and the mechanisms proposed to account for the counteradaptive response, varying from changes in enzyme activity to redundancy of receptors (reviewed in Way, 1978). Recent research on opioid tolerance and physical dependence seems to suggest that these hypotheses are not mutually exclusive and supportive data for several of the views appear to be emerging.

Using a cell culture of neurons derived from a neuroblastoma x glioma hybrid as a model system, Sharma et al. (1975) demonstrated that incubation with morphine and other opioids produces a rapid inhibition of both basal and prostaglandin-E-stimulated (PGE-stimulated) adenylate cyclase, which in turn results in a decrease in the cellular content of cAMP. With continued incubation for 1-2 days the activity of both basal and PGE-stimulated adenylate activity measured in the presence of morphine had increased to baseline levels and the cellular cAMP levels returned to normal. With respect to this enzyme system, the cells had become tolerant. When the morphine is washed out, the activity of adenylate cyclase is found to be greater than normal and leads to a sharp increase in levels of cAMP. In terms of this model the cells are physically dependent and show a rebound effect upon withdrawal. The net effect is diagrammed in Figure 1. The same rebound increase in cellular levels of cAMP are seen if, while morphine is still present, the opioid antagonist naloxone is added to the medium. Similar findings are obtained when the cell culture is incubated with met-enkephalin.

Previously, Collier and Roy (1974) postulated that opioid effects on adenylate cyclase played a role in analgesia, tolerance, and physical dependence, and presented data from brain preparations showing morphine inhibition of PGE_1-stimulated adenylate cyclase. While this hypothesis has not been confirmed in its narrowest sense, a broad hypothesis that opioids affect cyclic nucleotide systems that are related to the mechanisms of neurohormonal and neurotransmitter regulation has substantial experimental support.

Evidence is also accumulating that chronic treatment with opioids induces supersensitivity in several distinct transmitter systems, as previously suggested by several groups (Jaffe and Sharpless, 1968; Collier and Roy, 1974; Herz and Schulz, 1978). The precise neurochemical mechanisms by which changes in sensitivity are produced in transmitter systems has been explored in several studies. For example, in the nigrostriatal dopaminergic system, the striatum of the rat has been dissected in terms of opiate receptor localization and dopamine involvement (Pollard et al., 1978). The results of this study lead to the conclusion that some opioid receptors are located presynaptically at dopamine nerve terminals and that the primary action of opioids on this system is an inhibition of dopamine release (resulting in decreased transmission) immediately after acute administration. This primary effect triggers the second phase, a compensatory and relatively longlasting increase in dopamine synthesis (which leads to increased transmission) mediated by a release of feedback inhibition. In tolerant and dependent animals, the compensatory mechanisms include a hypersensitivity of dopamine receptors. In abstinence, dopamine release is disinhibited to act on hypersensitive receptors magnifying activities that result from dopamine receptor occupation (Pollard et al., 1978). In studies using cholinergic drugs a cholinergic supersensitivity has been demonstrated in rats treated chronically with morphine (Glick and Cox, 1977). Supersensitivity to serotonin and PGE has been observed in isolated guinea pig ileum taken from tolerant animals (Herz and Schulz, 1978).

Opioids also inhibit the activity of adrenergic neurons in the locus coeruleus (Korf et al., 1974), and lesions in this area increase the analgesic action of morphine (Samanin et al., 1978). These and other findings suggested that noradrenergic neurons may also develop a change in sensitivity during chronic morphine treatment and that increased activity in noradrenergic systems might

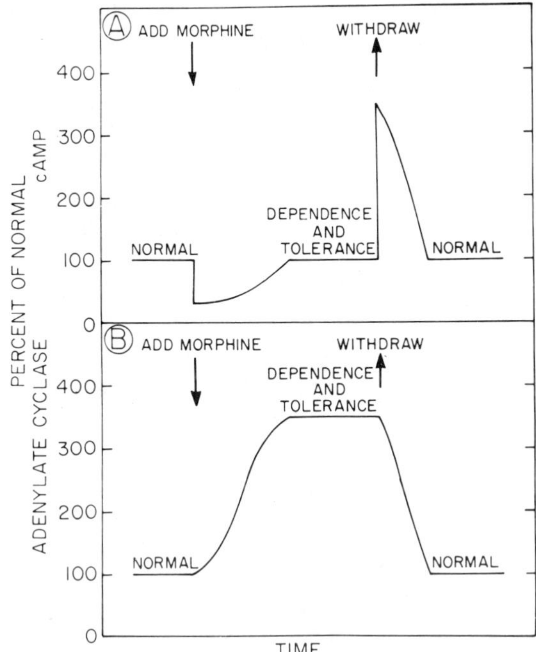

Figure 1 Model of the role of adenylate cyclase regulation in the development of morphine tolerance and dependence. Part A shows the effects of morphine upon cAMP levels, and part B the effects of the opiate upon adenylate cyclase activity as a function of time. (From Sharma et al., 1975.)

play a role in opioid withdrawal. The observation that certain α_2-adrenergic agonists such as clonidine also inhibit the activity of neurons in the locus coeruleus suggested that clonidine may be useful in suppressing withdrawal symptoms. Preliminary findings show that clonidine does suppress a number of withdrawal signs in dependent human subjects (Gold et al., 1978), confirming earlier findings in rats (Tseng et al., 1975). It has also been shown that in morphine-dependent rats, the microinjection of naloxone in the locus coeruleus induces increased firing of neurons and that this increased firing is suppressed by clonidine (Aghajanian, 1978).

It is worth noting that supersensitivity to neurotransmitters can also be induced by chronic treatment with drugs that are not subject to abuse (e.g., chronic treatment with anticholinergics or dopaminergic blockers produces increased sensitivity to cholinergic agonists and dopamine, respectively). Since it appears that morphine can inhibit the release of a number of neurotransmitters (acetylcholine, dopamine, norepinephrine), its effects probably involve some basic mechanism common to neuronal function. The transmembrane transport of calcium ions may be such a common mechanism. Calcium ion antagonizes morphine analgesia and morphine prevents the uptake of Ca^{2+} into brain slices and synaptosomes. Acutely, morphine depletes whole-brain and intrasynaptosomal levels of calcium, and the Ca^{2+} levels are increased in synaptosomes from tolerant-dependent animals (reviewed in Way, 1978).

A refinement of the mechanism by which opioids affect dopamine release involves the calcium-dependent regulator (CDR) protein. The reaction of morphine with the opioid presynaptic receptor in rat striatum triggers the release of CDR protein from the synaptic membrane into the cytoplasm, where it binds to free calcium, thus reducing available calcium (Hanbauer and Gimble, 1978). Since the activity of the rate-limiting enzyme in dopamine biosynthesis, tyrosine hydroxylase, is related to calcium with a concentration below normal as optimal, dopamine synthesis is increased by a lower calcium level. In addition, changes in ion permeability through membranes involve the phosphorylation of membrane proteins. The activation of membrane protein kinase by calcium requires CDR for full activation (Schulman and Greengard, 1978), an effect abolished by adding opioids to the kinase assay (Clouet et al., 1978). In striatal synaptic membranes from tolerant rats the activity of protein kinase in phosphorylating several membrane proteins is considerably reduced (O'Callaghan et al., 1979).

The need for protein synthesis during the development of tolerance to chronic opioid exposure is suggested by the inhibitory effect on tolerance produced by the administration of agents that inhibit protein and ribonucleic acid biosynthesis (reviewed by Clouet, 1978). One group of brain proteins that are likely to be involved in tolerance and dependence are the endogenous opioid peptides and their precursor proteins. Pituitary endorphins have been shown to arise from a large polypeptide (31 kdaltons) that is also the precursor of β-lipotropin and corticotropin (Roberts and Herbert, 1977). The precursor molecules for brain enkephalins are not yet known, although Undenfriend and his colleagues have described the isolation from striatum of large molecular weight proteins that possess opioid activity when subjected to digestion by a proteolytic enzyme (Lewis et al., 1978). Enkephalins are synthesized in brain in vivo (Yang et al., 1978) and in brain slices (Hughes et al., 1978) from radiolabeled precursor amino acids. If the inhibitor cycloheximide is added to the slices during the first 2 hr of synthesis, the amount of newly synthesized radiolabeled enkephalin is greatly reduced (McKnight et al., 1978). Other species of proteins that may be synthesized at altered rates in response to chronic opioid treatment are those involved in the transmission of the nerve impulse.

Another important consideration in comparing the effects of a single dose of a drug with those during chronic drug treatment is the cellular localization of the drug. The opioid receptor has been localized on the surface of the neuronal membrane, as have the immediate biochemical responses to the drug such as the release of neurotransmitters, the transmembrane transport of ions, and the modulation of the activity of membrane enzymes. The long-term effects that may require the synthesis of RNA or protein must be intracellular events. By analogy with other polypeptide hormones that have actions on cell surface and within cells, endogenous and exogenous opioids might be expected to have actions within neuronal cells. There is some biochemical evidence that opioids act intracellularly as well as on the cell surface (reviewed in Lee et al., 1978). For example, nuclear chromatin from morphine-dependent animals exhibits greater DNA template activity than chromatin from untreated animals. Chronic morphine treatment increases the phosphorylation of specific nuclear chromatin proteins in brain. In addition, the RNA synthetic activity in brain nuclei has been separated into three polymerases, one of which is reduced in activity morphine-dependent animals. β-Endorphin has the same effect as morphine in increasing DNA template activity (Lee et al., 1978).

From immunohistofluorescence studies it seems quite clear that β-endorphin and the enkephalins are found both at the membrane and within neuronal cells and their processes (Johansson et al., 1978). Although the radioautographic techniques used to localize exogenous opioids are not as precise as the immunofluorescence techniques, opioid drugs also seem to be within neuronal cells as well as at the cell surfaces (Watanabe et al., 1976). Studies on the entrance of nonopioid polypeptide hormones into their target cells suggest that the hormones enter the cells with their membrane receptors. The role played by intracellular membrane receptor/ligand complexes may be one or more of several possibilities: to prevent the proteolytic degradation of the hormones; to enable the receptor protein to be degraded by lysosomal enzymes; or to translate surface ligand/receptor binding into intracellular action by the active component, the receptor.

Although the number of opioid receptors has not been altered experimentally, in other transmitter systems the number of receptors changes as the ligand availability changes (Schwartz et al., 1978). The intracellular localization of opioids has theoretical importance for opioid dependence because it provides a mechanism that allows a differentiation of the immediate effects of the drug from the long-term effects. The results of these studies and many others indicate that adaptation at the cellular or functional level is widespread in opioid-tolerant and physically dependent animals. No changes have been found, however, in either the number or the affinities of opioid receptors in brain during chronic morphine treatment (Simon, 1978). The levels of met-enkephalin and leu-enkephalin in rat striatum or hypothalamus as measured by specific antibodies are not altered (Childers et al., 1978). Increases in β-endorphin levels in rat plasma have been found after acute morphine treatment and in physically dependent animals during naloxone-precipitated withdrawal (Höllt et al., 1978). However, since opioids produce an increased release of ACTH from the pituitary, and since, in the rat, ACTH and β-endorphin arise from the same 31-Kdalton precursor in pituitary and are released simultaneously into the plasma (Chretien et al.,

1978; Guillemin, 1978), the increase in β-endorphin may be a response to stress rather than a specific aspect of opioid withdrawal. The levels of endogenous opioids in plasma have not been examined systematically as yet in humans. β-endorphin is present at low levels in plasma of normal human subjects (Wardlaw and Frantz, 1978; Akil et al., 1979). When vasopressin is used to stimulate release of ACTH, there is a sharp rise in β-LPH, but no rise in β-endorphin (Suda et al., 1978).

Collier and Francis (1978) reviewed the evidence that is supportive of the various theories of tolerance and physical dependence. They concluded that to some degree each of them explains some of the phenomena of dependence and that they are complementary rather than competitive frameworks.

IX. VULNERABILITY AND DEPENDENCE

In societies in which the use of a drug is generally acceptable, as is the case with tobacco, those experimenters who go on to become heavy, dependent users differ in terms of personality from those who do not; but the overlap is great. Where even the use of a drug is viewed as being highly deviant, as in the case with illicit opioids in Western countries, experimenters differ from their peers in a number of ways. They tend to come from larger families with more intrafamily conflict, more parental criminality and alcoholism, to have experienced the loss of a parent, to report themselves as being less academically successful, more depressed or bored, and to have used other legal and illegal drugs (alcohol, tobacco, marijuana, and amphetamines) before experimenting with opioids. There is often evidence of delinquency, and the use of the drug appears to be imbedded in a general pattern of deviancy and alienation from cultural norms (reviewed by Platt and Labate, 1976; Jaffe, 1977; Jessor and Jessor, 1977; and Martin, 1978).

Epidemiological studies make it quite clear that not all who experiment with opioids become casual users and not all who use become dependent (O'Donnell et al., 1976). There are a number of possibilities that may account for such differences: dependence is more likely to develop in those who continue to use either because they find the opioid effects more reinforcing or because they are less concerned about the adverse consequences of continued use. Alternately, those who find other nonpharmacological sources of reinforcement less satisfying or less available are more likely to continue use. In turn, there are several possibilities that might account for observed differences in the reinforcing effects among individuals. For some, the hedonic effect might be more intense; for others, the major effect might be a "normalizing" relief from some dysphoria or internal aversive state that antedates the drug experiences. Still others might have a greater sensitivity to the development of the early stages of physical dependence. Any one of these possibilities could be viewed as an antecedent vulnerability to dependence which in turn might have its origins in genetically determined biochemical differences or in life experiences or both. There are probably numerous ways in which sociological and environmental factors could alter the reinforcing effects of opioids. Even diet may play a role: Dietary changes can alter brain levels of neurotransmitters such as acetylcholine and serotonin. Such changes are sufficient to modify the responses to painful stimuli and to opioid drugs (Lytle et al., 1978).

In early clinical work with opioid addicts it was noted that a significant percentage exhibited alcoholism or depression prior to opioid dependence. Chein and his colleagues, writing about adolescent drug users in 1964, described those most vulnerable to becoming heroin addicts as those expressing pessimism, unhappiness, and futility. More recent work shows that a very significant percentage of heroin addicts and patients maintained on methadone score high on standard depression inventories and exhibit clinical signs of depression (for references, see Weissman et al., 1976). Among young people entering a therapeutic community, high scores on MMPI depression scales are correlated with early dropout rates and, presumably, relapse (DeLeon et al., 1973). Thus, there is ample evidence pointing to a role for depression in opioid dependence and relapse. What is unsettled are the origins of this depression and how this depression is related to other types of depression.

Early writers tended to attribute the pessimism, impulsivity, decreased self-esteem, and anhedonia of the opioid addict to the consequences of chaotic or distressing social and family conditions. However, many of these same signs and symptoms are seen among children diagnosed as hyperactive or as having minimal brain dysfunction (MBD) (Wood et al., 1976; Tarter et al., 1977). Recent observations that the male biological parents of children with MBD are more likely to exhibit alcoholism and sociopathy (Cantwell, 1972); that childhood MBD may be an antecedent to sociopathy (Guze, 1975), to alcoholism (Guze, 1975; Goodwin et al., 1975; Tarter et al., 1977), and to opioid use (Bihari, 1976); and that MBD may be genetically transmitted suggest that these associated conditions may be relevant to problems of opioid use and dependence. Wender hypothesized that MBD may persist into adulthood and that it represents a genetically transmitted physiological defect in monoamine metabolism in brain that produces hyperactivity, an inability to focus attention or inhibit irrelevant responses, and a diminished capacity for positive and negative affect. The latter is behaviorally manifested as a decreased response to both positive and negative reinforcement (Wood et al., 1976). Additionally, studies of the genetics of alcoholism in males, especially adoption studies in which the probands are adopted out in the first several weeks of life, and studies of half-siblings suggest that vulnerability to alcoholism in adults may be due more to a genetically transmitted disorder than to the effects of family role modeling or interpersonal relationships. While there are very few studies on the genetic vulnerability to developing opioid dependence, the high prevalence of depression, alcoholism, sociopathy, and MBD among opioid addicts (reviewed by Platt and Labate, 1976; Jaffe, 1977; Martin, 1978), and the studies suggesting that vulnerability to alcohol dependence may have genetic components (Goodwin et al., 1973,

1974) argue for a possibility of a genetic vulnerability in some instances of opioid dependence. Genetic differences in behavioral responses to opioids have been demonstrated in two strains of mice in studies that show two or more genetic loci controlling the behaviors (Baran et al., 1975). A strain difference in sensitivity of striatal adenylate cyclase to dopamine was found in the same strains of mice, with higher locomotor responses to opioids paralleling the higher sensitivity of the enzyme to dopamine (Oliverio et al., 1978).

Some of the disorders mentioned may contribute both directly and indirectly to a vulnerability to opioid dependence. For example, depression or hyperactivity (MBD) could lead to impaired performance and achievement in academic situations, further decreasing the individual's self-esteem and making him more susceptible to reinforcement by drug-using peers. In addition, the depressed or hyperactive young person might experience opioid effects as more reinforcing.

Dole and Nyswander (1968) seem to postulate that some opioid addicts have two related biochemical disorders—one which might predispose to an unusual response to opioid use and one which is the result of prolonged use and leads to "drug hunger" and relapse. Martin and his co-workers (1978) proposed a similar view but pointed out that the antecedent disorder probably manifests itself in mood and personality disturbances (hypophoria, decreased self-esteem). Goldstein (1976) and Snyder (1978) also speculated about a biochemical disorder antecedent to opioid use and that both this antecedent disorder and any longlasting disturbances induced by opioid use may involve the endogenous opioid system previously described. Thus far, the existence and the nature of such antecedent disorders remains unclear.

X. DRUG-INDUCED BIOLOGICAL CHANGES IN RELAPSE

It is now clear that the urge or craving to use an opioid drug bears a complex relationship to physical dependence and is highly dependent on environmental conditions.

The role of longlasting opioid-induced biological changes in relapse is still uncertain. Martin has termed the state which follows the acute or primary withdrawal syndrome "protracted" or "secondary" abstinence (Martin, 1972). Animal work also points to some long-lasting changes (Martin and Sloan, 1978; Bläsig et al., 1978).

At present the role of protracted abstinence in relapse is uncertain. It does appear that opioid addicts whether returning to their home communities after institutional detoxification or undergoing ambulatory withdrawal seem most vulnerable to relapse during the first few months of withdrawal. During this period they also appear to be more vulnerable to stress and to be more hypophoric and hypochondriacal (Martin, 1972). These are several hypotheses about this period of heightened vulnerability to stress and relapse. Factors postulated as contributions include conditioned craving or withdrawal effects (see below), social stress, relief of protracted abstinence per se, the desire for the original euphoric effects of opioids, and so on. Another possibility or mechanism, albeit a very speculative one, may be found in the observations that ACTH injected into the periaqueductal gray produces a withdrawal-like syndrome in naive rats (Jacquet, 1978) and that other polypeptide fragments of pituitary hormones (β-MSH and tetracosactin) antagonize the depressant effects of morphine in spinal cord and interfere with opioid binding (reviewed in Martin and Sloan, 1978). Conceivably, in withdrawn humans, stress could lead to the experience of acute withdrawal due to the release of ACTH or other pituitary polypeptides, but there is no experimental evidence that this is the case. The tendency of some ex-addicts to function well in therapeutic communities and of many to "mature out" of addiction suggests that protracted abstinence has a finite duration or that it plays a limited role in relapse.

XI. LEARNING AND CONDITIONING IN DEPENDENCE AND RELAPSE

Several researchers have emphasized the role of learning in the genesis of dependence and relapse (Wikler, 1973). The learning model postulates that different mechanisms may come into play at different stages of the drug-using cycle. Within this framework reinforcement of opioid use by approval of peers in a deviant subculture is soon replaced by the primary positive reinforcing action of the opioid drugs on drug-sensitive reward systems in the brain. Very soon in the process of regular use (perhaps a matter of hours, and certainly within days), the counteradaptive changes induced in the CNS by opioids create another source of reinforcement: the dysphoria of the early withdrawal syndrome. Wikler (1973) postulates that this source of reinforcement (withdrawal) develops relatively early in the course of opioid use, and is not readily apparent to the observer, and may not even be appreciated cognitively by the user, but may be experienced only as a craving. Antecedent psychopathology is not a necessary condition for this process, although it may act to accentuate the initial responses to opioids or the subtle dysphoria of withdrawal.

In his integrated theory of dependence, Wikler (1973) emphasized an additional learning paradigm: the classical conditioning of withdrawal phenomena to a variety of internal and external stimuli. The removal of the opioid drug from its receptor is viewed as the unconditioned stimulus for eliciting withdrawal. The previously neutral stimuli which can become linked to the withdrawal phenomena (i.e., become conditioned stimuli) may be either in the external environment or interoceptive (events and emotional states producing cues within the body). There are both animal and human data showing that opioid withdrawal phenomena can be conditioned to environmental stimuli (O'Brien et al., 1977; Schuster, 1978; Lal et al., 1978).

Within this framework the notion of craving or "needing a fix" weeks or months after withdrawal may be due to reactivation of withdrawal symptoms by previously conditioned exteroceptive or interoceptive stimuli. The addict does not differentiate between conditioned and unconditioned withdrawal, but experiences both as craving or a need for the drug. Often the response to the experience of craving is to use an opioid, thereby reinitiating the process. Yet, in a number of studies, conditions associated with drug use and drug availability are much more effective in eliciting craving than those associated with withdrawal. In the studies of O'Brien et al., (1977), addicts were asked to rank the situations most likely to cause craving. The situations ranking highest were those directly associated with drug use—being offered drugs by a friend, seeing someone else "shoot up." In their studies of the effects of antagonists on heroin self-administration, Mirin and Meyer and colleagues also observed a relationship between environmental circumstances and craving (1976). Craving was highest when the subject knew that the drug was available for use and when the subjects perceived that they were not taking the antagonist and would be able to experience the acute heroin effects. Theoretically, certain emotional states (anxiety, depression, anger) can become stimuli which elicit conditioned withdrawal and/or craving for an opioid drug.

In explaining the genesis of dependence and relapse the learning model allows for but does not emphasize antecedent vulnerability, drug use as self-medication (to ameliorate depression or dysphoric states that are independent of opioid use), or drug use to suppress a state of protracted abstinence. It is clear that if such conditions are present, they would not invalidate the contributions of learning but would provide still additional sources of reinforcement. As was the case with theories of physical dependence, each of the views of the etiology of the behavioral syndromes of dependence and relapse may have some validity.

XII. CONCLUSIONS

This review of selected biological factors that may play a role in the various stages of opioid use, dependence, and relapse does not imply that social and psychological factors are not important in the etiology of opioid abuse. Indeed, some of the described concepts such as differences in vulnerability to opioid use and abuse or the possible dysfunction of endogenous opioid systems in subjects susceptible to opioid abuse may include mechanisms through which external circumstances affect drug use; and concepts such as the similarity of anatomical sites and pathways for reward and the consolidation of memory or learning with those involved in opioid responses suggest mechanisms through which psychological factors may affect opioid abuse. It is difficult to make judgments as to which of the many factors contributes most to any given case of opioid abuse, which factors are within our present capacity to modify, and which factors require the acquisition of additional knowledge, but it is important to be able to do so in order to modify and improve the current treatment modalities for opioid addictions.

XIII. RECENT DEVELOPMENTS

Among the significant findings or clarifications published since this review was completed are the following:

Naloxone, once thought to be a pure opioid antagonist, alters the responses to nonopioids, including the degree of ethanol-induced behavioral impairment and intoxication in humans; the facilitation effect of chlordiazepoxide, ethanol, and amphetamine on intracranial self-stimulation (ICSS) in rats; ethanol self-administration by monkeys; and the severity of ethanol physical dependence in mice. Such findings suggest that endogenous opioids play a role in some of the actions of nonopioid substances, or that naloxone has other effects. An anti-GABA effect of naloxone has been proposed.

Endogenous opioids (enkephalins and endorphins) probably play a role in response to certain forms of pain and stress, since the analgesia produced by prolonged intermittent shock (but not by brief continuous shock) is antagonized by the antagonist naloxone. Endorphin levels have been measured in human CSF and plasma. In patients with chronic pain, stimulation of the periaqueductal gray produces increases in β-endorphin associated with relief of pain.

There have been improvements in the measurement of specific enkephalins and endorphins and improved mapping of their distribution and circuitry. It is now believed that the endorphins are produced in the brain as well as the pituitary; the independent localization of endorphins, met-enkephalin, and leu-enkephalin, along with recognition of differences of receptor affinities, supports the view that these substances may have distinct functions. Nevertheless, the role of endogenous opioids in the development of opioid dependence, in the manifestations of withdrawal, and in relapse have yet to be made clear.

These endogenous substances may also be involved in learning, since at lower-than-analgesic doses endogenous opioids increase the resistance to extinction of avoidance behavior; however, effects on other types of learning are varied and are not consistent among the several enkephalins and endorphins tested. Different effects may reflect actions at different subtypes of opioid receptors. Whether the substances act by altering the aversiveness of stimuli or by other mechanisms (e.g., release of vasopressin or other peptides known to affect memory) is uncertain.

REFERENCES

Aghajanian, G. K. (1978). Tolerance of locus coeruleus neurones to morphine and suppression of withdrawal response by clonidine. *Nature 276,* 186-188.

Akil, H., Watson, S. J., Barchas, J. D., and Li, C. H. (1979). β-Endorphin immunoreactivity in rat and human blood. Radio immunoassay, comparative levels and physiological alterations. *Life Sci. 24,* 1659-1666.

Baran, A., Shuster, L., Eleftheriou, S., and Bailey, D. W. (1975). Opiate receptors in mice. Genetic differences. *Life Sci. 17,* 633-640.

Beaumont, A., and Hughes, J. (1979). Biology of opioid peptides. *Ann. Rev. Pharmacol. Toxicol. 20,* 245-267.

Biggio, G., Corda, M. G., Casu, M., and Gessa, G. L. (1978). Striato-cerebellar pathway controlling cyclic GMP content in the cerebellum. Role of dopamine, GABA and enkephalins. In *Advances in Biochemical Psychopharmacology,* Vol. 18, *The Endorphins,* E. Costa and M. Trabucci (Eds.). Raven, New York, pp. 227-244.

Bihari, B. (1976). Drug dependency. Some etiological considerations. *American Journal of Drug and Alcohol Abuse 3,* 409-422.

Bläsig, J., Meyer, G., and Städele, M. (1978). Factors influencing the manifestation of dependence in rats. In *Factors Affecting the Action of Narcotics,* M. L. Adler, L. Manara, and R. Samanin (Eds.). Raven, New York, pp. 133-146.

Bloom, F., Battenberg, E., Rossier, J., Ling, N., and Guillemin, R. (1978). Neurons containing β-endorphin in rat brain exist separately from those containing enkephalin. Immunocytochemical studies. *Proc. Nat. Acad. Sci. USA 75,* 1591-1595.

Bradbury, A. F., Smyth, D. G., Snell, C. R., Birdsell, N. J. M., and Hulme, E. C. (1976). C-fragment of lipotropin has a high affinity for brain opiate receptors. *Nature 260,* 793-797.

Buchsbaum, M. S., Davis, G. C., and Bunney, W. E. (1977). Naloxone alters pain perception and somatosensory evoked potentials in normal subjects. *Nature 270,* 620-622.

Cannon, J. R., Liebeskind, J. C., and Frenk, H. (1978). Neural and neurochemical mechanisms of pain inhibition. In *The Psychology of Pain,* R. Sternbach (Ed.). Raven, New York, pp. 27-47.

Cantwell, D. P. (1972). Psychiatric illness in families of hyperactive children. *Arch. Gen. Psychiatr. 27,* 414-421.

Catlin, D. H., Hui, K. K., Loh, H. H. and Li, C. H. (1978). β-Endorphin. Subjective and objective effects during narcotic abstinence in man. In *Advances in Biochemical Psychopharmacology,* Vol. 18, *The Endorphins,* E. Costa and M. Trabucchi (Eds.). Raven, New York, pp. 341-350.

Chein, I., Gerard, D. I., Lee, R. S., and Rosenfels, E. (1964). *The Road to H. Narcotics, Delinquency and Social Policy.* Basic Books, New York.

Childers, S. R., Schwartz, R., Coyle, J. T., and Snyder, S. H. (1978). Radioimmunoassay of enkephalins. Levels of methionine- and leucine-enkephalin in morphine dependent and kainic acid lesioned rat brains. In *Advances in Biochemical Psychopharmacology,* Vol. 18, *The Endorphins,* E. Costa and M. Trabucchi (Eds.). Raven, New York, pp. 161-174.

Chrétien, M., Crine, P., Lis, M., Gianoulakis, C., Gossard, F., Benjannet, S., and Seidah, N. G. (1978). Pulse-chase release of β-endorphin from a radioactive precursor in rat pars intermedia. In *Characteristics and Function of Opioids,* J. Van Ree and L. Terenius (Eds.). Elsevier North-Holland, Amsterdam, pp. 291-292.

Clouet, D. H. (1978). The role of brain proteins and peptides in opiate actions. In *Factors Affecting the Action of Narcotics,* M. L. Adler, L. Manara, and R. Samanin (Eds.). Raven, New York, pp. 379-386.

Clouet, D. H., O'Callaghan, J. P., and Williams, N. (1978). Inhibition of calcium-stimulated protein kinase activity in striatal synaptic membranes by opioids. In *Characteristics and Function of Opioids,* J. Van Ree and L. Terenius (Eds.). Elsevier North-Holland, Amsterdam, pp. 351-352.

Collier, H. O. J., and Francis, D. L. (1978). A pharmacological analysis of opiate tolerance and dependence. In *Life Sciences Research Report 8, The Bases of Addiction,* J. Fishman (Ed.). Dahlem Konferenzen, Berlin, pp. 281-298.

Collier, H. O. J., and Roy, A. C. (1974). Hypothesis. Inhibition of prostaglandin E sensitive adenyl cyclase as the mechanism of morphine analgesia. *Prostaglandins 7,* 361-376.

DeLeon, G., Skodel, A., and Rosenthal, M. (1973). Pheonix House. Changes in psychopathological signs of resident drug addicts. *Arch. Gen. Psychiatry 28,* 131-142.

Dole, V. P., and Nyswander, M. E. (1968). Methadone maintenance and its implications for theories of narcotic addiction. In *The Addictive States,* A. Wikler (Ed.). Williams and Wilkins, Baltimore.

Dupont, A., Cusan, L., Garon, M., Labrie, F., and Li, C. H. (1977). β-Endorphin. Stimulation of GH release in vivo. *Proc. Nat. Acad. Sci. USA. 74,* 358-359.

Esposito, R., and Kornetsky, C. (1977). Morphine lowering of self-stimulation thresholds: lack of tolerance with long term administration. *Science 195,* 189-191.

Fibiger, H. C. (1978). Drugs and reinforcement mechanisms. A critical review of catecholamine theory. *Ann. Rev. Pharmacol. Toxicol. 18,* 37-56.

George, R., and Kokka, N. (1976). The effects of narcotics on growth hormone, ACTH and TSH secretion. In *Tissue Responses to Addictive Drugs,* D. H. Ford and D. H. Clouet (Eds.). Spectrum, Holliswood, New York, pp. 527-540.

Glick, S. D., and Cox, R. D. (1977). Change in morphine self-administration after brain stem lesions. *Psychopharmacology 52,* 151-156.

Glick, S. D., and Cox, R. D. (1978). Changes in morphine self-administration after tel-diencephalon lesions in rats. *Psychopharmacology 57,* 283-288.

Glick, S. D., Cox, R. D., and Crane, A. M. (1975). Changes in morphine self-administration and morphine dependence after lesions of the caudate nucleus in rats. *Psychopharmacology 41,* 219-224.

Gold, M. E., Redmond, D. C., and Kleber, H. D. (1978) Clonidine blocks acute opiate-withdrawal symptoms. *Lancet 2* (September 16, #8090), 599-602.

Goldberg, S. R. (1970). Relapse to opioid dependence. The role of conditioning. In *Drug Dependence,* R. T. Harris, W. M. McIsaac, and C. R. Schuster (Eds.). University of Texas Press, Austin, pp. 170-197.

Goldstein, A. (1976). Opioid peptides (endorphins) in pituitary and brain. *Science 193,* 1081-1086.

Goodwin, D. W., Schulsinger, F., Hermansen, L., Guze, S. B., and Winokur, G. (1973). Alcohol problems in adoptees raised apart from alcoholic biological parents. *Arch. Gen. Psychiatr. 28,* 238-243.

Goodwin, D. W., Schulsinger, F., Moller, N., Hermansen, L., Winokur, G., and Guze, S. B. (1974). Drinking problems in adopted and nonadopted sons of alcoholics. *Arch. Gen. Psychiatr. 31,* 164-169.

Goodwin, D. W., Schulsinger, F., Hermansen, F. et al. (1975). Alcoholism and the hyperactive child syndrome. *J. Nerv. Ment. Dis. 160,* 349-353.

Gorodetsky, C. W. (1974). Assays of antagonist activity of narcotic antagonists in man. In *Narcotic Antagonists,* M. L. Braude, L. S. Harris, E. L. May, J. P. Smith, and J. E. Villarreal (Eds.). Raven, New York, pp. 291-298.

Grevert, P., and Goldstein, A. (1978). Endorphins: Naloxone fails to alter experimental pain in humans. *Science 199,* 1093-1095.

Guillemin, R. (1978). β-lipotropin and endorphins. Implications of current knowledge. *Hosp. Prac. (November),* 53-60.

Guze, S. B. (1975). The validity and significance of the clinical diagnosis of hysteria (Briguet's syndrome). *Am. J. Psychiatr. 32,* 138-141.

Hanbauer, I., and Gimble, J. (1978). Regulation of striatal dopaminergic neurons by opiate receptors. *Fed. Proc. 37,* 238.

Herz, A., and Schulz, R. (1978). Changes in neuronal sensitivity during the addictive processes. In *Life Sciences Research Report 8, The Bases of Addiction,* J. Fishman (Ed.). Dahlem Konferenzen, Berlin, pp. 375-394.

Hökfelt, T., Ljungdahl, A., Terenius, L., Elde, R., and Nilsson, G. (1977). Immunohistochemical analyses of peptide pathways possibly related to pain and analgesia: enkephalin and substance P. *Proc. Nat. Acad. Sci. USA. 74,* 3081-3085.

Höllt, V., Przewlocki, R., and Herz, A. (1978). β-Endorphin-like immunoreactivity in plasma, pituitaries and hypothalamus of rats following treatment with opiates. *Life Sci. 23,* 1057-1066.

Hughes, J., Smith, T. W., Kosterlitz, H. W., Fothersgill, L. A., Morgan, B. A., and Morris, H. R. (1975). Identification of two related pentapeptides from the brain with potent opiate agonist activity. *Nature 258,* 577-579.

Hughes, J., Kosterlitz, H. W., and McKnight, A. T. (1978). The incorporation of H^3-leucine into the enkephalins of striatal slices of guinea-pig brain. *Br. J. Pharmacol. 59,* p. 396.

Jacquet, Y. F. (1978). Opiate effects after adrenocorticotropin or β-endorphin injection in the periaqueductal gray matter of rats. *Science 201,* 21032-1034.

Jaffe, J. H. (1977). Factors in the etiology of drug use and drug dependence. Two models: opiate use and tobacco use. In *Rehabilitation Aspects of Drug Dependence,* A. Schecter (Ed.). CRC Press, Cleveland, pp. 23-68.

Jaffe, J. H., and Martin, W. R. (1980). Opioid analgesics and antagonists. In *The Pharmacological Basis of Therapeutics.* A. G. Gilman and L. S. Goodman (Eds.). Macmillan, New York, pp. 494-534.

Jaffe, J. H. and Sharpless, S. (1968). Pharmacological denervation supersensitivity in the central nervous system. A theory of physical dependence. In

The Addictive States, A. Wikler (Ed.). Williams and Wilkins, Baltimore, pp. 226-240.

Jessor, R., and Jessor, S. L. (1977). *Problem Behavior and Psychosocial Development: A Longitudinal Study of Youth.* Academic, New York.

Johansson, O., Hökfelt, T., Elde, R. P., Schultzberg, M., and Terenius, L. (1978). Immunohistochemical distribution of enkephalin neurons. In *Advances in Biochemical Psychopharmacology,* Vol. 18, *The Endorphins,* E. Costa and M. Trabucchi (Eds.). Raven, New York, pp. 51-70.

Jones, R. (1978). Naloxone-induced mood and physiologic changes in normal volunteers. In *Endorphins in Mental Illness,* E. Usdin and W. E. Bunney (Eds.). Macmillan, London.

Kalant, H. (1978). Behavioral aspects of addiction. Group report. In *Life Sciences Research Report 8, The Bases of Addiction,* J. Fishman (Ed.). Dahlem Konferenzen, Berlin, pp. 463-495.

Korf, J., Bunney, B. S., and Aghajanian, G. K. (1974). Noradrenalin neurons. Morphine inhibition of spontaneous activity. *Eur. J. Pharmacol. 25,* 165-169.

Kosterlitz, H. W., and Hughes, J. (1978). Development of concepts of opiate receptors and their ligands. In *Advances in Biochemical Psychopharmacology,* Vol. 8, *The Endorphins,* E. Costa and M. Trabucchi (Eds.). Raven, New York, pp. 31-44.

Lal, H., Miksic, S., and Drawbaugh, R. (1978). Influence of environmental stimuli associated with narcotic administration on narcotic actions and dependence. In *Factors Affecting the Action of Narcotics,* M. L. Adler, L. Manara, and R. Samanin (Eds.). Raven, New York, 643-668.

Lee, N. M., Loh, H. H., and Li, C. H. (1978). Morphine and β-endorphin on RNA synthesis. In *Advances in Biochemical Psychopharmacology,* Vol. 18, *The Endorphins,* E. Costa and M. Trabucchi (Eds.). Raven, New York, pp. 278-288.

Leibeskind, J. C., Guilbaud, G., Besson, M., and Oliveras, J. L. (1973). Analgesia from electrical stimulation of the periaqueductal gray matter in the cat. Behavioral observations and inhibitory effects on spinal cord interneurons. *Brain Res. 50,* 441-446.

Lewis, R. V., Stein, S., Gerber, L. D., Rubenstein, M., and Udenfriend, S. (1978). High molecular weight opioid-containing proteins in striatum. *Proc. Nat. Acad. Sci. USA 75,* 4021-4023.

Li, C. H. (1964). Lipotropin, a new active peptide from pituitary glands. *Nature 201,* 924-926.

Li, C. H., and Chung, D. (1976). Isolation and structure of an untriakontapeptide with opiate activity from camel pituitary glands. *Proc. Nat. Acad. Sci. USA 73,* 1145-1148.

Lotti, V., Kokka, N., and George, R. (1969). Pituitary activation following intrahypothalamic microinjection of morphine. *Neuroendocrinology 4,* 326-332.

Lytle, L. D., Phebus, L., Fisher, L. A., and Messing, R. B. (1978). Dietary effects on analgesic drug potency. In *Factors Affecting the Action of Narcotics,* M. L. Adler, L. Manara, and R. Samanin (Eds.). Raven, New York, 543-564.

Martin, W. R. (1978). Chemotherapy of narcotic addiction. In *Handbook of Experimental Pharmacology: Drug Addiction,* Vol. 1. W. R. Martin (Ed.). Springer-Verlag, Berlin, pp. 279-318.

Martin, W. R. (1972). Pathophysiology of narcotic addiction. Possible role of protracted abstinence in relapse. In *Drug Abuse,* C. D. J. Zarafonetis (Ed.). Lea and Febiger, Philadelphia, pp. 153-159.

Martin, W. R. (Ed.). (1978). *Handbook of Experimental Pharmacology: Drug Addiction,* I Vol. 1. Springer-Verlag, Berlin.

Martin, W. R., and Sloan, J. W. (1978). Neuropharmacology and neurochemistry of subjective effects, analgesia, tolerance and dependence produced by narcotic analgesics. *Handbook of Experimental Pharmacology, Drug Addictions,* Vol. 1. W. R. Martin (Ed.). Springer-Verlag, Berlin, pp. 143-158.

Martin, W. R., Jasinski, D. R., Haertzen, C. A., Kay, D. C., Jones, B. E., Mansky, P. A., and Carpenter, R. W. (1973a). Methadone. A reevaluation. *Arch. Gen. Psychiatry 28,* 286-295.

Martin, W. R., Jasinski, D. R., and Mansky, P. A. (1973b). Naltrexone. An antagonist for the treatment of heroin dependence. *Arch. Gen. Psychiatr. 28,* 784-791.

Martin, W. R., Eades, C. G., Thompson, J. H., Huppler, R. E., and Gilbert, P. E. (1976). The effects of morphine and nalorphine-like drugs in the nondependent and morphine-dependent chronic spinal dog. *J. Pharmacol. Exp. Ther. 197,* 517-532.

Martin, W. R., Haertzen, C. A., and Hewett, B. B. (1978). Psychopathology and pathophysiology of narcotic addicts, alcoholics and drug abusers. In *Psychopharmacology: A Generation of Progress,* M. A. Lipton, A. DiMascio, and K. F. Killam (Eds.). Raven, New York.

Mayer, D. J., and Hayes, R. L. (1975). Stimulation-produced analgesia. Development of tolerance and cross tolerance to morphine. *Science 188,* 941-943.

McAuliffe, W. E., and Gordon, R. A. (1974). A test of Lindesmith's theory of addiction. The frequency of euphoria among long-term addicts. *Am. J. Sociol. 79,* 795-840.

McKnight, A. T., Hughes, J., and Kosterlitz, H. W. (1978). Synthesis of enkephalins in striatal slices of guinea-pig brain. In *Characteristics and Function of Opioids,* J. Van Ree and L. Terenius (Eds.). Elsevier/North-Holland, Amsterdam, pp. 259-270.

McMillan, D. W., and Morse, W. H. (1967). Some effects of morphine and morphine antagonists of schedule-controlled behavior. *J. Pharmacol. Exp. Ther. 157,* 175-184.

Mello, N. K., and Mendelson, J. H. (1978). Behavior pharmacology of human alcohol, heroin and marihuana use. In *Life Sciences Research Report 8, The Bases of Addiction,* J. Fishman (Ed.). Dahlem Konferenzen. Berlin, pp. 133-156.

Mirin, S. M., Meyer, R. E., and McNamee, H. B. (1976). Psychopathology and mood during heroin use. *Arch. Gen. Psychiatr 33,* 1503-1508.

Mushlin, B. E., and Cochin, J. (1976). Some effects of agonists and antagonists on the development of tolerance and dependence. In *Tissue Response to Addictive Drugs,* D. H. Ford and D. H. Clouet (Eds.). Spectrum, Hollis-wood, New York, pp. 435-445.

O'Brien, C. P., Testa, T., O'Brien, T. J., Brady, J. P., and Wells, B. (1977). Conditioned narcotic withdrawal in humans. *Science 195,* 1000-1002.

O'Brien, C. P. (1975). Experimental analysis of conditioning factors in human narcotic addiction. *Pharmacol. Rev. 27,* 533-543.

O'Callaghan, J. P., Williams, N., and Clouet, D. H. (1979). The effect of morphine on the endogenous phosphorylation of synaptic plasma membrane proteins of rat brain. *J. Pharmacol. Exp. Thera. 208* (in press).

O'Donnell, J. A., Voss, H. L., Clayton, R. R., Slatin, G. T., and Room, R. G. W. (1976). Young men and drugs. A nationwide survey. In *National Institute on Drug Abuse Research Monograph 5* (ADM 76-311), National Technical Information Service, Springfield, Virginia.

Oliverio, A., Castellano, C., Racani, F., Spano, P. F., Trabucchi, M., and Cattebene, F. (1978). Genetic aspects of narcotic action. In *Factors Affecting the Action of Narcotics,* M. L. Adler, L. Manara, and R. Samanin (Eds.). Raven, New York, pp. 7-18.

Pang, C. N., and Zimmerman, E. (1975). Effects of morphine on plasma levels of LH, TSH and prolactin in ovariectomized rats. *Anatom. Rec. 181,* 444-452.

Pert, A. (1978). Central sites involved in opiate actions. In *Life Sciences Research Report 8, The Bases of Addiction,* J. Fishman (Ed.). Dahlem Konferenzen, Berlin, pp. 299-332.

Pickens, R., Meisch, R. A., and Dougherty, J. A. (1968). Chemical interactions in metamphetamine reinforcement. *Psychol. Rep. 23,* 1267-1270.

Platt, J. J. and Labate, C. (1976). *Heroin Addiction: Theory, Research and Treatment.* Wiley, New York.

Pollard, H., Llorens, C., Schwartz, J. C., Gros, C., and Dray, F. (1978). Localization of opiate receptors and enkephalins in the rat striatum in relationship with the nigrostriatal dopaminergic system. Lesion studies. *Brain Res. 151,* 392-398.

Pomeranz, B., and Chiu, D. (1976). Naloxone blockade of acupuncture analgesia. Endorphin implicated. *Life Sci. 19,* 1757-1762.

Rivier, C., Vale, W., Ling, N., Brown, M., and Guillemin, R. (1977). Stimulation in vivo of the secretion of prolactin and growth hormone by β-endorphin. *Endocrinology 100,* 238-241.

Roberts, J. L., and Herbert, E. (1977). Characterization of a common precursor to corticotropin and β-lipotropin peptides and their arrangement relative to corticotropin in the precursor synthesized in a cell-free system. *Proc. Nat. Acad. Sci. USA 74,* 5300-5304.

Robins, L. A. (1974). *The Vietnam Drug User Returns.* Special Action Office Monograph Series A, No. 2, U. S. Government Printing Office, Washington.

Rolls, E. T., Kelly, P. H., and Shaw, S. G. (1974). Noradrenalin, dopamine and brain stimulation reward. *Pharmacol. Biochem. Behav. 2,* 735-740.

Samanin, R., Miranda, F., and Mennini, T. (1978). Serotonergic mechanisms of narcotic action. In *Factors Affecting the Action of Narcotics,* M. L. Adler, L. Manara, and R. Samanin (Eds.). Raven, New York, pp. 523-541.

Sandberg, D. E., and Segal, M. (1978). Pharmacological analysis of analgesia and self-stimulation elicited by electrical stimulation of catecholamine nuclei in rat brain. *Brain Res. 152,* 529-532.

Schulman, H., and Greengard, P. (1978). Calcium-dependent protein phosphorylation system in membranes from various tissues, and its activation by the "calcium-dependent regulator." *Proc. Nat. Acad. Sci. USA 75,* 5432-5436.

Schuster, C. R. (1978). Theoretical basis of behavioral tolerance. Implications of the phenomenon for problems of drug abuse. In *Behavioral Tolerance: Research and Treatment Implications,* N. A. Krasnegor (Ed.). NIDA Research Monograph 18, U. S. Government Printing Office, Washington, D. C., pp. 4-17.

Schwartz, J. C., Costenin, J., Martres, M. P., Protais, P., and Baudry, M. (1978). Modulation of receptor mechanisms in the CNS. Hyper- and hypo-sensitivity to catecholamines. *Neuropharmacology 17,* 665-685.

Segal, M., and Bloom, F. E. (1976). The action of norepinephrine in the rat hippocampus III. Hippocampal cellular responses to locus coeruleus stimulation. *Brain Res. 107,* 499-511.

Shaar, C. J., Frederickson, R. C. A., Dininger, N. B., and Jackson, L. (1977). Enkephalin analogues and naloxone modulate the release of GH and prolactin. Evidence for regulation by an endogenous peptide in brain. *Life Sci. 21,* 853-860.

Sharma, S. K., Klee, W. A., and Nirenberg, M. (1975). Dual regulation of adenylate cyclase account for narcotic dependence and tolerance. *Proc. Nat. Acad. Sci. USA 72,* 3092-3096.

Shorr, J., Foley, K., and Spector, S. (1978). Presence of non-peptide morphine-like compound in human cerebrospinal fluid. *Life Sci. 23,* 2057-2062.

Simantov, R., Kuhar, M. J., Uhl, G. R., and Snyder, S. H. (1977). Opioid peptide enkephalin. Immunohistochemical mapping in rat central nervous system. *Proc. Nat. Acad. Sci. USA 74,* 2167-2171.

Simon, E. J. (1978). In vitro studies on opiate receptors and their action. In

Factors Affecting the Action of Narcotics, M. L. Adler, L. Manara, and R. Samanin (Eds.). Raven, New York, pp. 193-206.

Simon, E. J., and Hiller, J. M. (1978). The opiate receptors. *Ann. Rev. Pharmacol. Toxicol. 18,* 371-394.

Snyder, S. H. (1978). The opiate receptor and morphine like peptides in the brain. *Am. J. Psychiatr. 135,* 645-652.

Snyder, S. H., and Childer, S. R. (1979). Opiate receptors and opioid peptides. *Ann. Rev. Neurosci. 2,* 35-64.

Spealman, R. D., and Goldberg, S. R. (1978). Drug self-administration by laboratory animals. Control by schedules of reinforcement. *Ann. Rev. Pharmacol. Toxicol. 18,* 313-340.

Stein, L., and Belluzzi, J. D. (1978). Brain endorphins and the sense of well being. A psychobiological hypothesis. In *Advances in Biochemical Psychopharmacology,* Vol. 18, E. Costa and M. Trabucchi (Eds.). Raven, New York, pp. 299-311.

Stein, L., Belluzzi, J. D., and Wise, C. D. (1976). Norepinephrine self-stimulation pathways. Implication for long-term memory and schizophrenia. In *Brain Stimulation Reward,* A. Wauquiver and E. T. Rolls (Eds.). Elsevier, New York, pp. 277-334.

Stimson, G. V., Oppenheimer, E., and Thorley, A. (1978). Seven year follow-up of heroin addicts. Drug use and outcome. *Br. Med. J. 1,* 1190-1192.

Suda, T., Liotta, A. S., and Krieger, D. T. (1978). β-Endorphin is not detectable in plasma from normal human subjects. *Science 202,* 221-223.

Tarter, R. E., McBride, H., Buonopane, N., and Schneider, D. U. (1977). Differentiation of alcoholics. *Arch. Gen. Psychiatr. 34,* 761-768.

Terenius, L. (1978). Significance of endorphins in endogenous antinociception. In *Advances in Biochemical Psychopharmacology,* Vol. 18, *The Endorphins,* E. Costa and M. Trabucchi (Eds.). Raven, New York, pp. 321-332.

Thompson, T., and Young, A. M. (1978). Relevance of animal models for human addiction. In *Life Sciences Research Report 8, The Bases of Addiction,* J. Fishman (Ed.). Kahlem Konferenzen. Berlin, pp. 119-132.

Tseng, L. F., Loh, H. H., and Wei, E. T. (1975). Effects of clonidine on morphine withdrawal signs in the rat. *Eur. J. Pharmacol. 30,* 93-99.

Tseng, L. F., Loh, H. H., and Li, C. H. (1976). β-Endorphin as a potent analgesic by intravenous injection. *Nature 263,* 239-241.

Vaillant, G. E. (1973). A 20-year follow-up of New York narcotic addicts. *Arch. Gen. Psychiatr. 29,* 237-255.

Verebey, K., Volavka, J., and Clouet, D. (1978). Endorphins in psychiatry. An overview and a hypothesis. *Arch. Gen. Psychiatr. 35,* 877-888.

Wardlaw, S. L., and Frantz, A. G. (1979). Measurement of β-Endorphin in human plasma. *J. Clin. Endocrinol. Metab. 48,* 176-180.

Watanabe, M., Diab, I. M., Schuster, C. R., and Roth, L. J. (1976). H^3-morphine localization in brain. In *Tissue Responses to Addictive Drugs,* D. H. Ford and D. H. Clouet (Eds.). Spectrum, Holliswood, New York, pp. 49-60.

Way, E. L. (1978). Common and selective mechanisms in drug dependence. In *Life Sciences Research Report 8, The Bases of Addiction.* J. Fishman (Ed.). Dahlem Konferenzen: Berlin, pp. 333-352.

Way, E. L., and Bhargava, H. N. (1976). Assessment of the role of acetylcholine in morphine analgesia, tolerance and dependence. In *Tissues Response to Addictive Drugs,* D. H. Ford and D. H. Clouet (Eds.). Spectrum, Holliswood, New York, pp. 237-253.

Wei, E., and Loh, H. H. (1976). Physical dependence on opiate-like peptides. *Science 193,* 1262-1263.

Weissman, M. M., Slobertz, F., Prusoff, B., Mezritz, M., and Howard, P. (1976). Clinical depression among narcotic addicts maintained on methadone in the community. *Am. J. Psychiatr. 133,* 1434-1438.

Wikler, A. (1965). Conditioning factors in opiate addiction and relapse. In *Narcotics,* D. M. Wilner and G. G. Kassebaum (Eds.). McGraw-Hill, New York, pp. 85-110.

Wikler, A. (1973). Dynamics of drug dependence. Implications of a conditioning theory for research and treatment. *Arch. Gen. Psychiatr. 28,* 611-619.

Wise, R. A. (1978). Catecholamine theories of reward. A critical review. *Brain Res. 152,* 215-247.

Wood, D. R., Reimherr, F. W., Wender, P. H., and Johnson, G. E. (1976). Diagnosis and treatment of minimal brain dysfunction in adults. *Arch. Gen. Psychiatr. 33,* 1453-1460.

Wüster, M., Loth, P., and Schulz, R. (1978). Characterization of opiate-like material in blood and urine. In *Advances in Biochemical Psychopharmacology,* Vol. 18, *The Endorphins,* E. Costa and M. Trabucchi (Eds.). Raven, New York, pp. 313-320.

Yang, H-Y. T., Hong, J. S., Fratta, W., and Costa, E. (1978). Rat brain enkephalins. Distribution and biosynthesis. In *Advances in Biochemical Psychopharmacology,* Vol. 18, *The Endorphins,* E. Costa and M. Trabucchi (Eds.). Raven, New York, pp. 149-159.

8

Memory and Memory Disorders: A Biological and Neurologic Perspective

Larry R. Squire and Werner T. Schlapfer*
Veterans Administration Medical Center
San Diego, California and
University of California at San Diego School of Medicine
La Jolla, California

**Present Affiliation:* Veterans Administration Medical Center, Livermore, California.

I. INTRODUCTION

Study of the biology of memory is predicated on the belief that the changes in behavior we call memory are stored as changes in neuronal interactions in the brain. Although the precise nature of these changes is not yet understood, a good deal is known about the morphology, physiology, and biochemistry of neurons and about the ways in which neurons can change the way they communicate with one another.

Examples of neuronal plasticity are of great interest for understanding how memory might work in the whole animal. By identifying the various ways in which neurons can alter their effective connectivity as a function of their past activity, we can discover the various control points or plastic elements of neuronal connections and thereby identify specific candidates for memory mechanisms.

A good deal has also been learned about memory by studies of whole animals. Since the mammalian brain is very complex, consisting of at least 10^{10} neurons and 10^{14} synaptic connections, direct study of the biological basis of memory storage in the behaving animal is not feasible. However, it has been possible to demonstrate neuronal plasticities that result from behavioral events, to identify specific brain regions and biochemical events that appear to be important in information storage, and to identify at a "systems analysis" level some general features of how the brain accomplishes information storage.

Some things are remembered for only a short time. Other things are remembered for a long time, even for years. It has therefore seemed reasonable to suppose that neurons might possess different types of plastic properties that could endure for different lengths of time. The kind of mechanism required to store information for only a few seconds might be quire different from the kind of mechanism required to store information for years. Changes underlying short-term memory must be established rapidly but could be rapidly reversible. Changes underlying long-term memory could develop gradually, but must be quite stable.

The discussion that follows will consider long-term memory mechanisms, short-term memory mechanisms, and some general principles about plasticity that emerge from these considerations. With this framework in mind, we can then ask what kind of memory disorders occur and what additional information these disorders provide as to the biology of memory.

II. LONG-TERM MEMORY MECHANISMS

A. Biochemistry: Inhibitors of Protein Synthesis

It is important to note that the lifetime of a memory in the nervous system need not necessarily be limited by the lifetime of any particular chemical substance. The formation of memory probably depends on a chain of events. If the final stage in this chain of events results in actual morphological changes in the synaptic region, then the constituent elements of the synaptic regions could be continually replaced without destroying the memory.

Because of its importance in many cellular regulatory processes, it has seemed reasonable to think that protein synthesis might be involved in memory in some way. Protein synthesis could be involved in memory in two fundamentally different ways: (1) newly synthesized proteins could code information, such that different protein molecules represent different memories; (2) newly synthesized proteins could be part of a series of events that results in a change in synaptic efficacy along particular neuronal pathways. By this latter view, specificity of information is conferred by where synaptic efficacy is altered rather than by which protein molecules are synthesized. This idea is rather appealing because it means that the nervous system could use the same protein molecules wherever changes in synaptic efficacy occur.

One approach to studying the possible role of protein synthesis in memory has been to use drugs that inhibit brain protein synthesis and to ask what effect such drugs have on learning and on memory (Squire and Barondes, 1972; Squire and Barondes, 1974). Several drugs are available, such as cycloheximide and anisomycin, which inhibit brain protein synthesis by about 95% and which are fully reversible after a few hours. Since most brain proteins have half-lives of several days, this period of inhibition is not long enough to seriously affect life-sustaining metabolic events, and mice given such drugs tolerate them very well. In a typical behavioral experiment, cerebral protein synthesis is inhibited in mice by about 95% just before or after training in a simple task that requires mice to escape footshock by touching the smaller of two metal objects. Normally, mice learn this task rather quickly and then can remember the habit for a week or

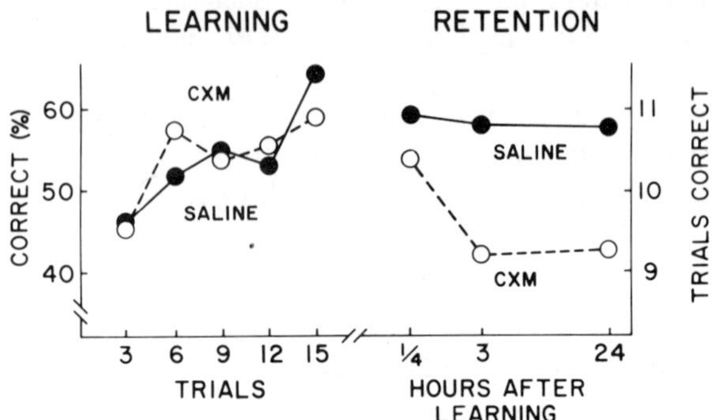

Figure 1 Following inhibition of 90-95% brain protein synthesis by cycloheximide (CXM), mice acquire a discrimination habit at a normal rate (left panel). Amnesia develops gradually during the hours after learning and is complete by 3 hours (right panel). (Based on data obtained from Squire and Barondes, 1972, 1973.)

more. When brain protein synthesis is markedly inhibited, initial learning is normal but amnesia develops gradually after training and can be clearly observed within a few hours (Fig. 1). This basic finding has been obtained in rodents, birds, and fish using a variety of inhibitors and learning tasks.

The finding that acquisition during a brief training experience is normal despite inhibition of 95% brain protein synthesis argues strongly that synthesis of new protein is not required for initial acquisition of a new task and suggests that biochemical events other than protein synthesis must be involved in the initial learning process. Additional studies have been necessary to evaluate fully the effect of these drugs on long-term memory. For example, the possibility that animals are made sick by the drug and that sickness is responsible for amnesia is ruled out by showing that mice given the drug 30 min after training and then tested later show no impairment. Thus, to be effective the drug must be present during the time of training or during the minutes after training. It has also been possible to dissociate a variety of side effects of these drugs from their effects on memory (Spanis and Squire, 1978). These effects on memory have now been demonstrated with three agents, cycloheximide, anisomycin, and puromycin, all of which potently inhibit brain protein synthesis but by different mechanisms and with different side effects. Emetine and pactamycin, two other inhibitors of protein synthesis that do not cross the blood brain barrier sufficiently to inhibit brain protein synthesis to a great extent, do not cause amnesia (Dunn et al., 1976).

Although definitive conclusions from behavioral pharmacological studies are not possible, all available evidence is consistent with the hypothesis that brain protein synthesis during or shortly after training is required for the formation of long-term memory. The proteins whose synthesis is required for long-term memory could occur (1) in those neurons whose connectivity must be changed in order to store memory and/or (2) in neurons that do not directly participate in the information storage network but that instead have the capability of influencing connectivity between other neurons.

B. Biochemistry: Correlates of Experience

Another strategy for studying the biochemical aspects of long-term memory has been to try to measure biochemical events that occur in the brain during learning. One method has been to measure the extent of incorporation of radioactive precursors into brain macromolecules during a training experience (Rose et al., 1976; Shashoua, 1978). Using this approach, increased incorporation of amino acids into protein and nucleotides into RNA have been correlated with various training experiences in rat, fish, and chick. For example, chicks exposed to an imprinting stimulus 18-24 hr after hatching exhibited increased incorporation of [^{3}H]uracil into brain RNA and of [^{3}H] lysine into brain protein, compared to chicks kept in darkness or exposed only to diffuse light (Rose et al., 1976).

One difficulty with this approach has been that the measurements are sensitive to changes in blood flow and to changes in metabolism of the precursor material, so that it is often difficult to know whether synthesis of macromolecules has been altered. In some cases, however, the effect appears to be limited to only a few molecular species having certain molecular weights (Shashoua, 1977a,b), and such results do suggest that macromolecular synthesis was stimulated by environmental events. Another perhaps even more difficult problem concerns what aspect of the environment is responsible for the observed biochemical events. For example, these events could be caused by nonspecific features of the environment, such as stress or activity. Alternatively, they could be caused by quite specific features of training, such as the acquisition of certain kinds of information. A variety of clever control procedures have been designed to address these questions (Rose et al., 1976; Shashoua, 1976a).

Chicks given imprinting training exhibited increased incorporation of radioactive substances into macromolecules during training but not during subsequent retention trials, and split-brain chicks exhibited these changes only in the hemisphere exposed to the imprinting stimulus (Rose et al., 1976). Similarly, fish learning to swim upright in a float-training task exhibited increased incorporation into RNA and protein only during learning and not during a retention test 24 hours later. Moreover, increased incorporation was not observed in fish that attempted to learn a similar but insoluble task, or in fish that mastered the task but did not show long-term retention (Shashoua,

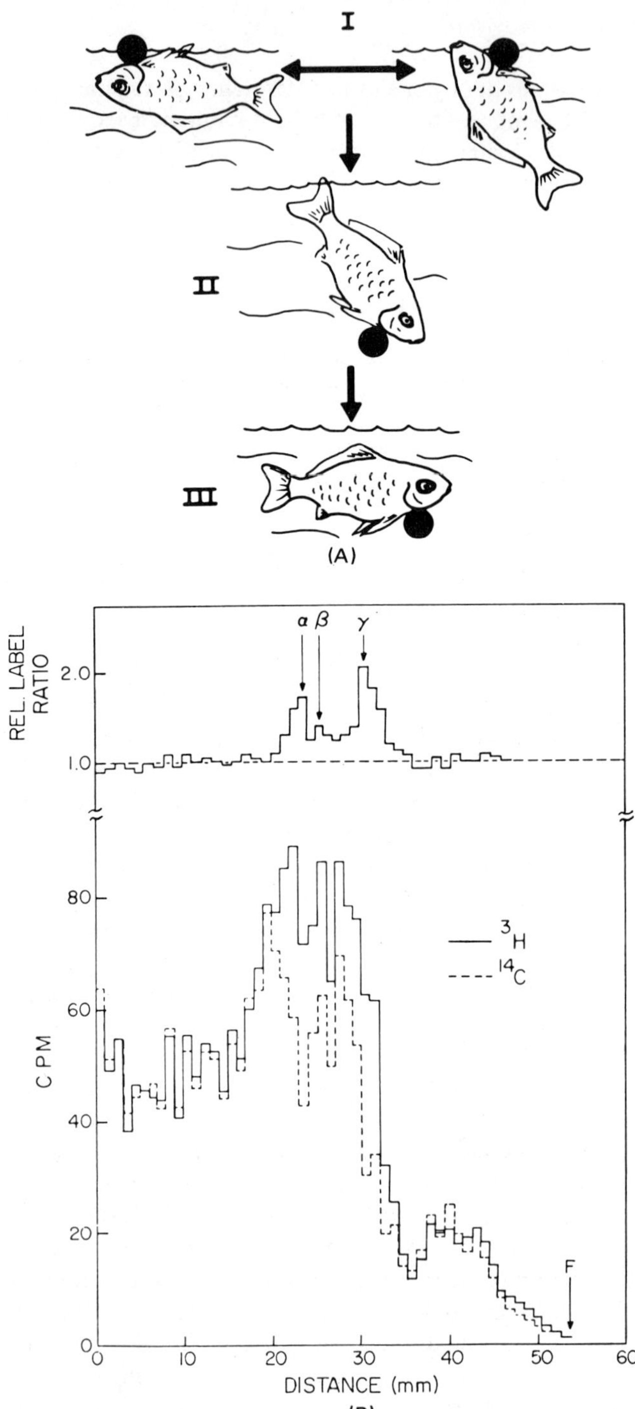
I
II
III
(A)
REL. LABEL RATIO
α
β
γ
2.0
1.0
80
60
40
20
0
CPM
^3H
^{14}C
F
0
10
20
30
40
50
60
DISTANCE (mm)
(B)

1976). Although these control procedures do rule out some kinds of nonspecific effects, it is usually conceded that it is not possible to control for every aspect of a training event so as to isolate completely the process of information acquisition.

Further studies in the fish using the float-training task (Fig. 2) have indicated that the changes in incorporation into RNA and protein are specific and do not involve all brain RNA or protein (Shashoua, 1976a,b, 1977a,b). In the case of protein, incorporation of radioactive precursors is increased specifically in three cytoplasmic proteins (designated α, β, γ) having molecular weights of 37,000, 32,500, and 26,000, respectively. Immunological studies of one of these substances (β) suggest that it is localized to approximately 15,000 cells that lie primarily near the ventricles. Several lines of evidence have suggested that the identified cells may be nonneuronal. It has been proposed that this material is secreted from glial cells during training and then plays a role, elsewhere in the brain, in altering synaptic connectivity. Since it is usually assumed that memory is the result of changes along a few discrete and perhaps anatomically disparate pathways, the synthesis of proteins α, β, and γ presumably do not represent the laying down of information, but instead reflect the synthesis of substances that have a role in altering synaptic efficacy along specific pathways.

C. Biochemistry: Induction of Specific Protein Synthesis

The evidence seems quite strong that macromolecular synthesis is required for the formation of long-term memory. However, very little is known about how synaptic activity results in macromolecular synthesis. Since sensory information about experience of the external world enters the central nervous system coded as electrical signals (action potentials and synaptic potentials), the transformation of bioelectric information into enduring alterations in the function of neurons is a necessary step in memory formation.

What mechanisms are available to neurons for this transformation? At many synapses, the transmitter-receptor interaction sets into motion a sequence of biological steps. The best-studied examples involve cyclic nucleotides as second messenger molecules (e.g., Nathanson, 1977). This scheme postulates that some neurotransmitters (in particular the biogenic amines dopamine,

---

Figure 2 (A) In the float-training task, a polystyrene float is sutured to the ventral surface of a goldfish, causing it to swim upside down (I). During a period of learning requiring about 5 hr, animals adapt to the float and gradually assume a horizontal posture (III). (From Shashoua, 1978.) (B) Following this training procedure, experimental fish were labeled with [^{3}H]valine and untrained fish with [^{14}C]valine. Cytoplasmic proteins were separated on a polyacrylamide-SDS gel. The highest ^{3}H/^{14}C ratios coincided with three bands of increased incorporation (α, β, and γ). (From Shashoua, 1977b.)

norepinephrine, and serotonin but probably others as well) activate receptors on the external cell surface which are coupled through the cell membrane to enzymes that catalyze the formation of cyclic nucleotides (in particular cyclic adenosine monophosphate, cAMP; but possibly also cyclic guanidine monophosphate, cGMP). These cyclic nucleotides in turn stimulate enzymes (protein kinases) which can phosphorylate specific proteins and thereby alter their function. It has also been shown that histones (proteins associated with DNA) can be phosphorylated by cAMP-dependent protein kinases (Langan, 1973). Phosphorylated histones might then expose genes for transcription and translation into proteins. In this way cAMP could be an intermediary in the induction of specific protein synthesis.

For example, stimulation of the adrenergic neuronal input to rat pineal gland triggers synthesis of the enzyme N-acetyltransferase in the pineal gland, presumably by way of a cAMP-activated protein kinase (Klein, 1974). Other examples of transsynaptic induction of de novo protein synthesis in the nervous system have also been described. A particularly interesting case is the specific induction of the enzyme tyrosine hydroxylase in adrenal gland or sympathetic ganglia by synaptic activation (Costa et al., 1974). Behavioral manipulation (cold stress) can also induce tyrosine hydroxylase. Tyrosine hydroxylase is the rate-limiting enzyme in the synthesis of the neurotransmitters dopamine and norepinephrine, and changes in the amount of this enzyme could presumably lead to enduring changes in the amount of transmitter in the postsynaptic cell. It is not completely clear as to whether or not cAMP is involved in the induction of tyrosine hydroxylase (Oesch et al., 1975).

The nature of the proteins whose synthesis is required for long-term memory is not yet known but could be of several types: (1) enzymes that regulate neurotransmitter metabolism or enzymes that are involved in other aspects of neuronal function, (2) receptor molecules, and (3) structural proteins.

D. Morphological Changes

It is now known that the morphology of neurons is not fixed, but can be influenced by a variety of natural and artificial conditions. This type of plasticity has been the basis for proposals that changes in neuronal morphology may ultimately be the basis for long-term information storage. Such morphological changes would presumably require the induction of specific protein synthesis, possibly mediated by cyclic nucleotides.

Perhaps the best-known example of this type of plasticity comes from studies of brain anatomy in animals who have been reared in complex environments (Rosenzweig et al., 1972). Rats reared for 15-30 days in large group cages filled with toys exhibited thicker cortices, particularly in the occipital region, compared with rats reared in standard laboratory cages. These changes occurred

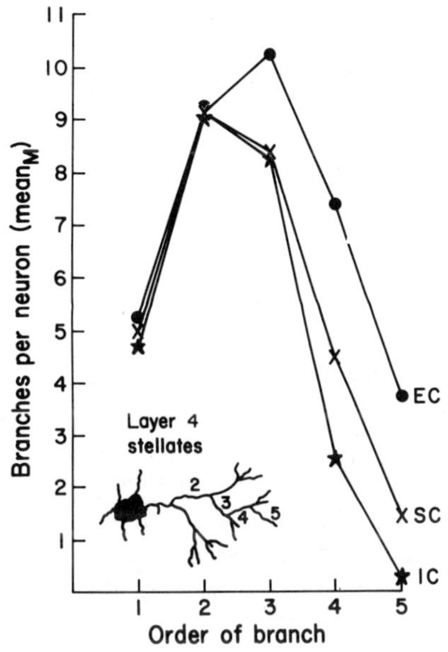

Figure 3 Mean number of dendritic branches of each order in occipital cortical neurons of rats reared for 30 days under complex (EC), social (SC), or isolated (IC) conditions. Enriched rats had significantly greater branching in 3rd, 4th, and 5th order dendritic branches. [Reprinted with permission from F. R. Volkmar and W. T. Greenough (1972). *Science 176,* 1445-1447. Copyright 1972 by the American Association for the Advancement of Science.]

together with an increase in size of neurons, but not their number, and an increase in the number of glial cells.

Subsequent studies have looked for possible changes in neuronal morphology that could have implications for synaptic connectivity. Rats reared in a complex environment have increased branching of dendrites in layers II, IV, and V of the visual cortex (Volkmar and Greenough, 1972) (Fig. 3). These results mean that the arborization patterns of dendritic fields, and thus their opportunity for synaptic interactions, can be increased by experience. Similar though smaller effects on dendritic branching can be produced in adult rats by daily maze training for 25 days. Although it is not clear as to what aspect of training is responsible for greater dendritic branching, the results clearly indicate that in adults relatively natural environmental events can alter the potential wiring diagram of the brain. These changes in neuronal morphology produced by complex environment seem similar in many respects to differences between light-reared and dark-reared animals. Cats reared in the dark during the first 6 weeks of life exhibited smaller neurons in the visual cortex, higher neuronal density, and a smaller number of synapses per neuron (Cragg, 1975a). Apparently, the neuropil develops less extensively in the deprived animal and opportunity for connectivity is thereby diminished.

Another kind of morphological plasticity that can result from relatively natural perturbations is alterations in synaptic contact size. Following rearing in enriched environments, a small but significant increase in synaptic length could be observed in rat visual cortex (West and Greenough, 1976; Bennett, 1976). It is not clear as to whether there is an average increase in the contact size of preexisting synapses or the establishment of new synapses that are on average larger than preexisting ones. In any case, synaptic length appears to be another dimension of morphology readily affected by experience.

E. Sprouting of Axon Collaterals

When less natural kinds of perturbations are studied, still other examples of neuronal plasticity can be observed. Following a unilateral lesion of entorhinal cortex in young or adult rats, which subsequently causes degeneration of its projection to the granule cells of the dentate gyrus, other inputs that ordinarily terminate on the dendrites of the same cells now sprout axon collaterals and spread out to occupy vacated synaptic sites (Lynch and Cotman, 1975; Lynch and Wells, 1978). This reaction seems to begin about 5 days postlesion and then proceeds rapidly to completion during the subsequent 48 hr (Lynch et al., 1977). As a result the wiring diagram of this region appears to be permanently altered (Fig. 4). Collateral sprouting has also been reported in the septum. Following section of fornical fibers from hippocampus to septum, there is expansion of the septal projection from the medial forebrain bundle (Moore, 1976).

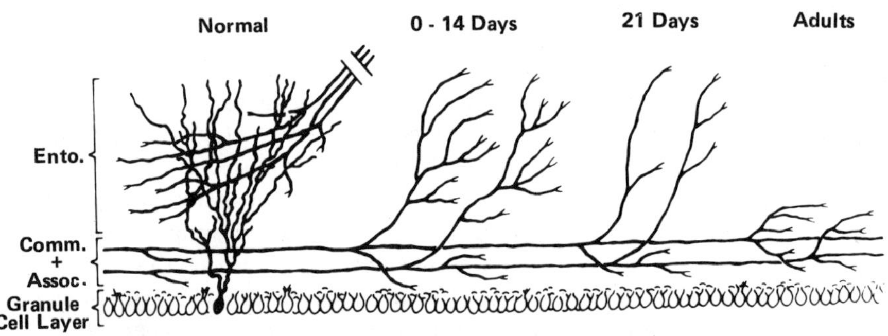

Figure 4 In the normal case (left), cells in the granular layer of rat dentate gyrus receive inputs from ipsilateral pyramidal cells (assoc.), from contralateral pyramidal cells (comm.), and from the ipsilateral entorhinal cortex (ento.). Following destruction of the entorhinal inputs, the commissural and association projections extend outward to occupy a greater portion of the dendritic tree. Collateral sprouting is greater when the experiment is performed on very young animals (0-14 days old) than on older animals. (From Lynch and Wells, 1978.)

In addition, ablation of the superior colliculus in the newborn hamster results in increased innervation of the lateral geniculate body and an anomalous projection to the lateral posterior nucleus of the thalamus (Schneider, 1973). Thus when one source of synaptic connections is removed, remaining ones can sprout new terminals and invade the vacated space. This sequence of events has also been studied extensively in sensory nerve of amphibians (Diamond et al., 1976). In the case of the hamster, the anomalous projection can support forms of visually guided behavior (Schneider, 1979).

F. Plasticity of Synaptic Connectivity in the Visual System

An example of a kind of plasticity that involves more natural conditions can be observed in the visual system of the developing kitten (Wiesel and Hubel, 1965; Hubel and Wiesel, 1970). Normally, neurons in the visual cortex of the cat are binocular and can be influenced to some extent by input from both eyes (Fig. 5). The majority of cortical cells respond to some extent to input from each eye. A minority of cells respond exclusively to input from either the left or the right eye. The visual experience of the kitten during a few critical weeks early in life is capable of altering the responsiveness of cortical cells and their binocular characteristics. Thus when kittens are reared with the left eye covered, as adults they have cortical cells that are driven almost exclusively by the experienced eye. Since there are apparently few or no cells that cannot be driven at all, nor is there histological evidence of cellular atrophy, the conclusion has been that neuronal connectivity has been altered by monocular deprivation such that cells that would ordinarily have been responsive to the covered eye come to be responsive instead to the experienced eye.

That this result reflects interaction between the inputs from each eye is demonstrated by another experiment in which kittens are reared with both eyes covered (Wiesel and Hubel, 1965). In this case there is some reduction in the number of cells that will respond to visual stimulation but there is no change in the binocular characteristics of the responsive cells. These results indicate that the effect of deprivation of visual experience in one eye depends on what is happening to the other eye. Ordinarily, axons carrying visual information from each eye appear to compete for postsynaptic cells, and simultaneous activity or inactivity to the two inputs is required to maintain binocularity. It is interesting to note that the critical period for these effects of unilateral eye closure (about the 4th week of life) corresponds to the time when synapse formation in the visual cortex is occurring at its peak rate (Cragg, 1975b). Thus, the result of competitive interaction between inputs from each eye could conceivably express itself in how many synapses are formed. Synapses would not necessarily need to be unmade to account for these findings. It is not yet known what kind

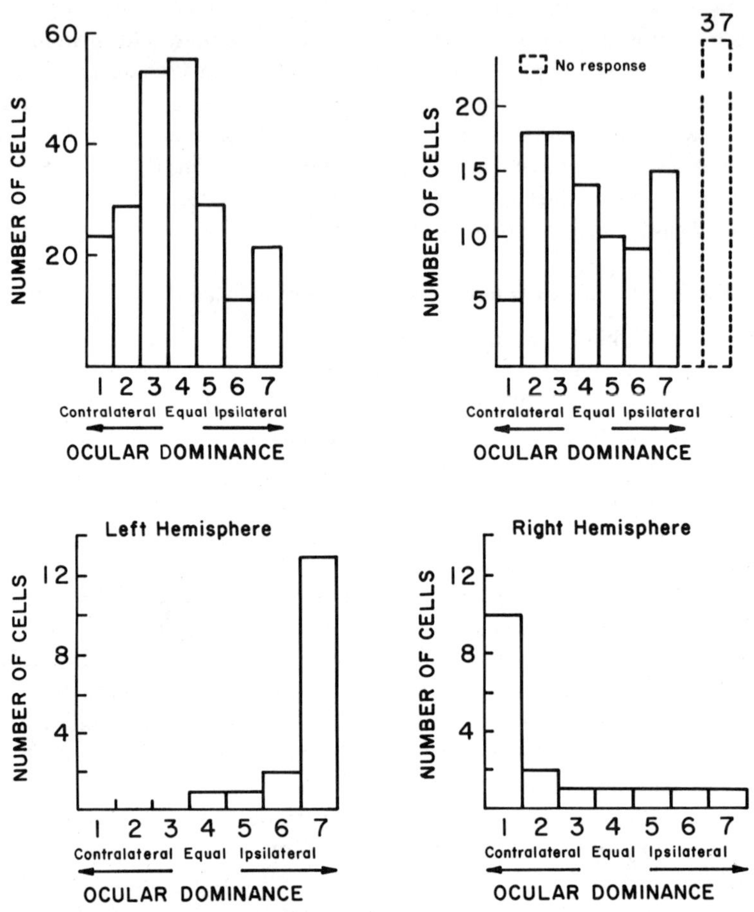

Figure 5 (top left) Ocular dominance distribution of 223 cells recorded from striate cortex of normal adult cats. Cells in groups 1 and 7 were driven by only one eye. In groups 2-3 and 5-6, cells were driven better by one eye than the other. In group 4, both eyes have about equal influence. (bottom) Ocular dominance distribution of 32 cells recorded from the left and right striate cortex of a cat without visual experience in the right eye from 9 weeks to 6 months of age. The vast majority of cells responded only to stimulation from the experienced eye. (top right) Ocular dominance distribution of 126 cells recorded from four cats that had been deprived of visual experience in both eyes from about 2 weeks to 3 months of age. Thirty-seven cells did not respond to visual stimulation. In contrast to the effects after unilateral eye closure, both eyes could drive cortical cells. (From Wiesel and Hubel, 1963, 1965.)

of synaptic events underlie the influence that visual input has on cortical cells. Yet it seems reasonable to suppose that morphological changes occur in the terminal field of the geniculostriate projections, since monocular deprivation leads to a shrinkage of the cortical columns that ordinarily receive input from the deprived eye and an expansion of the cortical columns that ordinarily receive input from the experienced eye (Hubel et al., 1976). In any case, the increased influence of the experienced eye does not result from atrophy of neurons responsive to the deprived eye. If the experienced eye is covered soon enough after the critical period, the influence of the formerly deprived eye on cortical cells can be reestablished and can even become dominant (Blakemore, 1974).

These studied taken together describe a type of plasticity that depends on an interaction between two inputs that converge on a common target. In this respect, findings in the visual system have some formal similarities to collateral sprouting. In both cases, when the influence of one input is diminished, a remaining input increases its influence.

G. Pruning and Reorganization of Synaptic Connections

Another kind of plasticity involves the attrition of synaptic connections. The possibility that more synapses may be present early in life than ultimately survive into adulthood has been considered in several species. For example, the number of distal dendritic spines in mouse visual cortex reaches a peak at about 19 days of age and then falls (Ruiz-Marcos and Valverde, 1969). Synaptic terminals on spinal motoneurons of kittens that are present at birth appear to be eliminated during the first 3 weeks of life (Ronnevi and Conradi, 1974).

In rat peripheral nervous system, each immature muscle fiber is supplied by multiple axons. In the adult state, each muscle fiber receives only one axon (Brown et al., 1976). The transition from immaturity to the adult stage occurs such that the number of motor axons is preserved, but the number of fibers contacted by each axon is reduced.

Sometimes synapse elimination occurs together with a reorganization of connections. In the lateral geniculate of neonatal hamster, axons from the contralateral eye arrive first and occupy their own terminal fields as well as the terminal field that will eventually be occupied by the ipsilateral projection. After the ipsilateral projection arrives a few days later, the contralateral projection reorganizes to achieve appropriate segregation of contralateral and ipsilateral terminal fields. It is not clear whether this is accomplished by eliminating the excessive portion of the contralateral projection or by rerouting it to form a denser projection at the correct location (So et al., 1978).

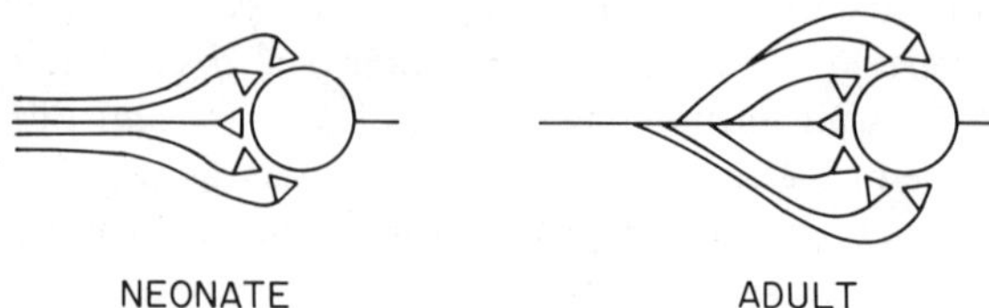

Figure 6 In the submandibular ganglion of neonatal rat (left), cells receive input from an average of five separate preganglionic fibers. By adulthood (right), a reorganization of synaptic connections has occurred such that there is an increase in the total number of synaptic terminals per cell, but they generally arise from a single presynaptic fiber. (Based on data reported by Lichtman, 1977.)

A particularly interesting example of synaptic reorganization during development has been described in the submandibular ganglion of rat (Lichtman, 1977). During the first week of life, cells in the ganglion are innervated by an average of five preganglionic nerves. In the following weeks, there is a gradual elimination of multiple innervation so that by 5 weeks most ganglion cells are innervated by only one preganglionic fiber. During the same time period, there is a gradual increase in the number of synaptic profiles per neuronal perimeter (Fig. 6). Taken together, the results suggest that during development some inputs are lost whereas the potential influence of the remaining inputs is strengthened. These results thus constitute still another example of competitive interaction between afferents for synaptic sites. As in the case of the visual system and collateral sprouting considered above, when the synaptic activity of some inputs is diminished, remaining input can increase its potential influence on the postsynaptic cell.

The examples described above indicate that the nervous system has a number of ways of responding to natural and artificial perturbations. These include synthesis of macromolecules which might alter synaptic activity, formation of larger synapses or more synapses, increased arborization of dendritic trees, sprouting of axonal collaterals, and attrition of synapses.

Whereas these have been the best studied, it is possible to imagine other ways that neuronal pathways could alter their connectivity in an enduring way. For example, changes in excitation threshold could occur as a result of membrane alterations at the spike initiator zone (e.g., Woollacott and Hoyle, 1977) or changes could occur that affect the pattern of spike propagation at axon branch points (Chung et al., 1970; Raymond and Lettvin, 1978). Note that plasticity need not necessarily depend on changes at the synapse itself, so long as the result of a plastic change is to alter the connectivity between cells.

One property shared by many of the mechanisms considered here is competitive interaction between neurons. Axon terminals may normally compete for synaptic sites. When the ability of one set of axons to affect the postsynaptic cell is diminished either artificially or naturally, the remaining axons can sometimes increase their influence on postsynaptic cells. All these mechanisms have been illustrated largely outside the context in which one would ordinarily use terms such as "learning" or "memory." Although some of the examples of plasticity described here are based on studies with whole animals, the relationship between these plasticities and memory is still indirect. It seems reasonable to suppose that the strategy that the nervous system has evolved for storing memory may involve some or all of these plasticities, but a definitive conclusion about the neuronal basis of long-term memory must await further study.

III. SHORT-TERM CHANGES

A. Modulation of Synaptic Efficacy

All the putative mechanisms for stable, long-term memory discussed above would require some time to be established. This fact means that other mechanisms must be available to hold information while the long-term changes are developing. Mechanisms for short-term information storage are indeed available in the nervous system. Many synapses vary the effectiveness of their transmission as a function of the recent history of stimulation, i.e., they "remember" previous events. Some synapses show synaptic depression, i.e., the synaptic potential decreases in amplitude with repetitive stimulation. Others show facilitation, i.e., the synaptic potential increases in amplitude with repetitive stimulation. At some synapses, both depression and facilitation occur with different time courses: A synapse may facilitate first, and then depress during continuous stimulation, or a synapse may depress first and then facilitate (Fig. 7) (Schlapfer et al., 1976). The degree of depression and facilitation is usually frequency-dependent, i.e., a certain synapse may show depression at one frequency and facilitation at another.

Following a period of repetitive stimulation the synaptic potentials at many synapses can be potentiated for a relatively long time (Fig. 7). This post-tetanic potentiation may last tens of minutes and up to hours in some cases (e.g., Hubbard, 1963; Rosenthal, 1969; Schlapfer et al., 1976). In the mammalian hippocampus, long-term potentiation is observed which can last for days (Bliss and Lømo, 1973). However, it is not yet clear whether this latter phenomenon is the same as short-term post-tetanic potentiation.

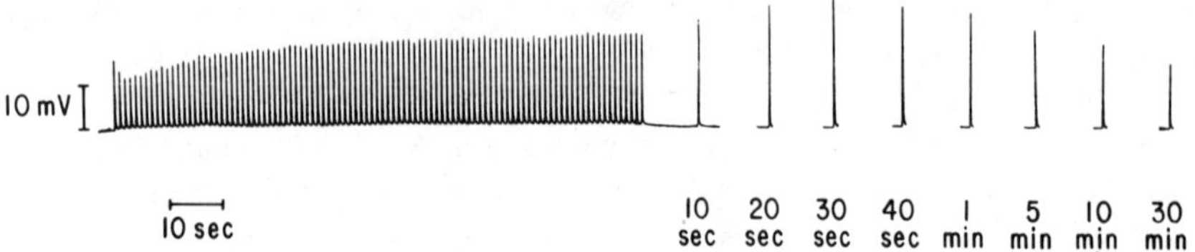

Figure 7 Synaptic depression, facilitation, and post-tetanic potentiation (PTP) at a synapse in the abdominal ganglion of *Aplysia californica.* Trace shows excitatory postsynaptic potentials recorded with an intracellular electrode in cell R15 during and after repetitive stimulation of the right visceropleural connective. Depression at the beginning of and facilitation of the synaptic potential during a train of 100 pulses at 1/sec are illustrated. After cessation of the train, PTP occurs in response to single-test pulses and endures for about 30 min. (From Schlapfer et al., 1976.)

Short-term synaptic plasticities have been extensively studied in several systems (e.g., Hubbard, 1963; Magleby and Zengel, 1975; Schlapfer et al., 1976). In the best studied cases it has been found that they are based on stimulus-dependent alterations in transmitter release rather than on postsynaptic modulations in receptor sensitivity. These variations in transmitter release depend in turn on changes in the availability of transmitter substance (depletion or mobilization) and/or on changes in the efficacy of the transmitter release mechanism.

These phenomena represent biological mechanisms for short-term information storage that could be used to construct a system that learns and remembers. The next section considers ways in which some of these mechanisms are actually used by animals to store information.

B. Cellular Analysis of Simple Forms of Learning

One approach to the biology of learning and memory has been to search for relatively simple nervous systems and simple kinds of learning. Invertebrates are particularly well suited for analysis of the neuronal circuitry underlying behavioral change. The analysis of short-term habituation in the crayfish (Zucker, 1972b; Krasne, 1976,1978) and in *Aplysia californica* (Kandel, 1976) has been particularly fruitful. Other examples are reviewed by Krasne (1976).

C. Habituation

Sufficiently strong tactile stimulation of the crayfish abdomen leads to a tail flip and then escape. The escape response habituates in response to repeated

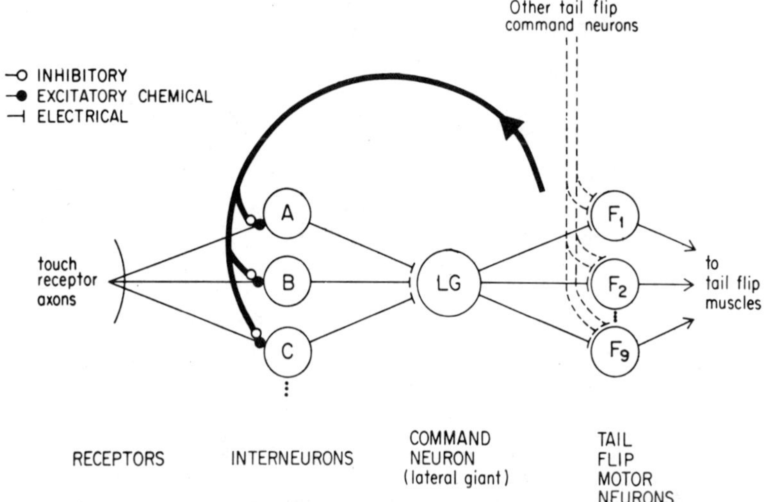

Figure 8 Basic neuronal circuit underlying behavioral habituation of the tail flip escape reflex in crayfish. Habituation occurs by synaptic depression between sensory neurons (touch receptors) and interneurons (A, B, C, etc.). The pathway indicated by the bold line can protect the labile synapses from depression by presynaptically inhibiting the terminals of the touch receptor axons. Dashed lines represent other input by which tail flip motor neurons can be activated. (From Krasne, 1978.)

tactile stimulation. The essential elements of the neuronal circuit for this reflex have been mapped and are shown diagrammatically in Figure 8. Sensory neurons make excitatory connections to interneurons. These interneurons excite command neurons (LG) that in turn excite the motor neurons. During behavioral habituation the synapses between the sensory neurons and the interneurons undergo depression, i.e., the synaptic potential decreases with repeated stimuli. Other synapses between sensory neurons and motor neurons seem unperturbed (Zucker, 1972b).

Tactile stimulation of the siphon of *Aplysia* with a jet of water results in the withdrawal of the gill. After a few seconds the gill gradually relaxes. With repeated tactile stimulation the response decreases and finally vanishes. With daily training sessions (4 sessions with 10 trials each) habituation develops more rapidly and on subsequent days even the first presentation of the stimulus elicits a weaker response. After 5 days of training evidence of retention can be observed for as long as 26 days.

The neuronal pathways underlying this reflex have been studied in detail (Kandel, 1976). The elementary circuit is a monosynaptic pathway subserved by

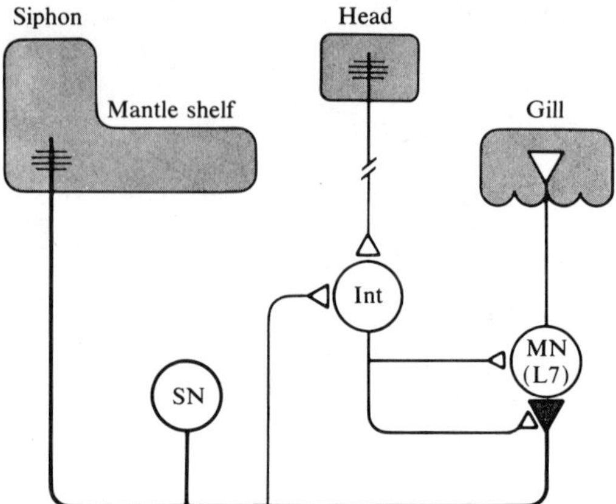

Figure 9 Simplified schematic representation of the neuronal circuit underlying short-term behavioral habituation of the gill withdrawal reflex in *Aplysia californica.* Only one sensory neuron (SN), interneuron (Int), and motor neuron (L7) is shown. Each cell represents a population of cells thought to be connected as shown here. The site of habituation is the synapse between the sensory neuron and the motor neuron. Repetitive activation of this path leads to a decrease in the amplitude of the synaptic potential in cell L7 (synaptic depression). Activation of the interneurons by strong stimulation of the neck or head region results in dishabituation, i.e., heterosynaptic facilitation of the sensory neuron-motor neuron path. (From Kandel et al., 1975; see also Kandel, 1976.)

a number of parallel sensory and motor neurons. During behavioral habituation, the synapses between the sensory neurons and the motor neurons exhibit depression. Synaptic depression has been analyzed especially carefully in motor neuron L7 (see Fig. 9).

In both of these well-studied cases of habituation in crayfish and *Aplysia* the plastic change has proved to be depression of the synapse between the sensory neuron and its follower cell. Further analysis has indicated in both cases that synaptic depression is based upon a gradual reduction in transmitter release (Zucker, 1972a; Kandel, 1976).

Behavioral habituation does not always depend on changes at just one group of synapses. The escape reflex of cockroach evoked by air puffs to the anal antennas is disynaptic (Zilber-Gachelin and Chartier, 1973a,b). The neuronal circuit underlying habituation in this case involves connections from sensory neurons to interneurons and then to motor neurons. Both groups of synapses are labile and undergo depression upon repeated stimulation.

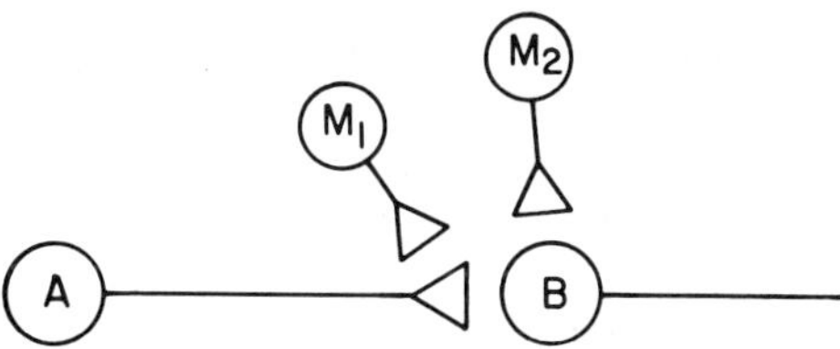

Figure 10 Hypothetical synaptic interaction between two neurons A and B with heterosynaptic modulators M_1 (acting presynaptically) and M_2 (acting postsynaptically). This scheme illustrates possible ways by which modulation could occur for synaptic plasticities that develop in the path AB. Modulation could also occur from a distance by hormonal action.

D. Extrinsic Control of Plasticities

In addition to these examples of plasticity, which occur along the altered pathways, synaptic efficacy can also be modulated heterosynaptically by changes that occur outside the altered pathway (Kandel, 1976; Krasne, 1978). Figure 10 schematically represents two hypothetical neurons, A and B, connected by a synapse. A third neuron, M, acts as a modulator, either presynaptically (M_1) by affecting transmitter release from cell A or postsynaptically (M_2) by affecting the receptor sensitivity or membrane properties of cell B. The efficacy of transmission between neurons A and B can be decreased (heterosynaptic inhibition) (e.g., Tauc, 1965; Kennedy et al., 1974) or increased (heterosynaptic facilitation) (Kandel and Tauc, 1964) by the modulator, M_1 or M_2. Such mechanisms can be used to regulate or alter behavioral plasticity.

For example, the habituation of both crayfish tail flip reflex and *Aplysia* gill withdrawal can be modulated. Crayfish can prevent maladaptive habituation of the escape reflex that would ordinarily result from tactile stimulation received during normal swimming. The labile synapses in the escape reflex pathways are protected from habituation during normal swimming by presynaptic inhibition (Krasne and Bryan, 1973), which decreases transmitter release from the sensory neurons and thereby prevents transmitter depletion (Fig. 8).

Another example is dishabituation, a mechanism by which behavioral habituation is invalidated by a novel stimulus. In the gill withdrawal reflex of *Aplysia*, the habituated response can be dishabituated by a strong stimulus to the neck region (Kandel, 1976). Cellular analysis has revealed that the labile synapses between the sensory neurons and the motor neurons receive a heterosynaptic facilitatory input that can increase transmitter release from the sensory neurons and thus restore the response (Fig. 9). Heterosynaptic inputs can also decrease the duration of posttetanic potentiation and thus influence the memory of a synapse for past events (Woodson et al., 1976). Whereas this form of modulation has not yet been linked to behavior, it provides another interesting way to modulate synaptic plasticity. Taken together, these examples illustrate the capability of the nervous system to control the development and expression of plasticity.

From this discussion of short-term plasticities, a number of general principles emerge: (1) plasticities can emerge as subtle alterations in already existing synaptic pathways; (2) in the case of the gill withdrawal response, for example, plasticity occurs in the same pathways that are hard-wired for the performance of the response; (3) at the synaptic level, there exist control systems that can regulate synaptic plasticities. Thus most disruptions of neuronal activity that would affect the plasticity itself would of necessity affect the hard-wired response (e.g., gill withdrawal). Disruptions of neural activity that disrupt only the control systems could in principle affect only plasticity without affecting performance of the response under study. As the following sections will illustrate, these mechanisms apply as well to long-term memory in higher animals.

IV. MEMORY AND MEMORY DYSFUNCTION

A. Memory Storage Loci

In long-term mammalian memory it has never been possible to dissociate the location of memory storage from the location of those mental operations required to perform the task under study. For example, memory for the delayed alternation task in monkeys can be effectively destroyed by excising a small amount of cortical tissue along the depths and banks of the middle third of the sulcus principalis in the frontal lobe (Butters and Pandya, 1969). Yet it is not correct to conclude that memory for delayed alternation is stored in this region, since the excision also makes the animal unable to ever learn the task again. The defect cannot reflect a general memory impairment, since even monkeys with much larger lesions in the frontal lobes can learn and remember a variety of visual discriminations (Warren and Akert, 1964). It is possible that this region is involved both in performing the delayed response task and in storing memory for the results of this activity. In any case the brain regions that store memory for this task have not been clearly separated from brain regions required to perform the task.

In *Aplysia* memory for gill withdrawal habituation involves alterations in synaptic connectivity along the same pathways that are normally involved in performing the task. Perhaps this principle is preserved in vertebrates, so that memory involves synaptic alterations along neuronal pathways that ordinarily have a role in the behavior of the animal. By this view, there is no reason to believe in the existence of memory centers or memory neurons. The distribution of memory for new information may be as broad as the distribution of the neuronal machinery needed to perceive, think about, and act on this information.

B. Association of Memory Defects with Other Cognitive Defects

Given this working hypothesis about memory and brain function, one might expect that disorders of learning and memory would never occur in isolation but would always occur in the context of a general impairment affecting many functions, i.e., whenever dysfunction occurs in a neural network, one might expect that those behaviors normally subserved by the network would be impaired along with the capacity of the network to exhibit plasticity. This pattern of dysfunction is in fact commonly observed.

Learning and memory disorders that occur in psychiatric and neurological patients usually occur in the context of impaired cognitive abilities. For example, mental retardation affects a wide spectrum of mental functions, including memory. Profound mental retardation in children is associated with a marked reduction in dendritic spines on cortical neurons (Purpura, 1974). Similarly, normal aging involves a wide variety of neuronal changes including a gradual loss of cells, a loss of dendritic mass in cortical neurons (Sheibel and Sheibel, 1975), abnormal EEG (Obrist, 1972), and diminished capacity for certain types of neurophysiological plasticity (Landfield and Lynch, 1977). Aging is also associated with measurable loss in a variety of cognitive tasks, particularly those requiring speed (Jarvik et al., 1973). Although complaints about memory dysfunction may be particularly prominent in aged persons (Kahn et al., 1975), dysfunction of memory (Craik, 1977) occurs together with cognitive impairment.

C. Dissociation of Memory Defects from Other Defects

Having noted that defects of memory are commonly associated with other cognitive defects, we can next ask whether memory can ever be disturbed in isolation. It turns out that disorders of memory can occur in a relatively pure form in the absence of any discernible cognitive defects. Such disorders appear to reflect the loss of control systems needed for the establishment of enduring memory. Though not as common as the type considered above, these disorders have been studied extensively and have provided a great deal of information about the biology of memory. The following examples illustrate how amnesia can occur as a circumscribed defect. The first two examples are the noted cases H.M. and N.A. The third is the amnesic defect associated with Korsakoff's syndrome.

D. Case H. M.

In 1953, at the age of 27, H. M. sustained a radical bilateral excision of the medial temporal region for relief of intractable epilepsy. The regions excised during surgery included the anterior two-thirds of the hippocampus, the para-

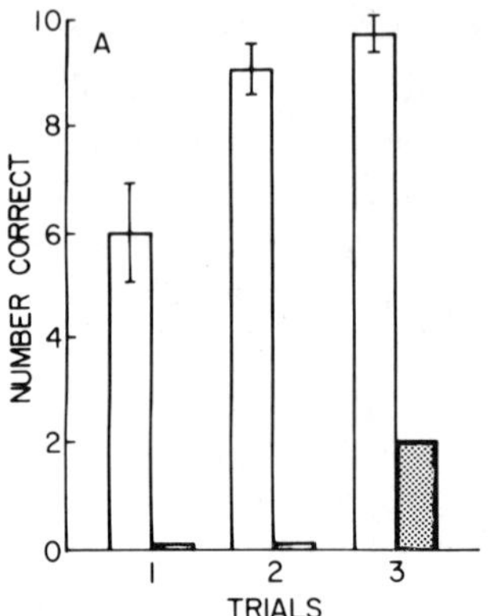

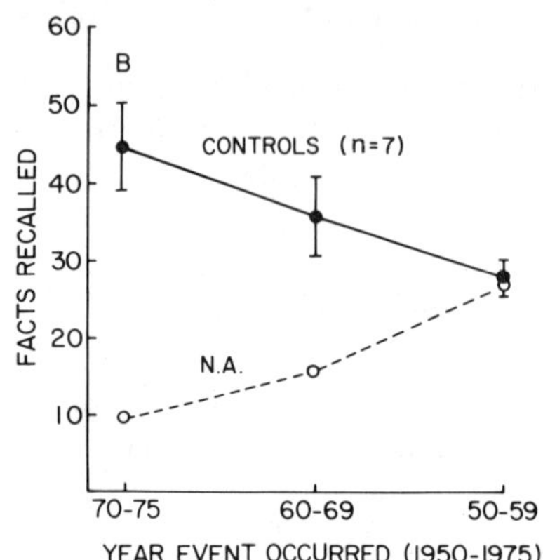

Figure 11 (A) Paired associate learning of ten noun pairs over three trials by the amnesic patient N.A. and seven control subjects. (B) Recall of details about public events that occurred 1950-1959, 1960-1969, and 1970-1975. N. A. became amnesic in 1960. (Reprinted with permission from Squire and Slater, 1978.)

hippocampal gyrus, uncus, and amygdala (Scoville and Milner, 1957). Following surgery, H. M. exhibited an above-average intellectual capacity and intact immediate memory. By contrast, he exhibited a marked impairment in the ability to learn new material that has continued to the present time (Milner, 1972). Extensive formal testing has confirmed that this patient has severely limited ability to acquire new information and that he has little knowledge of events that have occurred since his operation in 1953. However, his knowledge of events that occurred in the 1930s and in the 1940s appears normal (Marslen-Wilson and Teuber, 1976).

E. Case N. A.

In 1960, at the age of 22, N. A. sustained a stab wound to the diencephalic region just to the left of midline as the result of a fencing accident. Since his accident, N. A. has exhibited a marked amnesia, worse for verbal material than for nonverbal material. Yet N. A. recently scored 124 in IQ and surpassed control subjects in many perceptual and cognitive tests (Teuber et al., 1968; Squire and Slater, 1978). By contrast, his ability to acquire new information is severely limited and he has been unable to work since his accident. Formal testing indicates that his knowledge of events that have occurred since his accident is deficient, but his knowledge of events that occurred in the 1950s is quite good (Fig. 11) (Squire and Slater, 1978). Recent neurologic studies indicate that this individual sustained damage to the left dorsal thalamic region in an area corresponding to the position of the dorsal medial nucleus (Squire and Moore, 1979).

F. Korsakoff's Psychosis

Korsakoff's syndrome is a neurologic disease associated with chronic alcoholism and believed to be caused by thiamine deficiency. In its chronic form patients are amnesic and sometimes confabulatory, but they can perform normally on tests of general intelligence (Talland, 1965). The amnesia associated with Korsakoff's syndrome is not as pure as that observed in the two cases described above. Performance is affected on some cognitive tests, particularly those that seem to demand complex and rapid perceptual integration. As assessed by formal tests, these patients are able to achieve little new learning and may have little knowledge of events that have occurred during the last few years (Butters and Cermak, 1975).

Extensive documentation of the neuropathology of Korsakoff's disease has indicated that the mammillary bodies, the dorsal medial nucleus of the thalamus, and the terminal aspects of the fornix are the most affected structures. It is not yet entirely clear as to which structures are the most important. Based on a few cases with damage limited to the mammillary bodies who did not exhibit amnesia, it has been argued that damage to the dorsal medial thalamus may be critical for this syndrome (Victor et al., 1971). Yet cases have been reported with damage apparently limited to the mammillary bodies who did exhibit amnesia (Delay and Brion, 1969). Whatever the contribution of the mammillary bodies to diencephalic amnesia, the finding that the patient N. A. has damage in the dorsal thalamic region (Squire and Moore, 1979) indicates that damage in the dorsal thalamus is at least sufficient to cause amnesia.

The finding that memory for events that occurred prior to amnesia can be relatively unaffected compared to memory for events that happened since the onset of amnesia means that the hippocampus and the diencephalic midline are not the sites of memory storage. Rather, these regions appear to play a specific role in the formation of stable memories. Storage of memory must occur elsewhere. These regions appear to function as a control system that can regulate the establishment of plastic changes along other neuronal pathways in the nervous system.

It is well known that a variety of drugs can influence the formation of memory in animals when given shortly after training (Squire, 1981). Recent work has indicated that amines and hormones such as epinephrine, ACTH, and vasopressin may have a special role to play in the development of memory (Gold and McGaugh, 1978). It has been suggested that these substances influence memory by creating a brain state that is favorable for information storage. By this view, the consequences of training, and agents that can amplify these consequences, create a state that facilitates information storage (Gold and McGaugh, 1975; Kety, 1976). Perhaps the hippocampus and diencephalon are normally involved in mediating such nonspecific effects of an experience so that information storage can occur in cortical loci. It is interesting to speculate that these systems might have their phylogenetic roots in those control systems shown in invertebrates (Section II.D) to be capable of regulating synaptic plasticity.

V. MEMORY AND TIME

An additional characteristic of memory that provides clues about its biological basis is the fact that in amnesia recent events are lost more readily than remote events. The consolidation theory of memory, which developed out of this fundamental observation, states that memory is initially in a labile state and becomes progressively invulnerable to disruption with the passage of time (see McGaugh and Herz, 1972). It had traditionally been thought that consolidation was completed within a few minutes or hours after learning. Indeed, such a belief was consistent with the notion that some types of long-term plasticity could probably be established and would be able to replace short-term plasticities within a few minutes after learning. This notion was also consistent with the results of many studies in experimental animals showing that retrograde amnesia can occur when a disruptive agent is administered shortly after learning, but not when it is administered several hours after learning (McGaugh and Gold, 1976). It is now clear, however, that the gradient of retrograde amnesia can cover years rather than minutes or hours. It follows that the long-term memory storage system continues to change and becomes more resistant to disruption for years after learning occurs. These conclusions are based on a series of studies of patients receiving ECT for psychiatric illness.

ECT is known to cause anterograde and retrograde amnesia (Squire, 1977). Using remote memory tests designed to permit an equivalent sampling of past time periods (Squire and Slater, 1975), it has been possible to ask how far back in time the retrograde amnesia extends and across what time period differential resistance to amnesia can be demonstrated. Patients were asked questions about television programs that broadcast for only one season during the past several years. After ECT, patients exhibited amnesia for the names of programs broadcast 1-3 years previously, but no amnesia for programs braodcast 4-16 years previously (Fig. 12) (Squire et al., 1975; Squire and Cohen, 1979). These results indicated that resistance of long-term memory to disruption continues to develop for years after learning.

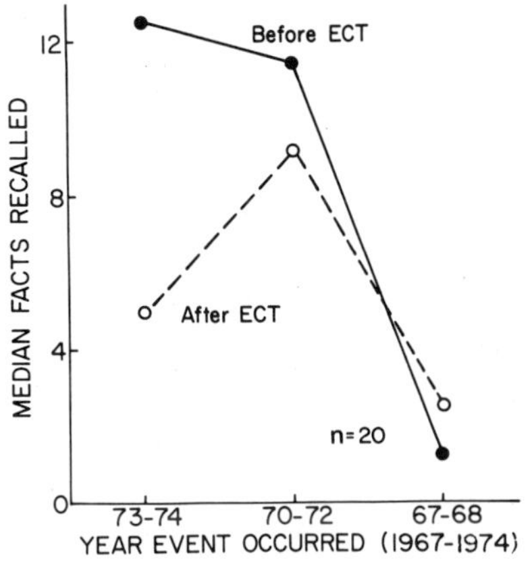

Figure 12 Number of facts recalled about former one-season television programs before and after electroconvulsive therapy (ECT). After five bilateral treatments there was a selective impairment in the ability to recall information about programs broadcase 1-2 years previously. Information acquired prior to that time was poorly remembered before ECT but was resistant to the amnesic effects of ECT. Resistance to disruption appears to develop for years after initial learning. (From Squire and Cohen, 1979.)

The interesting aspect of these gradual changes is that resistance develops while forgetting is occurring. As discussed previously, models of memory based on two neurons and one synapse cannot easily account for the gradual development of both forgetting and resistance (Squire, 1976). However, these phenomena are easily accounted for by a network of connections in which some elements are lost while those that remain get stronger. By this view the development of normal human memory over time bears formal similarities to many of the plasticities that have been proposed as candidates for long-term memory mechanisms. In the case of collateral sprouting (Section II.E), the removal of inputs on a target cell leads to an increase in the influence of remaining inputs. In the case of the visual system (Section II.F), the influence of an experienced eye on a cortical cell increases following the diminution of input via the other eye. In the case of development (Section II.G), when inputs are lost remaining ones can increase their potential influence on the postsynaptic cell. Thus, many of the putative mechanisms for long-term memory that have been studied in detail exhibit some type of competition and have the capability of responding to a loss of connections with an increase in the efficacy of remaining connections. In the case of human long-term memory, it is interesting to suppose that a similar mechanism might operate, and that forgetting and resistance might ultimately depend on competition (loss of effective connections and a compensatory gain in remaining connections) similar to what has been described in simpler experimental systems (see Fig. 13).

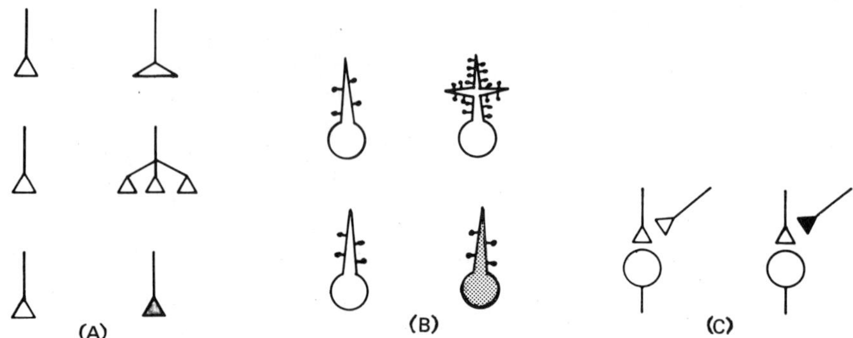

Figure 13 Summary of potential substrates of memory. (A) Alterations of synaptic terminals: top, larger (or smaller) synaptic contact area (Section II.D); middle, synaptic sprouting (or pruning) (Sections II.E, II.F); bottom, biochemical alterations (e.g. changes in transmitter synthesis or membrane properties) (Sections II.A, II.B, II.C). (B) Alterations of postsynaptic elements: top, changes in dendritic structure, branching spike number and/or spine geometry. (Sections II.D, II.G); bottom, biochemical alterations (e.g. receptor sensitivity, membrance properties, transsynaptic enzyme induction) (Sections II.A-II.C). (C) Alterations in modulatory inputs, changes in heterosynaptic inputs (could be based on any of the above alterations).

VI. SUMMARY

Neurons possess intrinsically plastic properties that can serve as a basis for short-term information storage. In invertebrates, where this capacity has been best studied, plasticities like low-frequency depression and heterosynaptic facilitation are involved in information storage and have a lifetime of minutes or hours. Invertebrates also possess control systems that can control the development and expression of these plasticities. In mammals, a variety of longlasting plasticities have been demonstrated that could conceivably serve as a basis for long-term information storage. Such storage may be initiated by protein synthesis and mediated by cAMP, and then result in morphological changes at synapses. A variety of such morphological changes have been demonstrated including changes in dendritic branching, number of dendritic spines, and synaptic contact size—but none of these has yet been clearly linked to behavioral memory.

As time passes after learning, long-term memory develops in such a way that resistance develops while forgetting occurs. With the passage of time, it is hypothesized that there is a reorganization of synaptic connections wherein the loss of one group of inputs is associated with an increase in the synaptic efficacies of others. There is precedent for such a program of reorganization in the phenomenon of collateral sprouting, in the effects of monocular deprivation in kittens, and in development. It seems possible that this sequence of reorganization may be pervasive in the nervous system. This sequence could be used during normal development to form genetically specified networks and then be continued into adulthood to permit these networks to remember and to forget.

Disorders of memory occur in two forms. Disruption of neuronal networks that are intrinsically plastic cause defects in memory along with other cognitive defects or cause defects in memory along with a more general loss of the ability to perform specific kinds of tasks. Disruption of neuronal networks that control plasticities cause defects in the ability to form new memories without causing defects in the ability to recall memories formed prior to the time of disruption.

ACKNOWLEDGMENT

This work was supported by the Medical Research Service of the Veterans Administration and by grants from the National Institute of Mental Health and the National Institutes of Health.

REFERENCES

Bennett, E. L. (1976). Cerebral effects of differential experience and training. In *Neural Mechanisms of Learning and Memory,* M. R. Rosenzweig and E. L. Bennett (Eds.). MIT Press, Cambridge, Mass., pp. 279-287.

Blakemore, C. (1972). Developmental factors in the formation of feature extracting mental neurons. In *The Neurosciences,* F. O. Schmitt and F. G. Worden (Eds.). Third study Program, MIT Press, Cambridge, Mass., pp. 105-113.

Bliss, T. V. P., and Lϕmo, T. (1973). Long-lasting potentiation of synaptic transmission in the dentate area of the anesthetized rabbit following stimulation of the perforant path. *J. Physiol. (London) 232,* 331-356.

Brown, M. C., Jansen, J. K. S., and Van Essen, D. (1976). Polyneuronal innervation of skeletal muscle in new-born rats and its elimination during maturation. *J. Physiol. 261,* 387-422.

Butters, N., and Cermak, L. S. (1975). Some analyses of amnesic syndromes in brain-damaged patients. In *The Hippocampus,* Vol. 2, R. L. Isaacson and K. Pribram (Eds.). Plenum, New York, pp. 377-409.

Butters, N., and Pandya, D. (1969). Retention of delayed-alteration: Effect of selective lesions of sulcus principalis. *Science 165,* 1271-1273.

Chung, S. H., Raymond, S. A., and Lettvin, J. Y. (1970). Multiple meaning in single visual units. *Brain Behav. Evol. 3,* 72-101.

Costa, E., Guidotti, A., and Hanbauer, I. (1974). Do cyclic nucleotides promote the trans-synaptic induction of tyrosine hydroxylase? *Life Sci. 14,* 1169-1188.

Cragg, B. G. (1975a). The development of synapses in kitten visual cortex during visual deprivation. *Exp. Neurol. 46,* 445-451.

Cragg, B. G. (1975b). The development of synapses in the visual system of the cat. *J. Comp. Neurol. 160,* 147-166.

Craik, F. I. (1977). Age differences in human memory. In: *Handbook of Psychology of Aging,* J. E. Birren and K. W. Schaie (Eds.). Van Nostrand, New York, pp. 384-420.

Delay, J. L. and Brion, S. (1969). *Le Syndrome de Korsakoff.* Masson, Paris.

Diamond, M. C., Lindner, B., Johnson, R., Bennett, E. L., and Rosenzweig, M. R. (1975). Differences in occipital cortical synapses from environmentally enriched, impoverished, and standard colony rats. *Int. J. Neurosci. 1,* 109-119.

Diamond, J., Cooper, E., Turner, C., and MacIntyre, L. (1976). Trophic regulation of nerve sprouting. *Science 193,* 371-377.

Dunn, A. J., Gray, H. E., and Iuvone, P. M. (1976). Protein synthesis and amnesia. Studies with emetine and pactamycin. *Pharmacol. Biochem. Behav. 6,* 1-4.

Gold, P. E., and McGaugh, J. L. (1975). A single-trace, two-process view of memory storage processes. In *Short-Term Memory,* J. A. Deutsch and D. Deutsch (Eds.). Academic, New York, pp. 356-378.

Gold, P. E., and McGaugh, J. L. (1978). Neurobiology and memory. Modulators, correlates and assumptions. In *Brain and Learning,* T. Teyler (Ed.). Greylock, New York, pp. 93-103.

Hubbard, J. I. (1963). Repetitive stimulation at the mammalian neuromuscular junction and the mobilization of transmitter. *J. Physiol. (London) 169,* 641-662.

Hubel, D. H., and Wiesel, T. N. (1970). The period of susceptibility to the physiological effects of unilateral eye closure in kittens. *J. Physiol. 906,* 416-436.

Hubel, D. H., Wiesel, T. N., and LeVay, S. (1976). Functional architecture of area 17 in normal and monocularly deprived Macacue monkey. In *Cold Spring Harbor Symposium Quantitative Biology 40,* 581-589.

Jarvik, L. F., Eisdorfer, E., and Blum, J. E. (1973). *Intellectual Functioning in Adults.* Springer, New York.

Kahn, R. L., Zarit, S. H., Hilbert, N. M., and Niedereke, G. (1975). Memory complaint and impairment in the aged. *Arch. Gen. Psychiatr. 32,* 1569-1573.

Kandel, E. R. (1976). *Cellular Basis of Behavior.* Freeman, New York.

Kandel, E. R., and Tauc, L. (1964). Mechanism of prolonged heterosynaptic facilitation. *Nature (London) 202,* 145-147.

Kandel, E. R., Brunell, M., Byrne, J., and Castellucci, V. (1975). A common presynaptic locus for the synaptic changes underlying short-term habituation and sensitization of the gill withdrawal reflex in Aplysia. Cold Spring Harbor Laboratory Symposium on Quantitative Biology XL: The Synapse, Cold Spring Harbor, N.Y., pp. 465-482.

Kennedy, D., Calabrese, R. L., and Wine, J. J. (1974). Presynaptic inhibition. Primary afferent depolarization in crayfish neurons. *Science 186,* 451-454.

Kety, S. S. (1976). The biogenic amines in the central nervous system. Their possible roles in arousal, emotion and learning. In *The Neurosciences,* F. O. Schmitt (Ed.). Second Study Program. Rockefeller University Press, New York, pp. 324-335.

Klein, D. C. (1974). Circadian rhythms in indole metabolism in the rat pineal gland. In *The Neurosciences,* F. O. Schmitt and F. G. Worden (Eds.). Third Study Program. MIT Press, Cambridge, Mass., pp. 509-515.

Krasne, F. B. (1976). Invertebrate systems as a means of gaining insight into the nature of learning and memory. In *Neural Mechanisms of Learning and Memory,* M. R. Rosenzweig and E. L. Bennett (Eds.). MIT Press, Cambridge, Mass., pp. 401-429.

Krasne, F. B. (1978). Extrinsic control of intrinsic neuronal plasticity. An hypothesis from work on simple systems. *Brain Res. 14,* 197-216.

Krasne, F. B., and Bryan, J. S. (1973). Habituation: Regulation through presynaptic inhibition. *Science 182,* 590-592.

Landfield, P. W., and Lynch, G. (1977). Impaired monosynaptic potentiation in in vitro hippocampal slices from aged, memory-deficient rats. *J. Gerontol. 32,* No. 5, 523-533.

Langan, T. A. (1973). Protein kinases and protein kinase substrates. In *Advances in Cyclic Nucleotide Research,* Vol. 3, P. Greengard and G. A. Robison (Eds.). Raven, New York, pp. 99-153.

Lichtman, J. W. (1977). Reorganization of synaptic connections in the rat submandibular ganglion during postnatal development. *Physiology 273,* 155-177.

Lynch, G., and Cotman, C. W. (1975). The hippocampus as a model for studying anatomical plasticity in the adult brain. In *The Hippocampus,* Vol. 1, R. L. Isaacson and K. Pribram (Eds.). Plenum, New York, pp. 128-154.

Lynch, G., and Wells, J. (1978). Neural anatomical plasticity and behavioral adaptability. In *Brain and Learning,* T. Teyler (Ed.). Greylock, New York, pp. 105-124.

Lynch, G., Gall, C., and Cotman, C. W. (1977). Temporal parameters of axon sprouting in the adult brain. *Exp. Neurol. 54,* 179-183.

Magleby, K. L., and Zengel, J. E. (1975). A quantitative description of tetanic and post-tetanic potentiation of transmitter release at the frog neuromuscular function. *J. Physiol. (London) 245,* 183-208.

Marslen-Wilson, W. D., and Teuber, H-L. (1975). Memory for remote events in anterograde amnesia. Recognition of public figures from newsphotographs. *Neuropsychologia 13,* 355-364.

McGaugh, J. L., and Gold, P. E. (1976). Modulation of memory by electrical stimulation of the brain. In *Neural Mechanisms of Learning and Memory,* M. R. Rosenzweig and E. L. Bennett, (Eds.). MIT Press, London, pp. 549-560.

McGaugh, J. L., and Herz, M. J. (1972). *Memory Consolidation.* Albion, San Francisco.

Milner, B. (1972). Disorders of learning and memory after temporal lobe lesions in man. *Clin. Neurosurg. 19,* 421-446.

Moore, R. Y. (1976). Synaptogenesis and the morphology of learning and memory. In *Neural Mechanisms of Learning and Memory,* M. R. Rosenzweig and E. L. Bennett (Eds.). MIT Press, London, pp. 340-347.

Müller, G. E., and Pilzecher, A. (1900). Experimentelle Beitrage zur Lehre Von Gedachetniss. *Z. Psychol. 1,* 1-288.

Nathanson, J. A. (1977). Cyclic nucleotides and nervous system function. *Physiol. Rev. 57,* 157-256.

Obrist, W. D. (1972). Problems of aging. In *Handbook of Electroencephalography and Clinical Neurophysiology,* A. Remond (Ed.). Vol. 6, Elsevier, Amsterdam, pp. 275-292.

Oesch, F., Otten, U., Mueller, R. A., Goodman, R., and Thoenen, H. (1975). Transsynaptic regulation of enzyme synthesis. In *Golgi Centennial Symposium,* M. Santini (Ed.). Raven, New York, pp. 503-513.

Purpura, D. P. (1974). Dendritic spine "dysgenesis" and mental retardation. *Science 186,* 1126-1128.

Raymond, S. A., and Lettvin, J. Y. (1978). After effects of activity in peripheral axons as a clue to nervous coding. In *Physiology and Pathobiology,* S. G. Waxman (Ed.). Raven, New York, pp. 203-225.

Ronnevi, L. O., and Conradi, S. (1974). Ultrastructural evidence for spontaneous elimination of synaptic terminals on spinal motoneurons in the kitten. *Brain Res. 80,* 335-339.

Rose, S. P. R., Hambley, J., and Haywood, J. (1976). Neurochemical approaches to developmental plasticity and learning. In *Neural Mechanisms of Learning and Memory,* M. R. Rosenzweig and E. L. Bennett (Eds.). MIT Press, London, pp. 293-307.

Rosenthal, J. (1969). Post-tetanic potentiation at the neuromuscular junction the frog. *J. Physiol. (London) 203,* 121-133.

Rosenzweig, M. R., Bennett, E. L., and Diamond, M. C. (1972). Clinical and anatomical plasticity of brain. Replications and extentions. In *Macromolecules and Behavior, 2nd Ed.,* J. Gaito (Ed.). Appleton-Century-Crofts, New York, pp. 205-207.

Ruiz-Marcos, A., and Valverde, R. (1969). The temporal evolution of dendritic spines in the visual cortex of normal and dark raised mice. *Exp. Brain Res. 8,* 284-294.

Schlapfer, W. T., Tremblay, J. P., Woodson, P. B. J., and Barondes, S. H. (1976). Frequency facilitation and post-tetanic potentiation of a unitary synaptic potential in *Aplysia californica* are limited by different processes. *Brain Res. 109,* 1-20.

Schneider, G. E. (1973). Early lesions of the superior colliculus. Factors affecting the formation of abnormal retinal connections. *Brain Behav. Evol. 8,* 73-109.

Schneider, G. E. (1979). Is it really better to have your brain lesion early? A revision of the "Kennard principle." *Neuropsychologia 17,* 557-583.

Scoville, W. B., and Milner, B. (1957). Loss of recent memory after bilateral hippocampal lesions. *J. Neurol. Neurosurg. Psychiatr. 20,* 11-21.

Shashoua, V. E. (1976a). Brain metabolism and the acquisition of new behaviors. I. Evidence for specific changes in the pattern of protein synthesis. *Brain Res. 111,* 347-364.

Shashoua, V. E. (1976b). Identification of specific changes in the pattern of brain protein synthesis after training. *Science 193,* 1264-1266.

Shashoua, V. E. (1977a). Brain protein metabolism and the acquisition of new patterns of behavior. *Proc. Nat. Acad. Sci. USA 74,* No. 4, 1743-1747.

Shashoua, V. E. (1977b). Brain protein metabolism and the acquisition of new behaviors. II. Immunological studies of the α, β, γ proteins of goldfish brain. *Brain Res. 122,* 113-124.

Shashoua, V. E. (1978). The goldfish as a model experimental animal for studies of biochemical correlates of the information storage process. In *Model Systems in Biological Psychiatry,* D. J. Ingle and H. M. Shein (Eds.). MIT Press, London, pp. 166-189.

Sheibel, M. E., and Sheibel, A. B. (1975). Structural changes in the aging brain. In *Aging,* Vol. 1, *Chemical Morphologic and Neurochemical Aspects in the Aging Central Nervous System,* H. Brody and J. M. Ordy (Eds.). Raven, New York, pp. 11-37.

So, K-F, Schneider, G. E., and Frost, D. O. (1978). Postnatal development of retinal projections to the lateral geniculate body in Syrian hamsters. *Brain Res. 142,* 343-352.

Spanis, C. W., and Squire, L. R. (1978). Elevation of brain tyrosine by inhibitors of protein synthesis is not responsible for their amnesic effects. *Brain Res. 139,* 384-388.

Squire, L. R. (1976). Amnesia and the biology of memory. In *Current Developments in Psychopharmacology,* Vol. 3, W. B. Essman and L. Valzelli (Eds.). Spectrum, New York, pp. 258-282.

Squire, L. R. (1977). Electroconvulsive therapy and memory loss. *Am. J. Psychiatr. 134,* 997-1001.

Squire, L. R. (1981). The pharmacology of memory: a neurobiological perspective. *Ann. Rev. Pharm. Toxicol. 21,* in press.

Squire, L. R., and Barondes, S. H. (1972). Variable decay of memory and its recovery in cycloheximide-treated mice. *Nat. Acad. Sci. USA 69,* 1416-1420.

Squire, L. R., and Barondes, S. H. (1973). Memory impairment during prolonged training in mice given inhibitors of cerebral protein synthesis. *Brain Res. 56,* 214-225.

Squire, L. R., and Barondes, S. H. (1974). Anisomycin, like other inhibitors of cerebral protein synthesis, impairs "long-term" memory of a discrimination task. *Brain Res. 66,* 301-308.

Squire, L. R., and Cohen, N. (1979). Memory and amnesia. Resistance to disruption develops for years after learning. *Behav. Neural Biol. 25,* 115-125.

Squire, L. R., and Moore, R. (1979). Dorsal thalamic lesion in a noted case of chronic memory dysfunction. *Ann. Neurol. 6,* 503-506.

Squire, L. R., and Slater, P. C. (1975). Forgetting in very long-term memory as assessed by an improved questionnaire technique. *J. Exp. Psychol. Human Learning and Memory 104,* 50-54.

Squire, L. R., and Slater, P. C. (1978). Anterograde and retrograde memory impairment in chronic amnesia. *Neuropsychologia 16,* 313-322.

Squire, L. R., Slater, P. C., and Chace, P. M. (1975). Retrograde amnesia. Temporal gradient in very long-term memory following electroconvulsive therapy. *Science 187,* 77-79.

Talland, G. A. (1965). *Deranged Memory.* Academic Press, New York.

Tauc, L. (1965). Presynaptic inhibition in the abdominal ganglion of *Aplysia. J. Physiol. (London) 181,* 282-307.

Teuber, H. -L., Milner, B., and Vaughn, H. G. (1968). Persistent anterograde amnesia after stab wound of the basal brain. *Neuropsychologia 6,* 267-282.

Victor, M., Adams, R. D., and Collins, G. H. (1971). *The Wernicke-Korsakoff Syndrome.* Davis, Philadelphia.

Volkmar, F. R., and Greenough, W. T. (1972). Rearing complexity affects branching of dendrites in the visual cortex of the rat. *Science 176,* 1445-1447.

Warren, J. M., and Akert, L. (1964). *The Frontal Granular Cortex and Behavior.* McGraw-Hill, New York.

West, R. W., and Greenough, W. T. (1972). Effects of environmental complexity on cortical synapses of rats. Preliminary results. *Behavior. Biol. 7,* 279-284.

Wiesel, T. N., and Hubel, D. H. (1963). Single cell responses in striate cortex of kittens deprived of vision in one eye. *J. Neurophysiol. 26,* 1003-1017.

Wiesel, T. N., and Hubel, D. H. (1965). Extent of recovery from the effects of visual deprivation in kittens. *J. Neurophysiol. 29,* 1029-1040.

Woodson, P. B. J., Tremblay, J. P., Schlapfer, W. T., and Barondes, S. H. (1976). Heterosynaptic inhibition modifies the presynaptic plasticities of the transmission process at a synapse in Aplysia californica. *Brain Res. 109,* 83-95.

Woollacott, M., and Hoyle, G. (1977). Neural events underlying learning in insects. Changes in pacemaker. *Proc. Res. Soc. (London) 195,* 395-415.

Zilber-Gachelin, N. F., and Chartier, M. P. (1973a). Modification of the motor reflex responses due to repetition of the peripheral stimulus in the cockroach. I. Habituation at the level of an isolated abdominal ganglion. *J. Exp. Biol. 59,* 359-381.

Zilber-Gachelin, N. F., and Chartier, M. P. (1973b). Modification of the motor reflex responses due to repetition of the peripheral stimulus in the cockroach. II. Conditions of activation of the motoneurons. *J. Exp. Biol. 59,* 383-403.

Zucker, R. S. (1972a). Crayfish escape behavior and central synapses. I. Neural circuit exciting lateral giant fiber. *J. Neurophysiol. 35,* 599-620.

Zucker, R. S. (1972b). Crayfish escape behavior and central synapses. II. Physiological mechanisms underlying behavioral habituation. *J. Neurophysiol. 35,* 621-637.

9

Biochemical Aspects of Neurotic Behavior

John R. Smythies
University of Alabama in Birmingham
Birmingham, Alabama

I. INTRODUCTION

In this review I interpret the term "neurotic behavior" to cover mainly aspects of anxiety, stress reactions, and flight/fight responses; other aspects of neurosis (i.e., depressive neurosis) are covered elsewhere in this volume. Besides, very little is known about any possible biochemical basis of other neurotic conditions such as obsessive-compulsive neurosis. The rapidly developing state of our knowledge concerning the biochemical basis of emotional reactions involves both certain gross anatomical areas of the brain (e.g., the amygdala, septum, hippocampus, hypothalamus) and particular biochemical systems (including GABA, glycine, serotonin, enkephalin, and somatostatin).

The neuroanatomical basis of anxiety is related to a hierarchically ordered system of complex limbic system circuits. These include areas of limbic cortex, the amygdala, the hippocampus and septal nuclei, parts of the hypothalamus, and the hypothalamopituitary-adrenal axis. This is organized generally into a stress-mediating system in which the nuclei of the amygdala are particularly important and a stress-reducing system in which the hippocampus and septum play a major role. We do not know how the higher reaches of this system are

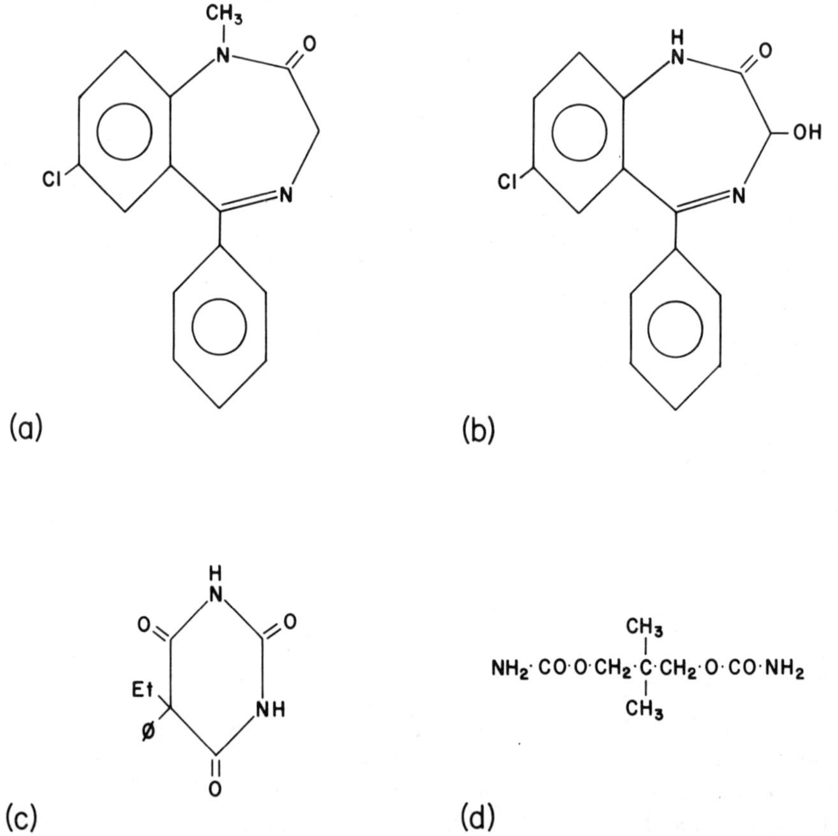

(a)

(b)

(c)

(d)

$NH_2 \cdot CO \cdot O \cdot CH_2 \cdot C(CH_3)_2 \cdot CH_2 \cdot O \cdot CO \cdot NH_2$

Figure 1 Formulas of some anxiolytics: (a) diazepam, (b) oxazepam, (c) phenobarbitone and (d) meprobamate.

biochemically organized, but evidence is being obtained as to the important influence of hypothalamic and pituitary hormone peptides directly on the brain itself via some form of collateral, or CSF, or blood form carrier systems. These pathways set in motion, via a direct action on the brain, behavioral patterns complementary to the peripheral effect of these hormones on their traditional target organs, (thyroid, adrenal, ovary, etc.). The development of our knowledge in this area forms one of the most promising and exciting areas of neuroscience.

Another area of advance is provided by studies of the mode of action of drugs that alleviate neurotic behavior, such as the benzodiazepines (Fig. 1a, b). This remarkable family of drugs has a wide spectrum of activities–antianxiety, anticonvulsant, muscle relaxant–and a vast amount of research has been carried out on their mechanism of action in these areas. Theories involving their action on serotonin systems (Stein et al., 1975), glycine (Young et al., 1974), GABA (Costa et al., 1976), somatostatin (Brown et al., 1977), catecholamines (Fuxe et al., 1975), and acetylcholine (Ladinsky et al., 1973) have been put forward.

The significance of biological research in neurosis is that modern biological psychiatry supports the concept that all aspects of behavior, both normal and abnormal, neuroses as well as psychoses, have biological aspects to their genesis and development. Most psychiatrists are familiar with the major role that biological factors, such as alterations in brain amine levels, play in the major psychoses, parkinsonism, etc., but their view of neuroses has tended to be dominated by psychodynamic concepts on the one hand and by learning theory on the other. Yet operational factors in neuroses of great importance include many limbic system functions as detailed in this chapter.

II. POSSIBLE MECHANISMS OF ACTION OF THE BENZODIAZEPINES

A. The GABA System

GABA (Fig. 2a) has two main types of action in the brain: (1) presynaptic inhibition and (2) postsynaptic inhibition. In (1) it depolarizes axon terminals and so prevents the release of their transmitters; in (2) it hyperpolarizes the membrane of the postsynaptic cell and so tends to inhibit its firing. The former mechanism is thought to be involved in the muscle relaxant properties of the benzodiazepines (Fig. 1a, b) and the latter, via an action on the cerebellum, in their production of ataxia. The exact mode of interaction between benzodiazepines and central anxiety mechanisms is not known. However, picrotoxin (an anti-GABA compound) (Fig. 2d) antagonizes the effect of benzodiazepines on conditioned emotional behavior in rats (Stein et al., 1973).

Costa and his co-workers (Costa et al., 1975) have conducted some experiments to quantify the anticonvulsant actions of a number of drugs including the benzodiazepines against a number of convulsant drugs of known site of action.

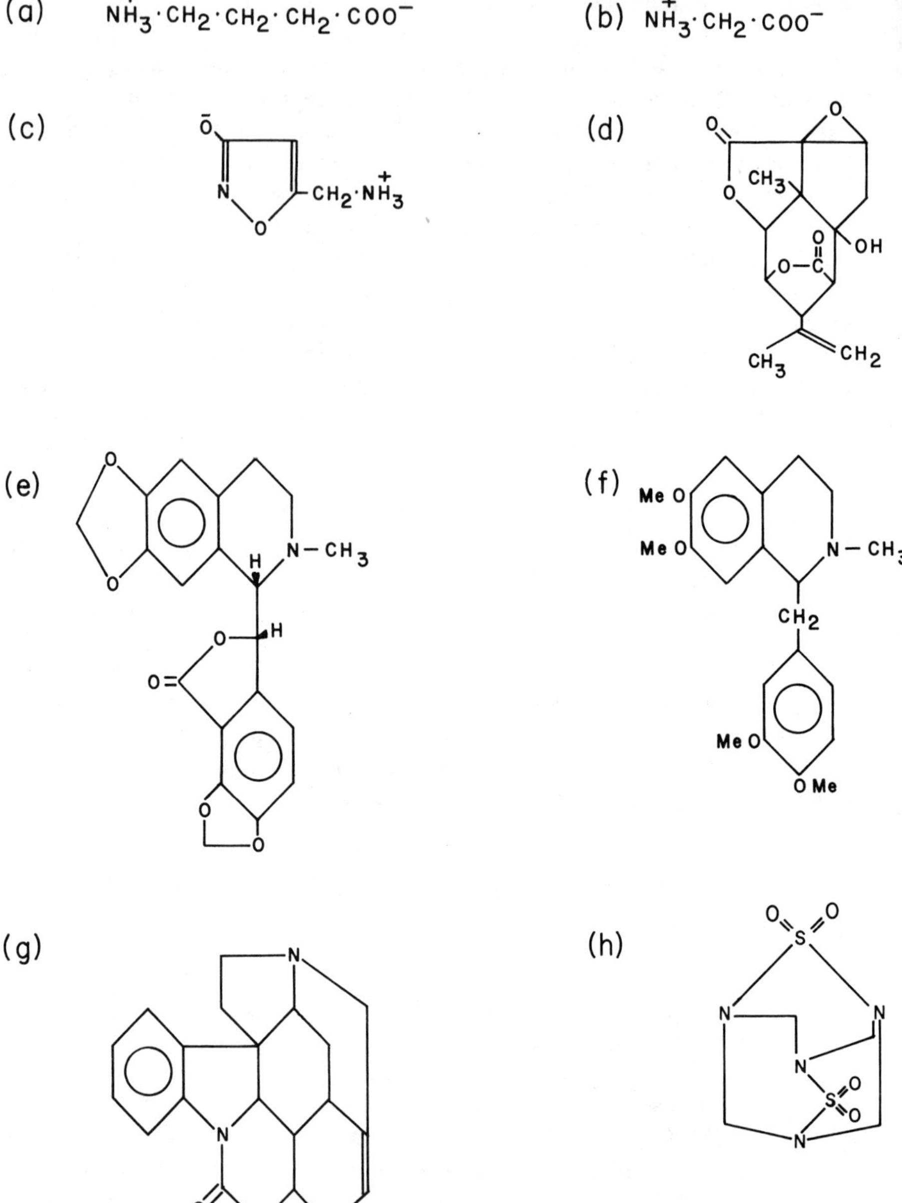

Figure 2 Some GABA- and glycine-active drugs: (a) GABA, (b) glycine, (c) muscimol (GABA agonist), (d) picrotoxinin (GABA antagonist), (e) bicuculline (GABA antagonist), (f) dendrobine (glycine antagonist), (g) strychnine (glycine antagonist), and (h) TETS (mixed GABA/glycine antagonist).

Benzodiazepines are much more effective against convulsions induced by isoniazid, thiosemicarbazide, and 3-mercaptropropionic acid (which act by a reduction in the synthesis of GABA), and by bicuculline (an anti-GABA compound) than they are against convulsions induced by strychnine (Fig. 2g), an antiglycine compound (Haefely et al., 1975). Since diazepam (Fig. 1a) does not prevent the reduction in brain GABA induced by isoniazid, one can assume that its anticonvulsant effect is due to some augmentation of existing GABA.

In the bullfrog sympathetic ganglia diazepam inhibits the post-tetanic potentiation (PTP) of fast excitatory postsynaptic potentials without changing the amplitude of a single shock-induced potential; since the former, but not the latter, is determined by presynaptic events, one may suppose that this action of diazepam is in the presynaptic area (Suria and Costa, 1973). GABA and diazepam depolarize preganglionic axon terminals. On the other hand picrotoxin failed to change the polarization of these terminals by itself, but antagonized the depolarizations produced by GABA and diazepam. However, isoniazid and thiosemicarbazide antagonized the depolarization induced by diazepam but not by GABA. This suggests that this presynaptic depolarziation induced by diazepam depends on de novo GABA synthesis.

In the cerebellum various stimuli lead to an increase of cyclic GMP (cGMP). This increase is inhibited by GABA, but not glycine or glutamate, injected intraventricularly, and it is increased by GABA-blocking agents. Diazepam (but not dilantin) is a very potent lowerer of cerebellar cGMP levels.

Another GABA system in the brain is the recurrent strionigral pathway that is inhibitory of the dopamine (DA) cells of the substantia nigra. Various tests indicate that benzodiazepines reduce the turnover rate of striatal dopamine by facilitating this recurrent strionigral pathway.

However, whereas these anatomical systems may be related to the anticonvulsant, muscle relaxant, and ataxia-producing components of benzodiazepine action, it is not clear whether this also applies to their antianxiety action.

It is important to distinguish between sedation and relieving anxiety. Barbiturates (Fig. 1c), it is thought, relieve anxiety by a nonspecific sedative action, whereas benzodiazepines at the appropriate dose level produce an anxiolytic effect in the absence of drowsiness and sedation. Animal experiments using a conditioned emotional response show that barbiturates reduce both punished and unpunished lever-pressing responses, whereas benzodiazepines reduce the former but not the latter. Tolerance develops to the sedative effect of the barbiturates and to the sedating aspect of the action of benzodiazepines, but not to their anxiolytic effect. This explains why patients on benzodiazepines often show an initial reaction of drowsiness that wears off in a few days. There is a similar dichotomy between the anxiolytic and muscle relaxant effects of different benzodiazepines and between their anticonvulsant and muscle relaxant properties as well. For example, diazepam is a very potent muscle relaxant, whereas other benzodiazepines are equally or more potent in their anxiolytic effect. Other benzodiazepines have stronger anticonvulsant than muscle relaxant properties. Likewise barbiturates are weak muscle relaxants. So it seems likely that these various effects of the benzodiazepines may be mediated via different mechanisms, possible via different receptors. Furthermore, the action of benzodiazepines as anxiolytics might be indirect, i.e., mediated by a second system; for example, they slow the turnover of serotonin, and serotonin receptor antagonists mimic the effects of benzodiazepines. Thus benzodiazepines may affect primarily a GABA system which in turn modulates a serotonin system (Costa et al., 1975), but it is the latter, not the former, that is the brain "substrate" for the anxiety.

If benzodiazepines really act by augmenting brain GABA, then one might suppose that a direct GABA agonist acting on GABA receptors would also have anxiolytic and sedative actions. Muscinol (Fig. 2c), found in *Amanita muscaria*, is a powerful GABA agonist. In human volunteers, however, the subjective experience of ~10 mg produced rather than alleviated anxiety, diminished concentration, and produced depersonalization and disorders of time perception. However, the anxiolytic effect of the benzodiazepines might depend on the simultaneous activation of GABA and glycine (and perhaps other systems). Thus a *pure* GABA agonist might well have different effects. Furthermore, benzodiazepines may modulate rather than activate GABA receptors (see Section II.E).

B. The Glycine System

GABA is the main inhibitory transmitter of the "higher" brain and glycine (Fig. 2b) fills this role for the spinal cord and part of the brain stem. Strychnine (Fig. 2g) acts by blocking glycine receptors. Benzodiazepines are potent displacers of strychnine from glycine receptors. Diazepam has an affinity for the glycine receptor equal to glycine itself. In general, there is a good correlation between the affinity for binding to glycine (or strychnine) receptors and the human clinical potency (relaxant) of a number of benzodiazepines (Snyder et al., 1977). Snyder suggested that benzodiazepines are glycine *agonists.* Thus benzodiazepines seem to act on both GABA and glycine systems and the former might be responsible for their sedative effects and the latter for their anxiolytic and muscle relaxant effects, possibly in conjunction with serotonin (and norepinephrine) systems as suggested above. However, it is also possible that the displacement of strychnine by benzodiazepines may have no functional significance since direct neurophysiological studies do not show any direct effect of benzodiazepines on glycine transmission in the spinal cord (Curtis et al., 1976).

C. The Serotonin System

Stein et al. (1977) recently extended their serotonin (5-HT) hypothesis of punishment and benzodiazepine action. The original hypothesis suggested that negative reinforcement is signaled in the brain by the release of 5-HT, just as the release of NE is supposed to signal positive reinforcement received. They suggested that benzodiazepines act directly by inhibiting 5-HT release systems. To support this hypothesis they quote the experiments of Graeff and Schoenfeld (1970), who showed that serotonin antagonists, such as methysergide and D-2-brom-LSD, have the same degree of punishment-reducing effects on pigeon operant behavior as diazepam. This was confirmed on rats with methysergide by Stein et al. (1973) and with cinanserin by Cook and Stepinwall (1975).

The serotonin-depleting agent PCPA has a similar effect (Wise et al., 1972) and the time course of brain 5-HT depletion and behavioral response have similar time courses. A similar marked but transitory effect was obtained in rats following the injection of 5,6-dihydroxytryptamine, which destroys 5-HT-containing terminals in the brain (Stein et al., 1975). Intraventricular injections of 5-HT antagonize the punishment-lessening effect of oxazepam on rat conditioned behavior; NE had the opposite effect (Stein et al., 1973). Stein et al. (1975) also showed that picrotoxin (2 mg/kg) will effectively block the effect of oxazepam on punished behavior without altering unpunished responses. Strychnine affected both types of response equally. Thus this evidence suggests that 5-HT is concerned with anxiety and that one effect, or one part of the effect, of benzodiazepines may be mediated via this system, possibly by a primary action on a GABA system.

D. Somatostatin

Very recently, a great deal of interest has been shown in the behavior-modifying effect of certain hypothalamic and pituitary peptides. For example, fragments of ACTH have been shown to modulate learning; LRH to initiate aspects of sexual behavior; TRF stimulates CNS centers capable of increasing motor activity and reverses pharmacologically induced sedation; angiotensin induces drinking behavior and so on. In the context of the cerebral basis of anxiety somatostatin is of particular interest since it has many of the properties of the benzodiazepines, producing sedation and decreasing seizure activity (Brown et al., 1977). It has even been suggested that benzodiazepines really act on the somatostatin receptor, which thus comes to bear the same relation to benzodiazepines as the enkephalin receptor does to morphine. The amino acid sequence of somatostatin is H-ala-gly-cys-lys-asn-phe-phe-trp-lys-thr-phe-thr-ser-cys-OH, with a disulfide bond linking the two cys. A Chou and Fasman analysis (Fasman et al., 1976) indicates the probability of a β-turn at 6-9 (i.e., phe, phe, trp, lys). Corey-Pauling-Kaltun (CPK) models indicate this would locate the aromatic rings of phe (6) and phe (7) in a steric relationship somewhat similar to the two aromatic rings of a benzodiazepine, and asn (5) to the NH. CO. system of the benzodiazepine. Thus, possibly benzodiazepines act as somatostatin agonists by filling part of the somatostatin receptor.

E. An Endogenous Ligand?

Recently it has been suggested that benzodiazepines act at a high-affinity binding site, possibly an allosteric binding site at the GABA receptor, at which the natural endogenous ligand was unknown. Möhler et al. (1979) published data suggesting that this endogenous ligand may be nicotinamide. This is isolatable from brain, binds to the high-affinity benzodiazepine receptor, and has a large number of neuropharmacological and psychopharmacological effects similar to those of benzodiazepines, including action on a variety of spinal cord reflexes. Where given locally, nicotinamide was equipotent to a potent benzodiazepine (RO 11-7800); this was indicated by tests designed to demonstrate anticonflict, anticonvulsant, antiaggressive, muscle relaxant, and hypnotic actions. Nicotinamide is usually thought of as a "vitamin" (B_3). However, it is not a vitamin at all; it is in fact the major metabolite of tryptophan in the body. Tryptophan metabolism is known to produce one certain mood-related neurotransmitter—serotonin—and one possible neurotransmitter or neuromodulator—tryptamine. Thus there is no reason that it should not give rise to another mood-related neuromodulator—nicotinamide—via the alternative kynurenine pathway. However, further work needs to be done to determine whether these effects of nicotinamide are only pharmacological or whether nicotinamide is really the endogenous ligand at the benzodiazepine receptor and thus a species of endogenous tranquilizer.

III. SIGNIFICANCE OF ANIMAL RESEARCH FOR INSIGHT INTO NEUROTIC BEHAVIOR

The significance of animal research for insight into neurotic behavior is that since Pavlov's time it has been recognized that models for certain aspects of human neuroses may be found in animal behavior. Counterparts of certain aspects of anxiety neuroses, depression, and compulsive neuroses may be found in animals, where the syndromes involved may be used as the basis for quantitative tests. Conditioned emotional response (CER) can be used as a model for anxiety; the "depressed" syndrome induced by reserpine has been used in research on depression; the stereotyped behavior patterns following the administration of amphetamine have been seen as the homologue of certain behavior patterns seen in obsessive-compulsive neurosis as well as schizophrenia. Naturally, these behaviors in animals differ in many respects from the human conditions. However, if they are homologous in some respect, their use in psychopharmacological, neuropharmacological, and brain stimulation and lesion research may throw out data, ideas, or hypotheses relevant to human illness. Also, of course, they are widely used in the pharmaceutical industry as a means of screening for new psychotropic agents.

IV. SPECULATION ON FUTURE DEVELOPMENTS

The inevitable progress of science implies that our knowledge of brain function in all its aspects will increase. This will include knowledge of the normal stress reaction, aberrations of the stress reaction, learning phenomena, and the neuroses, which may be regarded in part as an amalgam of stress and learning.

The disorders of the brain systems underlying neuroses must represent disturbances in an exceedingly complex system that will need many years of careful work to unravel. However, at any point it is possible that some new insight will be gained that will allow us to intervene therapeutically in the complex disorders that underlie neurosis: the "overactive" anxiety and stress systems as well as the inability to order thinking, emotional, and behavior patterns. The brain functions involved may include homeostatic neuronal feedback loops; transmitter synthesis; release, reuptake, and metabolism; "modulators" such as prostaglandins and polypeptides; DNA control; protein synthesis; axoplasmic transport; and so on. There is no reason that some day the pharmacological armamentarium of the psychiatry cannot be fully as extensive as that of general medicine today.

V. RECENT DEVELOPMENTS

Since this chapter was written, much information has been obtained concerning the specific benzodiazepine receptor in the brain. It now appears that the main action of benzodiazepines is to modulate the binding of GABA to its own receptor, in the allosteric sense. The GABA receptor complex is viewed as a triad with a chloride channel controlled by a GABA receptor, which in turn is modulated by a benzodiazepine receptor, the three acting as a single uniform mechanism. The identity of the natural endogenous ligand at the "benzodiazepine" receptor has not yet been finally determined, but candidates under active investigation include inosine, hypoxanthine, nicotinaminde, a nicotinamide metabolite, somatostatin, or a small peptide of the form gly-phe-phe, or even cyclo gly-phe-phe.

REFERENCES

Brown, M., Rivier, J., and Vale, W. (1977). Neurotropic actions of central nervous system peptides. *Proc. VIII Congr. Int. Soc. Psychoneuroendocrinology 37.*

Cook, L., and Stepinwall, J. (1975). Behavioral analysis of the effects and mechanisms of action of benzodiazepines. In *Mechanism of Action of Benzodiazepines,* E. Costa and P. Greengard (Eds.). Raven, New York, pp. 1-28.

Costa, E., Guidotti, A., and Mao, C. C. (1976). A GABA hypothesis for the action of benzodiazepines. In *GABA in Nervous System Function,* E. Roberts, T. N. Chase, and D. B. Tower (Eds.). Raven, New York, pp. 413-426.

Costa, E., Guidotti, C., Mao, C. C., and Suria, A. (1975). New concepts on the mechanism of action of benzodiazepines. *Life Sci. 17,* 167-186.

Curtis, D. R., Gaine, C. J. A., and Lidge, D. (1976). Benzodiazepines and central glycine transmitters. *Br. J. Pharmacol. 56,* 307-311.

Fasman, G. D., Chou, P. Y., and Adler, A. J. (1976). Prediction of the conformation of the histones. *Biophys. J. 16,* 1201-1238.

Fuxe, K., Agnati, L. F., Bolme, P., Hokfelt, T., Lidbrink, P., Ljungdahl, A., Perez de la Mova, M., and Ogven, S-O (1975). The possible involvement of GABA mechanisms in the action of benzodiazepines on central catecholamine neurons. In *Mechanism of Action of Benzodiazepines,* E. Costa and R. Greengard (Eds.). Raven, New York, 45-61.

Graeff, F. G., and Schoenfeld, R. I. (1970). Tryptaminergic mechanisms in punished and unpunished behavior. *J. Pharmacol. Exp. Ther. 173,* 277-283.

Ladinsky, H., Consolo, S., Peri, G., and Gavattini, S. (1973). Increase in mouse and rat brain acetylcholine levels by diazepam. In *The Benzodiazepines,* E. Mussini and L. O. Randall (Eds.). Raven, New York, pp. 241-242.

Möhler, H., Polc, P., Cumin, R., Pieri, L., and Kettler, R. (1979). Nicotinamide is a brain constituent with benzodiazepine-like actions. *Nature 278,* 563-565.

Snyder, S. H., Enna, S. J., and Young, A. B. (1977). Brain mechanisms associated with therapeutic actions of benzodiazepines. Focus on neurotransmitters. *Am. J. Psychiatry 134,* 662-665.

Stein, L., Wise, C. D., and Berger, B. D. (1973). Antianxury action of benzodiazepines. Decrease in activity of serotonin neurons in the punishment system. In *The Benzodiazepines,* S. Garattini and P. Greengard (Eds.). Raven, New York, pp. 299-326.

Stein, L., Wise, C. D., and Belluzzi, J. D. (1975). Effects of benzodiazepines on central serotonergic mechanisms. In *Mechanism of Action of Benzodiazepines,* E. Costa and P. Greengard (Eds.). Raven, New York, pp. 29-44.

Stein, L., Belluzzi, J. D., and Wise, C. D. (1977). Benzodiazepines. Behavioral and neurochemical mechanisms. *Am. J. Psychiatry 134*, 665-669.

Suria, A., and Costa, E. (1973). Benzodiazepines and post-tetanic potentiation in sympathetic ganglia of the bullfrog. *Brain Res. 50*, 235-239.

Wise, L., Berger, B. D., and Stein, L. (1972). Benzodiazepines anti-anxiety activity by reduction of serotonin turnover in brain. *Fed. Proc. 31*, 270.

Young, A. B., Zukin, S. R., and Snyder, S. H. (1974). Interaction of benzodiazepines with central nervous system glycine receptors. Possible mechanism of action. *Proc. Nat. Acad. Sci. USA 71*, 307-311.

10

Neurochemical Aspects of Aging in Humans

J. Mark Ordy
Tulane University
Covington, Louisiana

I. GERONTOLOGY, NEUROBIOLOGY, AND NEUROCHEMISTRY

A. Gerontology

Aging is a universal and inevitable scientific and social challenge confronting humanity. The lives of all multicellular organisms begin with conception, extend through development, maturity, senescence, and end in death. As an interdisciplinary science, gerontology now includes sociology, psychology, physiology, biochemistry, morphology, and pathology.

B. Neurobiology

As a hybrid discipline, neurobiology has undergone a remarkable expansion in recent years. The spectacular progress has occurred primarily in research on brain development rather than on aging. There has been an increasing scientific and social interest in aging. This is based in part on the significant increase in the proportion of the population over 65 in all industrial nations. Many of the human problems in aging include mental impairments and neurologic disorders. The increasing incidence of depressive states and diminished memory appear as serious personal and social consequences.

C. Neurochemistry

As one of the most recent disciplines, neurochemistry has begun to play a dynamic role in neuropsychology, neurophysiology, neuropharmacology, molecular neurobiology, and neuropathology. As a distinct new field, neurochemistry has included studies of (1) chemical composition, (2) metabolism, and (3) neurotransmission in the brain. Within a broader multidisciplinary "neuroscience framework," a neurochemistry of gerontology can contribute significantly to clarification of age-dependent changes in sensory, learning, memory, motivation, motor capacity and neuropathology. As yet, no satisfactory explanation of learning and memory is available in molecular, cellular, or neuronal network terms. It is widely accepted within an information processing network, that sensory information is transformed through short-term electrical and chemical events, with some of the information consolidated into long-term memory in chemical and/or anatomical circuits of the brain.

II. BRAIN AS "PACEMAKER" IN EVOLUTION OF LIFE-SPAN AND RATE OF AGING

Aging may be generalized throughout the body. Increasing attention has been directed toward the role of the brain and endocrine organs as "pacemakers" of aging. As interrelated control systems of the body, the brain plays a unique role in adaptation to the environment through reflexes, conditioning, and higher forms of learning. The endocrine organs play a key role in growth, reproduction, metabolism, homeostasis, and adaptation (Ordy and Kaack, 1976). Significant correlations have been established among life-span, brain size, and metabolism among species (Sacher, 1977; Cutler, 1976). By making organisms more independent of their environment, the brain and endocrines have played a critical role in the evolution of life in phylogeny by maintaining and extending the life-span (Sacher, 1975; Ordy and Kaack, 1976).

Current theories of aging range from genetic hypotheses of molecular neurobiology to concepts from mathematical or cybernetic information-processing models of the brain as an environmentally modifiable "adaptive control system" (Ordy and Schjeide, 1973). The brain is a repository for both inherited and acquired information. According to genetic hypotheses concerning DNA programs, maturity and aging represent an extension or direct consequence of a life-span ontogenetic program. The biochemical, anatomical, physiological, and behavioral characteristics of an organism are determined by codes of nucleotides stored in DNA. The DNA molecules specify, through RNA transcription and translation into specific proteins, not only the phylogenetic instructions for the life-span of a species, but also ontogenetic instructions for sequences and limits of structural and functional organization of the brain, forms of learning, adaptation, and possibly the subsequent decline in senescence. However, the brain is uniquely characterized not only by tissue interdependence, organizational complexity, and redundancy, but also by environmental modifiability. As an environmentally adaptive control system, the unique features of the brain are acquisition, storage, and retrieval of information, generally characterized as learning and memory. Sources of age decline in the brain can range from molecular error accumulation in DNA-programmed cell functions to DNA-environment interaction effects. Environmentally programmed influences on the brain include age-related changes in learning, memory, personality, role expectancies, and altered psychosocial relationships. It has been shown that the brain may retain chemical and morphological modifiability or "plasticity" from maturity to senescence (Ordy and Schjeide, 1973; Cotman and Scheff, 1979). Genetic and environmental interactions can influence the rate of change in the brain throughout the life-span.

III. AGING IN THE TOTAL ORGANISM: BIOCHEMISTRY AND NEUROCHEMISTRY

The organizational complexity essential to maintain life extends from molecular, cellular and organ to organism-environment levels. Many molecular, cellular, biochemical, physiological, and behavioral functions begin to decline long before the endpoint of death (Ordy, 1975a). There has been explosive progress in molecular biology. The prominent role of DNA, RNA, and protein as carriers of replicative and transcriptional information in each cell has quite naturally implicated them as primary sources of aging (Gershon and Gershon, 1976). The rates of aging appear to vary among organs, tissues, and their constituent cells. Cellular theories of aging have focused on mitotic capacity of cells. Significant age differences have been reported in in vitro cell-doubling potential of fibroblast cells obtained from young and old donors. The genetic mechanisms which reduce cell-doubling potential with age may be the same as those that reduce cell capacity with age in all somatic cells of the body (Hayflick, 1975). Even if applicable to organs with continuous or intermittant mitotic cells, the molecular error accumulation and the cell-doubling hypotheses would have least applicability, possibly limited to repair, to such organs as the brain with postmitotic cells, in which the life-span of neurons coincides with the individual's total life. Many other biological theories with single and multiple causes of aging have been proposed (Curtis, 1966; Rockstein, 1974; Shock, 1977).

Molecular theories appear prominent for three reasons: (1) the spectacular success of molecular biology, (2) the cell is the basic unit of structure and function in the organism, and (3) the range of maximum life-spans among species is greater than the range of individual life-spans within a species. Many sources of aging in the total organism are being examined. Some are considered primary, some secondary. Changes in some organs may either contribute to a greater extent than other organs to aging in the total organism, or they are of greater importance to humanity. Selected organs include the nervous system, endocrine glands, reproductive and immune systems (Cherkin et al., 1979). Theories of aging based on a "systems" approach are appealing for three reasons: (1) significant correlations have been established among life-span, brain-body size, and metabolism; (2) the brain and endocrines play a critical integrative role in the biochemistry and physiology of the total organism; (3) aging may represent breakdown of regulatory mechanisms; and (4) according to neurophysiological aggregate field hypothesis of brain function, molecules, organelles, single cells, and existing connections among groups of cells, even in specific pathways and centers of the brain, may have little or nothing to do with neuronal coding of information, learning, memory, or motor coordination. Functional activity in the brain depends on properties of tissue interdependence and global network capacity (John, 1972).

A. Effects of Aging in Other Organs and Total Organism on the Brain

Many cellular and extracellular changes occur throughout the total organism during aging (Kohn, 1971). Biochemical changes in the brain may influence cellular changes in other organs during aging. These cellular changes may in turn effect aging in the brain. The brain is frequently sensitive to and affected by a variety of metabolic disorders and hormonal imbalances that have an origin in other organs. The brain is a target for substrates, metabolites, and hormones. The increasing incidence of metabolic disorders and hormonal imbalances during aging can have significant effects on the brain (Cherkin et al., 1979). Cardiovascular diseases and hypertension can have significant effects on cerebral blood flow, metabolism, and psychological functioning (Thompson, 1976). Some psychological impairments have been related to cardiovascular diseases during aging (Abrahams, 1976). Subjects suffering from organic brain disease with mental impairments may also be afflicted by malnutrition, heart disease, stroke, hypertension, respiratory infections, alcoholism, cancer, and a variety of undiagnosed clinical conditions (van Praag and Kalverboer, 1972; Terry and Gershon, 1976).

B. Effects of Aging in Brain and Endocrines on Total Organism

Intrinsic DNA-programmed biochemical changes may occur throughout the total organism during aging. Biochemical changes in the brain and endocrines may be of special importance since breakdowns in the major integrative systems may in turn affect aging in the total organism. The brain plays a unique role in adaptation to the environment through reflexes, conditioning, and higher forms of learning. Through the release of hormones, the endocrine glands play a key role in growth, reproduction, metabolism, homeostasis, and reactivity to stress. The integration among all organs of the body in mammals takes place through cells specialized for communication. These cells respond to inputs by releasing chemical signals which are decoded in target organs. Communication among organs in mammals is based on two types of chemical signals: neurotransmitters and hormones. Neurotransmitters mediate chemical information transferred from input by sensory receptor neurons, to interneurons and finally to motor neurons affecting such effectors as muscles and glands. Neurotransmitter-receptor interactions determine excitatory or inhibitory influences on other neurons or on effectors. Hormones are distributed by the circulation to virtually every cell in the body. Hormonal influences on cells are decoded by tissue-specific receptors, including neuronal receptors localized in different regions of the brain (Roth, 1979).

IV. OBJECTIVES AND SCOPE OF THIS CHAPTER

The objectives of this chapter are to examine the effects of aging on behavior in relation to changes in electrical, chemical, morphological, and pathological changes in the human brain. Specific aims are as follows: (1) to examine age changes in such sensory processes of humans as vision, hearing, smell, taste, pain, touch, and vestibular function in relation to age changes in sensory pathways and centers of the brain; (2) to examine age changes in intellectual capacity, learning, short- and long-term memory in humans in relation to loss of brain cell populations in the human brain; (3) to examine age changes in such motor output functions as speed and accuracy of perceptual-motor skills, reaction times, and arousal in relation to age changes in skeletal muscles, the autonomic nervous system, neuroendocrines, and endocrine glands; (4) to examine age changes in sensory input leading to motor output in terms of electroencephalographic (EEG) measures and the bioelectric responses elicited by sensory stimulation and recorded as the averaged evoked potentials (AEP) and event related potentials (ERP) from the human brain; (5) to examine those age changes in chemical composition, metabolism, and neurotransmitters of the CNS-ANS that may be involved in impaired regulation of physiology and behavior during aging; (6) to examine some neurochemical aspects of psychiatric and neurological disorders, senile dementia, organic brain syndromes, and neuropathology; and (7) to examine prospects of intervention and modifiability in rate of aging in brain.

V. BRAIN MECHANISMS, BEHAVIOR, AND AGING

Evidence for the brain in evolution of life-span in phylogeny is based on significant correlations among life-span, brain size, and metabolism among different species. Evidence for the role of the brain as a pacemaker in the regulation of the rate of aging within a species is based on the following: (1) The brain plays a critical role in adaptation to the physical and social environment through reflexes, sensory processes, learning, memory, and more complex perceptual-motor skills. (2) Age-dependent neuropsychological changes may become noticeable to each individual since the brain mediates the sensory input from the physical and social environments into a motor output. (3) Mental activities, including sensory abilities, learning, memory, intelligence, perceptual and motor skills, may be altered imperceptibly during maturity but at a more rapid and noticeable rate during old age. The most prominent behavioral changes during aging in humans include: (1) sensory capacity declines gradually from the age of 30, possibly at different rates for different sensory modalities, (2) learning and short-term memory for new information decrease with age, whereas long-term memory appears relatively more intact, (3) there are changes in behavioral arousal, attention, motivation, and emotional reactivity, (4) age declines in speed and accuracy of complex perceptual-motor skills become greater with task complexity during aging, and (5) in personality, there is disengagement, rigidity, caution, and a reduction in psychosocial relationships (Botwinick, 1973; Woodruff and Birren, 1975; Birren and Schaie, 1977). Regarding brain mechanisms, behavior, and aging, it should be noted that many psychological studies deal with the effects of age on behavior in terms of age changes in stimulus (S) and response (R) relations, without reference to age changes in the organism (O), including the nervous system (Ordy, 1975b). There are also many studies in neurobiology that deal with structural, physiological, and chemical changes in the brain during aging without reference to behavior. The main attempt in this chapter is to examine how aging affects brain-behavior relationships in terms of age-dependent changes in sensory input leading to, or being correlated with, concomitant age decrements in learning, memory, and motor output. The focus emphasizes studies of age changes in sensory function, learning, and memory. Age changes in sensory input, learning, and motor output are considered in relation to evidence on differential loss of cell populations and chemical changes in different sensory, association, and motor regions of the brain. Evaluations of age changes in cell populations will include evidence based on histological, histochemical, and biochemical techniques used for mapping anatomical connections and chemical neurotransmitter pathways in the brain.

It seems likely that the anatomical organization illustrating the basic elements of sensory, association, and motor nervous circuits, particularly synaptic plasticity, can provide important clues concerning reduced cellular redundancy or reserve capacity in the brain during aging. For example, in brain ontogeny, reflex development has been related to Golgi I macroneurons and modifiable behavior and "memory" to Golgi II microneurons. The mammalian nervous system (NS) has been subdivided into the central nervous system (CNS), with the brain and the spinal cord; the peripheral nervous system (PNS), with 12 pairs of cranial and 31 pairs of spinal nerves; and the autonomic nervous system

(ANS), with the sympathetic and parasympathetic divisions. The "wiring diagram" of the NS includes receptor or afferent neurons (Golgi I), with long axons and cell bodies located outside the CNS; interneurons (Golgi II), with cell bodies and short axons located within the CNS; and efferent or motor neurons (Golgi I), with long axons and cell bodies located within the CNS (see Fig. 1).

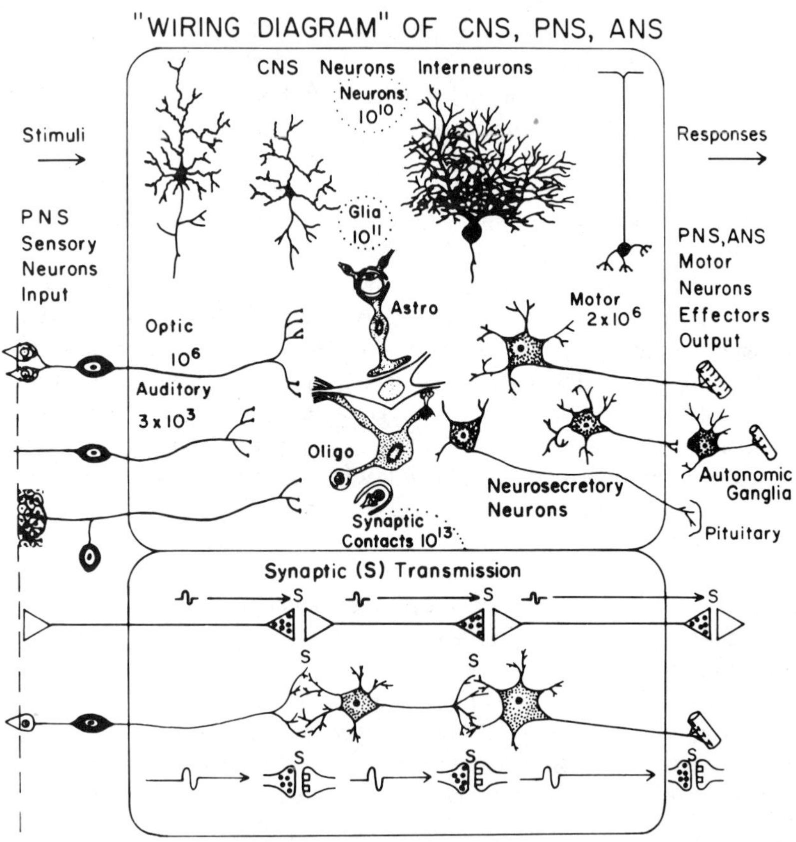

Figure 1 Basic wiring diagram of mammalian CNS, PNS, ANS, including role of synapse. [Modified from D. Bodian (1967). Neurons, circuits, and neuroglia. In *The Neurosciences,* G. C. Quarton, T. Melnechuk, F. O. Schmitt (Eds.). Rockefeller Univ., New York, p. 17, fig. 10. Reproduced with permission of author and publisher.]

A. Age Changes in Sensory Processes

Sensory systems of the brain are the links which connect all organisms with their external and internal environments. An understanding of the normal and pathological changes which occur in vision, audition, taste, smell, pain, touch, and vibration during the years from adulthood to senescence is essential for an understanding of major possible sources of age declines in learning and memory. Sensory systems also play a vital role in initiating, maintaining, and directing motor reflexes and perceptual-motor skills.

1. Vision

Many different visual functions increase during development, remain relatively constant throughout maturity, and then decrease, at first gradually and then more markedly during senescence. However, life-span changes in visual acuity, as functions, of luminance, contrast, frequency, and orientation, have not been examined in detail. Visual acuity values are based on limited samples reported in older studies. More recent findings of life-span changes in visual acuity for humans as function of luminance and contrast are illustrated in Figure 2. It seems important to note that visual acuity in humans reaches adult asymptotic levels by the age of 20, remains relatively constant only at high luminance and contrast until 50, declines at first gradually from 30 to 60 at low luminance and contrast, and then markedly from 60 to 90 years of age, even at high luminance and contrast. Age-dependent changes in such other visual functions as adaptation, flicker fusion frequency, color vision, and depth perception have also been described (Corso, 1975; Fozard et al., 1977; Ordy and Brizzee, 1979a).

2. Hearing

As in vision, there appears to be a loss in auditory acuity for loudness and pitch as a function of age. The capacity to discriminate high frequency decreases with age is relatively well known in the condition described as presbycusis. The early onset and rate of decline in auditory frequency discrimination appear to be similar to the early decline in visual acuity at low luminance and contrast. There is a relatively constant and gradual decline in auditory frequency discrimination or pitch from age 30 in humans (Corso, 1975; 1977).

3. Chemical Senses: Smell and Taste

As in vision and hearing, age declines appear in smell or olfaction as well as in taste or gustation. Age declines in smell and taste appear slowly by the late 50s and then more markedly after 60, as in visual and auditory acuity (Schiffman, 1979; Schiffman et al., 1979).

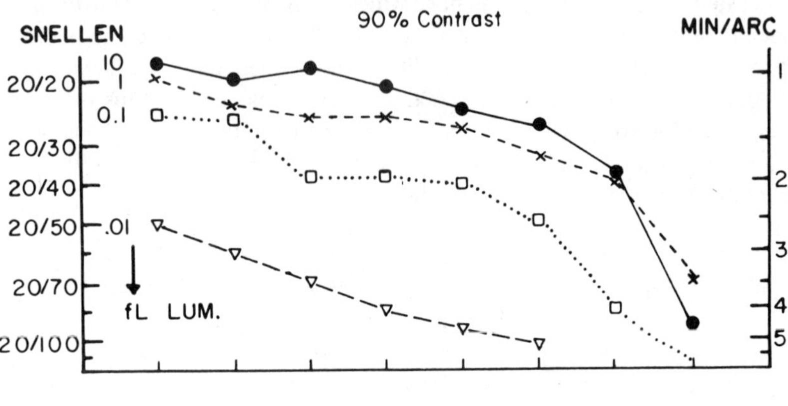

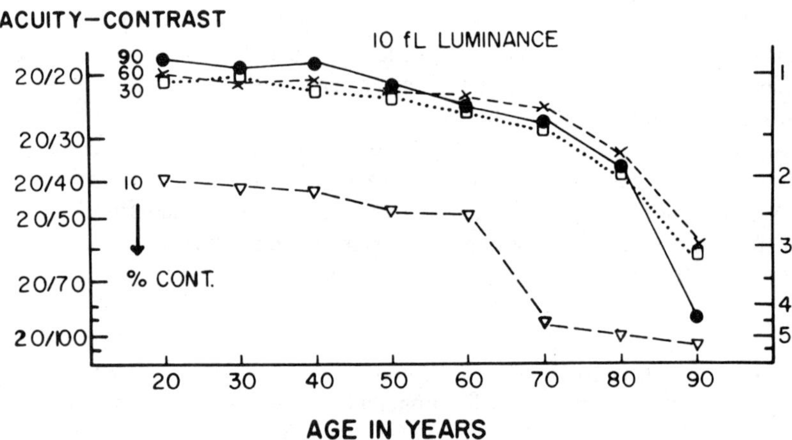

Figure 2 Life-span changes in human visual acuity at four luminance levels with 90% test letter contrast (top), and four levels of test letter contrast at 10 fl luminance (bottom). (Based on data reported by Richards, 1977.)

4. Pain

Regarding age changes in pain, the experimental findings are inconsistent. Some studies failed to observe threshold differences for pain up to 80 years. Other studies obtained data on earlier age changes in pain threshold (Corso, 1975).

5. Touch and Vibration

Only a few studies have been reported on age-dependent changes in sensory thresholds for touch and vibration. Thresholds for touch and vibration appear to increase with age, but the magnitude of increase depends on location on the body, sex, clinical condition, and a variety of other variables (Kenshalo, 1979).

6. Vestibular System

Because age samples in a few studies have been relatively small, age changes in vestibular functions of humans have not been reliably established. As in the loss of audible frequency discrimination based on cochlear degeneration, there may be saccular degeneration in the vestibular system which may result in vestibular disturbances during aging (Corso, 1975; Kenshalo, 1979).

The responses to peripheral sensory stimulation are restricted to localized primary cortical projection regions of the brain. Studies have shown that there is considerable chemical and morphological "plasticity" in the sensory pathways of the brain during development in response to environmental stimulation. Sensory stimulation may be essential for normal brain development. According to the cited studies of sensory processes and aging, there are significant decreases in sensory processes or links which connect the brain of organisms not only with their external but also their internal environments (Brizzee and Ordy, 1979). Compared with the young, old subjects have been considered to be in a state analogous to increasing sensory deprivation (Woodruff, 1975). Regarding the possible cellular basis of sensory loss, it seems relevant to note that the pattern of age-dependent declines in sensory and perceptual functions of humans includes differences in (1) time of onset and (2) rate of decline for different sensory modalities. The differences in the onset and rate of sensory loss among different modalities are probably based on differences in peripheral and central neural mechanisms. Recent studies have focused on age declines in convergent multimodal sensory integration, short-term memory, and stimulus-reward coupling centers in the cerebral cortex and limbic system (Ordy et al., 1980a). Considerably more information is available on age changes in peripheral sensory organs and receptor systems than on changes in sensory pathways and centers in the brain (Ordy and Brizzee, 1979b). In the eye, the lens thickens, the pupil narrows, and the ciliary and extraocular muscles atrophy, and the amplitude of accommodation decreases. All affect visual acuity. Loss of photoreceptors from the human retina has also been reported (Weale, 1978). In the ear, the average number of fibers in the cochlea has been estimated to be 32,500 at 30 years, and to decrease by 2000 fibers by 60 years of age (Ordy et al., 1979). In the nose and tongue, it has been estimated that there may be a loss of over 50% in the olfactory and taste receptors by the age of 70 in humans (Corso, 1975; Schiffman et al., 1979). It remains to be determined to what extent age differences in all sensory declines are attributable to (1) changes in peripheral organs and receptor systems, (2) number of afferent nerve fibers in sensory tracts, or (3) loss of cell populations in primary sensory projection and related association areas (Ordy and Brizzee, 1979b).

B. Age Changes in Learning, Memory, and Brain Cell Populations

According to many current views, the representation of information learning and memory constitute the most fundamental or unique characteristics of the brain. Learning has generally been defined as a relatively permanent change in behavior that is produced by reinforced practice. Since the "language" of neurons is electrochemical, almost all previous investigations of the neural correlates of learning have directed their attention to neurotransmitters and neuronal membranes, particularly the synapse, as a possible cellular site of plasticity during learning (Zornetzer, 1978). At present, there is little agreement as to which neural system in the cerebral cortex and limbic system may be involved in multimodal sensory integration, and stimulus-reward coupling involved in learning and memory. However, age declines in iconic memory for vision and echoic memory for audition have been related to a loss of cell populations in the visual (Devaney and Johnson, 1980) and auditory cortical areas, respectively. (Ordy and Brizzee, 1979a, Ordy et al., 1979).

Brain regions which have received increasing attention in sensory function, learning, and memory in relation to cell loss during aging are the multisensory centers of the cerebral cortex and the stimulus-reward coupling centers of the limbic system, particularly the hippocampus (Ordy et al., 1980b; Brizzee et al., 1980). The greatest redundancy and plasticity may be associated with these integration centers of the cerebral cortex and limbic system. Limbic structures have extensive connections not only with the cortex, but also with the midbrain reticular formation. Cortical-limbic connections indicate a role in coupling of learning and motivation. Limbic-reticular formation pathways suggest a role in attention and behavioral arousal. An examination of age changes in learning and memory in relation to cell loss encounters many methodological and theoretical difficulties involving cell redundancy and network capacity. Age declines in memory may be related to reduced sensory input, diminished learning capacity, altered motivation or arousal, impairment of motor coordination, or some combination of all these factors. (See Fig. 3 for neurobiology model of memory.)

Until recently, cell loss from the brain was estimated by descriptive, nonautomated methods (Brizzee et al., 1976). Also, according to statistical versus switchboard theories of learning and memory, cells and synaptic connections among groups of cells, even in specific pathways and centers, may have little or nothing to do with neuronal coding, learning, and memory (John, 1972). However, age declines in short-term memory have been related to significant loss of neurons and lipofuscin accumulation in the cerebral cortex and hippocampus of old rats (Ordy et al., 1978) and nonhuman primates (Brizzee et al., 1980).

Despite the formidable difficulties, the effects of age on intellectual functions have been studied extensively in humans. Most of the measureable intellectual abilities reach a peak in early adulthood and appear to decline in senescence. Declines in performance of perceptual-motor skills and nonverbal abilities appear greater and more rapid than in verbal abilities. Correlations between age and performance declines are higher than between age and verbal

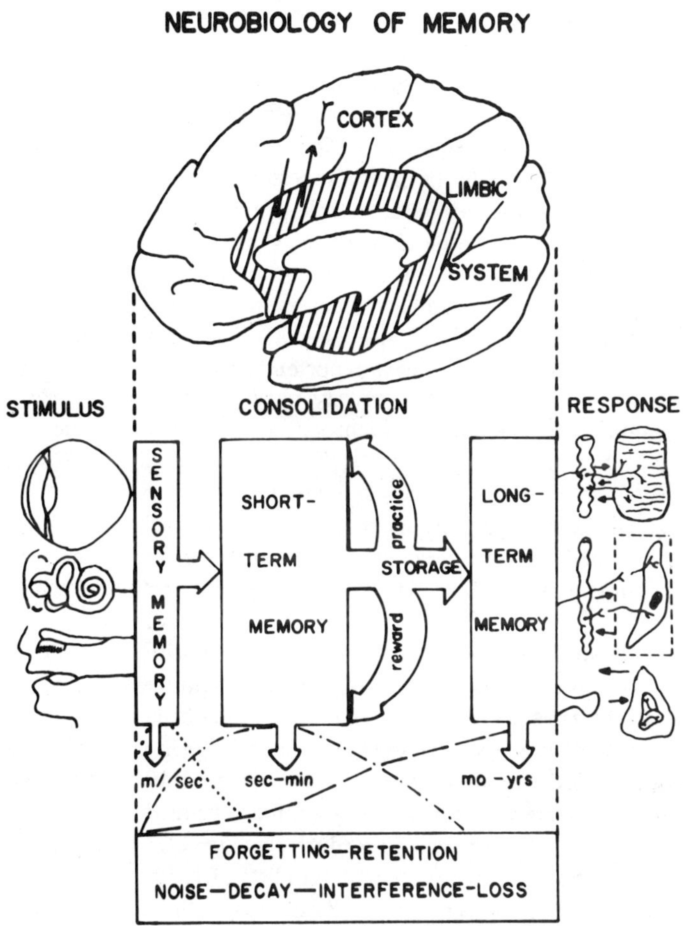

Figure 3 Three-stage neurobiology memory model: (1) sensory memory (SM) – modality-specific, milliseconds-seconds; (2) short-term memory (STM) – labile, polysensory memory, sensory imagery-semantic coding, seconds-minutes; (3) long-term memory (LTM) – chemical storage, months-years. [From J.M. Ordy, K. R. Brizzee, and T. R. Beavers (1980). Sensory function and short-term memory in aging. In *The Aging Nervous System,* G. J. Maletta and F. J. Pirozzolo (Eds.). Praeger, New York, pp. 40-78. Reproduced with permission of authors and publisher.]

abilities (Botwinick, 1977). However, generalizations concerning intellectual declines in old age have been obtained mainly from cross-sectional studies. Other longitudinal studies have cast some doubt on the validity of stereotyped views on deterioration of all intellectual functions in senescence (Shaie, 1975). Cross-sectional studies confound generation and cultural effects. They exaggerate the decline of intellectual functions in old age, and they include wide individual variation. Both stability of mental function and dramatic decline can be observed in persons even over the age of 70, depending upon the cognitive functions, status of the brain, general health, and overall physiological characteristics (Woodruff, 1975; Botwinick, 1977).

The effects of age on learning and memory in humans have also received considerable attention (Walsh, 1975; Arenberg and Robertson-Tchabo, 1977; Craik, 1977). Age differences have been reported in paired-associate and serial learning, meaningfulness, information processing, and short- and long-term memory. Information-processing models of sensory memory include iconic memory for vision and echoic memory for audition. There is considerable controversy concerning distinctions between short- and long-term memory (Craik, 1977). However, age differences in recent memory have been reported when experiments have been designed to evaluate how information presented once is maintained over a short period of time. These age declines in short-term memory have received increasing attention in both human and animal studies (Bartus, 1979a). According to common experiences reported by older subjects, memories of recent events appear to be poorly retained compared with memories of childhood and maturity (Bahrick et al., 1975). It has not yet been established definitely whether short-term memory does decline with age in humans if the tasks do not require divided attention, or reorganization (Craik, 1977). Some studies have shown that the rate with which information can be retrieved from short-term memory does decline. In a test procedure developed for short-term memory retrieval, subjects have been presented with lists of 1, 3, 5, and 7 digits and the time required to respond is measured. By increasing the number of items in the list and recording increases in time to reach a decision, the rate of retrieving items from short-term memory can be determined. Differences in response speed between shorter and longer lists reflect the rate at which items are retrieved from short-term memory. In general, the curves of older human subjects are steeper in slope than those of young and middle-aged subjects. It is presumed that older subjects retrieve information at a slower rate from short-term memory (Walsh, 1975). Studies have also shown that old subjects have difficulty retrieving information from long-term memory as indicated by comparisons between recognition and recall (Bahrick et al., 1975). Significant age differences in long-term memory have been reported in recall but not in recognition (Walsh, 1975). It is becoming increasingly apparent that significant age differences exist not onlv in short-term memory retrieval but also in recall in long-term memory. According to another study that provided an extension of the Wechsler WAIS Scale norms to older age groups, subtests that involve short-term memory show age declines with decreasing intelligence. Subtests for visual reproduction show age declines independent of intelligence. One-hour delayed recall of easy material and logical memory shows stability up to age 70 but declines rapidly thereafter (Cauthen, 1977). Earlier doubts concerning age-related loss of short-term memory were attributed to failure to control for possible increases in caution, rigidity, or response bias. Using signal detection methodology for control of possible age changes in response bias, significant decline in recognition, storage, and retrieval of short-term visual information processing have been reported in the elderly (Harkins et al., 1979).

Although morphological studies of cell enumeration in the brain have not been concerned with sensory function, learning, and memory, the counting or enumeration of cell populations in different regions of the human brain has a long history (Blinkov and Glazer, 1968). Of all the age-related morphological alterations in the human brain, including weight, volume, convolutions, etc., which have attracted the attention of neurobiologists, probably none has excited greater interest than cell loss. However, opinions still differ widely in regard to the (1) occurrence, (2) magnitude, and (3) rate of neuronal loss and possibly glial cell loss or increase in various regions of the brain with age. The greater discrepancy of published results may be due to difficulty in distinguishing small neuronal nuclei from glial nuclei, differences in histological methods, and in so-called quantitative histological techniques for enumeration of cell populations. Many errors in estimates of cell loss are inherent in limited sampling of specific regions, by a small number of sections from an organ with enormous neuronal and glial cell populations (Brizzee, 1975).

The above-cited methodological difficulties illustrate the necessary caution until morphometric studies can provide reliable quantitative values for neurons and glia in specific regions. However, there is preliminary evidence that morphological changes take place in the human brain during aging as follows. Total hemisphere volume for both men and women falls linearly from the age of 20 until 50. More gray matter is lost than white matter during this period. After 50, more white matter is lost than gray matter (Corsellis, 1976). Cell loss has been reported in the cerebral cortex of humans (Brody, 1976; Tomlinson and Henderson, 1976). There is also a loss of dendritic spines in neuropil of the cerebral cortex (Scheibel and Scheibel, 1975) and alterations occur in macroscopic and microscopic features of cerebral blood vessels (Fang, 1976). Despite this considerable evidence, it is still a matter of debate as to whether significant cell loss occurs in the brain during normal aging in the absence of cardiovascular or cerebrovascular diseases or other neuropathology (Brizzee, 1975). However, in subsequent sections of this chapter, evidence on age-dependent cell loss is also examined based on histochemical and biochemical techniques used for estimating cell loss in specific chemical pathways of the brain.

Direct correlational studies of sensory function, learning, memory, and cell loss have not been reported for humans. Such studies have been carried out in animal subjects. According to a recent review, an increasing number of studies have examined learning and memory in older animals (Walker and Hertzog, 1975), including nonhuman primates (Bartus, 1979a). Whereas age deficits are not prominent on simple discrimination or maze-learning tasks, deficits in learning increase with task complexity. The slower learning in old animals has been attributed to age-related impairments in short-term memory since with increased practice slow learners ultimately learn the task. Passive and active shock-elicited avoidance tasks have also been used to study learning and memory in rats. Using the Fisher 344 rat as an animal model, a number of recent studies have examined age changes in learning, memory, and electrical activity in relation to cell loss in the cerebral cortex and hippocampus. Using a one-trial passive avoidance task, it was established that retention or memory of a one-trial inhibitory avoidance task, as tested at 6 hr after training, declined more rapidly in 2-year-old compared to 1-year-old and 60-day-old rats (Gold and McGaugh, 1975). Using the same strain of rats, neurophysiological experiments have indicated considerable deficits in synaptic potentiation (Landfield et al., 1977) and in neuronal and astroglial degeneration in the hippocampus of old, memory-deficient rats (Landfield et al., 1978). Other studies have shown a loss of both axosomatic and axodendritic synapses in the hippocampus of old rats (Hasan and Glees, 1973; Bondareff and Geinisman, 1976). In two recent studies, life-span changes in learning and passive avoidance short-term memory were examined by behavioral tests in relation to neuron and glia packing density, and lipofuscin age pigment in visual cortex area 17, and the hippocampus of the Fisher 344 rat. Cell counts were determined by manual and by an automated, computer-programmed, image-analyzing system (Leitz-TAS). The rats were 11, 17, and 29 months old. According to statistical analyses (1) age declines in passive avoidance short-term memory at 6 hr were not related to age declines in passive avoidance learning or to age declines in other measures of behavioral performance; (2) age declines in learning and short-term memory of old rats were significantly correlated with age differences in neuron but not glia packing density in area 17 of the cerebral cortex; and (3) age decreases in neuron packing density and of cortical depth in area 17 occurred independent of, or prior to, possible age decreases in brain weight. In the second study, the age declines in short-term memory of old rats were also correlated significantly with age declines in neuron packing density and with lipofuscin accumulation in the CA1 zone of the hippocampus (Brizzee and Ordy, 1979). In the above-cited rat studies, observations for the direct correlational comparisons were made on the same subjects. The effects of age on short-term memory observed in the Fisher 344 rat appear to be similar to the memory deficits and cell loss reported in other animals (Walker and Hertzog, 1975), including old monkeys (Medin et al., 1973; Bartus, 1979a; Brizzee et al., 1980) and humans (Talland, 1968; Botwinick, 1973; Walsh, 1975; Brizzee, 1975).

C. Age Changes in Motor Output

Decreases in speed, accuracy, and strength of neuromuscular responses become prominent during senescence (Hassler, 1965). Age declines in speed and accuracy of perceptual-motor skills become particularly noticeable with increased task complexity during aging (Birren, 1965). Decreased psychomotor performance ranges from increases in visual, auditory, and choice or disjunctive reaction time, to age decrements in nerve conducting velocity, muscle strength, particularly in coordinated movements involving several muscle groups (Shock and Norris, 1970; Welford, 1977). Age declines in psychomotor performance may involve complex factors, not only in the nervous system and in muscles, but also in circulation, endocrine glands, elasticity of joints, skin, connective tissue, and total body composition. In the past, major age declines in psychomotor performance were more closely associated with changes in the CNS rather than the muscular system (Birren, 1965). On the motor output side, age changes in the "final common" extrapyramidal motor system, with its very limited redundancy of neuronal Betz cell populations (Hassler, 1965; Scheibel and Scheibel, 1975), and in the integrity of neuromuscular junctions connecting nerve and muscle fibers cannot be minimized (Gutmann and Hanzlikova, 1975). Recent evidence on other major sources of age changes in motor output include (1) emphasis on loss of skeletal muscle mass and protein metabolism, (2) changes in behavioral arousal, biofeedback conditioning, and other changes in the autonomic nervous system, and (3) changes in neuroendocrine and hormone imbalances during aging (Ordy and Kaack, 1976). The neuroendocrine system and the endocrine glands have now been added as a third major motor or effector system to the skeletal and autonomic systems (Mason, 1975).

1. Age Changes in Speed and Reaction Time

Decreases in speed and accuracy of behavior with age in humans and other animals are fundamental manifestations of aging (Birren, 1965; Welford, 1977). This is of great importance for interpreting almost all observations on the effects of aging on brain mechanisms and behavior. Conclusions concerning age changes in sensory input and all psychological variables, including such intervening variables as learning and memory, are ultimately inferences made from changes in some form of motor performance. Age increases in simple visual, auditory, or in more complex choice or disjunctive reaction time have played a prominent role in studies of behavior, aging, and the nervous system (Welford and Birren, 1965;

Marsh, 1976). The total reaction time to a visual and auditory stimulus or the so-called psychological refractory period may be related to the activity of receptor organs, their afferent pathways, the sensory projection areas, intracortical pathways, efferent pathways, and finally the effector muscles leading to reaction time of behavior (see Fig. 1). There is considerable evidence that there is a decrease in speed of initiation of response and reaction time in normal subjects and to a greater extent in those suffering from various categories of brain damage (Talland, 1965). It has been established that simple reaction time to auditory signals is significantly shorter than to visual signals. Studies have shown significant age differences in reaction time when light or sound was used as a warning signal. The effects of stimulus complexity and arousal on choice or disjunctive reaction time have also been examined during aging. In general, reaction time is longer in older than in younger subjects. If a warning signal is presented prior to the stimulus for eliciting reaction time, younger subjects benefit from the warning information as demonstrated by a faster reaction time. Older subjects benefit less and as the period between the warning and response signal increases, the benefits are lost in older subjects (Marsh, 1976). Figure 4 illustrates age changes in simple visual, simple auditory, and two-choice visual reaction time in humans.

2. Age Changes in Conduction Velocity of Nerve Fibers

Reaction time includes information transfer across synapses from sensory input leading to motor output. Numerous attempts have been made earlier to relate age declines in speed of reaction to age changes in conduction velocity of sensory and motor fibers. Other earlier studies have examined spinal synaptic delay involved in total reflex delay between afferent dorsal root input and efferent ventral root output (Botwinick, 1965). Studies have shown 10-15% decreases in the conduction velocity of nerve impulses from age 30 to age 80. In general, age decreases in conduction velocity of peripheral nerves have been considered to be

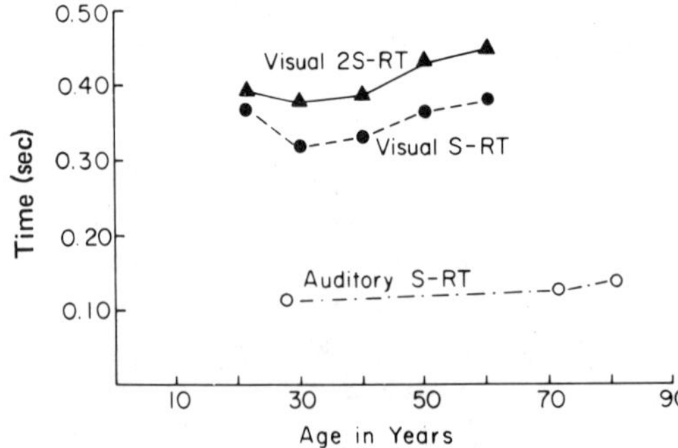

Figure 4 Life-span changes in visual auditory reaction time in humans. (Based on data reported by Talland, 1965 and Obrist, 1953.)

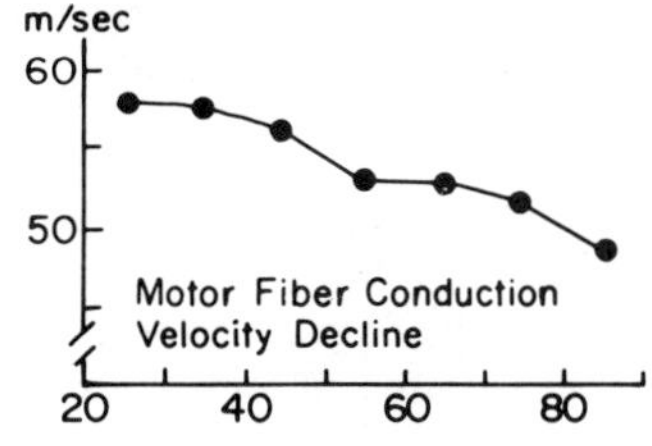

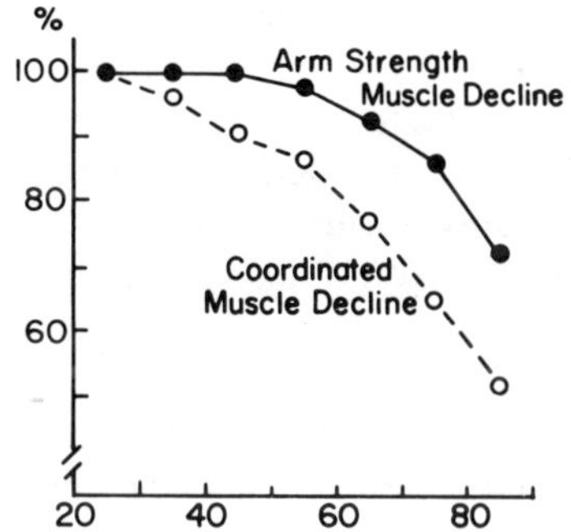

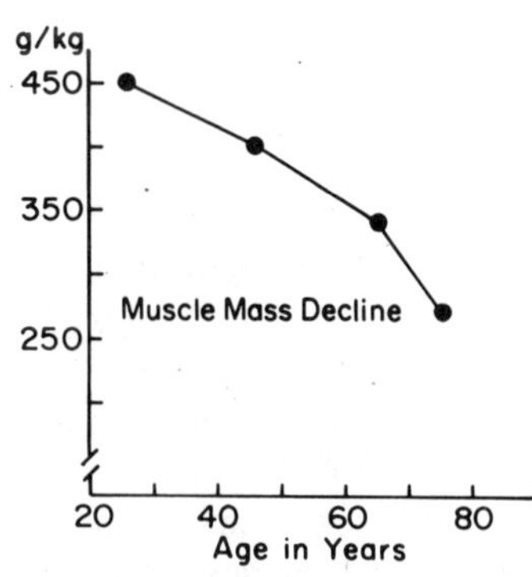

Figure 5 (top) Age declines in human ulnar motor nerve fiber conduction velocity in m/sec. (Based on data reported by Norris et al., 1953.) (middle) Age declines in arm muscle strength compared with greater decline of coordinated muscle movement by same muscle groups in cranking of an ergometer. (Based on data reported by Shock and Norris, 1970.) (bottom) Age declines in human muscle mass expressed in g/kg. (Based on data reported by Young et al., 1976.)

negligible and to play a relatively minor role in the age increases in reaction time. Age decreases in peripheral nerve conduction velocity are illustrated in Figure 5 (top).

3. Age Decreases in Muscle Strength and Mass

Another major source in the increase in reaction time and slowness of behavior during aging is the skeletal muscle system. As in the case of the brain, muscle tissue is composed of postmitotic cells. Skeletal muscle strength and tone peak between 20 and 30 years remain relatively constant until 50 and then decline at an accelerated rate. Age declines in muscle strength are greater in coordinated movement of the same muscle groups than those of component muscles. This is illustrated in Figure 5 (middle) comparing the age decline in simple arm strength with maximum power of cranking of an ergometer utilizing the same muscle groups (Shock and Norris, 1970). Some regeneration of muscle tissue is possible throughout the life-span. Skeletal muscle mass does decrease significantly from 30 to 80 years of age. Expressed in g/kg body weight, skeletal muscle in humans as a function of age decreases from a maximum of 452 g/kg at age 30 by 40% to 270 g/kg by age 70 (Young et al., 1976). Biochemical studies of body potassium and nitrogen have also indicated a reduction in body cell mass in humans (Parizkova et al., 1971). Skeletal muscle mass may account for 80% of the total body potassium and 50% of nitrogen content in humans. Figure 5 (bottom) illustrates age changes in muscle strength and muscle mass during aging in humans. Whereas the age declines in skeletal muscle strength and mass are considerable, the rate of decline can be altered significantly by such factors as nutrition, exercise, aerobic capacity, and general health (DeVries, 1975). Age changes in skeletal muscle depend on changes in trophic or innervation effects from the nervous system, changes in the cardiovascular and respiratory systems and body composition. Loss of the extremely limited number of the Betz motor neurons must result in significant alterations in transsynaptic regulation and innervation of skeletal muscle (Scheibel, 1979). Whatever the primary source of aging in the neuromuscular system, age declines of 50% from age 30 to 70 in skeletal muscle strength and mass must contribute significantly to behavioral declines during aging.

4. Age Changes in the Autonomic Nervous System

Age decreases in behavior of old subjects may also be due to lower activation, arousal, motivation, or emotional reactivity (Ellias and Ellias, 1977). There is an optimum level between under- and overarousal, described by a U-shaped function, and the efficiency of performance. One major source in the slowing of behavior with age and the longer reaction time may be that the old become less aroused, less alert, and perform more slowly. The ANS which is intimately involved in the regulation of arousal, motivation, and emotional reactivity has received considerable attention in aging (Frolkis, 1977). The ANS is part of the NS and innervates the viscera and glands as part of the homeostatic regulation of the internal environment. There are intricate relationships between arousal and sensory thresholds, learning, memory, and between autonomic activity and performance (Mason, 1975; de Wied, 1977). One interpretation of increased arousal is that sensory thresholds are lowered, more learning and memory takes place, and the reaction time becomes shorter, resulting in increased speed and accuracy of motor performance (Welford, 1977). Regarding the relationship of the ANS to the CNS in arousal, it has been proposed that activation and increased autonomic activity also increases the frequency of sensory nerve impulses which affect the EEG patterns, reflecting increased firing of cortical cells in response to greater stimulation and activation (Welford, 1965; Marsh and Thompson, 1977).

Many older subjects are underaroused as indicated by such measures of autonomic arousal as heart rate, galvanic skin response (GSR), skin conductance, and the EEG. However, by using such biochemical measures of ANS activity as cortisol and blood catecholamines, it has been shown that some older people are often overaroused and may also respond with tension, anxiety, and stress (Woodruff, 1975). There have been many studies on age differences in arousal, response speed, the EEG α cycle, and the physiological and biochemical output of the ANS (Welford and Birren, 1965; Thompson and Marsh, 1973; Marsh, 1976; Marsh and Thompson, 1977; Storrie and Eisdorfer, 1978). The evidence concerning age changes in the relationship between the CNS and ANS, and physiological and biochemical measures of arousal during aging remains conflicting. There may be an increasing desynchronization between the CNS and the ANS during aging. Using contingent negative variation (CNV) of averaged EEG cycles as measures of CNS activity and heart rate as a measure of ANS activity, it was shown that the older subjects were underaroused in terms of EEG or CNS activity and overaroused in terms of heart rate of ANS activity (Thompson and Marsh, 1973). One interpretation of CNS-ANS desynchronization with age has been that overarousal and increased ANS activity may be compensatory to the declining functional capacity of the brain, which may result from cell loss, particularly in such regions of the limbic system as the hippocampus and the hypothalamus (Ordy and Kaack, 1976; Finch, 1977).

5. Age Changes in Neuroendocrines, Endocrines, Hormones

The neuroendocrine system in the brain and the endocrine glands have recently been added to the skeletal and autonomic systems as a third major motor or effector system (Mason, 1975). Through the release of hormones, the endocrine glands play a key role in growth, reproduction, metabolism, homeostasis, and reactivity to stress. The integration between the brain and endocrines takes place through the limbic system, particularly hypothalamic nuclei, where neurons have been identified as neuroendocrine transducer cells. Neurons of the hippocampus and the hypothalamus are sensitive to hormones and form part of complex "feedback loops" involving the pituitary and endocrine organs. It has been proposed that anatomical connections as well as neural, neurohumoral, and hormonal linkages may provide important clues to the scope and complexity of psychoneuroendocrine relationships.

Figure 6 illustrates diagrammatically current views of relationships among the limbic system; pituitary, adrenals, and thyroid glands; gonads; and components of the autonomic nervous system. The figure includes a schematic outline of the established and proposed limbic and neuroendocrine components, neuroendocrine transducer cells, pituitary and endocrine target organs with the short

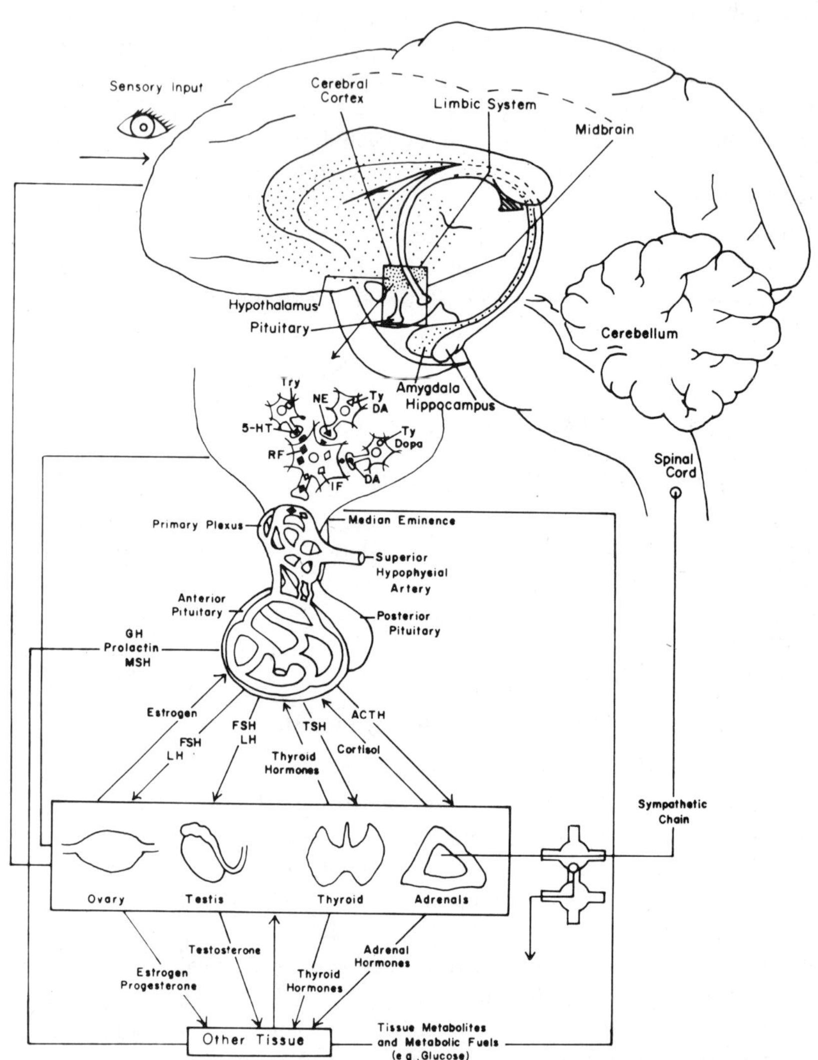

Figure 6 Schematic outline of the established and proposed interrelationships among limbic system, hypothalamus, neuroendocrine transducer cells, pituitary, endocrine target organs, and sympathetic adrenomedullary system. [Reproduced from J. M. Ordy and B. Kaack (1976). Psychoneuroendocrinology and aging in man. In *Special Review of Experimental Aging Research,* M. F. Elias, B. E. Eleftheriou, and P. K. Elias (Eds.). EAR, Inc., Bar Harbor, Me., pp. 255-302. Reproduced with permission of authors and of Beech Hill Publishing Company.]

and long closed and open feedback loops involved in the complex neuroendocrine regulation of pituitary and endocrine secretions. Since the sympathetic-adrenal medullary system is one of the oldest endocrine systems to be studied in homeostasis, emotional arousal, and reactivity to stress, it is also illustrated schematically in Figure 6.

The brain has received considerable attention in recent neurobiological studies of aging (Ordy and Brizzee, 1975; Terry and Gershon, 1976). Considerably less current information is available on life-span changes in neuroendocrines (Finch, 1977), endocrines (Andres and Tobin, 1977), hormones, behavior, and aging (Eisdorfer and Raskind, 1975; Elias and Elias, 1975; Kaack et al., 1975). However, the endocrine glands have a long history as focal points or sources of biological aging in terms of their role in (1) homeostasis and stress, (2) metabolism, and (3) reproduction. Due to the increasing mortality and decreasing adaptation to stress with age, it has been proposed that aging is caused by declines in capacity to resist repeated stresses and failure of the adrenal glands (Selye, 1970). It has been proposed that aging results from a general decline of cellular metabolism (Sanadi, 1977). This led to the belief that aging was primarily a result of alterations in the thyroid gland (Gregerman, 1967). Based on the assumption that the capacity of the sex glands or gonads to secrete appropriate amounts of sex hormones declined with age, the injection of gonadal extracts and the transplantation of gonads was proposed as a "cure for aging" in the earlier part of this century (McGrady, 1968; Talbert, 1977). Once the role of the pituitary as "master gland" became apparent in the regulation of all endocrine glands, impairments of the pituitary were proposed as primary sources of aging (Freeman, 1967). The vital roles of the hypothalamus and pituitary in homeostasis, metabolism, and reproduction have suggested to many investigators that the hypothalamus and pituitary may represent the basic biological "clocks" that regulate aging throughout the body (Everitt and Burgess, 1976; Finch, 1977; Frolkis, 1977).

Recently, more specific attention has been focused on neurotransmitters of limbic system neurons and their hormone receptors and on releasing factors (RF) and inhibitory factors (IF) of hypothalamic neuroendocrine transducer cells as regulators of pituitary and ultimately as regulators of target endocrines and their hormones during aging (Finch, 1973, 1975, 1977; Roth, 1979; Ordy and Kaack, 1976). It seems likely that age related hormone imbalances may have even more widespread effects than neurotransmitter imbalances as regulators of coordinated physiology and behavior. Life-span changes in sensory function, learning, and memory have been associated with cell loss from specific regions of the brain. More recently, hormones and catecholamines have been implicated as modulating influences on impairments in memory consolidation during aging (McGaugh et al., 1975). It has long been suspected that endocrine secretions may play a role not only in biological drives, motivation, and emotions, but also in learning and memory (de Weid, 1977). Pituitary ACTH and related peptides have been reported to enhance learning of fear-motivated behavior, whereas corticosteroids appear to facilitate its extinction (de Wied, 1974). Other studies have shown that the effects of hormones on cell function extend to molecular control mechanisms at the level of the nuclear genome (McEwen, 1973). According to some molecular theories of aging, the increasing errors with age in the transmission of information from DNA to RNA and protein synthesis represent the basic causes of cellular aging (Gershon and Gershon, 1976). In brief, it is apparent that hormones can play a ubiquitous and critical role in (1) cellular aging ranging from possible effects on molecular error accumulation in the genome with age, (2) age-dependent declines in neuroendocrines, endocrines, homeostasis metabolism, and reproduction, and (3) progressive impairments in memory consolidation, motivation, and emotions with age. It seems likely that hormones may play a critical role in bridging the gaps from molecular, cellular, regional, organ, and organismic levels of organization (Ordy and Kaack, 1976).

VI. NEUROPHYSIOLOGY, BRAIN AND AGING

There have been numerous studies and several comprehensive reviews of age changes in EEG measures in relation to reaction time, intellectual function, cerebral blood flow, metabolism, and clinical status from maturity to old age (Obrist and Busse, 1965; Thompson and Marsh, 1973; Marsh, 1976; Marsh and Thompson, 1977; Storrie and Eisdorfer, 1978). Sensory input may lead to desynchronization or EEG α blocking. It has been assumed that there must be some association between speed of information processing in reaction time at the behavioral level and changes in EEG activity. Several studies have found no relationship between measures of EEG and speed of reaction time in either young or old subjects. Other studies have shown EEG α slowing and increased reaction time during aging (Survillo, 1968). There are changes in sleep patterns with age. Other studies have examined the effects of age on EEG during sleep. Sleep patterns remain relatively stable throughout maturity, with some decrease in total sleep time during senescence. The effects of old age on EEG activity during sleep are markedly greater than on any other age changes in EEG characteristics (Prinz, 1976). Generally, although lacking quantification, it is now widely accepted that brain rhythms in the elderly, as reflected in the EEG, become slower, lower in amplitude, and less responsive to stimulation (Storrie and Eisdorfer, 1978).

In addition to EEG recordings, stimulus-evoked response techniques have been developed to study the brain's electrical activity in response to sensory stimulation. The average evoked potential (AEP) is the bioelectric response of the CNS elicited by specific sensory stimulation. In contrast to the spontaneous EEG, stimulus-evoked responses are under stimulus control and can provide information about age differences in speed of information processing in different

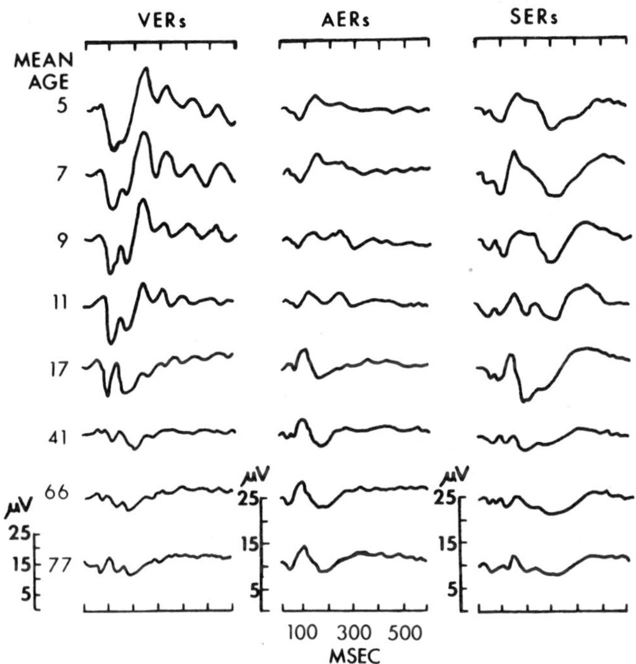

Figure 7 Age differences in neural transmission of sensory information, over multisynaptic pathways. Multisensory and concurrent declines in sensory information processing as reflected in visual evoked responses (VER), auditory evoked responses (AER), and somatosensory evoked responses (SER) in man. [From E. C. Beck, R. E. Dustman, and T. Schenkenberg (1975). Life-span changes in the electrical activity of the human brain as reflected in the cerebral evoked response. In *Neurobiology of Aging,* J. M. Ordy and K. R. Brizzee (Eds.). Plenum, New York, pp. 175-192. Reproduced with permission of authors and publisher.]

sensory systems, multisynaptic pathways, and cortical areas involved in the response. Visual, auditory, and somatosensory evoked potentials have characteristic latency, amplitude, and time patterns. Various evoked response components may also reflect involvement of specific cortical areas since significant correlations have been established between surface responses and firing patterns of individual cortical cells. Normative values for visual, auditory, and somatosensory evoked potentials have now been recorded from early childhood through age 85 (Beck et al., 1975, 1979). Whereas age changes in EEG do not become prominent until late in senescence, one striking contrast to EEG in the sensory evoked potential studies is that age differences in specific sensory AEP become apparent at age 40. However, the changes in visually evoked responses from

41 to 70 years are relatively small compared with those during brain development between 5 and 17 years. Major age changes in visual, auditory, and somatosensory evoked potentials are diminished amplitude and increased latency. Figure 7 illustrates a comparison of visual (VER), auditory (AER), and somatosensory (SER) AEP during maturation and aging in humans (Beck et al., 1975).

The findings in Figure 7 illustrate concomitant declines in neural transmission of visual, auditory, and somatosensory information over multisynaptic pathways from peripheral receptors to primary projection areas, probably a very important source of short-term memory impairment in the elderly (Ordy et al., 1980). Recently, even more promising Event Related Potentials (ERP) have been used for concurrent evaluation of sensory information processing, attention, short-term memory, choice reaction time, and decision processes from maturity to old age (Klorman et al., 1978). Significant aging effects have been reported in ERP components (Hansch, 1980). It seems likely that the ERP techniques will be used to examine age differences not only in sensory evoked potentials in relation to short-term sensory memory, but also to cerebral blood flow, metabolism, and cell loss in the brain. The ERP technique is also promising for examining age differences in sensory information processing in terms of hemispheric dominance, specialization, and interaction during aging (Hansch, 1980).

VII. AGE CHANGES IN CHEMICAL COMPOSITION, METABOLISM, AND NEUROTRANSMITTERS INVOLVED IN REGULATION OF PHYSIOLOGY AND BEHAVIOR

In contrast to the broader approach in the biochemistry of aging, the new field of neurochemistry exemplifies, by virtue of its subject matter, a more specific emphasis on one particular organ, the nervous system (Himwich, 1959; Hermann, 1971). Considerable progress has been made recently in clarification of neurochemical correlates involved in the regulation of physiology and behavior (Iversen, 1976). The historic antecedents of neurochemistry include (1) chemical composition and (2) metabolism in the brain. However, a major effort has been devoted to (3) the chemistry of synaptic transmission. Some reasons for this interest are (1) ultimately, the physiological "language" of neurons includes interactions of excitation and inhibition with information transfer at the synapse; (2) through its structural and functional asymmetry, neurotransmitters at the synapse provide not only the site of information transfer but also the possible site of plasticity; (3) the reliance on neurotransmitters is one important way in which the biochemistry and physiology of the brain differs from all other organs; (4) dramatic progress has been made in drug manipulation of neurotransmitters in relation to changes in physiology and behavior; and (5) on the basis of lesions or pathologies in anatomical or specific chemical pathways, significant correlations have been established among behavioral changes, physiology, and neurotransmitters (Iversen and Iversen, 1975a).

A. Age Changes in Chemical Composition

As chemical estimates of age declines in total brain capacity, the brain weight decreases by 17%, H_2O by 14%, dry weight by 22%, lipids by 26%, and protein by 29%, indicating a considerable loss of constituents from total brain weight (Ordy and Kaack, 1975; Ordy et al., 1975). DNA increases by 40% from 30 to 90 years. With the apparent exception of DNA and H_2O, the relative proportions of major chemical constituents of the human brain appear to remain approximately the same from 30 to 90 years. The proportionate increases in H_2O and DNA of 3-6%, respectively, may be attributed either to cross-sectional sampling errors or to real age differences that remain to be clarified. Based on electron micrographs, a significant decrease in extracellular space in the cerebral cortex of the rat has been reported from 20% of the total volume at 3 months to 10% in 26-month-old rats (Bondareff and Narotzky, 1972). However, the loss of neurons and decreased neuropil density have suggested an increase in extracellular space. Essentially, the age differences in weight and in the 10 main chemical constituents from 30 to 90 years may indicate a decreased brain capacity in humans.

Although "secular trends" suggest possible overestimation of this loss, a comparison of differences in brain capacity between these two cross-sectional age samples indicates a 17% loss of brain weight by 90 years of age. The water content of the human brain constitutes approximately 80% of the entire weight. Brain H_2O of the 350-g weight at birth is at least 90% and the proportion decreases to approximately 75% by age 30. It appears to increase slightly to 78% by age 90. The increase of H_2O from 75 to 78% may be due to a sampling error in cross-sectional age samples or to the possibility that white matter, with a lower H_2O content, may be lost to a greater extent than grey matter from age 50 to 90 (Corsellis, 1976). Of the total dry weight of 330 g at 30 years, lipids constitute 165 g or 50% of dry weight and decrease to 122 g or 47.5% by age 90. Proteins constitute 140 g or 42.2% dry weight at 30 and decrease to 100 g or 38.9% dry weight by 90 years. This increase in DNA has been attributed to neuronal pyknosis and increase in glia. Essentially, the age differences in weight and main chemical constituents indicate a decrease in total brain capacity in humans. Although regional and microchemical studies are essential, the reported age changes in weight and main chemical constituents suggest that the processes of aging in the brain are diffuse rather than associated with some particular chemical constituents (Ordy and Kaack, 1975). The rank order of age differences in the 10 main chemical constituents from an average 30-year-old adult (1450 g) and an average 90-year-old (1200 g) human brain are contained in Table 1.

Table 1 Rank Order of and Differences in 10 Main Chemical Constituents in the Average 30-Year-Old and 90-Year-Old Human Brain[a]

Rank	constituents	Brain wet weight (w.w.): 30 yr. 1450 g: 100%		Brain wet weight (w.w.): 90 yr. 1200 g: 83%		Abs dif wt 30-90		Rel dif ± % 30-90
		30 yr. 1450g	% or vol. ( )	90 yr. 1200 g	% or vol. ( )			
1	H_2O	1079	74.4 w.w.	928	77.3 w.w.	151	14	+2.9
	Dry weight (d.w.)	330	22.8 w.w.	257	21.4 w.w.	73	22	-1.4
2	Total lipids	165	50.0 d.w.	122	47.5 d.w.	43	26	-2.5
3	Total protein	140	42.4 d.w.	100	38.9 d.w.	40	29	-3.5
4	DNA	25	7.6 d.w.	35	13.6 d.w.	10	40	+6.0
5	Extracellular space		(20)		(10)			
6	CSF		(9)		?			
7	Blood		(3)		?			
8	Soluble organic substances: free amino acids, 34.25 mo/g	21	1.4 w.w.	?	?			
9	Inorganic salts, electrolytes (cations: Na, K, Ca; anions: C1)	14	1.0 w.w.	11.7	1.0 w.w.			0.0
10	Carbohydrates (glycogen)	6	0.4 w.w.	?	?			

[a]Values of the adult (30-year-old) and old (90-year-old) human brain weights and % or volume ( ) constituents of total mass are based on published references. The values are approximations since they do not include specifications of exact chronoligical age, sex, sample size, mean, standard deviation, or other statistics. *Source:* From Ordy and Kaack, 1975.

Recent studies of regional age changes in DNA, RNA, and protein content in the human brain from maturity to old age are few in number (Shelanski, 1976). Depending upon region, increases and decreases have been reported. Estimates of DNA content have been utilized as chemical indices of cell number. The RNA content of neurons is considerably higher than that of glial cells. RNA/DNA ratios have been used as chemical estimates of differential neuron/glial populations in different regions of the brain. Protein/DNA and protein/RNA ratios have been used as estimates of cellular protein concentrations and synthesis. Neurochemical and morphometric histological evaluations have been combined at the laminar and regional level in the human cerebral cortex to obtain concurrent chemical and anatomical indices of cell number during development. Thus far, these quantitative neurochemical-morphometric methods have not been utilized for studying the "chemoanatomical" changes in the human brain during aging (Hess and Pope, 1972).

Until recently, selective cell loss of different types of neurons and glia in specific regions of the brain was studied mainly with descriptive, or quantitative, histological techniques. With the development of histochemical, fluorescent, immunocytochemical, and biochemical techniques, considerable progress has been made in establishing the chemical identity of neurons and mapping chemical pathways in the brain (Iversen and Iversen, 1975a). Rapid progress is being made in mapping cholinergic, dopaminergic, noradrenergic, serotonergic, and GABAergic pathways in the brain. Current mapping of chemical pathways in the brain is based primarily on rodents, cats, and a few studies in nonhuman primates and humans. As yet, there are very few studies of cell loss and other age changes in specific chemical pathways of the human brain. Using synthetic enzymes and neurotransmitter concentrations as biochemical markers and estimates of cell number, selective loss of serotonergic and cholinergic neurons has been reported recently in discrete nuclei of the rat brain (Meek et al., 1977). Other evidence of age changes in neurotransmitters in the human brain is presented in Section VII.C. Figure 8 illustrates the presumptive neurotransmitter pathways in the primate brain. A better understanding of the effects of age on the brain depends on analysis in functionally distinct pathways and chemically identifiable cell groups (Finch, 1977).

B. Age Changes in Cerebral Circulation and Metabolism

As in all other organs, the basic functions of cerebral circulation are to provide substrates for energy metabolism, maintain the structural integrity of the organ, and remove products of metabolism. The blood content of the adult human brain comprises 3.0% of the brain volume (See Table 1). Average values for the brain of normal young males include (1) cerebral blood flow (CBF), 620 ml/kg per minute; (2) cerebral metabolic rate for oxygen ($CMRO_2$), 35 ml O_2/kg per minute; (3) glucose (CMRG), 5.4 mg/kg per minute. Normally, glucose is the

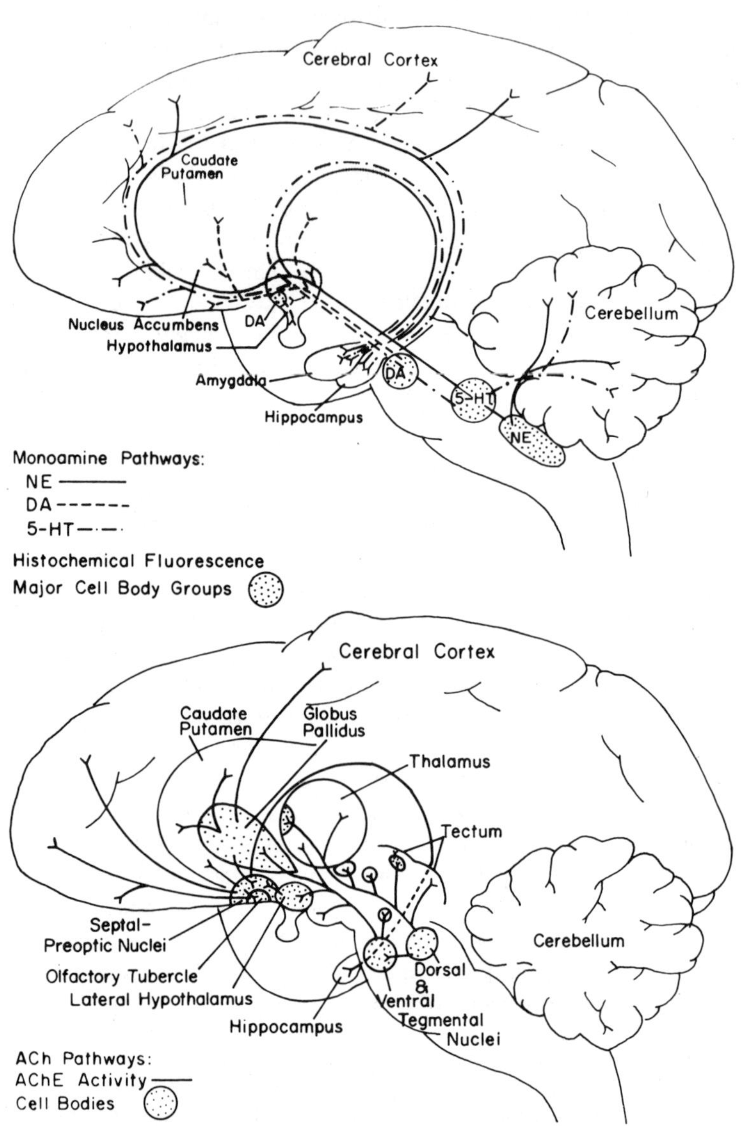

Figure 8 (top) Organization and distribution of chemical neurotransmitter pathways for norepinephrine (NE), dopamine (DA), and serotonin (5-HT) based on histochemical fluorescence, including location of cell body groups. (bottom) Presumptive acetylcholine (ACh) distribution, based on AChE with cell bodies.

exclusive energy substrate for the brain. Although only 1450 g or 2% of the average 70-kg human body, the brain utilizes over 15% of the total basal cardiac output, 20% of the basal O_2, and 20% of the total glucose consumption (Sokoloff, 1976). These high-energy requirements are essential for (1) maintenance and/or replacement of intracellular membranes, organelles, and possibly cells, (2) maintenance of ATPase-dependent potassium and sodium gradients in neuronal membranes for conduction of the action potential, and (3) synthesis, storage, release, and reuptake of neurotransmitters. Synaptic endings may consume as high as 40% of total O_2 (Siesjo et al., 1974). Over 90% of O_2 is utilized by mitochondria. The brain contains less than 1% of glucose and glycogen. Over 90% of glucose is oxidized in glycolysis. The remaining glucose carbon is incorporated into glycogen, lipids, amino acids, and protein. If they did occur, age changes in cerebral blood flow (CBF), O_2, and glucose should have significant consequences for sensory, learning and motor functions, electrical activity, neurotransmitters, and the structural integrity of the brain. However, the most widely cited conclusion, based on data in Table 2, has been that there is no significant age decline in CBF and $CMRO_2$ without disease (Sokoloff, 1975).

According to the data in Table 2, the significant increases in mean arterial blood pressure and cerebral vascular resistance even in the 71-year-old healthy subjects indicate that cardiovascular changes may occur as a primary aging process independent of disease. The 7% decline in CBF and 5% decline in $CMRO_2$ indicate an age trend but they are not significantly lower in the old healthy select group. However, cerebral glucose utilization (CMRG) was significantly reduced in this group. Normally, the brain uses O_2 and glucose in stoichiometric amounts and both may be used as measures of cerebral metabolic rate. The dissociation between O_2 and glucose in the healthy old group may represent a significant finding. The dissociation between O_2 and glucose in old age may involve utilization of ketone bodies in place of glucose. The use of ketone bodies may result from increased circulating fatty acids due to decreased use by diminished skeletal muscle mass (Sokoloff, 1975). However, ketone bodies are used by the brain only in starvation, diabetes, and high-fat diets. The significantly higher blood glucose values in the old age groups (see Table 2) appear inconsistent with the proposed metabolism of ketone bodies by the old brain in place of glucose. The most widely cited interpretation of the findings in Table 2 has been that there is no significant age decline in cerebral circulation and metabolism independent of disease (Sokoloff, 1975). However, this conclusion is based on the unresolved definition of normal aging, which includes only a highly select healthy old age group as representative of senescence rather than the heterogenous normal and disease age groups (2-7, Table 2) as being the more representative sample of senescence.

Evidence for relationships among CBF, O_2, glucose, and cell loss in the human brain is indirect. Normally, there is a close relationship between changes

Table 2 Summary of Age Differences in Cerebral Circulation and Metabolism Between Young and Old Men[a]

Independent-dependent variables	1 Normal young (NY) (15)	2 Normal old (NO) (26)	3 NO asymptomatic disease (15)	4 Hypertensive (HT) old (5)	5 Arteriosclerotic (5)	6 HT Arterio-sclerotic (4)	7 Chronic brain syndrome (10)
Age (years)	21	71[b]	73[b]	71[b]	73[b]	75[b]	72[b]
Mean arterial blood pressure (mm/Hg)	84.2 ±1.9	93.2[b] ±1.3	110.8[b] ±5.0	128.2[b] ±11.1	94.0[b] ±3.7	118.0[b] ±3.2	101.7[b] ±6.2
Cerebral blood flow (ml/100g/min)	62.1 ±2.9	57.9 ±2.1	52.1[b] ±2.5	55.4 ±5.5	48.5[b] ±4.2	48.5[b] ±4.9	48.5[b] ±3.8
Cerebral vascular resistance (mmHg/ml/100g/min)	1.29 ±.06	1.58[b] ±.07	2.05[b] ±.12	2.30[b] ±.11	1.78[b] ±.23	2.35[b] ±.21	2.11[b] ±.25
Cerebral metabolic rate oxygen (ml/100g/min)	3.51 ±.21	3.33 ±.08	3.22 ±.13	3.64 ±1.4	3.25 ±2.7	3.10 ±.29	2.72[b] ±.18
Cerebral metabolic rate glucose (mg/100g/min)	6.0 ±.7	4.6[b] ±.2	4.8[b] ±.4	5.6 ±.7	5.2 ±.5	4.0 ±.5	3.6[b] ±.6
Oxygen/glucose ratio (mM/mM)	5.5 ±.5	6.0 ±.2	5.7 ±.4	5.1 ±.5	5.3 ±.7	6.3 ±.4	5.7 ±.8
Blood glucose: (mg%)							
Arterial	83.2 ±3.3	88.0 ±1.7	90.4 ±4.8	86.2 ±2.8	99.6 ±13.0	80.6 ±1.6	92.1[b] ±2.1
Int. jug.	73.8 ±1.1	79.9[b] ±1.7	80.9 ±4.9	75.9 ±2.1	88.1 ±14.4	73.8 ±1.7	85.1[b] ±1.9

[a]Group ranks: normal young compared with select old without and with diseases. Numbers in parentheses are sample numbers.
[b]Mean values are significantly different from young controls ($P<.05$). *Source:* Data from Dastur et al., 1963.

in blood supply and changes in tissue demand for O_2 and substrates in different organs. From increased age differences in $(A\text{-}V)O_2$ in the brain of old subjects with asymptomatic vascular diseases, it has been concluded that if the brain cannot extract more O_2 per unit volume, ischemia may result with accelerated loss of brain cells. It has been widely accepted that neurons could only survive approximately 5 min of ischemia before cell death would occur. According to regional studies, neurons may cease to function at perfusion rates below 180 ml/kg per minute during temporary ischemia and then recover. Irreversible damage and cell death may occur at perfusion rates below 100 ml/kg per minute (Heiss et al., 1975). Other evidence on cerebral circulation, metabolism, vascular disease, ischemia, and cell loss in senile dementia has been reviewed (O'Brien, 1977).

Recent developments in radioisotope techniques have made it possible to monitor regional CBF in the human brain without intracarotid injection or other invasive methods. Measurement of CBF by inhalation of ^{133}Xe has made it possible to examine age changes in intellectual performance in relation to EEG, CBF, cerebral vascular resistance (CVR), and $CMRO_2$ in the left and right cerebral hemispheres, during normal aging as well as in psychiatric and neurologic disorders, senile dementia, and organic brain syndromes (Thompson, 1976). The most significant correlations have been established among age, intellectual deficits, EEG frequency, reduced CBF, $CMRO_2$, multi-infarcts, and Alzheimer's disease. Future studies will have to establish whether these significant correlations with age may occur independent of neuropathology.

C. Age Changes in Neurotransmitters

Knowledge of chemical transmission in the mammalian brain is considerable but far from complete. Recent efforts in the entire field of neurochemistry appear to be directed mainly to neurotransmitters in the mammalian brain rather than its chemical composition or metabolism. The most spectacular progress in neurochemical studies has been made on (1) identity of neurotransmitters in the CNS, (2) mapping of chemical pathways, and (3) role of neurotransmitters in the regulation of behavior (Iversen and Iversen, 1975b). However, values for neurotransmitters and their respective enzymes in the human brain are scarce and scattered throughout the literature. Also, neurotransmitter values in the literature are based more on anatomically rather than chemically defined pathways. Due to the development of new methods, age changes in sensory processes, learning, memory, and motor skills can now be studied in the normal human brain in relation to stimulus-elicited AEP, ERP, and CBF without reliance on invasive procedures. However, for neurochemical evaluations, fresh brain tissue is essential, particularly for assessment of energy substrates, for neurotransmitter concentrations, and their respective enzyme activities. Published values on chemical composition of the human brain are less variable since such constituents as myelin, lipids, and proteins remain relatively stable under proper conditions. Values for energy substrates, enzymes, and neurotransmitters are much more variable for the human brain due to rapid postmortem changes. These constituents are highly labile even after special precautions are taken in the processing of fresh tissue samples obtained from the human brain of accident victims or patients with neurologic disorders.

As indicated earlier, one major reason for the extremely high energy requirements of the brain is the synthesis, storage, release, and reuptake of neurotransmitters. Whether reduced supply of O_2 and glucose is primary and reduced demand due to cell loss is secondary, there are no oxygen stores in the brain and the supply of glucose is also extremely negligible. From recent studies of the effects of ischemic anoxia in humans, it is known that reductions in cerebral blood flow, oxygen, and glucose may result in mental impairments, neurologic deficits, EEG slowing, changes in evoked potentials, altered cAMP levels, reduced mitochondrial respiration, and, ultimately, irreversible cellular damage and possibly cell loss (Meyer et al., 1976). Although these high correlations are more characteristic for certain diseases than age alone, an increasing number of studies have indicated decreases in synthesizing enzyme activity, neurotransmitter concentration and turnover, and increases in catabolic enzyme activity within a particular neurotransmitter system during aging independent of disease (Finch, 1977; Domino et al., 1978). Other studies have suggested progressive imbalances, not only within a particular neurotransmitter system, but also among different neurotransmitter systems in the human brain during aging, particularly in a variety of neurologic disorders and in senile dementia (Samorajski and Hartford, 1980).

Based on earlier criteria for identifying acetylcholine (ACh) and norepinephrine (NE) as excitatory and inhibitory transmitters in the ANS, the following substances and their respective enzymes of synthesis and degradation have been tentatively identified as putative transmitters in the mammalian CNS: (1) ACh, cholineacetyltransferase (ChAc), and acetylcholinesterase (AChE); (2) the catecholamines NE and dopamine (DA) with the enzymes tyrosine hydroxylase (TH), DOPA decarboxylase (DDC), and monoamineoxidase (MAO); (3) serotonin (5-HT) with catechol-o-methyltransferase (COMT); and (4) the amino acids γ-aminobutyric acid (GABA), glutamic acid, and glycine. Table 3 contains a summary of neurotransmitters, the synthesizing and catabolizing enzymes for some regions of the adult human brain. These values have been obtained from sources scattered throughout the literature (Ordy and Kaack, 1975).

It has not been established as to whether cholinergic or monaminergic neurons are more vulnerable during normal aging, independent of disease. The life-span changes in cholinergic and monoaminergic transmitter concentrations and in their enzyme activities that have been reported in a few studies are based on brain tissue samples obtained from accident victims ranging in age from 1 to

Table 3 Neurotransmitters and Associated Enzymes in Adult Human Brain[a]

Neurotransmitter	Associated enzymes: Synthesis	Associated enzymes: Catabolism
Acetylcholine 0.5-0.6 μg/g (ACh) (human cerebral cortex)	Choline acetyltransferase 0.39 nmol/g/hr (ChAc) (human cortex)	Acetylcholinesterase 0.29 nmol/g/hr (AchE) (human cortex)
Dopamine 2.45-3.75 μg/g (DA) (human caudate)	DOPA decarboxylase 3.0 μmol/g/hr (DOD) (human caudate)	Dopamine β-hydroxylase 0.5 nmol/h/ml (DβH) (human CSF)
Norepinephrine 0.35-0.60 μg/g (NE) (human hypothalamus)	Dopamine β-hydroxylase 0.5 nmol/h/ml (DβH) (human CSF)	Catechol-O-methyltransferase 0.5 μmol/g/hr (COMT) (human hypothalamus)
Serotonin 0.2-0.23 μg/g (5-HT) (human hindbrain)	5-Hydroxytryptophan decarboxylase 3.0 nmol/g/hr (AAD) (human hypothalamus)	Monomine oxidase 8.4 μmol/g/hr (MAO) (human hypothalamus)
γ-Aminobutyric acid 3.1 μmol/hr/g (GABA) (human caudate)	Glutamic acid decarboxylase 1640 nmol/g/hr (GAD) (human hypothalamus)	GABA transaminase 9 nmol/kg/hr (GABA-T) (Monkey occipital cortex)
Glutamate 10 mmol/brain (mammalian brain)	Glutamate dehydrogenase 0.59 mg/ml (GD) (beef liver)	GAD 1640-1656 nmol/g/hr (human hypothalamus)

[a]Neurotransmitter and associated enzyme values for the adult human brain were selected from regions with highest content or as the only values available. Values are based on published references. *Source:* From Ordy and Kaack, 1975.

80 years, with no apparent history of neuropathology or other diseases. Thus far, life-span changes in ACh for humans have not been reported (Finch, 1977; Domino et al., 1978). Only two studies have reported on ACh values in the adult human brain. Postmaturity declines in ChAc and AChE activity have been reported for the human cerebral cortex. ChAc appears to decline and AChE increases with age. Small but statistically significant postmaturity declines in DA, NE, and 5-HT concentrations have also been reported for the caudate nucleus and for the hindbrain. Age-dependent declines in the activities of DOD, TH, and GAD in the substantia nigra, caudate nucleus, putamen, and hypothalamus of the human brain have also been reported. MAO has been reported to increase

and decrease in activity with old age depending upon region. Other age-dependent changes in enzyme activity associated with catecholamines, GABA, and ACh in various regions of the old human brain have also been reported recently (McGeer and McGeer, 1976). In general, the published findings indicate that neurotransmitter concentrations and synthesizing enzyme activities decrease, whereas catabolizing enzyme activities may increase or decrease depending upon transmitter system or region of the brain. Figure 9 illustrates the reported life-span changes in neurotransmitter concentrations and in the respective enzyme activities in some regions of the human brain.

Normal behavior and physiology depend upon a proper balance of excitatory and inhibitory neurotransmitter interactions in the brain. Depending upon the region of the brain, imbalances in neurotransmitters and their respective enzymes during aging appear as possible major sources of age-dependent declines in chemical pathways of the brain. Although such possible and progressive imbalances have not been explored in detail in the normal human brain during aging, they have been established in the brain of the chicken during development and aging. The synthesizing enzyme ChAc and the hydrolyzing enzyme AChE of ACh were determined during development, maturity, and aging in the cerebral cortex, optic lobes, cerebellum, and midbrain (Vernadakis, 1973). In the cerebral hemispheres, ChAc and AChE reach asymptotic levels by 3 months posthatching; but after 3 months, ChAc decreased up to 3 years; whereas AChE decreased up to 20 months and then reached high levels of activity at 3 years. It appears that in old age of 3 years, activities of the two cholinergic enzymes were at opposite extremes from what they were during development, since the synthesizing enzyme ChAc had a very low level of activity whereas the hydrolyzing enzyme AChE appears to be at a very high level of activity in the cortex. Since ChAc appears to be a more reliable index of ACh, the age-dependent declines in ChAc may reflect decreases in this synthesizing enzyme activity, loss of cholinergic neurons, or both. However, to establish more fully whether imbalances within any cholinergic pathway during aging represent a possible major source of age-dependent chemical decline in the brain, ACh levels, turnover, and ACh receptor alterations would have to be established. Decreases in rate-limiting enzyme activity accompanied by decrease in neurotransmitter concentration has been used as a biochemical index of cell loss. However, ChAc activity does not necessarily indicate the rate of ACh synthesis, since choline uptake, not ChAc activity, is the rate-limiting step to ACh synthesis. Figure 10 illustrates ChAc and AChE enzyme activity during development, maturity, and aging in the cerebral hemispheres of the chicken.

As in the case of possible imbalances within the cholinergic system in the cerebral cortex, imbalances among different types of neurotransmitters may be involved in processing of information from sensory input leading to motor output. The identification, based on specific criteria for chemical transmitters in

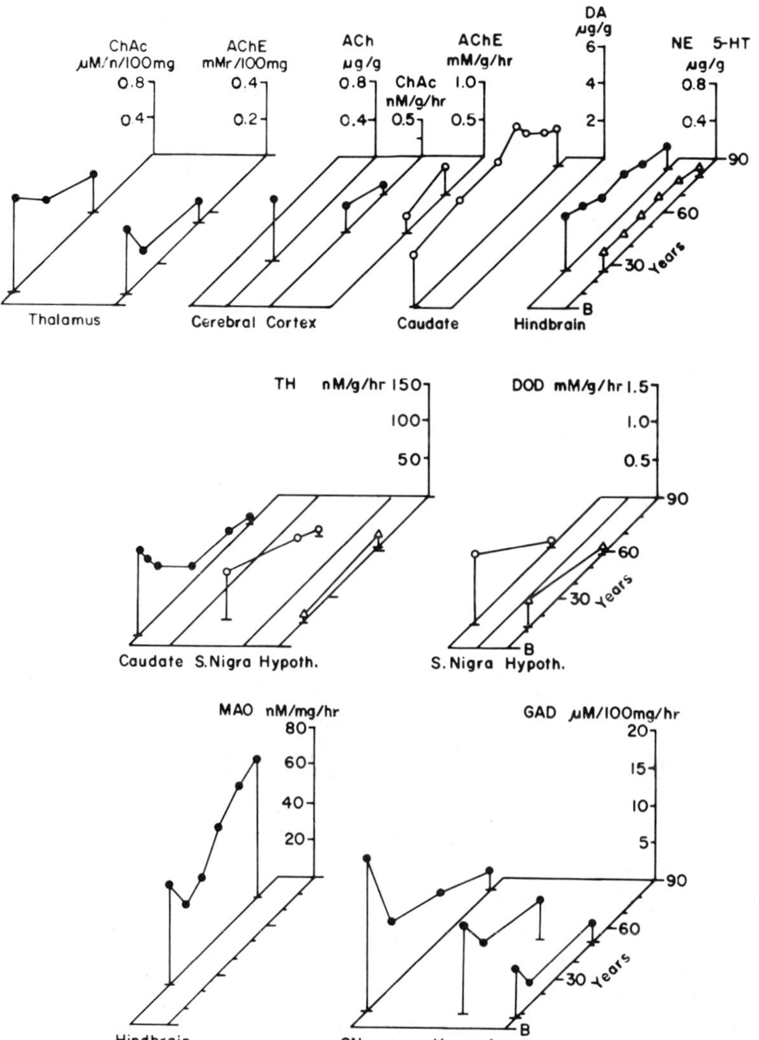

Figure 9 Life-span differences in neurotransmitters and enzymes in some regions of human brain, based on published references. [From J. M. Ordy and B. Kaack (1975). Neurochemical changes in composition, metabolism, and neurotransmitters in the human brain with age. In *Neurobiology of Aging,* J. M. Ordy and K. R. Brizzee (Eds.). Plenum, New York, pp. 253-286. Reproduced with permission of authors and publisher.]

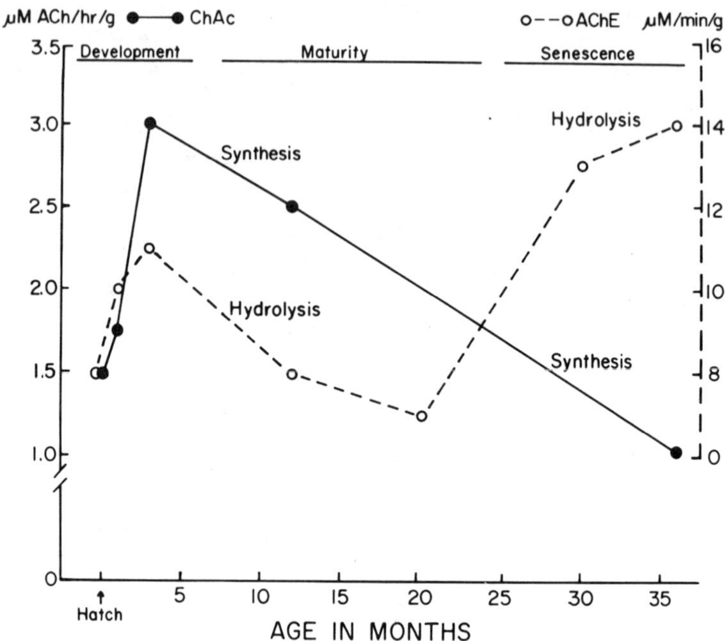

Figure 10 ChAc and AChE enzyme activity during development, maturity, and aging in the cerebral hemispheres of chicken. (Based on data reported by Vernadakis, 1973.)

the CNS, represents a relatively recent development. Criteria for identification of ACh and NE as excitatory and inhibitory transmitters, respectively, were first established in isolated motor ganglia of the ANS. Next ACh was identified as an excitatory transmitter at the neuromuscular junction. As yet the chemical identity of putative transmitters in receptor neurons or in most sensory pathways remains to be established. The thalamus represents the main relay station for all sensory pathways, except the olfactory, from sensory receptors to projection areas in the cortex. The enzyme glutamic acid decarboxylase (GAD) is involved in the synthesis of GABA, a possible neurotransmitter in the thalamus. Significant decreases of GAD in the thalamus during aging have suggested that loss of GABAergic neurons may play a role in the declining capacity to process sensory information in the main sensory relay system of the human brain during aging (McGeer and McGeer, 1976). Until recently, animal drug studies on learning and memory focused on cholinergic mechanisms and the cerebral cortex. DA and NE interactions in the limbic system, particularly the hypothalamus, were associated with drives and their reinforcement, emotional arousal, and other affective states. Sensory thresholds, learning, memory, and motor performance also depend on arousal, drives, and their reinforcement. Age changes in learning and memory may be associated not only with changes in cholinergic neurons in the cortex, but also with DA and NE neurons, particularly hypothalamic neuroendocrine transducer cells. Hormonal feedback effects also appear to be important by their influence on hormone receptors of neurons in the cortex and limbic system. Such cholinergic drugs as scopolamine and physostigmine have produced significant age-dependent effects on short-term memory, as determined in young and old human subjects (Drachman and Leavitt, 1974) and more recently in nonhuman primates (Bartus, 1979b). Significant but transient improvements in short-term memory have been reported after L-dopa treatment in Parkinsonian patients (Halgin et al., 1977). Animal drug studies have shown that drug inhibition by diethyldithiocarbamate (DDC), a dopamine B-hydroxylase inhibitor of NE but not DA, can affect not only arousal but also short-term memory in mice as determined in a single-trial passive avoidance test (Randt et al., 1971). On the motor output side, more progress has been made on neurotransmitter balances and interactions involved in the regulation of coordinated motor activity. Regulation of extrapyramidal motor functions depends on a balance between dopaminergic, cholinergic, and GABAergic activity. During aging, there may be a progressive imbalance among dopaminergic, cholinergic, and GABAergic neurotransmitters in the basal ganglia of humans resulting in the reported decreases in speed and accuracy of behavior.

Age declines in neurotransmitter function may be based either on loss of cholinergic or monoaminergic neurons, age changes in the functional state of the remaining neurons, or concomitant changes in both. Communication among neurons takes place in the neuropil. Cell loss may reduce network capacity by changing intercellular communication. According to deafferentation and denervation studies, neuronal input is essential for normal functioning of other neurons and effectors. Morphological studies have indicated loss of neurons in the cerebral cortex of humans, rhesus monkey, and rat (Brody, 1976; Brizzee, 1975; Ordy et al., 1976). Neurochemical studies have shown loss of cholinergic and monoaminergic neurons in different regions of the human brain (McGeer and McGeer, 1976). Physiologically, the language of neurons is based on interactions of excitation and inhibition. Selective loss of excitatory or inhibitory neurons would result in an imbalance among cholinergic-monoaminergic transmitters and less than optimum regulation of physiology and behavior. Figure 11 illustrates possible age-related neurotransmitter imbalances in physiology and behavior.

Elegant single-unit neuron iontophoretic studies of neuronal excitation, conduction, and transmission have been carried out in recent years in different regions of the mammalian brain. These single-unit electrochemical studies have been applied only recently to study possible age-dependent changes in excitation, conduction, and transmission in relation to chemical and morphological changes in single neurons (Rogers et al., 1980). Loss of dendritic spines with aging has been reported in the neuropil of the cerebral cortex of humans

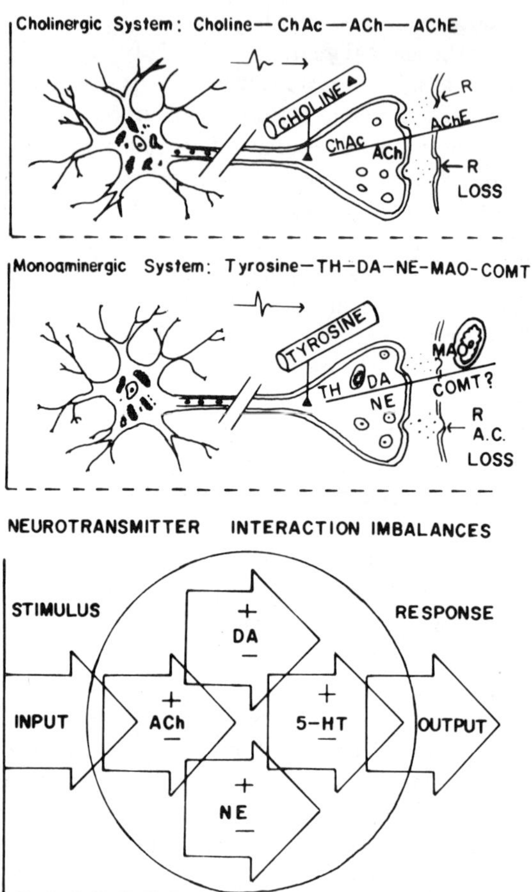

Figure 11 Possible age-dependent neurotransmitter-enzyme-receptor imbalances within cholinergic and monoaminergic systems, and also among cholinergic-monoaminergic interactions regulating physiology and behavior.

(Scheibel and Scheibel, 1975) and rat (Feldman, 1976). Decreases in axonal transport have also been reported (Ochs, 1973). At the single-unit neuron level, it seems possible that the age-dependent decreases in dendritic spines may result in decreases in "input"; intraneuronal accumulation of lipofuscin may produce declines in cell functional capacity; alterations in axon myelin lamellae and/or axon diameter may result in decreasing conduction velocity; and changes in neurotransmitters or their enzyme imbalances may result in decreases in synaptic neurotransmission. Figure 12 illustrates possible age-dependent changes in excitation, conduction, and transmission in single neurons associated with loss of dendrites, accumulation of lipofuscin, changes in axon characteristics and synaptic components.

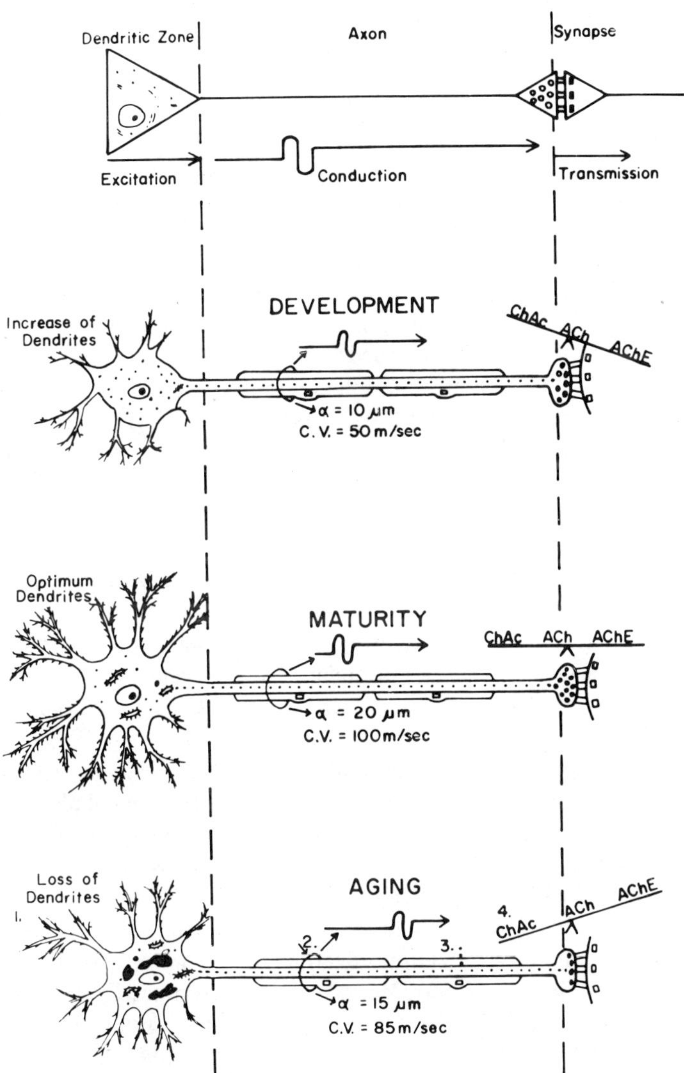

Figure 12 Model for age changes in neuron. Changes include loss of dendritic spines, lipofuscin pigment accumulation, loss of myelin lamellae, conduction velocity (C.V.), decreased transport of transmitter via neurotubules, imbalance in synthesizing and catabolizing enzymes.

VIII. NEUROCHEMICAL ASPECTS OF PSYCHIATRIC AND NEUROLOGIC DISORDERS, SENILE DEMENTIA, AND ORGANIC BRAIN SYNDROMES

Any review concerned with neurobiology and aging in humans is immediately confronted by (1) the presence and extent of the increasing incidence of mental impairments and brain disorders with age, (2) the differentiation of "normal" aging from brain pathology, and (3) the role of brain disorders in mortality in relation to mortality from such other major causes as vascular disease, malignancy, and immunological disorders. Recent volumes have examined psychopathology, brain physiology, and biochemistry (Shagass et al., 1977), biochemistry and neurologic disorders (Davison, 1976), hormones, behavior, and psychopathology (Sachar, 1976), and aging and dementia (Smith and Kinsbourne, 1977). Increasing social and physical isolation during aging undoubtedly influence the incidence of some mental impairments and neurologic disorders (Woodruff, 1975; Weg, 1975). As cited in this chapter, it has been relatively well established that there is decreasing stimulus input and sensory information processing in the brain during aging (Ordy and Brizzee, 1979). It has been suggested that increasing social and physical isolation may result in a state analogous to sensory deprivation. The effects of increasing social and physical isolation become superimposed on the normal age declines in sensory capacity that occur gradually and almost imperceptibly in different sensory modalities from maturity to old age. Recent studies of brain plasticity, memory, and aging have suggested that age declines in memory may be related to decreased biochemical and anatomical plasticity of the brain (Bennett and Rosenzweig, 1979). A very important but neglected issue in neurobiology of aging is the extent to which sensory stimulation is essential for the maintenance of the normal physiological, chemical, and morphological organization of the brain from maturity to old age. A sensory deprivation model of aging has been proposed (Woodruff, 1975).

There is an increased incidence of mental impairment, loss of memory, and depression in old age. Age declines in memory are related to reduced learning capacity, altered arousal or motivation, loss of motor coordination, or some combination of these factors. Mental capacity has generally been associated with the cerebral cortex and arousal, motivation, and reinforcement have been associated with the limbic and autonomic systems and endocrine organs. The most significant correlations among age decline and intellectual impairment, EEG, stimulus-evoked potentials (AEP), cerebral circulation, and metabolism have been reported in some psychiatric and neurologic disorders, senile dementia, and organic brain syndromes (Thompson, 1976). Similarly, the highest correlations among intellectual capacity, regional cerebral blood flow, and neurotransmitter imbalances have been reported in multiple infarct dementia and Altzheimer's disease (Meyer et al., 1976). Estimates of cell loss by biosynthetic enzyme activity and neurotransmitter concentration in biopsy tissue

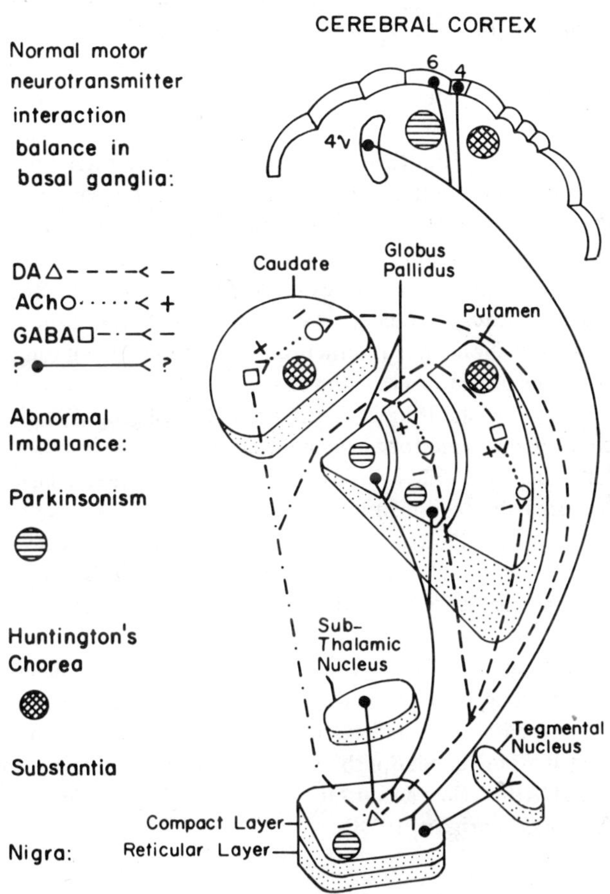

Figure 13 Imbalances among dopaminergic, cholinergic, and GABAergic transmitters in basal ganglia in parkinsonism and Huntington's chorea.

samples also indicate selective vulnerability or loss of cholinergic and GABAergic neurons from the cortex of patients suffering from Altzheimer's disease (Davison, 1976; Spillane et al., 1977). Impaired capacity to learn more complex tasks and defects in short-term memory consolidation become most prominent under hypoxic conditions. These learning and memory deficits improve after CO_2 administration. Depression and drug effects are also frequent manifestations in many cases of senile dementia and organic psychosis. The most prominent concomitant degenerative changes in the brain characterized physiologically, biochemically, and morphologically have been reported in the grey matter of the cerebral cortex and hippocampus. Age-dependent imbalances, not only in neurotransmitters, neuropeptides, particularly in output of neuroendocrine transducer cells, and also imbalances among circulating hormones that have the brain as target organ have now been identified as possible sources of aging and possibly the increasing incidence of brain diseases during aging (Ordy and Kaack, 1976).

In terms of motor output, considerable progress has been reported in clarification of imbalances among dopaminergic, cholinergic, and GABAergic systems in Parkinson's and Huntington's diseases (Barbeau, 1978). According to histochemical fluorescent studies, dopaminergic axons from the substantia nigra project to the caudate, putamen, and globus pallidum. Using immunohistochemical techniques for ChAc, it has been demonstrated that these structures, in turn, are found to contain cholinergic interneurons. From these basal ganglia nuclei, GABAergic neurons project back to the substantia nigra and other regions of the brain. In the normal adult brain circuits of the basal ganglia, a proper balance of these excitatory and inhibitory neuron interactions is essential for optimum motor performance. Even mild symptoms of Parkinson's disease have been associated with reduced striatal dopamine. In Huntington's chorea, the caudate appears more affected pathologically than the putamen. In this disorder, there is greater decrease in ChAc, and consequently ACh, in the caudate nuclei. Symptoms of Parkinson's disease and Huntington's chorea appear related not only to significant decreases in DA, or GAD, but each of these diseases appears related to specific patterns of imbalance between dopaminergic and cholinergic neurotransmitter interactions, or between dopaminergic and GABAergic interactions, respectively, in the basal ganglia (McGeer and McGeer, 1976). Figure 13 illustrates proposed anatomical relationships and imbalances among dopaminergic, cholinergic, and GABAergic transmitters in the basal ganglia in parkinsonism and Huntington's chorea (Barbeau, 1978).

IX. ENVIRONMENTAL MODIFIABILITY OF THE RATE OF AGING IN THE BRAIN

One of the most important questions with significant consequences to each individual and society is whether the structural and functional declines in the human brain are genetically fixed and inevitable; or whether there are prospects involving behavioral, pharmacological, and other biological strategies of intervention that can be used for modifying the rate of aging in the brain and ameliorating some of the brain disorders during senescence. Observations in human and animal studies suggest that a wide range of environmental variables can influence the brain, the rate of aging, and the average life-span. Major environmental variables that have been considered are nutrition, exercise, stress, drugs (particularly alcohol and tobacco), accidents (primarily the effects of head injury), radiation, infectious diseases, and immunological competence (Makinodan, 1979). Numerous studies have shown improved mental performance in the elderly as a result of improved cardiovascular and muscular fitness based on nutrition and exercise (Weg, 1975; DeVries, 1975). Another promising behavioral strategy for intervention includes biofeedback conditioning to reduce declining or maximize residual capacity in the older subjects (Woodruff, 1975). The effects of improved nutrition and exercise are more desirable since there are fewer side effects. However, due to promptness of effects, demand, expediency, and a great variety of other reasons, psychopharmacology constitutes an inevitable, although not necessarily a desirable, mode of intervention (Lehmann, 1979; Ordy, 1979). Clinically, greater knowledge of drug effects on the brain during aging is essential since drug "intoxication" is frequently mistaken for depression and mental impairment in dementia and organic syndromes. Finally, problems of polypharmacy, abuse, and overuse in any drug-dependent culture make it imperative to obtain a greater understanding of psychoactive drugs that affect mental capacity, electrical activity, cerebral circulation, metabolism, autonomic function, and cardiovascular physiology during aging (Eisdorfer and Fann, 1973; Ban, 1978; Ordy et al., 1980c).

X. RECENT DEVELOPMENTS

The findings reviewed in this chapter make it apparent that within a broader neuroscience framework, neurochemistry can contribute significantly to: (1) clarification of age differences in chemical composition, metabolism, and neurotransmitters of the brain, (2) changes in sensory, learning, memory, and motor capacities, and (3) increasing incidence of mental impairments and neurologic disorders with age. This neuroscience approach conceptualizes the brain as an organ that is uniquely specialized for the acquisition, storage, and retrieval of information, generally defined as learning and memory. Satisfactory explanations of sensory function, learning, and memory are not yet available in terms of specific molecular, physiological, chemical, and anatomical mechanisms. It is widely accepted that within an information processing framework, sensory function, learning, and memory include neurophysiological or electrical events, followed by neurochemical events, ultimately resulting in long-term memory based on chemical and/or anatomical changes in specific regions of the brain. Recent developments in neurobiology of aging include: (1) coupling of sensory function and short-term memory, (2) reality and significance of short-term memory impairment in the elderly, (3) development of three-stage, time-dependent, convergent multisensory, stimulus-reward coupling, neurobiology model of memory localized within the cerebral cortex and limbic system, (4) prospects of "nootropic" drug and dietary lecithin or choline precursor improvement of memory, mood, and cholinergic brain function in the elderly, and (5) alternative theoretical views of the brain, behavior, and aging.

Coupling of sensory function and short-term memory: Sensory function, learning, memory, and perceptual-motor skills are intimately related. Learning and memory depend first upon a sensory information input, registration, or acquisition stage. Information is received and transduced by modality specific sensory systems, passed on to short-term or primary memory (STM-PM)—which represents a limited store comprising items of sensory images or features—and followed by transfer of information to long-term or secondary memory (LTM-SM), which may be based on rehearsal and/or reinforcement (Marcer, 1974; Craik, 1977). Sensory memory (SM) is considered to be modality specific (i.e., iconic, echoic, etc.); its duration is presumed to be milliseconds, or at most a few seconds; and it decays rapidly with time (Crowder, 1978). Short-term memory, or so-called primary memory, is believed to occur across sensory modalities. Its duration may range from 2 to 30 seconds, and it may also decay promptly, due to interference or lack of reinforced practice (Deutsch and Deutsch, 1975). Although short-term memory represents only a small segment of learning or information processing, it may be of crucial importance for encoding, storage, and retrieval of all information. It may represent the basic control process for all thinking, remembering, and consciousness (Atkinson and Shiffrin, 1971).

Reality and significance of short-term memory impairment in the elderly: One of the more widely accepted views is that recent or short-term memory becomes impaired, whereas long-term memory for remote events remains relatively unimpaired (Marcer, 1974). In contrast to this widespread belief, recent authoritative reviews of short-term memory impairment in the elderly have concluded that (1) short-term or primary memory (PM) may be of less concern than long-term or secondary memory (SM) to the elderly, unless, memory, or information processing is conceptualized as "flowing from PM to SM (or even sensory memory to PM to SM)" (Botwinick, 1975); (2) short-term memory may not be impaired in the elderly, or "age differences in PM are negligible," if the sensory information is adequately perceived and registered, or provided that elderly subjects are not required to divide their attention between two sensory inputs, or to reorganize the material (Craik, 1977). There is considerable experimental evidence for negligible effects of age on some short-term memory tasks (Craik, 1977). Significant effects of age on short-term memory have also been demonstrated independent of age differences in sensory function, learning, motivation, and motor performance, particularly in animal studies (Ordy et al., 1978; Bartus, 1979a). However, recently, it has also been recognized that age declines in multisensory function, short-term memory, increased susceptibility to sensory interference, and decreased capacity to modify previously learned behavior may represent some of the more prominent characteristics of aged humans and nonhuman primates (Bartus, 1979a; Ordy et al., 1980a). Although theoretical views concerning the interpretation of short-term memory as a brief "organizing process," or as a "time-dependent, convergent multisensory, stimulus-reward coupling process in the cerebral cortex and limbic system" may differ, there is increasing evidence, based on signal detection methodology, that in the elderly, there may be a decreasing capacity to register, encode, store, and retrieve information over brief periods of time (Harkins et al., 1979). This has been demonstrated for visual short-term memory (Adamowicz, 1976), auditory short-term memory (Clark and Knowles, 1973), and particularly when visual and auditory stimuli are presented in combination (Craik, 1977, 1979). Consequently, it has been proposed that age declines in modality specific memory, and particularly in convergent multisensory information processing in multimodal sensory integration centers within the cerebral cortex and limbic system, must play an important role in short-term memory impairment during aging (Ordy et al., 1980a).

Development of three-stage, time-dependent, convergent multisensory, stimulus-reward coupling, neurobiology model of short-term memory within cerebral cortex and limbic system: Even though generally not concerned with neuronal networks of convergent multisensory integration and short-term memory, the more recent experimental literature on the effects of age on human memory has been interpreted within a three-stage information processing framework (Ordy et al., 1980a). However, the previous emphasis has been on short-term memory as a "brief organizing process," rather than on the specific sequence and duration of information flowing from sensory memory, to primary, or short-term memory, and then to long-term, or secondary memory (Craik, 1977). There is now considerable behavioral, physiological, chemical, pharmacological, and anatomical evidence in support of conceptualizing short-term memory as part of a "convergent multisensory, time-dependent, stimulus-reward coupling process," involving specific circuits in the cerebral cortex and in the limbic system (Ordy et al., 1980a).

Studies of sensory functions in the elderly have been restricted to a single sensory modality. They have focused on peripheral sense organs without reference to afferent pathways, convergent multisensory integration, and stimulus-reward coupling mechanisms within the cerebral cortex and limbic system. If reference was made to afferent pathways, it was generally assumed that they "terminate" in the primary sensory projection areas of the cerebral cortex. Recent studies have begun to place greater emphasis on convergent multisensory integration not only within the cerebral cortex but also in the limbic system, particularly the hippocampus as a multisensory and stimulus-reward coupling center of the brain (Swanson, 1979). According to recent studies, visual, auditory, and somatosensory inputs from respective sensory cortical areas relay convergent multisensory information to the entorhinal area, the hippocampus, medial dorsal thalamus, and principal gyrus of the frontal lobe. Neuroendocrine studies have identified neuropeptide and hormone receptors in hippocampal circuits which may provide for the coupling of convergent sensory information and also the reward properties of stimuli. Since the hippocampus has been implicated in convergent sensory integration, stimulus-reward coupling, spatial orientation, short-term memory, and in neuroendocrine regulation of endocrine and autonomic function, it has received increasing attention in aging (Brizzee and Ordy, 1979; Ordy et al., 1980a).

Prospects of nootropic, or mind-acting, drugs and dietary lecithin or choline precursor improvement of memory, mood, and cholinergic brain function in the elderly: The first compound of a new class of psychoactive drugs for which the term nootropic, or mind acting drug, was proposed for improvement of memory was piracetam. In the initial report it was claimed that the new drug promoted interhemispheric transfer of information, protected memory against amnestic agents, and facilitated EEG recovery after severe hypoxia, in doses which had no demonstrable effects on the limbic system, autonomic functions, and psychomotor behavior (Gieurgea, 1973). Subsequently, it was proposed that piracetam represents a new nootropic drug for selective improvement of learning and memory, through direct effects on telencephalic integration centers, without effects on autonomic nervous system activity or psychomotor behavior (Gieurgea, 1976). In addition to piracetam, such other compounds as hydergine, centrophenoxine, vincamine, and naftidrofuryl have been proposed as possible psychoactive drugs for improvement of memory in the elderly (Lehmann, 1979). Comprehensive reviews of clinical trials with these drugs have concluded that the effects on learning and memory in the elderly are equivocal (Lehmann, 1979; Ordy, 1979). Studies with animals have reported that so-called nootropic drugs may improve cerebral circulation, increase cerebral glucose metabolism, improve cellular metabolism through modification of enzyme activity, reduce the accumulation of lipofuscin, and possibly retard the loss of neurons in the brain (Lehmann, 1979). However, recent studies have reported that hydergine (Clemens and Fuller, 1978), and piracetam (Nybäck et al., 1979) alter serum prolactin levels in the rat, suggesting that CNS effects include blockade of dopamine receptors, similar to the effects of neuroleptic drugs with antipsychotic actions.

Significant advances in "mapping" of central acetylcholine and other neurotransmitter pathways, and new pharmacological evidence on the possible role of the cholinergic system in learning, memory, and affective states have enhanced interest in the cholinergic system (Goldberg and Hanin, 1976). An increasing number of researchers have examined the effects of such cholinergic drugs as physostigmine and atropine on learning and memory in relation to aging of human (Drachman, 1978) and nonhuman primates (Bartus, 1979b). Oral administration of choline and dietary intake of lecithin, the nutritional source of choline, have been reported to increase serum levels of choline, and also brain levels of choline and acetylcholine in some animal species (Cohen and Wurtman, 1976). Clinical trials, based on the "transmitter precursor strategy" for modifying the cholinergic system, have reported some cognitive improvements in patients treated for certain neuropsychiatric disorders with choline or lecithin

(Davis and Berger, 1979). In preliminary clinical trials, elderly patients with Alzheimer's disease showed improved orientation and mood after taking 5 or 10 g of choline per day for 4 weeks (Boyd et al., 1977). However, a more recent study with normal elderly subjects concluded that the effects on memory were negligible, and larger groups of normal elderly persons must be studied to determine whether or not quantifiable, significant improvements in human memory can be produced by increased dietary choline intake (Mohs et al., 1979). Since there is preliminary basic and clinical evidence that the cholinergic system may become impaired with age, cholinergic drugs and dietary supplements of choline and lecithin appear as inevitable and possibly useful agents and precursors for improving memory and cholinergic brain function in the elderly (Drachman, 1978; Wurtman and Growdon, 1979).

Alternative theoretical models of the brain, behavior, and aging: There is a considerable descriptive literature on the brain, behavior, and aging. Faced with complexity and gaps in knowledge, a number of alternative views or models have been proposed for major sources of aging in the brain. Theoretical models, both general and specific, deal with environmental or biological sources of aging in the brain, prospects of intervention, and modification of the rate of aging. According to the *life-span developmental model,* the alleged loss of intellectual capacity is currently attributed mainly to a biological decremental model of human subjects. However, age declines in intellectual capacity may be a myth. Cognitive declines are based on methodological artifacts which include confounding between maturational age and cultural cohort or secular trend effects (Schaie, 1977). Improved intellectual capacity due to secular trend benefits maximize or exaggerate age differences between currently young and old subjects. Age declines in intelligence, learning, and memory may be attributable primarily to such environmental factors as increasing social and physical isolation, decreased sensory stimulation, motivation, and inappropriate tests for remaining mental capacity. Age declines in learning and memory may be due primarily to these environmental factors rather than biological decremental processes in the brain. In contrast to the life-span developmental model, in the *neurobiology of aging model,* the brain is an information-processing organ with postmitotic or nonrenewable cells. Despite enormous redundancy and reserve capacity, there is an age decline in information-processing capacity of the brain extending from sensory input to learning, memory, and motor output. This functional decline may be due in part to an intrinsically programmed and selective loss of cells and their connectivity, such concomitant alterations as lipofuscin accumulation in remaining cells, decreasing neuronal plasticity, imbalances within and among neurotransmitters, neuropeptides, and ultimately reduced sensory, learning, memory, and motor capacity. Chronological age and biological age do not coincide. Genetic-environmental interactions may determine the onset and linear and/or exponential rate of decline in the brain from maturity to old age.

REFERENCES

Abrahams, J. P. (1976). Physiological correlates of cardiovascular diseases. In *Special Review of Experimental Aging Research,* M. F. Elias, B. E. Eleftheriou, and P. K. Elias (Eds.). EAR, Inc., Bar Harbor, Me., pp. 330-350.

Adamowicz, J. K. (1976). Visual short-term memory and aging. *J. Gerontol. 31,* 39-46.

Andres, R., and Tobin, J. D. (1977). Endocrine Systems. In *Handbook of the Biology of Aging,* C. E. Finch and L. Hayflick (Eds.). Van Nostrand, New York, pp. 357-378.

Arenberg, D., and Robertson-Tchabo, G. A. (1977). Learning and aging. In *Handbook of the Psychology of Aging,* J. E. Birren and K. W. Schaie (Eds.). Van Nostrand, New York, pp. 421-449.

Atkinson, R. C., and Schiffrin, R. M. (1971). The control of short-term memory. *Sci. Am. 224,* 82-90.

Bahrick, H. P., Bahrick, P. O., and Wittlinger, R. P. (1975). Fifty years of memory for names and faces: a cross-sectional approach. *J. Exp. Psych.: General 104,* 54-75.

Ban, T. A. (1978). Vasodilators, stimulants, and anabolic agents in the treatment of geropsychiatric patients. In *Psychopharmacology: A Generation of Progress,* M. A. Lipton, A. DiMascio, and K. F. Killam (Eds.). Raven, New York, pp. 1525-1533.

Barbeau, A. (1978). The last ten years of progress in the clinical pharmacology of extrapyramidal symptoms. In. *Psychopharmacology: A Generation of Progress,* M. A. Lipton, A. DiMascio, and K. F. Killam (Eds.). Raven, New York, pp. 771-776.

Bartus, R. T. (1979a). Effects of aging on visual memory, sensory processing, and discrimination learning in a nonhuman primate. In *Aging,* Vol. 10, *Sensory Systems and Communication in the Elderly,* J. M. Ordy and K. R. Brizzee (Eds.). Raven, New York, pp. 85-114.

Bartus, R. T. (1979b). Physostigmine and recent memory: effects in young and aged nonhuman primates. *Science 206,* 1087-1089.

Beck, E. C., Dustman, R. E., and Schenkenberg, T. (1975). Life-span changes in the electrical activity of the human brain as reflected in the cerebral evoked response. In *Neurobiology of Aging,* J. M. Ordy and K. R. Brizzee (Eds.). Plenum, New York, pp. 175-192.

Beck, E. C., Dustman, R. E., Blusewicz, M. J., and Cannon, W. G. (1979). Cerebral evoked potentials and correlated neurophysiological changes in the human brain during aging. A comparison of alcoholism and aging. In *Aging,* Vol. 10, *Sensory Systems and Communication in the Elderly,* J. M. Ordy and K. R. Brizzee (Eds.). Raven, New York, pp. 203-226.

Bennett, E. L., and Rosenzweig, M. R. (1979). Brain plasticity, memory, and aging. In *Aging* (Vol. 8): *Physiology and Cell Biology of Aging,* A. Cherkin, C. E. Finch, N. Kharasch, T. Makinodan, F. L. Scott, and B. S. Stiehler (Eds.). Raven, New York, pp. 141-150.

Birren, J. E. (1965). Age changes in speed of behavior. Its central nature and physiological correlates. In *Behavior, Aging and the Nervous System,* A. T. Welford and J. E. Birren (Eds.). Thomas, Springfield, Ill. pp. 191-216.

Birren, J. E., and Schaie, K. W. (Eds.). (1977). *Handbook of the Psychology of Aging,* Vol. 2. Van Nostrand, New York.

Blinkov, S. M., and Glazer, I. I. (1968). *The Human Brain in Figures and Tables.* Plenum, New York.

Bodian, D. (1967). Neurons, circuits, and neuroglia. In *The Neurosciences,* G. C. Quarton, T. Melnechuk, and F. D. Schmitt (Eds.). Rockefeller Univ., New York, p. 17, Fig. 10.

Bondareff, W., and Geinisman, Y. (1976). Loss of synapses in the dentate gyrus of the senescent rat. *Am. J. Anat. 145(1),* 129-136.

Bondareff, W., and Narotzky, R. (1972). Age changes in the neuronal micro-environment. *Science 176,* 1135-1136.

Botwinick, J. (1965). Theories of antecedent conditions of speed of response. In *Behavior, Aging and the Nervous System,* A. T. Welford and J. E. Birren (Eds.). Thomas, Springfield, Ill., pp. 57-87.

Botwinick, J. (1973). *Aging and Behavior.* Springer, New York.

Botwinick, J. (1975). *Aging and Behavior: a Comprehensive Integration of Research Findings,* 2nd ed. Springer, New York, pp. 311-322.

Botwinick, J. (1977). Intellectual abilities. In *Handbook of the Psychology of Aging,* J. E. Birren and K. W. Schaie (Eds.). Van Nostrand, New York, pp. 580-605.

Boyd, W. D., Grahan-White, J., Blackwood, G., Glen, I., and McQueen, J. (1977). Clinical effects of choline in Alzheimer senile dementia. *Lancet 2,* 711.

Brizzee, K. R. (1975). Gross morphometric analyses and quantitative histology of the aging brain. In *Neurobiology of Aging,* J. M. Ordy and K. R. Brizzee (Eds.). Plenum, New York, pp. 401-424.

Brizzee, K. R., and Ordy, J. M. (1979). Effects of age on visceral afferent components of the autonomic nervous system. In *Aging,* Vol. 10, *Sensory Systems and Communication in the Elderly.* J. M. Ordy and K. R. Brizzee (Eds.). Raven, New York, pp. 283-296.

Brizzee, K. R., Ordy, J. M., Hansche, J., and Kaack, B. (1976). Quantitative assessment of changes in neuron and glia cell packing density and lipofuscin accumulation with age in the cerebral cortex of a nonhuman primate *(Macaca mulatta).* In *Aging: Neurobiology of Aging,* R. Terry and S. Gershon (Eds.). Raven, New York, pp. 229-244.

Brizzee, K. R., Ordy, J. M., and Bartus, R. T. (1980). Short-term memory: localization of cellular changes within multimodal sensory regions in aged monkey brain. *J. Neurobiol. Aging 1*(1), 45-52.

Brody, H. (1976). An examination of cerebral cortex and brainstem aging. In *Aging: Neurobiology of Aging,* R. Terry and S. Gershon (Eds.). Raven, New York, pp. 177-182.

Cauthen, N. R. (1977). Extension of the Wechsler memory scale norms to older age groups. *J. Clin. Psychol. 33,* 208-211.

Cherkin, A., Finch, C. E., Kharasch, N., Makinodan, T., Scott, F. L., and Strehler, B. (Eds.) (1979). *Aging,* Vol. 8, *Physiology and Cell Biology of Aging,* Raven, New York.

Clark, L. E., and Knowles, J. B. (1973). Age differences in dichotic listening performance. *J. Gerontol. 28,* 173-178.

Clemens, J. A., and Fuller, R. W. (1978). Chemical manipulation of some aspects of aging. In *Pharmacological Intervention in the Aging Process,* J. Roberts, R. C. Adelman, and V. J. Cristofalo (Eds.). Plenum, New York, pp. 187-206.

Cohen, E. L., and Wurtman, R. J. (1976). Brain acetylcholine: increase after systematic choline administration. *Life Sci. 16,* 1095-1102.

Corsellis, J. A. N. (1976). Some observations on the Purkinje cell population and on brain volume in human aging. In *Aging: Neurobiology of Aging,* R. Terry and S. Gershon (Eds.). Raven, New York, pp. 205-210.

Corso, J. F. (1975). Sensory processes in man during maturity and senescence. In *Neurobiology of Aging,* J. M. Ordy and K. R. Brizzee (Eds.). Plenum, New York, pp. 119-144.

Cotman, C. W., and Scheff, S. W. (1979). Synaptic plasticity in the hippocampus in the aged rat. In *Aging,* Vol. 8, *Physiology and Cell Biology of Aging,* A. Cherkin, C. W. Finch, N. Kharasch, T. Makinodan, F. L. Scott, and B. Strehler (Eds.). Raven, New York, pp. 109-130.

Craik, F. I. M. (1977). Age differences in human memory. In *Handbook of the Psychology of Aging,* J. E. Birren and K. W. Schaie (Eds.). Van Nostrand, New York, pp. 384-420.

Craik, F. I. M. (1979). Human memory. In *Annual Review of Psychology,* Vol. 30, M. R. Rosenzweig and L. W. Porter (Eds.). Annual Reviews, Palo Alto, Calif., pp. 63-102.

Crowder, R. G. (1978). Sensory memory systems. In *Handbook of Perception,* E. C. Carterette and M. P. Friedman (Eds.). Academic, New York, pp. 239-260.

Curtis, H. J. (1966). *Biological Mechanisms of Aging.* Thomas, Springfield, Ill.

Cutler, R. G. (1976). Evolution of longevity in primates. *J. Hum. Ev. 5,* 169-202.

Dastur, D. K., Lane, M. H., Hansen, D. B., Kety, S. S., Butler, R. N., Perlin, S., and Sokoloff, L. (1963). Effects of aging on cerebral circulation and metabolism in man. In *Human Aging,* J. E. Birren, R. N. Butler, S. W. Greenhouse, L. Sokoloff, and M. R. Yarrow (Eds.). U. S. Department of Health, Education and Welfare, Washington, D. C., pp. 59-76.

Davis, K. L., and Berger, P. A. (Eds.) (1979). *Brain Acetylcholine and Neuropsychiatric Disease,* Plenum, New York.

Davison, A. N. (Ed.) (1976). *Biochemistry and Neurological Disease,* Blackwells, London.

Deutsch, D., and Deutsch, J. A. (1975). *Short-term Memory,* Academic, New York.

Devaney, K. O., and Johnson, H. A. (1980). Neuron loss in the Aging Visual Cortex of man. *J. Gerontol.* In press.

DeVries, H. A. (1975). Physiology of exercise and aging. In *Aging: Scientific Perspectives and Social Issues,* D. Woodruff and J. E. Birren (Eds.). Van Nostrand, New York, pp. 257-276.

de Wied, D. (1974). Pituitary-adrenal system hormones and behavior. In *The Neurosciences: Third Study Program,* F. O. Schmitt and F. G. Worden (Eds.). MIT Press, Cambridge, Mass., pp. 653-666.

de Wied, D. (1977). Behavioral effects of neuropeptides related to ACTH, MSH, and BLPH. *Ann. N. Y. Acad. Sci. 297,* 263-274.

Domino, E. F., Dren, A. T., and Giardina, W. J. (1978). Biochemical and neurotransmitter changes in the aging brain. In *Psychopharmacology: A Generation of Progress,* M. A. Lipton, A. DiMascio, and K. F. Killam (Eds.). Raven, New York, pp. 1507-1516.

Drachman, D. A. (1978). Central cholinergic system and memory. In *Psychopharmacology: A Generation of Progress,* M. A. Lipton, A. DiMascio, and K. F. Killam (Eds.). Raven, New York, pp. 651-662.

Drachman, D. A., and Leavitt, J. (1974). Human memory and the cholinergic system. A relationship to aging? *Arch. Neurol. 30,* 113-121.

Eisdorfer, C., and Fann, W. E. (1973). *Psychopharmacology and Aging,* Plenum, New York.

Eisdorfer, C., and Raskind, M. (1975). Aging, hormones and human behavior. In *Hormonal Correlates of Behavior,* B. F. Eleftheriou and R. L. Sprott (Eds.). Plenum, New York, pp. 369-394.

Elias, M. F., and Elias, P. K. (1975). Hormones, aging and behavior in infrahuman mammals. In *Hormonal Correlates of Behavior,* B. E. Eleftheriou and R. L. Sprott (Eds.). Plenum, New York, pp. 395-439.

Elias, M. F., and Elias, P. K. (1977). Motivation and Activity. In *Handbook of the Psychology of Aging,* J. E. Birren and K. W. Schaie (Eds.). Van Nostrand, New York, pp. 357-374.

Everitt, A. V., and Burgess, J. A. (1976). *Hypothalamus, Pituitary and Aging,* Thomas, Springfield, Ill.

Fang, H. C. H. (1976). Observations on aging characteristics of cerebral blood vessels, macroscopic and microscopic features. In *Aging: Neurobiology of Aging,* R. Terry and S. Gershon (Eds.). Raven, New York, pp. 155-166.

Feldman, M. L. (1976). Aging changes in morphology of cortical dendrites. In *Aging: Neurobiology of Aging,* R. Terry and S. Gershon (Eds.). Raven, New York, pp. 211-228.

Finch, C. E. (1973). Catecholamine metabolism in the brains of ageing male mice. *Brain Res. 52,* 261-276.

Finch, C. E. (1975). Aging and the regulation of hormones. A review in October, 1974. In *Explorations in Aging,* V. J. Cristofalo, J. Roberts, and R. C. Adelman (Eds.). Plenum, New York, pp. 229-238.

Finch, C. E. (1977). Neuroendocrine and autonomic aspects of aging. In *Handbook of the Biology of Aging,* C. E. Finch and L. Hayflick (Eds.). Van Nostrand, New York, pp. 262-280.

Fozard, L. F., Wolf, E., Bell, B., McFarland, R. A., and Podolsky, S. (1977). Visual perception and communication. In *Handbook of the Psychology of Aging,* Vol. 2, J. E. Birren and K. W. Schaie (Eds.). Van Nostrand, New York, pp. 497-534.

Freeman, J. T. (1967). Endocrinology in geriatrics. Historical background. In *Endocrines and Aging,* L. Gitman (Ed.). Thomas, Springfield, Ill., pp. 3-35.

Frolkis, V. V. (1977). Aging of the autonomic nervous system. In *Handbook of the Psychology of Aging,* J. E. Birren and K. W. Schaie (Eds.). Van Nostrand, New York, pp. 177-189.

Gershon, D., and Gershon, H. (1976). An evaluation of the "error catastrophe" theory of ageing in the light of recent experimental results. *Gerontology 22,* 212-219.

Gieurgea, C. (1973). The "nootropic" approach to the integrative activity of the brain. *Con. Reflex 8,* 108-115.

Gieurgea, C. (1976). Piracetam. Nootropic pharmacology of neurointegrative activity. In *Current Developments in Psychopharmacology,* Vol. 3, W. B. Essman and L. Valzelli (Eds.). Spectrum, New York, pp. 222-273.

Gold, P. E., and McGaugh, J. L. (1975). Changes in learning and memory during aging. In *Neurobiology of Aging,* J. M. Ordy and K. R. Brizzee (Eds.). Plenum, New York, pp. 145-158.

Goldberg, A. M., and Hanin, I. (Eds.). (1976). *Biology of Cholinergic Function.* Raven, New York.

Gregerman, R. I. (1967). The age-related alteration of thyroid function and thyroid hormone metabolism in man. In *Endocrines and Aging,* L. Gitman (Ed.). Thomas, Springfield, Ill., pp. 161-173.

Gutmann, E., and Hanzlikova, V. (1975). Changes in neuromuscular relationships in aging. In *Neurobiology of Aging,* J. M. Ordy and K. R. Brizzee (Eds.). Plenum, New York, pp. 193-208.

Halgin, R., Riklan, M., and Misiak, H. (1977). LevoDOPA, Parkinsonism and recent memory. *J. Nerv. Ment. Dis. 164,* 268-272.

Hansch, E. C., Syndulko, K., Pirozzolo, F. J., Cohen, S. N., Tourtellotte, W. W., and Potvin, A. R. (1980). Electrophysiological measurement in aging and dementia. In *The Aging Nervous System,* G. J. Maletta and F. J. Pirozzolo (Eds.). Praeger, New York, pp. 187-210.

Harkins, S. W., Chapman, C. R., and Eisdorfer, C. (1979). Memory loss and response bias in senescence. *J. Gerontol. 34,* 66-72.

Hasan, M., and Glees, P. (1973). Ultrastructural age changes in hippocampal neurons, synapses and neuroglia. *Exp. Gerontol. 8,* 75-83.

Hassler, R. (1965). Extrapyramidal control of the speed of behavior and its change by primary age processes. In *Behavior, Aging and the Nervous System,* A. T. Welford and J. E. Birren (Eds.). Thomas, Springfield, Ill., pp. 284-306.

Hayflick, L. (1975). Cell biology of aging. *Bioscience 25,* 629-637.

Heiss, W. D., Waltz, A. G., and Hayakawa, T. (1975). Neuronal function and local blood flow during experimental cerebral ischaemia. In *Blood Flow and Metabolism in the Brain,* A. M. Harper, W. B. Nennett, J. D. Miller, and J. O. Rowan (Eds.). Churchill-Livingston, Edinburgh, sec. 14.27.

Hermann, R. L. (1971). Aging. In *Handbook of Neurochemistry,* Vol. 5, Pt. B, *Metabolic Turnover in the Nervous System,* A. Lajtha (Ed.). Plenum, New York, pp. 481-488.

Hess, H. H., and Pope, A. (1972). Quantitative neurochemical histology. In *Handbook of Neurochemistry,* Vol. 7, *Pathological Chemistry of the Nervous System,* A. Lajtha (Ed.). Plenum, New York, pp. 289-328.

Himwich, H. E. (1959). Biochemistry of the nervous system in relation to the process of aging. In *The Process of Aging in the Nervous System,* J. E. Birren, H. A. Imus, and W. F. Windle (Eds.). Thomas, Springfield, Ill., pp. 101-112.

Iversen, S. D. (1976). *Behavioral Pharmacology,* Oxford, New York.

Iversen, S. D., and Iversen, L. L. (1975a). Chemical pathways in the brain. In *Handbook of Psychobiology,* M. S. Gazzaniga and C. Blakemore (Eds.). Academic, New York, pp. 141-152.

Iversen, S. D., and Iversen, L. L. (1975b). Central neurotransmitters and the regulation of behavior. In *Handbook of Psychobiology,* M. S. Gazzaniga and C. Blakemore (Eds.). Academic, New York, pp. 153-200.

John, E. R. (1972). Switchboard versus statistical theories of learning and memory. *Science 177,* 850-864.

Kaack, B., Ordy, J. M., and Trapp, B. (1975). Changes in limbic, neuroendocrine and autonomic systems, adaptation, homeostasis during aging. In *Neurobiology of Aging,* J. M. Ordy and K. R. Brizzee (Eds.). Plenum, New York, pp. 209-232.

Kenshalo, D. R., Sr. (1979). Changes in the vestibular and somesthetic systems as a function of age. In *Aging,* Vol. 10, *Sensory Systems and Communication in the Elderly,* J. M. Ordy and K. R. Brizzee (Eds.). Raven, New York, pp. 269-282.

Klorman, R., Thompson, L. W., and Ellingson, R. J. (1978). Event-related brain potentials across the life span. In *Event Related Brain Potentials in Man,* E. Callanag, R. Tenting, and S. H. Koslow (Eds.). Academic, New York, pp. 511-570.

Kohn, R. (1971). *Principles of Mammalian Aging,* Prentice-Hall, Englewood, N.J.

Landfield, P. W., Rose, G., Sandles, L., Wohlstadter, T. C., and Lynch, G. (1977). Patterns of astroglial hypertrophy and neuronal degeneration in the hippocampus of aged, memory-deficient rats. *J. Gerontol. 32,* 3-12.

Landfield, P. W., McGaugh, J. L., and Lynch, G. (1978). Impaired synaptic potentiation processes in the hippocampus of aged, memory-deficient rats. *Brain Res. 105,* 85-101.

Lehmann, H. E. (1979). Psychopharmacotherapy in psychogeriatric disorders. In *Brain Function in Old Age,* F. Hoffmeister and C. Muller (Eds.). Springer-Verlag, Berlin, pp. 456-479.

McEwen, B. S., Denef, C. J., Gerlach, J. L., and Plapinger, L. (1974). Chemical studies of the brain as a steroid hormone target tissue. In *The Neurosciences: Third Study Program,* F. O. Schmitt and F. G. Worden (Eds.). MIT, Cambridge, Mass., pp. 599-620.

McGaugh, J. L., Gold, P. E., VanBuskirk, R., and Haycock, J. (1975). Modulating influences of hormones and catecholamines on memory storage processes. In *Progress in Brain Research,* Vol. 42, *Hormones, Homeostasis and the Brain,* W. H. Gispen, T. B. van Wimersma Greidanus, B. Bohus, and D. De Wied (Eds.). Elsevier, Amsterdam, pp. 151-162.

McGeer, E., and McGeer, P. (1976). Neurotransmitter metabolism in the aging brain. In *Aging: Neurobiology of Aging,* R. Terry and S. Gershon (Eds.). Raven, New York, pp. 389-404.

McGrady, P. M. (1968). *The Youth Doctors,* Coward-McCann, New York.

Makinodan, T. (1979). Prevention and restoration of age-associated impaired normal immune functions. In *Aging,* Vol. 8, *Physiology and Cell Biology of Aging,* A. Cherkin, C. E. Finch, N. Kharasch, T. Makinodan, F. L. Scott, and B. S. Strehler (Eds.). Raven, New York, pp. 61-70.

Marcer, D. (1974). Aging and memory loss – role of experimental psychology. *Gerontol. Clin. 16,* 118-125.

Marsh, G. R. (1976). Electrophysiological correlates of aging and behavior. In *Special Review of Experimental Aging Research,* M. F. Elias, B. E. Eleftheriou, and P. K. Elias (Eds.). EAR, Inc., Bar Harbor, Me., pp. 165-180.

Marsh, G. R., and Thompson, L. W. (1977). Psychophysiology of aging. In *Handbook of the Psychology of Aging,* J. E. Birren and K. W. Schaie (Eds.). Van Nostrand, New York, pp. 219-248.

Mason, J. (1975). Emotion as reflected in patterns of endocrine integration. In *Emotions: Their Parameters and Measurement,* L. Levi (Ed.). Raven, New York, pp. 143-181.

Medin, D. L., O'Neil, P., Smeltz, E., and Davis, R. T. (1973). Age differences in retention of concurrent discrimination problems in monkeys. *J. Gerontol. 28,* 63-67.

Meek, J. L., Bertilsson, L., Cheney, D. L., Zsilla, G., and Costa, E. (1977). Aging-induced changes in acetylcholine and serotonin content of discrete brain nuclei. *J. Gerontol. 32,* 129-131.

Meyer, J. S., Welch, K. M. A., Titus, J. L., Suzuki, M., Kim, Han-Seob, Perez, F. I., Mathew, N. T., Gedye, J. L., Hrastnik, F., Miyakawa, Y., Achar, V. S., and Dodson, R. F. (1976). Neurotransmitter failure in cerebral infarction and dementia. In *Aging: Neurobiology of Aging,* R. Terry and S. Gershon (Eds.). Raven, New York, pp. 121-137.

Mohs, R. C., Davis, K. L., Tinklenberg, J. R., Pfefferbaum, A., Hollister, L. E., and Kopell, B. S. (1979). Cognitive effects of physostigmine and choline chloride in normal subjects. In *Brain Acetylcholine and Neuropsychiatric Disease,* K. L. Davis and P. A. Berger (Eds.). Plenum, New York, pp. 237-251.

Norris, A. H., Schock, N. W., and Wayman, I. H. (1953). Age changes in the maximum conduction velocity of motor fibres in human ulnar nerves. *J. Appl. Physiol. 5,* 589-593.

Nybäck, H., Wiesel, F. A., and Skett, P. (1979). Effects of piracetam on brain monoamine metabolism and serum prolactin levels in the rat. *Psychopharmacology 61,* 235-238.

O'Brien, M. D. (1977). Vascular disease and dementia in the elderly. In *Aging and Dementia,* W. L. Smith and M. Kinsbourne (Eds.). Spectrum, New York, pp. 77-90.

Obrist, W. D. (1953). Simple auditory reaction time in aged adults. *J. Psychol. 35,* 259-266.

Obrist, W. D., and Busse, E. W. (1965). The electroencephalogram in old age. In *Aging and the Brain,* C. Gaitz (Ed.). Plenum, New York, pp. 117-133.

Ochs, S. (1973). Effect of maturation and aging on the rate of fast axoplasmic transport in mammalian nerve. In *Progress in Brain Research,* Vol. 40, *Neurobiological Aspects of Maturation and Aging,* D. H. Ford (Ed.). Elsevier, Amsterdam, pp. 349-362.

Ordy, J. M. (1975a). Principles of mammalian aging. In *Neurobiology of Aging,* J. M. Ordy and K. R. Brizzee (Eds.). Plenum, New York, pp. 1-22.

Ordy, J. M. (1975b). The nervous system, behavior and aging; an interdisciplinary life-span approach. In *Neurobiology of Aging,* J. M. Ordy and K. R. Brizzee (Eds.). Plenum, New York, pp. 85-118.

Ordy, J. M. (1979). Geriatric psychopharmacology: drug modification of memory and emotionality in relation to aging in human and nonhuman primate brain. In *Brain Function in Old Age,* F. Hoffmeister and C. Muller (Eds.). Springer-Verlag, Berlin, pp. 435-455.

Ordy, J. M., and Brizzee, K. R. (Eds.) (1975). *Neurobiology of Aging: An Interdisciplinary Life-Span Approach.* Plenum, New York.

Ordy, J. M., and Brizzee, K. R. (1979a). Functional and structural age differences in the visual system of man and nonhuman primate models. In *Aging,* Vol. 10, *Sensory Systems and Communication in the Elderly,* J. M. Ordy and K. R. Brizzee (Eds.). Raven, New York, pp. 13-50.

Ordy, J. M., and Brizzee, K. R. (Eds.) (1979b). *Aging,* Vol. 10, *Sensory Systems and Communication in the Elderly.* Raven, New York.

Ordy, J. M., and Kaack, B. (1975). Neurochemical changes in composition, metabolism and neurotransmitters in the human brain with age. In *Neurobiology of Aging,* J. M. Ordy and K. R. Brizzee (Eds.). Plenum, New York, pp. 253-286.

Ordy, J. M., and Kaack, B. (1976). Psychoneuroendocrinology and aging in man. In *Special Review of Experimental Aging Research,* M. F. Elias, B. E. Eleftheriou, and P. K. Elias (Eds.). EAR, Inc., Bar Harbor, Me., pp. 255-302.

Ordy, J. M., and Schjeide, O. A. (1973). Univariate and multivariate models for evaluating long-term changes in neurobiological development, maturity and aging. In *Progress in Brain Research,* Vol. 40, *Neurobiological Aspects of Maturation and Aging,* D. H. Ford (Ed.). Elsevier, Amsterdam, pp. 25-51.

Ordy, J. M., Kaack, B., and Brizzee, K. R. (1975). Life-span neurochemical changes in the human and nonhuman primate brain. In *Aging: Clinical, Morphologic and Neurochemical Aspects in the Aging Central Nervous System,* H. Brody, D. Harman, and J. M. Ordy (Eds.). Raven, New York, pp. 133-190.

Ordy, J. M., Brizzee, K. R., Kaack, B., and Hansche, J. W. (1978). Age differences in short-term memory and cell loss in the cortex of the rat. *Gerontol. 24,* 276-285.

Ordy, J. M., Brizzee, R., Beavers, T., and Medart, P. (1979). Age differences in the functional and structural organization of the auditory system in man. In *Aging,* Vol. 10, *Sensory Systems and Communication in the Elderly,* J. M. Ordy and K. R. Brizzee (Eds.). Raven, New York, pp. 153-166.

Ordy, J. M., Brizzee, K. R., and Beavers, T. L. (1980a). Sensory function and short-term memory in aging. In *Advances in Neurogerontology,* Vol. 1, *The Aging Nervous System,* C. J. Maletta and F. J. Pirozzolo (Eds.). Praeger, New York, pp. 40-78.

Ordy, J. M., Brizzee, K. R., and Johnson, H. A. (1980b). Age differences in acuity, color vision, stereopsis, and iconic memory. Relation to cellular alterations in the retino-geniculo-striate pathway and limbic system. In *Aging and Human Visual Function,* Symposium, National Research Council, Washington, D. C., March 31-April 1, 1980.

Ordy, J. M., Brizzee, K. R., and Bartus, R. T. (1980c). Neuropharmacology: drug modification of memory and affect in relation to aging in human and nonhuman primate brain. In *Aging,* Vol. 16, *Clinical Pharmacology and the Aged Patient,* L. F. Jarvick, D. Greenblatt, and D. Harman (Eds.). Raven, New York. In Press.

Parizkova, J., Eiselt, E., Spryvarova, L., and Wachtlova, M. (1971). Body composition, aerobic capacity and density of muscle capillaries in young and old men. *J. Appl. Physiol. 31,* 323-325.

Prinz, P. N. (1976). EEG during sleep and waking states. In *Special Review of Experimental Aging Research,* M. F. Elias, B. E. Eleftheriou, and P. K. Elias (Eds.). EAR, Inc., Bar Harbor, Me., pp. 135-164.

Randt, C. T., Quartermain, D., Goldstein, M., and Anagnoste, B. (1971). Norepinephrine biosynthesis inhibition. Effects on memory in mice. *Science 172,* 498-499.

Richards, O. W. (1977). Effects of luminance and contrast on visual acuity, ages 16 to 90 years. *Am. J. Optom. Phys. Opt. 54,* 178-184.

Rockstein, M. (Ed.) (1974). *Theoretical Aspects of Aging.* Academic, New York.

Rogers, J., Silver, M. A., Shoemaker, W. J., and Bloom, F. E. (1980). Senescent changes in a neurobiological model system. Cerebellar Purkinje cell electrophysiology and correlative anatomy. *Neurobiol. Aging 1*(1), 3-12.

Roth, G. S. (1979). Hormone action during aging. Alterations and mechanisms. *Mech. Aging Devl. 9,* 497-514.

Sachar, E. J. (Ed.) (1976). *Hormones, Behavior and Psychopathology,* Raven, New York.

Sacher, G. A. (1975). Maturation and longevity in relation to cranial capacity in hominid evolution. In *Primate Functional Morphology and Evolution,* R. Tuttle (Ed.). Mouton, The Hague, pp. 417-441.

Sacher, G. A. (1977). Life table modification and life prolongation. In *Handbook of the Biology of Aging,* C. E. Finch and L. Hayflick (Eds.). Van Nostrand, New York, pp. 582-638.

Samorajski, T., and Hartford, J. (1980). Brain physiology of aging. In *Handbook of Geriatric Psychiatry,* E. W. Busse and D. G. Blazer (Eds.). Van Nostrand, New York, pp. 46-82.

Sanadi, D. R. (1977). Metabolic changes and their significance in aging. In *Handbook of the Biology of Aging,* C. E. Finch and L. Hayflick (Eds.). Van Nostrand, New York, pp. 73-98.

Schaie, K. W. (1975). Age changes in adult intelligence. In *Aging: Scientific Perspectives and Social Issues,* D. S. Woodruff and J. E. Birren (Eds.). Van Nostrand, New York, pp. 111-124.

Schaie, K. W. (1977). Quasiexperimental research designs in the psychology of aging. In *Handbook of the Psychology of Aging,* J. E. Birren and K. W. Schaie (Eds.). Van Nostrand, New York, pp. 39-58.

Scheibel, A. B. (1979). Aging in human motor control systems. In *Aging,* Vol. 10, *Sensory Systems and Communication in the Elderly,* J. M. Ordy and K. R. Brizzee (Eds.). Raven, New York, pp. 297-310.

Scheibel, M. E., and Scheibel, A. B. (1975). Structural changes in the aging brain. In *Aging: Clinical, Morphologic and Neurochemical Aspects in the Aging Central Nervous System,* H. Brody, D. Harmen, and J. M. Ordy (Eds.). Raven, New York, pp. 11-38.

Schiffman, S. (1979). Changes in taste and smell with age. Psychophysical aspects. In *Aging,* Vol. 10, *Sensory Systems and Communication in the Elderly,* J. M. Ordy and K. R. Brizzee (Eds.). Raven, New York, pp. 227-246.

Schiffman, S., Orlandi, M., and Erickson, R. P. (1979). Changes in taste and smell with age. Biological aspects. In *Aging,* Vol. 10, *Sensory Systems and Communication in the Elderly,* J. M. Ordy and K. R. Brizzee (Eds.). Raven, New York, pp. 247-268.

Selye, H. (1970). Stress and aging. *J. Am. Ger. Soc. 18,* 669-680.

Shagass, C., Gershon, S., and Friedhoff, A. J. (Eds.) (1977). *Psychopathology and Brain Dysfunction.* Raven, New York.

Shelanski, M. L. (1976). Neurochemistry of aging. Review and prospectus. In *Aging: Neurobiology of Aging,* R. Terry and S. Gershon (Eds.). Raven, New York, pp. 339-350.

Shock, N., and Norris, A. H. (1970). Neuromuscular coordinating as a factor in age changes in muscular exercise. In *Medicine and Sport,* Vol. 4, *Physical Inactivity and Aging,* D. Brunner and E. Jokl (Eds.). Karger, Basel, pp. 92-99.

Shock, N. W. (1977). Biological theories of aging. In *Handbook of the Psychology of Aging,* Vol. 1, J. E. Birren and K. W. Schaie (Eds.). Van Nostrand, New York, pp. 103-115.

Siesjo, B. K., Johannsson, H., Ljunggren, B., and Norberg, K. (1974). Cerebral utilization of nonglucose substrates and their effect in hypoglycemia. In *Brain Dysfunction in Metabolic Disorders,* F. Plum (Ed.). Raven, New York, pp. 75-110.

Smith, W. L., and Kinsbourne, M. (Eds.) (1977). *Aging and Dementia,* Spectrum, New York.

Sokoloff, L. (1976). Circulation and energy metabolism of the brain. In *Basic Neurochemistry,* G. J. Siegel, R. W. Albers, R. Katzman, and B. W. Agranoff (Eds.). Little, Brown, Boston, pp. 388-413.

Spillane, J. A., White, P., Goodhardt, M. J., Flack, R. H. A., Bowen, D. M., and Davison, A. N. (1977). Selective vulnerability of neurons in organic dementia. *Nature 266,* 558-559.

Storrie, M. C., and Eisdorfer, C. (1978). Psychophysiological studies in aging: a ten year review. In *Psychopharmacology: A Generation of Progress,* M. A. Lipton, A. DiMascio, and K. F. Killam (Eds.). Raven, New York, pp. 1489-1497.

Survillo, W. W. (1968). Timing of behavior in senescence and the role of the central nervous system. In *Human Aging and Behavior,* G. A. Talland (Ed.). Academic, New York, pp. 1-35.

Swanson, L. W. (1979). The hippocampus–new anatomical insights. *Trends in Neurosciences (January),* pp. 9-12.

Talbert, G. B. (1977). Aging of the reproductive system. In *Handbook of the Biology of Aging,* C. E. Finch and L. Hayflick (Eds.). Van Nostrand, New York, pp. 318-356.

Talland, G. A. (1965). Initiation of response, and reaction time in aging, and with brain damage. In *Behavior, Aging and the Nervous System,* A. T. Welford and J. E. Birren (Eds.). Thomas, Springfield, Ill., pp. 526-561.

Talland, G. A. (1968). Age and the span of immediate recall. In *Human Aging and Behavior,* G. A. Talland (Ed.). Academic, New York, pp. 92-129.

Terry, R., and Gershon, S. (Eds.) (1976). *Ageing: Neurobiology of Aging,* Raven, New York.

Thompson, L. W. (1976). Cerebral blood flow, EEG and behavior in aging. In *Aging: Neurobiology of Aging,* R. Terry and S. Gershon (Eds.). Raven, New York, pp. 103-120.

Thompson, L. W., and Marsh, G. R. (1973). Psychophysiological studies of aging. In *The Psychology of Adult Development and Aging,* C. Eisdorfer and M. P. Lawton (Eds.). American Psychological Ass., Washington, D. C., pp. 112-150.

Tomlinson, B. E., and Henderson, G. (1976). Some quantitative cerebral findings in normal and demented old people. In *Aging: Neurobiology of Aging,* R. Terry and S. Gershon (Eds.). Raven, New York, pp. 183-204.

van Praag, H. M., and Kalverboer, A. F. (Eds.). (1972). *Ageing of the Central Nervous System: Biological and Psychological Aspects,* Bohn, Haarlem.

Vernadakis, A. (1973). Comparative studies of neurotransmitter substances in the maturing and aging central nervous system of the chicken. In *Progress in Brain Research,* Vol. 40, *Neurobiological Aspects of Maturation and Aging,* D. H. Ford (Ed.). Elsevier, Amsterdam, pp. 231-244.

Walker, J., and Hertzog, C. (1975). Aging, brain function, and behavior. In *Aging: Scientific Perspectives and Social Issues,* D. S. Woodruff and J. E. Birren (Eds.). Van Nostrand, New York, pp. 152-178.

Walsh, D. A. (1975). Age differences in learning and memory. In *Aging: Scientific Perspectives and Social Issues,* D. S. Woodruff and J. E. Birren (Eds.). Van Nostrand, New York, pp. 125-151.

Weale, R. A. (1978). The eye and aging. *Interdiscipl. Topics Gerontol. 13,* 1-13.

Weg, R. B. (1975). Changing physiology of aging. Normal and pathological. In *Aging: Scientific Perspectives and Social Issues,* D. S. Woodruff and J. E. Birren (Eds.). Van Nostrand, New York, pp. 229-256.

Welford, A. T. (1965). Performance, biological mechanisms and age. A theoretical Sketch. In *Behavior, Aging and the Nervous System,* A. T. Welford and J. E. Birren (Eds.). Thomas, Springfield, Ill., pp. 3-20.

Welford, A. T. (1977). Motor performance. In *Handbook of the Psychology of Aging,* J. E. Birren and K. W. Schaie (Eds.). Van Nostrand, New York, pp. 450-496.

Welford, A. T., and Birren, J. E. (Eds.) (1965). *Behavior, Aging and the Nervous System,* Thomas, Springfield, Ill.

Woodruff, D. S. (1975). A physiological perspective of the psychology of aging. In *Aging: Scientific Perspectives and Social Issues,* D. S. Woodruff and J. E. Birren (Eds.). Van Nostrand, New York, pp. 170-200.

Woodruff, D. S., and Birren, J. E. (Eds.) (1975). *Aging: Scientific Perspectives and Social Issues.* Van Nostrand, New York.

Wurtman, R. J., and Growdon, J. H. (1979). Dietary control of central cholinergic activity. In *Brain Acetylcholine and Neuropsychiatric Disease,* K. L. Davis and P. A. Berger (Eds.). Plenum, New York, pp. 461-481.

Young, V. R., Winterer, J. C., Munro, H. N., and Scrimshaw, N. S. (1976). Muscle and whole body protein metabolism in aging, with special reference to man. In *Special Review of Experimental Aging Research,* M. F. Elias, B. E. Eleftheriou, and P. K. Elias (Eds.). EAR, Inc., Bar Harbor, Me., pp. 217-252.

Zornetzer, S. F. (1978). Neurotransmitter modulation and memory: a new neuropharmacological phrenology? In *Psychopharmacology: A Generation of Progress,* M. A. Lipton, A. DiMascio, and K. F. Killam (Eds.). Raven, New York, pp. 637-650.

11

Biochemical Aspects of Dementia

C. G. Gottfries
University of Göteborg, St. Jörgen's Hospital
Göteborg, Sweden

I. INTRODUCTION

Dementia means impairment of mental functions and is a condition which is often irreversible and progressive. Various diseases affecting the brain can cause dementia. The onset can be at any age, but is most common in older age groups; therefore, the old age dementias are considered most often in the concept of dementia disorders.

It may be difficult from the clinical point of view to delimit normal aging (physiological aging or orthoinvolution) from pathological aging (dementia disorders or pathoinvolution). Usually, normal aging is not associated with severe mental impairment. The reserve capacity of the brain may be reduced but the elderly can still cope with social life if not overly stressed. With abnormal involution mental impairment is pronounced and may cause total dependence.

With regard to structural and biochemical changes, normal aging has features in common with the dementia disorders. Therefore, the question of a continuity between normal involution and abnormal involution has not yet been settled.

The diseases that cause dementia in old age and which are usually included in the concept of abnormal involution can be split into two groups, namely, cerebrovascular diseases and degenerative disorders with no obvious vascular disease. The most common vascular diseases in old age are due to hypertension, which plays the most important role in the development of cerebral arteriosclerosis. It is now accepted that the dementia caused by vascular disease is due to infarctions or hemorrhage. Of these two pathological processes infarction seems the more common and the term *multi-infarct dementia* has been suggested (Hachinsky et al., 1974).

The nonvascular diseases are divided into senile dementia and presenile dementia. Senile dementia has its onset after 65 years of age. It is unclear as to whether senile dementia forms a homogeneous group and the distinction between senile dementia and presenile dementias is difficult and even impossible. It is obvious that the clinical diagnosis of senile dementia may be given to patients with presenile dementias with late onset and patients with somatic or neurologic diseases with mental impairment.

The presenile dementias are Alzheimer's disease and Pick's disease. Some textbooks also include Huntington's chorea and the spongioform encephalopathies (Jacob Creutzfeldt's disease). Huntington's chorea, however, is a hereditary disease with degeneration in the neostriatum and Jacob Creutzfeldt's disease is caused by a slow virus infection. It seems inappropriate to include these disorders in the group of presenile dementias. Alzheimer's disease has many features in common with senile dementia, but genetic investigations (Larsson et al., 1963) do not support the assumption that these are the same type of disorder. Nevertheless, many authors discuss these two disorders together, as is the case in this chapter.

Although there have been rapid advances in research on the neurochemistry of the human brain during the past decade, little is known about the neurochemistry of dementia conditions in old age.

II. SENILE DEMENTIA AND ALZHEIMER'S DISEASE

A. Histopathological Changes

Light as well as electron microscopy has shown up the morphological and histopathological characteristics of aging and dementia disorders. There structural changes, which can be found in the normal aging brain, are of the same type but more massive in Alzheimer's disease and senile dementia. This means that morphological changes are not specific in their nature, and in fact they have offered few clues as to the etiology and pathogenesis of dementia disorders (for reviews see Scheibel and Scheibel, 1975; Brizze et al., 1975).

The brain weight is significant lower and there is probably a loss of neurons in several parts of the brain in patients with Alzheimer's disease and senile dementias. There is also a reduction of dendrite number and extent (Wisniewski and Terry, 1973; Mehrain et al., 1975). It seems as if the total number of glial cells is unchanged.

The most prominent finding other than atrophy and cell loss is the formation of senile plaques and neurofibrillary tangles of Alzheimer type. Other histological findings include granulovacuolar degeneration, lipofuscin accumulation, and amyloid angiopathy.

1. *Senile Plaques*

Simchowitz (1911) introduced the term *senile plaque* for some degenerative changes in the human brain. Senile plaque is composed of a central core of amyloid with neuronal elements in the periphery in varying degrees of degenerative change (Divry, 1934). The outer margin can be a corona of glia. The source of senile plaques is unknown. It was supposed that these degenerative changes were related to occurrence of mental failure. Gellerstedt (1933) showed, however, that plaques could be found in the brains of old people without specific dementia disorders in as high a frequency as 84%. Studying 300 patients with psychiatric disorders of old age, Corsellis (1962) found senile plaque more often in those with organic disorders than in those with functional psychoses. In Alzheimer's disease and in senile dementia plaques are found in high concentrations throughout cortical regions and in the hippocampus.

In an investigation by Nikaido et al. (1972), patients with Alzheimer's disease and senile dementia were shown to have increased silicon in the cores and rims of the plaques. A still higher increase was found in plaques from patients with Down's syndrome. The results indicate that there is a focal increase of silicon in those dementia disorders that have degenerative changes in the form of senile plaques. The relationship between levels of silicon, aging, and dementia disorders is, however, unknown.

Roth et al (1966) have shown a relation between the number of plaques and mental impairment. Nondemented people have few plaques while severely impaired patients have a high frequency of senile plaques. Although the pathophysiological significance of the senile plaques is unclear, they are a characteristic of normal aging as well as of dementia disorders and there are only quantitative differences.

2. *Alzheimer's Neurofibrillary Tangles*

Alzheimer (1907) described in presenile dementia some degenerative neurofibrillary changes which now bear his name. The changes are thought to result from abnormal protein metabolism in the nerve cell. Neurofibrillary tangles consist of large numbers of tubules found as parallel bundles which fill the cytoplasmic envelope. The tubules are abnormal in size and have constrictions along their length (Terry, 1963; Terry and Wisniewski, 1970). It is believed that these changes cause an interruption of the axoplasmic flow (Suzuki and Terry, 1967). Tomlinson (1972) has shown these changes in normal aging, but only in the hippocampus. In Alzheimer's disease and senile dementia they are found in the hippocampus, and as the disease progresses these changes are also found in the cerebral cortex. Of interest is that these degenerative changes are not only a part of the pathological anatomy of senescence, senile dementia, and Alzheimer's disease, but are also associated with dementing changes in Pick's disease, the dementia complex found on Guam (Hirano et al., 1966), and postencephalitic parkinsonism (Greenfield and Bosancuet, 1953).

3. *Granulovacuolar Changes*

The granulovacuolar changes of Simchowitz (1911) are largely limited to the pyramid cells of the hippocampus. These vacuoles contain a small central granule. The cause of there structural changes and the nature of their contents are still unknown. The changes are rarely seen in normal aging, but may be very common in all hippocampal pyramid cells in Alzheimer's disease or in advanced senile dementia (Tomlinson, 1972).

4. *Lipofuscin and Amyloidosis*

A constant finding in normal aging is yellow, green, or brown fluorescent pigments called lipocromes or lipofuscin. Lipofuscin accumulates progressively in most neurons in the mammalian brain. Some pathological conditions in the brain are characterized by accumulation of lipofuscin pigments. Kuf's disease or generalized lipofuscinosis (Kornfelt, 1972) and neuronal ceroid-lipofuscinosis of Betten's disease (Zeman and Dyken, 1969) are disorders in which there is a large accumulation of lipofuscin. Kristenson and Sourander (1966) observed an increased amount of lipofuscin in metachromatic leukodystrophy and in Tay-Sachs disease. Whether the presence of lipofuscin in these diseases may have pathogenic importance for the function of the neuron is still unknown.

In the aging brain amyloid also accumulates which seems to occur mainly during senescence. While the lipofuscin accumulates in the cell bodies or processes, the amyloid is deposited extracellularly. In the senile plaque lipofuscin as well as amyloid tissue accumulates. Although lipofuscin pigmentation and amyloidosis are seen in normal aging, a more widespread amyloid angiopathy is found in Alzheimer's disease and in senile dementia (von Bogaert, 1970).

The presence of amyloid indicates involvement of immune mechanisms and some serum laboratory findings in patients with Alzheimer's disease are in line with this suggestion (Behan and Feldman, 1970). Kalter and Kelly (1975) showed that patients with Alzheimer's disease had elevated levels of IgM and IgA. Of interest is also the investigation of Cohen et al. (1976), who found positive correlations between serum levels of IgG and IgM and test scores measuring intellectual function in old people with no obvious dementia.

B. Neurotransmitters

The following substances and their associated enzyme of synthesis and degradation have been identified as transmitters in the mammalian brain:

Active amines	Related enzymes	Metabolites
Acetylcholine (ACh)	Cholinacetyltransferase (CAT)	Choline Acetate
	Acetylcholinesterase (AChE)	
Dopamine (DA)	Tyrosine hydroxylase (TH)	Homovanillic acid (HVA)
	Dopa decarboxylase (DOD)	
	Monoamine oxidase (MAO)	
	Catechol-o-methyl-transferase (COMT)	
Norepinephrine (NE)	Dopamine-β-hydroxylase	3-Methoxy-4-hydroxy-phenylglycol (MHPG)
	MAO	
	COMT	
5-Hydroxytryptamine (5-HT) (Serotonin)	Tryptophan hydroxylase	5-Hydroxyindoleacetic acid (5-HIAA)
	5-Hydroxytryptophan decarboxylase	
	MAO	
γ-Aminobutyric acid (GABA)	Glutamic acid decarboxylase	
	GABA transaminase	

1. Acetylcholine

In the cholinergic system it is accepted that CAT, the synthesizing enzyme, is a more reliable index of cholinergic activity than AChE, the hydrolyzing enzyme.

Experiments in chickens have shown an age-related decline in CAT whereas AChE increases (Vernadakis, 1973). AChE declines related to age have, however, been reported in rats (Hollander and Barrows, 1968; Ordy and Schjeide, 1973). A decline in CAT activity with age in rats was confirmed by McGeer et al. (1971a) and McGeer and McGeer (1976a). Meek et al. (1977) reported a reduced CAT activity in rat brains, but this was only true for the caudate nucleus while six other areas of the brain investigated showed no reduced CAT activity.

White et al. (1977) have investigated CAT activity and muscarin receptor binding sites post mortem in humans. In normal elderly people the receptor binding sites were decreased as compared to young people. In cortex from patients with dementia conditions of the senile type the CAT activity was reduced up to 44% of that of the age-matched control group. The reduction was most severe in cases where there were also morphological degenerative changes. Reduced CAT activity in dementia of the senile type was also found by Bowen et al. (1976), Davies and Maloney (1976), and Perry et al. (1977). These groups found no age-related decline in CAT activity. This was, however, found in the investigation by McGeer and McGeer (1976a) in postmortem investigations of human brains. Davies and Maloney (1976) studied AChE and found it reduced in senile dementia. In an attempt to get valid information about CAT activity in Alzheimer's disease, Spillane et al. (1977) examined cortical biopsies removed at craniotomi; they found at least a 50% reduction of CAT activity in this disease.

It seems reasonable to conclude from the data from biopsy and postmortem investigations that the presynaptic cholinergic system is affected in senile dementia and Alzheimer's disease. Of interest is a pharmacological study (Drachman and Leavitt, 1974) which suggests that the cholinergic system is involved in age-related memory disturbances in humans. It is also of interest to consider whether the reduced CAT activity in dementia disorders is secondary to reduced activity in dopaminergic systems (see below). DA, however, inhibits cholinergic activity and thus increased cholinergic activity should occur.

It can be questioned as to whether the CAT activity of brain tissue is a marker of the ACh turnover since choline uptake is the rate-limiting step in the ACh synthesis. In the investigations by Meek et al. (1977) in rats, no age-related changes in the brain tissue levels of Ch or ACh were found in any of the nuclei examined. Ch and ACh were estimated by mass fragmentography.

2. *The monoamines: Dopamine, Norepinephrine, and 5-Hydroxytryptamine*

Certain dominant techniques often become crucial determinants of the direction of progress. A histochemical method made it possible to visualize the monoamines DA, NE, and 5-HT (Carlsson et al., 1962). This has focused interest on monoamine functions in the brain. Studies in mental disorders strongly suggest that the estimation of the monoamines and their metabolites have given important information and it has been reported that biogenic amine levels may be decreased in affective disorders (Schildkraut, 1965; Coppen, 1967; Weil-Malherbe, 1972).

Several investigations have shown that catecholamine activity in the aged rat brain is reduced (Finch, 1973, 1976; Algeri et al., 1978). In the investigation by Algeri et al. (1978), a decrease in TH was supposed to be the cause of the reduced activity in catecholamine turnover in old age. The activities of TH as well as DOD have been examined post mortem in humans in the substantia nigra, the caudate nucleus, the putamen, and the hypothalamus. There were highly significant age-related decreases in TH and DOD in the substantia nigra, the caudate nucleus, and the putamen. The TH activity in the hypothalamus was, however, not altered with increasing age (Cote and Kremzner, 1974). In investigations by McGeer et al. (1971b) and McGeer and McGeer (1973) TH activity was investigated in six human subjects varying in age from 5 to 57 years, and the age-related decline was confirmed. As TH activity is the rate limiting step in the synthesis of catecholamines, the age-related reduced activity of TH is of special interest. In postmortem investigations of the human brain, age-related declines in DOD have also been reported by Lloyd and Hornykiewicz (1970).

Postmortem studies in humans have shown reduced levels of DA and NA related to age (Nies et al., 1973; Carlsson and Winblad, 1976; Robinson et al., 1977; Adolfsson et al., 1979a; Gottfries et al., 1979). In senile dementia and Alzheimer's disease monoamine metabolites in the brain are altered (Gottfries et al., 1968, 1969). The concentration of HVA was estimated in the caudate nucleus, the putamen and the globus pallidus in a control group and in dementia groups. The verification of the dementia groups was made at autopsy and the degree of dementia was measured post mortem with a rating scale. In the senile dementia group HVA was at a significantly lower concentration in the caudate nucleus, the putamen, and the globus pallidus, than the controls. In this investigation HVA brain levels were related to the degree of dementia according to the rating scale. The higher the degree of intellectual impairment the lower were the levels of HVA but such a relation was not seen in a multi-infarct dementia group. When the dementia disorders were split into a group of senile dementia and a group of Alzheimer conditions, the Alzheimer group had the significantly lower level of HVA; the estimations were made in the putamen and the caudate nucleus (Gottfries et al., 1968). In postmortem investigations reported by Gottfries et al. (1979) and Adolfsson et al. (1979b), DA and NE were significantly reduced in groups of senile dementia and Alzheimer's disease in some areas of the brain when compared with age-matched controls.

In the investigation by Adolfsson et al. (1979b), the level of NE in brain tissue was significantly negatively correlated to the degree of dementia, i.e. the lower the NE levels in the brain the more pronounced the intellectual impairment.

Bowen et al. (1974) studied DOD activity in postmortem samples from different brain regions. The patients included in the investigation suffered from senile dementia and were matched with controls. The results indicated that in the demented patients there was a reduction of DOD activity by 70-90%. The authors' interpretation of the findings was that the reduction of DOD indicates a fallout of dopaminergic neurons beginning at the synapse.

In animal experiments (Samorajski et al., 1971, Samorajski and Rolsten, 1973) 5-HT in mouse forebrain increased slightly with age but decreased in the rhesus monkey hypothalamus. Himwich and Himwich (1959) found an increase of 5-HT in the aging rat brain. In postmortem investigations Bertler (1961) found no significant differences in the levels of 5-HT in different regions of the brain when a 73-87 year age group was compared with younger groups. Relatively small but statistically significant decreases in 5-HT with age have been reported by Robinson et al. (1972). In the investigation by Gottfries et al. (1979), there were positive correlations between age and 5-HT levels in the hypothalamus, the mesencephalon, and the medulla oblongata, while there were significant negative correlations between age and 5-HT levels in the globus pallidus and the cortex gyrus hippocampus. These data are in line with data presented by MacLean et al. (1965) and Pare et al. (1969). Thus at present it seems relevant to assume age-related increased levels of 5-HT in the brainstem and decreased levels in cortical areas. The 5-HIAA levels tend to increase with age (Gottfries et al., 1979).

Determinations of acid monoamine metabolites such as HVA and 5-HIAA in the cerebrospinal fluid (CSF) provide valid information regarding the metabolism of the corresponding amines in the brain (Moir et al., 1970; Roos, 1970). Although the concentrations of HVA and 5-HIAA increase with age, in clinical groups of senile dementia and Alzheimer's disease the levels of HVA and 5-HIAA are reduced in the CSF (Gottfries et al., 1969). By using the probenecid test further information is available about the monoamine turnover in humans. Probenecid blocks the elimination of HVA and 5-HIAA from brain tissue to blood (Neff et al. 1964, 1967; Werdinius, 1966) and from CSF to blood (Guldberg et al., 1966; Olsson and Roos, 1968). Probenecid thus normally induces an increase in the concentration of the acid monoamine metabolites in the CSF which is related to the turnover of the monoamines in the brain. This test was performed in a series of 15 Alzheimer patients and the finding of impaired DA metabolism was confirmed (Gottfries et al., 1974). In this investigation the release of 5-HT seemed slightly impaired. The high levels of HVA and 5-HIAA in the CSF in normal aging (Bowers and Gerbode, 1968; Gottfries et al., 1971) can, of course, be interpreted as a sign of an increased turnover or release of DA respectively 5-HT in the brains of old people. This interpretation is, however, not in line with the brain tissue findings indicating a reduced turnover of catecholamines in the aged human brain. Another interpretation of the high levels of acid monoamine metabolites in CSF in the aged is that the aged have a reduced outflow through membranes which would indicate an age-related alteration in the membrane composition. This could account for the change in the turnover of neuronal catecholamine stores. The membranes of the synapses contain high proportions of fatty acids which may be vulnerable to lipid peroxidation from free radical attack during aging. There may be a change in the permeability properties of the membranes (Bishayee and Balasubramaninan, 1971).

To get information about monoamine metabolism in the CNS one can also study the activity in catabolic enzyme systems. MAO is the main deaminating enzyme for the monoamines and its activity increases with age in a number of species (Novick, 1961; Horita, 1967; Prange et al., 1967; Horita and Lowe, 1972). Robinson et al. (1972, 1977) studied MAO in human brains in post-mortem investigations and found a marked increase in the MAO activity (see Shih, 1975). An increase in MAO activity with age has also been shown in platelets and in plasma, using benzylamine as substrate. Evidence has been presented that MAO exists in at least two forms, MAO-A and MAO-B. The age-related increase in MAO in brain tissue has been confirmed by Gottfries et al. (1975) and in this investigation the relation between age and MAO-B was most evident. Robinson et al. (1972) have suggested that high MAO activity is important for mental disturbances in old age. The increased frequency of affective disorders in old age can eventually be caused by a high MAO activity. Of interest is that patients with dementia disorders of Alzheimer type have still higher brain MAO activity than age-matched controls and again it is MAO-B which is increased (Carlsson, 1979). Also platelet MAO activity in patients with Alzheimer's disease is increased when compared to age-matched controls (Adolfsson et al., 1978).

The increased MAO-B activity in normal aging and the still higher increase in patients with dementia disorders of Alzheimer type may indicate that this dementia disorder is an accelerated process of aging. The increased enzyme activity may be due to changes in membrane structures. Since MAO is partly dependent on the composition of its membranous environment for its activity (Ekstedt and Oreland, 1976; Houslay, 1977), such an increased rate of alteration in membrane structure may explain the increased MAO activity in Alzheimer patients. Another explanation for increased MAO activity may be that as a consequence of an accelerating decrease of protein-degrading enzyme activity there is a reduced breakdown of the enzyme MAO itself. This explanation has been suggested for the increase in MAO in aging rat heart (Della Corte and Callingham, 1977). A further explanation is that MAO-B (determined with β-phenylethylamine as substrate) is localized to extra neuronal cells, while MAO-A (determined with serotonin and partly with tryptamine as substrate) is localized to the neurons. In the old brain and in the dementias there may be a glial cell proliferation. The increased MAO-B activity therefore reflects an increased glial content in the brain tissue. This interpretation will then also explain why only MAO-B is increased and not MAO-A. One objective to this explanation, however, is that MAO-B in platelets is also increased, which cannot of course be explained by the glial cell proliferation. In view of the increased MAO activity in platelets it may be concluded that dementia of Alzheimer type is a systemic disease, localized not only to the central nervous system but also to other organs.

It is still debatable as to whether studies of neurotransmitters or their metabolites outside the CNS can give valid information about the turnover in the brain tissue. In an investigation by Fisher (1972), the urinary excretion of HVA was decreased in a group of demented patients compared with controls. Fisher also studied the excretion of 3-methoxy-4-hydroxymandelic acid and found its urinary excretion the same in dementia cases as in controls.

It has been suggested that aging and dementia disorders may bc rclated to deficiency in folic acid and in vitamin B12 (Read et al., 1965; Hurdle and Picton Williams, 1966; Carney, 1967; Shulman, 1967). As the rate-limiting step in the synthesis of catecholamines as well as serotonin is hydroxylation of the amino acids and as folate is the coenzyme of this process (Kaufman and Friedman, 1965; Gal et al., 1966; Grahame-Smith, 1967) a deficiency of folate could be the cause of the disturbed monoamine turnover. Shaw et al. (1971) made an investigation of patients with senile dementia but the results were disappointing. The authors found it unlikely that lack of folate in the demented patients is a significant factor in the amine metabolism.

To summarize the findings about aging and dementia disorders and metabolism of biogenic amines, it can be concluded that the CAT activity is reduced in senile dementia and Alzheimer's disease. Too few investigations are made to answer the question of whether Ch or ACh is reduced in these dementia disorders. In normal aging there is a decline of the activity of TH and DOD and the levels of DA and NE are reduced in the old human brain. In senile dementia and Alzheimer's disease there is still more serious reduction of the activity of DOD and also the levels of DA, NE, and HVA in brain tissue are pathologically reduced when compared with age-matched controls. The findings concerning the serotonin turnover are contradictory. Of interest is that in old age there is an increase of MAO activity. Preliminary results indicate that in Alzheimer's disease the increase of the MAO activity is significantly higher than in age-matched control groups.

It is of interest to note that in normal aging as well as in Alzheimer's disease and senile dementia the same type of neurochemical changes are found. Differences are not qualitative but quantitative.

It can, of course, be discussed as to whether the findings made in aging and dementia disorders have any pathogenetic importance or are only epiphenomenon that are secondary to other degenerative changes in the brain. There are indications, however, that the activity of CAT, which is reduced in Alzheimer's disease, parallels increasing senile morphological changes (Spillane et al., 1977). Bowen et al. (1974) found that there was a selective decline in the DOD while other enzyme systems in the human brain not were reduced, at least not to the same extent. In the investigations by Gottfries et al. (1968) and Adolfsson et al. (1979b) there are significant correlations between the degree of intellectual impairment and the reduction of the levels of HVA and NE. It can also be noticed that while the activity of catecholamines seems to decline, serotonin turnover is not reduced to the same degree. This supports the conclusion that the disturbed metabolism of ACh and catecholamines may have specific importance for normal aging as well as for senile dementia and Alzheimer's disease.

The increased levels of acid metabolites, HVA and 5-HIAA, in the CSF and the age-related increase of 5-HIAA levels in brain tissue support the assumption that in aging there is a reduced transport of these metabolites. This may indicate membrane disturbances in old age and it can be asked whether these membrane disturbances are also of importance for the disturbances in the amine turnover. Another question is whether the increased activity of MAO also can be related to membrane disturbances as this enzyme is bound to membranes. Of interest are the findings of Crapper et al. (1980) which also may indicate membrane disturbances. They found increased amounts of aluminum associated to cell nuclear structures in brain tissue from Alzheimer patients. A pathological metabolism of aluminum is suggested due to defects in blood-brain and cytoplasmic barriers, permitting aluminum to accumulate upon nuclear constituents.

3. *γ-Aminobutyric Acid*

GABA is considered to be an inhibiting transmitter in the CNS. The synthesizing enzyme is GAD. Most parts of the human brain have active amounts of GABA and GAD but there are regional differences (Tappaz et al., 1976; Okada, 1976; McGeer and McGeer, 1976b). GABA seems to be a regulator in the nigroneostriatal system where it inhibits DA activity (see Tarsy et al., 1975). Changes in GABA activity have been reported in parkinsonism and Huntington's chorea (Barbeau, 1973).

In an investigation of Bowen et al. (1974), the brains from patients with senile dementia were investigated post mortem for their GAD content. The activity of GAD was reduced by 72% in the dementia cases as compared with controls. The reduced activity of GAD was confirmed in an investigation by Bowen and Davison (1975). In the investigations mentioned above, GAD activity was reduced more in the cortex than in the caudate nucleus. The greater reduction of GAD in the cerebral cortex compared to basal ganglias is consistent with histopathological findings as senile plaques and neurofibrillary degenerations are found more in the cortex than in deep grey matter. Of interest, however, is the investigation by Spillane et al. (1977) wherein biopsy studies showed GAD activity unaffected. This investigation makes it unclear as to whether the earlier findings of reduced cortical GAD activity in Alzheimer's disease reflects the activity in the GABA-containing neurons. The reduction may be caused by reduced cerebral blood flow and/or a cerebral hypoxia before death (Bowen et al., 1976).

III. DEMENTIA DISORDERS AND PARKINSONISM

In parkinsonism Greenfield and Bosanquet (1953) reported morphological changes like Alzheimer's neurofibrillary tangles. Carlsson as early as 1959 proposed that DA was a transmitter in the CNS and that it could be involved in Parkinson's syndrome. By 1960 Ehringer and Hornykiewicz showed that the DA content of the caudate nucleus and putamen was reduced in Parkinson's disease and by 1961 Birkmayer and Hornykiewicz reported a beneficial effect on Parkinson akinesia when the patients were treated with L-dopa. As shown in investigations by Gottfries et al. (1969), the levels of HVA in the CSF in subjects with Alzheimer's disease are almost as low as those found in patients with parkinsonism. An obvious question is why patients with Alzheimer's disease do not show such serious movement disturbances as patients with parkinsonism. It must be borne in mind, however, that in parkinsonism—either the true Parkinson's disease or the parkinsonism type—many of the main symptoms such as tremor and akinesia are signs of an overfunction of the cholinergic system rather than of underfunction of the dopaminergic system (Hornykiewicz, 1968). In senile dementia and Alzheimer's disease findings suggest reduced activity in cholinergic functions also. Perhaps the reduced dopaminergic and cholinergic activities in the brains from patients with senile dementia and Alzheimer's disease can still balance each other but at a lower level than normals. More careful clinical studies have shown that up to 60% of patients with Alzheimer's disease have demonstrable movement disturbances of the Parkinson type (Pearce, 1974). Clinical investigations have also shown that in parkinsonism both movement disorder and dementia occur. In various clinical reports 12-53% of patients with parkinsonism have intellectual impairment (Pollack and Hornabrook; 1966; Mindham, 1970; Celesia and Wanamaker, 1972). This finding has, however, not been generally confirmed (Coppen et al., 1972). On the island of Guam a disease occurs in which parkinsonism and intellectual impairment are always combined.

These clinical investigations suggest some overlap between parkinsonism and some dementia disorders; a deficiency state in the catecholamine system may have pathogenetic importance for a spectrum of diseases varying from parkinsonism to dementia.

In parkinsonism it is well known that, although there is serious degeneration of the dopaminergic neurons in the substantia nigra, treatment with L-dopa is of great benefit to the patients. According to this treatment model patients with Alzheimer's disease and senile dementia might also respond to L-dopa.

Favorable results have been reported (Drachman and Stahl, 1975) but in a controlled investigation by Kristensen et al. (1977) the results were negative.

IV. PICK'S DISEASE

Clinical differentiation between Alzheimer's and Pick's diseases is difficult. Pick's disease is also characterized clinically by a progressing dementia. Pathologically a localized cerebral atrophy is found, most commonly in the frontal, temporal, and parietal lobes. The atrophy therefore has quite a different pattern from that seen in Alzheimer's disease, where cortical atrophy is more diffuse.

Light microscopy shows loss of neurons and gliosis. The cell loss is not only found in cortical grey matter but also in white matter and basal ganglia (Jervis, 1971). Affected neurons show swelling and pallor with loss of the intracytoplasmic nissl bodies (von Braunmühl, 1958). Senile plaques, neurofibrillary tangles, and granulovacuolar degeneration are rarely seen in brains from patients who have Pick's disease, but Hirano bodies may be seen (Hirano et al., 1968; Jervis, 1971). Genetic factors seem important in the etiology of Pick's disease (Sjögren et al., 1952).

Few investigations have concerned monoamine metabolism in Pick's disease. A reduction of muscarinic receptor binding sites was found in postmortem investigations of two cases with Pick's disease (White et al., 1977). Guard (1976) investigated a series of 17 patients with presenile dementias and included a probenecid test. In 13 patients with Alzheimer's disease the turnover rates of HVA and 5-HIAA were insignificantly diminished compared with normals. In four patients with Pick's disease the turnover rate of HVA was similar to normal whereas the turnover rate of 5-HIAA was insignificantly decreased.

In an investigation of Op Den Velde and Stam (1976), brain enzyme activities in patients with dementia disorders were studied. The material included one patient with Pick's disease in whom AChE activity was low and unspecific cholinesterase activity was high.

REFERENCES

Adolfsson, R., Gottfries, C. G., Oreland, L., Roos, B. E., and Winblad, B. (1978). Reduced levels of catecholamines in the brain and increased activity of monoamine oxidase in platelets in Alzheimer's disease: Therapeutic implications. In *Alzheimer's Disease: Senile Dementia and Related Disorders*, R. Katzman, R. D. Terry, and K. L. Bick (Eds.). Raven, New York, pp. 441-451.

Adolfsson, R., Gottfries, C. G., Roos, B. E., and Winblad, B. (1979a). Postmortem distribution of dopamine and homovanillic acid in human brain, variations related to age, and a review of the literature. *J. Neurol. Transm. 45*, 81-105.

Adolfsson, R., Gottfries, C. G., Roos, B. E., and Winblad, B. (1979b). Changes in the brain catecholamines in patients with dementia of Alzheimer type. *Br. J. Psychiatry 135,* 216-223.

Algeri, S., Bonati, M., Brunello, N., Ponzio, F., Stramentinoli, G., and Gualano, M. (1978). Biochemical changes in central catecholaminergic neurons of the senescent rats. In *Neuro-Psychopharmacology,* P. Deniker, C. Radouco-Thomas, and A. Villeneuve (Eds.). Proc. 10th Congr. Collegium International Neuro-Psychopharmacologicum, Quebec, July 1976, Pergamon, Oxford, pp. 1647-1654.

Alzheimer, A. (1907). Ueber eine eigenartige Erkrankung der Hirnrinde. Cbl. Nervenheilk Psychiat., *18,* 177-179. Cited in Torack, R. (1971), In *Dementia,* C. Wells (Ed.). F. A. Davis, Philadelphia.

Barbeau, A. (1973). Biochemistry of Huntington's chorea. *Advances in Neurology,* Vol. 1. Raven, New York, pp. 473-516.

Behan, P. O., and Feldman, R. G. (1970). Serum proteins, amyloid and Alzheimer's disease. *J. Am. Geriatr. Soc. 18,* 792-797.

Bertler, A. (1961). Occurrence and localization of catecholamines in the human brain. *Acta Physiol. Scand. 51,* 97-107.

Birkmayer, W., and Hornykiewicz, O. (1961). Der L-3-4-dioxyphenyl alanin (=DOPA)-effect bei der Parkinson-Akinese. *Wien. Klin, Wochenschr. 45,* 787-788.

Bishayee, S., and Balasubramaninan, A. S. (1971). Lipid peroxide formation in rat brain. *J. Neurochem. 18,* 909-920.

Bowen, D. M., and Davison, A. N. (1975). Extrapyramidal diseases and dementia. *Lancet 15,* 1199-1200.

Bowen, D. M., Flack, R. H. A., Smith, C. B., White, P., and Davison, A. N. (1974). Brain-decarboxylase activities as indices of pathological change in senile dementia. *Lancet 1,* 1247-1249.

Bowen, D. M., Smith, C. B., White, P., and Davison, A. N. (1976). Neurotransmitter-related enzymes and indices of hypoxia in senile dementia and other abiotrophies. *Brain 99,* 459-496.

Bowers, M. B., and Gerbode, F. A. (1968). Relationship of monoamine metabolites in human cerebrospinal fluid to age. *Nature (London) 219,* 1256-1257.

Brizze, K. R., Harkin, J. C., Ordy, J. M., and Kaack, B. (1975). Accumulation and distribution of lipofuscin, amyloid and senile plaques in the aging nervous system. In *Aging,* Vol. 1: *Clinical, Morphological, and Neurochemical Aspects in the Aging Central Nervous System,* H. Brody, D. Harman, and J. M. Ordy (Eds.). Raven, New York, pp. 39-78.

Carlsson, A. (1959). The occurrence, distribution and physiological role of catecholamines in the nervous system. *Pharmacol. Rev. 11,* 409-493.

Carlsson, A. (1979). The impact of catecholamine research on medical science and practice. In *Catecholamines: Basic and Clinical Frontiers,* E. Usdin, I. J. Kopin, and J. Barchas (Eds.). Pergamon, New York, pp. 4-19.

Carlsson, A., and Winblad, B. (1976). Influence of age and time interval between death and autopsy on dopamine and 3-methoxytyramine levels in human basal ganglia. *J. Neurol. Transm. 38,* 271-276.

Carlsson, A., Falck, B., and Hillarp. N. A. (1962). Cellular localization of brain monoamines. *Acta Physiol. Scand. 56 (Supplement 196).*

Carney, M. W. P. (1967). Serum folate values in 423 psychiatric patients. *Brit. Med. J. 4,* 512-516.

Celesia, G. G., and Wanamaker, W. M. (1972). Psychiatric disturbances in Parkinson's disease. *Dis. Nerv. Sys. 33,* No. 9, 577-583.

Cohen, D., Matsuyama, S. S., and Jarvik, L. F. (1976). Immunoglobulin levels and intellectual functioning in the aged. Short communication.

Coppen, A. (1967). The biochemistry of affective disorders. *Brit. J. Psychiatry 113,* 1237-1264.

Coppen, A., Metcalfe, M., Carroll, J. D., and Morris, J. G. L. (1972). Levodopa and L-tryptophan therapy in parkinsonism. *Lancet 1,* 654-658.

Corsellis, J. A. N. (1962). *Mental Illness and the Ageing Brain.* Oxford University Press, London.

Cote, L. J., and Kremzner, L. T. (1974). Changes in neurotransmitter systems with increasing age in human brain. *Abstr. Am. Soc. Neurochem.,* 83.

Crapper, D. R., Quittkat, S., Krishnan, S. S., Dalton, A. J., and De Boni, U. (1980). Intranuclear aluminum content in Alzheimer's disease, dialysis encephalopathy, and experimental aluminum encephalopathy. *Acta Neuropathol.* (Berl) 50, 19-24.

Davies, P., Maloney, A. J. F. (1976). Selective loss of central cholinergic neurons in Alzheimer's disease. *Lancet 2,* 1403.

Della Corte, L., and Callingham, B. A. (1977). The influence of age and adrenalectomy on rat heart monoamine oxidase. *Biochem. Pharmacol. 26,* 407-415.

Divry, P. J. (1934). De la nature de l'alteration fibrillaire d'Alzheimer. *J. Belge Neurol. Psychiatr. 34,* 197-201.

Drachman, D. A., and Leavitt, J. (1974). Human memory and the cholinergic system. *Arch. Neurol. 30,* 113-121.

Drachman, D. A., and Stahl, S. (1975). Extrapyramidal dementia and levodopa. *Lancet 1,* 809.

Ehringer, H., and Hornykiewicz, O. (1960). Verteilung von Noradrenalin im Dopamin (3-hydroxytyramin) im Gehirn des Menschen und ihr Verhalten bei Erkrankungen des extrapyramidalen Systems. *Klin. Wschr. 38,* 1236-1240.

Ekstedt, B., and Oreland, L. (1976). Effects of lipid-depletion on the different forms of monoamine oxidase in rat lever mitochondria. *Biochem. Pharmacol. 25,* 119-124.

Finch, C. E. (1973). Catecholamine metabolism in the brains of ageing male mice. *Brain Res. 52,* 261-276.

Finch, C. E. (1976). The regulation of physiological changes during mammalian aging. *Quart. Rev. Biol. 51,* 49-83.

Fisher, R. H. (1972). The urinary excretion of homovanillic acid and 4-hydroxy-3-methoxy mandelic acid in the elderly demented. *Geront. Clin. 14,* 172-175.

Gal, E. M., Armstrong, J. C., and Ginsberg, B. (1966). The nature of in vitro hydroxylation of L-tryptophan by brain tissue. *J. Neurochem. 13,* 643-654.

Gellerstedt, N. (1933). Zur Kenntnis der Hirnveranderungen bei der normalen Attersinvolution. *Uppsala Läk.F ören. F örh.* 38, 193.

Gottfries, C. G., Gottfries, I., and Roos, B. E. (1968). Disturbances of monoamine metabolism in the brains from patients with dementia senilis and Mb Alzheimer. *Exp. Med. Int. Congr. Ser. No. 180,* 310-312. (The present status of psychotropic drugs proceedings of the VIth In. Congr. C.I.N.P. Tarragona, April, 1968).

Gottfries, C. G., Gottfries, I., and Roos, B. E. (1969). The investigation of homovanillic acid in the human brain and its correlation to senile dementia. *Br. J. Psychiatry 115,* 563-574.

Gottfries, C. G., Gottfries, I., Johansson, B., Olsson, R., Persson, T., Roos, B. E., and Sjöström, R (1971). Acid Monoamine metabolites in human cerebrospinal fluid and their relations to age and sex. *Neuropharmacology 10,* 665-672.

Gottfries, C. G., Kjällqvist, A., Ponten, U., Roos, B. E., and Sundbärg, G. (1974). Cerebrospinal fluid pH and monoamine and glucolytic metabolites in Alzheimer's disease. *Br. J. Psychiatry 124,* 280-287.

Gottfries, C. G., Oreland, L., Wiberg, A., and Winblad, B. (1975). Lowered monoamine oxidase activity in brains from alcoholic suicides. *J. Neurochem. 25,* 667-673.

Gottfries, C. G., Roos, B. E., and Winblad, B. (1976). Monoamine and monoamine metabolites in the human brain post mortem in senile dementia. *Aktvel Geront. 6,* 429-435.

Gottfries, C. G., Adolfsson, R., Oreland, L., Roos, B. E., and Winblad, B. (1979). Monoamines and their metabolites and monoamine oxidase activity related to age and to some dementia disorders. In *Drugs and the Elderly. Perspectives in geriatric clinical pharmacology.* J. Crooks, and Stevenson, I.H. (Eds.). Proc. Symp. Ninewells Hospital, Dundee, 13-14 Sept. 1977, MacMillan, London, pp. 289-197.

Grahame-Smith, D. G. (1967). The biosynthesis of 5-hydroxytryptamine in brain. *Biochem. J. 105,* 351-360.

Greenfield, J. G., and Bosanquet, F. D. (1953). The brainstem in parkinsonism. *J. Neurol. Neurosurg. Psychiatry 16,* 213-226.

Guard, O., Renaud, B., and Chazot, G. (1976). Metabolism cérébral de la dopamine et de la sérotonine au cours des maladies d'Alzheimer et de Pick. Etude dynamique par le test au probénécide. *L'Encéphale 2,* 293-303.

Guldberg, H. C., Ashcroft, W. G., and Crawford, T. B. B. (1966). Concentrations of 5-hydroxyindoleacetic acid and homovanillic acid in the cerebrospinal fluid of the dog before and during treatment with probenecid. *Life Sci. 5,* 1571-1575.

Hachinsky, V. D., Lassen, N. A., and Marshall, J. (1974). Multi-infarct dementia. A cause of mental deterioration in the elderly. *Lancet 2,* 207-209.

Himwich, W. A., and Himwich, H. E. (1959). Neurochemistry of aging. In *Handbook of Aging and the Individual,* J. E. Birren (Ed.). University of Chicago Press, pp. 187-215.

Hirano, A., Malamud, N., Elizen, T. S., and Kurland, L. T. (1966). Amyotrophic lateral sclerosis and Parkinson-dementia complex on Guam. *Arch. Neurol. 15,* 35-51.

Hirano, A., Dembitzer, H. M., Kurland, L. T., and Zimmermann, H. M. (1968). The fine structure of some intraganglionic alterations. Neurofibrillary tangles, granulovacuolar bodies and "rod-like" structures as seen in Guam amyotrophic lateral sclerosis and Parkinsonism-Dementia complex. *J. Neuropath. Exp. Neurol. 27,* 167-182.

Hollander, J., and Barrows, C. G. (1968). Enzymatic studies in senescent rodent brains. *J. Gerontol. 23,* 174-179.

Horita, A. (1967). Cardiac monoamine oxidase in rat. *Nature (London) 215,* 411-412.

Horita, A., and Lowe, M. C. (1972). On the extraneuronal nature of cardiac monoamine oxidase in the rat. *Adv. Biochem. Psychopharmacol. 5,* 227-242.

Hornykiewicz, O. (1968). Gegenwärtiger Stand der biochemisch-pharmakologischen Erforschung des extrapyramidal-motorischen Systems. *Pharmakopsychiatrie, Neuro-Psychopharmakologie 1,* No. 1, Stuttgart, 6-17.

Houslay, M. D. (1977). A model for the selective mode of action of the irreversible monoamine oxidase inhibitors clorgyline and deprenil, based on studies of their ability to activate a Ca^{2+} –Mg^{2+} –ATPase in defined lipid environment. *J. Pharm. Pharmacol. 29,* 664-669.

Hurdle, A. D. F., and Picton Williams, T. C. (1966). Foliacid deficiency in elderly patients admitted to hospital. *Br. Med. J. 2,* 202-205.

Jervis, G. A. (1971). Pick's disease. In *Pathology of the Nervous System,* Vol. 2. J. Minckler (Ed.). McGraw-Hill, New York, pp. 1395-1404.

Kalter, S., and Kelly, S. (1975). Alzheimer's disease evaluation of immunologic indices. *NY State J. Med. (July)*, pp. 1222-1225.

Kaufman, S., and Friedman, S. (1965). Dopamine-β-hydroxylase. *Pharmacol. Rev. 17*, 71-100.

Kornfelt, M. (1972). Generalized lipofuscinosis (generalized Kuf's disease). *J. Neuropathol. Exp. Neurol. 31*, 668-682.

Kristensen, V., Olsen, M., and Theilgaard, A. (1977). Levodopa treatment of presenile dementia. *Acta Psychiat. Scand 55*, 41-51.

Kristenson, K., and Sourander, P. (1966). Occurrence of lipofuscin in inherited metabolic disorders affecting the nervous system. *J. Neurol. Neurosurg. Psychiatry 29*, 113-118.

Larsson, T., Sjögren, T., and Jacobsson, G. (1963). Senile dementia. A clinical sociomedical and genetic study. *Acta Psychiatr. Scand. (Supplement 167)*.

Lloyd, K., and Hornykiewicz, O. (1970). Occurrence and distribution of L-dopa decarboxylase in the human brain. *Brain Res. 22*, 426-428.

MacLean, R., Nicholson, W. J., Paré, C. M. B., and Stacey, R. S. (1965). Effect of monoamineoxidase inhibitors on the concentration of 5-hydroxytryptamine in the human brain. *Lancet 2*, 205-20[illegible]

McGeer, E. G., and McGeer, P. L. (1973). Some characteristics of brain tyrosine hydroxylase. In *New Concepts in Neurotransmitter Regulation*, A. J. Mandell (Ed.). Plenum, New York, pp. 53-69.

McGeer, E., and McGeer, P. L. (1976a). Neurotransmitter metabolism in the aging brain. In *Neurobiology of Aging*, R. D. Terry and S. Gershon (Eds.). Raven, New York, pp. 389-403.

McGeer, P. L., and McGeer, E. G. (1976b). Enzymes associated with the metabolism of catecholamines, acetylcholine, and GABA in human controls and patients with Parkinson's disease and Huntington's chorea. *J. Neurochem. 26*, 65-76.

McGeer, E. G., and Fibiger, H. C., McGeer, P. L., and Wickson, V. (1971a). Aging and brain enzymes. *Exp. Gerontol. 6*, 391-396.

McGeer, E. G., McGeer, P. L., and Wada, S. A. (1971b). Distribution of tyrosine hydroxylase in human and animal brain. *J. Neurochem. 18*, 1647-1658.

Meek, J. L., Bertilsson, L., Cheney, D. L., Zsilla, G., and Costa, E. (1977). Aging induced changes in acetylcholine and serotonin content of discrete brain nuclei. *J. Gerontol. 732*, 129-131.

Mehrain, P., Yamada, M., and Tarnowska-Dzidiszko, E. (1975). Quantitative study on dendrites and dendritic spines in Alzheimer's disease and senile dementia. In *Advances in Neurology*, Vol. 12. G. W. Kreutzberg, (Ed.). Raven, New York, pp. 453-458.

Mindham, R. H. S. (1970). Psychiatric symptoms in parkinsonism. *J. Neurol. Neurosurg. Psychiatry 33*, 187-191.

Moir, A. T. B., Ashcroft, G. W., Crawford, T. B. B., Eccleston, D., and Guldberg, H. C. (1970). Cerebral metabolites in cerebrospinal fluid as a biochemical approach to the brain. *Brain 93,* 357-368.

Neff, N. H., Tozer, T. N. and Brodie, B. B. (1964). A specialized transport system to transfer 5-HIAA directly from brain to blood. *Pharmacologist 6,* 194.

Neff, N. H., Tozer, T. N., and Brodie, B. B. (1967). Application of steady-state kinetics to studies of the transfer of 5-hydroxyindoleacetic acid from brain to plasma. *J. Pharmacol. Exp. Ther. 158,* 214-218.

Nies, A., Robinson, D. S., Davis, J. M., and Ravaris, C. G. (1973). Changes in monoamine oxidase with ageing and depression in man. *Psychopharmacology and Aging: Advances in Behavioral Biology,* C. Eisdorfer and W. E. Fann (Eds.). Plenum, New York, pp. 41-54.

Nikaido, T. J., Austin, J., Trueb, L., and Rinehart, R. (1972). Studies in ageing of the brain. II. Microchemical analyses of the nervous system in Alzheimer patients. *Arch. Neurol. 27,* 549-554.

Novick, W. J. (1961). The effect of age and thyroid hormones on the monoamine oxidase of rat heart. *Endocrinology 69,* 55-59.

Okada, Y. (1976). *GABA in Nervous System Function,* E. Roberts, T. N. Chase, and D. B. Tower (Eds.). Raven, New York, pp. 235-243.

Olsson, R., and Roos, B. E. (1968). Concentration of 5-hydroxyindoleacetic acid and homovanillic acid in the cerebrospinal fluid after treatment with probenecid in patients with Parkinson's disease. *Nature 219,* 502-503.

Op Den Velde, W., and Stam, F. C. (1976). Some cerebral proteins and enzyme systems in Alzheimer's presenile and senile dementia. *J. Am. Geriatr. Soc. 24,* No. 1, 12-16.

Ordy, J. M., and Schjeide, O. A. (1973). Univariate and multivariate models for evaluating long-term changes in neurobiological development, maturity and aging. In *Progress in Brain Research, Neurobiological Aspects of Maturation and Aging* Vol. 40, D. H. Ford (Ed.). Elsevier, Amsterdam, pp. 25-51.

Pare, C. M. B., Young, D. P. H., Price, K., and Stacey, R. S. (1969). 5-hydroxytryptamine, noradrenaline, and dopamine in brainstem, hypothalamus and caudate nucleus of controls and patients committing suicide by coalgas poisoning. *Lancet 25,* 133-135.

Pearce, J. (1974). Letter. Mental changes in parkinsonism. *Br. Med. J. 2,* 445.

Perry, E. K., Perry, R. H., Blessed, G., and Tomlinson, B. E. (1977). Necropsy evidence of central cholinergic deficits in senile dementia. Letters to the Editor, *Lancet 1,* 189.

Pollock, M., and Hornabrook, R. W. (1966). The prevalence, natural history and dementia of Parkinson's disease. *Brain 89,* 429-448.

Prange, A. Jr., White, J., Lipton, M., and Kirkead, A. M. (1967). Influence of age on monoamine oxidase and catechol-o-methyl-transferase in rat tissues. *Life Sci. 6,* 581-586.

Read, A. E., Gough, K. R., Pardoo, J. L., and Nicholas, A. (1965). Nutritional studies on the entrants to an old people's home, with particular reference to folic-acid deficiency. *Br. Med. J. 2,* 843-848.

Robinson, D. S., Davies, J. M., and Nies, A. (1972). Aging, monoamines, and monoamine oxidase levels. *Lancet 1,* 290-291.

Robinson, D. S., Sourkes, T. L., Nies, A., Harris, L. S., Spector, S., Bartlett, D. L., and Kaye, I. S. (1977). Monoamine metabolism in human brain. *Arch. Gen. Psychiatry 34,* 89-92.

Roos, B. E. (1970). Metabolites of the monoamines in the cerebrospinal fluid. Monoamines et noyaux gris centraux. Symposium Bel-Air IV, Geneva.

Roth, M., Tomlinson, B. E., and Blessed, G. (1966). Correlation between score for dementia and counts of senile plaques in cerebral grey matter of elderly subjects. *Nature (London) 209,* 106.

Samorajski, T., and Rolsten, C. (1973). Age and regional differences in the chemical composition of brains of mice, monkeys and humans. In *Progress in Brain Research,* Vol. 40, *Neurobiological Aspects of Maturation and Aging,* D. H. Ford (Ed.). Elsevier, Amsterdam, pp. 253-265.

Samorajski, T., Rolsten, C., and Ordy, J. M. (1971). Changes in behavior, brain and neuroendocrine chemistry with age and stress in C57B1/19 male mice. *J. Gerontol. 26,* 168-175.

Scheibel, M. E., and Scheibel, A. B. (1975). Structural changes in the aging brain. In *Aging,* Vol. 1, *Clinical, Morphologic, and Neurochemical Aspects in the Aging Central Nervous System,* H. Brody, D. Harman, and J. M. Ordy (Eds.). Raven, New York, pp. 11-37.

Schildkraut, J. J. (1965). The catecholamine hypothesis of affective disorders. A review of supporting evidence. *Am. J. Psychiatry 122,* 509-522.

Shaw, D. M., Macsweeney, D. A., Johnson, A. L., O'Keeffe, R., Naidoo, D., Macload, D. M., Jog, S., Preece, J. M., and Crowley, J. M. (1971). Folate and amine metabolites in senile dementia. A combined trial and biochemical study. *Psycholog. Med. 1,* 166-171.

Shih, J. C. (1975). *Multiple Forms of Monoamine Oxidase and Aging,* Vol. 1. H. Brody, D. Harman, and J. M. Ordy (Eds.). Raven, New York.

Shulman, R. (1967). A survey of vitamin B_{12} deficiency in an elderly psychiatric population. *Br. J. Psychiatry 113,* 241-251.

Simchowitz, T. (1911). Histologische Studien über die senile Demenz. *Histol. Histopathol. Arb. Grosshirnrinde 4,* 267-274.

Sjögren, T., Sjögren, H., and Lindgren, A. G. H. (1952). Morbus Alzheimer and morbus Pick. A genetic clinical and pathoanatomical study. *Acta Psychiatr. Scand. (Supplement 82).*

Spillane, J. A., White, P., Goodhardt, M. J., Flack, R. H. A., Bowen, D. M., and Davison, A. N. (1977). Selective vulnerability of neurones in organic dementia. *Nature,* 266, 558-559.

Suzuki, K., and Terry, R. D. (1967). Fine structural localization of acid phosphatase in senile plaques in Alzheimer's presenile dementia. *Acta Neuropathol. 8,* 276.

Tappaz, M. L., Brownstein, M. J., and Palkovits, M. (1976). Distribution of glutamate decarboxylase in discrete brain nuclei. *Brain Res. 89,* 160-165.

Tarsy, D., Pycock, C., Meldrum, B., and Marsden, C. D. (1975). Rotational behavior induced in rats by intranegral picrotoxin. *Brain Res. 89.* 160-165.

Terry, R. D. (1963). The fine structure of neurofibrillary tangles in Alzheimer's disease. *J. Neuropathol. Exp. Neurol. 22,* 629-642.

Terry, R. D. and Wisniewski, H. (1970). The ultrastructure of the neurofibrillary tangle and the senile plaque. In *Ciba Foundation Symposium on Alzheimer's Disease and Related Conditions,* G. E. W. Wolstenholm and M. O'Connor (Eds.). Churchill, London, pp. 95-104.

Tomlinson, B. E. (1972). Morphological brain changes in non-demented old people. In *Aging of the Central Nervous System,* H. M. van Praag and A. K. Kalverboorn (Eds.). Bohn, New York, pp. 38-57.

Weil-Malherbe, H. (1972). The biochemistry of affective disorders. In *Handbook of Neurochemistry,* Vol. 7, *Pathological Chemistry of the Nervous System,* A. Lajtha (Ed.). Plenum, New York, pp. 371-416.

von Bogaert, L. (1970). Cerebral amyloid angiopathy and Alzheimer's disease. In *Ciba Symposium: Alzheimer's Disease and Related Condition* G. Wolstenholme and Haeve O'Connor (Eds.). Church, London, pp. 95-104.

von Braunmühl, A. (1958). Alterserkrankungen des Zentralnervensystem. In *Hdbch. spez. path. Anat. XIII/1A,* O. Lubarsch, F. Henke, and R. Rössle (Eds.). Springer-Verlag, Berlin, pp. 337-539.

Werdinius, B. (1966). Effect of probenecid on the level of homovanillic acid in the corpus striatum. *J. Pharmacol. 18,* 546-547.

Vernadakis, A. (1973). Neuronal-glial interactions during development and aging. *Fed. Proc. 34,* 89-95.

White, P., Goodhardt, M. J., Keet, J. P., Hiley, C. R., Carrasco, L. H., and Williams, I. E. I. (1977). Neocortical cholinergic neurons in elderly people. *Lancet 1,* 668.

Wisniewski, H., and Terry, R. (1973). Morphology of the aging brain, human and animal. In *Neurological Aspects of Mutation and Aging.* D. H. Ford (Ed.). Elsevier, Amsterdam, pp. 167-186.

Zeman, W., and Dyken, P. (1969). Neuronal ceroid-lipofuscinosis (Batten's disease). Relationship to amaurotic family idiocy? *Pediatrics 44,* 570-573.

12

Biochemical Aspects of Mental Retardation

Norbert Herschkowitz
University of Berne
Berne, Switzerland

I. INTRODUCTION

Mental retardation can be caused by abnormal development or secondary destruction of brain structures. The normal functioning of the nervous system depends on the integrated and coordinated actions of neuronal circuits. The highly complex brain structures are formed and integrated as the result of a precisely timed sequence of metabolic events. The blueprint which regulates the formation of brain structures is genetically determined; however, exogenous factors can interfere during all periods of development.

Main phases of development include the *proliferation* of neurons and glial cells, the *migration* of these cells to their predetermined locations, the *differentiation* of the precursor cells to specific cells, and, finally, *cell death.*

Inborn errors of metabolism (mutations) and/or exogenous toxic factors which interfere with metabolism can lead to abnormal brain structures and nerve circuits, which can result in mental retardation.

It is important to note that until now we have very little knowledge of the *direct* connection between abnormal brain metabolism and abnormal behavior. Until the anatomical-metabolical basis of behavior is understood, the complete pathogenetic mechanisms of abnormal brain function are still a matter of conjecture.

The careful multidisciplinary study of mental retardation can further the understanding of the metabolic mechanisms involved in behavior.

The final goal of the enormous efforts undertaken today to identify and investigate the biochemical events leading to mental retardation is the prevention of this condition, which, depending on the sociomedical criteria applied, affects 3-10% of the population.

II. NORMAL BRAIN DEVELOPMENT

Periods of rapid development of brain structures—growth spurts—are periods of high metabolic activity. These are especially vulnerable to various noxes. The hypothesis put forward by Dobbing states that if a developmental process is restricted by any agent at the time of its fastest rate, this will not only delay the process but will restrict its ultimate extent, even when the restricting influence is removed and the fullest possible rehabilitation obtained (Dobbing, 1968).

Since the periods of rapid development are critical, the knowledge of the timing involved in brain development is of major importance. It must be taken into account that there are regional differences in brain with respect to periods of intense development and therefore regional differences in the time of vulnerability.

Proliferation of neurons usually takes place in brain between 15 and 25 weeks in gestation (WIG) (Dobbing and Sands, 1970). This information was gained by measuring DNA in brains during development. DNA estimation is, with some limitations, a good indicator for cell number and an overall indicator for a major period of neuroblast multiplication.

The "dogma" that there is no neuronal multiplication in the adult brain may have to be at least partially corrected. In the rat adult brain Kaplan and Hinds (1977) found evidence for neuronal proliferation in the hippocampus and in the olfactory bulb. Although the biological significance of this finding is not yet clear, it is important to be aware that neuronal proliferation may continue in the "mature" brain.

In the cortical area of the human brain formation and differentiation of neurons takes place very early. Molliver et al. (1973) could demonstrate synapses above and below the cortical plate between 8.5 and 15 WIG.

Migration of neuroblasts starts shortly after neuroblast multiplication, as early as 12 WIG (Evrad et al., 1978).

Differentiation of neurons takes place mainly after the cells have reached their destination. Purpura (1977) described maximal differentiation of neurons (formation of dendrites and spines) in the primary visual cortex between 29 and 33 WIG.

Differentiation of neurons (formation of dendrites, synapses, elongation of axons) takes place until approximately the 4th postnatal year.

Differentiation of oligodendrocytes leads to myelination of the axons. Myelination can be observed in the pyramidal tract and reticular formation at 25-30 WIG (Gilles et al., 1976). Myelination in the human brain as a whole takes place in a rapid period from birth until the 2nd postnatal year and a second, slow period which lasts until about the 15th year.

Brain development can be followed by biochemical "markers," i.e., structural proteins, lipids, or enzymes which are enriched in the particular structural element. DNA is localized in the nucleus of the cell and is a measure for the number of cells, provided that the majority of the cells are diploid. Metabolic interference with DNA metabolism can affect the number of cells formed.

Gangliosides are present in several membranes but are particularly enriched in the membranes of the synapses (Vanier et al., 1971). The increase in gangliosides during the period of neuronal differentiation may be correlated to the number of synapses formed. The lipids cerebroside and sulfatide and the myelin basic protein are localized in the myelin membrane. The degree of their increase in brain is correlated to the rate of myelin formation.

III. ABNORMAL BRAIN DEVELOPMENT

Inborn errors of metabolism or toxic agents which affect the metabolism of compounds involved in the formation or maintenance of brain structures can affect brain function in various ways and to various degrees, all leading to mental retardation. Our current knowledge of the molecular basis of human mental function is so small that it is not astonishing that very little is known about the molecular basis of mental retardation. In the group of inborn errors of metabolism an abnormal permanent metabolic process is present, and the primary enzymatic defect is known with its resulting biochemical consequences. This allows us to at least partially determine the "hierarchy of causes" which leads from the primary biochemical defects to secondary metabolic aberrations affecting certain brain structures and its neurophysiological dysfunctions. It is still a great step to the understanding of mental functions and mental retardation. The investigation of the inborn errors of metabolism leading to mental retardation allows us to study the dynamics of the processes and to try to correlate the timed sequence of metabolic-structural events with the sequence of clinical symptoms.

In this chapter the discussion of the biochemistry of mental retardation is therefore restricted to examples of inborn errors of metabolism leading to mental retardation.

IV. MENTAL RETARDATION RESULTING FROM INBORN ERRORS OF METABOLISM

Over 100 inborn errors of metabolism have so far been identified, of which at least 50 are connected with mental retardation. In a patient with mental retardation, the clinician can suspect an inborn error of metabolism when one or more of the following conditions are present:

1. Anamnestically no significant pre- or postnatal toxic factor is known.
2. Familiarity:
   a. Sibling of the patient has the same disease; possibility of a recessive disorder.

   b. Relatives of the patient in one family line are affected; possibility of a dominant disorder.
   c. Only males are affected; possibility of a sex X-linked mutation.
3. Progressive disorder: Anamnestically there is a regression of acquired abilities, e.g., loss of motor skills, loss of cognitive functions, changes in personality, progression of neurologic signs.
4. a. Signs of accumulation in several organs such as liver, spleen (hepatosplenomegaly), brain (macrocephaly), retina (cherry red spot), or skeleton.
   b. Accumulation of abnormal substances in kidney urinary output, inclusions in leukocytes and bone marrow cells.

The clinical history of the patient and his family is of primary importance for differential diagnosis. Are family members affected by the same or similar problems? Is there a possibility of consanguinity of the parents? Which family members are affected? Is there a sex prevalence? When did the clinical symptoms appear? What kind of symptoms came first? What is the clinical course of the disease? Which organ systems are involved?

Some information on the neural system primarily involved can be gained by studying the progression of the disorders:

1. Neuronal disorders usually begin with dementia and convulsions. These are followed by the symptoms of ataxia, spasticity, and Babinsky sign.
2. Myelin disorders usually begin with ataxia, spasticity, and Babinsky sign. These are followed by the symptoms of dementia and convulsions.

V. INBORN ERRORS OF AMINO ACID METABOLISM

Amino acids, the basic units in protein formation, either enter the brain from the circulation or are formed by metabolic processes within the brain.

There are systems known which transport acidic amino acids and others which transport basic amino acids. Amino acid levels in the blood may reflect intracerebral concentrations. This is true, for example, for tyrosine, glutamine, histidine, and phenylalanine. The serum levels of other amino acids, such as glutamate, lysine, and leucine, do not reflect brain concentrations.

Impairment of amino acid metabolism in the brain resulting in abnormal amino acid levels in the brain may affect protein synthesis.

Because some amino acids are putative neurotransmitters or precursors of neurotransmitter, an inborn error affecting amino acid metabolism may affect neurophysiological functions regulated by neurotransmitters. Furthermore, synapses which play a key role in brain functions are capable of synthesizing proteins from amino acid. Abnormal amino acid metabolism may therefore also affect synaptic structures and functions directly, leading to a clinical picture which may resemble an overall neuronal dysfunction.

A. Phenylketonuria

In 1934 Fölling described in a biochemical journal that he had found a high output of phenylpyruvic acid in the urine of 10 mentally retarded children. He suggested that there was a causative relationship between the abnormal phenylalanine metabolism and the mental retardation.

The development of new biochemical methods such as spectrophotometry and chromatography provided the basis for a rapid increase in knowledge of the underlying biochemical defect of this disease. In 1953 the enzymatic defect was found to be in the conversion of phenylalanine to tyrosine by Jervis and Udenfried and Boxxman. In 1954 the possibility of a dietary treatment of the disease to prevent or lessen mental retardation was demonstrated by Bickel and coauthors. In 1963, as the result of intensive biochemical investigation, tests were introduced which made possible screening for this disease soon after birth (Guthrie and Susi, 1963). The disease has an incidence of 1 in 13,000 to 1 in 24,000. No race or sex preference has been found.

In the classical form of phenylketonuria (PKU) there are no discrete features of the patient at birth (Pueschel and Rotteman (1976). After the first postnatal year, however, the clinical symptoms accumulate to the point where a diagnosis is usually made.

If untreated in the 1st year, a patient loses about 50 points of his EQ. There are no very specific clinical signs which lead to the diagnosis of PKU. At an age of 2-3 months a musty odor (phenylacetic acid) may be present. After the 1st year the developmental failure becomes evident: failure to learn to walk or talk and microcephaly. Hyperactivity, agressive behavior, tremor, and convulsions follow. There is muscular hypertonicity. The patients show a prominent maxilla with widened interdental spaces and decalcification of the long bones. The pigment dilution of hair and skin becomes more evident. Life expectancy is usually shortened.

The underlying defect in PKU is a reduction of the activity of the enzyme phenylalanine hydroxylase, which converts phenylalanine into tyrosine. In the case of decreased conversion, phenylalanine enters an alternate pathway. It will be converted to phenylpyruvic acid and to further derivatives. Phenylalanine and the products of the alternate pathway will accumulate in the body fluids. In normals phenylalanine levels are under 1 mg/100 ml plasma; in patients levels can range from 6 to 80 mg/100 ml. Most patients with the clinical signs of PKU have values over 20 mg/100 ml. There is some relationship between phenylalanine levels in the blood and phenylpyruvic acid in the urine.

A simple test introduced by Guthrie and Susi (1963), based on the estimation of phenylalanine in one drop of blood, will allow the estimation of phenylalanine concentration in the plasma. This test made it possible to screen newborns for high phenylalanine levels. When the result is positive, the diagnosis must be confirmed by additional tests, such as a phenylalanine-loading test by Blaskovic et al. (1974).

The pathogenetic mechanisms in PKU which lead to mental retardation are not yet fully understood. Protein synthesis is quantitatively decreased (Appel, 1966) and myelin lipid synthesis is inhibited by high levels of phenylalanine (Barlato et al., 1968). The reduced myelin formation may be of special importance during the period of myelination, which lasts until approximately age 15.

Secondary effects of the enzymatic deficiency and the accumulation of products include the decrease of melanine, which may explain the hypopigmentation. The observed decrease of serotonin (5-hydroxytryptamine) may be due to a secondary inhibition of the enzyme 5-hydroxytryptophan decarboxylase by the accumulated phenylalanine derivates. The metabolites may also inhibit the enzyme dopamine decarboxylase leading to decreased levels of epinephrine, norepinephrine, and dopamine. There is a further possibility that the accumulated substances inhibit the enzyme glutamic acid decarboxylase, which could lead to a decreased formation of γ-aminobutyric acid.

These disorders of neurotransmitter metabolism may be partly responsible for the abnormal behavior, the hyperactivity, and the seizures.

1. *Maternal Phenylketonuria*

Children of mothers with PKU may be affected at birth (Mabry et al., 1966). They may show intrauterine growth retardation and microcephaly. The mechanisms leading to the retardation are not understood. It is possible that increased phenylalanine levels in the circulating blood of the mother are toxic for the fetus, but there is no direct relationship between phenylalanine levels in the mothers' blood during pregnancy and mental retardation of the offspring (Fisch et al., 1966). Still, dietary treatment is recommended for mothers with PKU during pregnancy.

2. *Treatment*

The treatment consists of lowering phenylalanine intake during the most active period of brain development. Bickel et al. (1954) were the first to try this treatment by using an acid caseine hydrolyzate from which phenylalanine had been removed.

Later phenylalanine was added in limited amounts to the diet because phenylalanine is an essential amino acid necessary for development. There are now several preparations commercially available which contain carbohydrates, fats, vitamins, and minerals in adequate amounts. The treatment is monitored by frequent measurement of phenylalanine levels in the blood, which are usually kept at 3-7 mg/100 ml (normal levels would be 1-2 mg/100 ml). The requirements and the tolerance for phenylalanine have to be determined for each patient individually by frequent serum determinations. The usual requirement for children with PKU is 15-30 mg phenylalanine/kg per day.

It is important that treatment is started as early as possible and closely monitored by clinical and biochemical observation in specialized centers. It is not yet clear as to when to stop the treatment. For now this is usually done between 8 and 10 years. At this age brain development, especially myelination, is not finished, but the main active period is over; and numerous difficulties in treating children of school age with the diet as well as secondary psychological problems may become a very serious disadvantage.

It is not yet completely known how effective the treatment of PKU is in preventing mental retardation. Under optimal conditions of both diet and education and with the onset of the treatment at an age of under 2 months, near-normal to normal EQ may be achieved. There are, however, not yet enough longitudinal studies which encompass the school time. It is obvious that these studies will be very difficult to undertake and will require careful interpretation. However, in order to optimize treatment and to determine when to discontinue the diet, these longitudinal studies are a great necessity.

B. Maple Syrup Urine Disease

Maple syrup urine disease affects about 1 child in 120,000-250,000 born alive. Since several enzymes involved in a functional complex are affected, different phenotypes of the disease are possible and the clinical picture therefore varies greatly.

In the classical form the first clinical symptoms appear around the 2nd week of life starting with apathy, failure to thrive, followed later by high-pitched crying, apnea, decreasing or disappearance of the Moro reflex, convulsions, and coma. Death or severe cerebral damage can be the consequence. The body fluids smell like maple syrup or curry. The amino acids leucine, isoleucine, and valine are elevated in serum and urine. Concomitant hypoglycemia can occur. The enzyme defect is the reduction of the capability for oxidative decarboxylation of the three-branched chain ketoacids. It can be detected in liver tissue as well as in leukocytes or in fibroblasts. This makes a prenatal diagnosis possible.

If untreated for several months, there is a clear reduction in myelin, possibly due to reduced synthesis of myelin components. As these children do not tolerate normal protein intake, therapy must begin immediately: Protein intake must stop. Hypoglycemia and acidosis have to be corrected. Peritoneal dialysis is sometimes necessary for the removal of toxic metabolites. Lipids and carbohydrates must be given to provide enough calories. Later protein intake may be resumed; the amount tolerated must be determined individually by monitoring amino acid levels. In addition, synthetic amino acid mixtures which do not contain valine, leucine, and isoleucine are used. Dietary restrictions may be necessary during the entire life (Bachmann and Baumgartner, 1978; Bachmann and Nyhan, 1978).

C. Nonketotic Hyperglycinemia

Nonketotic hyperglycinemia is caused by the deficiency of the glycine cleavage system, which is reduced in the liver and lacking in the brain of affected children. Glycine levels can be raised up to 3-fold in plasma and up to 20-fold in the CSF, indicating high brain tissue levels. Death may occur in the 1st days or weeks of life. If a child survives this phase, severe mental retardation, generalized seizures, and muscular hypertonia may develop. Various treatments have been tried: dietary restriction, administration of sodium benzoate, supplying the coenzyme, use of glycine-binding agents, and ventriculoperitoneal shunting. The results have been doubtful.

Gitzelmann et al. (1977) tried a new approach in the treatment of this disease. Glycine is a putative neurotransmitter of small inhibitory neurons in the brain stem and spinal cord. The hypothesis is that the pathogenetic mechanism of the nonketotic hyperglycinemia is the blocking of certain synapses by excessive glycine. Strychnine, which has a very high affinity for the glycine receptor, is therefore a glycine antagonist and could offset some of the effects of excessive glycine. One child was treated from the 7th month for at least 12 months with oral strychnine, 3 mg/day. The drug caused improvement of muscle tone, motoricity, vigilance, and social behavior. A temporary withdrawal of strychnine produced after 24 hr a prompt loss of interest in the surroundings and floppiness. After 36 hr the patient was almost motionless; tendon reflexes were nearly absent. After the strychnine therapy was resumed, the child was again active and showed normal muscle tone and reflexes. After 12 months of treatment (18 months of age), no negative side effects have been observed. The psychomotor development of this child is not normal, but his development has proceeded further than that of his 9½-year-old affected brother who was only treated with antiepileptics. It is possible that an earlier treatment with strychnine will augment the therapeutic success.

Many questions remain open, particularly as to the long-term effect of the strychnine application, but the results until now warrant further clinical investigations. This treatment is a good example of the collaboration between clinical medicine and basic research.

VI. INBORN ERRORS OF SPHINGOLIPID METABOLISM

Sphingolipids are complex lipids with a common structure. The variability of the sphingolipids is due to differences in the fatty acids and especially the carbohydrates. The great variation of the glycolipids can be compared to that of glycoproteins. Sphingolipids occur in membranes in the central nervous system, and when their degradation is affected their accumulation may lead to mental retardation. Normally the lipids are degraded by specific hydrolases in intracellularly located lysosomes. This allows a stepwise degradation. The mutation affects primarily one enzyme protein by reducing its degradative activity against a main substrate and maybe also against several structurally similar compounds. The molecule which is not degraded accumulates in the enlarged lysosomes. This can be seen as vacuoles in the leukocytes and in cells in the bone marrow; it can also lead to enlargement of the organs, e.g., hepatosplenomegaly or megacephaly. The accumulation of lipids in the retina cells changes their translucence, except at the macula. This causes a conspicuous macula which is seen as a cherry red spot.

It is interesting to note that the total weight increase of an organ in which a substance accumulates is more than the weight increase due to the accumulated substances; however, no conclusive explanation has been given for this observation. In order to identify the primary enzyme defect, it is necessary to ensure that the reduced enzyme activity does not result from the presence of an inhibitor or the lack of a cofactor. Of special importance is the estimation of the enzyme activity in the obligate heterozygotes, where an intermediate enzyme activity should be observed.

If the primary enzyme activity defect can be established, then it will be diagnostically important to know whether the affected enzyme activity can be detected in serum, leukocytes, fibroblasts, or urine. If the detection of the defect is possible in the fibroblasts, then a prenatal diagnosis in cultured amniotic fluid cells around the 20th week in gestation is a possibility.

Some recent reviews which deal with problems of diagnosis and pathogenetic mechanisms are cited (O'Brien, 1978; Brady, 1978a,b; Pilz et al., 1978; Adachi et al., 1978).

A. GM_1 Gangliosidosis

1. GM_1 Gangliosidosis Type 1

Symptoms are present from birth on in GM_1 gangliosidosis type 1. There are feeding problems and the newborn is hypotonic. Convulsions may occur. There is a rapid deterioration after 1 year leading to blindness, deafness, and spastic quadriplegia. The face is coarse, there may be edema, gingiva hypertrophy, and macroglossy. The signs of accumulation are often present (hepatosplenomegaly and cherry red spot in the retina). In X rays the picture of dysostosis multiplex is seen. Death from pneumonia usually occurs.

The basic defect is the deficiency of the enzyme β-galactosidase, which degrades GM_1 ganglioside. The diagnosis can be made from leukocytes or cultured fibroblasts, or prenatally from amniotic fluid cells. Heterozygotes can be detected. GM_1 gangliosides are accumulated in the brain and in visceral organs. Glycoproteins and mucopolysaccharides accumulate in viscera and in bones.

2. *GM_1 Gangliosidosis Type 2*

In gangliosidosis type 2 the clinical symptoms start later and the progress is slower. An initial symptom is often ataxia, which is observed at 1 year. Once the first symptoms appear, a loss of acquired abilities occurs, i.e., loss of speech and coordinated movements. Convulsions can occur after the 1st year. Pneumonia usually leads to death between 3 and 10 years of age. In contrast to the type 1, there is no coarsening of the face, no hepatosplenomegaly, and no cherry red spot in the retina. Radiological changes of the skeleton are not prominent.

GM_1 ganglioside is stored in brain, but usually not in the viscera. Glycoproteins accumulate in the viscera. β-galactosidase activity in cells is low. Prenatal diagnosis and heterozygote detection are possible.

3. *Other Acid β-Galactosidase Deficiencies With or Without Mental Retardation*

There are several disorders known which show low β-galactosidase activity with quite different phenotypes. There can be minimal skeletal involvement with a slow progressive neurologic disease. There have been patients reported with moderate bone involvement and moderate neurologic impairment. A third phenotype is manifested in a patient N. R., who showed no mental impairment, but rather severe skeletal deformities (O'Brien et al., 1976). No differences in the enzyme activities between the different phenotypes can be observed by using artificial substrate in the enzyme assay. However, with natural substrates differences in enzyme activities can be observed. Using GM_1 ganglioside as substrate, GM_1 gangliosidosis type 1 shows an enzyme activity which is 0.4-0.7% of the normal value. Type 2 has an activity which is 1.9-5.3% of the normal. The biological effect of these differences is difficult to assess, but it is possible that these differences may be rate limiting at low activity and lead to differences in the rate of accumulation. This could influence the rate of deterioration in a disease. In the patient N. R., who had no brain involvement, the enzyme activity against GM_1 ganglioside was 7% but that against the glycoprotein only 1.4% of the mean. This may explain the fact that the skeleton (glycoproteins) was affected and the brain (gangliosides) apparently not.

B. GM_2 Gangliosidosis

1. GM_2 Type 1 (Tay-Sachs Disease)

An early symptom (at a few weeks of age) of Tay-Sachs disease is a startle response to noise without any habituation. Also, motor weakness can be observed at 3 months of age. After 1 year, psychomotor deterioration progresses rapidly and at 1½ years a state of decerebrate rigidity, blindness, deafness, and convulsions is reached. There is frequently a cherry red spot in the retina and macrocephaly due to introcerebral accumulation and fibrosis. The patients usually die of pneumonia at about 2-4 years.

The frequency of this disease is higher among Ashkenazy Jews originating from the Balkan region and Poland than the rest of the population. Mortality records in the United States indicate a heterozygote frequency for Tay-Sachs disease in Ashkenazy Jews of about .027 and .0029 for non-Jewish individuals (O'Brien, 1978).

The basic defect is a deficiency of the enzyme hexosaminidase (Okada and O'Brien, 1969; Okada et al., 1971) (possessing both β-D, N-glucosaminidase and β-D, N-galactosaminidase activity). The result is an accumulation of GM_2 ganglioside. Hexosaminidase consists of two isoenzymes, hexosaminidase A and B. In Tay-Sachs disease the isoenzyme A is nearly absent.

Diagnosis of the homozygote and heterozygote can be done in serum, leukocytes, or cultivated fibroblasts. A prenatal diagnosis is possible using amniotic fluid cells. The serum test allows an accurate genotype assignment in about 96% of those tested. Four percent remain doubtful and can be tested with leukocytes or fibroblasts which allow a reliability of about 99% (Kaback and Zeiger, 1972). False positive values for "heterozygotes" in serum tests can be observed in women taking oral contraceptives, in pregnant women, in women with diabetes mellitus or diseases with tissue destruction, such as myocardial infarction or pancreatitis. In those situations leukocyte measurement will avoid false positive values. The enzymatic diagnosis should be made only in centers which have enough experience to avoid as many of the various pitfalls as possible. Under these circumstances genetic counseling is possible and a great help for families and individuals at risk.

2. GM_2 Type 2 (Sandhoff's Disease)

The clinical picture of Sandhoff's disease is very similar to that of Tay-Sachs disease. The enzymatic defect is, however, different: The two isoenzymes hexosaminidase A and B are deficient. This can be diagnosed in all tissues using artificial or natural substrates. Prenatal diagnosis is possible.

3. GM_2 Type 3 (Juvenile GM_2 Gangliosidosis)

The first prominent symptom of juvenile GM_2 gangliosidosis is ataxia, usually occurring between 2 and 6 years of age. The disease progresses with spasticity and athetoid movements, loss of speech, and minor motor seizures. Blindness develops late in this disorder quite in contrast to Tay-Sachs and Sandhoff's disease. Death occurs between 5 and 15 years. Neither hepatosplenomegaly, skeletal deformities, lymphocyte vacuoles, nor inclusions in the cells of the bone marrow have been described.

Batten-Spielmeer-Vogt disease may have sometimes been wrongly diagnosed as this disorder. However, in that disease early visual disturbances and macular degeneration are prominent features, in contrast to the juvenile GM_2 gangliosidosis. In several patients the enzymatic defect was found to be a partial deficiency in hexosaminidase A. This is more prominent when the natural substrate GM_2 ganglioside is used instead of the artificial substrate. There have been reports of healthy adults with hexosaminidase A and A+B deficiency (Vidgoff et al., 1973; Dreyfuss et al., 1977). As more investigations are made, more and more variant forms are being detected, each one requiring a complete individual study.

4. *Pathogenetic Considerations in Gangliosidosis*

Why do these diseases lead to abnormal mental development? The fact that some substances accumulate in lysosomes does not alone explain the consequences to brain functions. Gangliosides are localized in synapses, but in accumulative disorders with ganglioside storage in lysosomes synapses do not seem profoundly affected.

The main reason for our lack of knowledge is the fact that we do not know enough about the molecular basis of psychomotor function, and therefore we cannot correlate the molecular effects of a mutation to the mental aberrations. On the other hand, the careful multidisciplinary study of these rare diseases involving all branches of the neurosciences may help considerably to gain a better understanding of the basic mechanisms of normal mental function. Once the pathogenetic mechanisms of diseases are better known, then prophylactic and therapeutic measures can be applied rationally.

Recent studies by Purpura and Suzuki (1976) in cerebral biopsy tissue using Golgi stainings has brought new insights. In GM_2 gangliosidosis type 2 (Sandhoff's), large, thick processes were found to emerge from the nerve cell body. These were found to be axons which contained masses of stored material and membranes. These meganeurites are studded with spines, some of which are in postsynaptic relationship to presynaptic endings. Also, in Tay-Sachs disease meganeurites have been found in small- and medium-size pyramidal neurons. The meganeurites may have a surface which surpasses that of the neuronal body. The increased membrane surface area can decrease whole neuronal input resistance. This attenuates potentials elicited in the somatodendritic membrane of storage neurons more than in normal neurons. In addition, the abnormal neuronal geometry may affect normal integration of somatodendritic inputs, leading to the formation of aberrant synapses.

The abnormal synapses formed on meganeurites are close to the initial axonal segment. This may affect neuronal excitability to a greater extent than normal axodendritic synapses. These features together may lead to neuronal dysfunction. In addition to this, other pathogenetic mechanisms are possible: The increase in neuronal size due to the meganeurite formation may lead to a decrease of dendritic spines and synapses in normal locations and may produce functionally deafferent cortical neurons.

All these considerations are speculative; however, they are a step in the direction of trying to understand the molecular basis of neuronal function and dysfunction.

C. Metachromatic Leukodystrophy

1. Late Infantile Form

The autosomal recessive disease metachromatic leukodystrophy (MLD) results from a decrease in the activity of the lysosomal enzyme sulfatidase, which leads to the accumulation of the lipid sulfatide.

The clinical symptoms start around 1 year of age with ataxia. The child who has learned to walk becomes unsteady. There is a general hypotonia and weakness or absence of deep tendon reflexes (Hagberg, 1963). After about 1-2 years the child can neither walk nor stand; there is a marked dysarthria and asphasia. There may now be a muscular hypertonicity and intermittent pain in arm and legs. Some months later the child can no longer sit and is quadriplegic. There may be bulbar paresis, which makes feeding difficult. The children are no longer capable of speech but may be able to smile in response. In the final stage, which is reached about 1/4-3½ years later, the children are blind and without voluntary movement. This stage may go on for years. Patients have been known to live in this decerebrated stage for more than 7 years. The late infantile form of metachromatic leukodystrophy has a frequency of about 1 in 40,000 live births.

2. Juvenile Form

In the juvenile form, development may be normal until about the age of 5 years. Then gait disturbances are the first symptom. At 7 years the child may be unable to stand without support and may be bedridden at about 9 years. Speech may be impossible at this stage, but patients can still recognize family members.

3. Adult Form

In contrast to the late infantile and juvenile forms, the adult form does not start with gait disturbances, which are a "myelin" symptom (see page 443) but with psychosis and dementia, which are "neuronal" symptoms (see page 443).

The onset of clinical symptoms is between 19 and 40 years. The initial symptoms are similar to those found in schizophrenia or organic dementia. The IQ of patients, which was normal prior to the onset of the disease, may drop to values of 50-60. In a very protracted course a patient died 44 years after the onset of the disease (Raizin et al., 1968). Short courses of the disease have, however, also been described with a duration of only 1½ years.

Later in the progression of the disease motor symptoms appear such as general slowness and clumsiness. Deep-tendon reflexes are hyperactive and muscular tone is increased. However, nerve conduction velocity may be slow. There may be a slight truncal ataxia, nystagmus, and intention tremor. In the later stage generalized convulsions appear, and the patient is severely deteriorated, incontinent, and mute.

4. Biochemical Tests

In all three forms the diagnosis can be further confirmed by examining the urine: There is an absence or decrease of the enzyme sulfatidase or arylsulfatase A (ASA). Also, sulfatide is frequently found in the urine. To confirm the diagnosis, ASA is estimated in the leukocytes or cultivated fibroblasts of the patient. The heterozygote condition can be determined by examining leukocytes or cultivated fibroblasts. Prenatal diagnosis of the fetus is possible with cultured amniotic fluid cells (Wiesmann et al., 1975). In the patient nerve conduction velocity is decreased, and the histological and histochemical examination of a peripheral nerve shows metachromasia (abnormal staining due to accumulation of sulfatide) and demyelination.

5. Pathogenetic Mechanisms

a. Localization of Accumulation in Organs

The enzyme defect of ASA is expressed in all cells. Accumulation of sulfatide or a similar substrate, however, only occurs in organs in which sulfatide or any of the substrates of ASA is synthesized (Table 1). The accumulation of substrates may or may not affect the organ functions.

The evidence of functional impairment of an organ depends on the tests used, among other factors, and where now no impairments are known, functional abnormalities may become evident with refined testing procedures. In principle Table 1 shows that the organ localization of functional impairment depends on whether the enzyme defect is present in an organ in which the equivalent substance degraded by the enzyme is synthesized.

b. Onset of Clinical Symptoms

Late infantile, juvenile, and the adult form seem to be genetically distinct forms of ASA deficiency. In one family only one type of the disease is

Table 1 Pathogenetic Mechanisms of Arylsulfatase A Deficiency

Organ	Enzyme defect	Substrate synthesis	Substrate accumulation	Functional impairment
CNS	+	+	+	+
PNS	+	+	+	+
Kidney	+	+	+	–
Gall bladder	+	+	+	+
Liver	+	+	+	–
Pancreas	+	+	+	–
Heart	+	–	–	–
Spleen	+	–	–	–
Lung	+	–	–	–
Testis	+	+	+	–
Leukocytes	+	–	–	–
Fibroblasts	+	–	–	–
Amnion cells	+	–	–	–

observed. The measurement of the enzyme ASA using artificial substrate in cultivated fibroblasts shows in all three forms the same decrease of enzyme activity and does not make it possible to distinguish the three forms.

Kihara et al. (1973) used the natural substrate sulfatide and checked the degradation of ^{35}S-labeled sulfatide in cultivated fibroblasts. This was added to the medium and pinocytosed. Under these experimental conditions the three forms showed a clear distinction: Fibroblasts from patients with the late infantile form degraded the least sulfatide, about 4% of that of normal fibroblasts; fibroblasts from patients with the juvenile form degraded about 6-9%; and fibroblasts from the adult form about 25%.

If the finding in the fibroblasts of the three types of metachromatic leukodystrophy corresponds to the values in the tissue of the nervous system, then these differences found may be of importance for the clinical development of the disease. It suggests that the onset of the disease and its rate of progress depends on the residual activity of the enzyme and consequently on the rate of accumulation of nondegraded compounds. In our own studies (Wiesmann et al., 1972) we found that fibroblasts of the obligate heterozygotes degrade about 30% of the [^{35}S] sulfatide degraded by normals. This is probably a decrease of enzyme activity such that sulfatide degradation is not impaired in such a way as to cause accumulation of sulfatide and functional disturbances. Below that activity the degree of degradation may be correlated with the rate of accumulation of sulfatide or other substrates. Therefore, it is possible that in the late infantile form the accumulation of sulfatides and other substances is fast and the progress of the disease likewise rapid. The accumulation rate in the juvenile form is lower, leading to a slower course. In the adult form there is a very slow accumulation affecting a mature brain. It was possible to correct the sulfatide degradation defect in the cultured fibroblasts of the patients by adding enriched sulfatidase preparations to the culture medium. This temporarily increased the intracellular enzyme activity (Wiesman et al., 1972; Kihara et al., 1973).

Another explanation for the different time course in the three types of the disease is that there may be other pathways of sulfatide metabolism than those known today.

c. Effect of Myelin

The pathogenetic mechanism of the demyelination in MLD is not yet clear: The question arises as to whether there is an accumulation of a toxic substance which leads to the demyelination, since the sulfatide itself does not seem to be toxic.

In MLD there is also a deficiency of an enzyme which degrades psychosinsulfate (Eto et al., 1974). It is known for psychosine that this substance is cytotoxic. It is possible that the accumulation of psychosine sulfate is also cytotoxic, affecting oligodendrocytes and Schwann cells, leading to demyelination.

D. Globoid Cell Leukodystrophy (Krabbe's Disease)

Krabbe's disease results from a deficiency of the lysosomal enzyme galactosylceramide-β-galactosidase, which impairs the degradation of galactosylceramide or galactocerebroside. The very rare disease starts at about 3-6 months with irritability and psychomotor retardation. It progresses into spastic quadriparesis, blindness, and deafness. At 1 year tube feeding may be required, and the patients respond poorly to stimuli. Children rarely live more than 2 years.

There are patients with the same enzymatic defect who show the first symptoms late in childhood. These symptoms are visual impairment and difficulties in walking. The diagnosis can be made by estimating galactosylceramide-β-galactosidase in leukocytes and fibroblasts. Heterozygotes can be diagnosed; prenatal diagnosis is possible.

The main pathological finding is the marked decrease of myelin in brain. Clinically, there is often a relative microcephaly. In the white matter there are globoid cells which are PAS-positive, indicating the presence of carbohydrate-containing material.

Despite the defect of degradation of cerebroside, there is no accumulation of cerebroside found. There is also a profound lack of myelin alone with a significant decrease in the number of oligodendrocytes. The peripheral nervous system is not as severely affected. Suzuki and Suzuki (1978) evaluated the several facts known in this disease and tried to formulate a pathogenetic mechanism: The enzyme defect reduces the degradation of a lipid, cerebroside, which is almost exclusively located in myelin. After birth, when the formation of meylin together with cerebroside synthesis is increased, significant accumulation of cerebroside occurs. This undegraded cerebroside leads to the globoid cell reaction, which has been shown to be a unique feature of galactocerebroside.

The reason for the profound loss of oligodendrocytes is still unclear. It could be shown that the defective enzyme does degrade psychosine (sphingosine galactose) to sphingosine. In Krabbe's disease this degradation is impaired, and there is an increase in psychosine in the brain. Psychosine with its free amino group is known to be very cytotoxic. Since psychosine formation occurs almost exclusively in the oligodendrocytes where cerebroside is accumulated, these cells may be destroyed and therefore accumulated cerebroside is lost. Upon loss of cerebroside, no further myelin can be synthesized.

This hypothesis could explain the unique features of this disease: presence of globoid cells, decreased amount of myelin, decreased number of oligodendrocytes, and lack of cerebroside accumulation.

E. Niemann-Pick Disease

In the autosomal recessive disorder Niemann-Pick disease, the activity of a lysosomal enzyme sphingomyelinase is decreased, leading to the accumulation of a phospholipid, sphingomyelin.

1. *Clinical Course*

a. Type A: Neuronopathic Form

The first symptoms are seen soon after birth. The affected children have feeding difficulties and the psychomotor development is severely retarded from the beginning on. Liver and spleen are enlarged at 6 months of age (Fredrickson and Sloan, 1978). Skin in exposed areas may show an olive coloration. A cherry red spot in the retina is present in 30-50% of the cases. Large waxy cells are found in the bone marrow, which stain for lipid and phosphorus. Later in the course of the disease there is a progressive loss of learned capabilities. Death usually occurs in the 3rd year of life. This disease is prevalent in Ashkenazy Jews.

b. Type B: Chronic Form Without Nervous System Involvement

In this form there is enlargement of liver and spleen in the 1st year of life; however, there is no impairment of psychomotor function. The lungs are often diffusely infiltrated, and the patients tend to have frequent pneumonias. Foam cells are found in the bone marrow.

c. Type C: Chronic Neuronopathic Form

The patients develop normally for about 1-2 years, then a slow progressive deterioration is observed. Acquired verbal behavior deteriorates, and moderate ataxia becomes manifest. There is a gradual loss of all psychomotor skills. Grand mal seizures may occur. Liver and spleen are less affected than in the forms A and B. The patients usually die between 5 and 15 years.

2. Pathogenetic Mechanisms

The sphingomyelinase defect can be found in tissue obtained by biopsy or autopsy, also in cultured fibroblasts and in leukocytes. It is possible to detect heterozygotes in cultivated fibroblasts (Brady, 1972) and diagnose the disease prenatally in cultured amniotic fluid cells. Different biochemical studies in Niemann-Pick disease have made it possible to better understand the basis of the observed phenotypes. Using natural substrates, various authors found that the activity of sphingomyelinase in liver of patients with type A was 0-9% and type B 15-20% that of normals (Brady et al., 1966; Brady, 1973).

In the type C disease sphingomyelinase activity in fibroblasts is 50-63% that of normals (Gal et al., 1975).

Isoelectric focusing has made it possible to distinguish two isoenzyme forms of sphingomyelinase: form I and form II in the liver of normals (Callahan and Khalil, 1975). In cultured fibroblasts of patients with form A there is a virtual absence of both sphingomyelinase isoenzymes, in form B the activity of both isoenzymes is found to be decreased. In form C only isoenzyme I is found.

In form A it seems that the near absence of isoenzymes I and II affects both the nervous systems and the visceral organs. In form B there may be enough residual activity left to maintain a normal function of the nervous system. In form C there is an absence of isoenzyme II; this may lead mainly to damage in the nervous system.

In the enlarged organs the substance which is increased most is the lipid sphingomyelin. In the spleen the increase of sphingomyelin can be about 25 times that of the normal in type A and about 6 times in type B. There is a wide range in type C. Lymph nodes show considerable sphingomyelin accumulation. There is only a moderate accumulation of sphingomyelin in the grey matter of the brain in type A and less in the white matter. There is no accumulation of sphingomyelin in the brains of patients with types B and C. In addition, cholesterol is also accumulated in liver in type A and even more so in spleen. Other lipids such as gangliosides can be accumulated, but these changes are probably due to the agglomeration of membranes in the lysosomes.

The pathogenetic mechanism in type C in unclear because there is no significant sphingomyelin accumulation in brain; however, brain function is severely affected.

F. Gaucher's Disease

Gaucher's disease is an autosomal recessive disorder. The activity of the lysomal enzyme glucocerebrosidase is decreased, which affects glucocerebroside degradation.

Type 1: Chronic nonneuronopathic form. This is the most frequent form, with an increased incidence in Ashkenazy Jews. The central nervous system is not involved. There is an enlargement of the liver and spleen; the bones and the lungs are also involved.

Type 2: Acute neuronopathic form. Nervous system dysfunction may become apparent shortly after birth or at the age of 6-7 months, with hypertonicity-retroflexion of the head, dysphagia, and laryngeal stridor. There may be seizures. The patients die at about 9 months.

Type 3: Subacute neuronopathic form. In this form the clinical signs manifest themselves after infancy, with hypertonicity, coordination difficulties, strabismus, and convulsions. This type has also been described in adults with mental retardation, grand mal seizures, tremor, and gait difficulties (Miller et al., 1973). Sometimes the bones are also involved.

In all three forms lipid-laden histiocytes (Gaucher cells) are found in the reticuloendothelial system. The structure and ultrastructure of these cells often permits a tentative diagnosis of Gaucher's disease.

1. Pathogenetic Mechanisms

Glucocerebrosidase activity, frequently measured with an artificial substrate as β-glucosidase, is significantly lowered in Gaucher's disease. Since this enzyme degrades glucocerebroside, the effect of the low enzyme activity is an accumulation of glucocerebroside. The three forms of Gaucher's disease cannot be clearly distinguished by different levels of residual activity of β-glucosidase. Also, not all the brains of patients obtained by autopsy with the neuronopathic form show distinct accumulations of cerebroside. However, it is interesting to note that an increased percentage of glucocerebroside was found in the brain of a child with type 2 Gaucher rather than galactocerebroside, as is usually the case.

2. Diagnosis

The enzymatic defect can be found in leukocytes and cultured fibroblasts, preferably by using the natural substrate glucocerebroside. The detection of heterzygotes for Gaucher's disease is possible by assaying the enzyme activity in leukocytes and fibroblasts. Prenatal diagnosis is also possible in cultured anmiotic fluid cells.

3. *Treatment*

Enzyme replacement has been tried with some success (Brady, 1978a). An encouraging observation (Belchetz et al., 1977) reported that intermittent infusions of glucocerebrosidase from human placenta over a period of 13 months reduced the size of the enlarged liver of a patient as confirmed by whole-body scan. This indicates a decrease of the accumulated material by the enzyme replacement. This was, however, in an adult patient with nonneuronal Gaucher's disease. It is not yet known whether enzyme replacement would also be beneficial in the neuronal forms.

VII. MUCOPOLYSACCHARIDOSIS

Mucopolysaccharidosis denotes a group of several diseases caused by abnormal lysosomal degradation of mucopolysaccharides. In recent years, important progress has been achieved in elucidating the basic enzymatic defects. As a result of this progress, the pathogenetic mechanisms of the disease are better understood; accurate diagnosis, genetic counseling, and prenatal diagnosis have become possible; and the first steps in the direction of future treatment of the disease have been made (Neufeld and Frantantoni, 1970). The disorders are progressive; the accumulation of mucopolysaccharides and other substances can take place in several organs. As a consequence of faulty degradation, mucopolysaccharides accumulate in parenchymal and mesenchymal tissue.

In the brains of patients with mental retardation, mucopolysaccharides are accumulated mostly in perivascular regions (Constantopoulas et al., 1978). In the neurons lipids are stored (Constantopoulos and Dekafan, 1978). The accumulation of lipids is probably the result of a secondary inhibition of lipid degrading enzymes resulting from the accumulation of mucopolysaccharides. The exact reason for the mental retardation is not clear. Either:

1. The accumulated mucopolysaccharides in blood vessels play a role in the blood-brain barrier and thus alter neuronal metabolism, or
2. Primary accumulation of mucopolysaccharides inhibits mostly lipid-degrading enzyme activity leading to an accumulation of gangliosides and by that to neuronal dysfunction. Neuronal lipid accumulation and reduced β-galactosidase activity was already found in a 22-WIG fetus affected with mucopolysaccharidosis (Wiesman et al., unpublished results).

Both mechanisms individually or combined may help to explain mental retardation in mucopolysaccharidosis.

The enzymatic defects of most classical mucopolysaccharidoses are known and are expressed in cultured fibroblasts or amniotic fluid cells as faulty degradation of sulfated mucopolysaccharide or as the enzyme defect itself (Table 2) leukocytes can also be used to detect heterozygotes. Fragments of partially degraded mucopolysaccharides are excreted into the urine of the patient. This fact is a help in clinical diagnosis. McKusic et al. (1965, 1972) classified the different mucopolysaccharidoses according to biochemical and clinical criteria.

A. Mucopolysaccharidosis I-H (Hurler's Syndrome)

Children with Hurler's syndrome develop normally until the age of 1 year. Then progressive mental and somatic deterioration starts, usually leading to death at an age of under 10 years. The facies becomes coarse (gargoylism). There is progressive clouding of the cornea. Liver and spleen are enlarged. There are extensive skeletal abnormalities. Typical is the widening of the medial clavicle and a hypoplastic broad-hooked vertebra at the apex of the dorsal lumbar gibbus. Growth almost stops at 2-3 years. The joints become stiff. The deposition of stored material in the heart valves and coronaries can lead to cardiac insufficiency, coronary infarction, and early death. Frequently deafness occurs as a result of conductive and neurosensory failure. Mucopolysaccharides and gangliosides accumulate in the brain.

B. Mucopolysaccharidosis I-S (Scheie's Syndrome)

In Scheie's syndrome α-L-iduronidase activity is also deficient as in Hurler's syndrome. The patients have corneal clouding, deformities of the hands, heart involvement, but no mental impairment. Neither mucopolysaccharides nor gangliosides accumulate in the brain (Table 2), possibly because of a higher residual activity of the enzyme. It is tempting to correlate the presence and absence of mental retardation in Hurler's and Scheie's syndromes with the presence and absence of mucopolysaccharide and ganglioside accumulation in the brain.

The mutation may be of an allelic type affecting the same gene as in Hurler's syndrome, but not at the same location. This leads to an altered enzyme, which is, however, different from the mutant α-L-iduronidase in Hurler's syndrome.

C. Mucopolysaccharidosis II (Hunter's Syndrome)

There are two important differences between Hurler's and the Hunter's syndromes: Hunter's syndrome is an X-linked recessive mutation affecting only males and there is no corneal clouding. With regard to mental retardation, there is a severe and a mild form. In the severe form death may occur before age 15; in the mild form there may be a normal life-span. The enzymatic defect is a deficiency of the enzyme iduronate sulfatase. Different types of mutations on the X-chromosome may explain the different clinical forms.

Table 2 Enzymatic Defects of Mucopolysaccharidoses

Type	Syndrome	Enzymatic defect	Mental retardation	Mucopoly-saccharid accumulation	Perivascular lesions	Neuronal storage (gangliosides)
Mucopolysaccharidosis I-H	Hurler's	α-L-Iduronidase	+++	+++	++	+++
Mucopolysaccharidosis I-S	Scheie's	α-L-Iduronidase	–	+	+	(+)
Mucopolysaccharidosis II-s	Hunter's, severe	Iduronate sulfatase	++	++	++	+++
Mucopolysaccharidosis II-m	Hunter's, mild	Iduronate sulfatase	+			+++
Mucopolysaccharidosis III-A	Sanfilippo A	Heparan-N-sulfatase	+++	+++	++	
Mucopolysaccharidosis III-B	Sanfilippo B	N-Acetyl-α-D-glucosaminidase	+++			
Mucopolysaccharidosis IV	Morquio's	Hexosamine-6-sulfatase	–			
Mucopolysaccharidosis VI-s	Maroteaux-Lamy's severe	Arylsulfatase B	–			
Mucopolysaccharidosis VI-i	Maroteaux-Lamy's interm.	Arylsulfatase B	–			
Mucopolysaccharidosis VI-m	Maroteaux-Lamy's mild	Arylsulfatase B	–			
Mucopolysaccharidosis VIII	β-Glucoronidase	β-glucoronidase	Variable			

D. Mucopolysaccharidosis III (Sanfilippo Syndrome)

In contrast to mucopolysaccharidosis I and II, stiffness of the joints and skeletal abnormalities are less severe in Sanfilippo syndrome. There is no corneal clouding. The mental functions are severely affected and clearly evident by school age. Death usually occurs at age 20. The mucopolysaccharide heparan sulfate may not be as elevated in the urine as in mucopolysaccharidosis type I and II. The disease results from the deficient degradation of the heparan sulfate. Four enzymes are involved in this degradation. Two enzyme deficiencies are known thus far: heparan-N-sulfatase and N-acetyl-α-D-glucosaminidase.

The two forms are not clinically distinguishable. This is probably because the two different enzymatic defects lead to the accumulation of the same substance.

E. Treatment of Mucopolysaccharidosis

Based on the observations of Fratantoni et al. (1969) that cocultivation of fibroblasts from Hurler and Hunter patients results in a correction of the degradation defect, it became clear that lysosomal enzymes leave the cells and can be taken up from other fibroblasts. These correction experiments led to the clinical trial of transplanting histocompatible fibroblasts as a long-term source of lysosomal enzymes for replacement therapy in three patients with Hunter's syndrome (Dean et al., 1979).

The three patients were HLA-compatible with the sibling donors, against whom no mixed-leukocyte reaction was detected, and 2×10^8 cultured fibroblasts from the donor were injected into the patients subcutaneously as a cell suspension. During the observation time of 2½-3¾ years, all three patients showed increased enzyme levels in serum and leukocytes. The increase in enzyme activity was accompanied by an increased degradation of mucopolysaccharides as measured in the urine.

For ethical reasons the three patients selected for this experimental treatment were all severely affected, both physically and mentally, at the beginning of the treatment. None of the patients showed consistent changes in joint mobility or liver and spleen size as a consequence of the therapy. However, during the observation time of over 3 years there was no further deterioration as would be expected from the natural history of the disease. One patient, who was observed for 3¾ years, showed at the beginning of the treatment a developmental age of 1 year 10 months. After the 3¾ years his developmental age was over 2 years and not further deteriorated, as would have been expected.

In order to affect mental development, fibroblast treatment must probably start at an early age before irreversible changes in the brain have taken place. It is also possible that this type of treatment works well only when the pathological changes are due primarily to vascular pathology. It has not yet been shown that circulating enzymes from the transplanted fibroblasts leave the arteries and enter the brain. Therefore, this treatment may not apply to other lysosomal disorders in which the damage is directly in the neuronal or glial structures and not in the arteries.

VIII. MUCOLIPIDOSIS II (I-CELL DISEASE)

Patients with this autosomal recessive disorder resemble patients with Hurler's syndrome, but they show no mucopolysacchariduria. From birth on there are clinical signs present: bone lesions, gargoylism, umbilical and inguinal hernia, thoracic deformities, and hyperplastic gums. Somatic and mental deterioration is rapid, and most of the patients die before the age of 10.

Not all the organs are affected in the same way. The mesenchymal tissues are the most severely affected. Fibroblasts, chondrocytes, Schwann cells, glomerulus cells, vascular cells, and peripheral neurons show inclusions. The accumulation in Kupfer cells, hepatocytes, bone marrow cells, leukocytes, and cortical neurons is variable.

Cultured fibroblasts show a deficiency of several lysosomal enzymes intracellularly and increased levels of the same enzymes in the culture medium (Wiesmann et al., 1971a). Based on those findings, the extracellular fluids in a patient were tested for the activity of lysosomal enzymes. The same enzymes which showed elevated activities in the medium of cultured fibroblasts also showed elevated activities in serum, plasma, and CSF (Wiesmann et al., 1971b). The estimation of lysosomal enzymes in urine and plasma is now an easy diagnostic tool.

Hickman and Neufeld (1972) found that lysosomal enzymes from media in which I-cell fibroblasts were grown were only one-fifth to one-tenth as effective as their normal counterparts in experiments that involved uptake of the enzymes from the medium.

This led to the hypothesis that a common recognition site on the lysosomal glycoproteins may be affected, which further affects the intracellular localization of these enzymes. The exact nature of the defect is not yet known.

The "I-cell story" shows two interesting aspects: Basic research, which is interested in the localization of lysosomal enzymes in cultured fibroblasts, can lead to direct practical clinical applications. In addition, the profound study of a very rare disease can reveal important new aspects of general biological interest: Recognition of molecules to cell surfaces plays an important role in, for example, hormonal target cell interaction, drug cell uptake, and viral infection of specific cells. With the help of the I-cell model, important contributions can be made to the solution of these important problems.

IX. CONCLUSIONS

The basic structure of brain consists of neurons supported by astrocytes and myelinated by oligodendroglial cells. Mental retardation may be caused by abnormal metabolism of neurons and/or glial cells. Conditions affecting myelination or the maintenance of myelin will lead to disturbances of nerve conduction and to secondary neuronal dysfunction. This may be expressed in delayed psychomotor development or in motor-mental deterioration. The impaired neuronal function may also lead to sensory deprivation, which creates a vicious circle aggravating mental retardation.

Conditions which primarily affect the neurons may impair the formation and maintenance of synaptic membranes. As a result, neurotransmitter formation, release, and turnover may be disturbed, leading to a dysfunction in the neuronal circuitry. In a general way this may be the basis of mental retardation. The mentally retarded patient is greatly disturbed in his interaction with his environment. In the normal child this interaction leads to a perfection in performance, while in the retarded child the abnormal interaction may aggravate the effects of the primary biochemical defects.

The study of rare inborn errors of metabolism which lead to mental retardation can provide useful models for studying basic mechanisms of mental function and dysfunction. Our knowledge of brain function is a mosaic with many missing pieces. Each additional piece of information helps to complete the picture and increases our knowledge of causes and pathogenetic mechanisms leading to the clinical expression of the different forms of mental retardation. This knowledge is the basis for any treatment of the causes of mental retardation and a necessary step toward the goal of its prevention.

REFERENCES

Adachi, M., Schneck, L., and Volk, B. W. (1978). Progress in investigations of sphingolipidosis. *Acta Neuropathol. 43,* 1-18.

Appel, S. H. (1966). Inhibition of proteinsynthesis. An approach to the biochemical basis of neurological dysfunction in the aminoaceduria. *Ann. N.Y. Acad. Sci. 29,* 63.

Bachmann, C., and Nyhan, W. (1978). Disorders of amino acid metabolism. In *Medical Aspects of Mental Retardation,* 2nd ed., Ch. C. Carter (Ed.). Thomas, Springfield, Ill.

Bachmann, C., and Baumgartner, R. (1978). In *Aminosäuren une ihre Metaboliten,* C. Bachmann, Ewerbeck, H., Joppich, G., Kleinhauser, E., Rossi, E., and Stalder, G. R. (Eds.). Paediatrie in Praxis und Klinik. Thieme Verlag, Stuttgart, F. R. G.

Belchetz, P. E., Braidmann, I. P., and Crawley, J. C. W. (1977). Gregoriadis, G. *Lancet 2,* 116-117.

Barbato, L., Barbato, I. W. M., and Homanaka, A. (1968). The in vivo effect of high level of phenylalanine on lipids and RNA of the developing rabbit brain. *Brain Res. 7,* 399.

Bickel, H., Gerrard, J., and Hickmans, E. M. (1954). The influence of phenylalanine intake on the chemistry and behavior of a phenylketonuria child. *Acta Paediat. 43,* 64.

Blaskovic, M. E., Schaeffler, G. E., and Hack, S. (1974). Phenylalanaemia. Differential diagnosis *Arch. Dis. Child. 49,* 835-843.

Brady, R. O. (1972). Biochemical and metabolic basis of familial sphingolipidosis. *Semin. Hematol. 9,* 273.

Brady, R. O. (1973). The abnormal biochemistry of inherited disorders of lipid metabolism. *Fed. Proc. 32,* 1660.

Brady, R. O. (1978). Sphingolipidosis. *Ann. Rev. Biochem. 47,* 687-713.

Brady, R. O. (1978b). Inherited metabolic diseases and pathogenesis of mental retardation. *Ann. Biol. Clin. 36,* 113-119.

Brady, R. O., Kaufer, J. N., Mock, M. B., and Fredrickson, D. S. (1977). The metabolism of sphingomyelin. *Proc. Nat. Acad. Sci. USA 44,* 366.

Callahan, J. W., and Khalil, M. (1975). Sphingomyelinase in human tissues. *Ped. Res. 9,* 914.

Constantopoloulos, G., McComb, R. D., and Dekaban, A. (1976). Neurochemistry of the mucopolysaccharidoses. *J. Neurochem. 26,* 901-908.

Constantopoulos, G., and Dekaban, A. (1978). Neurochemistry of the mucopolysaccharidoses. *J. Neurochem. 30,* 965-973.

Dean, M. F., Sterens, R. L., Muir, H., Benson, P. F., Button, L. R., Anderson, R. L., Boylston, A., and Mowbray, J. (1979). Enzyme replacement therapy by fibroblast transplantation. *J. Clin. Invest. 63,* 138-145.

Dobbing, J. (1968). In *Applied Neurochemistry,* A. N. Davison and J. Dobbing (Eds.). Blackwell, Oxford, pp. 287-316.

Dobbing, J., and Sands, J. (1970). Timing of neuroblast multiplication in developing human brain. *Nature 226,* 639-640.

Dreyfuss, J. C., Prenarn, L., and Svennerholm, L. (1977). Absence of hexoseaminidase A and B in a normal adult. *N. Engl. J. Med. 292,* 61.

Eto, Y., Wiesmann, U., and Herschkowitz, N. (1974). Sulfogalactosyl-sphingosine sulfatase. Characteristics of the enzyme and its deficiency in metachromatic leukodystrophy in human cultured skin fibroblasts. *J. Biol. Chem. 249,* 4955.

Evrard, P., Caviness, V. S., Prats-Vinas, J., and Lyon, G. (1978). The mechanism of arrest of neuronal migration in the Zellweger malformation. *Acta Neuropathol. 41,* 109-117.

Fisch, R. O., Walker, W. A., and Anderson, J. A. (1966). Prenatal and postnatal developmental consequences of maternal phenylketonuria. *Pediatrics 37,* 979.

Fölling, A. (1934). Ueber Ausscheidung von Phenylbrenztraubensäure im Harn als Stoffwechselanomalie in Verbindung mit Imbezillität. *Hoppe Seylers Z. Physiol. Chem. 227,* 169.

Frantantoni, J. C., Hall, C. W., and Neufeld, E. F. (1969). Hurler and Hunter syndrome. Mutual correction of the defect in cultured fibroblasts. *Science 162,* 570.

Frederickson, D. S., and Sloan, H. R. (1978). *Sphingomyelin Lipidosis in the Metabolic Basis of Inherited Disease,* 3rd ed. J. B. Stanbury, J. B. Wyngaarden, and D. S. Fredrickson (Eds.). McGraw-Hill, New York, p. 783.

Gal, A., Brady, R. O., Hibberty, S. R., and Pentechev, P. G. (1975). A practical chromogenic procedure for the detection of homocygotes and heterocygous carriers of Niemann-Pick disease. *N. Engl. J. Med. 293,* 632.

Gilles, F. H., Dooling, E., and Fulchiero, A. (1976). Sequence of myelination in the human fetus. *Trans. Am. Neurol. Ass. 101,* 244-246.

Gitzelmann, R., Steinmann, B., Otten, A., Dummermuth, G., Herdan, M., Reubi, J. C., and Cuénod, M. (1977). Nonketotic hyperglycinemia treated with strychnine a glycine receptor antagonist. *Paediat. Acta 32,* 517-525.

Guthrie, R., and Susi, A. (1963). A simple phenylalanine method for detecting phenylketonuria in large populations of newborn infants. *Pediatrics 32,* 338.

Hagberg, B. (1963). Clinical symptoms, signs and tests in metachromatic leucodystrophy. In *Brain Lipids and the Lipoproteins and the Leucodystrophies,* J. Folch-Pi and H. Bauer (Eds.). Elsevier, Amsterdam, pp. 134-146.

Hall, C. W., and Neufeld, E. F. (1973). α-L-Iduronidase activity in cultured skin fibroblasts and amniotic fluid cells. *Arch. Biochem. Biophys. 158,* 817-821.

Hickman, S., and Neufeld, E. F. (1972). A hypothesis for I-cell disease. *Biochem. Biophys. Res. Commun. 49,* 992-999.

Jervis, G. (1953). Phenylpyruvic oligophrenia deficiency of phenylalanine oxidizing system. *Proc. Soc. Exp. Biol. Med. 82,* 514.

Kaback, M. M., and Zeiger, R. S. (1972). Heterozygote detection in Tay-Sachs disease. In *Sphingolipids, Sphingolipidosis and Allied Disorders,* B. W. Volk, and S. M. Aronson (Eds.). Plenum, New York, p. 613.

Kaplan, M., and Hinds, J. W. (1977). Neurogenesis in the adult rat. *Science 197,* 1092-1096.

Kihara, H., Porter, M. T., and Fluharly, A. (1973). Enzyme replacement in cultured fibroblasts from metachromatic leucodystrophy. In *Enzyme Therapy in Genetic Disease,* D. Bergsma, R. J. Desnick, R. W. Berulohr, and W. Krivit (Eds.). Williams and Wilkin, Baltimore, for the National Foundation, March of Dimes, p. 19.

Mabry, C. C., Denniston, J. C., Nelson, T. L., and Cern, C. D. (1966). Maternal phenylketonuria. A cause of mental retardation in children without metabolic defect. *N. Engl. J. Med. 275,* 1331.

McKusic, V. A. (1972). *Heritable disorders of connective tissue,* 4th ed. Moshy, St. Louis, pp. 521-686.

McKusic, V. A., Kaplan, D., Wise, D., Hanley, W. B., Suddarth, S. B., Sevick, M. E., and Maumenee, A. V. (1965). The genetic mucopolysaccharidoses. *Medicine 44,* 445.

Miller, J. D., McCluer, R., and Kaufer, J. N. (1973). Gaucher disease. Neurologic disorder in adult siblings. *Ann. Intern. Med. 78,* 833.

Molliver, M. E., Kostovic, I., and van der Loos, H. (1973). The development of synapsies in cerebral cortex of the human fetus. *Brain Res. 50,* 403-407.

Neufeld, E. F., and Frantantoni, J. C. (1970). Inborn errors of mucopolysaccharide metabolism. *Science 169,* 141-146.

O'Brien, J. S. (1978). The gangliosidosis. In *The metabolic basis of inherited disease,* 4th ed. J. S. Stanbury, J. B. Wyngaarden, and D. S. Fredrick (Eds.). McGraw-Hill, New York.

O'Brien, J. S., Gugler, E., Giedion, A., Wiesmann, U., Herschkowitz, N., Meier, C., and le Roy, J. (1976). Spondyloepiphyseal dysplasia, corneal clouding, normal intelligence and β-galactosidase deficiency. *Clin, Genet. 9,* 495.

Okada, S., and O'Brien, J. S. (1969). Tay-Sachs disease. Generalized absence of a β-B-N-acetylhexoseaminidase component. *Science 165,* 698.

Okada, S., Veath, M. L., le Roy, J., and O'Brien, J. S. (1971). Ganglioside GM_2 storage disease. *Am. J. Hum. Genet. 23,* 55.

Pilz, H., Heipertz, R., and Seidel, D. (1978). Clinical, preclinical and prenatal diagnosis of congenital sphingolipidosis by determining lysosomal hydrolases. *Fortschr. Neurol. Psychiat. 46,* 207-221.

Pueschel, S. M., and Rotteman, K. J. (1976). Birth weight analysis of children with phenylketonuria. *Pediat. Res. 10,* 419.

Purpura, D. (1977). In *Fetal and Infant Brain,* S. R. Berenburg (Ed.). Martinus Niyhoff, The Hague, p. 54-79.

Purpura, D. P., and Suzuki, K. (1976). Distortion of neuronal geometry and formation of aberrant synapses in neuronal storage disease. *Brain Res. 116,* 1-21.

Roizin, L., Scheinesson, G., and Eros, G. (1968). Comparative histological and histochemical studies of infantile and adult metachomatic leucodystrophy. *Pathol. Eur. 3,* 286.

Suzuki, K., and Suzuki, Y. (1978). Galactosylceramide lipidosis. In *The Metabolic Basis of Inherited Disease,* J. B. Stanbury, J. B. Wyngaarden, and D. S. Fredrickson (Eds.). McGraw-Hill, New York.

Udenfried, S., and Bessmann, S. P. (1953). The hydroxylation of phenylalanine and antipyrene in phenylpyruvic oligophrenia. *J. Biol. Chem. 203,* 961.

Vanier, M. T., Holm, M., Oehmann, R., and Svennerholm, L. (1971). Developmental profiles of gangliosides in human and rat brain. *J. Neurochem. 18,* 581-592.

Vidgoff, J., Bust, N. R., and O'Brien, J. S. (1973). Absence of β-N-acetyl-D-hexoseaminidase A activity in a healthy woman. *Am. J. Hum. Genet. 25,* 372.

Wiesmann, U., Lighthody, J., Vasella, F., and Herschkowitz, N. (1971). Multiple lysosomal enzyme deficiency due to enzyme leakage? *N. Engl. J. Med. 284,* 109.

Wiesmann, U., Vasella, F., and Herschkowitz, N. (1971b). I-cell disease. Leakage of lysosomal enzymes into extracellular fluids. *New Engl. J. Med. 285,* 1090-1091.

Wiesmann, U., Rossi, E. E., and Herschkowitz, N. (1972). Correction of the defective sulfatide degradation in cultured fibroblasts from patients with metachromatic leucodystrophy. *Acta Paediatr. Scand. 61,* 296-302.

Wiesmann, U., Meier, C., Spycher, M. A., Schmid, W., Bischoff, A. Gautier, E., and Herschkowitz, N. (1975). Prenatal metachromatic leucodystrophy. *Helv. Paediatr. Acta 30,* 31-42.

13

Modulation of Behavior by Neuropeptides: Modes of Action and Clinical Prospects

Henk Rigter and Henk van Riezen
Organon International B.V.,
Oss, The Netherlands

I. INTRODUCTION

This chapter is devoted to a review of developments in a recent branch of the neurosciences: the study of neurotropic effects of peptides. Independent of their endocrine effects, many peptide hormones exert direct actions on the central nervous system (CNS). This has been established for a variety of pituitary hormones on the basis of several lines of evidence (de Wied, 1969; Kastin et al., 1975a; van Wimersma Greidanus and de Wied, 1976). CNS effects of pituitary hormones can still be demonstrated after extirpation of relevant endocrine target organs. Furthermore, a dissociation of endocrine and CNS activities is apparent from the finding that some fragments or analogs of these peptide hormones virtually lack the endocrine properties but do possess the CNS-modulating properties of the parent substances. In addition, direct application of pituitary hormones or related peptides to specific brain areas often duplicates the effects of systemic administration.

Pituitary hormones and related peptides are not the only class of peptides with neurotropic properties. For instance, hypothalamic hormones, i.e., hypophysiotropic-releasing and release-inhibiting factors, appear to exert effects on brain other than their effects on the pituitary gland (Prange et al., 1975; Plotnikoff and Kastin, 1977). Furthermore, a number of presumptive or actual hormones of the gastrointestinal tract and the pancreas have also been identified in a variety of brain areas (Pearse, 1976), suggesting that these peptides play a role in CNS processes, too. Even peptides of nonmammalian origin, e.g., from amphibian skin, may modulate CNS processes in mammals. At least 12 classes of nonmammalian peptides can be distinguished; some of these peptides structurally resemble the amino acid sequences of peptides common to mammalian brain and intestine (Bertaccini, 1976).

We will use the term *neuropeptides* for all the various peptides with CNS effects resulting in behavioral alterations. We will discuss a large body of data indicating that neuropeptides may be involved in the regulation and modulation of a huge variety of behavioral responses. Biochemical and physiological findings will be summarized whenever they may be of relevance for the understanding of the behavioral data. For the sake of clarity we do not attempt to review all the available experimental results. Instead, we present exemplary peptide effects which are pertinent to the field of biological psychiatry. We will therefore highlight the results of studies of peptides whose potential psychotropic properties have been examined in humans, i.e., ACTH 4-10, TRH, PLG, and endorphins.

II. ADRENOCORTICOTROPIC HORMONE (ACTH) AND RELATED PEPTIDES

A. Animal Studies

The extraendocrine behavioral effects of ACTH-like peptides have been studied extensively. Pioneering work has been done by de Wied and associates. Their early studies have been reviewed by de Wied (1969). These investigators started to study the behavior of rats in active avoidance tests. An example of an active avoidance paradigm is the shuttlebox test. The shuttlebox apparatus used by de Wied consists of two compartments separated by a hurdle. A buzzer is used to warn the animal of an impending electric shock to the feet. The rat can avoid the shock if it responds within 5 sec by jumping over the hurdle to the other side of the box. After an average time interval of 1 min a second trial is started by sounding the warning signal again, and so on. De Wied showed that ablation of the anterior lobe of the pituitary gland impaired the ability of rats to acquire the shuttlebox response. Adenohypophysectomy results in physical debilitation which in part may account for the behavioral deficiency seen in the shuttlebox test. Thus, a hormone replacement therapy consisting of cortisone, testosterone, and thyroxin normalized acquisition in adenohypophysectomized rats (de Wied, 1969). In addition, however, a more specific role is reserved for ACTH. This hormone also restores performance of (adeno)hypophysectomized animals in the shuttlebox test. This ameliorative action does not solely depend on the ability of ACTH to release steroids from the adrenal cortex. The fragment ACTH 4-10 is virtually devoid of adrenocorticotropic activity and it does not alleviate the physical malaise that occurs after removal of the pituitary. Yet ACTH 4-10 still shares the parent hormone's property of restoring deficient shuttlebox acquisition in hypophysectomized rats. Many subsequent studies have revealed that this behavioral activity of ACTH, ACTH 4-10, and related fragments and analogs is mediated through a direct action on the brain (see Section II.B).

Various explanations are possible to account for the restorative action of ACTH and related peptides on the acquisition of the shuttlebox response in hypophysectomized animals. First, ACTH may enhance motility, thereby increasing the chance that a treated animal will "shuttle" over the hurdle. This possibility is disproven by the finding that ACTH 4-10 does not increase the number of intertrial responses, i.e., shuttles in the absence of the warning signal displayed by hypophysectomized rats (Bohus et al., 1973). Second, pain sensitivity may be changed after hypophysectomy and an ACTH-induced normalization of pain perception may account for the amelioration of shuttlebox performance. Although ablation of the pituitary enhances responsiveness of rats to electric shock, ACTH 1-10 does not restore this altered responsiveness to normal (Gispen et al., 1970). Third, it is possible that hypophysectomy interferes with memory consolidation and that this memory deficit is normalized by ACTH. Indeed, there are some indications that ACTH and ACTH 4-10 may influence memory consolidation (Flood et al., 1976; Gold and McGaugh, 1977). However, the available evidence indicates that ACTH certainly has no indispensable role in memory consolidation (Rigter and van Riezen, 1978). This is illustrated by an experiment by Bohus (1973). Hypophysectomized rats were trained in the shuttlebox during a period of 14 days. Placebo-treated rats showed the usual acquisition deficit: This group of animals never scored more than an average of 50% avoidance responses. The behavioral deficit was reversed by ACTH 4-10. The peptide was only given during the first week of the study. In this time period, ACTH 4-10-treated animals attained a performance level of 80% avoidances, which suggests that relevant information had been stored in memory. In the second week of the experiment ACTH 4-10 was no longer administered and performance declined gradually to the level of the placebo-treated control group. If treatment with ACTH 4-10 had normalized memory consolidation, there is no apparent reason that cessation of treatment after formation of memory had taken place would have led to a progressive deterioration of performance.

A fourth possibility is that ACTH restores a motivational deficit in hypophysectomized rats. For instance, in the above-mentioned study of Bohus and co-workers, the effect of ACTH 4-10 could be interpreted as a temporary normalization of fear motivation. There are indeed many data which indicate that ACTH-like peptides may influence motivation in operated as well as intact animals (de Wied, 1977). One prominent effect of ACTH-like peptides in intact rats is a delay of extinction. In the shuttlebox, for example, extinction can be measured by continuing the presentation of the warning signal without delivering electric shock. Treatment with ACTH or related peptides during this period retards extinction, i.e., the animals persevere in responding to the signal despite the absence of punishment (de Wied, 1969). This effect has not only been found in tests involving extinction of shock-motivated responses but also when food-motivated or sexually motivated behavior was studied (Garrud et al., 1974; Bohus et al., 1975). Consequently, a possible motivational effect of ACTH-like peptides is not restricted to fear motivation.

It should be noted that ACTH and related peptides certainly do not induce generalized changes in motivation. De Wied (1977) refined the motivation hypothesis by stating that ACTH and related peptides enhance arousal in response to motivationally relevant cues. This formulation comes quite close to the view expressed by Kastin and co-workers that ACTH-like peptides facilitate attention.

This latter group of investigators has conducted many studies on the behavioral actions of α-melanocyte-stimulating hormone (α-MSH). α-MSH is composed of the first 13 amino acids in ACTH with an acetyl group in front. Behavioral tests have generally yielded similar results for ACTH or ACTH 4-10 and α-MSH, e.g., correction of deficient shuttlebox acquisition in hypophysectomized rats (de Wied, 1969) and delay of extinction of various responses (Garrud et al., 1974; Kastin et al., 1974; Rigter and Popping, 1976). The attention hypothesis has been developed to account for the effect of α-MSH on the ability of rats to reverse an acquired response tendency (Sandman et al., 1972; Sandman et al., 1973). Rats were trained to choose a white door rather than a black door in order to escape or avoid electric shock. During subsequent reversal learning the rats were required to respond to the black door. α-MSH-treated animals did not show consistent improvement of original learning but displayed greater ease in acquiring the reversal task than control animals. The investigators proposed that α-MSH had helped the rats during original training to pay attention to the relevant cues of the problem, including the black door.

Another line of research has addressed the possibility that ACTH-like peptides influence retrieval from memory. Studies of amnesia may serve as an example. Amnesia can be induced in rats by a variety of agents, e.g., carbon dioxide, electroconvulsive shock, and protein synthesis inhibitors. With the exception of protein synthesis inhibitors, amnesic agents are usually administered immediately after acquisition of a response. Amnesia is assessed at a subsequent retrieval test which is usually given at least 24 hr after acquisition. ACTH-like peptides attenuate amnesia induced by different agents. Most studies agree that this antiamnesic effect is most marked when peptide treatment is given shortly before the retrieval test (for recent reviews, cf. Rigter and van Riezen, 1978; 1979).

In conclusion, ACTH-like peptides exert behavioral actions. Various explanations have been offered to account for these effects. These explanations make use of such closely related but ill-defined concepts as motivation, attention, and retrieval. Probably these views are not incompatible. For instance, memory retrieval involves attentional and motivational components. As yet, the proposed modes of action of ACTH-like peptides may best be regarded as provisional descriptions of (some of) the behavioral effects of these substances.

B. Physiological and Biochemical Aspects

ACTH-like peptides modulate behavior through direct actions on the brain. Several studies suggest that the nucleus parafascicularis of the thalamus may be a site of action of these peptides. Microinjections of ACTH 4-10 into the posterior thalamic area, including the parafascicular nuclei, mimic the inhibitory effect of systemic administration on extinction of an avoidance response. Bilateral lesions in the parafascicular area render rats unresponsive to this behavioral influence of ACTH 4-10 and α-MSH (van Wimersma Greidanus et al., 1975). Similarly, ACTH 4-10 is ineffective in retarding extinction in rats bearing lesions in the anterodorsal hippocampus and the rostral septum (van Wimersma Greidanus and de Wied, 1976). These data indicate that the integrity of midbrain limbic structures is a prerequisite for the behavioral actions of ACTH-like peptides.

The importance of the septum for the mediation of behavioral activity of ACTH and related substances is further suggested by the finding that radioactively labeled Org 2766 is preferentially taken up by septal nuclei (Verhoef et al., 1977). Org 2766 is a very potent, orally active ACTH 4-9 analog with the typical behavioral profile of ACTH-like peptides (Greven and de Wied, 1973; Rigter et al., 1976). The anatomical data find some support in electrophysiological investigations. Urban (1977) induced hippocampal θ activity in rats by electrical stimulation of the reticular formation. Treatment with ACTH 4-10 accelerated θ activity; this was attributed to an increase in excitability of the θ-generating reticuloseptohippocampal circuit. Kastin and coworkers found that α-MSH and β-MSH produce species-dependent changes in EEG recorded from occipital cortex (Kastin et al., 1975a). For instance, α-MSH appeared to facilitate the late components of evoked potentials in the occipital cortex of cats (Kastin et al., 1975b). On the other hand, ACTH 4-10 diminishes the amplitudes of the afterdischarge of visual evoked responses in rats. This latter effect has been interpreted as a specific increase in vigilance (Wolthuis and de Wied, 1976). For a more detailed review of the electrophysiological effects of ACTH-like peptides, the reader is referred to Urban (1977) and Bohus and de Wied (1977).

Information of the effects of ACTH and related peptides on brain amines is still sketchy and confusing. Increases in noradrenaline turnover in rat brain have been reported by Versteeg (1973) and Leonard (1974). Increments in cerebral dopamine turnover have also been found in ACTH 4-10-treated rats and mice (Leonard, 1974; Dunn et al., 1976) but, surprisingly, α-MSH and β-MSH seem to be inactive in this respect (Spirtes et al., 1975; Dunn et al., 1976). A series of studies attempted to relate one of the behavioral effects of ACTH 4-10 to alterations in brain biochemistry. It was shown in rats that acquisition of a passive avoidance response was paralleled by a rise in hippocampal serotonin levels persisting for at least 24 hr. This increase was not observed in animals rendered amnesic with carbon dioxide. ACTH 4-10, but not ACTH 11-24, was able to reinstate the rise in hippocampal serotonin (Ramaekers et al., 1978).

It is generally assumed that peptide hormones interact with receptors at the membranes of effector cells, thus producing increases in intracellular cyclic adenosine monophosphate (cAMP). The cyclic nucleotide, in turn, triggers a train of biochemical processes within the effector cell. Although the data for ACTH-like peptides are not completely conclusive (reviewed by Gispen et al., 1977), there is evidence that changes in cAMP may underlie at least some of the behavioral actions of these peptides. Thus ACTH 1-10 has been found to increase cAMP levels in slices from rat posterior thalamus, including the parafascicular nuclei (Wiegant and Gispen, 1975). α-MSH has been reported to raise cAMP levels in the occipital cortex of normal and hypophysectomized rats (Christensen et al., 1976). These findings do not exclude the possibility that ACTH-related peptides exert cAMP-independent effects. For instance, a recent study showed that cAMP and ACTH 1-24 both altered in vitro phosphorylation of rat brain membrane proteins but different protein bands were involved in the effects of these substances (Zwiers et al., 1976).

Changes in cAMP may be reflected in changes in brain macromolecule metabolism. Hypophysectomized rats have deficient brain RNA and protein metabolism (Gispen and Schotman, 1973), which suggests that pituitary principles are involved in the regulation of these processes. ACTH 1-24 stimulates the incorporation of uridine in brain stem RNA of rats. This effect is probably related to the corticotrophic property of this peptide since the endocrine inert amino acid sequence ACTH 1-10 is inactive in this respect (Schotman et al., 1976). The available data suggest that behaviorally active ACTH-like peptides influence brain macromolecule metabolism at the translational rather than the transcriptional level. Thus, chronic treatment with ACTH 1-10, but not with ACTH 11-24, reversed the deficit of hypophysectomized rats in the incorporation of radioactive leucine into brain stem proteins (Schotman et al., 1972). This effect is general in nature, i.e., not restricted to particular protein species (Reith et al., 1975). Furthermore, there is ample evidence that ACTH-like peptides enhance cerebral protein synthesis in intact animals, too (reviewed by Gispen et al., 1977; Dunn, 1976).

C. Studies in Humans

The animal data suggest that a peptide like ACTH 4-10 may be able to ameliorate deficient mental performance of humans. Several groups of investigators have attempted to assess in humans the effects of ACTH 4-10 on a variety of psychological functions. Gaillard and Sanders (1975) administered 15 mg ACTH 4-10 to healthy young volunteers. The peptide improved performance of the subjects on a continuous reaction time task demanding a sustained level of attention. In the course of the 30-min session placebo-treated subjects showed an increasing number of lapses in performance as evidenced by occasional high reaction times. Peptide-treated subjects did not display as many lapses, indicating that they were probably mentally less fatigued.

In another study ACTH 4-10 was found to delay the development of electroencephalographic signs of habituation in a "go-no go" reaction time task (Miller et al., 1974). Volunteers were requested to respond to a go signal by pressing a lever and to refrain from pressing when the no go signal was presented. ACTH 4-10-treated subjects habituated normally to the no go signal but, in contrast to the control group, showed no habituation to the go signal. This was taken as evidence for a peptide-induced enhancement of selective attention. In a subsequent double-blind crossover experiment, volunteers were tested on a continuous performance task. When in this task the relative frequency of occurrence of a relevant stimulus was decreased, ACTH 4-10 reduced both the number of errors of omission, i.e., failures to respond to relevant stimuli, and errors of commission, i.e., responses to irrelevant stimuli. This finding was interpreted as an improvement of attention. EEG data (visual evoked potentials) were consistent with a peptide-induced activation of the diffuse thalamic projection system (Miller et al., 1976).

ACTH 4-10 may also enhance attention in the mentally retarded (Sandman et al., 1976). Adult retardates were trained on a visual discrimination task and subsequently on reversal, intradimensional, and extradimensional shifts. The visual stimuli differed on two dimensions, e.g., color and shape. If during original acquisition the subjects had learned to choose between stimuli on basis of their color (e.g., red versus green) and to disregard their shape, color remained the relevant dimension during reversal training (e.g., green instead of red). On the intradimensional shift, a new set of stimuli with new colors and shapes was presented, color still being the relevant cue (e.g., blue). The extradimensional shift required the subject to ignore the previously relevant cue (color) and begin to respond on the basis of shape. Peptide-treated subjects showed improved performance on reversal and both forms of shift learning. These results were ascribed to an ACTH 4-10-induced facilitation of attention.

The studies reviewed above are most pertinent for the attention/motivation hypothesis. Although the effects in these investigations were often small, the picture emerges that ACTH 4-10 may improve attention in humans and may be useful as a treatment for disorders of attention. In addition, ACTH 4-10 may influence other aspects of human mental performance, too, but the available data are not consistent enough to draw even tentative conclusions. For instance, some effects on learning and memory have been described but the evidence is far from conclusive. Dose of the peptide, nature of the subject population, and characteristics of the memory test seem to be important variables (Sandman et al., 1975; Dornbush and Nikolovski, 1976; Ferris et al., 1976; Miller et al., 1976).

III. THYROTROPIN-RELEASING HORMONE (TRH)

A. Animal Pharmacology

The hypothalamus controls the secretion of anterior pituitary hormones by the release of peptide hormones into the pituitary portal system. One of these hypothalamic hormones is pGlu-His-Pro-NH_2. On the basis of its ability to stimulate the secretion of thyrotropin, this tripeptide has been called thyrotropin-releasing hormone (TRH) or thyrotropin-releasing factor. In addition, TRH has other endocrine properties, including the ability to induce the release of prolactin (Vale et al., 1977).

Of interest for the present discussion is that TRH has CNS effects independent of its role in the control of pituitary functions. This is already suggested by the presence of TRH in brain areas other than the hypothalamus (Brownstein et al., 1974). TRH has been studied in a number of animal models with assumed predictive value as to the nature of psychotropic effects of drugs. The first CNS activity to be reported for TRH was established in the dopa potentiation test. This test has been proposed as a screening tool for the detection of antidepressant drugs (Everett, 1966) but its suitability for this purpose is doubtful (Berendsen et al., 1976). The dopa potentiation test assesses increases in locomotor activity and irritability of animals treated with dopa and a monoamine oxidase inhibitor. TRH appeared to potentiate these responses; this effect is consistent with possible antidepressant properties of the peptide (Plotnikoff et al., 1972; Huidobro-Toro et al., 1974). The nonendocrine character of this effect is apparent from the finding that TRH still potentiates dopa-induced responses after ablation of a variety of endocrine organs, e.g., the pituitary and thyroid glands (Plotnikoff,1975; Plotnikoff et al., 1974). TRH has also been examined in an animal model of parkinsonism (Plotnikoff and Kastin, 1977). Oxotremorine induces Parkinson-like symptoms, including tremors, in mice. TRH was unable to antagonize the effects of oxotremorine. A third animal model was used by Plotnikoff and Kastin (1977). This model is based on the observation that the increases in motor activity and stereotyped behavior of monkeys following treatment with methamphetamine resemble symptoms of schizophrenia. TRH appeared to protect rhesus monkeys against the behavioral effect of methamphetamine.

Other experimental data suggest that TRH may have psychostimulant properties similar to amphetamine. Thus, TRH produces behavioral excitation, EEG desynchronization, and hyperthermia in rabbits (Kruse, 1975; Horita et al., 1976). Both amphetamine and TRH are known to reduce the sedation produced by barbiturates (Breese et al., 1974). TRH tends to stimulate motility although it is less active and consistent in this respect than amphetamine (Segal and Mandell, 1974; Breese et al., 1974; Goujet et al., 1975). There are, however, also clear-cut pharmacological differences between TRH and amphetamine. For instance, neuroleptics, such as chlorpromazine and haloperidol, block amphetamine-induced excitation and hyperthermia in rabbits, but do not alter the effects produced by TRH (Horita et al., 1976). TRH antagonizes the sedative properties of ethanol whereas amphetamine has the opposite effect (Breese et al., 1974).

The biochemical basis of the CNS effects of TRH is far from clear. TRH may modify some aspects of brain noradrenaline metabolism. The peptide does not affect whole-brain levels of noradrenaline (Plotnikoff, 1975; Green et al., 1976) or uptake of this amine by brain tissue (Horst and Spirt, 1974; Reigle et al., 1974), but a general finding has been that TRH produces a small but consistent enhancement of cerebral noradrenaline turnover (Constantinidis et al., 1974; Keller et al., 1974; Horst and Spirt, 1974). However, it is improbable that this activation of a noradrenergic system is associated with all pharmacological effects of TRH. Thus, administration of noradrenaline to mice mimics the TRH reduction of barbiturate-induced narcosis and ethanol-induced hypothermia (Breese et al., 1975; Cott et al., 1976) but, unlike TRH, the amine fails to influence narcosis produced by ethanol.

The activity of TRH in the dopa potentiation test suggests that the peptide may also alter brain dopaminergic functions. TRH has no effect on whole-brain dopamine concentrations (Plotnikoff, 1975). However, turnover studies indicate that TRH may decrease cerebral dopamine turnover. TRH probably acts presynaptically since the peptide does not interfere with the pharmacological actions of the postsynaptic dopamine receptor stimulant apomorphine (Green et al., 1976). In contrast, TRH may act postsynaptically at serotonergic neurons. This is suggested by the finding that TRH does not affect brain tryptophan and serotonin levels and brain serotonin turnover in rats, but does potentiate a syndrome of hyperactivity produced by pharmacological stimulation of postsynaptic serotonin receptors (Green and Grahame-Smith, 1974). The picture is even further complicated by the finding that interactions exist between TRH and brain cholinergic and GABAergic systems (Cott et al., 1976; Cott and Engel, 1977).

The postulate that cAMP is the second messenger of TRH has been examined by Cohn and co-workers (1976). The effects of TRH, dibutyryl cAMP, and the combination of both substances on barbiturate-induced sedation was studied in rats. A simple additive or synergistic interaction between TRH and dibutyryl cAMP was not found. The data therefore failed to support that cAMP is involved in the regulation of at least this particular CNS effect of TRH.

In conclusion, animal pharmacology provides crude indications that TRH may be useful as a treatment for depression and/or schizophrenia. In addition, TRH may have stimulant properties; however, its pharmacological profile is different from that of amphetamine. The physiological significance of these pharmacological effects of the peptide remains obscure. The fact that TRH is able to reverse the depressant CNS effects of a variety of drugs may be taken as an indication that TRH modulates generalized arousal. Green and Grahame-Smith (1974) proposed that the peptide increases overall sensitivity of neurons to excitatory stimuli. In view of the heterogeneity of the pharmacological and biochemical data, though, it is improbable that a single mode of action can be evoked to explain all actions of TRH.

B. Studies in Humans

A few studies have attempted to demonstrate psychotropic effects of TRH in normal volunteers. In a first double-blind investigation TRH or placebo was intravenously administered to women and mood changes were assessed using both subjective reports and ratings by two independent observers. TRH produced a pronounced elevation of mood (Wilson et al., 1973). The blind character of this study has been doubted on the basis of the assumption that subjects may be able to discriminate TRH from placebo since the peptide, when given intravenously, produces somatic side effects (Betts et al., 1976). This difficulty can be overcome if oral doses of TRH are employed. Betts and co-workers therefore administered the peptide in a single oral dose. Subjects of this double-blind crossover study were female students. TRH had no effect on subjective reports of mood change and on conventional objective mood measurements. However, an etiological analysis of videotaped interviews with the subjects showed peptide-induced changes in nonverbal behavior, such as facial expressions. The authors concluded that TRH may have a mild psychotropic effect in a euphoriant direction although they emphasized that more experiments are needed to substantiate this conclusion (Betts et al., 1976).

The contingent negative variation (CNV) is a special type of cortical evoked response reflecting the degree of alertness and arousal of the subject. This electroencephalographic phenomenon has been proposed as an objective measure of CNS effects of psychotropic drugs. The magnitude of the CNV is increased by stimulants and decreased by central depressant drugs (Ashton et al., 1976). This group of investigators studied the action of TRH, given as an infusion, in normal subjects and found it to be ineffective in altering CNV magnitude.

In summary, the results of these studies do not provide consistent evidence that TRH has psychotropic actions in normal subjects. There are some indications that the peptide may have a mild stimulant effect associated with mood elevation and euphoria.

The possibility that TRH may have more pronounced actions in patients has been examined in a large number of clinical studies. In particular, attempts have been made to establish whether TRH has antidepressant properties. Itil (1975a) examined the effect of TRH on cerebral biopotentials recorded from the scalp of depressed patients and analyzed by computer. The data suggest a stimulant action of the peptide, similar to amphetamine and a "stimulant" antidepressant like protriptyline.

Early reports of trials of TRH in mental depression were optimistic. Transient improvement of depressed patients was observed after infusion (Kastin et al., 1972; Prange et al., 1972) or oral administration of the peptide (Van der Vis-Melsen and Wiener, 1972). The antidepressant effect was rapid in onset, i.e., alleviation of symptoms became apparent within hours rather than days. However, many subsequent studies have failed to confirm the original findings (reviewed by Ehrensing and Kastin, 1976; and Mountjoy, 1976). The available data are difficult to compare as studies differed with respect to dosage, route of administration, duration of treatment, and types of patient. In some trials TRH was given as an adjunct to conventional treatments such as tricyclic antidepressants or electroconvulsive shock; in other trials TRH was administered alone. Despite these differences in design, however, failures to establish antidepressant activity of TRH are so numerous that the conclusion is warranted that this peptide is not a generally effective antidepressant. The possibility cannot be excluded, though, that TRH may be helpful in the treatment of a subgroup of depressed patients (Prange et al., 1975; Furlong et al., 1976). The available data indicate that if such a subgroup exists, it is not readily identifiable. However, this possibility certainly merits further investigation.

Independent of its possible applicability as a therapeutic agent, TRH may also be of diagnostic value in mental depression. A recent review shows that depressed patients frequently, but not always, display a blunted thyrotropin response to challenge by intravenously administered TRH. This deficit cannot be accounted for by primary changes in the pituitary or thyroid glands but seems often to result from a disruption of hypothalamic regulatory function. In addition, depressed patients may show other abnormalities in pituitary responses to TRH, such as changes in growth hormone and prolactin release (Loosen et al., 1976). The thyrotropin response deficit seems unrelated to type or severity of depression, nor does it consistently predict the degree of therapeutic effect of TRH. Most patients who demonstrate the thyrotropin fault during depression do not correct it upon clinical recovery (Hollister et al., 1976; Loosen et al., 1976). The relevance of the flattened thyrotropin response for the diagnosis, understanding, and treatment of depression remains to be clarified. An important lead for further investigations is the possibility that failure of the thyrotropin response to normalize during clinical recovery of the patient may be indicative of imminent clinical relapse (Kirkegaard et al., 1975).

TRH has also been subjected to clinical trials in schizophrenia. The present position here is much the same as outlined above for depression. Initial reports of Wilson and his colleagues (cf. Prange et al., 1975) indicated that TRH had a favorable effect in groups of schizophrenics. Improvement was seen within 6 hr after injection and lasted on average about a week. Subsequent studies, however, either failed to demonstrate a beneficial action of TRH (Clark et al., 1975; Lindström et al., 1977) or even found a deterioration of psychotic symptoms (Bigelow et al., 1975; Davis et al., 1975). It should be noted that in the original investigations of Wilson and co-workers the patients had been highly selected; each had shown good response to phenothiazines and had been off medication for several weeks before the TRH study was started. It is therefore possible that only a particular subgroup of schizophrenics is responsive to TRH treatment.

Lastly, a few preliminary studies should be mentioned. Since animal pharmacology has provided evidence that TRH may influence cerebral dopaminergic systems, Lakke and colleagues decided to examine the role of TRH as a possible dopamine-activating agent in Parkinson patients. However, the peptide did not affect Parkinson symptomatology and mood in these subjects (Lakke et al., 1974). Furthermore, some remarkable observations have been reported by Tiwary and co-workers. A mentally deficient boy greatly improved his disorganized behavior after treatment with TRH (Tiwary et al., 1972) and in two hyperkinetic children an immediate focusing of attention was noted (Tiwary et al., 1975). These findings require confirmation.

In summary, there is no consistent evidence that TRH has therapeutic value for a variety of behavioral disorders. TRH is not a generally effective antidepressant or antipsychotic compound. Its efficacy in subgroups of patients remains to be established. In addition, the applicability of TRH as a diagnostic tool should further be investigated.

IV. PRO-LEU-GLY-NH_2 (PLG)

A. Animal Pharmacology

The tripeptide Pro-Leu-Gly-NH_2 has been isolated from ovine hypothalamus (Nair et al., 1971). This tripeptide is identical to the tail amino acid sequence of oxytocin and, in fact, there is evidence that Pro-Leu-Gly-NH_2 can be cleaved from oxytocin by a hypothalamic enzyme (Celis et al., 1971). Pro-Leu-Gly-NH_2 is active in some assays for MSH-release inhibiting activity and therefore has also been designated MIF-I (MSH-release inhibiting factor). There is uncertainty, though, as to whether Pro-Leu-Gly-NH_2 can be considered to be the principal MSH-release inhibiting factor (cf. Vale et al., 1977) and we therefore prefer to use the abbreviation PLG.

The experimental approach used to assess CNS effects of PLG has some features in common with the approach followed for TRH. Thus, PLG has also been studied in animal tests which are possible models of psychiatric disorders. The peptide potentiates dopa in mice pretreated with a monoamine oxidase inhibitor, suggesting that it may have antidepressant activity in humans (Plotnikoff et al., 1971; Huidobro-Toro et al., 1974). The activity of PLG to potentiate dopa-induced responses is not lost after ablation of the pituitary or a variety of other endocrine organs (Plotnikoff, 1975). In contrast to TRH, however, PLG does not potentiate 5-hydroxytryptophan in mice (Huidobro-Toro et al., 1974; Plotnikoff, 1975). PLG is active in an assumed animal model of parkinsonism: the peptide protects both intact and hypophysectomized mice against tremors and other Parkinson-like symptoms induced by oxotremorine. The effectiveness of the peptide in this test has been demonstrated using a variety of routes of administration, including the oral one, and single as well as subchronic treatments. Moreover, PLG is not only active in its own right; it also potentiates the reduction of oxotremorine effects by a minimally active dose of dopa (Plotnikoff and Kastin, 1977).

Since PLG does not have any substantial anticholinergic action (Plotnikoff and Kastin, 1977), the most likely basis for its described pharmacological actions would be an interaction with central dopamine mechanisms. However, studies with PLG in tests capable of measuring dopamine stimulation have not yielded consistent results. If PLG was capable of activating central dopamine receptors, it would be expected to produce stereotyped behavior. Such an effect has been found in the cat (North et al., 1973) but not in the rat (Cox et al., 1976). It is possible that PLG, though not a dopamine receptor stimulant in its own right, may sensitize CNS receptors to dopamine or dopamine-like drugs. Such an effect would show up in a potentiation of CNS actions of drugs like apomorphine, amphetamine, and dopa. As mentioned above, PLG has been demonstrated to potentiate dopa in the dopa potentiation test and in the oxotremorine test. PLG also potentiates the facilitatory effect of apomorphine on aspects of sexual behavior of male rats (Kastin, 1975b). On the other hand, PLG does not affect the stereotyped behavior induced in rats by amphetamine, apomorphine, or dopa + monoamine oxidase inhibitor (Cox et al., 1976). Similarly, PLG does not stimulate locomotor activity of rodents, nor does it potentiate the hyperactivity induced by methamphetamine (Kastin et al., 1975; Cox et al., 1976). Species differences may contribute to the lack of consistency of the data, as suggested, for instance, by the cat/rat difference with respect to the peptide's ability to produce stereotypy and by the finding that PLG does stimulate locomotor activity in monkeys (Crowley and Hydinger, 1976).

Van Ree and de Wied (1977a,b) demonstrated that PLG facilitates in rats development of tolerance to morphine and self-administration of heroin. According to these authors, learning processes are involved in the development of tolerance and the acquisition of self-administering behavior. It is therefore possible that these exciting findings can be attributed to a modulation of underlying learning processes by PLG. The effects of PLG on tolerance and self-administration are the more remarkable as the dose in these studies was only 5 μg/kg. In the vast majority of the investigations that we have reviewed in this section much higher doses were used, i.e., in the range of 0.1-50 mg/kg.

Little is known about alterations in levels or turnover rates of neurotransmitters after treatment with PLG, making it difficult at present to relate PLG-produced biochemical changes to behavioral actions of the peptide. In view of the pharmacological data, it is not surprising that most biochemical studies have attempted to determine if PLG interacts with brain dopaminergic systems. However, biochemical investigations have failed to yield consistent evidence in favor of effects of the peptide on dopamine levels or metabolism in whole brain or brain areas. Friedman et al. (1973) stated that PLG decreases endogenous levels of dopamine in the striatum of intact rats and enhances the in vitro synthesis of tritiated dopamine from tritiated tyrosine in slices of striatum. The increased striatal dopamine synthesis did not persist in hypophysectomized animals and, therefore, cannot be related to the extrapituitary CNS effects of PLG. In contrast to the study of Friedman and co-workers, other groups of investigators have found no signs of altered whole-brain or striatal steady-state levels of dopamine in PLG-treated rodents. Similarly, PLG failed to affect whole-brain or striatal levels of homovanillic acid (Kostrzewa et al., 1975; Plotnikoff, 1975; Cox et al., 1976). In addition, various other parameters of brain dopaminergic function have been examined. Administration of PLG did not change in rats the active uptake of tritiated dopamine by synaptosome-rich homogenates of the striatum, nor did the peptide alter tyrosine hydroxylase or dopa decarboxylase activity in the striatum or substantia nigra (Kostrzewa et al., 1976). Nevertheless, it is possible that with the use of more sophisticated dissection techniques, subtle actions of PLG on dopaminergic function in specific brain areas can be established. This is illustrated by a recent study in which small samples of rat brain tissue were examined (Versteeg et al., 1978). Intracerebroventricularly administered PLG appeared to accelerate dopamine disappearance induced by the tyrosine hydroxylase inhibitor α-methyl-*p*-tyrosine; this effect was restricted to the caudate nucleus.

Plotnikoff (1975) found whole-brain levels of noradrenaline to be unaltered in PLG-treated mice. This was confirmed in rats: in this study PLG did not consistently change noradrenaline content in various brain areas of intact or hypophysectomized animals (Kostrzewa et al., 1975). However, there are a few indications that PLG may influence the rate of disappearance of noradrenaline after treatment with α-methyl-*p*-tyrosine. An increased rate of noradrenaline disappearance has been observed by Kostrzewa in the midbrain of both intact and hypophysectomized PLG-treated rats (Kostrzewa et al., 1975). A more detailed dissection of this midbrain area revealed that PLG may both decrease and increase noradrenaline disappearance. In particular, a reduction was noted in the A9 region and an enhancement in the A8 region. The A8 and A9 regions contain the cell bodies of the nigrostriatal dopamine neurons (Versteeg et al., 1977).

In conclusion, animal experiments provide crude indications that PLG may have antidepressant and/or antiparkinsonian activity in humans. In addition, PLG may facilitate tolerance to and self-administration of addictive drugs. Dopaminergic mechanisms may be involved in the mediation of CNS effects of PLG but the available pharmacological and biochemical data are inconsistent and inconclusive. Most biochemical changes produced by PLG seem to be restricted to the nigrostriatal system. This is in keeping with the finding that after injection of tritiated PLG into a rat brain ventricle, there is specific localization of radioactivity, among other brain areas, in the striatum (Pelletier et al., 1975).

B. Studies in Humans

PLG may have CNS effects in normal subjects as suggested by the observation that the peptide produced EEG changes in healthy volunteers (Itil, 1975b). The computer-analyzed EEG profile of a low dose of PLG (50 mg) resembled that of amitriptyline, whereas higher dosages (1000 and 1500 mg) produced an amphetamine-like stimulatory effect. These findings accord with animal data: A high dose of 30 mg/kg of PLG stimulated the EEG of the rabbit (Kastin et al., 1975).

The indication derived from animal experiments that PLG may have antiparkinsonian activity has been submitted to clinical trial. Additional arguments which prompted the initiation of studies in humans, came from reports that exogenous β-MSH may exacerbate parkinsonism (Cotzias et al., 1967) and that circulating β-MSH levels may be increased in Parkinson patients (Shuster et al., 1973). Clinical investigations with PLG were started by Barbeau and associates. In a follow-up trial this group of investigators found that an intravenous bolus of 200 mg PLG greatly potentiated the ameliorative action of dopa on motor performance of patients. This combined treatment not only amended motility but also improved intellectual functioning (Barbeau et al., 1976).

These results have partly been replicated in subsequent studies. Woods and Chase (1973) confirmed that PLG possesses nontoxic modest antiparkinsonian acitivity. An intravenous dose of 20 mg produced a mild and transient reduction of tremors and slightly attenuated rigidity. In contrast to the claim of Barbeau and co-workers, however, PLG tended to aggravate rather than reduce preexisting dopa-induced dyskinesias; this effect was of a temporary nature. A positive action of PLG on some symptoms of Parkinson's disease has also been described by Fischer et al. (1974). PLG (30 mg) was injected intravenously, either acutely or daily during a 14-day period. A slight improvement of some features of the clinical status was observed: notably, tremors were reduced, whereas akinesia and rigidity remained virtually unaltered. Psychometric tests revealed significant mood elevation, particularly in patients who displayed a reduction of tremors after PLG treatment. In fact, these authors suggested that the slight antiparkinsonian activity of the peptide was secondary to its mood-brightening effect. Results of another investigation also indicate that PLG may elevate mood in Parkinson patients (Gerstenbrand et al., 1975). In this trial, intravenous doses as high as 400 mg/day were administered for 10 days. The pattern of antiparkinsonian activity of PLG differed somewhat from that reported in other studies. Amelioration of symptoms was evident with respect to akinesia and rigidity and less in regard to tremors.

In most of the trials mentioned in this survey PLG was administered intravenously. The preliminary investigation of Barbeau (cf. Barbeau et al., 1976) provided an indication that oral treatment with PLG may also be effective. This expectation was not borne out in a better controlled double-blind trial. A gradually increasing dose of the peptide was given orally to 20 Parkinson patients. At lower dose levels PLG tended to amend the clinical status of the subjects but the ultimate dose of 1.5 g/day was clearly ineffective (Barbeau et al., 1976). It is possible that the oral route is not adequate for the establishment of clinical effects of PLG. Alternatively, it may be that clinical effects of the peptide are dose-related, lower doses being more effective than higher ones.

This latter possibility is supported by the above-mentioned report that low (50 mg) and high (1000 and 1500 mg) oral doses of PLG produced qualitatively different changes in the EEG of normal subjects (Itil, 1975b). A dose-related action of the peptide is also suggested by results of studies in depressed patients (Ehrensing and Kastin, 1976). In these latter double-blind investigations the majority of subjects treated daily for 5-9 days with an oral dose of 60 or 75 mg PLG displayed substantial improvements, whereas patients receiving 150 or 750 mg/day did not benefit from PLG treatment in comparison with placebo control groups. A subsequent study confirmed these findings of beneficial effects in depression (Ehrensing and Kastin, 1978).

In summary, the data reviewed suggest that PLG may have dose-related antiparkinsonian and antidepressant activity in humans. This general conclusion is supported by the results of most clinical trials but there are some discrepancies between studies which need to be clarified. The ameliorative action of the peptide in Parkinson's disease has been slight in the majority of trials but can perhaps be improved when more is known about the most adequate route of administration and schedule of treatment. It remains to be ascertained if the reported positive effects of PLG afford a sufficiently firm basis to be able to apply the peptide in the treatment of Parkinson's disease and/or mental depression.

V. ENDORPHINS

A. Animal Studies

In Section II we described behavioral activities of ACTH-like peptides. There is evidence that ACTH is physiologically related to another hormone, i.e., lipotropic hormone (β-lipotropin or β-LPH). β-LPH is a polypeptide with 91 residues, comprising the amino acid sequence of ACTH 4-10 (= β-LPH 47-53). β-LPH has been isolated from the pituitary glands of a variety of species, including humans (Li and Chung, 1976). In the rat pituitary, ACTH and β-LPH are stored in the same secretory granules and both hormones are released together (Pelletier et al., 1977). In addition, the distribution of ACTH-like immunoreactivity in rat brain parallels that of β-LPH and is altered by specific lesions in a similar fashion (Watson et al., 1978). These findings accord with the proposal that ACTH and β-LPH have a common precursor (Mains et al., 1977).

β-LPH, in turn, may be the precursor of several endorphins. Endorphins are opioid peptides which share the affinity of opiates, such as morphine, for specific receptors within the central and peripheral nervous systems. Therefore these peptides are considered to be the endogenous ligands for these receptors. A number of endorphins have been isolated from brain and pituitary tissues of a variety of animal species (Hughes et al., 1975; Simatov and Snyder, 1976; Guillemin et al., 1976). These peptides have been termed methionine^5-enkephalin (met-enkephalin = β-LPH 61-65); α-endorphin (= β-LPH 61-76); γ-endorphin (= β-LPH 61-77); and β-endorphin (= β-LPH 61-91). In addition to met-enkephalin, another opioid pentapeptide has been identified, i.e., leucine^5-enkephalin (leu-enkephalin).

The endorphins derive their name from the endogenous ligand concept (endorphin: from endogenous morphine). However, it now appears that endorphins cannot simply be considered as endogenous morphines. If this were the case, one would expect that the brain distribution of endorphins would run parallel to the distribution of the morphine-sensitive opiate receptors. Opiate receptors can be demonstrated by biochemical, or autoradiographic assessment of the stereospecific binding of radioactive opiates to neuronal membranes (Snyder, 1977). Indeed, there is a rough correlation between the distribution of the enkephalins in most brain regions and the presence of opiate receptors but there are apparent differences, too. For instance, the medial thalamus in the monkey and the cortex in the rat have high numbers of opiate receptors but contain little, if any, enkephalin (Simatov et al., 1976; Watson et al., 1977). Furthermore, as will be discussed below, there are clear pharmacological differences between endorphins and morphine. The picture is further complicated by findings suggesting that different endorphins may have different functions. Thus, the distribution of β-endorphin deviates from that seen for met- and leu-enkephalin in rat brain (Bloom et al., 1978). In addition, there are several types of opiate receptors and β-endorphin and the enkephalins can be distinguished on the basis of their differential affinity for these receptors (Lord et al., 1977).

The widespread brain distribution of the enkephalins (Elde et al., 1976; Yang et al., 1977), the multiplicity of opiate receptors, and the possible functional differences between various endorphins all point to the involvement of opioid peptides in the regulation of a variety of behaviors. We will limit this discussion to responses of potential relevance to (1) pain management and (2) treatment of affective disorders.

When administered intracerebroventricularly, high doses of the enkephalins produce a weak and transient analgesia; systemic injection of these pentapeptides is virtually ineffective in this respect (Belluzzi et al., 1976; Büscher et al., 1976; Frederickson, 1977). The lack of activity following systemic administration and the small effects seen following central administration have been attributed to the rapid enzymatic cleavage of the enkephalins. Structural modifications aimed at increasing metabolic stability have yielded potent enkephalin analogs producing longlasting analgesia (Frederickson, 1977; Hill et al., 1978). Of the opioid peptides identified so far, β-endorphin possesses the greatest antinociceptive potency. When injected into the cerebral ventricles, β-endorphin results in a longlasting analgesia; the potency of this peptide is greater than that of morphine (Gráf et al., 1977; Loh and Li, 1977). The analgesic activity of the endorphins is mediated through opiate receptors since the antinociceptive effects are reversed by the opiate antagonist naloxone (Frederickson, 1977; Loh and Li, 1977). As with morphine, tolerance and dependence are associated with continuous infusion or repeated injection of β-endorphin or the enkephalins. Thus, rats chronically intracerebroventricularly treated with β-endorphin manifest attenuated analgesia and some cross-tolerance to the antinociceptive action of morphine (van Ree et al., 1976) and withdrawal signs upon challenge with naloxone (Wei and Loh, 1976).

In spite of the antinociceptive activities found for endorphins and analogs, it is doubtful whether the physiological function of the opioid peptides includes induction of the type of analgesia produced by morphine. If that were true, it would mean that naloxone, as an antagonist of opioid peptide systems, should have dramatic effects when given in situations in which the organism confronts painful stimuli. However, naloxone has remarkably few effects in normal (morphine-naive) animals. Although there is evidence that naloxone can cause a decrease in pain threshold (hyperalgesia) in morphine-naive animals (Jacob et al., 1974; Frederickson, 1977), this effect is not robust enough to be readily replicated (Goldstein et al., 1976). Naloxone has also been examined for its ability to block analgesia induced by a variety of nonpharmacological treatments. The efficacy of naloxone may depend on the nature of the elicited analgesia but, in general, the effects obtained have been variable and weak. Thus, naloxone has been reported to partially block analgesia induced by electrical stimulation of the periaqueductal gray, a midbrain area implicated in pain perception (Akil et al., 1978), but again, this result is not easily reproducible (Yaksh et al., 1976). Similarly, naloxone has been found to incompletely block analgesia resulting from severe stress (Akil et al., 1978). Interestingly, analgesia can also be elicited in animals by electroacupuncture. In a study in mice the action of acupuncture was blocked by naloxone (Pomeranz and Chiu, 1976).

In conclusion, opioid peptides are able to modulate pain perception. However, the relative inactivity of naloxone in morphine-naive animals argues against an exclusive role of endorphins in the regulation of any response to pain. Presumably, other pain modulatory mechanisms exist and these may compensate for a naloxone-induced blockade of endorphin systems. The relative lack of activity of naloxone also indicates that subjects are not dependent on their own endorphins. If so, the administration of the opiate antagonist would be expected to result in withdrawal symptoms. Such an effect has not been demonstrated. Kosterlitz and Hughes (1978) concluded that the endorphins are well sequestered in their stores. The conditions under which the opioid peptides are normally released are not yet understood but it is probably that, once released, the endorphins are sufficiently rapidly inactivated so that opiate receptors are only transiently exposed and tolerance and dependence cannot therefore develop.

There are a few data bearing on the issue that endorphins, or a lack of endorphins, may be related to psychopathological states. Jacquet and Marks (1976) injected endorphins into the periaqueductal grey of rats and, in the case of β-endorphin, observed diminution or abolition of reflexes, immobile cataleptic-like postures, and sedation. The animals could often be "molded" in bizarre positions and maintain awkward postures for a long time. Met-enkephalin, leu-enkephalin, or α-endorphin produced this behavioral syndrome in an attenuated form but only when given in relatively high doses. Jacquet and Marks (1976) likened the syndrome seen after treatment with β-endorphin to the catalepsy induced by neuroleptics. Accordingly, these authors suggested that β-endorphin may be an endogenous neuroleptic and that its reduced availability may be significant in the etiology of certain forms of psychopathology.

However, evidence contrary to this conclusion has been obtained by Bloom et al. (1976) and Segal et al. (1977). These investigators also found that small amounts of β-endorphin, injected into the cerebrospinal fluid or into the periaqueductal gray, produced a behavioral syndrome similar in some aspects to that described by Jacquet and Marks (1976). However, two features of the β-endorphin syndrome were not seen after treatment with the neuroleptic drug haloperidol, i.e., extreme muscular rigidity and loss of righting reflex. Moreover, naloxone was able to reverse the actions of β-endorphin but not those of haloperidol. Therefore, the syndrome induced by β-endorphin seems to be different from the catalepsy caused by neuroleptics. In fact, Bloom and Segal stated that the behavioral state produced by β-endorphin is reminiscent of some aspects of schizophrenia. Accordingly, they proposed that derangements in endorphin systems may lead to signs and symptoms of mental illness (Bloom et al., 1976; Segal et al., 1977).

The supposition of Bloom and Segal implies that an antagonist of endorphins, e.g., naloxone, should have therapeutic value in the treatment of mental illness. A few animal data bear on this issue. As discussed above, naloxone has surprisingly few pharmacological effects. However, there are indications that naloxone may share some of the properties of conventional neuroleptics. Conventional neuroleptics are known to antagonize certain actions of agents that increase cerebral dopaminergic functions. The dopamine receptor stimulant apomorphine, for instance, elicits in mice stereotyped climbing along the walls of a test cage; this stereotypy is reduced or abolished by neuroleptics. Naloxone was found to have a similar effect but only when low doses of apomorphine were used; the opiate antagonist was unable to overcome the stereotypy produced by higher doses of apomorphine (Rigter et al., 1978). The limited antagonism of apomorphine-induced climbing suggests that naloxone may have weak or restricted antipsychotic activity. However, naloxone is not easily comparable to conventional neuroleptics. In general, these latter drugs influence dopaminergic function predominantly by blocking postsynaptic receptors, whereas naloxone seems to interact with dopaminergic systems at the presynaptic level (Harris et al., 1977).

The search for β-LPH fragments with antipsychotic properties has received a new impetus from the work of de Wied and associates. These authors found differential actions of β-endorphin and α-endorphin, on one hand, and γ-endorphin and des-tyr[1]-γ-endorphin, on the other, on extinction of an active avoidance response and consolidation of a passive avoidance response in rats. This differential activity led to an experiment to test the effect of des-tyr[1]-γ-endorphin in an animal model used for screening of potential neuroleptics, i.e., the "grip test." The peptide appeared to be active. The authors suggested that des-tyr[1]-γ-endorphin, or a closely related neuropeptide, is an endogenous antipsychotic with a profile more specific than that of haloperidol (de Wied et al., 1978a).

B. Physiological and Biochemical Aspects

A substance is considered to be a neurotransmitter when it fulfills a set of criteria regarding production, storage, release, receptor action, and inactivation. Evidence in favor of a neurotransmitter role of endorphins has been summed up by Frederickson (1977) in five points:

1. Endorphins are present in specific brain areas in association with stereospecific receptors and are localized in nerve terminals [cf. Section V.A; and Frederickson (1977)].
2. Synthesis of enkephalins from labeled ($[^3]$glycine) precursor has been observed in rat brain (Clouet and Ratner, 1976).
3. A highly effective enzymatic system for inactivation of the pentapeptide enkephalins exists in brain (Hambrook et al., 1976); the longer endorphins are relatively resistant to the action of brain exopeptidases but are degraded by endopeptidases (Hughes and Kosterlitz, 1977).
4. Evidence has been obtained for release of endorphins (Frederickson, 1977; Guillemin, 1977).
5. Endorphins may be inhibitory neurotransmitters since microiontophoretic application of these peptides generally results in a depression of the activity of single neurons in a variety of brain areas. How-

ever, excitation has also been observed. Many, but not all, of the depressant and excitatory actions of endorphins can be reversed by naloxone, suggesting opiate receptor involvement. Some of the actions of endorphins in microiontophoretic studies have been attributed to a postsynaptic mechanism (Bradley et al., 1976; Gent and Wolstencroft, 1976; Zieglgänsberger and Fry, 1976; Nicoll et al., 1977). However, there is also evidence for presynaptic actions of endorphins (see below).

Neurotransmitter action involves activation or inactivation of specific receptors which are coupled to membrane conductance. The time course of such action is in the order of milliseconds to seconds and is subject to desensitization. A recent report throws doubt on the concept that endorphins are neurotransmitters. This study employed mouse spinal neurons grown in tissue culture. Leu-enkephalin-depressed glutamate evoked responses in a noncompetitive manner; the effect of the peptide did not fade or desensitize during sustained application. The results were taken as support for a *neuromodulatory* action of the peptide functionally distinct from the operation of the conventional neurotransmitter classes. Neuromodulation was defined as the alteration of synaptic-receptor-coupled membrane conductances without direct activation of such conductances (Barker et al., 1978), thus modulating stimulus-effect relationships.

Enkephalins have been found in brain areas implicated in pain perception, such as the periaqueductal grey, the nucleus spinalis trigemini and the dorsal horn of the spinal cord (Cuello, 1978; Johansson et al., 1978). These areas also contain opiate receptors (Simantov et al., 1976; Lamotte et al., 1976). The fact that dorsal root section (rhizotomy) does not affect enkephalin levels in spinal cord suggests that these peptides are contained in interneurons. The opiate receptors in this region presumably are located presynaptically on primary afferent nerve terminals of pain conveying substance P neurons (Lamotte et al., 1976; Cuello, 1978). The picture thus arises that enkephalin interneurons in the spinal cord make axoaxonic contacts with substance P neurons; enkephalin may modulate pain perception by inhibition of substance P release.

However, enkephalins are also present in brain areas not directly involved in pain perception. An example is the corpus striatum. The corpus striatum is also rich in opiate receptors. Roughly one-third of these receptors are presynaptically located on terminals of the nigrostriatal dopaminergic tract; another one-third is presumably associated with neurons intrinsic to the striatum (perhaps cholinergic or GABAergic in nature); and the last one-third may be presynaptically located on fibers from cortical neurons (Pollard et al., 1977a; Childers et al., 1978; Costa et al., 1978).

Opiate receptors have also been identified on mesolimbic dopaminergic neurons (Pollard et al., 1977b). Following destruction of dopaminergic cell bodies in the midbrain of rats, binding of radioactively labeled naloxone to membranes from septum and nucleus accumbens was markedly decreased. It was estimated that most opiate receptors in the septum and 50-79% of the opiate receptors in the nucleus accumbens are located on dopaminergic nerve terminals.

The anatomical evidence of endorphin-dopamine interactions finds some support in biochemical data. Thus, β-endorphin has been shown to inhibit in vitro the potassium-stimulated release of dopamine from rat striatal slices; met-enkephalin was inactive in this respect (Loh et al., 1976). Intracerebroventrical injection of the metabolically stable enkephalin analog D-ala^2-met-enkephalinamide produces an increase in striatal dopamine metabolites in rats, suggestive of enhanced dopamine turnover (Algeri et al., 1977); a similar effect has been reported for β-endorphin (Van Loon and Kim, 1977). D-ala^2-met-enkephalinamide also increases striatal dopamine metabolite levels when directly administered into the striatum. This effect persists after destruction of striatal postsynaptic receptors with kainic acid (Biggio et al., 1978). The fact that only part of the opiate receptors are associated with dopaminergic neurons indicates that endorphins probably also affect neurotransmitters other than dopamine. Indeed, in addition to the above mentioned endorphin-substance P interactions, met-enkephalin has been found to reduce the release of noradrenaline from slices of rat occipital cortex (Taube et al., 1976) and β-endorphin has been shown to alter the turnover rate of acetylcholine in a variety of rat brain areas (Costa et al., 1978). This variety of interactions between endorphins and neurotransmitters, the possible functional differences between endorphins, and the multiplicity of opiate receptors all point to a complex involvement of endorphins in the regulation of normal behavior and, possibly, in the development of psychopathological behavior.

C. Studies in Humans

Analogous to our discussion of animal data, we will first outline some results in humans bearing on the analgesic properties of opioid peptides and then proceed with survey of preliminary evidence relating these peptides to affective disorders.

As in animals, naloxone alone has few actions in healthy humans. Thus, Grevert and Goldstein (1978) have reported that naloxone fails to alter experimental pain or mood in humans. Pain was produced by either ischemia or cold-water immersion. There were no effects of the opiate antagonist on subjective pain ratings, finger plethysmograph recordings, or responses to mood-state questionnaires. The authors concluded that these laboratory procedures apparently do not activate any functionally significant pain attenuating or mood-altering effects of endorphins. The possibility that naloxone may reverse experimentally induced analgesia has also been examined. Similar to what we have noted for animals, the efficacy of naloxone in this respect may depend on the nature of the analgesia. Goldstein and Hilgard (1975) failed to alter analgesia induced by hypnosis. Electrical stimulation of the brain is sometimes used to obtain pain relief in patients with intractable persistent pain; such pain relief has been found to be blocked by naloxone (Hosubuchi et al., 1977). Also, pain relief resulting from peripheral electroacupuncture has been reported to be reversible by naloxone in several subjects (Sjölund and Eriksson, 1976).

As outlined in Section V.A, opioid peptides probably exert a modulatory influence on pain processes. This influence is not readily observable in normal animals, perhaps due to the existence of compensatory modulatory mechanisms. However, it is important to distinguish between acute and chronic pain. In particular, Terenius and co-workers (1977) have proposed that the role of endorphins in pain processes might be more pronounced in chronic pathological pain. This concept is supported by the above-mentioned ability of naloxone to reverse pain relief in some patients. Further evidence in favor of this hypothesis has recently been reviewed by Terenius (1978). In several of their studies, Terenius and associates have isolated endorphins from lumbar cerebrospinal fluid (CSF) of patients. Subjects with chronic organic pain generally had low CSF endorphin levels in comparison with healthy volunteers or patients with so-called psychogenic pain. Measurements of endorphin levels in lumbar CSF before and after intracerebral electrical stimulation indicated that those patients that responded to the stimulation by manifesting naloxone-reversible pain relief also responded with an elevation in endorphin levels. This finding has been confirmed by a group of workers who sampled CSF from the cerebral ventricles (Akil et al., 1978). These studies yield the first demonstration of in vivo release of endogenous opioid peptides in humans.

Direct evidence for analgesic activity of endorphins in humans is provided by a report of pain relief in cancer patients following initiation of intravenous infusion of β-endorphin (Catlin et al., 1977). Two subjects reported good analgesia and mild improvement in mood; these reports were corroborated by independent observers. A third subject reported minimal pain relief but the observer noted evidence of moderate analgesia. Clearly, no generalizations can be made from this single trial with a limited number of patients but the results are encouraging enough to warrant further research.

Naloxone has also been employed as a tool in studies inspired by the concept that opioid peptides may be involved in affective disorders. In an initial single-blind trial by Gunne et al. (1977) a low dose of naloxone (0.4 mg intravenous) reversed auditory hallucinations in four out of six chronic paranoid schizophrenics.

Similarly, Orr and Oppenheimer (1978) found that naloxone (0.4 mg) blocked auditory hallucinations in a single patient. Interestingly, this subject had earlier experienced relief from hallucinations by self-administration of morphine and heroin. The authors suggested that both morphine and naloxone might have acted as competitive inhibitors of an endorphin fraction possibly present in excess in the patient. It is noteworthy in this respect that in previous centuries morphine has been used as an antipsychotic. It fell into disfavor with the recognition of its addictive properties (Comfort, 1977).

Several attempts to replicate the naloxone effect, using more sophisticated experimental designs, yielded negative results (Janowsky et al., 1977; Kurland et al., 1977; Volavka et al., 1977). Davis et al. (1977) noted that naloxone significantly improved only one of the target symptoms of schizophrenia ("unusual thought content"). These authors did not observe a diminution of hallucinations. In all these trials relatively low intravenous doses of naloxone were used (generally between 0.4 and 1.2 mg) and in most of these trials the patients were observed for only a brief period of time after infusion (15 min to 1 hr). In two subsequent double-blind crossover studies higher intravenous doses of the opiate antagonist were given (1.2-4.0 mg and 10.0 mg, respectively) and the subjects were observed for at least several hours (Herz et al., 1978; Watson et al., 1978). In both of the latter two studies a subpopulation of subjects gave evidence of transient relief or diminution of schizophrenic symptoms, including hallucinations. The naloxone effect was often delayed, i.e., was most pronounced 1 hour or several hours after injection.

The designs of these first studies of the antipsychotic potential of naloxone in humans are not easily comparable. Differences in patient selection, continuation or discontinuation of conventional medication, dose, and time of observation may account for the differences in results. Some data suggest that a subpopulation of patients may benefit from treatment with high doses of naloxone. That a high dose is required may mean that an opiate receptor is involved for which naloxone has relatively low affinity. However, it is also possible that the effect of naloxone was indirect, e.g., through a reversal of the stress associated with participation in a trial. Underlining the complexity of the naloxone data is the report by Gitlin and Rosenblatt (1978), who report that in two schizophrenic patients naloxone administration was consistently followed by abstinence-like effects, but not by therapeutic effects. The authors suggest that these data may indicate that withdrawal from endogenous opiates (endorphines) may have been observed in these patients and suggest to use the procedure as a test for (a subpopulation of) schizophrenia.

Naloxone has also been given to patients with endogenous depression (Terenius et al., 1977). There was no indication that the drug relieved depression. The doses used were rather low, however (0.4-0.8 mg thrice each day; subcutaneous or intramuscular).

Another experimental approach has been the analysis of endorphins in lumbar CSF. In one study (Lindström et al., 1978), six out of nine schizophrenics showed enhanced endorphin levels with returned to normal or slightly supranormal values after treatment with neuroleptics or propranolol. This decrease was accompanied by clinical improvement in four of the six responding patients. Since not every untreated schizophrenic had elevated endorphin levels, the authors suggested that patients with increased endorphin levels might constitute a subpopulation of schizophrenia. CSF endorphin levels were also elevated in four manic-depressive subjects. In three out of four patients with puerperal psychosis, an increase in endorphin levels was seen in the acute drug-free stage. After successful treatment with electroconvulsive shock and/or neuroleptics, the endorphin levels were within the normal range.

In a second study (Terenius et al., 1977), patients with endogenous depression also gave evidence of increased endorphin levels in lumbar CSF. Taken together, these results show that in at least a subpopulation of patients a variety of affective disorders are reflected in abnormal endorphin levels in CSF. The nature of the relation between affective state and endorphin levels remains to be established. An interpretation that altered endorphin functions are a contributing factor in the etiology of affective disorders is as yet premature.

The results of two preliminary clinical trials with endorphins have been published to date. Kline and associates administered β-endorphin intravenously (1.5-8.0 mg) to three schizophrenic and three depressed patients. On first injection, the peptide appeared to rapidly worsen the cognitive difficulties of the schizophrenic subjects and to just as rapidly improve the mood of the depressed patients. A repeat injection 12-13 days later was remarkably less effective, except in one schizophrenic subject. This latter patient was the only one who was without conventional medication at the time of the repeat trial. After the second treatment with β-endorphin, he was talkative and energetic; this episode was followed by a period in which this patient reported fatigue. The feelings of fatigue could be reversed by naloxone (Kline et al., 1977).

Clearly, this pilot study raises many questions. For instance, the qualitatively and quantitatively different responses on second treatment with β-endorphin need to be elucidated. It can be safely concluded, however, that β-endorphin is active in humans. The therapeutical potential of this peptide certainly merits further investigation.

In another pilot trial des-tyr^1-γ-endorphin (1 mg/day) was given intramuscularly to six chronically schizophrenic patients who were completely or partly resistant to conventional neuroleptics. Conventional neuroleptics were withdrawn 1 week before treatment with the peptide was initiated. All six subjects improved when given des-tyr^1-γ-endorphin. The improvement during the first few days of treatment was followed by a relapse in three patients. In the other three patients psychotic symptoms returned only several days after discontinuation of peptide treatment (Verhoeven et al., 1978a). A second double-blind study confirmed these findings (Verhoeven et al., 1978b).

In summary, clinical data obtained with naloxone (although variable in nature) are preliminary data obtained with two endorphins suggest that some endorphins may have therapeutic potential in the treatment of schizophrenia and/or depression. Again, we wish to emphasize that one cannot speak of *the* endorphins or *the* opiate receptor. Pharmacological differences between various endorphins, their differential affinity for a variety of "opiate" receptors, all indicate that different representatives of this class of neuropeptides are involved in the mediation of different types of normal and perhaps pathological behavior. This field of research undoubtedly will expand beyond classical concepts of opiate agonist and antagonist activities.

VI. CLOSING REMARKS

Research on behavioral effects of neuropeptides is rapidly expanding. Within the limits of the present chapter it is impossible to review all available data. Instead, we have restricted ourselves to a discussion of experimental findings in regard to several neuropeptides, i.e., ACTH 4-10, TRH, PLG, and the endorphins, which reached the stage of human pharmacology. It is even unfeasible to survey the results of all studies that dealt with these neuropeptides. We therefore selectively reviewed those data which in our opinion are most relevant to illustrate possible modes of action of these neuropeptides and their potential applicability in biological psychiatry.

A few points should be stressed in this respect. Most peptides exert more than one behavioral action. Consequently, many assays fail to discriminate between the activities of peptides with distinctly different chemical structures. As yet, only a limited number of neuropeptides have been examined in a sufficiently large battery of animal tests to allow a conclusion as to the nature and relative importance of their behavioral effects in animals. The use of only a few tests for the evaluation of CNS activity of peptides clearly poses some problems. A subject in a test situation is usually quite restricted in its behavioral repertoire, which entails that behavioral changes assessed in that particular test may be caused by a variety of factors. Conversely, the lack of effect of a peptide in a behavioral assay does not mean that this peptide is not involved or has no influence on the regulation of that particular behavioral response. There may be many reasons why a peptide fails to induce a perceptible behavioral change (van Riezen et al., 1977). For instance, many peptides are metabolically rather instable and may therefore fail to reach CNS receptors in sufficient quantity after systemic or even intracerebroventricular administration.

Using a large battery of tests and different experimental techniques facilitates profiling of CNS activities for a particular peptide. It then appears that, despite considerable overlap in activities, different neuropeptides often exert different patterns of actions. The next question then to be answered is that of the physiological significance of the various effects of a peptide. The dose needed to induce a particular effect is an important factor in this respect. We have emphasized those actions of ACTH 4-10, TRH, PLG, and the endorphins which may be prospective of the clinical use of these peptides. However, a change in research interests may lead to the discovery of new actions of these peptides and, consequently, new applications.

Even if the nature and significance of peptide-induced behavioral changes have been ascertained, many questions remain to be answered. The present survey shows that many physiological and biochemical processes have been implicated in the actions of neuropeptides. The diversity of reported effects makes it probable that a variety of mechanisms are involved in the actions of even one peptide. It has been postulated that there exist peptidergic neurons which synthesize at least one specific peptide (Zetler, 1976). Such peptides could act as neurotransmitters, i.e., short-term mediators of chemical transmission, or as neuromodulators, i.e., regulators of membrane properties and synaptic efficacy. This latter function may also be served by peptides which are not synthesized by peptidergic neurons (Nicoll, 1975). These concepts are attractive and worthy of further investigations but as yet the evidence is insufficient.

This survey indicates that neuropeptides exert direct brain effects, resulting in behavioral changes. Results from human studies are generally consistent with animal findings. Although we believe that these conclusions are warranted, it is also apparent that many effects of the peptides discussed are small and/or controversial. It should be realized that neuropeptide research for the greater part is still in its infancy and many inherent methodological problems are not yet completely solved. On the other hand, one may expect that future studies will lead to the detection of more specific or more potent behavioral activity of peptides.

REFERENCES

Akil, H., Watson, S. J., Berger, P. A., and Barchas, J. D. (1978). Endorphins, β-LPH, and ACTH. Biochemical, pharmacological, and anatomical studies. In *The Endorphins: Advances in Biochemical Pharmacology,* Vol. 18. E. Costa and M. Trabucchi (Eds.). Raven, New York, pp. 125-139.

Algeri, S., Calderini, G., Consolazione, A., and Garattini, S. (1977). The effect of methionine-enkephalin and D-alanine methionine-enkephalinamide on the concentration of dopamine metabolites in rat striatum. *Eur. J. Pharmacol. 45,* 207-209.

Ashton, H., Millman, J. E., Telford, R., Thompson, J. W., Davies, T. F., and Hall, R. (1976). An electroencephalographic investigation of short-term effects of three hypothalamic hormones (TRH, LH/FSH-RH, GH-RIH) in normal subjects. *Br. J. Clin. Pharmacol. 3,* 423-531.

Barbeau, A., Gonce, M., and Kastin, A. J. (1976). Neurologically active peptides. *Pharmacol. Biochem. Behav. 5, (Supplement 1),* 159-163.

Barker, J. L., Neale, J. H., Smith, T. G., Jr., and Macdonald, R. L. (1978). Opiate receptor model of amino acid responses suggests novel form of neuronal communication. *Science 199*, 1451-1453.

Belluzzi, J. D., Grant, N., Garsky, V., Sarantakis, D., Wise, C. D., and Stein, L. (1976). Analgesia induced in vivo by central administration of enkephalin in rat. *Nature 260*, 625-626.

Berendsen, H., Leonard, B. E. and Rigter, H. (1976). The action of psychotropic drugs on DOPA induced behavioural responses in mice. *Arzneim. Forsch. (Drug Research) 26*, 1686-1689.

Bertaccini, G. (1976). Active polypeptides of nonmammalian origin. *Pharmacol. Rev. 28*, 127-177.

Betts, T. A., Smith, J., Pidd, S., Mackintosh, J., Harvey, P., and Finucane, J. (1976). The effects of thyrotropin releasing hormone on measures of mood in normal women. *Br. J. Clin. Pharmacol. 3*, 469-473.

Bigelow, L. B., Gillin, J. C., Semal, S., and Wyatt, R. J. (1975). Thyrotropin-releasing hormone in chronic schizophrenia. *Lancet 2*, 869-870.

Biggio, G., Casu, M., Corda, M. G., Di Bello, C., and Gessa, G. L. (1978). Stimulation of dopamine synthesis in caudate nucleus by intrastriatal enkephalins and antagonism by naloxone. *Science 200*, 552-554.

Bloom, F., Segal, D., Ling, N., and Guillemin, R. (1976). Endorphins. Profound behavioral effects in rats suggest new etiological factors in mental illness. *Science 194*, 630-632.

Bloom, F. E., Rossier, J., Battenberg, E. L. F., Bayon, A., French, E., Henriksen, S. J., Siggins, G. R., Segal, S., Browne, R., Ling, N., and Guillemin, R. (1978). β-Endorphin. Cellular localization, electrophysiological and behavioral effects. In *The Endorphins: Advances in Biochemical Pharmacology*, Vol. 18. E. Costa and M. Trabucchi (Eds.). Raven, New York, pp. 89-109.

Bohus, B., Gispen, W. H., and de Wied, D. (1973). Effect of lysine vasopressin and ACTH 4-10 on conditioned avoidance behavior of hypophysectomized rats. *Neuroendocrinology 11*, 137-143.

Bohus, B., and de Wied, D. (1980). Pituitary-adrenal system hormones and adaptive behavior. In *General, Comparative and Clinical Endocrinology of the Adrenal Cortex*, Vol. 3, I. Chester Jones and I. W. Henderson (Eds.). Academic, London. In press.

Bohus, B., Hendrickx, H. H. L., van Kolfschoten, A. A., and Krediet, T. G. (1975). Effect of ACTH 4-10 on copulatory and sexually motivated approach behavior in the male rat. In *Sexual Behavior: Pharmacology and Biochemistry*, M. Sandler and G. L. Gessa (Eds.). Raven, New York, pp. 269-275.

Bradley, P. B., Briggs, I., Gayton, R. J., and Lambert, L. A. (1976). Effects of microiontophoretically applied methionine-enkephalin on single neurones in rat brain stem. *Nature 261,* 425-426.

Breese, G. R., Cott, J. M., Cooper, B. R., Prange, A. J. Jr., and Lipton, M. A. (1974). Antagonism of ethanol narcosis by thyrotropin releasing hormone. *Life Sci. 14,* 1053-1063.

Breese, G. R., Cott, J. M., Cooper, B. R., Prange, A. J., Jr., Lipton, M. A., and Plotnikoff, N. P. (1975). Effects of thyrotropin releasing hormone (TRH) on the actions of pentobarbital and other centrally acting drugs. *J. Pharmacol. Exp. Ther. 196,* 594-604.

Brownstein, M. J., Palkovits, M., Saavedra, J. M., Bassiri, R. M., and Utiger, R. D. (1974). Thyrotropin-releasing hormone in specific nuclei of rat brain. *Science 185,* 267-269.

Büscher, H. H., Hill, R. C., Römer, D., Cardinaux, F., Closse, A., Hauser, D., and Pless, J. (1976). Evidence for analgesic activity of enkephalin in the mouse. *Nature 261,* 423-425.

Catlin, D. H., Hui, K. K., Loh, H. H., and Li, C. H. (1977). Pharmacologic activity of beta-endorphin in man. *Comm. Psychopharmacol. 1,* 493-500.

Celis, M. E., Taleisnik, S., and Walter, R. (1971). Regulation of formation and proposed structure of the factor inhibiting the release of melanocyte-stimulating hormone. *Proc. Nat. Acad. Sci. USA 68,* 1428-1433.

Childers, S. R., Schwarz, R., Coyle, J. T., and Snyder, S. H. (1978). Radioimmunoassay of enkephalins. Levels of methionine- and leucine-enkephalin in morphine-dependent and kainic acid lesioned rat brains. In *The Endorphins: Advances in Biochemical Pharmacology,* Vol. 18, E. Costa and M. Trabucchi (Eds.). Raven, New York, pp. 161-173.

Christensen, C. W., Hartston, C. T., Kastin, A. J., Kostrzewa, R. M., and Spirtes, M. A. (1976). Investigations on α-MSH and MIF-I effects on cyclic AMP levels in rat brain. *Pharmacol. Biochem. Behav. 5, (Supplement 1),* 117-120.

Clark, M. L., Paredes, A., Costiloe, J. D., and Wood, F. (1975). Synthetic thyroid releasing hormone (TRH) administered orally to chronic schizophrenic patients. *Psychopharmacol. Comm. 1,* 191-200.

Clouet, D. H. and Ratner, M. (1976). The incorporation of H^3-glycine into enkephalins in the brains of morphine treated rats. In *Opiates and Endogenous Opioid Peptides,* H. Kosterlitz (Ed.). Elsevier, Amsterdam, pp. 71-78.

Cohn, M. L., Cohn, M., Krzysik, B. A., and Taylor, F. H. (1976). Regulation of behavioral events by thyrotropin releasing factor and cyclic AMP. *Pharmacol. Biochem. Behav. 5, (Suppelement 1),* 129-133.

Comfort, A. (1977). Morphine as an antipsychotic. Relevance of a 19th-century therapeutic fashion. *Lancet 1,* 448-449.

Constantinidis, J., Geissbühler, F., Gaillard, J. M., Hovaguimian, Th., and Tissot,

R. (1974). Enhancement of cerebral noradrenaline turnover by thyrotropin-releasing hormone. Evidence by fluorescence histochemistry. *Experientia 30,* 1182.

Costa, E., Fratta, W., Hong, J. S., Moroni, F., and Yang, H.-Y. T. (1978). Interactions between enkephalinergic and other neuronal systems. In *The Endorphins: Advances in Biochemical Pharmacology,* Vol, 18, E. Costa and M. Trabucchi (Eds.). Raven, New York, pp. 217-226.

Cott, J., and Engel, J. (1977). Antagonism of the analeptic activity of thyrotropin-releasing hormone (TRH) by agents which enhance GABA transmission. *Psychopharmacology 52,* 145-149.

Cott, J., Breese, G. R., Cooper, B. R., Barlow, T. S., and Prange, Jr., A. J. (1976). Investigations into the mechanism of reduction of ethanol sleep by thyrotropin-releasing hormone (TRH) *J. Pharmacol. Exp. Ther. 196,* 594-604.

Cotzias, G. C., Van Woert, M. H., and Schiffer, L. M. (1967). Aromatic amino acids and modification of Parkinsonism. *N. Engl. J. Med. 276,* 374-379.

Cox, B., Kastin, A. J., and Schnieden, H. (1976). A comparison between a melanocyte stimulating hormone inhibitory factor (MIF-I) and substances known to activate central dopamine receptors. *Eur. J. Pharmacol. 36,* 141-147.

Crowley, T. J., and Hydinger, M. (1976). MIF, TRH, and similian social and motor behavior. *Pharmacol. Biochem. Behav. 5 (Suppelement 1),* 79-87.

Cuello, A. C. (1978). Enkephalin and substance P containing neurons in the trigeminal and extrapyramidal systems. In *The Endorphins: Advances in Biochemical Pharmacology,* Vol. 18, E. Costa and M. Trabucchi (Eds.). Raven, New York, pp. 111-123.

Davis, G. C., Bunney, W. E., DeFraites, E. G., Kleinman, J. E., van Kammen, D. P., Post, R. M., and Wyatt, R. J. (1977). Intravenous naloxone administration in schizophrenia and affective illness. *Science 197,* 74-77.

Davis, K. L., Hollister, L. E., and Berger, P. A. (1975). Thyrotropin-releasing hormone in schizophrenia. *Am. J. Psychiatry 132,* 951-953.

de Wied, D. (1969). Effects of peptide hormones on behavior. In *Frontiers in Neuroendocrinology, 1969,* W. F. Ganong and L. Martini (Eds.). Oxford University Press, New York, pp. 97-140.

de Wied, D. (1977). Peptides and behavior. *Life Sci. 20,* 195-204.

de Wied, D., Bohus, B., van Ree, J. M., Kovács, G. L., and Greven, H. M. (1978a). Neuroleptic-like activity of [des-Try^1]-γ-endorphin in rats. *Lancet 1,* 1046.

de Wied, D., Kovács, G. L., Bohus, B., van Ree, J. M., and Greven, H. M. (1978b). Neuroleptic activity of the neuropeptide β-LPH$_{62\text{-}77}$ ([Des-Tyr^1]-γ-endorphin; DTγE). *Eur. J. Pharmacol. 49,* 427-436.

Dornbush, R. L., and Nikolovski, O. (1976). ACTH 4-10 and short-term memory. *Pharmacol. Biochem. Behav. 5, (Supplement 1),* 69-72.

Dunn, A. J. (1976). Biochemical correlates of training experiences. A discussion of the evidence. In *Neural Mechanisms of Learning and Memory,* M. R. Rosenzweig and E. L. Bennett (Eds.). MIT Press, Cambridge, Mass., pp. 311-320.

Dunn, A. J., Iuvone, P. M., and Rees, H. D. (1976). Neurochemical responses of mice to ACTH and lysine vasopressin. *Pharmacol. Biochem. Behav. 5, (Supplement 1),* 139-145.

Ehrensing, R. H., and Kastin, A. J. (1976). Clinical investigations for emotional effects of neuropeptide hormones. *Pharmacol. Biochem. Behav. 5 (Supplement 1),* 89-93.

Ehrensing, R. H., and Kastin, A. J. (1978). Dose-related biphasic effect of prolyl-leucyl-glycinamide (MIF-I) in depression. *Am. J. Psychiatry 135,* 562-566.

Elde, R., Hökfelt, T., Johansson, O., and Terenius, L. (1976). Immunohistochemical studies using antibodies to leucine-enkephalin. Initial observation on the nervous system of the rat. *Neuroscience 1,* 349-351.

Everett, G. M. (1966). The DOPA response potentiation test and its use in screening for antidepressant drugs. *Excerpta Med. Int. Cong. Ser.,* No. 122, 164-167.

Ferris, S. H., Sathananthan, G., Gershon, S., Clark, C., and Moshinsky, J. (1976). Cognitive effects of ACTH 4-10 in the elderly. *Pharmacol. Biochem. Behav. 5 (Supplement 1),* 73-78.

Fischer, P. A., Schneider, E., Jacobi, P., and Maxion, H. (1974). Effect of melanocyte-stimulating hormone-release inhibiting factor (MIF) in Parkinson's syndrome. *Eur. Neurol. 12,* 360-368.

Flood, J. F., Jarvik, M. E., Bennett, E. L., and Orme, A. E. (1976). Effects of ACTH peptide fragments on memory formation. *Pharmacol. Biochem. Behav. 5 (Supplement 1),* 41-51.

Frederickson, R. C. A. (1977). Enkephalin pentapeptides. A review of current evidence for a physiological role in vertebrate neurotransmission. *Life Sci. 21,* 23-42.

Friedman, E., Friedman, J., and Gershon, S. (1973). Dopamine synthesis. Stimulation by a hypothalamic factor. *Science 182,* 831-832.

Furlong, F. W., Brown, G. M., and Beeching, M. F. (1976). Thyrotropin-releasing hormone. Differential antidepressant and endocrinological effects. *Am. J. Psychiatry 133,* 1187-1190.

Gaillard, A. W. K., and Sanders, A. F. (1975). Some effects of ACTH 4-10 on performance during a serial reaction task. *Psychopharmacologia (Berlin) 42,* 201-208.

Garrud, P., Gray, J. A., and de Wied, D. (1974). Pituitary-adrenal hormones and extinction of rewarded behaviour in the rat. *Physiol. Behav. 12,* 109-119.

Gent, J. P., and Wolstencroff, J. H. (1976). Effects of methionine-enkephalin and leucine-enkephalin compared with those of morphine on brainstem neurones in the cat. *Nature 261,* 426-427.

Gerstenbrand, V. F., Binder, H., Kozma, C., Pusch, S., and Reisner, T. (1975). Infusion Therapie mit MIF (Melanocyte inhibiting factor) beim Parkinson-syndrom. *Wien. Klin. Wochenschr. 87,* 822-823.

Gispen, W. H., and Schotman, P. (1973). Pituitary-adrenal system, learning and performance. Some neurochemical aspects. In *Drug Effects on Neuroendocrine Regulation, Progress in Brain Research,* Vol. 39, E. Zimmermann, W. H. Gispen, B. Marks, and D. de Wied (Eds.). Elsevier, Amsterdam, pp. 443-459.

Gispen, W. H., van Wimersma Greidanus, Tj. B. and de Wied, D. (1970). Effects of hypophysectomy and ACTH 1-10 on responsiveness to electric shock in rats. *Physiol. Behav. 5,* 143-147.

Gispen, W. H., van Ree, J. M., and de Wied, D. (1977). Lipotropin and the central nervous system. *Int. Rev. Neurobiol. 20,* 209-250.

Gitlin, M., and Rosenblatt, M. (1978). Possible withdrawal from endogenous opiates in schizophrenics. *Am. J. Psychiatry 135,* 377-378.

Gold, P. E., and McGaugh, J. L. (1977). Hormones and memory. In *Neuropeptide Influences on the Brain,* L. H. Miller, C. A. Sandman, and A. J. Kastin (Eds.). Raven, New York, pp. 127-144.

Goldstein, A., and Hilgard, E. R. (1975). Failure of the opiate antagonist naloxone to modify hypnotic analgesia. *Proc. Nat. Acad. Sci. USA 72,* 2041-2043.

Goldstein, A., Pryor, G. T., Otis, L. S., and Larsen, F. (1976). On the role of endogenous opioid peptides. Failure of naloxone to influence shock escape threshold in the rat. *Life Sci. 18,* 599-604.

Goujet, M. A., Simon, P., Chermat, R., and Boissier, J. R. (1975). Profile de la T. R. H. en psychopharmacologie expérimentale. *Psychopharmacologia (Berlin) 45,* 87-92.

Gráf, L., Cseh, G., Barát, E., Rónai, A., Székely, J. I., Kenessey, A., and Bajusz, S. (1977). Structure-function relationships in lipotropins. *Ann. NY Acad. Sci. 297,* 63-82.

Green, A. R., and Grahame-Smith, D. G. (1974). TRH potentiates behavioural changes following increased brain 5-hydroxytryptamine accumulation in rats. *Nature 251,* 524-526.

Green, A. R., Heal, D. J., Grahame-Smith, D. G., and Kelly, P. H. (1976). The contrasting actions of TRH and cycloheximide in altering the effects of centrally acting drugs. Evidence for the non-involvement of dopamine sensitive adenylate cyclase. *Neuropharmacology 15,* 591-599.

Greven, H. M. and de Wied, D. (1973). The influence of peptides derived from ACTH on performance. Structure activity studies. In *Drug Effects on*

Neuroendocrine Regulation, Progress in Brain Research, Vol. 39, E. Zimmermann, W. H. Gispen, B. H. Marks, and D. de Wied (Eds.). Elsevier, Amsterdam, pp. 429-442.

Grevert, P., and Goldstein, A. (1978). Endorphins. Naloxone fails to alter experimental pain or mood in humans. *Science 199,* 1093-1095.

Guillemin, R., Ling, N., and Burgus, R. (1976). Endorphines, peptides d'origine hypothalamique et neurohypophysaire à activité morphinomimétique. Isolement et structure moléculaire de l'α-endorphine. *Comptes Rendus de l'Academie des Sciences (Paris) 282,* 783-785.

Guillemin, R., Vargo, T., Rossier, J., Minick, S., Ling, N., Rivier, C., and Bloom, F. (1977). β-Endorphin and adrenocorticotropin are secreted concomitantly by the pituitary gland. *Science 197,* 1367-1369.

Gunne, L. -M., Lindström, L., and Terenius, L. (1977). Naloxone-induced reversal of schizophrenic hallucinations. *J. Neur. Transm. 40,* 13-19.

Hambrook, J. M., Morgan, B. A., Rance, M. J., and Smith, C. F. C. (1976). Mode of deactivation of the enkephalins by rat and human plasma and rat brain homogenates. *Nature 262,* 782-783.

Harris, R. A., Snell, D., Loh, H. H., and Way, E. L. (1977). Behavioral interactions between naloxone and dopamine agonists. *Eur. J. Pharmacol. 43,* 243-246.

Herz, A., Bläsig, J., Emrich, H. M., Cording, C., Pirée, S., Kölling, A., and von Zerssen, D. (1978). Is there some indication from behavioral effects of endorphins for their involvement in psychiatric disorders? In *The Endorphins, Advances in Biochemical Pharmacology,* Vol. 18, E. Costa and M. Trabucchi (Eds.). Raven, New York, pp. 333-339.

Hill, R. C., Roemer, D., and Buescher, H. H. (1978). Some pharmacological properties of FK 33-824, a stable orally active analogue of methionine enkephalin, In *The Endorphins, Advances in Biochemical Pharmacology,* Vol. 18, E. Costa and M. Trabucchi (Eds.). Raven, New York, pp. 211-215.

Hollister, L. E., Davis, K. L., and Berger, P. A. (1976). Pituitary response to thyrotropin-releasing hormone in depression. *Arch. Gen. Psychiatry 33,* 1393-1396.

Horita, A., Carino, M. A., and Smith, J. R. (1976). Effects of TRH on the central nervous system of the rabbit. *Pharmacol. Biochem. Behav. 5, (Supplement 1),* 111-116.

Horst, W. D., and Spirt, N. (1974). A possible mechanism for the anti-depressant activity of thyrotropin releasing hormone. *Life Sci. 15,* 1073-1082.

Hosubuchi, Y., Adams, J. E., and Linchitz, R. (1977). Pain relief by electrical stimulation of the central grey matter in humans and its reversal by naloxone. *Science 197,* 183-186.

Hughes, J., and Kosterlitz, H. W. (1977). Opioid peptides. *Br. Med. Bull. 33,* 157-161.

Hughes, J., Smith, T. W., Kosterlitz, H. W., Fothergill, L. A., Morgan, B. A., and Morris, H. R. (1975). Identification of two related pentapeptides from the brain with potent opiate agonist activity. *Nature 258,* 577-579.

Huidobro-Toro, J. P., Scotti de Carolis, A., and Longo, V. G. (1974). Action of two hypothalamic factors (TRF, MIF) and of angiotensin II on the behavioral effects of L-DOPA and 5-hydroxytryptophan in mice. *Pharmacol. Biochem. Behav. 2,* 105-109.

Itil, T. M. (1975a). Effects of steroid hormones and hypothalamic hormones on human brain function. In *Neuropsychopharmacology,* J. R. Boissier, H. Hippius, and P. Pichot (Eds.). Excerpta Medica, Elsevier, Amsterdam, pp. 672-682.

Itil, T. M. (1975b). New psychotropic drug trials in Turkey. *Psychopharmacol. Bull. 11,* 5-10.

Jacob, J. J., Tremblay, E. C., and Colombel, M. -C. (1974). Facilitation de réactions nociceptives par la naloxone chez la souris et chez le rat. *Psychopharmacologia (Berlin) 37,* 217-223.

Janowsky, D. S., Segal, D. S., Abrams, A., Bloom, F., and Guillemin, R. (1977). Negative naloxone effects in schizophrenic patients. *Psychopharmacology 53,* 295-297.

Jacquet, Y. F. and Marks, N. (1976). The C-fragment of β-lipotropin. An endogenous neuroleptic or antipsychotogen? *Science 194,* 632-635.

Johansson, O., Hökfelt, T., Elde, R. P., Schultzberg, M., and Terenius, L. (1978). Immunohistochemical distribution of enkephalin neurons. In *The Endorphins: Advances in Biochemical Pharmacology, Vol. 18,* E. Costa and M. Trabucchi (Eds.). Raven, New York, pp. 51-70.

Kastin, A. J., Ehrensing, R. H., Schalch, D. S., and Anderson, M. S. (1972). Improvement in mental depression after administration of thyrotropin-releasing hormone. *Lancet 2,* 740-742.

Kastin, A. J., Dempsey, G. L., LeBlanc, B., Dyster-Aas, K., and Schally, A. V. (1974). Extinction of an appetitive operant response after administration of MSH. *Horm. Behav. 5,* 135-139.

Kastin, A. J., Sandman, C. A., Stratton, L. O., Schally, A. V., and Miller, L. H. (1975a). Behavioral and electrographic changes in rat and man after MSH. In *Hormones, Homeostasis and the Brain, Progress in Brain Research,* Vol. 42, W. H. Gispen, Tj. B. van Wimersma Greidanus, B. Bohus and D. de Wied (Eds.). Elsevier, Amsterdam, pp. 143-150.

Kastin, A. J., Plotnikoff, N. P., Sandman, C. A., Spirtes, M. A., Kostrzewa, R. M., Paul, S. M., Stratton, L. O., Miller, L. H., Labrie, F., Schally, A. V., and Goldman, H. (1975b). The effects of MSH and MIF on the brain. In *Anatomical Neuroendocrinology,* W. E. Stumpf, and L. E. Grand (Eds.). Karger AG, Basel, pp. 290-297.

Keller, H. H., Bartholini, G., and Pletscher, A. (1974). Enhancement of cerebral noradrenaline turnover by thyrotropin-releasing hormone. *Nature 248,* 528-529.

Kirkegaard, C., Norlem, N., Lauridsen, U. B., Bjorum, N., and Christiansen, C. (1975). Protirelin stimulation test and thyroid function during treatment of depression. *Arch. Gen. Psychiatry 32,* 1115-1118.

Kline, N. S., Li, C. H., Lehmann, H. E., Lajtha, A., Larki, E., and Cooper, T. (1977). β-Endorphin-induced changes in schizophrenic and depressed patients. *Arch. Gen. Psychiatry 34,* 1111-1113.

Kosterlitz, H. W. and Hughes, J. (1978). Development of concepts of opiate receptors and their ligands. In *The Endorphins: Advances in Biochemical Pharmacology,* Vol. 18, E. Costa and M. Trabucchi (Eds.). Raven, New York, pp. 31-44.

Kostrzewa, R. M., Kastin, A. J., and Spirtes, M. A. (1975). α-MSH and MIF-I effects on catecholamine levels and synthesis in various rat brain areas. *Pharmacol. Biochem. Behav. 3,* 1017-1023.

Kostrzewa, R. M., Spirtes, M. A., Klara, J. W., Christensen, C. W., Kastin, A. J., and Joh, T. H. (1976). Effects of L-prolyl-L-leucyl-glycine amide (MIF-I) on dopaminergic neurons. *Pharmacol. Biochem. Behav. 5 (Supplement 1),* 125-127.

Kruse, H. (1975). Thyrotropin releasing hormone. Interaction with chlorpromazine in mice, rats and rabbits. *J. Pharmacologie* (Paris) *6,* 249-268.

Kurland, A. A., McCabe, O. L., Hanlon, T. E., and Sullivan, D. (1977). The treatment of perceptual disturbances in schizophrenia with naloxone hydrochloride. *Am. J. Psychiatry 134,* 1408-1410.

Lakke, J. P. W. F., van Praag, H. M., van Twisk, R., Doorenbos, H., and Witt, F. G. J. (1974). Effects of administration of thyrotropin-releasing hormone in Parkinsonism. *Clin. Neurol. Neurosurg. 3,* No. 4, 192-197.

Lamotte, C., Pert, C. B., and Snyder, S. H. (1976). Opiate receptor binding in primate spinal cord. Distribution and changes after dorsal root section. *Brain Res. 112,* 407-412.

Leonard, B. E. (1974). The effect of two synthetic ACTH analogues on the metabolism of biogenic amines in the rat brain. *Arch. Internationales de Pharmacodynamie et Thérapie 207,* 242-253.

Li, C. H., and Chung, D. (1976). Primary structure of human β-lipotropin. *Nature 260,* 622-624.

Lindström, L. H., Gunne, L. -M., Ost, L. -G., and Persson, E. (1977). Thyrotropin-releasing hormone (TRH) in chronic schizophrenia. A controlled study. *Acta Psychiatr. Scand. 55,* 74-80.

Lindström, L. H., Widerlöv, E., Gunne, L. -M., Wahlström, A., and Terenius, L. (1978). Endorphins in human cerebrospinal fluid. Clinical correlations to some psychotic states. *Acta Psychiatr. Scand. 47,* 153-164.

Loh, H. H. and Li, C. H. (1977). Biological activities of β-endorphin and its related peptides. *Ann. NY Acad. Sci. 297,* 115-128.

Loosen, P. T., Prange, Jr., A. J., Wilson, I. C., and Lara, P. O. (1976). Pituitary responses to thyrotropin releasing hormone in depressed patients. A review. *Pharmacol. Biochem. Behav. 5 (Supplement 1),* 95-101.

Lord, J. A. H., Waterfield, A. A., Hughes, J., and Kosterlitz, H. W. (1977). Endogenous opioid peptides. Multiple agonists and receptors. *Nature 267,* 495-499.

Mains, R. E., Eipper, B. A., and Ling, N. (1977). Common precursor to corticotropins and endorphins. *Proc. Nat. Acad. Sci. USA 74,* 3014-3018.

Miller, L. H., Kastin, A. J., Sandman, C. A., Fink, M., and Van Veen, W. J. (1974). Polypeptide influences on attention, memory and anxiety in man. *Pharmacol. Biochem. Behav. 2,* 663-668.

Miller, L. H., Harris, L. C., van Riezen, H. and Kastin, A. J. (1976). Neuroheptapeptide influence on attention, memory in man. *Pharmacol. Biochem. Behav. 5 (Supplement 1),* 17-21.

Mountjoy, C. Q. (1976). The possible role of thyroid and thyrotrophic responses in depressive illness. *Postgrad. Med. J. 52 (Supplement 3),* 103-107.

Nair, R. M. G., Kastin, A. J. and Schally, A. V. (1971). Isolation and structure of hypothalamic MSH release-inhibiting hormone. *Biochem. Biophys. Res. Comm. 43,* 1376-1425.

Nicoll, R. A. (1975). Peptide receptors in CNS. In *Handbook of Psychopharmacology,* Vol. 4, L. L. Iversen, S. D. Iversen, and S. H. Snyder (Eds.). Plenum, New York, pp. 229-263.

Nicoll, R. A., Siggins, G. R., Ling, N., Bloom, F. E., and Guillemin, R. (1977). Neuronal actions of endorphins and enkephalins among brain regions. A comparative microiontophoretic study. *Proc. Nat. Acad. Sci. USA 74,* 2584-2588.

North, R. B., Harik, S. I., and Snyder, S. H. (1973). L-prolyl-L-leucyl-glycinamide (PLG). Influences on locomotor and stereotyped behavior of cats. *Brain Res. 63,* 435-439.

Orr, M., and Oppenheimer, C. (1978). Effect of naloxone on auditory hallucinations. *Br. Med. J. 1,* 481.

Pearse, A. G. E. (1976). Peptides in brain and intestine. *Nature 262,* 92-94.

Pelletier, G., Labrie, F., Kastin, A. J., Coy, D., and Schally, A. V. (1975). Autoradiographic localization of radioactivity in rat brain after intraventricular or intracarotid injection of ^{3}H-L-prolyl-L-leucyl glycinamide. *Pharmacol. Biochem. Behav. 3,* 671-674.

Pelletier, G., Leclerc, R., Labrie, F., Cote, J., Chretien, M., and Lis, M. (1977). Immunohistochemical localization of β-lipotropic hormone in the pituitary gland. *Endocrinology 100,* 770-776.

Plotnikoff, N. P. (1975). Prolyl-leucyl-glycine amide (PLG) and thyrotropin-releasing hormone (TRH). DOPA potentiation and biogenic amine studies. In *Hormones, Homeostasis and the Brain, Progress in Brain Research,* Vol. 42, W. H. Gispen, Tj. B. van Wimersma Greidanus, B. Bohus and D. de Wied (Eds.). Elsevier, Amsterdam, pp. 11-23.

Plotnikoff, N. P., and Kastin, A. J. (1977). Neuropharmacological review of hypothalamic releasing factors. In *Neuropeptide Influences on the Brain,* L. H. Miller, C. A. Sandman and A. J. Kastin (Eds.). Raven, New York, pp. 81-108.

Plotnikoff, N. P., Kastin, A. J., Anderson, M. S., and Schally, A. V. (1971). DOPA potentiation by a hypothalamic factor, MSH release-inhibiting hormone (MIF). *Life Sci. 10,* 1279-1283.

Plotnikoff, N. P., Prange, Jr., A. J., Bresse, G. R., Anderson, M. S., and Wilson, I. C. (1972). Thyrotropin releasing hormone. Enhancement of DOPA activity by a hypothalamic hormone. *Science 178,* 417-418.

Plotnikoff, N. P., Prange, Jr., A. J., Breese, G. R., and Wilson, I. C. (1974). Thyrotropin releasing hormone. Enhancement of DOPA activity in thyroidectomized rats. *Life Sci. 14,* 1271-1278.

Pollard, H., Llorens-Cortes, C., and Schwartz, J. C. (1977a). Enkephalin receptors on dopaminergic neurons in rat striatum. *Nature 268,* 745-747.

Pollard, H., Llorens, C., Bonnet, J. J., Costentin, J., and Schwartz, J. C. (1977b). Opiate receptors on mesolimbic dopaminergic neurons. *Neurosci. Lett. 7,* 295-299.

Pomeranz, B., and Chiu, D. (1976). Naloxone blockade of acupuncture analgesia. Endorphin implicated. *Life Sci. 19,* 1757-1762.

Prange, Jr., A. J., Wilson, I. C., Lara, P. P., Alltop, L. B., and Breese, G. R. (1972). Effects of thyrotropin-releasing hormone in depression. *Lancet 2,* 999-1002.

Prange, Jr., A. J., Wilson, I. C., Breese, G. R., and Lipton, M. A. (1975). Behavioral effects on hypothalamic releasing hormones in animals and men. In *Hormones, Homeostasis and the Brain, Progress in Brain Research,* Vol. 42, W. H. Gispen, Tj. B. van Wimersma Greidanus, B. Bohus and D. de Wied (Eds.). Elsevier, Amsterdam, pp. 1-9.

Ramaekers, F., Rigter, H., and Leonard, B. E. (1978). Parallel changes in behaviour and hippocampal monoamine metabolism in rats after administration of ACTH-analogues. *Pharmacol. Biochem. Behav. 8,* 547-551.

Reigle, T. G., Avni, J., Platz, P. A., Schildkraut, J. J., and Plotnikoff, N. P. (1974). Norepinephrine metabolism in the rat brain following acute and chronic administration of thyrotropin releasing hormone. *Psychopharmacologia (Berlin) 37,* 1-6.

Reith, M. E. A., Schotman, P., and Gispen, W. H. (1973). Incorporation of ^{3}H-leucine into brainstem protein fraction. The effect of a behaviorally active, N-terminal fragment of ACTH in hypophysectomized rats. *Neurobiol. 5,* 355-368.

Rigter, H., Berendsen, H., and Crabbe, J. C. (1978). Activity of naloxone in an animal test predictive of clinical antipsychotic activity. In *Characteristics and Function of Opioids,* J. M. van Ree and L. Terenius (Eds.). Elsevier, Amsterdam, pp. 441-442.

Rigter, H., Janssens-Elbertse, R., and van Riezen, H. (1976). Reversal of amnesia by an orally active ACTH 4-9 analog (Org 2766). *Pharmacol. Biochem. Behav. 5 (Supplement 1),* 53-58.

Rigter, H., and Popping, A. (1976). Hormonal influences on the extinction of conditioned taste aversion. *Psychopharmacologia* (Berlin) *46,* 255-261.

Rigter, H., and van Riezen, H. (1978). Hormones and memory. In *Psychopharmacology: A Generation of Progress,* M. A. Lipton, A. DiMascio and K. F. Killam (Eds.). Raven, New York, pp. 677-689.

Rigter, H., and van Riezen, H. (1979). Pituitary hormones and amnesia. In *Current Development in Psychopharmacology,* Vol. 5, W. B. Essman and L. Valzelli (Eds.). Spectrum, New York, pp. 67-124.

Sandman, C. A., Miller, L. H., Kastin, A. J., and Schally, A. V. (1972). Neuroendocrine influence on attention and memory. *J. Comp. Physiol. Psychol. 80,* 54-58.

Sandman, C. A., Alexander, W. D., and Kastin, A. J. (1973). Neuroendocrine influences on visual discrimination and reversal learning in the albino and hooded rats. *Physiol. Behav. 11,* 613-617.

Sandman, C. A., George, J., Nolan, J. D., van Riezen, H., and Kastin, A. J. (1975). Enhancement of attention in man with ACTH/MSH 4-10. *Physiol. Behav. 15,* 427-431.

Sandman, C. A., George, J., Walker, B. B., Nolan, J. D., and Kastin, A. J. (1976). Neuropeptide MSH/ACTH 4-10 enhances attention in the mentally retarded. *Pharmacol. Biochem. Behav. 5 (Supplement 1),* 23-28.

Schotman, P., Gispen, W. H., Jansz, H. S., and de Wied, D. (1972). Effects of ACTH analogues on macromolecule metabolism in the brainstem of hypophysectomized rats. *Brain Res. 46,* 349-362.

Schotman, P., Reith, M. E. A., van Wimersma Greidanus, Tj. B., Gispen, W. H., and de Wied, D. (1976). Hypothalamic and pituitary peptide hormones and the central nervous system. With special reference to the neurochemical effects of ACTH. In *Molecular and Functional Neurobiology.* W. H. Gispen (Ed.). Elsevier, Amsterdam, pp. 309-344.

Segal, D. S., and Mandell, A. J. (1974). Differential behavioral effects of hypothalamic polypeptides. In *The Thyroid Axis, Drugs, and Behavior,* A. J. Prange, Jr. (Ed.). Raven, New York, pp. 129-133.

Segal, D. S., Browne, R. G., Bloom, F., Ling, N., and Guillemin, R. (1977). β-Endorphin. Endogenous opiate or neuroleptic? *Science 198,* 411-414.

Shuster, S., Thody, A. J., Goldlamali, S. K., Burton, J. L., Plummer, N., and Bates, D. (1973). Melanocyte-stimulating hormone and parkinsonism. *Lancet 1,* 463-464.

Simantov, R., and Snyder, S. H. (1976). Isolation and structure identification of a morphine-like peptide "enkephalin" in bovine brain. *Life Sci. 18,* 781-788.

Simantov, R., Kuhar, M. J., Pasternak, G. W., and Snyder, S. H. (1976). The regional distribution of a morphine-like factor enkephalin in monkey brain. *Brain Res. 106,* 189-197.

Sjölund, B., and Eriksson, M. (1976). Electro-acupuncture and endogenous morphines. *Lancet 2,* 1085.

Snyder, S. H. (1977). The brain's own opiates. *Chem. Eng. News 48,* 26-35.

Spirtes, M. A., Kostrzewa, R. M., and Kastin, A. J. (1975). α-MSH and MIF-I effects on serotonin levels and accumulation in various rat brain areas. *Pharmacol. Biochem. Behav. 3,* 1011-1015.

Taube, H. D., Borowski, E., Endo, T., and Starke, K. (1976). Enkephalin. A potential modulator of noradrenaline release in rat brain. *Eur. J. Pharmacol. 38,* 377-380.

Terenius, L. (1978). Significance of endorphins in endogenous antinociception. In *The Endorphins: Advances in Biochemical Pharmacology,* Vol. 18, E. Costa and M. Trabucchi (Eds.). Raven, New York, pp. 321-332.

Terenius, L., Wahlström, A., and Ågren, H. (1977). Naloxone (Narcan$^{(R)}$) treatment in depression. Clinical observations and effects on CSF endorphins and monoamine metabolites. *Psychopharmacology 54,* 31-33.

Tiwary, C. M., Frias, J. L., and Rosenbloom, A. L. (1972). Response to thyrotropin in depressed patients. *Lancet 2,* 1086.

Tiwary, C. M., Rosenbloom, A. L., Robertson, M. F., and Parker, J. C. (1975). Effects of thyrotropin-releasing hormone in minimal brain dysfunction. *Pediatrics 56,* 119-121.

Urban, I. (1977). Electrophysiological correlates of behaviorally active neuropeptides: Influence on hippocampal theta rhythm and paradoxical sleep. Ph.D. Thesis, University of Utrecht.

Urban, I., and de Wied, D. (1978). Neuropeptides. Effects on paradoxical sleep and theta rhythm in rats. *Pharmacol. Biochem. Behav. 8,* 51-59.

Vale, W., Rivier, C., and Brown, M. (1977). Regulatory peptides of the hypothalamus. *Ann. Rev. Physiol. 39,* 473-527.

van der Vis-Melsen, M. J. E., and Wiener, J. D. (1972). Improvement in mental depression with decreased thyrotropin response after administration of thyrotropin-releasing hormone. *Lancet 2,* 1415.

van Loon, G. R., and Kim, C. (1977). Effect of β-endorphin on striatal dopamine metabolism. *Res. Comm. Chem. Pathol. Pharmacol. 18,* 171-174.

van Ree, J. M., and de Wied, D. (1977a). Effect of neurohypophyseal hormones on morphine dependence. *Psychoneuroendocrinology 2,* 35-41.

van Ree, J. M., and de Wied, D. (1977b). Modulation of heroin self-administration by neurohypophyseal principles. *Eur. J. Pharmacol. 43,* 199-202.

van Ree, J. M., de Wied, D., Bradbury, A. F., Hulme, E. C., Smyth, D. G., and Snell, C. R. (1976). Induction of tolerance to the analgesic action of lipotropin C-fragment. *Nature 264,* 792-794.

van Riezen, H., Rigter, H., and Greven, H. M. (1977). Critical appraisal of peptide pharmacology. In *Neuropeptide Influences on the Brain,* L. H. Miller, C. A. Sandman, and A. J. Kastin (Eds.). Raven, New York, pp. 11-28.

van Wimersma Greidanus, Tj. B., Bohus, B., and de Wied, D. (1975). CNS sites of action of ACTH, MSH and vasopressin in relation to avoidance behavior. In *Anatomical Neuroendocrinology,* W. E. Stumpf and L. D. Grant (Eds.). Karger, Basel, pp. 284-289.

Van Wimersma Greidanus, Tj. B., and De Wied, D. (1976). Dorsal hippocampus. A site of action of neuropeptides on avoidance behavior? *Pharmacol. Biochem. Behav. 5 (Supplement 1),* 29-33.

Verhoef, J., Palkovits, M., and Witter, A. (1977). Distribution of a behaviorally highly potent ACTH 4-9 analog in rat brain after intraventricular administration. *Brain Res. 126,* 89-104.

Verhoeven, W. M. A., van Praag, H. M., Botter, P. A., Sunier, A., van Ree, J. M., and de Wied, D. (1978). [Des-tyr^1]-γ-endorphin in schizophrenia. *Lancet 1,* 1046-1047.

Verhoeven, W. M. A., van Praag, H. M., van Ree, J. M., and de Wied, D. (1979). Improvement of schizophrenic patients following Des-Tyr-γ-endorphin treatment. *Arch. Gen. Psychiatry 35,* 294-298.

Versteeg, D. H. G. (1973). Effects of two ACTH-analogs on noradrenaline metabolism in rat brain. *Brain Res. 49,* 483-485.

Versteeg, D. H. G., Tanaka, M., de Kloet, E. R., van Ree, J. M., and de Wied, D. (1978). Prolyl-leucyl-glycinamide (PLG). Regional effects on α-MPT-induced catecholamine disappearance in rat brain. *Brain Res. 143,*561-566.

Volavka, J., Mallya, A., Baig, S., and Perez-Cruet, J. (1977). Naloxone in chronic schizophrenia. *Science 196,* 1227-1228.

Watson, S. J., Akil, H., Sullivan, S., and Barchas, J. D. (1977). Immunocytochemical localization of methionine enkephalin. Preliminary observations. *Life Sci. 21,* 733-738.

Watson, S. J., Berger, P. A., Akil, H., Mills, M. J., and Barchas, J. D. (1978a). Effects of naloxone on schizophrenia. Reduction in hallucinations in a subpopulation of subjects. *Science 201,* 73-76.

Watson, S. J., Richard III, C. W., and Barchas, J. D. (1978b). Adrenocorticotropin in rat brain. Immunocytochemical localization in cells and axons. *Science 200,* 1180-1182.

Wei, E., and Loh, H. (1976). Physical dependence on opiate-like peptide. *Science 193,* 1262-1263.

Wiegant, V. M., and Gispen, W. H. (1975). Behaviorally active ACTH analogues and brain cyclic AMP. *Exp. Brain Res. 23 (Supplement),* 219.

Wilson, I. C., Prange, Jr., A. J., Lara, P. P., Alltop, L. B., Stikeleather, R. A., and Lipton, M. A. (1973). Psychobiological responses of normal women. I. Subjective experiences. *Arch. Gen. Psychiatry 29,* 15-21.

Wolthuis, O. L. and de Wied, D. (1976). The effect of ACTH analogues on motor behaviour and visual evoked responses in rats. *Pharmacol. Biochem. Behav. 4,* 273-278.

Woods, A. C., and Chase, T. N. (1973). M.I.F.: Effect of levodopa dyskinesias in man. *Lancet 2,* 513.

Yang, H. -Y. T., Hong, J. S., and Costa, E. (1977). Regional distribution of leu and met enkephalin in rat brain. *Neuropharmacology 16,* 303-307.

Yaksh, T. L., Yeung, T. C., and Rudy, T. A. (1976). An inability to antagonize with naloxone the elevated nociception thresholds resulting from electrical stimulation of the mesencephalic central grey. *Life Sci. 18,* 1193-1198.

Zetler, G. (1976). The peptidergic neuron. A working hypothesis. *Biochem. Pharmacol. 25,* 1817-1818.

Zieglgänsberger, W., and Fry, J. P. (1976). Actions of enkephalin on cortical and striatal neurones of naive and morphine tolerant/dependent rats. In *Opiates and Endogenous Opioid Peptides,* H. W. Kosterlitz (Ed.). Elsevier, Amsterdam, pp. 231-238.

Zwiers, H., Veldhuis, H. D., Schotman, P., and Gispen, W. H. (1976). ACTH, cyclic nucleotides, and brain protein phosphorylation in vitro. *Neurochem. Res. 1,* 669-677.

14

Neuropeptides: A New Dimension in Biological Psychiatry

Herman M. van Praag and Willem M. A. Verhoeven
Academic Hospital
State University of Utrecht
Utrecht, The Netherlands

I. SIGNIFICANCE OF NEUROPEPTIDES IN BIOLOGICAL PSYCHIATRY

In the past 20 years, research into biochemical determinants of disturbed behavior has focused mainly on the central monoamines (MA) (van Praag 1978; see also Chapter 3 in this volume). There were sound reasons for this.

1. Effective methods were evolved for determination of MA metabolites in cerebrospinal fluid (CSF) and peripheral body fluids.
2. The so-called probenecid technique enhanced the instructive value of determining these compounds in the CSF.
3. The degradation of MA is a "linear" process. MA metabolites are degradation products and have no precursor function in MA synthesis. The level of MA metabolites therefore reflects to some extent the rate of degradation of the mother substances in a given region.
4. Several enzymes involved in MA metabolism are measurable in peripheral blood (monoamine oxidase, catechol-O-methyltransferase, and dopamine-β-hydroxylase).

Other central transmitters did not fulfill these criteria, or did so only to a lesser extent. An example is acetylcholine. Choline is both precursor and metabolite of acetylcholine. Moreover, choline is not utilized exclusively for central acetylcholine synthesis. Finally, determination of these compounds in CSF has until recently been difficult and cumbersome. We were in fact able to demonstrate that determination of choline in CSF warrants no reliable conclusion about the acetylcholine turnover in the central nervous system (CNS) (Klaver et al., 1979).

The discovery of the neuropeptides was of importance to biological psychiatry for two reasons. The first is a general reason: Neuropeptides represent a new principle in neurobiology, the principle of hormone-like compounds produced in the brain whose target is their own source of production, i.e., the brain. The second is a specific biological psychiatric reason: The neuropeptides added a new dimension to human brain and behavior research, beside the MA dimension. This new dimension as such seems amply to merit investigation, but in addition raises the question as to whether (and, if so, how) neuropeptide and MA systems are related. The first question is discussed in this chapter. On the second question there are (as yet) no adequate (human) data.

II. NEUROPEPTIDES

A. Definition

Proteins consist of a random number of amino acids linked by a peptide bond. Peptides are small proteins which consist of at least 2 and usually no more than 40 amino acids. Longer chains are as a rule called proteins, but there are no firm agreements on this point.

Neuropeptides are peptides produced and active in the CNS. Some neuropeptides also show peripheral endocrine activity but their effect on the CNS is independent of this; it is *direct.* This direct effect on the CNS can give rise to behavior changes.

It is with these neuropeptides that this chapter is concerned. It does not claim comprehensiveness but confines itself to those peptides that (1) influence behavior via a direct effect on the CNS and (2) have already been tested in human subjects. The references to the literature concern review articles whenever possible.

B. Discovery of the Neuropeptides

Three independent lines of research have led to the discovery of behavior-active neuropeptides (de Wied, 1977a; Schally, 1978; Guillemin, 1978; Hughes, 1979; Nemeroff and Prange, 1978).

1. *Pituitary hormones.* Certain pituitary hormones—specifically adrenocorticotropic hormone (ACTH), melanocyte-stimulating hormone (MSH), vasopressin, and oxytocin—exert an influence on mnestic and motivational processes. Since derivatives which lack peripheral endocrine activity retain their effects on behavior, it seemed plausible that these effects are based on a direct effect on the CNS.
2. *Releasing and inhibiting factors.* These hormones occur in the hypothalamus and control the release of anterior pituitary hormones. Research into thyrotropin-releasing hormone (TRH) in depressions (Prange et al., 1972) revealed that peptides of this group can develop effects on behavior. Behavior research has since been carried out, not only with TRH but also with some other hypothalamic hormones such as luteinizing-hormone-releasing hormone (LH-RH) and the growth hormone release-inhibiting factor (somatostatin).
3. *Endorphins (and enkephalins).* The discovery of these peptides followed that of the so-called opiate receptors in the brain. The existence of these receptors prompted the question of the nature of the physiological candidates for these receptors. This led first to the discovery of two pentapeptides—methionine enkephalin and leucine enkephalin, mainly localized in the brain—followed by the discovery

of a few larger peptides, called endorphins. There are three known endorphins which, in order of diminishing size, are known as β-, γ- and α-endorphin. β-Endorphin is localized mainly in the pituitary gland and to a lesser extent in the brain.

III. PITUITARY HORMONES

A. Vasopressin and Oxytocin

1. General Data

Vasopressin and oxytocin are mainly produced in the cell bodies of two hypothalamic nuclei: the supraoptic and the paraventricular nucleus. They are stored in so-called neurosecretory granules, and these are then transported along the axons of these neurons to, and stored in, cells of the posterior pituitary lobe. Oxytocin influences lactation and uterine contractions. Vasopressin inhibits renal water excretion and, in larger doses, increases blood pressure. Vasopressin is released not only into the peripheral circulation but also into the hypothalamic-pituitary vascular system. This suggests that it may influence the function of the anterior pituitary lobe.

Vasopressin is also found in the medial eminence, but the function of this pool is still obscure; nor is it known how vasopressin reaches this site. Vasopressin is released not only into the systemic and local circulation but also into the CSF, via which it could reach various brain structures. An alternative possibility is that it is transported via axons of the neurosecretory cells in the paraventricular and the supraoptic nucleus.

2. Data from Animal Experiments: Memory Research

de Wied et al. (1976a) demonstrated that resection of the posterior pituitary lobe (including the middle lobe) in rats leads to disturbances in avoidance learning, specifically in the capacity to fix these new behavioral patterns in the memory (consolidation). The rate at which behavior is learned (the acquisition), however, is not affected. In other words, rats deprived of the neurohypophysis learn normally but the extinction of what they have learned is accelerated: they "forget" more quickly. There are indications, moreover, that the retrieval of stored information is also disturbed in these animals. These phenomena can be reversed with the aid of vasopressin and with vasopressin derivatives without peripheral endocrine activity, e.g., desglycinamide lysine vasopressin, a pituitary peptide endogenous in pigs.

Vasopressin has a comparable effect in intact rats: It inhibits the extinction of conditioned behavior, a long-term effect which may persist for several days after a single injection. The first hours after the learning trial are essential for the effect of vasopressin. This effect is most marked within the 1st hr, and disappears within 6 hr. When retrograde amnesia is provoked in rats with an intact brain, e.g., with the aid of electroshocks or by carbon dioxide inhalation, restoration of memory can be facilitated with vasopressin.

The physiological involvement of vasopressin in mnestic and learning processes is clinched by the following two experiments. In rabbits, specific antivasopressin antibodies can be provoked. When given intracerebrally to rats, this antiserum neutralizes cerebral vasopressin. These animals display the above described consolidation defects. Peripherally administered antiserum does not produce this effect. This suggests that the effect of vasopressin on memory is based on a direct influence on the CNS (van Wimersma Greidanus and de Wied, 1976).

The second experiment was carried out on rats of the Brattleboro strain by de Wied et al. (1975a). These rats have a genetic defect in vasopressin production and consequently suffer from diabetes insipidus. In addition, they were found to show marked mnestic disorders which could be reversed with the aid of vasopressin.

The effect of the second posterior pituitary hormone (oxytocin) on the learning of avoidance behavior is the opposite that of vasopressin (van Ree et al., 1978a). Oxytocin administration leads to dimished consolidation and retrieval, rendering the animals amnesic, so to speak, for the aversive experience. Inversely, intraventricular injection of oxytocin antiserum facilitates the learning of avoidance behavior.

Posterior pituitary hormones thus prove to be closely involved both in the acquisition of new types of behavior and in the extinction of established ones. It therefore seems likely that their activity plays a role in the individual's ability to maintain himself in his life environment.

3. *Data from Animal Experiments: Addiction Research*

Apart from the effects of vasopressin in learning processes, there are reports on a second series of behavior effects of this peptide in animals which may have medical significance: effects on opiate addiction behavior (van Ree et al., 1978b). Des-glycinamide^9-arginine^8-vasopressin (DG-AVP) reduces intravenous self-administration of heroin in rats, both when subcutaneously and when intraventricularly injected. Antivasopressin antibodies which neutralize the effect of endogenous vasopressin have the opposite effect. The effectiveness of the vasopressin analog appears to be of a long-term nature. It therefore looks as if the specific rewarding effect of heroin in animals is reduced by vasopressin.

Another effect of vasopressin on addiction behavior is accelerated habituation to the effects of morphine and related compounds (Krivoy et al., 1974; van Ree et al., 1978b; Hoffman et al., 1978). In the absence of vasopressin (rats with diabetes insipidus or normal rats treated with vasopressin antiserum), on the other hand, the development of tolerance is delayed. The development of tolerance has been compared with a learning process. This vasopressin effect may therefore come under the same denominator as the above described facilitation of consolidation and inhibition of extinction of conditioned behavior. The former effect seems to hold promises for the treatment of addicts; the latter, however, would be therapeutically undesirable.

Oxytocin exerts no significant influence on heroin self-administration. Its effect on the development of tolerance is similar to that of DG-AVP; it facilitates this development. In this respect, oxytocin was found to be five times as potent as DG-AVP (van Ree et al., 1978b).

4. *Human Studies*

In a few recent human studies the effect of vasopressin (about 14 IU/day) on learning and memory processes was studied by means of psychometric tests (Table 1). On the basis of a controlled study of 23 volunteers (aged 60-65), Legros et al. (1978) reached the conclusion that vasopressin (administered as nasal spray) improved attention, concentration, learning, and memory. Oliveros et al. (1978), Blake et al. (1978), and LaBoeuf et al. (1978) described the effect of vasopressin in a total of eight patients with an amnesic syndrome. Oliveros observed a favorable effect on memory functions in patients with post-traumatic amnesia. Blake observed no effect in patients with disturbed memory functions as a result of alcoholism. LaBoeuf et al. (1978) observed marked improvement of memory functions in two patients with a Korsakoff syndrome. Further investigations will have to show whether vasopressin treatment is of clinical significance in amnesia and other memory disorders with an

Table 1 Behavioral Studies with Vasopressin in Humans

Study	Diagnosis	*N*	Design	Dosage	Result
Blake, 1978	Korsakoff's syndrome	2	Open	16 IU daily, 15 or 21 days	
LaBoeuf, 1978	Korsakoff's syndrome	2	Double-blind	22.5 IU daily, 14 days	Improvement of memory and concentration
Legros, 1978	Volunteers with memory disorders, age 50-65 years	12	Double-blind	16 IU daily 3 days	Improvement of memory, concentration, and attention
Oliveros, 1978	Post-traumatic amnesia, alcoholic amnesia	3 1	Double-blind	11-15 IU daily 7-21 days	Improvement of memory and mood
Total		20			+18

anatomically intact cerebral substrate. To avoid side effects, moreover, it would be advisable to use a vasopressin analog without peripheral endocrine effects.

So far, one study has focused on the effect of vasopressin in heroin addicts. In the vasopressin group, the number of heroin administrations was significantly smaller than that in the placebo group (van Ree, personal communication). Follow-up studies will have to show whether there are also influences on tolerance development, which might cause the gain made with one hand to be lost with the other.

Patients with acute psychoses and a high degree of anxiety were found to have increased plasma vasopressin concentrations as compared with nonpsychotic patients with a high degree of anxiety and with normal controls (Raskind et al., 1978). Anxiety is therefore probably not the cause of this phenomena, the significance of which remains obscure. There have been speculations on the possible involvement of vasopressin in the pathogenesis of depressions (Gold et al., 1978), but no experimental data have so far been presented.

As pointed out, the effect of oxytocin on conditioned behavior is the opposite of the effect of vasopressin. The latter facilitates consolidation of new information, whereas the former facilitates its repression, the extinction. We considered the fact that there are categories of psychiatric patients with memory traces that lead to entirely dysfunctional, repetitive behavior. Typical examples are patients with obsessive-compulsive disorders. Extinction of the memory traces in question might produce a therapeutically desirable effect. We are now studying the effect of oxytocin on compulsive behavior and our preliminary results indicate that compulsive activities are less frequent during oxytocin medication than during placebo administration (Kraaimaat et al., unpublished results).

B. Adrenocorticotropic Hormone (ACTH)

1. General Data

ACTH is produced by the basophilic cells in the anterior pituitary lobe and released into the blood stream. It stimulates the adrenal cortex to increased hormone release, especially of glucocorticosteroids. Its effect on aldosterone secretion is small. ACTH release in turn is stimulated by the corticotropin-releasing factor (CRF) from the hypothalamus. CRF is produced in neurosecretory cells, transported via the axons of these cells to the blood vessels which connect the hypothalamus with the anterior pituitary lobe, and hence via the blood to the ACTH-producing cells. The structure of CRF is still unknown. In rats, ACTH is found also in the basal hypothalamus and the medial eminence.

ACTH consists of 39 amino acids. The amino acid sequence of this molecule is in part found also in β-lipotropin (β-LPH). β-LPH has been known for some time as a pituitary hormone involved in fat mobilization in the periphery (Li 1964), and is probably the mother substance of the endorphins and met-enkephalin. It has recently been established that β-LPH and ACTH originate from a common mother molecule (Nakanishi et al., 1979).

The first 13 amino acids of ACTH (ACTH 1-13) are identical to α-melanocyte-stimulating hormone (α-MSH) (Fig. 1).

2. *Data from Animal Experiments*

Rats deprived of the anterior pituitary lobe learn conditioned behavior less readily and "forget" more quickly what they have learned (de Wied et al., 1975a). This disorder cannot be reversed with corticosteroids but can effectively treated with ACTH and ACTH fragments without corticotropic activity, e.g., ACTH 4-10. This ACTH fragment also occurs in β-LPH (β-LPH 47-53) and in both melanocyte-stimulating hormones: α-MSH and β-MSH (α-MSH 4-10 and β-MSH 11-17). The amino acid sequence ACTH 4-7 is the smallest behavior-active ACTH fragment.

When given to intact rats, ACTH and its behavior-active fragments exert but little influence on the acquisition of conditioned behavior, but they do delay its extinction. This applies to conditioned avoidance behavior but equally to sexual and food-rewarded behavior. The effect of these compounds is brief (hours) if compared with that of vasopressin (days) (de Wied, 1977b).

Other behavioral effects of ACTH observed in rats were increased arousal, attentive ability, and increased motivational value of external clues (Donovan, 1978). These effects probably enable animals treated with ACTH peptides to retain new information more easily.

Intrathecal or intraventricular (not intravenous) administration of ACTH leads to frequent yawning and stretching in test animals (Bertolini et al., 1975). The significance of this syndrome is not clear, but it is conceivable that it suppresses sleep and therefore relates to the positive effects of ACTH on attention. Moreover, animals thus treated show frequently repeated erections, ejaculations, and copulation movements without seeking increased contacts with females.

	1	8	9	10	11	12	13	14	15	16	17	18	19	20	21	22
β-MSH	Ala.....	Pro	Tyr	Arg	Met	Glu	His	Phe	Arg	Try	Gly	Ser	Pro	Pro	Lys	Asp
		1	2	3	4	5	6	7	8	9	10	11	12	13		
α-MSH		Ser	Tyr	Ser	Met	Glu	His	Phe	Arg	Try	Gly	Lys	Pro	Val	NH_2	
		1	2	3	4	5	6	7	8	9	10	11	12	13		39
ACTH		Ser	Tyr	Ser	Met	Glu	His	Phe	Arg	Try	Gly	Lys	Pro	Val	....	Phe

Figure 1 Common amino acid sequences in corticotropin-related peptides. ACTH 4-10 = α-MSH 4-10 = β -MSH 11-17. ACTH 1-13 = α-MSH 1-13. (From Prange et al., 1978.)

3. Human Studies

Only ACTH 4-10 has so far been studied, both in normal volunteers are in aged patients with memory disorders (Table 2). In the former category, there were indications of a general arousal effect and improved concentration of attention. The fragment reduces performance deficits during serial reaction time tasks, delays the development of electroencephalographic signs of habituation, increases the arousal level, and improves short-term memory (Miller et al., 1974; Kastin et al., 1975; Gaillard and Sanders, 1975; Dornbush and Nikolovski, 1976; van Riezen et al., 1977).

It can be concluded from two controlled studies that ACTH can be valuable also in aged patients with slight deterioration based on organic cerebral lesions. Ferris et al. (1976) reported improvement of cognitive functions, Branconnier et al. (1979) placed more emphasis on motor and affective effects than on cognitive effects. Subjects experienced a reduction of depression and confusion and increased vigor. This evidence of increased vigor was supported behaviorally by a delay in the onset of increased latency in reaction time. The findings also indicated that retrieval from memory may be enhanced by ACTH 4-10. Although significant, these effects were not very pronounced. Further investigation will have to show whether ACTH 4-10 has true therapeutic significance.

According to Small et al. (1977), ACTH 4-10 has no effect on memory disorders caused by electroshock therapy (EST). The strength of this compound may after all be more that it increases the level of arousal—resulting in improved mood level, motivation, and selective attention—than that it improves memory functions per se. If so, then the compound would in fact much more useful in the treatment of patients with mild senile organic brain syndromes than in "pure" memory disorders such as those observed after EST or after head injuries.

C. Melanocyte-Stimulating Hormone (MSH)

1. General Data

The pituitary gland contains two melanocyte-stimulating hormones: α-MSH, which consists of 13 amino acids, and β-MSH, which consists of 22 amino acids. The first 13 amino acids of ACTH are identical to the α-MSH molecule (Fig. 1). The minimal chain which still shows MSH activity consists of the amino acids 4-10 of the α-MSH molecule. As mentioned in Section III.B.2, the amino acid sequence of this heptapeptide also occurs in ACTH, β-LPH, and β-MSH. Both α-MSH and β-MSH are found in the pars intermedia of the pituitary gland, as well as in the hypothalamus.

MSH plays no role in the mammalian pigment metabolism. Its function is in fact unknown. It is remarkable, moreover, that the hypothalamus contains an

Table 2 Behavioral Studies with ACTH 4-10 in Humans

Study	Diagnosis	*N*	Dosage (single-dose)	Results
Gaillard and Sanders, 1975	Volunteers 21-29 years	18	30 mg s.c.	Improvement of general motivation and activation
Dornbush and Nikolovski, 1976	Volunteers 63-70 years	9	15-60 mg s.c.	Improvement of visual reaction time
Sannita, 1976	Volunteers 19-29 years	12	60 mg i.v.	Improvement of level of attention
Miller, 1977	Volunteers 21-35 years	20	30 mg s.c.	No effect
Sandman, 1977	Volunteers 21-23 years	11	15 mg i.v. during 2 hr	Improvement of level of attention
Rapoport, 1976	Children with learning difficulties	20	30 mg i.v.	No effect
Will, 1978	Geriatric volunteers complaining of memory loss, 65-80 years	22	15 mg s.c.	No effect
Braconnier, et al., 1979	Organic brain syndrome >60 years	18	30 mg s.c.	Improvement of affective state and retrieval from memory
Total	Volunteers	70		+50
	Organic brain syndrome	60		+18

MSH release-inhibiting factor (MSH-RIF), but that vessels which could transport this product from hypothalamus to pars intermedia of the pituitary gland have not been identified.

2. *Data from Animal Experiments*

Like ACTH and its fragment ACTH 4-10, α-MSH and β-MSH are able to reverse memory and learning disorders resulting from extirpation of the anterior pituitary lobe. When given intrathetically or intracerebrally, they also provoke the previously mentioned yawning and stretching syndrome (see III.B.2) (van Wimersma Greidanus, 1977).

3. *Human Studies*

Cotzias et al. reported in 1967 that MSH aggravates the symptoms of Parkinson's disease. It therefore seemed plausible that a substance which inhibits MSH release, e.g., MSH-RIF, might have a therapeutic effect on this disease. It was also observed that MSH-RIF vigorously potentiates dopamine (DA) effects (Donovan, 1978). For these two reasons MSH-RIF was given to Parkinson patients (Fischer et al., 1974) and found to be therapeutically effective. The same was observed in depressions (Ehrensing and Kastin, 1974), but these experiments have not yet been repeated and confirmed. Nor is it known whether these MSH-RIF effects are produced via MSH release or based on a direct influence on the CNS.

IV. RELEASING AND INHIBITING HORMONES FROM THE HYPOTHALAMUS

A. Thyrotropin-Releasing Hormone (TRH)

1. *General Data*

TRH was the first pituitary-regulating hormone whose chemical structure was identified. It is a tripeptide which was named TRH in view of its ability to enhance the release of thyroid-stimulating hormone (TSH, thyrotropin) by the anterior pituitary lobe. It was later found that TRH also increases prolactin release, but it is still uncertain whether this is a physiological effect.

This hormone is found not only in the medial eminence but also in other parts of the hypothalamus and outside it, e.g., in the cerebral cortex, cerebellum brain stem, and CSF. The hypothalamus contains in fact no more than 20% of the total amount of TRH in the brain. The TRH concentration is relatively high in brain parts which are also rich in monoamines.

2. *Motives for Behavior Research with TRH*

Interest in a possible effect of TRH on certain types of disturbed behavior was aroused by the following observations.

The Prange group had demonstrated (Prange et al., 1969) that the thyroid hormone T_3 potentiates the therapeutic effect of the tricyclic antidepressant imipramine (Tofranil). The pituitary thyroid-stimulating hormone TSH produced a similar potentiating effect (Prange et al., 1970). This prompted the question of the possible effect of TRH in depressions. The urgency of this question was further increased by a number of observations made in animal experiments.

When given to rats and mice treated with the monoamine oxidase (MAO) inhibitor pargyline, L-dopa has a central stimulating effect (hyperactivity, increased aggressiveness, and irritability). Antidepressants potentiate this dopa effect. This phenomenon is used in screening potential antidepressants. TRH proved to behave like an antidepressant in this test, even in animals deprived of pituitary gland or thyroid (Plotnikoff et al., 1972). This TRH effect is therefore independent of the pituitary-thyroid axis, and is probably based on a direct influence of TRH on the brain.

Moreover, TRH antagonizes the sedative and hypothermal effects of various central depressants such as barbiturates, chloralhydrate, chlorpromazine (Largactil), and diazepam (Valium). This effect, too, persists in animals deprived of the pituitary gland. Thyroid hormones lack this potency. TRH analogs which lack the ability to enhance TSH release do antagonize sedatives (Prange et al., 1978). This warrants the conclusion that the analeptic potency of TRH is independent of its endocrine effects.

Finally, it was found that TRH potentiates the behavior effects resulting from an excess of serotonin in the brain (Green and Grahame-Smith, 1974). In addition, indications were found that TRH increases the release of noradrenaline from the presynaptic nerve terminals (Horst and Spirt, 1974). In view of the monoamine (MA) hypothesis on the pathogenesis of depressions, a serotonin- and/or noradrenaline-potentiating compound can be expected to have an antidepressant effect.

3. *TRH in Depressions*

Two publications which appeared in 1972 (Prange et al.; Kastin et al.) presented promising data on the use of TRH in depressions. In a double-blind crossover design, the former authors treated 10 women with unipolar depressions with a single dose of 0.6 mg TRH and reported a favorable effect within a few hours. The depression scores diminished by about 50%. The (partial) therapeutic effect persisted some considerable time (about a week). Kastin et al. (1972), using the same design, treated four women and one man with manic-depressive illness (depressed type) and involutional depression. On three consecutive days they were given 500 μg TRH by intravenous injection. Four showed pronounced improvement, and the fifth improved moderately. In three patients the favorable effect persisted for several days.

A fairly large series of studies has since been devoted to the effect of TRH in depressions. However, they show a marked diversity of design, dosage scheme, measuring methods, type of patients, etc. This material is therefore too heterogeneous to warrant a definite conclusion, and we have to confine ourselves to a few general, more tentative conclusions (Prange et al., 1978; Nemeroff et al., 1979).

1. The results obtained with orally given TRH are disappointing. Perhaps no effective blood concentration was attained, for TRH is degraded fairly rapidly in blood. The half-value time is about 2 min. Should absorption of TRH from the intestine be gradual, then the rate of degradation is possibly higher than the rate of absorption.
2. The majority of the authors observed that TRH had a psychopharmacological effect if given by rapid intravenous injection. However, the effect is described not so much as antidepressant but rather in terms of decrease in tension, increase in energy, enhanced capacity to cope with feelings, etc. In terms of effect, therefore, TRH seems to resemble a central stimulant more than a traditional antidepressant.
3. The conclusion given in item 2 is supported by findings in normal test subjects, in whom TRH induces relaxation, mild euphoria, and a sense of increased energy. This effect develops also if TRH administration is preceded by administration of thyroid hormone in order to block the TSH response of the pituitary gland. The behavior effects, therefore, are probably based on the activity of TRH per se.
4. The TRH effect in depressions is brief and of little significance therapeutically.
5. Hardly any research has been done into the question whether there exists a "TRH-susceptible" subgroup of depressions which can be distinguished in biochemical or psychopathological terms from "TRH-insusceptible" patients. Yet such research would be of interest; most authors intimate that, if TRH has any effect, only some of the depressive patients notice it. MA research in depressions has revealed the concept of the biochemical and endocrinological classifiability of depressions (see Chapter 3 of this volume). These variables should be taken into account in analyzing the results of antidepressant medications, particularly if they involve compounds with an effect on central MA metabolism.
6. TRH potentiates the effect of tricyclic antidepressant amitriptyline in no way. This shows that the thyroid-stimulating effect of TRH plays no role in its psychopharmacological effect, for the thyroid hormone T_3 does potentiate the effect of this antidepressant.

4. TRH in Schizophrenic Psychoses

An endogenous substance is not likely to have a specific therapeutic effect in a given syndrome, unless this involves a deficiency. There are no indications of TRH deficiency in depressions. This is why TRH has also been used in other psychiatric disorders, and more specifically in schizophrenic psychoses (Prange et al., 1978).

The number of available studies is too small, and their design not sufficiently perfect, to warrant definite conclusions as yet. The impression gained from the available data is that TRH can have a favorable effect on autistic, inert, reticent patients. In this category of patients, too, there is evidently a mild stimulating and euphorizing effect. As in the case of depression, this effect has been reported often to persist for days after discontinuation of medication.

5. *TRH in Parkinson's Disease*

The compound has proved ineffective against neurologic symptoms (Lakke et al., 1974), but a shift toward optimism and a sense of well-being has been repeatedly reported (Chase et al., 1974).

6. *Conclusions*

TRH exerts an influence on human behavior. In normal test subjects and in several categories of psychiatric patients it has a mild stimulating and activating effect. It is not a specific antidepressant.

B. Luteinizing-Hormone-Releasing Hormone (LH-RH)

LH-RH stimulates both the release of LH and that of follicle-stimulating hormone (FSH) from the anterior pituitary lobe. We do not know whether a separate FSH-releasing hormone also exists. LH-RH is localized chiefly in the hypothalamus but small amounts are found also in periventricular tissue.

In animal experiments this releasing factor has been demonstrated to have three behavioral effects: activation of sexual behavior (Moss et al., 1975), antagonism of barbiturate effects such as sedation and hypothermia (Bisette et al., 1976), and inhibition of the extinction of active avoidance behavior (de Wied et al., 1975b). Female rats show their sexual willingness by assuming a lordotic posture and lifting the hindquarters. Small amounts of LH-RH (s.c.) provoke this behavior, even in animals without pituitary gland or ovaries (Donovan, 1978), evidently via an extrapituitary mechanism. Human studies have been scanty. In a recent controlled study (McAdoo et al., 1978), 12 healthy male volunteers were given 500 μg LH-RH by continuous infusion. Psychological tests yielded indications of a slight increase in reaction speed and level of attention a few hours after administration. A decrease in anxiety and fatigue was likewise observed. Doering et al. (1977), however, observed no effect of LH-RH on mood and behavior in a study of human volunteers. Nor did it have a therapeutic effect in depression and impotence (Benkert, 1975).

C. Growth Hormone Release-Inhibiting Factor (Somatostatin)

This hormone inhibits not only the release of growth hormone (GH) by the anterior pituitary lobe but also the TRH-induced release of TSH. It is localized not only in the hypothalamus but also in other brain areas (e.g., midbrain, brain stem, cerebral cortex) and also outside the CNS (e.g., stomach, pancreas, and intestine). Over 60% of the somatostatin in the brain is localized outside the hypothalamus.

GH secretion diminishes to immeasurable values after division of the hypophyseal stalk. It is therefore unlikely that somatostatin inhibits GH secretion tonically, i.e., continuously.

Test animals treated by somatostatin infusion show less motor activity and an increased sensitivity to the sedative, sleep-inducing effect of barbiturates. This effect is observed also in hypophysectomized animals. Direct application of somatostatin to hippocampus or cerebral cortex induces a complex pattern of motor symptoms such as tremors, stereotyped movements, and ataxia. Behavioral effects in human subjects have not yet been studied.

D. MSH Release-Inhibiting Factor

The tripeptide Pro-Leu-Gly (PLG) inhibits the release of melanocyte-(pigment cell) stimulating hormone (MSH) from the pituitary gland. Apart from PLG, a tetrapeptide (Pro-His-Arg-Gly) has been isolated from hypothalamic tissue which shows about 20% of the effect of PLG on MSH release. PLG is therefore sometimes referred to as MIF-I, while the tetrapeptide is called MIF-II. PLG is believed to be enzymatically split off from oxytocin in the hypothalamus.

PLG is effective in the pargyline/dopa model (see Section IV.A.2), even in hypophysectomized animals. It increases the rate of synthesis of central dopamine but not that of noradrenaline or serotonin. This dopamine effect, however, requires the presence of the pituitary gland (Prange et al., 1978).

Human studies have already been briefly mentioned in Section III.C.3. The results can be summarized in the statement that PLG seems to have a mild antidepressant effect and also exerts a favorable influence on the motor pathology in Parkinson patients. However, the available data are limited and do not always result from methodologically well-designed research. Conclusions would therefore be premature.

V. ENDORPHINS

A. General Data

The discovery of the endorphins resulted from the following observations:

1. The mammalian CNS proved to contain receptors with a high affinity for morphine and related compounds and insensitive to any of the known neurotransmitters (Pert and Snyder, 1973; Simon et al., 1973; Terenius, 1973).

2. Pain can be alleviated in test animals by electrical stimulation of certain brain areas. This stimulation-induced analgesia can be antagonized with a morphine antagonist such as naloxone (Mayer et al., 1971; Akil et al., 1976).

These observations seemed to suggest the existence of an endogenous ligand for these so-called opiate receptors. Within a remarkably short time, two such compounds were isolated from the brain and identified (Hughes, 1975; Terenius, 1975). They were pentapeptides named enkephalins: methionine-enkephalin (met-enkephalin) and leucine-enkephalin (leu-enkephalin).

After the discovery of the enkephalins, the search for other peptides with opiate-like effects was further intensified by the fact that the amino acid sequence of met-enkephalin proved to be present in the 91-amino-acid pituitary hormone β-lipotropin (β-LPH). This research led to the discovery of β-endorphin (β-LPH 61-91) (Li and Chung, 1976), which consists of the terminal 31 amino acids of β-LPH, γ-endorphin (β-LPH 61-77), and α-endorphin (β-LPH 61-76) (Fig. 2).

All endorphins and enkephalins except leu-enkephalin, therefore, are β-LPH fragments. The endorphins—the larger β-LPH fragments—are chiefly found in the pituitary gland, like β-LPH itself. The enkephalins on the other hand are found almost exclusively in the brain. Neurons and pituitary cells with β-endorphin also contain β-LPH and ACTH. The brain contains neurons with β-endorphin as well as with enkephalin. There are sound reasons to assume that, in these cells, they play a role in impulse transmission (Snyder and Childers, 1979). In the following, *endorphins* is a collective term for endorphins in the strict sense and enkephalins.

B. Interest in Endorphins in Psychiatry

Endorphins have attracted psychiatric attention from the start. The following factors contributed to this:

1. High endorphin concentrations are found in brain areas involved in pain conduction, motor activity, and, probably, regulation of mood and affects (Snyder and Childers, 1979).
2. Opiates have a distinct effect on pain threshold, mood, and level of psychological integration. A similar effect could be expected of the "endogenous morphines."
3. Patients whose medial thalamus was electrically stimulated to alleviate chronic pain showed increased enkephalin-like activity in the CSF (Akil et al., 1978a).
4. Stress increases the release of ACTH as well as β-endorphin by the pituitary gland (Guillemin et al., 1977; Watson et al., 1979).

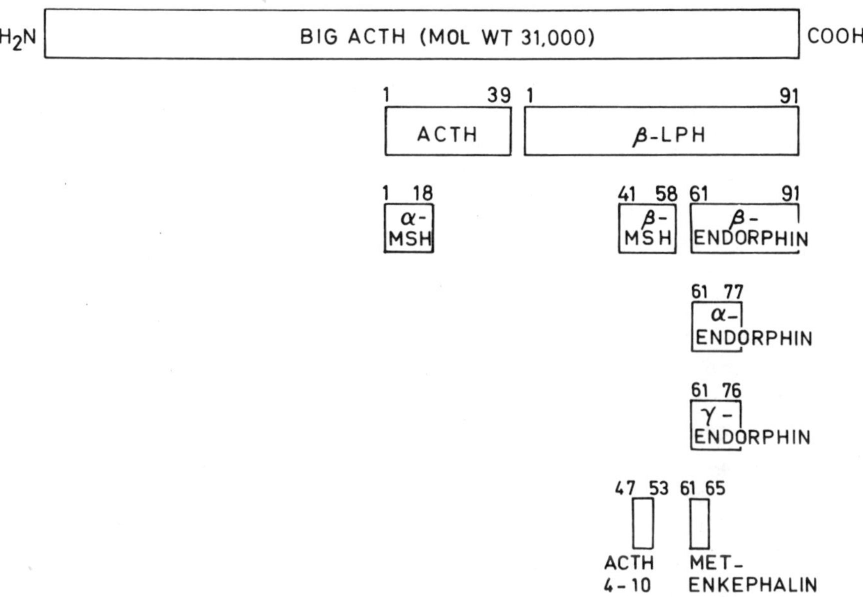

Figure 2. Precursor relationships of corticotropins and pituitary endorphins. The 31,000 molecular weight peptide "big ACTH" contains within its sequence the entire ACTH and β-lipotropin (β-LPH) molecules, which appear to be located next to each other. Within the ACTH molecule lies the sequence of α-MSH, while the sequence of β-MSH and the sequence of β-endorphin are contained within the structure of β-LPH. The sequence of the fourth through tenth amino acids of ACTH is contained within the β-LPH sequence, so that this portion of the ACTH molecule is repeated twice within the big ACTH precursor. The sequence of γ-endorphin, α-endorphin, and met-enkephalin is contained within that of β-endorphin. Supposedly α- and γ-endorphins are formed from β-endorphin. There is no evidence that β-endorphin is the precursor of met-enkephalin in the brain. (From Snyder and Childers, 1979).

5. β-Endorphin exerts an unmistakable influence on animal behavior. In large doses, it gives rise to a catatonia-like condition with motor retardation (Jacquet and Marks, 1976; Bloom et al., 1976; Snyder 1978).

Clinical endorphin research has so far fanned out in the following directions. Research into the endorphin concentration in body fluids (specially, CSF and dialysate after hemodialysis); the effects of (1) morphine (and endorphin) antagonists and (2) endorphin or endorphin derivatives in psychiatric patients. The following is a brief survey of these activities.

C. Endorphin Research in Psychiatric Patients

1. Endorphins in Human Cerebrospinal Fluid

Terenius and Wählström (1975a) isolated two endorphin fractions (opiate-like material) from human CSF. Neither of these fractions is identical to any of the endorphins now known.

The concentrations of these fractions were determined in 13 patients with schizophrenic and 7 with manic-depressive psychoses (Terenius et al., 1976, 1977; Lindström et al., 1978). An increased fraction I endorphin concentration was found in the schizophrenic patients. It was normalized by neuroleptic medication which resulted in reduction of psychotic symptoms. In the manic patients, an increased fraction I endorphin fraction was found during the manic phase. A correlation between fraction II endorphin and clinical symptoms was not demonstrable.

The β-endorphin concentration in the CSF was found to be markedly increased in patients with acute schizophrenic psychoses, whereas in chronic psychotic patients it was normal to slightly decreased (Domschke et al., 1979). Loeber et al. (1979) demonstrated the presence of α- and γ-endorphin in human CSF. Whether their concentrations can show changes in psychiatric patients has yet to be established.

2. Morphine Antagonists

Opiate antagonists block opiate receptors and have therefore been used in efforts to establish the (patho)physiological significance of endorphins, at least so far as their effects are produced via opiate receptors. The two pure opiate antagonists naloxone and naltrexone (with a slightly more prolonged effect and, unlike naloxone, orally administrable) have been used in human studies. Naltrexone has a dysphoric effect in normal test subjects (Mendelson et al., 1979). In psychiatric patients, these compounds have been studied mostly in schizophrenic and manic syndromes (Table 3).

In three double-blind crossover studies (Emrich et al., 1977; Watson et al., 1978; Akil et al., 1978b), 20, 11, and 8 patients with schizophrenic psychoses were given naloxone intravenously. In a total of 26 patients the psychotic symptoms (specifically the acoustic hallucinations) showed transient reduction 2-7 hr after the injection. In a single-blind study (Gunne et al., 1977), a similar effect was observed in 4 out of 6 patients. In two uncontrolled studies involving 5 and 3 schizophrenic patients, respectively (Mielke and Gallant, 1977; Gitlin and Rosenblatt, 1978), no effect was observed after oral administration of 250 mg and 50-100 mg naltrexone per day. In four controlled studies involving 14, 7, 8, and 20 patients with schizophrenic psychoses (Davis et al., 1977; Volavka et al., 1977; Janowsky et al., 1977; Hertz et al., 1978), no clinically demonstrable effect of naloxone was found.

Reduction of manic symptoms was demonstrated in 16 out of a total of 24 patients involved in two double-blind controlled studies (Janowsky et al., 1978; Judd et al., 1978). In both, 20 mg naloxone was given by continuous drip within 20 min: the maximum effect developed 15-30 min after the drip and lasted 1-2 hr. A pilot study of five patients with vital depressions (Terenius et al., 1977) revealed no effect of naloxone on the depressive symptoms.

In a recent study in the context of a WHO project we focused on the effect of naloxone on acoustic hallucinations and manic symptoms (Verhoeven et al., 1979a). In a double-blind placebo-controlled design, 10 patients were given a single injection of 20 mg naloxone subcutaneously. Five patients had verifiable acoustic hallucinations in the context of a schizophrenic psychosis, and the other five showed manic symptoms in the context of either a bipolar depression or a (schizophrenic) psychosis. All had already received neuroleptic medication without complete therapeutic success; the neuroleptic maintenance therapy was continued during the naloxone treatment. The symptoms of the manic patients were scored with the aid of the Brief Psychiatric Rating Scale and the Biegel-Murphy Mania Rating Scale, while those of the schizophrenic patients were scored with the aid of the Brief Psychiatric Rating Scale and a hallucination scale. In all cases, moreover, a checklist of individual symptoms was completed on the basis of a complete Present State Examination Interview.

This controlled study disclosed no demonstrable influence of naloxone on any of the psychopathological symptoms scored, and in particular no influence on acoustic hallucinations and/or manic symptoms.

To conclude: Only three out of eight controlled clinical trials (Emrich et al., 1977; Watson et al., 1978; Akil et al., 1978b) revealed a demonstrable favorable effect of naloxone which consisted of transient reduction to disappearance of acoustic hallucinations. Some 30% of the 107 patients so far treated with naloxone responded to this medication. Unlike neuroleptics, naloxone has no effect on serum prolactin (Lal et al., 1979). Dopamine receptors in the tubero-infundibular system are therefore not blocked. There are sound reasons to assume that the therapeutic effect of neuroleptics depends on their ability to block dopamine receptors (van Praag, 1977, in press). So far as naloxone has antipsychotic properties, therefore, this effect is produced via another mechanism.

The two controlled clinical studies of Janowsky et al. (1978) and Judd et al. (1978) revealed transient reduction of manic symptoms in 16 out of a total of 24 patients (Table 3). One controlled study (Verhoeven et al., 1980) produced negative results. We conclude tentatively from these data that there could exist a subgroup of psychotic patients or that there are psychotic symptoms that are susceptible to opiate antagonists. However, further definition of this range of indications is not yet possible.

Table 3 Effects of Naloxone in Schizophrenic and Manic Syndromes

Study	Diagnosis	*N*	Neuroleptic Medication	Design	Dosage naloxone[a]	Result	Duration	Attenuation of Symptoms
Emrich et al., 1977	Schizophrenia	20	–2 +18	Double-blind crossover	4.0 mg i.v.	+12	2-7 hr.	Auditory hallucinations
Watson et al., 1978	Schizophrenia	11	–6 +5	Double-blind crossover: 9 single-blind: 2	10 mg i.v.	+6	3-6 hr:4 48 hr: 2	Auditory hallucinations
Akil et al., 1978	Schizophrenia	8	–4 +4	Double-blind crossover	10 mg i.v.	+8	75-90 min	Auditory hallucinations
Gunne, 1976	Schizophrenia	6	+6	Single-blind	0.4 mg i.v.	+4	1-6 hr	Auditory hallucinations
Kurland et al., 1977	Schizophrenia	12	+12	Double-blind	0.4-1.2 mg i.v.	–		
Mielke and Gallant, 1977	Schizophrenia	5	–5	Open	naltrexone 250 mg 9 days	–		
Gitlin and Rosenblatt, 1978	Schizophrenia	3	–1 +2	Single-blind	naltrexone 50-100 mg 15 days		–	

Davis et al., 1977	Schizophrenia	14	−9 +5	Double-blind	0.4-10 mg i.v.		–	
Volavka et al., 1977	Schizophrenia	7	+7	Double-blind	0.4 mg i.v.		–	
Janowsky et al., 1977	Schizophrenia	8	+8	Double-blind crossover	1.2 mg i.v.		–	
Hertz et al., 1978	Schizophrenia	20	−20	Double-blind crossover	4.0 mg i.v.		–	
Janowsky et al., 1978	Manic syndrome	12	−3 +9	Double-blind crossover	20 mg i.v. (infusion)	+12	30-90 min	Manic symptoms
Judd et al., 1978	Manic syndrome	12	−12	Double-blind crossover	20 mg i.v. (infusion)	+4	0.5-2 hr	Manic symptoms
Verhoeven et al., 1979	Schizophrenia Manic syndrome	5 5	+10	Double-blind	20 mg s.c.	–		
Total	Schizophrenia, manic syndrome	119 29				+30 +16	2-7 hr 0.5-2 hr	Auditory hallucinations, symptoms

[a]So far only single-administration studies have been carried out.

3. *Dialysate Studies*

In 1977 Wagemaker and Cade described a favorable effect of long-term hemodialysate of dialyzed schizophrenic patients. It is believed to be β-endorphin in studies in which dialysis and sham dialysis are compared. A conclusion on the therapeutic validity of this method in schizophrenic patients would be premature.

Plamour et al. (1977) isolated a hitherto unknown peptide from the dialysate of dialyzed schizophrenic patients. It is believed to be β-endorphin in which the methionine in the 5 position has been replaced by leucine (βH-leu^5-endorphin), a sensational possibility which implies the possibility of a correlation between disorders of endorphin metabolism and schizophrenic psychoses. However, Lewis et al. (1979) recently reported that they had been unable to isolate a peptide of the above-mentioned structure from the hemodialysate of two schizophrenic patients.

D. Therapeutic Applications of Endorphins and Endorphin Derivatives

1. *β-Endorphin*

In an open study without a clearly defined protocol, a total dose of 9 mg β-endorphin–distributed over 4 days–was injected intravenously in five patients with schizophrenic psychoses and two with depressions (unipolar and bipolar, respectively) (Kline et al., 1977). The following psychotropic effects were observed: The injection was followed within a few minutes by an activating, anxiolytic, and antidepressant effect which persisted for 2-3 hr; a degree of drowsiness developed 2-4 hr after injection; about 12 hr after injection of β-endorphin, a therapeutic effect was observed which was characterized by reduction of the psychotic or depressive symptoms and lasted 1-10 days.

2. *Des-Tyrosine-γ-Endorphin (DTγE)*

a. Theoretical Background

Most endorphins–β-endorphin, α-endorphin, met-enkephalin, and leu-enkephalin–have the following properties:

1. They are morphinomimetics. Elimination of the terminal tyrosine molecule in position 6 leads to loss of the morphinomimetic characteristics.
2. They are able to delay the extinction ("forgetting") of conditioned behavior (e.g., conditioned active and passive avoidance behavior). This effect is independent on the opiate receptors because it persists after blockade of these receptors by means of naloxone.

One endorphin deviates from this general pattern: γ-endorphin (de Wied et al., 1978). It does have morphinomimetic properties but facilitates extinction instead of retention of new information. In this respect it behaves like the traditional neuroleptics of, say, the phenothiazine and butyrophenone series. If the terminal tyrosine molecule is split off (thus producing DTγE), then

1. The molecule loses its morphinomimetic characteristics, and
2. Its facilitating effect on the extinction of conditioned behavior is intensified.

Apart from its suppressive effect on conditioned behavior, DTγE has other properties in common with traditional neuroleptics, e.g., a positive grip test. In some ways its profile differs from that of traditional neuroleptics. For example, DTγE has no effect on gross behavior in an open field, nor does it antagonize the effects of apomorphine and amphetamine–compounds with a dopamine-potentiating capacity.

In biochemical terms, too, there is a similarity between neuroleptics and DTγE. Both types of compound increase the dopamine turnover in certain brain areas. With the neuroleptics, this effect is probably secondary to blockade of postsynaptic dopamine receptors. Exactly how DTγE increases the dopamine turnover remains to be established (Versteeg et al., 1979).

In view of the similarities between DTγE and the traditional neuroleptics we decided to study this peptide in patients with schizophrenic psychoses.

b. Clinical Research

So far, DTγE has been used in one open and one controlled study, involving a total of 14 patients (Verhoeven et al., 1978, 1979a) with recurrent schizophrenic and schizo-affective psychoses. Twelve had been hospitalized at least 6 months when the study started and were still psychotic despite medication with adequate doses of neuroleptics. The remaining two were treated with DTγE for acute schizophrenic psychosis immediately after admission. They had had no neuroleptics prior to admission. In the past, they had been repeatedly hospitalized with an acute psychotic episode.

In the first open pilot study, six patients were given a single intramuscular dose of 1 mg DTγE/day for 7 days. In the second study (a double-blind crossover design), six patients received 1 mg DTγE by intramuscular injection per day for 8 days. In the first study, neuroleptics were discontinued one week before DTγE injections were started. In the second study, neuroleptic maintenance was continued.

The six patients in the first study all showed marked exacerbation of the psychotic symptoms after discontinuation of neuroleptics. From the 4th day of DTγE medication on, three patients showed reduction of psychotic symptoms; these symptoms were entirely absent from the 6th day through the 3rd week

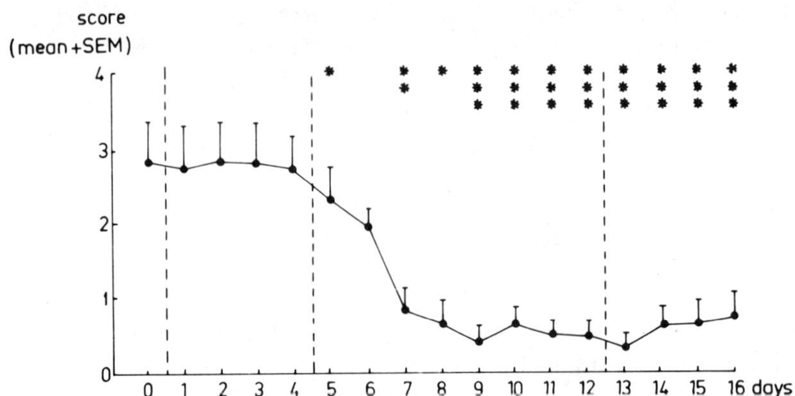

Figure 3 Summary of data obtained in the controlled (des-tyr')-γ-endorphin study. Days 1-4 refer to days preceding (des-tyr')-γ-endorphin treatment (days 5-12), followed by placebo treatment (days 13-16). Mean score of six patients was plotted versus days of treatment. Vertical bars indicate SEM. Student's paired t test was used to compare individual values on a given day to those obtained on day 4, * indicates $P < .05$; **, $P < .01$; *** $P < .005$. (From Verhoeven et al., 1979b).

after discontinuation of DTγE. Two of these three patients showed recurrence of psychotic symptoms after the 3rd week (the follow-up on the 3rd patient had to be discontinued when she was transferred to another hospital). The remaining three patients showed reduction of psychotic symptoms on days 3 and 4 of the medication, but from the 5th day on became psychotic again with severe agitation and aggressiveness. DTγE was then discontinued and neuroleptic medication reinstituted.

In the second study, progressive reduction of psychotic symptoms was observed from the first day of DTγE medication (Fig. 3). Four of the six patients became psychotic again 4-10 days after discontinuation of treatment, but their symptoms seemed less severe than those prior to DTγE medication. The remaining two patients remained free from psychotic symptoms. The same double-blind crossover design was used for the two acutely psychotic drug-free patients treated with DTγE immediately after admission. Both showed reduction of psychotic symptoms from the 3rd day of medication and, from the 6th day on, both remained free from psychotic symptoms for some considerable time (a few months).

All patients treated with DTγE seemed to show improved emotional responsiveness. No extrapyramidal, cardiovascular, or gastrointestinal side effects were observed.

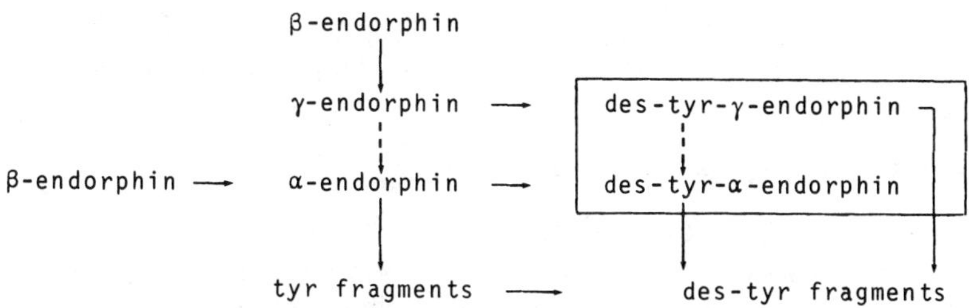

Figure 4 Schematic representation of the fragmentation of β-endorphin. (From de Wied, 1978.)

c. Interpretation of Clinical DTγE Data

Like γ-endorphin, DTγE has recently been demonstrated in human CSF (Loeber et al., 1979). It therefore seems plausible that this compound is normally formed in the brain, probably from γ-endorphin. Like α-endorphin, γ-endorphin is a split product of β-endorphin (Fig. 4).

It is conceivable that DTγE is antipsychotic because the patients involved are suffering from a DTγE deficiency (de Wied, 1978). Such a deficiency could in principle develop in two ways: be deficient formation of DTγE from β-endorphin or by accelerated conversion to α-endorphin. This hypothesis is now being investigated in our endorphin research. If arguments to support it were found, this would mean (1) that a disturbed endorphin metabolism plays a role in the pathogenesis of (some types of) schizophrenic psychoses and (2) that treatment with DTγE can be regarded as a form of substitution therapy.

A similar development, i.e., treatment of a psychiatric syndrome with endogenous substances in which the brain is probably deficient, has occurred in the field of depressions. The use of the serotonin precursor 5-hydroxytryptophan in the treatment and prevention of certain types of vital depression can probably be so regarded (see Chapter 3 of this volume).

In three patients in the first, open study, initial improvement was followed by marked psychotic exacerbation with intensive agitation and aggressiveness. In principle, there are two possible explanations. First, the exacerbation may have resulted from discontinuation of neuroleptics. Second, it may have been due to the DTγE medication. In the context of the latter possibility the following hypothesis might be advanced: the exogenous (administered) DTγE is unusually quickly converted to DTαE, and DTαE is responsible for the exacerbation. This seems a reasonable hypothesis because De Wied (personal communication) demonstrated that, at least in animals, DTαE has amphetamine-like properties; and central stimulants are known to be able to induce psychoses or exacerbate existing psychoses. That this complication did not develop in the second experiment could have been due to the fact that neuroleptic maintenance therapy was continued during the DTγE study in these patients. Verification of this hypothesis has to be postponed until reliable methods are evolved to determine DTγE and its split products in body fluids.

3. FK 33-824: A Synthetic Met-Enkephalin

FK33-824 is a met-enkephalin derivative synthesized by Sandoz, with the following amino acid sequence: Tyr-D-Ala-Gly-Mephe-Met(O)-ol. The amino acid sequence of met-enkephalin is Tyr-Gly-Gly-Phe-Meth. FK33-824 differs from met-enkephalin in (1) replacement of glycine by d-alanine, (2) N-methylation of phenylalanine, (3) alteration of methionine by oxidizing its sulfur to sulfoxide and conversion of the carboxyl to a carbinol.

Jorgensen et al. (1979) used FK33-824 in nine patients with chronic psychoses: eight chronic schizophrenics and one patient with alcohol hallucinosis. The patients had been hospitalized 7-15 years. Their medication was continued but in addition they received, in a single-blind design, intramuscular injections of 1, 2, and 3 mg of this peptide on three consecutive days. An unmistakable therapeutic effect was observed in six patients. Four of them showed a striking effect against hallucinations ("voices") and an increased sense of well-being: "they felt better than they had for years." In two patients there was no effect on the hallucinations but the patients became more open and spontaneous, more freely speaking than usual, and euphoric. The effect persisted until 4-7 days after the last injection.

A rebound effect was observed (as it was after DTγE) in three patients. Initial improvement in these patients was followed by exacerbation, which in turn was followed by improvement. The DTγE patients who showed exacerbation were given neuroleptics to control it, and consequently it was not established whether their rebound effect was transient.

Unlike DTγE, FK33-824 has retained its terminal tyrosine molecule and therefore possesses morphinomimetic properties; it is therefore uncertain whether its therapeutic effect is based on these properties or on a genuine, opiate-receptor-independent antipsychotic action.

VI. CONCLUSIONS

1. Until recently it was thought that pituitary hormones occurred only in the pituitary gland and had a solely peripheral endocrine function. It has been established, however, that several pituitary hormones and their fragments are found also outside the pituitary and also exert a direct influence on the CNS, as manifested by their effects on certain types of behavior.

Neuropeptides derived from ACTH, vasopressin, and oxytocin prove to influence motivation and learning and memory processes in animals. ACTH fragments have a short-term effect and probably play a role in attention and motivation, whereas vasopressin fragments have a long-term effect, specifically on memory processes, which is expressed in improved consolidation and retrieval. Oxytocin has the opposite effect and could therefore be regarded as an amnestic peptide. Vasopressin fragments also tend to reduce addictive behavior to heroin in rats. The clinical significance of these ACTH- and vasopressin-derived neuropeptides could therefore lie on the one hand in the treatment of cerebral disorders accompanied by disturbed memory function (which may in part be due to a diminished function of these hormonal systems) and on the other hand in the control of addiction to heroin and other morphine-like substances.

Clinical research has so far been scanty, but preliminary results are encouraging and indicate that conclusions based on animal experiments would also seem to have a certain validity for human individuals.

2. Of the releasing and inhibiting factors, the same can be said as of the pituitary hormones. They were believed to occur exclusively in the hypothalamus and solely to have a regulating function with regard to hormone release by the anterior pituitary lobe. It has recently been found, however, that they also occur in the CNS outside the hypothalamus and can exert a direct influence on the CNS, resulting in changes in behavior.

It is to be noted that modest therapeutic effects have only been demonstrated with TRH and PLG: TRH has a brief, slight central stimulant effect, and PLG slightly alleviates the symptoms in Parkinson's disease and depression. The clinical effects of the peptides of this group have so far been disappointing, perhaps because the proper indications have not yet been defined.

3. Since 1975 the identification of the endorphins, which can perhaps be regarded as neurotransmitters or neuromodulators, has given the field of psychoneuroendocrinology a new dimension. Animal experiments have shown that, in addition to a morphinomimetic effect, the endorphins exerts an unmistakable influence on behavior which may or may not be mediated by opiate receptors.

Therapeutic effects have so far been obtained with β-endorphin, DTγE (a split product of γ-endorphin), and FK33-824 (a synthetic met-enkephalin derivative). However, the clinical data available are still far too limited to warrant any definite conclusion. So far, observations on DTγE have been the most interesting in scientific terms. This is an endogenous, natural peptide in the brain, with properties also found in the pharmacological action profile of "true" neuroleptics. It is therefore conceivable that DTγE, or a compound closely related to it, is an endogenous "antipsychotic" and that a DTγE deficiency based on disturbed endorphin metabolism contributes to the pathogenesis of (certain types of) schizophrenia. The heuristic value of this theory is quite substantial, because it generates a number of hypotheses that can be clinically tested, provided reliable methods can be evolved to separate and measure endorphins in body fluids.

REFERENCES

Akil, H., Mayer, D. J., and Liebeskind, J. C. (1976). Antagonism of stimulation produced analgesia by naloxone, a narcotic antagonist. *Science 191,* 961-962.

Akil, H., Richardson, D. E., Hughes, J., and Barchas, J. D. (1978a). Enkephalin-like material elevated in ventricular cerebrospinal fluid of pain patients after analgetic focal stimulation. *Science 201,* 463-465.

Akil, H., Watson, S. J., Berger, Ph.A., and Barchas, J. D. (1978b). Endorphins, β-LPH, and ACTH. Biochemical, pharmacological and anatomical studies. In *Advances in Biochemical Psychopharmacology,* Vol. 18., E. Costa and M. Trabucchi (Eds.). Raven, New York, pp. 125-317.

Benkert, O. (1975). Effects of hypothalamic releasing hormones in depression and sexual impotence. *Excerpta Med. Int. Congr. Ser. 359,* 663-671.

Bertolini, A., Gessa, G. L., and Ferrari, W. (1975). Penile erection and ejaculation. A central effect of ACTH-like peptides in mammals. In *Sexual Behavior: Pharmacology and Biochemistry,* M. Sandler and G. L. Gessa (Eds.). Raven, New York, pp. 247-257.

Bisette, G., Nemerhoff, C. B., Loosen, P. T., Prange, Jr., A. J., Breese, G. R., and Lipton, M. A. (1976). Comparison of the potency of TRH, ACTH 4-10 and related peptides to reverse pentobarbital-induced narcosis and hypothermia. In *Hypothalamus and Endocrine Function,* F. Labrie, J. Meites, and G. Pelletier (Eds.). Proc. Int. Symp. Hypothalamus and Endocrine Functions, Quebec City, Canada, September 1975. Plenum, New York, pp. 478-479.

Blake, D. R., Dodd, M. J., and Grimley Evans, J. (1978). Vasopressin in amnesia. *Lancet 1,* 608.

Bloom, F., Segal, D., Ling, N., and Guillemin, R. (1976). Endorphins. Profound behavioral effects in rats suggest new etiological factors in mental illness. *Science 194,* 630-632.

Branconnier, R. J., Cole, J. O., and Gardos, G. (1979). ACTH 4-10 in the amelioration of neuropsychological symptomatology associated with senile organic brain syndrome. *Psychopharmacology 61,* 161-165.

Chase, T. N., Woods, A. C., Lipton, M. A., and Morris, C. E. (1974). Hypothalamic releasing factors and Parkinson disease. *Arch. Neurol. 31,* 55-56.

Davis, G. C., Bunney, W. E. Jr., DeFraites, E. G., Kleinman, J. E., van Kammen, D. P., Post, R. M., and Wyatt, R. J. (1977). Intravenous naloxone administration in schizophrenia and affective illness. *Science 197,* 74-76.

de Wied, D. (1977a). Peptides and behavior. *Life Sci. 20,* 195-204.

de Wied, D. (1977b). Behavioral effects of neuropeptides related to ACTH, MSH, and β-LPH. *Ann. NY Acad. Sci. 297,* 263-274.

de Wied, D. (1978). Psychopathology as a neuropeptide dysfunction. In *Characteristics and Function of Opioids,* Vol. 4, J. M. van Ree and L. Terenius (Eds.). Elsevier/North-Holland, Amsterdam, pp. 113-123.

de Wied, D., Bohus, B., and van Wimersma Greidanus, Tj.D. (1975a). Memory deficit in rats with heriditary diabetes insipidus. *Brain Res. 85,* 152-156.

de Wied, D., Witter, A., and Greven, H. M. (1975b). Behaviourally active ACTH analogues. *Biochem. Pharmacol. 24,* 1463-1468.

de Wied, D., van Wimersma Greidanus, Tj.B., Bohus, B., Urban, I., and Gispen, W. H. (1976). Vasopressin and memory consolidation. In *Perspectives in Brain Research,* Vol. 4, Progress in Brain Research. M. A. Corner and D. F. Swaab (Eds.). Elsevier/North-Holland Biomedical Press, Amsterdam, pp. 181-194.

de Wied, D., Kovacs, G., Bohus, B., van Ree, J. M., and Greven, H. M. (1978). Neuroleptic activity of the neuropeptide β-LPH 62-77 ([des-tyr[1]]γ-endorphin; DTγE). *Eur. J. Pharmacol. 49,* 427-436.

Doering, G. H., McAdoo, B. C., Kraemer, H. C., Brodie, H. K. H., Dessert, N. J., and Hamburg, D. A. (1977). Psychological effects of gonadotropin-releasing hormone in the adult male. In *Neuroregulators and Psychiatric Disorders,* D. A. Hamburg, D. Barchas, E. Usdin (Eds.). Oxford University Press, New York, pp. 267-275.

Domschke, W., Dickschas, A., and Mitznegg, P. (1979). CSF β-endorphin in schizophrenia. *Lancet 1,* 1029.

Donovan, D. T. (1978). The behavioral actions of hypothalamic peptides. A review. *Psycholog. Med. 8,* 305-316.

Dornbush, R. L., and Nikolovski, O. (1976). ACTH 4-10 and short-term memory. In *The Neuropeptides: Pharmacology, Biochemistry and Behavior,* Vol. 5. C. A. Sandman, L. H. Miller and A. J. Kastin (Eds.). Phoenix, New York, pp. 69-72.

Ehrensing, R. H., and Kastin, A. J. (1974). Melanocyte-stimulating hormone-release inhibiting hormone as an antidepressant. *Arch. Gen. Psychiatr. 30,* 63-65.

Emrich, H. M., Cording, C., Pirée, S., Kölling, A., von Zerssen, D., and Herz, A. (1977). Indication of an antipsychotic action of the opiate antagonist naloxone. *Pharmakopsychiatrie 10,* 265-270.

Ferris, S. H., Sathananthan, G., Gershon, S., Clark, C., and Moshinsky, J. (1976). Cognitive effects of ACTH 4-10 in the elderly. In *The Neuropeptides: Pharmacology, Biochemistry and Behavior,* Vol. 5. C. A. Sandman, L. H. Miller and A. J. Kastin (Eds.). Phoenix, New York, pp. 73-78.

Fischer, P. A., Schneider, E., Jacobi, P., and Maxion, H. (1974). Effect of melanocyte-stimulating hormone-release inhibiting factor (MIF) in Parkinson's syndrome. *Eur. Neurol. 12,* 360-368.

Gaillard, A. W. K., and Sanders, A. F. (1975). Some effects of ACTH 4-10 on performance during a serial reaction task. *Psychopharmacologia 42,* 201-208.

Gitlin, M., and Rosenblatt, M. (1978). Possible withdrawal from endogenous opiates in schizophrenics. *Am. J. Psychiatr. 135,* 377-378.

Gold, Ph.W., Goodwin, F. K., and Rens, V. I. (1978). Vasopressin in affective illness. *Lancet 2,* 1233-1235.

Green, A. R., and Grahame-Smith, D. G. (1974). TRH potentiates behavioral changes following increased brain 5-hydroxytryptamine accumulation in rats. *Nature 251,* 524-526.

Guillemin, R. (1978). Peptides in the brain. The new endocrinology of the neuron. *Science 202,* 390-402.

Guillemin, R., Vargo, T., Rossier, J., Minick, I., Ling, N., Rivier, C., Vale, W., and Bloom, F. (1977). β-Endorphin and adrenocorticotropin are secreted by the pituitary gland. *Science 197,* 1367-1369.

Gunne, L. -M., Lindström, L., and Terenius, L. (1977). Naloxone-induced reversal of schizophrenic hallucinations. *J. Neurol. Transm. 40,* 13-19.

Hertz, A., Bläsig, J., Emrich, H. M., Cording, C., Pirée, S., Kölling, A., and von Zerssen, D. (1978). Is there some indication from behavioral effects of endorphins for their involvement in psychiatric disorders? *Advances in Biochemical Psychopharmacology,* Vol. 18. E. Costa and M. Trabucchi (Eds.). Raven, New York, pp. 333-339.

Hoffman, P., Ritzmann, R. F., Walter, R., and Tabakoff, B. (1978). Arginine vasopressin maintains ethanol tolerance. *Nature 276,* 614-616.

Horst, W. D., and Spirt, N. (1974). A possible mechanism for the anti-depressant activity of thyrotropin-releasing hormone. *Life Sci. 15,* 1073-1082.

Hughes, J. (1975). Isolation of an endogenous compound from the brain with pharmacological properties similar to morphine. *Brain Res. 88,* 295-308.

Hughes, J. (1979). Opioid peptides and their relatives. *Nature 278,* 394-395.

Jacquet, Y. F., and Marks, N. (1976). The C-fragment of β-lipotropin. An endogenous neuroleptic or antipsychotogen. *Science 194,* 632-635.

Janowsky, D. S., Segal, D. S., Bloom, F., Abrams, A., and Guillemin, R. (1977). Lack of effect of naloxone on schizophrenic symptoms. *Am. J. Psychiatr. 134,* 926-927.

Janowsky, D. S., Judd, L. L., Huey, L., Roitman, N., Parker, D., and Segal, D. (1978). Naloxone effects on manic symptoms and growth-hormone levels. *Lancet 2,* 320.

Jorgensen, A., Fog, R., and Veilis, B. (1979). Synthetic enkephalin analogue in treatment of schizophrenia. *Lancet 1,* 935.

Judd, L. L., Janowsky, D. S., Segal, D. S., Leighton, Ph.D., and Huey, L. (1978). Naloxone related attenuation of manic symptoms in certain bipolar depressives. In *Characteristics and Function of Opioids,* Vol. 4. J. M. van Ree and L. Terenius (Eds.). Elsevier/North-Holland, Amsterdam, pp. 173-175.

Kastin, A. J., Ehrensing, R. H., Schalch, D. S., and Anderson, M. S. (1972). Improvement in mental depression with decreased thyrotropin response after administration of thyrotropin-releasing hormone. *Lancet 2,* 740-742.

Kastin, A. J., Sandman, C. A., Stratton, L. O., Goldman, H., Schally, A. V., and Miller, L. H. (1975). Influences of MSH on behavioral and electrographic correlates of attention, memory and anxiety in rat and man. In *Hormones, Homeostasis and the Brain,* Vol. 42. Progress in Brain Research. W. H. Gispen, T. B. van Wimersma Greidanus, B. Bohus, and D. de Wied (Eds.). Elsevier, Amsterdam, pp. 143-150.

Kastin, A. J., Coy, D. H., Jacquet, J., Schally, A. V., and Plotnikoff, N. P. (1978). CNS effect of somatostatin. *Metabolism 27* (supplement 1), 1247-1252.

Klaver, M. M., Flentge, F., Nienhuis-Kuiper, H. E., and van Praag, H. M. (1979). The origin of CSF choline and its relation to acetylcholine metabolism in brain. *Life Sci. 24,* 231-236.

Kline, N. S., Li, C. H., Lehmann, H. E., Lajtha, A., Laski, E., and Cooper, T. (1977). β-Endorphin-induced changes in schizophrenic and depressed patients. *Arch. Gen. Psychiatry 34,* 1111-1113.

Krivoy, W. A., Zimmerman, E., and Lande, S. (1974). Facilitation of development of resistance to morphine analgesia by desglycinamide^9-lysine vasopressin. *Proc. Nat. Acad. Sci. USA 71,* 1852-1856.

Kurland, A. A., McCabe, O. L., Hanlon, Th. E., and Sullivan, D. (1977). The treatment of perceptual disturbances in schizophrenia with naloxone hydrochloride. *Am. J. Psychiatr. 134,* 1408-1410.

LaBoeuf, A., Lodge, J., and Eames, P. G. (1978). Vasopressin and memory in Korsakoff syndrome. *Lancet 2,* 1370.

Lakke, J. P. W. F., van Praag, H. M., van Twisk, R., Doorenbos, H., and Witt, F. G. J. (1974). Effects of administration of thyrotropin releasing hormone in Parkinsonism. *Clin. Neurol. Neurosurg. 3,* 1-5.

Lal, S., Nair, N. P. V., Cervantes, P., Pulman, J., and Snyder, H. (1979). Effects of naloxone or levallorphan on serum prolactin concentrations and apomorphine induced growth hormone secretion. *Acta Psychiatr. Scand. 59,* 173-179.

Legros, J. J., Gilot, P., Seron, X., Claessens, J., Adam, A., Moeglen, J. W., Audibert, A., and Berchier, P. (1978). Influence of vasopressin on learning and memory. *Lancet 1,* 41.

Lewis, R. V., Gerber, L. D., Stein, S., Stephen, R. L., Grosser, B. I., Velick, S. F., and Udenfriend, S. (1979). On βH-Leu^5-Endorphin and schizophrenia. *Arch. Gen. Psychiatry 36,* 237-239.

Li, C. H. (1964). Lipotropin, a new active peptide from pituitary glands. *Nature 201,* 924.

Li, C. H., and Chung, D. (1976). Isolation and structure of an untriakontapeptide with opiate activity from camel pituitary glands. *Proc. Nat. Acad. Sci. USA 73,* 1145-1148.

Lindström, L. H., Widerlöv, E., Gunne, L. -M., Wahlström, A., and Terenius, L. (1978). Endorphins in human cerebrospinal fluid. Clinical correlations to some psychotic states. *Acta Psychiatr. Scand. 57,* 153-164.

Loebar, J., Verhoef, J., Burbach, J. P. H., and van Ree, J. M. (1979). Endorphins and related peptides in human cerebrospinal fluid. *Abstr. Acta Endocrinol. Congr.,* Munich.

Lundbaek, K. (1978). Somatostatin. Clinical importance and outlook. *Metabolism 27, (Supplement 1),* 1463-1469.

Mayer, D. J., Wolfe, T. L., Akil, H., Cardner, B., and Liebeskind, J. C. (1971). Analgesia from electrical stimulation in the brainstem of the rat. *Science 174,* 1351-1354.

McAdoo, B. C., Doering, C. H., Kraemer, H. C., Dessert, N., Brodie, H. K. H., and Hamburg, D. A. (1978). A study of the effects of gonadotropin-releasing hormone on human mood and behavior. *Psychosom. Med. 40,* 199-209.

Mendelson, J. H., Ellingboe, J., Keuhule, J. C., and Mello, N. K. (1979). Effects of naltrexone on mood and neuroendocrine function in normal adult males. *Psychoneuroendocrinology 3,* 231-236.

Mielke, D. H., and Gallant, D. M. (1977). An oral opiate antagonist in chronic schizophrenia. A pilot study. *Am. J. Psychiatry 134,* 1430-1431.

Miller, L. H., Kastin, A. J., Sandman, C. A., Fink, M., and van Veen, W. J. (1974). Polypeptide influences on attention, memory and anxiety in man. *Pharmacolog. Biochem. Behav. 2,* 663-668.

Miller, L. H., Fisher, C. S., Groves, G. A., Rudrauff, M. E., and Kastin, A. J. (1977). MSH/ACTH 4-10 influences on the CAR in human subjects: a negative finding. *Pharmacolog. Biochem. Behav. 7,* 417-419.

Moss, R. L., McCann, S. M., and Dudley, C. A. (1975). Releasing factors and sexual behavior. In *Hormones, Homeostasis and the Brain,* Vol. 42. Progress in Brain Research, W. N. Gispen, Tj.B. van Wimersma Greidanus, B. Bohus and D. de Wied (Eds.). Elsevier, Amsterdam, pp. 37-46.

Nakanishi, S., Inone, A., Kita, T., Nakamura, M., Chang, A. C. J., Cohen, S. N., and Numa, S. (1979). Nucleotide sequence of cloned CDNA for bovine corticotropin-β-lipotropin precursor. *Nature 278,* 423-427.

Nemeroff, Ch.B., and Prange, A. J. (1978). Peptides and psychoneuroendocrinology. *Arch. Gen. Psychiatry 35,* 999-1010.

Nemeroff, Ch.B., Loosen, P. T., Bisette, G., Manberg, P. J., Wilson, I. C., Lipton, M. A., and Prange, A. J. (1979). Pharmaco-behavioral effects of hypothalamic peptides in animals and man. Focus on thyrotropin-releasing hormone and neurotensine. *Psychoneuroendocrinology 3,* 279-310.

Oliveros, J. C., Jandali, M. K., Timsit-Berthier, M., Remy, R., Benghezal, A., Audibert, A., and Moeglen, J. M. (1978). Vasopressin in amnesia. *Lancet 1,* 42.

Palmour, R. M., Ervin, F. R., and Wagemaker, H. (1977). Characterization of a peptide derived from the serum of psychiatric patients. *Abstr. Soc. Neurosci. 7,* 32.

Pert, C. B., and Snyder, S. H. (Johns Hopkins) (1973). Opiate receptor. Demonstration in nervous tissue. *Science 179,* 1011-1014.

Plotnikoff, N. P., Prange, Jr., A. J., Breese, G. R., Anderson, M. S., and Wilson, I. C. (1972). Thyrotropin releasing hormone. Enhancement of DOPA activity by a hypothalamic hormone. *Science 178,* 417-418.

Prange, A. J., Wilson, I. C., Rabon, A. M., and Lipton, M. A. (1969). Enhancement of imipramine antidepressant activity by thyroid hormone. *Am. J. Psychiatry 126,* 457-469.

Prange, A. J., Wilson, I. C., Knox, A., McClane, T. K., and Lipton, M. A. (1970). Enhancement of imipramine by thyroid stimulating hormone: clinical and theoretical implications. *Am. J. Psychiatry 127,* 191-199.

Prange, Jr., A. J., Lara, P. P., Wilson, I. C., Alltop, L. B., and Breese, G. R. (1972). Effects of thyrotropin-releasing hormone in depression. *Lancet 1,* 999-1002.

Prange, A. J., Nemeroff, Ch.B., Lipton, M. A., Breese, J. R., and Wilson, I. C. (1978). Peptides and the central nervous system. In *Handbook of Psychopharmacology. Biology of Mood and Antianxiety Drugs,* Vol. 13, L. L. Iversen, S. D. Iversen, and S. H. Snyder (Eds.). Plenum, New York.

Raskind, M. A., Weitzman, R. E., Orenstein, H., Fisher, D. A., and Courtney, N. (1978). Is antidiuretic hormone elevated in psychosis? *Biol. Psychiatr. 13,* 385-390.

Rapoport, J. L., Quin, P. O., Copeland, A. P., and Burg, C. (1976). ACTH 4-10: Cognitive and behavioral effects in hyperactive learning-disabled children. *Neuropsychobiology 2,* 291-296.

Sandman, C. A., George, J., McCanne, T. R., Nolan, J. D., Kaswan, J., and Kastin, A. J. (1977). MSH/ACTH 4-10 influences behavioral and physiological measures of attention. *J. Clin. Endocrinol. Metab. 44,* 884-891.

Sannita, W. G., Irwin, P., and Fink, M. (1976). EEG and task performance after ACTH 4-10 in man. *Neuropsychobiology 2,* 283-290.

Schally, A. V. (1978). Aspects of hypothalamic regulation of the pituitary gland. *Science 202,* 18-28.

Simon, E., Hiller, J. M., and Edelman, I. (1973). Stereospecific binding of the potent narcotic analgesic (^{3}H) etorphine to rat brain homogenate. *Proc. Nat. Acad. Sci. USA 70,* 1947-1949.

Small, J. G., Small, I. F., Milstein, V., and Dian, D. A. (1977). Effects of ACTH 4-10 on ECT-induced memory dysfunctions. *Acta Psychiatr. Scand. 55,* 241-250.

Snyder, S. H. (1978). The opiate receptor and morphine-like peptides in the brain. *Am. J. Psychiatry 135,* 645-652.

Snyder, S. H., and Childers, S. R. (1979). Opiate receptors and opioids peptides. *Ann. Rev. Neurosci. 2,* 35-64.

Terenius, L. (1973). Characteristics of the "receptor" for narcotic analgesics in synaptic plasma membrane fraction from rat brain. *Acta Pharmacol. Toxicol. 33,* 377-384.

Terenius, L., and Wählström, A. (1975). Search for an endogenous ligand for the opiate receptor. *Acta Physiol. Scand. 94,* 74-81.

Terenius, L., and Wählström, A. (1975a). Morphine-like ligand for opiate receptors in human CSF. *Life Sci. 16,* 1759-1764.

Terenius, L., Wählström, A., Lindström, L., and Widerlöv, E. (1976). Increased CSF levels of endorphins in chronic psychosis. *Neurosci. Lett. 3,* 157-162.

Terenius, L., Wählström, A., and Agren, H. (1977). Naloxone (Narcan[R]) treatment in depression. Clinical observations and effects on CSF endorphins and monoamine metabolites. *Psychopharmacology 54,* 31-33.

van Praag, H. M. (1977). The significance of dopamine for the mode of action of neuroleptics and the pathogenesis of schizophrenia. *Br. J. Psychiatry 130,* 463-474.

van Praag, H. M. (1978). Amine hypotheses of affective disorders. In *Handbook of Psychopharmacology. Biology of Mood and Antianxiety Drugs,* Vol. 13, L. L. Iversen, S. D. Iversen, and S. H. Snyder (Eds.). Plenum, New York, pp. 184–294.

van Praag, H. M. (in press). Observations within and beyond the boundaries of catecholamine research in psychosis. *Int. J. Neurol.*

van Ree, J. M., Bohus, B., Versteeg, D. H. G., and de Wied, D. (1978a). Neurohypophyseal principles and memory processes. *Biochem. Pharmacol. 27,* 1793-1800.

van Ree, J. M., Dorsa, D. M., and Colpaert, F. C. (1978b). Neuropeptides and drug dependence. In *Characteristics and Function of Opioids,* Vol. 4. J. M. van Ree and L. Terenius (Eds.). Elsevier/North-Holland, Amsterdam, pp. 1-13.

van Riezen, H., Rigter, H., and de Wied, D. (1977). Possible significance of ACTH fragments for human mental performance. *Behav. Biol. 20,* 311-324.

van Wimersma Greidanus, Tj. B. (1977). Effects of MSH and related peptides on avoidance behavior in rats. *Front. Hor. Res. 4,* 129-139.

van Wimersma Greidanus, Tj. B., and de Wied, D. (1976). Modulation of passive-avoidance behavior of rats by intracerebroventricular administration of antivasopressin serum. *Behav. Biol. 18,* 325-333.

Verhoeven, W. M. A., van Praag, H. M., Botter, P. A., Sunier, A., van Ree, J. M., and de Wied, D. (1978). (des-tyr[1])-γ-endorphin in schizophrenia. *Lancet 1,* 1046-1047.

Verhoeven, W. M. A., de Jong, J. T. V. M., and van Praag, H. M. (1979a). The effects of naloxone on psychotic symptoms. In *Proc. 20th Dutch Fed. Meet.* p. 435.

Verhoeven, W. M. A., van Praag, H. M., van Ree, J. M., and de Wied, D. (1979b). Improvement of schizophrenic patients by treatment with (des-tyr[1])-γ-endorphin (DTγE). *Arch. Gen. Psychiatry 36,* 294-298.

Versteeg, D. H. G., de Kloet, E. R., and de Wied, D. (1979). Effects of α-endorphin, β-endorphin and (des-tyr[1])-γ-endorphin on α-MPT-induced catecholamine disappearance in discrete regions of the rat brain. *Brain Res.*, in press.

Volavka, J., Mallya, A., Baig, S., and Perez-Cruet, J. (1977). Naloxone in chronic schizophrenia. *Science 196,* 1227-1228.

Wagemacker, H., and Cade, R. (1977). The use of hemodialysis in chronic schizophrenia. *Am. J. Psychiatry 134,* 684-685.

Watson, S. J., Berger, Ph.A., Akil, H., Mills, M. J., and Barchas, J. D. (1978). Effects of naloxone on schizophrenia. Reduction in hallucinations in a subpopulation of subjects. *Science 201,* 73-76.

Watson, S., Akil, H., Berger, Ph.A., and Barchas, J. D. (1979). Some observations on the opiate peptides and schizophrenia. *Arch. Gen. Psychiatr. 36,* 35-41.

Will, J. C., Abuzzahab, F. S. Sr., and Zimmerman, R. L. (1978). The effects of ACTH 4-10 versus placebo in the memory of symptomatic geriatric volunteers. *Psychopharmacology Bull. 14,* 25-26.

15

Opiate Peptides and Brain Function

Agu Pert, Candace B. Pert, Glenn Craig Davis,* and William E. Bunney, Jr.
National Institute of Mental Health
Bethesda, Maryland

**Present Affiliation:* The University of Tennessee Center for the Health Sciences, Memphis, Tennessee

I. INTRODUCTION

How do morphine, heroin, methadone, Darvon, and all the other opiates work in the brain to produce their myriad effects? Research originally intended to answer this question has unearthed a whole new brain system which may turn out to be relevant to some psychiatric and neurologic diseases. The search for the mechanism of action of opiates began with the notion that all opiate effects were initiated by the binding of the drug to some tissue constituent called a "receptor." The opiate receptor was thought to consist of a concave surface made especially to fit and accommodate all of those opiates known to be pharmacologically active.

II. THE OPIATE RECEPTOR

In 1973, it became possible for the first time to actually measure the up to then hypothetical opiate receptor recognition sites. This was accomplished by using highly radiolabeled opiates and allowing them to bind to membranes prepared from rat brain. The radiolabeled opiate which did not bind tightly was rapidly washed away and the opiate that "stuck" to the tissue was counted by standard liquid scintillation methodology (Simon et al., 1973; Pert and Snyder, 1973; Terenius, 1973). The evidence that the opiate receptors which mediated the pharmacological response to opiates were indeed under study was overwhelming; potent opiate narcotics like etorphine and morphine required only very low doses of drug to displace the radiolabeled ligand in the test tube, while opiates that were known to be very weak, such as Darvon, required concentrations several orders of magnitude higher to achieve the same degree of displacement of the radioactive tracer. Even more striking was the stereospecificity of opiate receptor binding as it was measured in the test tube. For nearly 20 years medicinal chemists had reported a very striking feature of opiate pharmacology. The morphine molecule was rigid and stiff so that only opiates with the structure analogous to morphine were pharmacologically active. For example, synthetic L-morphine, the enantiomer or mirror image of the form of morphine that comes naturally from the poppy, was found to be virtually inert when it was first synthesized in the 1950s (Gates and Tschudi, 1956). In every case, the inactive opiates were unable to displace radioactive opiate tracer unless they were present in concentrations several thousand fold above the concentration of their active enantiomeric pair.

The study of opiate receptor binding in the test tube provided an important piece of the puzzle of the opiate antagonists. Opiate antagonists such as naloxone, nalorphine, diprenorphine, and naltrexone are drugs with a very similar structure to the opiate agonists. They, however, have the ability to block and even reverse the actions of the opiates with morphine-like effects. There is one important difference between opiate agonists and antagonists in terms of in vitro binding. The sodium ion has a completely opposite effect on the binding of opiate antagonists than it has on the binding of opiate agonists (Pert et al., 1973; Pert and Snyder, 1974). The sodium ion seems to promote the binding of opiate antagonists while simultaneously decreasing the binding of opiate agonists. Opiate receptors, in fact, seem to have the ability to interconvert between two conformations, one which binds more tightly to agonists and one which binds more tightly to antagonists (Simon et al., 1976; Pert and Garland, 1978).

While no one knew for certain, it seemed logical that these very specific opiate receptor sites were present for some purpose, not just in the hope that they would have a chance encounter with the product of an opium poppy. The brain itself must contain a morphine-like substance whose normal function is to interact with opiate receptors in brain. In 1974, John Hughes electrified scientists working in this area by announcing that he was in the process of purifying a substance from the brains of stockyard animals which acted just like morphine in the guinea pig ileum and the mouse vas deferens—its activity could even be blocked or reversed by the opiate antagonist naloxone. It took over a year before this opiate substance could be structurally identified as two pentapeptides, met- and leu-enkephalin (Hughes et al., 1975).

A. Structure-Activity Relationships

The announcement of the structure touched off a wave of excitement as various investigators successfully reproduced the effects of morphine by using the enkephalins. It quickly became apparent, however, that when met- and leu-enkephalin were microinjected into rat brain at the very site where morphine had been shown to produce a potent analgesia, the enkephalins turned out to be very weak and short-acting (Chang et al., 1976; Pert, 1976; Beluzzi et al., 1976). The problem was due to enkephalin's lability; it was very rapidly degraded by enzymes found in brain to an inactive form (Hambrook et al., 1976). When D-ala^2-met-enkephalin was synthesized, it was found to resist the enzymes found in brain while retaining its ability to bind tightly to opiate receptors (Pert et al., 1976). This analog proved to be a very potent opiate-like analgesic with a long-time course of action similar to that of morphine (Pert, 1976). Literally hundreds of analogs have since been prepared and studied for their activity in various tests which are sensitive to opiates. The tyrosine residue, which is analogous to the α ring and amino group of the morphine molecule itself, is unable to withstand any modification without a very large loss in activity (Chang et al., 1976). The substitution of any D-amino acid in the two position produces a nondegradable analog with the affinity for the opiate receptor preserved to various degrees, the D-ala substituent being the most potent (Miller et al., 1979). The five position of enkephalin can be tampered with considerably and much activity still remains. There are even some active tetrapeptides (Miller et al., 1979).

With the discovery of met- and leu-enkephalin, it was immediately noticed that β-lipotropin, a hormone that had been discovered more than 10 years previously (Li et al., 1965), contained the same sequence as met-enkephalin at residues 61-65. In a very short time, several groups had shown that β-endorphin, the 61-91 fragment of β-lipotropin isolated from pituitary gland (Bradbury et al., 1976; Guilleman et al., 1976; Li and Chung, 1976) had potent morphine-like activity. β-Endorphin was originally touted to be hundreds of times more active than morphine in some studies. It is now shown to be only a few times more active than morphine and the metabolically stable enkephalin analogs. Much of its potency is related to its ability to resist enzymatic degradation (Pert et al., 1976). Its importance lies not so much as a pharmacological agent, but as the naturally occurring hormonal form of enkephalin (see below).

B. Synthesis and Degradation

In general, small peptides are synthesized by cleavage from larger precursor peptides. At this time, the synthesis of opiate peptides has been studied carefully only in a pituitary tumor cell line (Maines et al., 1977; Roberts and Herbert, 1977). These investigators have shown that a very large (31K) precursor protein is first synthesized which subsequently gives rise to β-lipotropin and β-endorphin. The situation in brain, however, is less clear-cut. β-lipotropin seems to be located in all cells that contain β-endorphin (Watson et al., 1978). This suggests that in brain as well as pituitary, β-endorphin is cleaved from a larger precursor, perhaps β-lipotropin. Identification in brain of the very large (31K) protein whose entire structure has recently been determined has been reported. Neurons that contain met- or leu-enkephalin appear to be devoid of β-endorphin, but contain a long peptide precursor with repeating met- and leu-enkephalin sequences (4:1) and heterogeneous "spacers" which have been most completely characterized in adrenal gland extracts (Lewis et al., 1980).

Like many small biologically active peptides, enkephalin can be shown to be degraded by a number of specific protease enzymes. The question as to how enkephalin is inactivated in a physiological situation is, however, unclear at this time. Since the tyrosine residue on the N terminal is so critical for activity, cleavage of the terminal tyrosine by an aminopeptidase would be a very "sensible" way to terminate the activity of enkephalin. Brain membranes in fact contain a great deal of this type of aminopeptidase activity. However, no one has yet been able to demonstrate an enkephalin-inactivating mechanism which is present in some opiate-receptor-rich brain regions and not others. The finding that the D^2 analogs of enkephalin are resistant to degradation suggests, in fact, that the physiological inactivation of enkephalin is due to the cleavage of the internal tyrosine. It is only a matter of time before further study will reveal the nature of the synthetic and degradative enzymes in the enkephalinergic neurons. The development of drugs which inhibit enkephalin synthesis and breakdown is sure to follow.

C. Is Enkephalin a Neurotransmitter?

At this time, enkephalin fills most of the criteria required to identify it as a CNS neurotransmitter. It has been shown to be released from tissue slices by potassium (Iversen et al., 1978; Hughes et al., 1978). It is localized in synaptosomal fractions (Simantov et al., 1976). Its heterogenous localization in discrete brain regions and particularly its appearance on beaded axons after visualization by immunohistofluorescent techniques (Hokfeldt et al., 1977; Uhl et al., 1979) suggest that it is indeed a neurotransmitter. At most synapses, enkephalin appears to act as an inhibitory neurotransmitter (Bradley et al., 1978). Enkephalin and active opiates as well appear to slow the firing rate of the neurons onto which they are iontophoresed. Zieglgänsberger and Bayerl (1976) suggested that the mechanism of this action is the blockade of the influx of sodium which is normally triggered by an excitatory neurotransmitter. This neurophysiological observation might be related to the differential effect of the sodium ion on agonist and antagonist binding if, as we suspect, the opiate receptor is closely associated with a specific sodium ionophore.

If enkephalin is a neurotransmitter, opiate receptors almost certainly represent their postsynaptic receptors. We already have some information about the cellular distribution of opiate receptors. Receptors on the dorsal root axons and the vagal afferents disappear after lesioning these tracts and so possess a "presynaptic localization," strategically located for blocking neurotransmitter release (Lamotte et al., 1976; Atweh and Kuhar, 1977).

Assuming that enkephalin is indeed a neurotransmitter, it must mediate certain brain functions in various regions of the brain. The potent behavioral effects of morphine are in fact clues to the role of the endogenous opiate peptides since morphine is, quite simply, an "enkephalinomimetic." Opiate antagonists such as naloxone presumably block enkephalinergic neuronal activity; thus their effects can be interpreted as due to a reversal of basal enkephalin activity.

D. Neuronal Pathways in Brain Containing Opiate Peptides

Early studies using opiate receptor binding techniques (Kuhar et al., 1973; Hiller et al., 1973) as well as autoradiography (Pert et al., 1976; Atweh and Kuhar, 1977a-c) illustrated that opiate receptors enjoy a very distinct and heterogeneous distribution in brain. The highest receptor concentrations are generally associated with either extrapyramidal structures (striatum, globus pallidus, substantia nigra) or limbic midbrain or forebrain structures (amygdala, hippocampus, septal region, various hypothalamic nuclei, and the periaqueductal gray matter). Other structures that have been found to be high in opiate receptor concentration are the locus coeruleus (the origin of ascending noradrenergic neurons), the interpeduncular nucleus, and the medial thalamus. In the spinal cord, the substantia gelatinosa of the dorsal horn has been found to be strikingly high in opiate binding. Opiate receptors appear to be strategically localized on these structures to receive input from opiate-peptide-containing neurons.

Studies utilizing radioimmunoassays and the immunocytochemical techniques have revealed the presence of opiate peptides in brain as well as the pituitary. These two systems appear to be independent since hypophysectomy does not alter the levels of brain peptides while it does drastically decrease plasma levels (Rossier et al., 1977). There also appear to be two independent opiate peptide systems in brain—one encoded by β-endorphin and the other by met- or leu-enkephalin. While the β-endorphin-encoded neuronal pathways seem to be rather restricted in origin and distribution, the enkephalin-coded systems are much more ubiquitous in brain (Elde et al., 1976; Bloom et al., 1978; Watson et al., 1978; Jacobowitz et al., 1979; Miller et al., 1979; Uhl et al., 1979).

III. BEHAVIORAL AND PHYSIOLOGICAL EFFECTS OF OPIATES AND OPIATE PEPTIDES

The initial interaction of opiates with their specific neuronal membrane binding sites or receptors prompts a cascade of neuronal events leading to changes in pain perception, motor behavior, mood, and other affective and autonomic responses. The heterogeneous and distinct distribution of opiate receptors and opiate peptides in brain suggests that opiate-containing neurons are strategically located to modulate or influence specific neuronal actions that underlie these unique pharmacological responses. Thus, the pharmacological effects of opiates simply appear to reflect the true physiological functions of the endogenous opiate peptides in specific brain regions of systems. An understanding of the functions of endogenous opiates in brain can be achieved by evaluating the precise pharmacological effects of opiates or opiate peptides or their antagonists.

IV. ANALGESIC SITES AND MECHANISMS

One of the most profound effects of opiates is their ability to induce an analgesic state. Opiates appear to exert their analgesic effects through three different mechanisms: (1) by inhibiting primary afferents in the dorsal horn, (2) by inhibiting somatosensory afferents at supraspinal levels, and (3) by activating descending inhibitory pathways.

A. Supraspinal Sites of Opiate Analgesia

Studies in which opiates have been microinjected into discrete brain regions in the rat and monkey have revealed that the analgesic actions are quite circumscribed anatomically (Herz et al., 1970; Jacquet and Lajtha, 1974; Pert and Yaksh, 1974; Takagi et al., 1976). Potent analgesic effects have been found following direct injections of morphine into the periaqueductal gray matter of the midbrain, the nucleus gigantocellularis of the pontine reticular formation, and some regions of the medial thalamus.

One important observation concerning brain regions that appear to mediate opiate analgesia (i.e., PAG, reticular formation, and medial thalamus) is the fact that they all receive input from the anterolateral pathways that presumably carry pain information. This correspondence has prompted Pert and Yaksh (1974) to suggest that opiates may induce analgesia by specifically interfering with the processing of pain in these terminal areas of the pain pathways and preventing the access of pain information into limbic structures which mediate the affective and motivational components of the pain experience.

The periaqueductal-periventricular gray matter, medial thalamus, and nucleus gigantocellularis have all been implicated in mediating the aversive quality of pain by a number of findings (Nashold et al., 1969; Casey, 1971; Anderson and Mahon, 1971; Anderson and Pearl, 1977). Recent electrophysiological studies have in fact indicated an inhibitory role for morphine and enkephalin in these brain regions for both spontaneous (Frederickson and Norris, 1976; Bradley et al., 1976) and pain-induced (Haigler, 1976; Hill et al., 1976) activation.

Another important observation regarding the brain regions which seem to be involved in opiate analgesia is the high density of opiate receptors associated with these areas. This indicates that opioid peptide systems must play an important role in modulating pain in those areas which receive pain input.

B. Descending Inhibitory Mechanisms

Although inhibition of neuronal activity at the terminal regions of the ascending pain pathways may contribute to opiate analgesia, there is considerable evidence that the actions of opiates on supraspinal structures may also activate descending spinal pathways that interfere with pain processing by inhibiting dorsal horn cells.

Shiomi and Takagi (1974) recently proposed that the analgesic effects of opiates in the brainstem are mediated by the activation of descending noradrenergic pathways, presumably originating from area A1, which inhibit dorsal horn cells concerned with nociception. Others have proposed that opiate analgesia is determined primarily by the activation of descending serotonergic mechanisms originating from the nucleus raphe magnus (RM) in the brainstem (Proudfit and Anderson, 1975; Basbaum et al., 1976; Mayer and Price, 1976). There is considerable evidence to support the latter proposition. Proudfit and Anderson (1975) and Yaksh et al. (1977) demonstrated that lesions of the RM (the origin of descending serotonergic fibers) antagonize the analgesic effects of morphine. Basbaum et al. (1976) reported that lesions of the dorsolateral funiculus, which contains the descending fibers from the RM, also inhibited the analgesic effects of morphine.

The possibility that the RM is involved in opiate analgesia has also received support from recent electrophysiological studies. Electrical stimulation of the RM has been reported by a number of investigators to produce analgesia (Oliveras et al., 1975; Proudfit and Anderson, 1975) as well as inhibit dorsal horn cells (Fields et al., 1977) concerned with processing nociceptive information. In addition, Anderson et al. (1977) and Haighler (personal communication) found systemically administered morphine to increase the spontaneous activity of RM cells.

It is proposed that the direct inhibitory actions of morphine in the PAG and NGC inhibit both inhibitory neurons, which descend to the RM releasing them from inhibition, and excitatory neurons, which ascend to high limbic and diencephalic structures.

C. Direct Spinal Actions

A number of investigators have reported direct effects of morphine on dorsal horn cells, especially those that have been implicated in processing and transmitting nociceptive information (lamina I and V cells) and on cells in the anterolateral pathways. Besson et al. (1973) found that phenoperidine inhibited spontaneous activity of nociceptive responses induced by natural or electrical stimulation of lamina V cells in spinal cats. More recently, LeBars et al. (1976) reported that morphine suppressed lamina V neurons activated by C and A δ-fiber (pain) stimulation but had no effect on neuronal activation by A α

stimulation. Similar findings have been reported by other laboratories (Kitahata et al., 1974).

Direct iontophoretic applications of opiates and opioid peptides to dorsal horn cells have also been found to depress activity. Zieglgansberger and Bayerl (1976), employing both extra- and intracellular recording techniques, found that microiontophoretically applied morphine inhibited the spontaneous activity of lamina V cells as well as their induced activation by glutamate or tactile stimulation. Furthermore, both morphine and levorphonal depressed the activity of spinal neurons without influencing the resting membrane resistance and potential. The authors postulated that opiates block neuronal depolarization by impairing the sodium ion influx mechanism at the postsynaptic membrane. Direct spinal actions of opiates have also been suggested by recent behavioral data. Yaksh and Rudy (1976) reported that injections of morphine into the subarachnoid space of the spinal cord produces analgesia in the rat.

Since the highest spinal concentrations of opiate receptors is found in the substantia gelatinosa, it is likely that opiates, as well as enkephalin, exert part of their analgesic effects at this level. Whether the inhibitory action of opiates in the spinal cord is presynaptic or postsynaptic to the primary afferents is still a matter of debate, however (Zieglgänsberger and Bayerl, 1973; Mudge et al., 1978).

Thus there appear to be both spinal and supraspinal sites of action of opiates involved in opiate analgesia. The spinal actions appear to be direct. The origin of the enkephalinergic neurons in the spinal cord, however, is not known at the present and may, in fact, be supraspinal. The supraspinal actions of opiates, on the other hand, appear to inhibit neurons involved in the processing of pain information at terminal levels of the anterolateral pain pathways and to activate descending inhibitory systems by disinhibition.

D. Function of Enkephalinergic Pain Suppression System

The presence of enkephalinergic terminals and opiate receptors in central nervour system regions that are involved in processing pain information suggests that the brain contains an endogenous pain suppression mechanism. There are two possible functions for such a mechanism: (1) it may simply be part of a tonically active inhibitory system—possibly part of a negative feedback loop, or (2) enkephalinergic neurons may be phasically activated by certain environmental conditions of endogenous factors.

Mayer and Liebeskind (1974) demonstrated that potent analgesia could be induced in rats during electrical stimulation of the periaqueductal gray matter—an enkephalin-rich area that is a critical focus for opiate-induced analgesia. Analgesia induced by focal brain stimulation (SPA) has been subsequently demonstrated by other investigators in a number of species (Balagura and

Ralph, 1973; Liebeskind et al., 1973; Oliveras et al., 1975; Lewis and Gebhart, 1977). Most important, however, is the finding that naloxone partially antagonizes SPA in laboratory animals (Akil et al., 1976; Oliveras et al., 1977), although not invariantly (Pert and Walter, 1976: Yaksh et al., 1976). More recently, Hosabuchi et al. (1977) have reported that electrical stimulation of the periventricular gray matter in six human patients produced long-term relief from intractable pain. This analgesic effect of brain stimulation was also significantly antagonized by the administration of 0.2-1 mg of naloxone. The antagonism of SPA by naloxone has led a number of investigators to conclude that SPA is mediated by the release of enkephalin in the midbrain which presumably activates descending inhibitory pathways to the dorsal horn of the spinal cord.

Manipulations other than direct electrical stimulation of the enkephalin-rich brain regions have also been postulated to induce analgesia by the release of enkephalin on the activation of enkephalinergic pathways. Hayes et al. (1978) recently found that acute stress produces analgesia in rats. Madden et al. (1977) reported that acute stress induced by electrical shock to the feet increased levels of opioid peptides in brain (as measured by the opiate receptor assay) with concurrent decreases in pain responsiveness in the rat. These authors concluded that stressful stimuli may recruit pain-inhibitory mechanisms in the central nervous system, bringing about alterations in enkephalins with concurrent or subsequent changes in responses to pain. This hypothesis was particularly attractive considering the fact that both β-endorphin and ACTH are contained in the same prohormone and are released concomitantly during stress (Rossier et al., 1977). Subsequent studies (using more specific radioimmunoassays), however, failed to find increases in either enkephalin (Fratta et al., 1977) or β-endorphin (Rossier et al., 1977) levels in brain following stress. In addition, while the plasma levels do increase following stress, they are still several magnitudes too low to account for the analgesic effects that are seen following this manipulation (Tseng et al., 1976). However, most damaging to the position that stress-induced analgesia is mediated entirely by endorphins is the finding that it is relatively resistant to antagonism or inhibition by naloxone (Hayes et al., 1978; DeWald and Pert, 1978). Thus, while stress does mobilize β-endorphin release from the pituitary, the primary function of this release is apparently not to produce inhibition of pain transmission. The partial reversal of acupuncture analgesia by naloxone in humans (Mayer et al., 1977) has also been used to support the notion that enkephalins may be involved in this phenomenon. Recently, naloxone was also reported to antagonize electro-acupuncture analgesia in mice (Pomeranz and Chin, 1976) as well as peripheral electroanalgesia in rats (Woolf et al., 1977), again suggesting the mediation of these phenomena by enkephalins.

Interestingly, naloxone has also been reported to antagonize antinociceptive effects induced by other drugs and manipulations not directly related to opiates such as physostigmine (Harris et al., 1969), cannabinol analogs (Bloom et al., 1975), nitrous oxide (Berkowitz et al., 1977), intracerebral acetylcholine (Pedigo et al., 1975), and intracerebral lanthanum ions (Harris et al., 1976). Since it is unlikely that the analgesic actions of these compounds are mediated through the opiate receptor, which is highly specific (Pert and Snyder, 1973), there are only two possibilities: either (1) these compounds release enkephalin or (2) the apparent antagonism is related to decreased nociceptive thresholds per se produced by naloxone.

E. Naloxone-Induced Hyperalgesia

There is, in fact, considerable evidence that naloxone is a weak hyperalgesic. Jacob et al. (1974) were the first to report that naloxone enhanced nociceptive reactions in rats. Although other investigators have not consistently observed naloxone hyperalgesia (El-Sobky et al., 1976; Goldstein et al., 1976; Grevert and Goldstein, 1977; North, 1978), a number of recent reports found that naloxone does reduce pain thresholds in both animals (Berntson and Walker, 1977; Fredrickson et al., 1977) and humans (Buchsbaum et al., 1977; Levine et al., 1978).

Since naloxone alone does appear to be an active hyperalgesic under certain circumstances, naloxone reversal of analgesia induced by various manipulations (e.g., focal brain stimulation, acupuncture, drugs) is only a necessary and clearly not a sufficient criterion for concluding that endogenous opiate peptides underlie these analgesic manipulations. To conclusively demonstrate a link between various analgesic phenomena and the endogenous opioids would require the demonstration that enkephalin is released in those brain regions that mediate opiate analgesia during the analgesic manipulation in question. Such studies will undoubtedly be forthcoming.

The rather subtle and elusive nature of naloxone hyperalgesia makes it difficult to conceive that endogenous opioids are very important in a tonically active pain suppression system or that they are even activated or released by pain input. It must be that the endogenous opioids are activated predominantly by some other mechanisms or variable. The question as to what factors activate the endogenous opioid systems concerned with modulating pain is a most exciting research issue, one which may lead to more efficacious ways of dealing with acute and chronic pain.

V. EUPHOROGENIC SUBSTRATES OF OPIATE ACTION

Relatively little is known regarding the neural substrates that underly the euphorogenic or rewarding actions of opiates. Two basic approaches have been employed to study the brain mechanisms that may mediate these opiate effects. One approach has attempted to localize brain regions critical to opiate self-administration behavior with lesioning techniques. The other has employed self-stimulation procedures to analyze the effects of opiates on the reward pathways of the brain.

A. Self-Administration

Lesions of the ventral noradrenergic bundle (Lewis et al., 1976), medial forebrain bundle (Glick and Charap, 1973), ventrolateral hypothalamus (Arnit et al., 1973), and cingulate cortex (Trafton and Marques, 1971) have been found to decrease the consumption of opiates in addicted animals. Although some investigators have attempted to relate these findings to addictive mechanisms, it is still not clear whether such lesions interfere with opiate intake due to effects on reward mechanisms or on escape or avoidance behavior (i.e., animals increasing intake of opiates to attenuate withdrawal symptoms).

More recently, Glick and his colleagues have reported a series of studies in which lesion effects were assessed on self-administration behavior in animals that were not apparently addicted (i.e., they were not showing withdrawal symptoms during a drug-free weekend period). Lesions of the caudate nucleus were found to decrease self-administration response rates and to lower the threshold dose at which the rewarding effects of morphine could be detected (Glick et al., 1975). These effects were interpreted to imply that the destruction of this structure had increased the sensitivity of rats to the rewarding properties of morphine. Most recently, the same investigators (Glick and Cox, 1977) found that lesions of the substantia nigra (origin of the dopaminergic input into the caudate nucleus) also increased the rewarding effects, while lesions to the medial raphe nucleus decreased the rewarding effects assessed in this fashion. Dorsal raphe and locus ceruleus lesions had no effect. Although the rats were not showing any overt withdrawal signs following 2 weeks of morphine injections, they may still have been addicted sufficiently so that at least part of their behavior could have been motivated by an attempt to escape from or avoid aversive consequences of abstinence. It would be more convincing to demonstrate that lesions interfere with the acquisition of self-administration behavior.

B. Electrical Self-Stimulation

Electrical self-stimulation refers to the phenomenon that animals will learn to deliver small amounts of electrical current to certain regions of the brain (usually the ascending catecholamine systems) through chronically implanted electrodes. In humans, electrical stimulation of these regions has been reported to be pleasant or even euphoric (Heath, 1964). Considerable evidence has accumulated to implicate these reward pathways as neural substrates underlying the euphorogenic effects of sympathomimetics as well as hedonistic behaviors (Stein, 1968). This has suggested to some that opiate euphorogenic actions may also be mediated through the activation of these reward pathways (Pert and Hulsebus, 1975; Bush et al., 1976; Esposito and Kornetsky, 1977).

Opiates have been reported to have complex effects on self-stimulation rates in rats. While low doses appear to increase response rates (Glick and Rapoport, 1974), high doses cause an initial depression followed 2-3 hr later by facilitation (Lorens and Mitchell, 1974; Pert, 1975; Bush et al., 1976). Tolerance develops rapidly to the depressant effects while tolerance has seldom been found for the excitatory effects. It seems that the facilitatory effects of high doses of opiates on self-stimulation may be masked by depressant actions in the midbrain and hindbrain which may not be related to their rewarding properties.

The effects of opiates on self-stimulation behavior (from most brain regions) do not appear to involve a direct action on the reward pathways; rather, they seem to be mediated indirectly through the catecholamine systems. In this regard, Pert and Hulsebus (1975) reported that pretreatment of animals with α-methyl-*p*-tyrosine (AMPT) (a tyrosine hydroxylase inhibitor) antagonized the facilitatory effects of opiates on self-stimulation. Interestingly, AMPT has also been reported to decrease self-administration behavior of opiates (Davis and Smith, 1973). It is suggested that opiates increase self-stimulation by enhancing the evoked release of catecholamines along the reward pathways and that this action underlies some of the rewarding or euphorogenic action of opiates.

Belluzzi and Stein (1977), however, suggested an alternative mechanism for the rewarding effects of opiates and endogenous opioid peptides. Based on the ability of naloxone to antagonize self-stimulation from the PAG, these investigators have proposed that endogenous opioid peptide pathways mediate the "drive-reducing" reward function, which corresponds to the state of satisfaction or well-being associated with goal attainment. Catecholamines, on the other hand, are postulated to mediate the "drive-inducing" reward function, or the process by which goal-seeking behavior is motivated or steered. It is too early to decide as to the validity of this interesting proposition.

VI. NEURAL SUBSTRATES UNDERLYING EFFECTS OF OPIATES ON MOTOR BEHAVIORS

In addition to their analgesic effects, opiates also have profound effects on motor behaviors. This is not surprising since extrapyramidal and mesolimbic structures, which have been shown to have important functions in regulating motor activity, are among the highest in opiate receptor and enkephalin concentrations (see above).

Small doses of morphine produce increases in spontaneous locomotor activity, while large doses cause an initial depression and catalepsy (Babbini and Davis, 1972; Costall and Naylor, 1973), which is followed by excitation (Babbini and Davis, 1972). These psychomotor as well as cataleptic effects of opiates have generally been ascribed to their actions on various components of the nigrostriatal dopamine system (Kuschinsky, 1976; Lal, 1976). Specifically, it has been proposed that some of the motor effects of opiates like those of neuroleptics are due to their direct actions on striatal dopamine (DA) neurons (Kuschinsky, 1976).

Neuroleptics have been postulated to induce catalepsy by blocking the DA receptors in the striatum. This initial blockade of post-synaptic DA receptors has been thought to produce a compensatory increase in the activity of DA neurons via a feedback mechanism (Carlsson and Lindqvist, 1963), which results in an apparent increase in release, synthesis, and metabolism of DA in the striatum (Hornykiewicz, 1966). Several parallels seem to exist between the actions of opiates and neuroleptics on the dopaminergic systems. Morphine as well as other opiate agonists have also been found to increase DA synthesis as measured by their ability to increase the conversion of radioactive tyrosine into DA in the striata as well as the mesolimbic components of DA brain regions (Clouet and Ratner, 1970; Smith et al., 1972; Carenzi et al., 1975; Bloom et al., 1976; Gauchy et al., 1973). Likewise, opiates also accelerate depletion of brain DA after catecholamine synthesis inhibition (Gunne and Jonsson, 1969; Sugrue, 1974; Moleman and Bruinvels, 1976), which has been interpreted as resulting from increased activity within the ascending DA neurons. Opiates also increase striatal as well as mesolimbic levels of homovanillic acid (HVA), a major metabolite of DA (Laverty and Sharman, 1965; Sasame et al., 1972; Kuschinsky and Hornykiewicz, 1972; Ahtee, 1973; Papeschi et al., 1975; Westerink and Korf, 1975). Increased striatal HVA has also been recently observed after intraventricular injections of β-endorphin (Berney and Hornykiewicz, 1977) and D-ala^2-met-enkephalin (Algeri et al., 1977) as well as after direct intranigral injections of D-ala^2-met-enkephalin (Biggio et al., 1978).

In addition to the similarities between the effects of neuroleptics and other opiates on the synthesis and metabolism of DA in the striatum, both classes of compounds have been found to increase the spontaneous activity of the DA zona compacta neurons in the substantia nigra (Bunney et al., 1973; Iwatsubo and Clouet, 1977; Nowycky, 1976). In the case of neuroleptics, this effect has also been interpreted as due to a compensatory increase in neuronal activity via a feedback mechanism which is activated by DA blockade in the striatum (Bunney et al., 1973).

Considering these striking similarities between the actions of opiates and neuroleptics on the DA system, it is not surprising that several authors have proposed that the cataleptic actions of opiates may likewise be related to an inhibition of dopaminergic transmission in the striatum (Sasame et al., 1972; Lal, 1975; Kuschinsky, 1976). Recently, however, several important differences emerged between the actions of these two classes of drugs which make this hypothesis less attractive. First, it appears certain that opiates do not inhibit DA transmission by interacting directly with postsynaptic DA receptors. Carenzi et al. (1975) found that while both neuroleptics and morphine increased the turnover of DA in the striatum, there were clear differences in their actions on DA-stimulated adenylate cyclase. Haloperidol was found to block the in vitro activation of adenylate cyclase by DA, while morphine was entirely ineffective in this respect. More recently, Leysen et al. (1977) showed that opiate agonists do not have a significant affinity for the DA receptor as demonstrated by their inability to inhibit neuroleptic binding. While opiates do not block DA receptors directly, it is possible that an inhibition of DA transmission could be achieved through a different mechanism. Pollard et al. (1977), for example, recently demonstrated the presence of opiate receptors on DA terminals in the striatum and suggested that opiates may induce catatonia by inhibiting the release of DA. Arbilla and Langer (1978), however, failed to find any inhibition of potassium-stimulated release of DA by either morphine or β-endorphin in striatal slices.

Kuschinsky and Hornykiewicz (1973), on the other hand, suggested that opiates may influence DA metabolism directly in the presynaptic neuron by diverting newly synthesized DA from storage sites to sites of catabolism by some unspecified mechanism. The increased breakdown of newly formed DA would then result in a deficiency of this amine at the receptor sites. Carenzi et al. (1975) also suggested that opiate-induced catatonia could be attributable to a defect in the stimulation of postsynaptic receptors in the striatum resulting from an impairment of the extraneuronal release of DA.

Although the effects of opiates on the disposition of DA in the striatum have been tied to their cataleptic actions in a correlative fashion, it seems that they may not be related to this opiate-induced behavior at all. If both opiates and neuroleptics induce catalepsy by inhibiting DA transmission in the striatum, then lesions of this structure should have similar effects on the cataleptic actions of both classes of drugs. Costall and Naylor (1973), however, found that while lesions of the caudate-putamen as well as the globus pallidus reduced or abolished haloperidol-induced catalepsy, morphine catalepsy was enhanced by the same lesions. Nakamura et al. (1973) also found increases in morphine-induced catalepsy after destruction of the DA terminals in the rat striatum with 6-hydroxydopamine. Koffer et al. (1978) recently reported similar interactive effects between striatal lesions and opiate or neuroleptic catalepsy. These authors concluded that while the striatum appears to be a primary site of action of neuroleptic drugs in the production of catalepsy, opiate cataleptic effects may be mediated through other structures.

More direct evidence concerning the brain sites which mediate neuroleptic and opiate cataleptic effects comes from studies in which these compounds have been injected directly into various brain sites. Costall et al. (1972) found that injections of haloperidol into the caudate-putamen as well as the globus pallidus produce catalepsy. Pert (1978) recently found that while injections of chlorpromazine into the caudate nucleus produce catalepsy in rats, morphine was entirely ineffective. Morphine, on the other hand, was effective in inducing catatonia when it was injected into the periaqueductal gray matter and, to a lesser degree, following injections into the globus pallidus. Injections of chlorpromazine into the periaqueductal gray matter, on the other hand, were ineffective. Thus it appears that while opiates do affect DA disposition in the striatum, their catatonic actions are mediated predominantly through the periaqueductal gray matter in the midbrain.

There are relatively few studies that have attempted to analyze the complex effects of opiates on spontaneous locomotor activity. Recently, Pert and Sivit (1977) reported that injections of morphine and enkephalin into the nucleus accumbens (a dopaminergic terminal area of the mesolimbic dopamine system) produce increases in spontaneous activity in rats without motor depression. Injections of apomorphine into the same region also increased activity. However, the increases produced by apomorphine and morphine could be dissociated pharmacologically and it was suggested that there are two parallel systems in the forebrain that regulate locomotor activity, one encoded by enkephalin and the other by dopamine. Using microinjection techniques, Pert et al. (1979) extended the analysis of opiates on motor behavior to other brain structures. Injections into the PAG, ventral thalamus, globus pallidus, and hippocampus decreased locomotor activity while injections into the substantia nigra produced increased horizontal activity which was accompanied by stereotypic behavior. Injections into the amygdala, lateral hypothalamus, ventral tegmentum, and reticular formation were relatively ineffective.

Thus, in addition to modulating the transmission and integration of somatosensory information, enkephalinergic systems also appear to be involved in regulating motor output. That at least some components of these systems may be tonically active has recently been demonstrated by the ability of naloxone to decrease motor output of rats (Pert et al., 1978). On the other hand, it is possible that enkephalinergic neurons impinging on these motor pathways are activated by the same environmental or endogenous conditions that activate enkephalinergic neurons which inhibit the sensation of pain. The inhibition of pain, as well as conservation of energy, by decreased motor output would seem to have adaptive value in response to stress in life-threatening situations.

VII. TEMPERATURE-REGULATORY EFFECTS

Opiate agonists as well as antagonists exert complex effects on body temperature. In a number of species, including human beings, opiate agonists have been found to decrease body temperature. In the rat body temperature effects appear to be dose-dependent. Low doses of morphine as well as enkephalin produce hyperthermia, while higher doses induce hypothermia (Lotti et al., 1965b, 1966). The cat also exhibits a hyperthermic response to low doses of morphine (Banerjee et al., 1968).

Such effects on core temperature appear to be centrally mediated. First, N-methylmorphine, which does not pass into the brain readily, elicits hypothermia when injected intracerebrally but not when injected systemically (Foster et al., 1967). Second, intraventricular injections of morphine produce hyperthermia in cats which is antagonized by prior pretreatment with nalorphine (Banerjee et al., 1968).

A number of attempts have been made to localize the temperature effects by direct brain injections. Lotti et al. (1965a, b) found that injections of morphine into the preoptic and anterior hypothalamus produced a dramatic decrease in core temperature of rats. In addition, injections of nalorphine into the preoptic region were found to antagonize the hypothermic effects of systemically administered morphine (Lotti et al., 1965b). These investigators concluded that the changes in core temperature are due to the actions of opiate agonists on the rostral hypothalamic thermoregulatory centers.

It seems likely that an additional function of enkephalin, at least in mammals, is to modulate body temperature. In addition, enkephalinergic systems modulating body temperature appear to be tonically active to some degree since opiate antagonists have been shown to modify this response (Herz and Blasig, 1978). Enkephalins may also be involved in regulating temperature in response to some environmental input. Herz and Blasig (1978) have in fact found that naloxone inhibited emotionally induced hyperthermia in rats.

VIII. CARDIOVASCULAR AND RESPIRATORY EFFECTS

Morphine has been shown to produce both hypo- and hypertensive effects in cats following systemic administration (Kayalp and Kaymakcalan, 1966). Bolme et al. (1978) recently reported that centrally administered morphine and β-endorphin in rats induce an initial dose related hypertensive response which is followed 10-15 min later by a hypotensive phase. The hypotensive phase was also associated with a significant heart rate decrease. Laubie et al (1977) also found similar effects in the chloralosed dog following intracisternal injections of β-endorphin and D-ala^2-met-enkephalin.

Considering these findings, it is interesting to note that opiate receptors, as well as enkephalin terminals (see above), are highly localized in neural structures involved in cardiovascular reactions (e.g., nucleus tractus, solitarius, nucleus intercalatus, dorsal nucleus of the vagus, and nucleus ambiguus). Perhaps enkephalinergic neurons in these hindbrain nuclei play an important role in central cardiovascular control. Florez and Mediavilla (1977), however, proposed that the cardiovascular as well as respiratory effects of opiates are determined by their actions on sites located on the ventral surface of the brain rather than on the pontomedullary centers. These investigators found a short latency depression of respiration, ventilation, and heart rate following applications of met-enkephalin to the ventral region of the medulla. The precise sites and mechanisms of action of opiates and opioid peptides in regulating respiration and cardiovascular functions still remains to be elucidated.

A. Opiate Peptides and the Regulation of Pituitary Function

Both β-endorphin and enkephalin are localized in the region of the neuropituitary axis (Watson et al., 1978; Bloom et al., 1978). They appear to play a role in regulating the circulating hormonal levels of both prolactin and growth hormone. Morphine and the opiate peptides release growth hormone and prolactin, the effects being specifically reversed by opiate antagonists. Moreover, an enkephalinergic "tone" appears to contribute to the resting levels of these two hormones since opiate antagonist can actually diminish growth hormone and prolactin levels. Enkephalinergic modulation of prolactin and growth hormone release is at the hypothalamic level (Guidotti and Grandison, 1979). It has long been known that opiates can suppress ovulation by blocking the surge of luteinizing hormone (LH) release. Naltrexone has been shown to cause spikes of LH release accompanied by intense "inappropriate" sexual feelings in male human volunteers (Mendelson et al., 1978). The interaction between opiate peptides and vasopressin is less clear; vasopressin has been shown to release β-endorphin from a pituitary cell line (Allen et al., 1978). Furthermore, rats forced to drink 2% saline solution rapidly show depleted pituitary levels of β-endorphin, and Brattleboro rats which lack vasopressin also lack β-endorphin (Klee et al., 1977; Pert and Shibuya, 1978).

1. Endorphin as a Hormone

There is little doubt that in addition to the whole enkephalin-β-endorphin neuronal network in the CNS, the pituitary gland stores huge quantities of β-endorphin for release into the bloodstream to act at opiate receptors in peripheral tissue. Pert et al. (1976) first demonstrated the presence of an opiate substance circulating in human plasma which disappeared from rat blood upon hypophysectomy. Guillemin (1977) demonstrated that β-endorphin can be found in rat blood. Interestingly, its levels appear to rise and fall concomitantly with ACTH, which shares its common precursor molecule, pro-opiocortin (Udenfriend et al., 1978). It should be emphasized that the highest levels of β-endorphin achieved thus far (after the stress of a broken tibia or adrenalectomy) are still so low (about 5×10^{-10} M) that they are not sufficient to have a big effect on target receptors in the periphery. However, human plasma endorphin levels in the functionally significant nanomolar range can be detected by radioreceptor assay (Naber et al., 1980). Blood contains surprisingly high enkephalin levels (Clement-Jones et al., 1980) as well as heterogeneous radioreceptor-active, radioimmunoinert longer ekephalins derived from adrenal gland (Lewis et al., 1980).

A very recent finding (Margulis et al., 1978) suggests that pituitary β-endorphin has an important role to play in modulating feeding behavior. A rat and mouse strain of obese animals have a twofold higher concentration of β-endorphin in the fat animals compared to their lean litter mates. Moreover, circulating plasma levels of β-endorphin are higher in the obese rats and naloxone specifically abolishes overeating in the obese animals. Target opiate receptors in the periphery presently include those that line the gastrointestinal tract, the vas deferens, the pancreas, and the kidney, but more careful study in this area will probably reveal additional opiate receptor target areas.

IX. SLEEP

Opiates have long been thought to influence sleep. The term *narcotic,* in fact, reflects the early feeling that opiates produce sleep. Acute administration of morphine and heroin decreases the number and duration of rapid eye movement (REM) sleep periods and increases sleep correlates of arousal (such as α waves, muscle tension, non-REM light sleep) in humans (Kay et al., 1969; Lewis et al., 1970). Chronic administration of morphine also produces increases in arousal and decreases in REM duration, though partial tolerance to these effects develops (Kay, 1975). Thus these sleep effects contrast with the commonly held notion that the opiates are sedatives. Because of the sleep effects of narcotic analgesics and the recent suggestion that endogenous opiate-like substances play a role in sleep (King et al., 1976), naloxone effects on sleep parameters have been studied (Davis et al., 1977). In six young, healthy male subjects, no significant differences in sleep parameters were found when naloxone and placebo nights were compared.

X. ROLE OF OPIATE PEPTIDES IN MENTAL DISORDERS

In this chapter we have described the newly discovered opiate peptides as potentially important in pain regulation and as mediators of reward mechanisms, temperature regulators, neural substrates for motor behaviors, and possibly endocrine effectors. Could dysfunction of opioid peptide mechanisms underly any psychiatric disorder? Several theoretical arguments have been advanced in support of endorphin participation in mental illness. As reviewed earlier, the distribution of opiate receptors and endogenous opioid peptides is associated with limbic and motor regions of brain, regions felt to be functionally altered in some psychiatric illnesses. Many known neurotransmitters are present in these anatomical areas and as yet there is no proof of abnormal neuronal functioning. The most common argument advanced in support of a potential role of endorphins in mental illness is that opiates and endorphins produce behaviors which mimic the symptoms associated with major psychoses. The similarity of pharmacologically induced behaviors to psychiatric symptoms, while intriguing and worthy of investigation, is neither necessary nor sufficient to link alterations of endorphins to mental illness. Similar behaviors are produced by a wide range of diversely acting compounds. In this section we discuss strategies for studying the role of endogenous opioids in humans and neurochemical studies in schizophrenia, depression, and mania.

A. Studying Endorphins and Psychiatric Disorders

The administration of opioid peptides would provide direct evidence of their actions. The safety of most opioid peptides has yet to be determined and is a major impediment to human investigation. Met- and leu-enkephalin are rapidly degraded and thus parenteral administration is unlikely to reveal their actions. As discussed earlier, meth-enkephalin may be modified by D-ala^2-met-enkephalin, which slows its enzymatic degradation and thus might be useful in human studies if it proved safe in toxicology studies. β-Endorphin has been administered to humans in several studies (Kline et al., 1977; Angst et al., 1979) but may not enter the brain in sufficient concentrations to produce central effects.

The most common method of studying endorphin function in humans has been the administration of specific narcotic antagonists such as naloxone and naltrexone. Since narcotic antagonists block and reverse most of the effects of endorphins, their actions have been interpreted to reflect the blockade or reversal of peptide-mediated behaviors. This strategy required that the behavior studied be under the tonic influence of endorphins. Furthermore, it is not clear that narcotic antagonists block all of the specific actions of opioid peptides.

Another strategy for determining peptide functions is their measurement in plasma, urine, cerebrospinal fluid, and tissue specimens. Currently, there are no reports of specific assays for the opioid peptides in humans. Investigators are developing radioimmunoassays for opioid peptides which are both specific and sensitive.

1. Schizophrenia

Psychotomimetic reactions produced by narcotics and narcotic antagonists led to the suggestion that similar psychotic symptoms might be associated with an excess of opioid peptides in the CNS. The report of Gunne et al. (1977) that 0.4 mg of naloxone eliminated auditory hallucinations in four of six chronic schizophrenics stimulated studies on the effects of antagonists in schizophrenia. Emrich et al. (1977) and Watson et al. (1978) confirmed a significant but small effect of naloxone on auditory hallucinosis, while many other studies have been unable to produce such a therapeutic effect (Davis et al., 1977; Volavka et al., 1977; Kurland et al., 1977; Janowsky et al., 1977; Mielke and Gallant, 1977; Gitlin and Rosenblatt, 1978). In these negative studies, a wide range of schizophrenic symptoms were examined and a wide range of naloxone doses were utilized.

Kline et al. (1977) administered β-endorphin in an open trial and reported persistent improvement in 1-2 weeks after a single dose in several schizophrenic patients. Attempts to replicate this study in blind and placebo-controlled studies are currently underway.

The resemblance of behavioral states induced by endorphins in rats to human catatonia and neuroleptic-induced catalepsy prompted some investigators (Bloom et al., 1976; Jacquet and Marks, 1976) to suggest testing of narcotic antagonists in catatonic states. Many substances produce neuromuscular effects similar to catatonia and thus a catatonic-like effect of endorphins does not in itself implicate them as mediators of the effect. In fact, in one study (Davis et al., 1977), the variable "mannerisms and posturing" failed to improve after naloxone in 14 schizophrenic patients.

Cerebrospinal fluid taken by lumbar puncture from patients with schizophrenia has been analyzed for opiate binding (Terenius et al., 1976; Lindstrom et al., 1978). Untreated schizophrenic patients had increased opiate binding when compared to nonpatient controls. While these findings are exciting, they should be interpreted with caution. Neither β-endorphin nor met-enkephalin was present in these CSF fractions and the significance of the finding awaits identification of these CSF fractions.

2. *Depression*

Cyclazocine, a mixed narcotic agonist-antagonist, was reported to have a clinical antidepressant action in one study (Fink et al., 1970). In animal models used for testing efficacy of antidepressants, opiate antagonists show some similarities to commonly used antidepressants (Doggett et al., 1975). In another study of primary affective illness, depressed state, acute administration of 0.4-6 mg of naloxone failed to improve the depressed mood of a few affectively ill patients (Davis et al., 1977). Lindstrom et al. (1978) reported elevation of an opiate-binding fraction of CSF in manic-depressive illness as well as in schizophrenia as discussed earlier.

Kline et al. (1977) reported improvement in the symptoms of depression after acute administration of β-endorphin. Angst et al. (1979) reported switches to mania or hypomania in four of six subjects given β-endorphin.

3. *Mania*

There are a number of similarities in manic symptoms and endorphin-induced behaviors. Mania is an illness characterized by heightened activity, arousal, pressured speech, elevated mood, and pain tolerance. In animals, low doses of opiates cause hyperactivity and heightened arousal. In humans, opiates cause euphoria and are potent analgesics. As already described, endorphins play a role in regulating pain appreciation. Some manics are more pain-tolerance than age- and sex-matched controls (Davis et al., 1978).

Three groups have reported the effects of naloxone on mania (Davis et al., 1977; Janowsky et al., 1977; Emrich et al., 1977). Davis et al. (1977) administered 0.4-30 mg of naloxone to four patients in the manic phase of manic-depressive illness. In one of the four patients a clinical effect was observed. This patient reported that her "thoughts were slowed," that she had "difficulty finding words," and that "a blanket was pulled over my mind" in three of three high-dose trials (20-30 mg single dose), in one of three moderate-dose trials (10 mg), and in zero of three placebo trials. The patient spontaneously reported this effect at ½ hr after naloxone injection and its disappearance at 2-3 hr after naloxone injections. Janowsky et al. (1977) reported dramatic generalized antimanic effects of naloxone in several of seven patients administered 20 mg, while Emrich et al. (1977) were unable to demonstrate any naloxone-induced behavior changes in two manic patients using doses of 4 and 24.8 mg, respectively. Thus there have been suggestive behavioral effects of naloxone in a few manic patients in two of three studies.

XI. CONCLUSIONS

It seems incredible that a brain substance that was totally unheard of just 6 years ago is now being furiously studied and invoked to explain everything from analgesia to obesity. If we have learned anything from the discovery of opiate receptors and their natural peptide ligands, it is how little we really know about the constituents of the brain. In the long run, it is entirely possible that the enkephalin story will be most valuable as an inspiration for digging out other receptors for psychoactive substances and their endogenous ligands. For example, the valium receptor has already been identified (Squires and Braestrup, 1977; Mohler and Okada, 1977) and the search is on for the putative endogenous ligand for this receptor which might serve as an anxiety-producing or anxiety-reducing substance. Many novel peptides, including bombesin, VIP, CCK, and bradykinin, are only beginning to be carefully studied for their role in brain. In our eagerness to "explain" behavior, let us not be too eager to attribute everything to the opiate peptides and their receptors! And yet, the possibility that the brain's own morphine can create alterations in behavior, mood, and consciousness has captured the imaginations of all of us.

REFERENCES

Ahtee, L. (1973). Catalepsy and stereotyped behaviour in rats treated chronically with methadone. Relation to brain homovanillic acid content. *J. Pharm. Pharmacol. 25,* 649-651.

Akil, H., Mayer, D. J., and Liebeskind, J. C. (1976). Antagonism of stimulation-produced analgesia by naloxone, a narcotic antagonist. *Science 191,* 961-962.

Algeri, S., Calderini, G., Consalazione, A., and Garattini, S. (1977). The effect of methionine-enkephalin and D-alanine methionine-enkephalinamide on the concentration of dopamine metabolites in rat striatum. *Eur. J. Pharmacol. 45,* 207-209.

Allen, R., Herbert, E., Shibuya, H., and Pert, C. B. (1978). Release of β-endorphin from pituitary tumor cells. *Proc. Nat. Acad. Sci. USA.* In press.

Amit, Z., Corcoran, M. E., Amir, S., and Urca, G. (1973). Ventral hypothalamic lesions block the consumption of morphine in rats. *Life Sci. 13,* 805-816.

Anderson, K. V., and Mahan, D. E. (1971). Increased pain thresholds following combined lesions of thalamic nuclei centrum medianum and centralis lateralis. *Psychonom. Sci. 23,* 113-114.

Anderson, K. V., and Pearl, G. S. (1977). Long term increases in nociceptive thresholds following lesions in feline nucleus reticularis gigantocellularis. In *Advances in Pain Research and Therapy,* J. J. Bonica and D. Albe-Fessand (Eds.). Raven, New York.

Anderson, S. D., Basbaum, A. I., and Fields, H. L. (1977). Response of medullary raphe neurons to peripheral stimulation and to systemic opiates. *Brain Res. 123,* 363-368.

Angst, J., Autenrieth, V., Brem, F., et al. (1979). Preliminary results of treatment with β-endorphin in depression. In *Endorphins and Mental Health Research.* E. Usdin, W. E. Bunney, Jr., and N. S. Kline (Eds.). McMillan, London.

Arbilla, S., and Langer, S. Z. (1978). Morphine and β-endorphin inhibit release of noradrenaline from cerebral cortex but not of dopamine from rat striatum. *Nature 271,* 559-561.

Atweh, S. F., and Kuhar, M. J. (1977a). Autoradiographic localization of opiate receptors in rat brain. I. Spinal cord and lower medulla. *Brain Res. 124,* 53-67.

Atweh, S. F., and Kuhar, M. J. (1977b). Autoradiographic localization of opiate receptors in rat brain. II. The brain stem. *Brain Res. 129,* 1-12.

Atweh, S. F., and Kuhar, M. J. (1977c). Autoradiographic localization of opiate receptors in rat brain. III. The telencephalon. *Brain Res. 134,* 393-405.

Babbini, M., and Davis, W. M. (1972). Time-dose relationships for locomotor activity effects of morphine after acute or repeated treatment. *Br. J. Pharmacol. 46,* 213-224.

Balagura, S., and Ralph, T. (1973). The analgesic effect of electrical stimulation of the diencephalon and mesencephalon. *Brain Res. 60,* 369-379.

Banerjee, V., Feldberg, W., and Lotti, V. S. (1968). Effects on body temperature of morphine and ergotamine injected into cerebral ventricles of cats. *Br. J. Pharmacol. Chemother. 32,* 523-530.

Basbaum, A. I., Clanton, C. H., and Fields, H. L. (1976). Opiate and stimulus-produced analgesia: functional anatomy of a medullospinal pathway. *Proc. Nat. Acad. Sci. USA 73,* 4685-4688.

Belluzzi, J. D., and Stein, L. (1977). Enkephalin may mediate euphoria and drive-reduction reward. *Nature 266,* 556-558.

Belluzzi, J. D., Grant, N., Garsky, V., Sarantakis, D., Wise, C. D., and Stein, L. (1976). Analgesia induced "in vivo" by central administration of enkephalin in rat. *Nature 260,* 625-626.

Berkowitz, B. A., Finck, D. A., and Ngai, S. H. (1977). Nitrous oxide analgesia: reversal by naloxone and development of tolerance. *J. Pharmacol. Exp. Ther. 203,* 539-547.

Berney, S., and Hornykiewicz, O. (1977). The effect of β-endorphin and met-enkephalin on striatal dopamine metabolism and catalepsy: comparison with morphine. *Comm. Psychopharmacol. 1,* 597-604.

Berntson, G. G., and Walker, J. M. (1977). Effect of opiate receptor blockade on pain sensitivity in the rat. *Brain Res. Bull. 2,* 157-159.

Biggio, G., Carn, M., Corda, M. G., Di Bello, C., and Gessa, G. L. (1978). Stimulation of dopamine synthesis in caudate nucleus by intrastriatal enkephalins and antagonism by naloxone. *Science 200,* 552-554.

Bloom, A. S., Dewey, W. L., Harris, L. S., and Brasins, K. (1975). Brain catecholamines and the antinociceptive action of (±)9-Nor-9B-OH-hexahydrocannabinol. *Neurosci. Abstr. 1,* 375.

Bloom, F., Battenberg, E., Rossier, J., Ling, N., and Guillemin, R. (1978). Nuerons containing β-endorphin in rat brain exist separately from those containing enkephalin: immunocytochemical studies. *Proc. Nat. Acad. Sci. USA 75,* 1591-1595.

Bloom, F., Segal, D., Ling, N., and Guillemin, R. (1976). Endorphins. Profound behavioral effects in rats suggest new etiological factors in mental illness. *Science 194,* 630-632.

Bloom, F. E., Rossier, J., Battenberg, E. L. F., Bayon, A., French, E., Henricksen, S. J., Siggins, G. R., Ling, N., and Guillemin, R. (1979). β-Endorphin. Cellular localization, electrophysiological and behavioral effects. In *Endorphins and Mental Health Research,* E. Usdin, W. E. Bunney Jr., and N. S. Kline (Eds.). MacMillan, London, In press.

Bolme, P., Fuxe, K., Agnati, L. F., Bradley, R., and Smythies, J. (1978). Cardiovascular effects of morphine and opioid peptides following intracisternal administration in chloralose-anesthetized rats. *Eur. J. Pharmacol. 48,* 319-324.

Bradbury, A F., Fedlberg, W. F., Smyth, D. G., and Snell, C. R. (1976). Lipotropin C-fragment. An endogenous peptide with potent analgesic activity. In *Opiates and Endogenous Opioid Peptides,* H. W. Kosterlitz (Ed.). North-Holland, Amsterdam, pp. 9-18.

Bradley, P. B., Briggs, I., Gayton, R. J., and Lambert, L. A. (1976). Effects of microiontophoretically applied methionine-enkephalin on single neurons in rat brainstem. *Nature 261,* 425-426.

Bradley, P. B., Gayton, R. J., and Lambert, L. A. (1978). Electrophysiological effects of opiates and opioid peptides. In *Centrally Acting Peptides,* J. Hughes (Ed.). MacMillan, London, pp. 215-229.

Buchsbaum, M. S., Davis, G. C., and Bunney, W. E., Jr. (1977). Naloxone alters pain perception and somatosensory evoked potentials in normal subjects. *Nature 270,* 620-622.

Bunney, B. S., Walters, J. R., Roth, R. H., and Aghajanian, K. (1973). Dopaminergic neurons. Effects of antipsychotic drugs and amphetamine on single cell activity. *J. Pharmacol. Exp. Ther. 185,* 560-571.

Bush, H., Bush, M. F., Miller, M. A., and Reid, L. (1976). Addictive agents and intracranial stimulation. Daily morphine and lateral hypothalamic self-stimulation. *Physiol. Psychol. 4,* 79-85.

Carenzi, A., Guidotti, A., Revuelta, A., and Costa, E. (1975). Molecular mechanisms in the actions of morphine and viminol (R_2) on rat striatum. *J. Pharmacol. Exp. Ther. 294,* 311-318.

Carlsson, A., and Lindqvist, M. (1963). Effect of chlorpromazine and haloperidol on formation of 3-methoxytyramine and normetanephrine in mouse brain. *Acta Pharmacol. Toxicol. 20,* 140-144.

Chang, J. -K., Fong, B. T. W., Pert, A., and Pert, C. B. (1976). Opiate receptor affinities and behavioral effects of enkephalin. Structure-activity relationship of ten synthetic peptide analogues. *Life Sci. 18,* 1473-1482.

Clement-Jones, V., Lowry, P. J., Rees, L. H., Besser, G. M. (1980). Met-enkephalin circulates in human plasma *Nature 283,* 295-297.

Clouet, D. H., and Ratner, M. (1970). Catecholamine biosynthesis in brains of rats treated with morphine. *Science 168,* 854-855.

Costall, B., and Naylor, R. J. (1973). Neuroleptic and non-neuroleptic catalepsy. *Arz. Forsch. 23,* 674-683.

Costall, B., Naylor, R. J., and Olley, J. E. (1972). Catalepsy and circling behaviour after intracerebral injections of neuroleptic, cholinergic and anticholinergic agents into the caudate-putamen, globus pallidus and substantia nigra of rat brain. *Neuropharmacology 11,* 645-663.

Davis, W. M., and Smith, S. G. (1973). Blocking of morphine based reinforcement by alpha-methyltyrosine. *Life Sci. 12*, 185-191.

Davis, G. C., Bunney, W. E., Jr., DeFraites, E. G., Kleinman, J. E., van Kammen, D. P., Post, R. M., and Wyatt, R. J. (1977a). Intravenous naloxone administration in schizophrenia and affective illness. *Science 197*, 74-77.

Davis, G. C., Duncan, W. C., Gillin, J. C., and Bunney, W. E., Jr. (1977b). Failure of naloxone to affect human sleep. *Comm. Psychopharmacol. 1*, 489-492.

Davis, G. C., Buchsbaum, M. S. and Bunney, W. E., Jr. (1978). Analgesia to painful stimuli in affective illness. *Proc. Am. Psychiatric Ass.*, Atlanta, Georgia.

Davis, G. C., Bunney, W. E., Jr., Buchsbaum, M. S., DeFraites, E. G., Duncan, W., Gillin, J. C., van Kammen, D. P., Kleinman, J., Murphy, D. L., Post, R. M., Reus, V., and Wyatt, R. J. (1979). The use of narcotic antagonists to study the role of endorphins in normals and psychiatric patients. In *Endorphins and Mental Health Research*. E. Usdin, W. E. Bunney, Jr., and N. S. Kline (Eds.). MacMillan, London, pp. 000.

De Wald, L., and Pert, A. (1978). The role of the pituitary in stress-induced analgesia. *Physiol. Behav.* In press.

Doggett, N. S., Reno, H., and Spencer, P. S. J. (1975). Narcotic agonists and antagonists as models for potential antidepressant drugs. *Neuropharmacology 14*, 507-515.

Elde, R., Hakfelt, T., Johansson, O., and Terenius, L. (1976). Immunohistochemical studies using antibodies to leucine-enkephalin. Initial observations on the nervous system of the rat. *Neuroscience 1*, 349-351.

El-Sobky, A., Dostrovsky, J. O. and Wall, P. D. (1976). Lack of effect of naloxone on pain perception in humans. *Nature 263*, 783-784.

Emrich, H. M., Cording, C., Piree, S., Kolling, A., von Zerssen, D., and Herz, A. (1977). Indication of an antipsychotic action of the opiate antagonist naloxone. *Pharmakopsychiatrie 10*, 265-270.

Esposito, R., and Kornetsky, C. (1977). Morphine lowering of self-stimulation thresholds. Lack of tolerance with long-term administration. *Science 195*, 189-191.

Fields, H. F., Basbaum, A. I., Clanton, C. H., and Anderson, S. D. (1977). Nucleus raphe magnus inhibition of dorsal horn neurons. *Brain Res. 126*, 441-453.

Fink, M., Simeon, J., Itil, T. M., and Freedman, A. M. (1970). Clinical antidepressant activity of cyclazocine—a narcotic antagonist. *Clin. Pharmacol. Ther. 11*, 41-48.

Florez, J., and Mediavilla, A. (1977). Respiratory and cardiovascular effects of met-enkephalin applied to the ventral surface of the brain stem. *Brain Res. 138*, 585-590.

Foster, R. S., Jenden, D. J., and Lomax, P. (1967). A comparison of the pharmacologic effects of morphine and N-methyl morphine. *J. Pharmacol. 157,* 185-195.

Fratta, W., Yang, H-Y.T., Hong, J., and Costa, E. (1977). Stability of met-enkephalin content in brain structures of morphine-dependent or foot shock-stressed rats. *Nature 268,* 452-453.

Frederickson, R. C. A., Burgis, V., and Edwards, J. D. (1977). Hyperalgesia induced by naloxone follows diurnal rhythm in responsivity to painful stimuli. *Science 198,* 756-758.

Frederickson, R. C. A., and Norris, F. H. (1976). Enkephalin-induced depression of single neurons in brain areas with opiate receptors. Antagonism by naloxone. *Science 194,* 440-442.

Gates, M., Tschudi, G. (1956). The synthesis of morphine. *J. Am. Chem. Soc. 78,* 1380-1393.

Gauchy, C., Agid, Y., Glowinski, J., and Cheramy, A. (1973). Acute effects of morphine and dopamine synthesis and release and tyramine metabolism in the rat striatum. *Eur. J. Pharmacol. 22,* 311-319.

Gitlin, M., and Rosenblatt, M. (1978). Possible withdrawal from endogenous opiates in schizophrenics. *Am. J. Psychiatry 135,* 377-378.

Giudotti, A., and Grandison, L. (1979). Participation of endorphins inthe regulation of pituitary function. In *Endorphins and Mental Health Research,* E. Usdin, W. E. Bunney Jr., and N. S. Kline (Eds.). MacMillan, London.

Glick, S. D., and Charap, A. D. (1973). Morphine dependence in rats with medial forebrain bundle lesions. *Psychopharmacologia 30,* 343-348.

Glick, S., and Rapaport, G. (1974). Tolerance to the facilitatory effect of morphine on self-stimulation of the medial forebrain bundle in rats. *Res. Comm. Chem. Pathol. Pharmacol. 9,* 647-752.

Glick, S. D., and Cox, R. D. (1977). Changes in morphine self-administration after brainstem lesions in rats. *Psychopharmacologia 52,* 151-156.

Glick, S. D., Cox, R. S., and Crane, A. M. (1975). Changes in morphine self-administration and morphine dependence after lesions of the caudate nucleus in rats. *Psychopharmacologia 41,* 219-224.

Goldstein, A., Pryor, G. T., Otis, L. S., and Larren, E. (1976). On the role of endogenous opioid peptides. Failure of naloxone to influence shock escape threshold in the rat. *Life Sci. 18,* 599-604.

Grevert, P., and Goldstein, A. (1977). Effects of naloxone on experimentally induced ischemic pain and on mood in human subjects. *Proc. Nat. Acad. Sci. USA 74,* 1291-1294.

Guillemin, R., Ling, N., and Burgus, R. (1976). Endorphins, peptides, d'origine hypothalamique et neurohypophysaire a'activite morphinomimetique. Isolement et structure moleculaire de l'alpha-endorphine. *Comptes Rendus Hebdomadaires des Saences de l'Academie des Sciences (Paris) 282,* 783-785.

Guillemin, R., Vargo, T., Rossier, J., Minick, S., Ling, N., Rivier, C., Vale, W., and Bloom, F. (1977). β-Endorphin and adrenocortocitropin are secreted concomitantly by the pituitary. *Science 197,* 1367-1369.

Gunne, L.-M. and Jonsson, J. (1969). Effects of morphine intoxication on brain catecholamine neurons. *J. Eur. Pharmacol. 5,* 338-342.

Gunne, L.-M., Lindstrom, L., and Terenius, L. (1977). Naloxone-induced reversal of schizophrenic hallucinations. *J. Neural Transm. 40,* 13-19.

Haigler, H. J. (1976). Morphine. Ability to block neuronal activity evoked by a nociceptive stimulus. *Life Sci. 19,* 841-858.

Hambrook, J. M., Morgan, B. A., Rance, M. J., and Smith, C. F. C. (1976). Mode of deactivation of the enkephalins by rat and human plasma and rat brain homogenates. *Nature 262,* 782-783.

Harris, L. S., Dewey, W. L., Homes, J. F., Kennedy, J. S., and Parr, H. (1969). Narcotic-antagonist analgesics: interactions with cholinergic systems. *J. Pharmacol. Exp. Ther. 169,* 17-22.

Harris, R. A., Loh, H. H., and Way, E. L. (1976). Antinociceptive effects of lanthanum and cerium in nontolerant and morphine tolerant-dependent animals. *J. Pharmacol. Exp. Ther. 196,* 288-297.

Hayes, R. L., Bennett, G. J., Newlan, P. G., and Mayer, D. J. (1978). Behavioral and physiological studies of non-narcotic analgesia in the rat elicited by certain environmental stimuli. *Brain Res.* In press.

Heath, R. G. (1964). *The Role of Pleasure in Behavior.* Harper and Row, New York.

Herz, A., Albus, K., Metys, T., Schubert, P., and Teschemacher, H. J. (1970). On the central sites for the antinociceptive action of morphine and fentanyl. *Neuropharmacology 9,* 539-551.

Hiller, J. M., Pearson, J., and Simon, E. J. (1973). Distribution of stereospecific binding of the potent narcotic analgesia etorphine in the limbic system. *Res. Comm. Chem. Pathol. Pharmacol. 6,* 1052-1062.

Hokfeldt, T., Elde, R., Johanson, O., Luft, R., Nilsson, G., and Arimura, A. (1976). Immunohistochemical evidence for separate populations of somatostatin-containing and substance P-containing primary afferent neurons in the rat. *Neuroscience 1,* 131-136.

Hornykiewicz, O. (1966). Dopamine (3-hydroxytryptamine) and brain function. *Pharmacol. Rev. 18,* 925-964.

Hosabuchi, Y., Adams, J. E., and Linchitz, R. (1977). Pain relief by electrical stimulation at the central gray matter in humans and its reversal by naloxone. *Science 197,* 183-186.

Hughes, J., Smith, T. W., Kosterlitz, H. W., Fothergill, L. A., Morgan, B. A., and Morris, H. R. (1976). Identification of two related pentapeptides from the brain with potent opiate agonist activity. *Nature 258,* 577-580.

Hughes, J., Kosterlitz, H. W., McKnight, A. T., Sara, R. P., Lord, J. A. H., and Waterfield, A. A. (1978). Pharmacological and biochemical aspects of the enkephalins. In *Centrally Acting Peptides,* J. Hughes (Ed.). MacMillan, London, pp. 179-193.

Irwin, S., Houde, R. W., Bennett, D. R., Hendershot, L. C., and Seevers, M. H. (1951). The effects of morphine, methadone and meperidine on some reflex responses of spinal animals to nociceptive stimulation. *J. Pharmacol. Exp. Ther. 101,* 132-143.

Iversen, L. L., Iversen, S. D., Bloom, F. E., Vargo, T., and Guillemin, R. (1978). Release of enkephalin from rat globus pallidus in vitro. *Nature 271,* 679-681.

Iwatsubo, K., and Clouet, D. H. (1977). Effects of morphine and haloperidol on the electrical activity of rat nigrostriatal neurons. *J. Pharmacol. Exp. Ther. 202,* 429-436.

Jacob, J. J., Tremblay, E. C., and Colombel, M. C. (1974). Facilitation de reactions nociceptives par la naloxone chez la sowis et chez le rat. *Psychopharmacologia 37,* 217-222.

Jacobowitz, D. M., Silver, M. A., and Saden, W. (1979). Mapping of the localization of leucine-enkephalin-containing axons and cell bodies of the rat forebrain. In *Endorphins in Mental Health Research,* E. Usdin, W. E. Bunney Jr., and N. S. Kline (Eds.). MacMillan, London.

Jacquet, Y., and Lajtha, A. (1974). Paradoxical effects after microinjection of morphine in the periaqueductal gray matter in the rat. *Science 185,* 1055-1057.

Jacquet, Y., and Marks, N. (1976). The C-fragment of beta-lipotropin. An endogenous neuroleptic or antipsychotic? *Science 194,* 632-635.

Janowsky, D., Judd, L., Huey, L., Roitman, N., Parker, D., and Segal, D. (19xx). Naloxone effects on manic symptoms and growth hormone levels. *Lancet 2,* No. 320, 8084.

Janowsky, D. S., Segal, D. S., Bloom, F., Abrams, A., and Guillemin, R. (1977). Lack of effect of naloxone on schizophrenic symptoms. *Am. J. Psychiatry 134,* 926-927.

Kay, D. C. (1975). Human sleep during chronic morphine intoxication. *Psychopharmacologia (Berlin) 44,* 117-124.

Kay, D. C., Eisenstein, R. B., and Jasinski, D. R. (1969). Morphine effects on human REM state, waking state and NREM sleep. *Psychopharmacologia (Berlin) 14,* 404-416.

Kayalp. S. O., and Kaymacklon, S. (1966). A comparative study of the effects of morphine in unanaesthetized and anaesthetized cats. *Br. J. Pharmacol. 26,* 196-204.

King, C. D., Masserano, J. M., Santos, N., and Byrne, W. (1976). Endorphine causes naloxone-reversible hyposomnia in cats. Presented at the 16th Ann. Meet. APSS, Cincinnati, Ohio.

Kitahata, L. M., Kosaka, Y., Taub, A., Bonikos, K., and Hoffert, M. (1974). Lamina-specific suppression of dorsal-horn unit activity by morphine sulfate. *Anesthesiology 41,* 39-48.

Klee, W. A., Mata, M. N., and Gainer, H. (1977). Effect of dehydration on endogenous opiate content of the rat neuro-intermediate lobe. *Life Sci. 21,* 1159-1162.

Kline, N. S., Li, C. H., Lehmann, H. E., Lajtha, A., Laski, E., and Cooper, T. (1977). β-Endorphin-induced changes in schizophrenic and depressed patients. *Arch. Gen. Psychiatry 34,* 1111-1112.

Koffer, K., Berney, S., and Hornykiewicz, O. (1978). The role of the corpus striatum in neuroleptic and narcotic-induced catalepsy. *Eur. J. Pharmacol. 47,* 81-86.

Kuhar, M. J., Pert, C. B., and Snyder, S. H. (1973). Regional distribution of opiate receptor binding in monkey and human brain. *Nature 245,* 447-450.

Kurland, A. A., McCabe, O. L., Hanlon, T. E., and Sullivan, D. (1977). The treatment of perceptual disturbances in schizophrenia with naloxone hydrochloride. *Am. J. Psychiatry 134,* 1408-1410.

Kuschinsky, K. (1976). Actions of narcotics on brain dopamine metabolism and their relevance for "psychomotor" effects. *Arz. Forsch. 26,* 563-567.

Kuschinsky, K., and Hornykiewicz, O. (1972). Morphine catalepsy in the rat: relation to striatal dopamine metabolism. *Eur. J. Pharmacol. 19,* 119-122.

Kuschinsky, K., and Hornykiewicz, O. (1973). Effects of morphine on striatal dopamine metabolism. Possible mechanism of its opposite effect on locomotor activity in rats and mice. *Eur. J. Pharmacol. 26,* 41-50.

Lal, H. (1975). Narcotic dependence, narcotic action and dopamine receptors. *Life Sci. 17,* 483-496.

Laubie, M., Schmitt, H., Vincent, M., and Remond, G. (1977). Central cardiovascular effects of morphinomimetic peptides in dogs. *Eur. J. Pharmacol. 46,* 67-71.

Laverty, R., and Sharman, D. F. (1965). Modification by drugs of the metabolism of 3, 4-dihydroxyphenylethylamine, noradrenalin and 5-hydroxytryptamine in the brain. *Br. J. Pharmacol. 24,* 20-26.

LeBars, D., Guilbaud, G., Jurna, I., and Besson, J. M. (1976). Differential effects of morphine on responses of dorsal horn lamina V type cells elicited by A and C fibre stimulation in the spinal cat. *Brain Res. 115,* 518-524.

Levine, J. D., Gordon, N. C., Jones, R. T., and Fields, H. L. (1978). The narcotic antagonist naloxone enhances clinical pain. *Nature 272,* 826-827.

Lewis, M. J., Costa. J. L., Jacobowitz, D. M., and Margules, D. L. (1976). Tolerance, physical dependence and opioid-seeking behavior. Dependence on diencephalic norepinephrine. *Brain Res. 107,* 156-165.

Lewis, R. V., Stern, A. S., Kimura, S., Stem, S., and Udenfriend, S. (1980). An about 50,000 dalton protein in adrenal medulla: A common precursor of met- and leu-enkephalin. *Science 208,* 1459-1461.

Lewis, S. A., Oswald, C., Evans, J. I., Akindale, M. S., and Tamprett, S. L. (1970). Heroin and human sleep. *Electroencephalog. Clin. Neurophysiol. 28,* 374-381.

Lewis, V. A., and Gebhart, G. F. (1977). Evaluation of the periaqueductal central gray (PAG) as a morphine specific locus of action and examination of morphine-induced and stimulation-produced analgesia at coincident PAG loci. *Brain Res. 124,* 283-303.

Leysen, J., Tollenaere, J. P., Koch, M. H. J., and Laduron, P. (1977). Differentiation of opiate and neuroleptic receptor binding in rat brain. *Eur. J. Pharmacol. 43,* 253-267.

Li, C. H., and Chung, D. (1976). Primary structure of human beta-lipotropin. *Nature 260,* 622-624.

Li, C. H., Barnafi, L., Chretien, M., and Chung, D. (1965). Isolation and amino-acid sequence of β-LPH from sheep pituitary glands. *Nature 208,* 1093-1095.

Liebeskind, J. C., Guilbaud, G., Besson, J. M., and Oliveras, J.-L. (1973). Analgesia from electrical stimulation of the periaqueductal gray matter in the cat: behavioral observations and inhibitory effects on spinal cord interneurons. *Brain Res. 50,* 441-446.

Lindstrom, L. H., Widerlov, E., Gunne, L.-M., Wahlstrom, A., and Terenius, L. (1978). Endorphins in human cerebrospinal fluid. Clinical correlations to some psychotic states. *Acta Psychiatr. Scand. 47,* 253-264.

Lorens, S. A., and Mitchell, C. L. (1974). Influence of morphine on lateral hypothalamic self-stimulation in the rat. *Psychopharmacologia 32,* 271-277.

Lotti, V. J., Lomax, P., and George, R. (1965a). N-allylnormorphine antagonism of the hypothermic effect of morphine in the rat following intracerebral and systemic administration. *J. Pharmacol. 150,* 420-425.

Lotti, V. J., Lomax, P., and George, R. (1965b). Temperature responses in the rat following intracerebral microinjection of morphine. *J. Pharmacol. 150,* 135-139.

Lotti, V. J., Lomax, P., and George, R. (1966). Acute tolerance to morphine following systemic and intracerebral injection in the rat. *Int. J. Neuro-pharmacol. 5,* 35-42.

Madden, J., Akil, H., Patrick, R. L., and Barchas, J. D. (1977). Stress-induced parallel changes in central opioid levels and pain responsiveness in the rat. *Nature 265,* 358-360.

Maines, R. E., Eipper, B. A., and Ling, N. (1977). Common precursor to corticotropins and endorphins. *Proc. Nat. Acad. Sci. USA 74,* 3014-3018.

Margules, D. L., Moisset, B., Lewis, M. J., Shibuya, H., and Pert, C. B. (1978). β-Endorphin is associated with overeating in genetically obese mice (ab/ab) and rats (fa/fa). *Science. In press.*

Mayer, D. J., and Liebeskind, J. C. (1974). Pain reduction by focal electrical stimulation of the brain. An anatomical and behavioral analysis. *Brain Res. 68,* 73-93.

Mayer, D. J., and Price, D. D. (1976). Central nervous system mechanisms of analgesia. *Pain 2,* 379-404.

Mayer, D. J., Price, D. D., and Rafie, A. (1977). Antagonism of acupuncture analgesia in man by the narcotic antagonist naloxone. *Brain Res. 121,* 368-372.

Mendelson, J. H., personal communication.

Mielke, D. H., and Gallant, D. M. (1977). An oral opiate antagonist in chronic schizophrenia. A pilot study. *Am. J. Psychiatry 134,* 1430-1431.

Miller, R. J., Meltzer, H. Y., and Fang, V. S. (1979). The distribution and pharmacology of the enkephalins. In *Endorphins and Mental Health Research,* E. Usdin, W. E. Bunney Jr., and N. S. Kline (Eds.). MacMillan, London.

Mohler, H., and Okada, T. (1977). Benzodiazepine receptor. Demonstration in central nervous system. *Science 198,* 849-851.

Moleman, P., and Bruinvels, J. (1976). Morphine catalepsy in relation to striatal and extrastriatal dopamine. *Prog. Neuropsychopharmacol. 1,* 101-106.

Mudge, A. W., Leeman, S. E., and Fischbodi, G. D. (1979). Effect of enkephalin on sensory neurons in cell culture. Inhibition of substance P release and reduction of inward calcium currents. In *Endorphins and Mental Health Research,* E. Usdin, W. E. Bunney, Jr., and N. S. Kline (Eds.). MacMillan, London.

Naber, D., Pickar, D., Dionne, R. A., Bowie, D. L., Ewels, B. A., Moody, T. W., Soble, M. G. and Pert, C. B. (1980). Assay of endogenous opiate receptor ligands in human CSF and plasma. *Substance and Alcohol Action/Abuse.* Vol. 1, pp. 113-118.

Nakamura, K., Kuntzman, R., Maggio, A., and Cormey, A. H. (1973). Decrease in morphine's analgesic action and increase in its cataleptic action by 6-hydroxydopamine injected bilaterally into caudate and putamen areas. *Neuropharmacology 12,* 1153-1160.

Nashold, B. S., Wilson, W. P., and Slaughter, D. G. (1969). Sensations evoked by stimulation in the midbrain of man. *J. Neurosurg. 30,* 14-24.

North, M. A. (1978). Naloxone reversal of morphine analgesia but failure to alter reactivity to pain in formalin test. *Life Sci. 22,* 295-302.

Nowycky, M. C. (1976). Central dopaminergic neurons. Studies of neuronal activity and transmitter dynamics after chronic drug treatments. Ph.D. Dissertation, Yale University, New Haven, Conn.

Oliveras, J. L., Redjemi, F., Guilbaud, G., and Besson, J. M. (1975). Analgesia induced by electrical stimulation of the inferior centralis nucleus of the raphe in the cat. *Pain 1,* 136-145.

Papeschi, R., Theiss, P., and Herz, A. (1975). Effects of morphine on the turnover of brain catecholamines and serotonin in rats—acute morphine administration. *Eur. J. Pharmacol. 34,* 253-261.

Pedigo, N., Derney, W. L., and Harris, L. S. (1975). Determination and characterization of the antinociceptive activity of intraventricularly administered acetylcholine in mice. *J. Pharmacol. Exp. Ther. 193,* 845-852.

Pert, A. (1975). Effects of opiates on rewarding and aversive brain stimulation in the rat. *Proc. 37th Ann. Meet. Committee for Drug Dependence,* National Academy of Sciences USA.

Pert, A. (1976). Behavioral pharmacology of D-alanine^2-methionine-enkephalin amide and other long-acting opiate peptides. In *Opiates and Endogenous Opioid Peptides,* H. W. Kosterlitz (Ed.). North-Holland, Amsterdam, pp. 87-94.

Pert, A. (1978). Effects of opiates and opioid peptides on the nigro striatal dopamine system. In *Opioids, Developments in Neuroscience,* Vol. 4. J. Van Ree and L. Terenius (Eds.). Elsevier/North-Holland, Amsterdam. In press.

Pert, A., and Yaksh, T. (1974). Sites of morphine induced analgesia in the primate brain. Relation to pain pathways. *Brain Res. 80,* 134-140.

Pert, A., and Hulsebus, R. (1975). Effect of morphine on intracranial self-stimulation behavior following brain amine depletion. *Life Sci. 17,* 19-20.

Pert, A., and Walter, M. (1976). Comparison between naloxone reversal of morphine and electrical stimulation induced analgesia in the rat mesencephalon. *Life Sci. 19,* 1023-1032.

Pert, A., and Sivit, C. (1977). Neuroanatomical focus for morphine and enkephalin-induced hypermotility. *Nature 265,* 645-647.

Pert, A., DeWald, L. A., Liao, H., and Sivit, C. (1979). Effects of opiates and opioid peptides on motor behaviors. Sites and mechanisms of action. In *Endorphins and Mental Health Research,* E. Usdin, W. E. Bunney, Jr., and N. S. Kline (Eds.). MacMillan, London.

Pert, C. B., and Snyder, S. H. (1973). Properties of opiate-receptor binding in rat brain. *Proc. Nat. Acad. Sci. USA 70,* 2243-2247.

Pert, C. B., and Snyder, S. H. (1974). Opiate-receptor binding of agonists and antagonists affected differentially by radium. *Mol. Pharmacol. 10,* 868-879.

Pert, C. B., and Garland, B. L. (1978). The mechanism of opiate agonist and antagonist action. In *Hormone Receptors,* Vol. 2. L. Birnbaum and B. W. O'Malley (Eds.). Academic, New York.

Pert, C. B., and Shibuya, H. (1978). Depletion of pituitary β-endorphin by forced drinking of 2% NaCl. In preparation.

Pert, C. B., Pasternak, G., and Snyder, S. H. (1973). Opiate agonists and antagonists discriminated by receptor binding in brain. *Science 182,* 1359-1361.

Pert, C. B., Kuhar, M. J., and Snyder, S. H. (1976a). Opiate receptor. Autoradiographic localization in rat brain. *Proc. Nat. Acad. Sci. USA 73,* 3729-3733.

Pert, C. B., Pert, A., and Tallman, J. F. (1976b). Isolation of a novel endogenous opiate analgesic from human blood. *Proc. Nat. Acad. Sci. USA 73,* 2226-2230.

Pert, C. B., Bowie, D. L., Fong, B. T. W., and Chang, J.-K. (1976c). Synthetic analogues of met-enkephalin which resist enzymatic destruction. In *Opiates and Endogenous Opioid Peptides,* H. W. Kosterlitz (Ed.). North-Holland, Amsterdam, pp. 79-86.

Pert, C. B., Pert, A., Chang, J.-K., and Fong, B. T. W. (1976d). [D-Ala^2]-met-enkephalinamide. A potent, long-lasting synthetic pentapeptide analgesic. *Science 194,* 330-332.

Pollard, H., Lllarens-Cortes, C., and Schwartz, J. C. (1977). Enkephalin receptors on dopaminergic neurons in rat striatum. *Nature 268,* 745-747.

Pomeranz, B., and Chiu, D. (1976). Naloxone blockade of acupuncture analgesia: endorphins implicated. *Life Sci. 19,* 1757-1762.

Proudfit, H. K., and Anderson, E. G. (1975). Morphine analgesia. Blockade by raphe magnus lesions. *Brain Res. 98,* 612-618.

Roberts, J. L., and Herbert, E. (1977). Characterizations of a common precursor to corticotropin and β-lipotropin. Cell-free synthesis of the precursor and identification of corticotropin peptides in the molecule. *Proc. Nat. Acad. Sci. USA 74,* 4826-4830.

Rossier, J., French, E. D., Rivier, C., Ling, N., Guillemin, R., and Bloom, F. (1977a). Foot-shock induced stress increases β-endorphin levels in blood but not brain. *Nature 270,* 618-620.

Rossier, J., Vargo, T. M., Minick, S., Ling, N., Bloom, F., and Guillemin, R. (1977b). Independent variation of β-endorphin and enkephalin levels in rat brain regions. *Proc. Nat. Acad. Sci. USA 74,* 5162-5165.

Sasame, H. A., Perez-Cruet, J., Di Chiara, G., Tagliamonte, A., Tagliamonte, P., and Gessa, G. L. (1972). Evidence that methadone blocks dopamine receptors in the brain. *J. Neurochem. 19,* 1953-1957.

Shiomi, H., and Takagi, H. (1974). Morphine analgesia and the bulbospinal noradrenergic system. Increase in the concentration of normetanephrine in the spinal cord of the rat caused by analgesics. *Br. J. Pharmacol. 52,* 519-526.

Simon, E. J., Hiller, J. M., and Edelman, I. (1973). Stereospecific binding of the potent narcotic analgesic [^{3}H] etorphine to rat brain homogenate. *Proc. Nat. Acad. Sci. USA 70,* 1947-1949.

Smith, C. B., Sheldon, M. I., Bednarczyk, J. H., and Villarreal, J. F. (1972). Morphine-induced increases in the incorporation of ^{14}C-tyramine into ^{14}C-dopamine and ^{14}C-norepinephrine in the mouse brain. Antagonism by naloxone and tolerance. *J. Pharmacol. Exp. Ther. 180,* 547-557.

Squires, R. I., and Braestrup, C. (1977). Benzodiazepine receptor in rat brain. *Nature 266,* 732-734.

Stein, L. (1968). Chemistry of reward and punishment. In *Pharmacology: A Review of Progress, 1957-1967,* D. H. Efron (Ed.). U. S. Government Printing Office, Public Health Service #1836, Washington, D.C., pp. 105-123.

Sugrue, M. F. (1974). The effects of acutely administered analgesics on the turnover of noradrenalin and dopamine in various regions of the rat brain. *Br. J. Pharmacol. 52,* 159-165.

Takagi, H., Doi, T., and Akaike, A. (1976). Microinjections of morphine into the medial part of the bulbar reticular formation in rabbit and rat. Inhibitory effects on lamina V cells of spinal dorsal horn and behavioral analgesia. In *Opiates and Endogenous Opioid Peptides,* H. W. Kosterlitz (Ed.). North-Holland, Amsterdam, pp. 191-198.

Terenius, L. (1973). Characterization of the "receptor" for narcotic analgesics in synaptic plasma membrane fraction from rat brain. *Acta Pharmacol. Toxicol. 33,* 377-384.

Terenius, L., Wahlstrom, A., Lindstrom, L., and Widerlov, E. (1976). Increased CSF levels of endorphins in chronic psychosis. *Neurosci. Lett. 3,* 157-162.

Trafton, C. L., and Marques, P. R. (1971). Effects of septal area and cingulate cortex lesions on opiate addiction behavior in the rat. *J. Comp. Physiol. Psychol. 75,* 277-285.

Tseng, L. F., Loh, H. H., and Li, C. H. (1976). Beta-endorphin as a potent analgesic by intravenous injection. *Nature 263,* 239-240.

Udenfriend, S., Rubinstein, M., and Stein, S. (1978). A reevaluation of the opioid peptides present in the central nervous system utilizing microfluorometric procedures. In *Endorphins and Mental Health Research,* E. Usdin, W. E. Bunney, Jr., and N. S. Kline (Eds.). MacMillan, New York. In press.

Uhl, G., Kuhar, M. J., Goodman, R. R., and Snyder, S. H. (1979). Histochemical localization of the enkephalins. In *Endorphins and Mental Health Research,* E. Usdin, W. E. Bunney, Jr., and N. S. Kline (Eds.). MacMillan, London.

Volavka, J., Mallya, A., Barg, S., and Perez-Cruet, J. (1977). Naloxone in chronic schizophrenia. *Science 196,* 1227-1228.

Watson, S. J., Berger, P. A., Akil, H., Mills, M. J., and Barchas, J. D. (1978). Effects of naloxone on schizophrenia. Reduction in hallucinations in subpopulation of subjects. *Science 201,* 73-76.

Watson, S. J., Akil, H., and Barchas, J. D. (1978). Immunohistochemical and biochemical studies of the enkephalins, β-endorphins and related peptides. In *Endorphins and Mental Health Research,* E. Usdin, W. E. Bunney, Jr., and N. S. Kline (Eds.). MacMillan, London.

Westerink, B. H. C. and Korf, J. (1975). Influence of drugs on striatal and limbic homovanillic acid concentrations in the rat brain. *Eur. J. Pharmacol. 33,* 31-40.

Woolf, C. J., Barrett, G. D., Mitchell, D., and Myers, R. A. (1977). Naloxone-reversible peripheral electroanalgesia in intact and spinal rats. *Eur. J. Pharmacol. 45,* 311-314.

Yaksh, T. L. and Rudy, T. A. (1976). Analgesia mediated by a direct spinal action of narcotics. *Science 192,* 1357-1358.

Yaksh, T. L., Yeung, J. C., and Rudy, T. A. (1976). An inability to antagonize with naloxone the elevated nociceptive thresholds resulting from electrical stimulation of the mesencephalic central gray. *Life Sci. 18,* 1193-1198.

Yaksh, T. L., Plant, R. L. and Rudy, T. A. (1977). Studies on the antagonism by raphe lesions of the antinociceptive actions of systemic morphine. *Eur. J. Pharmacol. 41,* 399-408.

Zieglgänsberger, W., and Bayerl, H. (1976). The mechanism of inhibition of neuronal activity by opiates in the spinal cord of the cat. *Brain Res. 115,* 111-128.

16

Biochemical Determinants of Parkinson's Disease

Oleh Hornykiewicz
Institute of Biochemical Pharmacology
University of Vienna, Vienna, Austria

I. INTRODUCTION

Clinical and Morphological Features of Parkinson's Disease

Parkinson's disease is a chronic and progressive degenerative disease of the central nervous system. Clinically, Parkinson's disease is a classic example of a dysfunction of the basal ganglia, notably the striatum (caudate nucleus + putamen), globus pallidus, and the associated nuclei. The various signs of basal ganglia dysfunction can be reduced to three cardinal extrapyramidal motor symptoms: tremor (shaking) at rest, cogwheel ("plastic") rigidity (stiffness) of the skeletal musculature, and akinesia, i.e., difficulty in initiating movements or modifying ongoing motor activity. These main symptoms usually are present, in varying degrees, in any of the three main etiological subgroups of Parkinson's disease, i.e., idiopathic Parkinson's disease (etiology unknown), postencephalitic parkinsonism (sequelae of von Economo's lethargic encephalitis), and the senile arteriosclerotic variety (Calne, 1970). The most consistent morphological brain lesion in Parkinson's disease is degeneration of the melanin-containing neurons in the compact zone of the substantia nigra (and, to a lesser degree, other melanin-containing brainstem nuclei, e.g., locus coeruleus) (Hassler, 1938). The biochemical basis for this selective cell death in Parkinson's disease is unknown.

The exact role of the substantia nigra for the functioning of the basal ganglia is not yet understood. Anatomically, this midbrain region occupies a strategic position, being situated between the higher subcortical extrapyramidal brain centers of the basal ganglia and the reticular formation of the brainstem and spinal cord (see Fig. 1). Experimental lesions of the substantia nigra in laboratory animals reproduce some of the main symptoms of Parkinson's disease, especially akinesia (Poirier and Sourkes, 1965).

II. BIOCHEMISTRY OF THE BASAL GANGLIA

Neurochemically Characterized Fiber Connections

For the understanding of the molecular pathology of Parkinson's disease the most important biochemical feature of the basal ganglia is their high content of several biologically active substances, especially dopamine (DA), acetylcholine (ACh), serotonin (5-HT), noradrenaline (NA), γ-aminobutyric acid (GABA), substance P, and enkephalin (Fonnum and Walaas, 1979). Figure 1 shows diagrammatically the most important neurochemically defined neuronal systems within the basal ganglia complex. Of these intraneuronally localized putative neurotransmitters, DA has attained a special significance. The DA found in high concentrations in the caudate nucleus and putamen is mostly confined to one well-defined pathway originating in the melanin-containing neurons of the

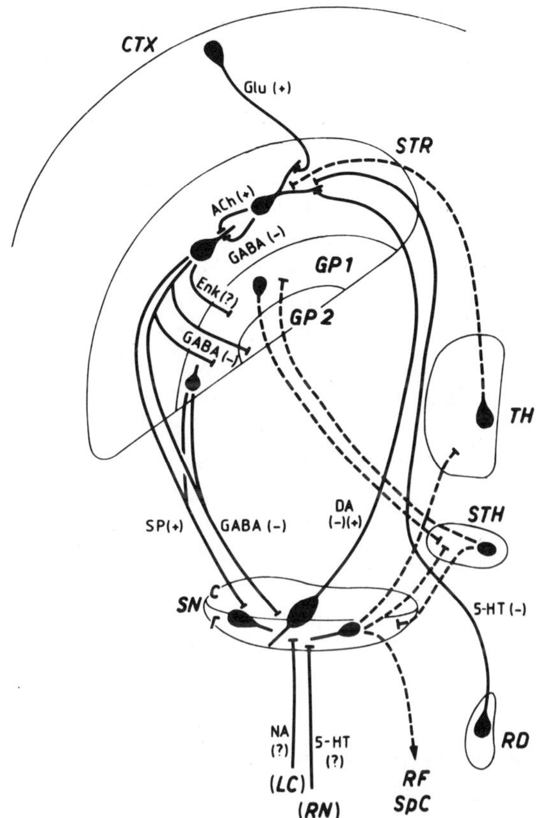

Figure 1 Simplified representation of the most important neurotransmitter systems within the basal ganglia complex. Those neurons (in the striatum and substantia nigra) that are shown to give rise to more than one neurochemically defined (or questionable) pathway have to be visualized as representing distinct and separate neuronal systems. The probable neurophysiological effects of the indicated putative neurotransmitters are: (+) excitatory; (-) inhibitory. Abbreviations: ACh = acetylcholine; CTX = cortex cerebri; DA = dopamine; Enk = enkephalin(s); GABA = γ-aminobutyric acid; Glu = glutamic acid; GP 1 = globus pallidus, external part; GP 2 = globus pallidus, internal part; 5-HT = serotonin; LC = locus coeruleus; NA = noradrenaline; RD = dorsal raphe nucleus; RF = reticular formation of the lower brainstem; RN = raphe nuclei; SN^c_r = substantia nigra, compact/reticular zone; SpC = spinal cord; STH = subthalamic nucleus; STR = striatum (caudate + putamen); TH = thalamus. (?) = the neurophysiological effect of a putative neurotransmitter, or the origin of the fiber system, not yet established. Dashed lines indicate pathways whose chemical neurotransmitters have not yet been identified.

compact zone of the substantia nigra and terminating (mostly synaptically) in the striatal nuclei (Fuxe et al., 1970). The neuronal systems containing ACh seem to be mostly intrinsic to the striatum, being part of the extensive striatal interneuronal networks. Neuropharmacological observations suggest that in the striatum the dopaminergic and cholinergic systems are functionally interdependent, a proper balance between them being essential for the proper functioning of these brain centers. Dopaminergic hyperactivity or cholinergic hypoactivity result in increased locomotion, hyperkinetic behavior, and hypotonia of the skeletal musculature; in contrast, DA deficiency or cholinergic hyperactivity in the striatum produce akinesia, rigidity of the skeletal muscles, and tremor (Hornykiewicz, 1972). As far as is known at present, the striatum gives rise to two distinct types of GABA neurons: GABAergic interneurons, and two efferent systems, a striatopallidal and a striatonigral pathway. The functional significance of these striatal GABA systems has not yet been fully elucidated; there is evidence that one of the possible functions of that division of the striatonigral GABA pathway terminating in the rostral portions of the substantia nigra is to inhibit the activity of the nigrostriatal DA pathway, possibly by way of a negative feedback mechanism (James and Starr, 1978).

In addition to these neuronal systems, the basal ganglia receive several inputs from the lower brainstem and the thalamus, including serotonergic and noradrenergic fiber systems as well as massive cortical, partly glutamatergic, projections.

III. BIOCHEMICAL DETERMINANTS OF PARKINSON'S DISEASE

A. Striatal Dopamine Deficiency

It has been mentioned that the main morphological lesion in Parkinson's disease is the loss of the melanin-containing neurons in the compact zone of the substantia nigra; these neurons are identical with the neurons giving rise to the nigral DA pathway innervating the striatum. Consequently, the main neurochemical feature of Parkinson's disease is a severe decrease in DA levels within the nigrostriatal (and pallidal) system (Ehringer and Hornykiewicz, 1960) (see Table 1). The striatal DA deficiency is accompanied by a decrease in homovanillic acid (HVA), DA's main metabolite (Bernheimer and Hornykiewicz, 1965) (see Table 1) as well as the DA-synthesizing enzymes tyrosine hydroxylase and dopa decarboxylase (Lloyd et al., 1975; Nagatsu et al., 1977). These alterations of the striatal dopaminergic system are characteristic of Parkinson's disease regardless of its etiology. The only determinant of the severity of the striatal DA deficiency is the degree of cell loss of the DA- (and melanin-) containing neurons in the substantia nigra (Bernheimer et al., 1973).

Table 1 Neurochemistry of Parkinson's Disease: Levels of DA, HVA, NA, 5-HT (all in μg/g); Activity of Glutamate Decarboxylase (in nmol CO_2/100 mg protein/2 hr); Specific Binding of [^{3}H]haloperidol to Membrane Preparations ([^{3}H]HAL) (in fmol/mg protein) in Some Regions of Basal Ganglia and Limbic Forebrain

Brain region		DA[a]	HVA[a]	Mol ratio DA/HVA	[^{3}H]HAL[b]	NA[c]	5-HT[d]	GAD[e]
Caudate nucleus	C[f]	4.52±0.63(8)	6.08±0.51(8)	1.2	42± 3(7)	0.12±0.02(9)	0.33(6)	1,318±185(13)
	P[g]	1.60±0.26(4)	2.30±0.56(4)	1.4	63±12(5)	–	0.12(5)	641(2)
Putamen	C	5.37±0.70(8)	11.40±1.63(8)	2.0	44± 5(7)	0.13±0.02(9)	0.32(6)	1,243±220(13)
	P	0.50±0.10(4)	2.06±0.44(4)	4.1	69± 4(9)	–	0.14(5)	583(2)
Subst. nigra	C	0.46(13)	2.32(7)	4.7	–	0.23±0.05(9)	–	1,273±306(13)
	P	0.07(10)	0.41(9)	5.4	–	0.11±0.03(3)	–	526(2)
Nucl. accumbens	C	3.79±0.82(8)	4.38±0.64(8)	1.1	–	1.29±0.14(7)	–	–
	P	1.61±0.28(4)	3.13±0.13(3)	1.9	–	0.52±0.11(4)	–	–
Lat hypothal.	C	0.51±0.08(4)	1.96±0.28(3)	3.6	–	1.25±0.09(8)	–	–
	P	<0.03(2)	1.03±0.23(3)	–	–	0.36±0.07(3)	–	–
Parolfact. gyr.	C	0.35±0.09(4)	0.98(2)	2.6	–	0.14±0.11(5)	–	–
	P	<0.03(2)	–	–	–	–	–	–

‡

[a]From Price et al. (1978); [b]from Lee et al. (1978); [c]from Farley and Hornykiewicz (1976); [d]from Bernheimer et al. (1961); [e]from Lloyd and Hornykiewicz (1973); [f]C = controls; [g]P = Parkinson's disease. Except for the column "Mol ratio DA/HVA," the figures in all other columns indicate the mean value ± sem, with number of analyzed brains in parentheses.

B. Compensatory Mechanisms Elicited by the Striatal Dopamine Deficiency

As expected, the dopaminergic denervation of the Parkinsonian striatum elicits two important compensatory mechanisms, namely, (1) overactivity of the remaining DA neurons and (2) denervation-type supersensitivity of the striatal postsynaptic DA receptors. The presence of these functionally very important compensatory mechanisms can be concluded from observations showing that (1) in the Parkinsonian striatum, the ratio DA/HVA is shifted in favor of the metabolite (Bernheimer and Hornykiewicz, 1965) (see Table 1), indicating an increased turnover (= synthesis and release) of DA in the remaining neurons (Hornykiewicz, 1966); and (2) the specific binding (in vitro) of [^{3}H] haloperidol and other DA receptor blockers (tagging the postsynaptic DA rcccptors) sccms to be significantly increased in the parkinsonian striatum, especially putamen (see Table 1), indicating an increased number, or increased affinity, of the postsynaptic DA receptor sites (Lee et al., 1978). The existence of this (denervation-type) supersensitivity of the parkinsonian striatum is supported by clinicopharmacological observations indicating that (1) patients with more severe symptoms (akinesia) and consequently higher degrees of striatal DA deficiency usually react more sensitively to L-dopa than patients with milder symptoms (Bernheimer et al., 1973); and (2) only in parkinsonian subjects low (therapeutic) doses of L-dopa produce hyperkinetic-dyskinetic side effects of striatal origin.

C. Relationship Between Striatal Dopamine Deficiency and Parkinsonian Symptomatology

Of crucial importance for the specificity of the striatal DA deficiency in Parkinson's disease is the demonstration that there exists a close cause-effect relationship between the striatal DA decrease and the severity of the parkinsonian symptoms. In this respect, the following observations are particularly relevant: (1) in a case with hemiparkinsonism the neurochemical changes were more pronounced in the striatum contralateral to the affected side of the body (Barolin et al., 1964); (2) the degree of striatal DA and HVA deficiency was found to be positively correlated with the severity of symptoms, notably akinesia (Bernheimer et al., 1973); and (3) functional replacement of the missing DA by its immediate precursor L-dopa (which in contrast to DA penetrates the blood-brain barrier) is highly efficacious in improving the main clinical features of Parkinson's disease, especially akinesia (Birkmayer and Hornykiewicz, 1961; Barbeau et al., 1962; Cotzias et al., 1967).

D. Compensated and Decompensated Stages of Parkinson's Disease

An important quantitative aspect of the neurochemical pathology of Parkinson's disease is that the diseased striatum can effectively compensate lower degrees of DA deficiency, with the overall result that the condition will remain clinically silent. This most likely explains the observation that even mild, clinically just detectable symptoms were observed to be associated with a disproportionately high degree of striatal DA deficiency (Bernheimer et al., 1973). It seems that the decrease of striatal DA has to exceed the 70-80% mark (i.e., only 20-30% of DA remaining) in order to produce clinically manifest symptoms. Thus, from a neurochemical point of view, Parkinson's disease can be subdivided into two stages (Hornykiewicz, 1973): (1) the compensated, clinically latent stage during which the remaining DA neurons can offset functionally the progressive decrease in striatal DA and (2) the stage of decompensation, i.e., the clinically overt syndrome which manifests itself only when the degree of striatal DA deficiency exceeds the compensatory capacity of the affected basal ganglia. It is obvious that the mentioned overactivity of the remaining DA neurons as well as the supersensitivity of the (denervated) DA receptors must play an important role for the functional compensation. From the above neurochemical considerations it follows that the main goal of a specific drug therapy of Parkinson's disease—such as the DA substitution by L-dopa or other direct-acting DA-mimetic drugs—will be to revert the decompensated stage of the striatal DA deficiency to the stage of functional compensation (Hornykiewicz, 1974).

E. Other Basal Ganglia Neurotransmitter Systems in Parkinson's Disease

In view of the interdependence of the striatal dopaminergic and cholinergic mechanisms (see Section II.A), the striatal DA deficiency in Parkinson's disease may be expected to result in a relative cholinergic predominance. This tipping of the DA-ACh balance in favor of ACh may aggravate the symptoms (such as rigidity and akinesia) primarily due to the striatal DA deficiency. This secondary cholinergic predominance probably explains the (modest) clinical effectiveness of anticholinergic agents in Parkinson's disease.

The deficiency of DA in the nigrostriatal neuron system is the most prominent and functionally most significant neurochemical abnormality in Parkinson's disease. However, in addition, several other putative neurotransmitter systems seem to be deranged in this disorder (see Table 1). Thus, the striatal levels of 5-HT (Bernheimer et al., 1961; Rinne et al., 1974) as well as the activity of the GABA-synthesizing enzyme glutamate decarboxylase (GAD) (Bernheimer and Hornykiewicz, 1962; McGeer et al., 1971; Lloyd and Hornykiewicz, 1973; Rinne et al., 1974) are significantly subnormal. Similarly, the concentration of NA in several forebrain regions, including the nucleus accumbens, is reduced in Parkinson's disease (Farley and Hornykiewicz, 1976). Whereas the reduction of NA may be due to loss of NA-containing neurons in lower brainstem nuclei, especially the locus coeruleus, no anatomical substrate is known for the changes of the striatal 5-HT and GAD. Since both the 5-HT and GABA neurons seem to supress the activity of the nigrostriatal DA system, it is possible that the changes of these two inhibitory systems are functional in nature, intended to release from inhibition the already reduced DA system (Hornykiewicz, 1976).

F. Therapeutic Efficacy of L-dopa in Parkinson's Disease

From the clinical point of view, the most significant consequence of the recent advances in neurochemistry of Parkinson's disease has been the introduction of L-dopa as a potent and specific, although mostly symptomatic, pharmacotherapeutic agent for Parkinson's disease (Birkmayer and Hornykiewicz, 1961; Barbeau et al., 1962; Cotzias et al., 1967). L-dopa's high therapeutic efficacy probably is greatly determined by, and dependent on, three factors: (1) preservation of a critical minimum number of DA (and possibly 5-HT) terminals in the striatum containing the enzymatic machinery for the conversion of L-dopa to DA (i.e., dopa decarboxylase); (2) the compensatory overactivity of the remaining nigrostriatal DA neurons; and (3) the development of (denervation) supersensitivity to DA of the striatal postsynaptic DA receptors. These factors ensure that (1) large amounts of DA are formed from the administered L-dopa and released at the terminals of the overactive remaining nigrostriatal DA neurons and (2) after diffusion into the vicinity of the terminals, the newly formed DA produces an augmented physiological response at the supersensitive DA receptor sites (Hornykiewicz, 1974).

IV. LIMBIC DOPAMINE IN PARKINSON'S DISEASE: BRIDGE BETWEEN NEUROLOGY AND BIOLOGICAL PSYCHIATRY

In addition to the severe depletion of DA in the striatal nuclei, there is in Parkinson's disease a decrease of DA levels in several regions of the limbic forebrain (see Table 1). These regions include the nucleus accumbens (septi), the lateral hypothalamus, and the parolfactory gyrus (Brodmann area 25) (Price et al., 1978). These limbic DA changes are noteworthy in several respects. From a pharmacological point of view, and in analogy to the striatal DA, the accumbens

DA system seems to subserve a "kinetic" function in the brain. Thus, pharmacological manipulations of the accumbens DA levels produce marked changes in (loco)motor behavior (Pijnenburg et al., 1976; Iversen and Koob, 1977). The role of accumbens DA in motor function makes it likely that in addition to the role played by the striatal DA deficiency, the DA deficiency in the nucleus accumbens will significantly contribute to some motor deficits, especially akinesia, in Parkinson's disease (Price et al., 1978).

In addition to these recently uncovered motor functions of the limbic forebrain, disturbances of limbic function have long been implicated in affective disorders as well as some behavioral abnormalities seen in schizophrenic patients (MacLean, 1970). These possibilities suggest that in Parkinson's disease the observed disturbances of DA metabolism in some of the limbic forebrain regions, especially the lateral hypothalamus and the parolfactory gyrus, may be an important etiological factor for the affective disturbances often presented by patients with Parkinson's disease. In respect to schizophrenia, recently a functional hyperactivity of limbic DA mechanisms (including the possibility of abnormally sensitive DA receptors) has been considered (Matthysee, 1974; Snyder, 1974). If pursued logically, this hypothesis seems to imply that because of the decreased limbic DA (and HVA) levels in Parkinson's disease, the incidence of schizophrenic symptoms should be abnormally low in this disorder. Although there do not seem to exist any large-scale studies, recently the appearance of schizophrenic symptomatology in a small group of patients with a long-standing history of Parkinson's disease has been reported (Crow et al., 1976). It is to be expected that further studies along these lines will help to bridge the current gap between neurology and biological psychiatry, shedding light on many neurochemically as yet poorly defined disturbances of brain function.

REFERENCES

Barbeau, A., Sourkes, T. L., and Murphy, G. (1972). Les catecholamines dans la maladie de Parkinson. In *Monoamines et Systeme Nerveux Central,* J. de Ajuriaguerra (Ed.). Georg, Geneva and Masson, Paris, pp. 246-262.

Barolin, G. S., Bernheimer, H., and Hornykiewicz, O. (1964). Seitenverschiedenes Verhalten des Dopamins (3-Hydroxytyramin) im Gehirn eines Falles von Hemiparkinsonismus. *Schweiz. Arch. Neurol. Psychiatry 94,* 241-248.

Bernheimer, H., and Hornykiewicz, O. (1962). Das Verhalten einiger Enzyme im Gehrin normaler und Parkinson-kranker Menschen. *Arch. Exp. Pathol. Pharmak. 243,* 295.

Bernheimer, H., and Hornykiewicz, O. (1965). Herabgesetzte Konzentration der Homovanillinsäure im Gehirn von Parkinsonkranken Menschen als

Ausdruck der Störung des zentralen Dopaminstoffwechsels. *Klin. Wschr. 43,* 711-715.

Bernheimer, H., Birkmayer, W., and Hornykiewicz, O. (1961). Verteilung des 5-Hydroxytryptamins (Serotonin) im Gehirn des Menschen und sein Verhalten bei Patieten mit Parkinson-Syndrom. *Klin. Wschr. 39,* 1056-1059.

Bernheimer, H., Birkmayer, W., Hornykiewicz, O., Jellinger, K., and Seitelberger, F. (1973). Brain dopamine and the syndromes of Parkinson and Huntington. *J. Neurol. Sci. 20,* 415-455.

Birkmayer, W., and Hornykiewicz, O. (1961). Der L-Dioxyphenylalanin (= L-DOPA)–Effekt bei der Parkinson-Akinese. *Wien. Klin. Wschr. 73,* 787-788.

Calne, D. B. (1970). *Parkinsonism.* Arnold, London, pp. 1-136.

Cotzias, G. C., Van Woert, M. H., and Schiffer, L. M. (1967). Aromatic amino acids and modification of parkinsonism. *N. Engl. J. Med. 276,* 374-379.

Crow, T. J., Johnstone, E. C., and McClelland, H. A. (1976). The coincidence of schizophrenia and parkinsonism. Some neurochemical implications. *Psychol. Med. 6,* 227-233.

Ehringer, H., and Hornykiewicz, O. (1960). Verteilung von Noradrenalin und Dopamin (3-Hydroxytyramin) im Gehirn des Menschen und ihr Verhalten bei Erkrankungen des extrapyramidalen Systems. *Klin. Wschr. 38,* 1236-1239.

Farley, I. J., and Hornykiewicz, O. (1976). Noradrenaline in subcortical brain regions of patients with Parkinson's disease and control subjects. In *Advances in Parkinsonism,* W. Birkmayer and O. Hornykiewicz (Eds.). Basle, Editiones Roche, pp. 178-185.

Fonnum, F., and Walaas, I. (1979). Localisation of neurotransmitter candidates in neostriatum. In *The Neostriatum,* I. Divac and R. G. E. Öberg (Eds.). Pergamon, Oxford, pp. 53-69.

Fuxe, K., Hökfelt, T., and Ungerstedt, U. (1970). Morphological and functional aspects of central monoamine neurons. *Int. Rev. Neurobiol. 13,* 93-126.

Hassler, R. (1938). Zur Pathologie der Paralysis agitans und des postenzephalitischen Parkinsonismus. *J. Psychol. Neurol.* (Lpz.) *48,* 387-476.

Hornykiewicz, O. (1966). Dopamine (3-hydroxytyramine) and brain function. *Pharmacol. Rev. 18,* 925-962.

Hornykiewicz, O. (1972). Biochemical and pharmacological aspects of akinesia. In *Parkinson's Disease,* Vol. 1, J. Siegfried (Ed.). Huber, Bern, pp. 128-149.

Hornykiewicz, O. (1973). Parkinson's disease. From brain homogenate to treatment. *Fed. Proc. 32,* 183-190.

Hornykiewicz, O. (1974). The mechanisms of action of L-dopa in Parkinson's disease. *Life Sci. 15,* 1249-1259.

Hornykiewicz, O. (1976). Neurohumoral interactions and basal ganglia function and dysfunction. In *The Basal Ganglia,* M. D. Yahr (Ed.). Raven, New York, pp. 269-278.

Iversen, S. D., and Knoob, G. F. (1977). Behavioral implications of dopaminergic neurons in the mesolimbic system. *Adv. Biochem. Psychopharmacol. 16,* 209-214.

James, T. A., and Starr, M. S. (1978). The role of GABA in the substantia nigra. *Nature 275,* 229-230.

Lee, T., Seeman, P., Rajput, A., Farley, I. J., and Hornykiewicz, O. (1978). Receptor basis for dopaminergic supersensitivity in Parkinson's disease. *Nature 273,* 59-61.

Lloyd, K. G., Davidson, L., and Hornykiewicz, O. (1975). The neurochemistry of Parkinson's disease. Effect of L-dopa therapy. *J. Pharmacol. 195,* 453-464.

Matthysse, S. (1974). Schizophrenia. Relationships to dopamine transmission, motor control, and feature extraction. In *The Neurosciences,* Third Study Program, F. O. Schmitt and F. G. Worden (Eds.). MIT Press, Cambridge, pp. 733-737.

McGeer, P. L., McGeer, E. G., Wada, J. A., and Jung, E. (1971). Effects of globus pallidus lesions and Parkinson's disease on brain glutamic acid decarboxylase. *Brain Res. 32,* 425-431.

MacLean, P. (1970). The limbic brain in relation to the psychoses. In *Physiological Correlates of Emotion,* P. Black (Ed.). Academic, New York, pp. 129-146.

Nagatsu, T., Kato, T., Numata (Sudo), Y., Ikuta, K., Sano, M., Nagatsu, I., Kondo, Y., Inagaki, S., Iizuka, R., Hori, A., and Narabayashi, H. (1977). Phenylethanolamine N-methyltransferase and other enzymes of catecholamine metabolism in human brain. *Clin. Chem. Acta 75,* 221-232.

Pijnenburg, A. J. J., Honig, W. M. M., Van der Heyden, J. A. M., and Van Rossum, J. M. (1976). Effects of chemical stimulation of the mesolimbic dopamine system upon locomotor activity. *Eur. J. Pharmacol. 35,* 45-58.

Poirier, L. J., and Sourkes, T. L. (1965). Influence of the substantia nigra on the dopamine content of the striatum. *Brain 88,* 181-192.

Price, K. S., Farley, I. J., and Hornykiewicz, O. (1978). Neurochemistry of Parkinson's disease. Relation between striatal and limbic dopamine. *Adv. Biochem. Psychopharmacol. 19,* 293-300.

Rinne, U. K., Sonninen, V., Rickkinen, P., and Laaksonen, H. (1974). Dopaminergic nervous transmission in Parkinson's disease. *Med. Biol. 52,* 208-217.

Snyder, S. H. (1974). Catecholamines as mediators of drug effects in schizophrenia. In *The Neurosciences,* Third Study Program, F. O. Schmitt and F. G. Worden (Eds.). MIT Press, Cambridge, pp. 721-732.

17

Huntington's Chorea

Edward D. Bird* and Leslie L. Iversen
University of Cambridge Medical School, Addenbrooke's Hospital
Cambridge, England

**Present affiliation:* McLean Hospital, Belmont, Massachusetts, Harvard Medical School and Massachusetts General Hospital, Boston, Massachusetts.

I. INTRODUCTION

The basic neurotransmitter defects in clinical disorders involving the basal ganglia are being clarified through the analysis of postmortem brain from patients dying with these disorders. The discovery of a defect in dopamine production in Parkinson's disease and the relief of symptoms by L-dopa therapy has stimulated interest in the neurochemical findings in Huntington's chorea. This is a dominantly inherited disorder with progressive degeneration of nerve cells throughout the whole brain, with the most severe atrophy occurring in the basal ganglia. Huntington (1872) had observed families with this disorder in his father's practice and wrote a very clear description of this disorder the year he graduated in medicine at Columbia University. The onset of involuntary movements is heralded by occasional facial twitching, starting in middle life and followed by a progressive increase in twisting movements affecting the whole body. After about 15 years the patient is bedridden and usually dies of bronchopneumonia. This disorder is called Huntington's *disease* in the United States to acknowledge other clinical manifestations which may occur at various stages of the disease without choreiform movements.

Psychiatric abnormalities similar to those seen in schizophrenia may occur some 10-15 years before the onset of choreiform movements. This is more likely to appear in families in which the onset of the chorea occurs at an earlier age than usual. Such patients may have visual hallucinations and paranoia, and communication may be difficult. They may exhibit a catatonic posture and are often admitted to a psychiatric hospital with a diagnosis of schizophrenia if the psychiatrist has no knowledge of chorea in the family.

Dementia rarely occurs before the onset of choreiform movements but is commonly seen after the onset of chorea and runs a progressive course. It is not as severe when chorea has its onset late in life. The appearance of dementia in the last 5 years of the illness is associated with a more rapidly progressive clinical deterioration.

Epilepsy may occur when the onset of the disease is very early. One patient who died at the age of 5½ years had the typical histopathological changes of Huntington's chorea and the neurochemical abnormalities were similar to those described below for adult chorea. Rigidity is a feature often seen in young cases (Westphal, 1905); however, many adult cases now being kept alive as a result of antibiotic treatment for their frequent bouts of pneumonia often have severe rigidity in the late stages of their disease.

Histopathological findings will vary at different stages of the disease. The earliest change is a loss of small cells, particularly in the caudal caudate and putamen (Bruyn, 1968). These small cells may be GABA-containing and/or cholinergic interneurons. Progressive loss of small cells in more rostral regions of the basal ganglia is associated with a loss of larger cells. There is an extreme degree of basal ganglia atrophy in the rapidly progressive juvenile form of the

Table 1 Neurochemical Determinations in the Caudate Nucleus of Huntington's Chorea and Control Brain

Assay	Control	Chorea	*P*
GAD[a]	43.1 ± 2.8 (111)	16.5 ± 2.0 (91)	<.001
CAT[a]	184 ± 9.5 (89)	105 ± 16.2 (60)	<.001
T-OH[a] (tyrosine hydroxylase)	24.7 ± 5.3 (23)	33.5 ± 10.6 (22)	n.s.
Dopamine[b]	24.7 ± 4.1 (32)	15.4 ± 2.5 (33)	<.05
5-HT[c]	0.50 ± 0.15 (23)	0.69 ± 32 (15)	n.s.
Substance P[d]	3.7 ± 0.8 (18)	3.5 ± 0.6 (19)	n.s.

[a]μmol/g protein.
[b]μg/g protein.
[c]μg/g (wet weight).
[d]nmol/g protein.

disease (Campbell et al., 1961) and in the adult cases kept alive for long periods in hospital. The neurochemical changes in these cases are not only associated with loss of neurons but also reflect the consequences of an increased density of the remaining neurons.

II. γ-AMINOBUTYRIC ACID

A rational neurochemical explanation for choreiform movements was discovered when Perry et al. (1973) found a significant decrease in the neuroinhibitory neurotransmitter γ-aminobutyric acid (GABA) and Bird et al. (1973) found a large decrease in the biosynthetic enzyme for GABA, glutamic acid decarboxylase (GAD) in the caudate nucleus, putamen, globus pallidus, and substantia nigra of choreic postmortem brain (see Table 1). In other brain areas such as frontal cortex, hypothalamus, and hippocampus there was no significant decrease in GAD activity (Bird and Iversen, 1974,1976). The loss of GABA and GAD from basal ganglia tissue has been confirmed by several other studies (McGeer et al., 1973; Stahl and Swanson, 1974; Urquhart et al., 1975) and remains a most consistent finding in our own work which now extends to a series of more than 150 choreic brains. The loss of GAD appears to represent a biochemical reflection of progressive basal ganglia atrophy in the disease, since the decrease in GAD activity is not as great in those choreic patients who die earlier than expected in the course of their disease.

Table 2 Neurotransmitter Receptor Binding in Huntington's Chorea and Control Brain Tissue (pmol/mg protein)

Receptor	GABA	Muscarinic acetylcholine	5-HT
Caudate			
Control	0.15 ± 0.01 (16)	1.36 ± 0.05 (16)	0.085 ± 0.005 (5)
Chorea	0.11 ± 0.01 (15)	0.65 ± 0.08[a] (15)	0.057 ± 0.005[b] (5)
Frontal cortex			
Control	0.36 ± 0.01 (16)	0.73 ± 0.05 (16)	0.12 ± 0.01 (6)
Chorea	0.39 ± 0.03 (15)	0.66 ± 0.05 (15)	0.14 ± 0.02 (4)
Substantia nigra			
Control	0.018		
Chorea	0.033[c]		

[a] = $P < .001$.
[b] = $P < .025$.
[c] = $P < .01$.

A complication in interpreting GAD results obtained from human post-mortem brain samples is that GAD activity is considerably reduced (approximately 50%) in patients dying after prolonged terminal illness. This effect is seen in all brain regions (Spokes, 1979) and has an important bearing on the data obtained from patients dying with Huntington's chorea, in whom sudden deaths are uncommon. Thus, if data from Huntington's chorea are compared with those from control subjects who died after prolonged illness, the changes in GAD observed are somewhat less marked than if all control data are used; the reduction in GAD is, nevertheless, a consistent feature and is restricted to basal ganglia regions.

The GABA concentration in CSF samples from choreic patients has been found to be decreased when compared with controls (Glaeser et al., 1975), but the decrease does not appear to correlate with the length of illness (Wastek et al., 1977). Since it would appear that the decrease in GAD activity in the basal ganglia is slowly progressive in Huntington's chorea, it seems unlikely that GABA CSF concentrations will be useful as a predictive test for "at risk" subjects.

Using a technique for measuring the density of GABA receptors which involves the measurement of the bicuculline-sensitive binding of radioactively labled GABA to synaptic membrane fragments, Enna et al. (1976) found that the density of such receptors in choreic tissues was normal or even increased (see Table 2). This, therefore, provides a stimulus to search for GABA-like agents that might cross the blood-brain barrier and inhibit the choreiform movements.

More recent studies, however, by Lloyd et al. (1977) and by Iversen et al. (1978) show a substantial decrease in the density of GABA binding sites in basal ganglia tissue from Huntington's chorea patients. The results obtained were very variable, with some samples showing essentially normal densities of GABA sites, and others very low values. The individual variability perhaps explains why no differences in GABA binding were observed in our earlier studies, and suggests that GABA therapy may be applicable only to some Huntington's patients.

Mapping neurotransmitters within the substantia nigra provides some understanding of the abnormal movements of Huntington's chorea and their response to neuropharmacological agents. In the rostral region of the substantia nigra the dopaminergic neurons which contain melanin pigment are localized within the zona compacta, and the activity of tyrosine hydroxylase and the concentration of dopamine is normally twice as high in this region as the zona reticulata. GAD activity and GABA concentration, however, are greater in the zona reticulata, where most of the GABA-containing striatonigral afferents terminate (Fig. 1).

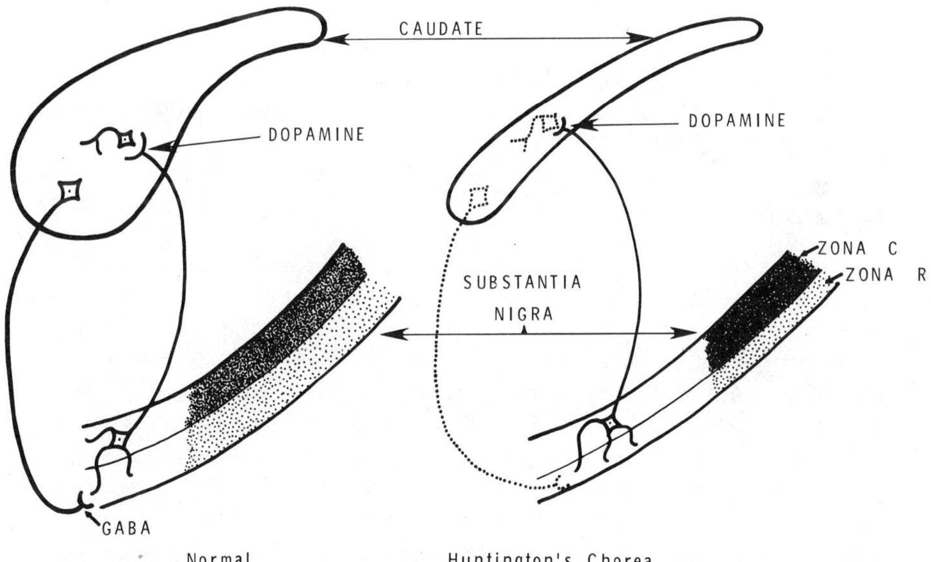

Figure 1 Schematic representation of the striatal-nigral connections showing dopaminergic pathways from the zona compacta to the striatum and GABAergic pathways from the striatum to the zona reticulata in both the control and choreic brain.

In Huntington's chorea, the whole brainstem is reduced in size and the substantia nigra appears more darkly pigmented than usual, and on cross-section the zona reticulata is more atrophic than the zona compacta. GAD activity in the whole substantia nigra is reduced by 75%, whereas the activity of tyrosine hydroxylase, the density of GABA receptors, and the concentration of dopamine per unit tissue weight are increased, sometimes twofold. This increase, however, no doubt reflects the increased density of dopaminergic cell bodies secondary to the loss of other neurons in this region. The total volume of the choreic substantia nigra is reduced by about 50% (Spokes, unpublished data; see also Fig. 1).

III. DOPAMINE

As suggested above, the dopamine cell bodies in the substantia nigra appear to remain intact in Huntington's chorea (Forno and Jose, 1973). The amount of dopamine found at terminals of these neurons in the putamen is not significantly decreased although there is a significant decrease of dopamine in the caudate nucleus (Bernheimer and Hornykiewicz, 1973; Bird and Iversen, 1974) (see Table 1). A great deal of attention has been directed to measurements of dopamine and its metabolite homovanillic acid (HVA) in Huntington's chorea because choreiform movements appear to reflect an overactivity of CNS dopamine mechanisms. The failure to find increased dopamine or HVA in either the postmortem choreic brain or in CSF samples from choreic patients (Curzon et al., 1972) led to the suggestion that the postsynaptic receptor for dopamine was hyperresponsive (Klawans, 1970).

IV. ACETYLCHOLINE

The marker enzyme for cholinergic neurons, choline acetyltransferase (CAT), was found to be decreased in the caudate and putamen of choreic brain but not to the same degree as GAD (see Table 1). There was no significant decrease in CAT activity in other regions of the brain where normally the CAT activity is less than a tenth of the activity in the putamen. Several choreic cases had normal CAT activity in basal ganglia and in such cases the decrease in GAD activity was not as marked as usual (Bird and Iversen, 1974,1976). McGeer et al. (1973) and Aquilonius et al. (1975) also reported a decrease in CAT activity in choreic brain and have each had a choreic case with normal CAT activity. We found that CAT correlated directly with GAD activity in the choreic tissues and noted that normal CAT activity but decreased GAD activity usually occurred in patients who died suddenly at an early stage of the disease.

The density of muscarinic acetylcholine receptors was measured in the postmortem choreic and control brain, and was found to be diminished by 50%

in the basal ganglia but not in frontal cortex (see Table 2) (Hiley and Bird, 1974; Enna et al., 1976).

V. 5-HYDROXYTRYPTAMINE

The cell bodies for serotoninergic neurons are located in the midbrain raphe nuclei with terminals in the basal ganglia. Bernheimer and Hornykiewicz (1973) found an increase in serotonin (5-hydroxytryptamine or 5-HT) concentration in both the central grey area that contains the raphe nuclei and the basal ganglia of choreic brain. The numbers of brains analyzed, however, were small. We also found increased 5-HT in these regions (Curzon and Bird, 1977) (see Table 1). Increased 5-HT concentration appears to be inversely related to the GAD concentration, suggesting that with more severe degeneration of GABA neurons there is a greater density of serotoninergic nerve terminals.

On the other hand, Enna et al. (1976) found that the density of 5-HT receptors was significantly decreased in choreic brain in the caudate nucleus, putamen, and globus pallidus but normal in the frontal cortex (see Table 2).

VI. 5-HYDROXYTRYPTOPHAN

The synthesis of 5-HT in the brain is dependent on the amount of free tryptophan in plasma and on concentrations of competing plasma amino acids (Fernstrom and Wurtman, 1972). The increased concentrations of serotonin in choreic brain might, therefore, be due to the decreased plasma concentrations of leucine, isoleucine, and valine in choreic patients (Perry et al., 1969). The decrease in free tryptophan concentration in plasma of choreic subjects (Phillipson and Bird, 1977) may reflect an increased transport of tryptophan out of the plasma compartment *into* brain and other tissues.

VII. MELATONIN

The involuntary movements of chorea disappear during sleep, and it is therefore important to consider neurochemical variations during sleep. Melatonin is synthesized in the pineal gland from 5-hydroxytryptamine by the enzymes serotonin-N-acetyltransferase (SNAT) and hydroxyindole-O-methyltransferase (HIOMT). Both melatonin and the synthetic enzymes exhibit a nyctohemeral rhythm in the rat (Axelrod et al., 1965) and human pineal gland (Smith et al., 1977). Concentrations of the pineal synthetic enzymes and plasma melatonin are highest at 0200 hr. In postmortem choreic pineal glands and in plasma from living choreic patients there was no significant difference in either the concentration of melatonin and activity of SNAT and HIOMT or in the nyctohemeral rhythm when compared to controls (Gonsalkorale, personal communication).

VIII. SUBSTANCE P

The undecapeptide substance P is highly concentrated in the human substantia nigra (Lembeck and Zetler, 1962; Duffy et al., 1975; Gale et al., 1977). In the substantia nigra and globus pallidus of postmortem choreic brain the substance P (SP) concentration is significantly decreased (Kanazawa et al., 1977; Gale et al., 1977). In animals, lesions in the striatum lead to a decreased concentration of SP and GAD activity in the substantia nigra, suggesting that cell bodies of SP- and GABA-containing neurons in the striatum project to terminals in the substantia nigra (Emson et al., 1976). In Huntington's chorea, cell body degeneration in the striatum probably produces the changes in SP and GAD in substantia nigral terminals.

IX. GROWTH HORMONE

The neurons producing the various peptide-releasing factors in the hypothalamus appear to be under some regulation by dopamine, noradrenaline, and 5-hydroxytryptophan (5-HTP) (Wurtman, 1971). Since the abnormal movements in chorea may be due to excessive dopamine activity, one might expect alterations in the release of hypothalamic releasing factors that are controlled by dopamine. Plasma growth hormone (GH) concentrations have been shown to be increased by the administration of L-dopa to normal subjects (Boyd et al., 1970). This effect of L-dopa is assumed to be at the level of the hypothalamus, but might also be in the pituitary gland. L-dopa may inhibit the production and/or release of the hypothalamic peptide somatostatin. The concentration of growth hormone in plasma is increased in choreics (Phillipson and Bird, 1976), with a greater increase in GH in response to L-dopa in choreics compared to controls (Podolsky and Leopold, 1974). Associated with the increase, in GH, plasma-fasting free fatty acids (FFA) are also increased in choreic patients (Phillipson and Bird, 1977). The concentrations of growth hormone are not as high as those seen in acromegaly and therefore tissue changes are not apparent. Free fatty acids can inhibit the glycolytic enzyme phosphofructokinase (PFK), an enzyme that we have found to be significantly depressed in choreic brain tissue (Ramadoss et al., 1976). The overall metabolic effect of these changes in Huntington's chorea will require further investigation.

X. GONADOTROPIC RELEASING FACTOR

It has been known for some time that choreic women have more children than their nonchoreic siblings. Menorrhagia is a significant problem in a number of women and sexual activity in some women is so demanding that their husbands plead for some medication to dampen their wives' libido. The large number of illegitimate offspring as a result of this sexual activity only compounds the problem of the preservation of the abnormal gene within the population.

Gonadotropic releasing factor (GnRF) given to female rats will produce mounting behavior (Moss and McCann, 1973) and GnRF given to men for infertility increases libido (Mortimer et al., 1974). GnRF is produced by cells in the preoptic region of the hypothalamus whose axons project to the median eminence for storage before release. We measured GnRF by radioimmunoassay in the hypothalamus and median eminence of postmortem choreic and control brain and found that there was a significant increase in the concentration of GnRF in the female choreic brain, but not in the male choreic tissue (Bird et al., 1976).

The GnRF cell bodies in the preoptic region of the hypothalamus appear to be stimulated by noradrenaline from the noradrenergic axons that have been found in that region. There are also dopaminergic axons whose cell bodies are in the arcuate nucleus and whose axons terminate close to the terminals of GnRF neurons in the median eminence. The relationship between dopamine and noradrenaline in the control of GnRF, however, is not entirely clear.

XI. PHARMACOLOGY

Agents that interfere with the CNS effects of dopamine are still the drugs of choice in Huntington's chorea. Agents commonly used include central dopamine depletors such as tetrabenazine (Nitoman) and dopamine-blocking drugs such as the phenothiazines and the butyrophenones. Patients early in the course of their disease probably do not need any drugs and in general when these drugs are given the amounts prescribed tend to be excessive. Tetrabenazine can cause depression, and this can be an even more difficult problem for the family. The patients themselves know their future having seen the progressive downhill course in their parents, so they generally like to stay alert as long as possible and dislike drugs that suppress their faculties. When they are alert they often manage their chorea and walking fairly well.

As new neurochemical discoveries are made, new therapeutic agents are evaluated. Choreic patients are anxious to take new drugs and will often show some improvement initially due to the placebo effect, which explains the frequent preliminary reports of the success of various drugs in Huntington's chorea and the frequent disappointments on long-term follow-up.

The discovery that GABA receptors are normal in some choreic patients provides some stimulus to administer GABA or a GABA-like drug. GABA itself will not cross the blood-brain barrier. Imidazole-4-acetic acid, a naturally occurring metabolite of histamine, stimultes postsynaptic GABA receptors (Van Balgooy et al., 1972), but a trial using this drug did not appear promising (Shoulson et al., 1975).

Recent interest has been shown in a drug, sodium n-dipropylacetate (Epilim), that increases the GABA concentration in animal brain by inhibiting the metabolizing enzyme GABA glutamic acid transaminase (GABA-T) (Godin et al., 1969). Initial reports on trials using this drug, however, do not seem encouraging (Shoulson et al., 1976; Bachman et al., 1977). There has been some progress in the development of an animal model to test various pharmacological agents that might be useful for Huntington's chorea (Coyle and Schwarcz, 1976). The unilateral injection of a glutamic acid analog, kainic acid, into the rat striatum resulted in neurochemical changes that are similar to those described above for the postmortem brain of Huntington's chorea. Preliminary pharmacological data using such an animal model has been produced by Coyle et al. (1977). The injection of another GABA transaminase inhibitor, γ-acetylynic GABA, intraperitoneally in kainate-lesioned animals led to a threefold increase in GABA concentration in the striatum and ipsilateral nigra.

There is still hope that such investigations will provide a suitable agent for the alleviation of the symptoms of Huntington's chorea, although the primary cause of cell death in the basal ganglia still remains elusive.

XII. SUMMARY

Huntington's chorea, a dominantly inhibited disorder, usually presents with abnormal movements at middle age but may present with epilepsy at an early age or schizophrenic-like behavior in the second and third decades. Progressive dementia occurs in most cases but is not very prominent in the elderly choreic. The atrophy seen at postmortem is consistent with the widespread loss of function throughout the brain, the greatest degree of atrophy occurring in the basal ganglia. The neurochemical defects that have been found thus far are largely confined to the basal ganglia. The greatest loss appears to be the decrease in function of the neuroinhibitory GABAergic neurons with some loss of cholinergic function in some cases. Other neurons that appear to have their cell bodies in the striatum such as substance-P-containing neurons are also affected. However, dopaminergic and serotoninergic neurons that have their terminals in the striatum do not appear to be affected by the disease process.

Receptor studies on postmortem choreic brain indicate decreases in the density of GABA receptors and of cholinergic and serotonin receptors in basal ganglia.

Endocrinological studies reveal increased plasma growth hormone and increased concentration of gonadotrophic releasing factor in the hypothalamus, two findings that are consistent with the general increase in dopaminergic activity in choreic brain. Neuroleptic agents may reduce the violent movements but can cause depression.

Hopefully, the development of more specific agents directed toward the neurochemical defects in this disorder will in the future give symptomatic relief to those suffering from this devastating disease.

REFERENCES

Aquilonius, S. M., Eckerhas, S. A., and Sundwall, A. (1975). Regional distribution of choline acetyltransferase in human brain. Changes in Huntington's chorea. *J. Neurol. Neurosurg. Psychiatry 38,* 669-677.

Axelrod, J., Wurtman, R. J., and Snyder, S. (1965). Control of hydroxyindole-o-methyltransferase activity in the rat pineal gland by environmental lighting. *J. Biol. Chem. 240,* 949-954.

Bachman, D. S., Butler, I. J., and McKhann, G. M. (1977). Long-term treatment of juvenile Huntington's chorea with dipropylacetic acid. *Neurology* (Minneapolis) *27,* 193-197.

Bernheimer, H., and Hornykiewicz, O. (1973). Brain amines in Huntington's chorea. In *Advances in Neurology,* Vol. 1, *Huntington's Chorea,* A. Barbeau, T. N. Chase, and G. W. Paulson (Eds.). Raven, New York, pp. 525-531.

Bird, E. D., and Iversen, L. L. (1974). Huntington's chorea. Post-mortem measurement of glutamic-acid decarboxylase, choline acetyltransferase and dopamine in basal ganglia. *Brain 97,* 457-472.

Bird, E. D. and Iversen, L. L. (1976). Neurochemical Findings in Huntington's chorea. In *Essays in Neurochemistry and Neuropharmacology,* M. B. H. Youdim, W. Lovenberg, D. F. Sharman, and J. R. Lagnado (Eds.). Wiley, London, pp. 177-195.

Bird, E. D., Chiappa, S. A., and Fink, G. (1976). Brain immunoreactive gonadotropin-releasing hormone in Huntington's chorea and in nonchoreic subjects. *Nature 260,* 536-538.

Bird, E. D., Mackay, A. V. P., Rayner, C. N., and Iversen, L. L. (1973). Reduced glutamic-acid decarboxylase activity of post-mortem brain in Huntington's chorea. *Lancet 1,* 1090-1092.

Boyd, A. E. III., Lebovitz, H. E., and Pfeiffer, J. B. (1970). Stimulation of growth hormone secretion by l-dopa. *N. Engl. J. Med. 283,* 1425-1429.

Bruyn, G. W. (1968). Huntington's chorea. Historical, clinical and laboratory synopsis. In *Handbook of Clinical Neurology,* Vol. 6, *Diseases of the Basal Ganglia.* North-Holland, Amsterdam, pp. 278-298.

Campbell, A. M. G., Corner, B., Norman, R. M., and Urich, H. (1961). The rigid form of Huntington's disease. *J. Neurol. Neurosurg. Psychiatry 24,* 71-77.

Coyle, J. T., and Schwarcz, R. (1976). Lesion of striatal neurones with kainic acid provides a model for Huntington's chorea. *Nature 263,* 244-246.

Coyle, J. T., Schwarcz, R., Bennett, J. P., and Campochiaro, P. (1977). Clinical neuropathologic and pharmacologic aspects of Huntington's disease. Correlates with a new animal model. In *Progress in Neuropsychopharmacology.* Vol. 1, pp. 13-30.

Curzon, G., and Bird, E. D. (1981). Concentration of 5-hydroxytryptamine in post-mortem choreic brain. In preparation.

Curzon, G., Gumpert, J., and Sharpe, D. (1972). Amine metabolites in the cerebrospinal fluid in Huntington's chorea. *J. Neurol. Neurosurg. Psychiatry 35,* 514-519.

Duffy, M. J., Wong, J., and Powell, D. (1975). Stimulation of adenylate cyclase activity in different areas of the human brain by substance P. *Neuropharmacology 14,* 615-618.

Emson, P. C., Kanazawa, I., Cuello, A. C., and Jessell, T. M. (1976). Substance P pathways in rat brain. *Biochem. Soc. Trans. 5,* 187-190.

Enna, S. J., Bird, E. D., Bennett, J. P., Bylund, D. B., Yamamura, H. I., Iversen, L. L., and Snyder, S. H. (1976). Huntington's chorea. Changes in neurotransmitter receptors in the brain. *New Engl. J. Med. 294,* 1305-1309.

Fernstrom, J. D., and Wurtman, R. J. (1972). Brain serotonin content. Physiological regulation by plasma amino acids. *Science 178,* 414-416.

Forno, L. S., and Jose, G. (1973). Huntington's chorea. A pathological study. In *Advances in Neurology,* Vol. 1, *Huntington's Chorea,* A. Barbeau, T. N. Chase, and G. W. Paulson (Eds.). Raven, New York, pp. 453-470.

Gale, J. S., Bird, E. D., Spokes, E., and Jessell, T. M. (1978). Human brain substance P. Distribution in controls and Huntington's chorea. *J. Neurochem. 30,* 633-634.

Glaeser, B. S., Hare, T. A., Vogel, W. H., Olewiler, D. B., and Beasley, B. L. (1975). Low GABA levels in C.S.F. in Huntington's chorea. *N. Engl. J. Med. 292,* 1029-1030.

Godin, Y., Heiner, L., Mark, J., and Mandel, P. (1969). Effects of Di-n-propylacetate, an anticonvulsive compound, on GABA metabolism. *J. Neurochem. 16,* 869-873.

Hiley, C. R., and Bird, E. D. (1974). Decreased muscarinic receptor concentration in post-mortem brain in Huntington's chorea. *Brain Res. 80,* 355-358.

Huntington, G. (1872). On chorea. *Med. Surg. Rep. 26,* 317-321.

Iversen, L. L., Bird, E. D., Spokes, E. S., Nicholson, S. H., and Suckling, C. J. (1978). Agonist specificity of GABA binding sites in human brain and GABA in Huntington's disease and schizophrenia. In *GABA Neurotransmitters,* P. Krogsgaard-Larsen (Ed.). Alfred Benzon Symposium 12, 179-190. Munksgaard, Copenhagen.

Kanazawa, I., Bird, E. D., O'Connell, R., and Powell, D. (1977). Evidence for a decrease in substance P content of substantia nigra in Huntington's chorea. *Brain Res. 120,* 387-392.

Klawans, H. L. (1970). A pharmacologic analysis of Huntington's chorea. *Eur. Neurol. 4,* 148-163.

Lembeck, F., and Zetler, G. (1962). Substance P. A polypeptide of possible physiological significance, especially within the nervous system. *Int. Rev. Neurobiol. 4,* 159-215.

Lloyd, K. G., Dreksler, S., and Bird, E. D. (1977). Alterations in ^{3}H-GABA binding in Huntington's chorea. *Life Sci. 21,* 747-754.

McGeer, P. L., McGeer, E. G., and Fibiger, H. C. (1973). Choline acetylase and glutamic acid decarboxylase in Huntington's chorea. *Neurology* (Minneapolis) *23,* 912-917.

Mortimer, C. H., Besser, G. M., Hook, J., and McNeilly, A. S. (1974). Intravenuous, intramuscular, subcutaneous and intranasal administration of LH/FSH-RH. The duration of effect and occurrence of asynchronous pulsatile release of LH and FSH. *Clin. Endocrinol. 3,* 19-25.

Moss, R. L., and McCann, S. M. (1973). Induction of mating behaviour in rats by luteinizing hormone releasing factor. *Science 181,* 177-179.

Perry, T. L., Hansen, S., and Kloster, M. (1973). Huntington's chorea, deficiency of gamma aminobutyric acid in brain. *N. Engl. J. Med. 288,* 337-342.

Perry, T. L., Hansen, S., Diamond, S., and Stedman, D. (1969). Plasma amino acid levels in Huntington's chorea. *Lancet 1,* 806-808.

Phillipson, O. T., and Bird, E. D. (1976). Plasma growth hormone concentration in Huntington's chorea. *Clin. Sci. Mol. Med. 50,* 551-554.

Phillipson, O. T., and Bird, E. D. (1977). Plasma glucose, non-esterified fatty acids and amino acids in Huntington's chorea. *Clin. Sci. Mol. Med. 52,* 311-318.

Podolsky, S., and Leopold, N. A. (1974). Growth hormone abnormalities in Huntington's chorea. Effect of L-dopa administration. *J. Clin. Endocrinol. Metab. 39,* 36-39.

Ramadoss, C. S., Uyeda, K., and Johnston, J. M. (1976). Studies on the fatty acid activation of phosphofructokinase. *J. Biol. Chem. 251,* 98-107.

Shoulson, I., Chase, T. N., Roberts, E., and Van Balgooy, J. N. A. (1975). Huntington's disease. Treatment with imidazole-4-acetic acid. *N. Engl. J. Med. 293,* 504-505.

Shoulson, I., Kartzinel, R., and Chase, T. N. (1976). Treatment with dipropylacetic acid and gamma-aminobutyric acid. *Neurology* (Minneapolis) *26,* 61-63.

Smith, J. A., Padwick, D., Mee, J. X., Minneman, K. P., and Bird, E. D. (1977). Synchronous nyctohemeral rhythms in human blood melatonin and in human post-mortem pineal enzyme. *Clin. Endocrinol. 6,* 219-225.

Spokes, E. G. S. (1980). Neurochemical alterations in Huntington's chorea. A study of post-mortem brain tissue. *Brain 103,* 179-210.

Stahl, W. L., and Swanson, P. D. (1974). Biochemical abnormalities in Huntington's chorea brains. *Neurology* (Minneapolis) *24,* 813-819.

Urquhart, N., Perry, T. L., Hansen, S., and Kennedy, J. (1975). GABA content and glutamic acid decarboxylase activity in brain of Huntington's chorea patients and control subjects. *J. Neurochem. 24,* 1071-1075.

Van Balgooy, J. N. A., Marshall, F. D., and Roberts, E. (1972). Metabolism of intracerebrally administered histidine and imidazolacetic acid in mice and frogs. *J. Neurochem. 19,* 2341-2353.

Wastek, G. J., Stern, L. Z., Yamamura, H. I., and Enna, S. J. (1977). Cerebrospinal fluid GABA in Huntington's disease. *Trans. Am. Soc. Neurochem. 8,* No. 2, Denver, Colorado, March 1977.

Westphal, A. (1905). Case Report. *Zbl. Nervenheilk 28* (ns. 16), 674-675.

Wurtman, R. J. (1971). Brain monoamines and endocrine function. *Bull. Neurosci. Res. Prog. 9,* 175-273.

18

Kindling Models for the Progressive Development of Psychopathology: Sensitization to Electrical, Pharmacological, and Psychological Stimuli

Robert M. Post and James C. Ballenger*
National Institute of Mental Health
Bethesda, Maryland

**Present affiliation:* University of Virginia Medical School, Charlottesville, Virginia.

I. INTRODUCTION

Precise description of progressive and sequential changes in psychopathology has long been a focal point for psychiatrists interested in the relationship of symptom development to underlying biological mechanisms. In this chapter, we will explore several apparently unrelated models and mechanisms for the development of increasingly severe behavioral pathology with the unifying theme that temporal factors and repeated exposure to critical stimuli, be they drugs, electrical stimulation of the brain, or even psychosocial stresses, are important determinants of the progression in behavioral disturbances.

Perhaps the most extensively explored example of increasingly severe behavioral abnormalities produced by a drug over time is that of the psychomotor stimulants. It has been well documented in clinical and laboratory data that the behavioral effects of acute and chronic administration of psychomotor stimulants are markedly different. In humans acute effects include both euphoria and dysphoria, but a paranoid psychosis may evolve following prolonged high-dose administration. Similarly, in animal studies with the psychomotor stimulants, increasing behavioral pathology may be observed following repeated administration of the same dose over time. Hyperactivity gives way to progressively more constricted stereotyped behavior and behavioral inhibition, social withdrawal, hyper- or hyporeactivity to stimuli, and catalepsy.

A variety of mechanisms at the synapse, particularly involving the catecholamine systems, have been proposed to explain such chronic and progressive phenomena. In addition, a kindling-like mechanism has been suggested (Post et al., 1975). Kindling was first described by Goddard et al. (1969); it refers to the progressive development of electrical after-discharges following repeated stimulation of a given brain site with an initially subthreshold current. This eventually leads to increasingly complex behavioral and electrical manifestations and finally culminates in a major motor seizure to this previously subthreshold stimulation. We will explore various aspects of this kindling model which seem relevant to the progressive development of behavioral pathology in a group of psychopathological state including temporal lobe epilepsy, alcohol withdrawal, and the functional psychoses. Several critical variables highlighted by the kindling paradigm include the intermittency of stimulation and appropriate frequency and intensity necessary to produce the cumulative kindling effect. The relevance of these characteristics to several psychopathological states will be explored.

It has long been recognized that many patients with temporal lobe epilepsy develop prominent behavioral disturbances, at times resembling those seen in manic-depressive illness or schizophrenia. While there is controversy about the relative incidence of such psychopathology in patients with temporal lobe epilepsy compared with other types of seizure, there is general agreement that psychiatric sequelae emerge only years after the onset of seizures and may progressively develop in relation to the duration of the seizure disorder or the interval between seizures. We suggest that the kindling model may help conceptualize the role of repeated and intermittent excitation of temporal and limbic structures in the development of a variety of psychopathological responses.

In a similar fashion, we will also present the model that each episode of alcohol *withdrawal*, with its concomitant increased excitatory foci in a number of brain sites, serves as a repeated stimulus to potentially "kindle" behavioral pathology and possibly central nervous system neurotransmitter changes (Ballenger and Post, 1978a; Ballenger et al., 1979). Consistent with this formulation are diverse clinical and laboratory data suggesting that the severity of alcohol withdrawal symptoms progressively increases with repeated episodes of alcohol withdrawal. Alcohol withdrawal seizures and delirium tremens appear to be late-developing phenomena which are related, at least in part, to the duration of alcohol abuse and presumably, the number of prior alcohol withdrawal episodes.

Finally, we will review a number of possible clinical and theoretical implications of such kindling-like mechanisms for the functional psychoses. In particular, these progressive and kindling-like models are offered with the hope that they may usefully direct clinical and experimental approaches to critical variables such as time course, duration, and interval between critical stimuli, neurotransmitter and neurohumoral systems involved, and possible new treatment strategies.

II. PSYCHOMOTOR STIMULANTS: BEHAVIORAL SENSITIZATION WITH CHRONIC ADMINISTRATION

A wealth of clinical and experimental data support the observations that chronic high doses of amphetamine-like psychomotor stimulants in susceptible individuals may produce a paranoid psychosis that is difficult to distinguish from schizophrenia (Griffith et al., 1970; Gunne et al., 1972; Angrist et al., 1974; also see

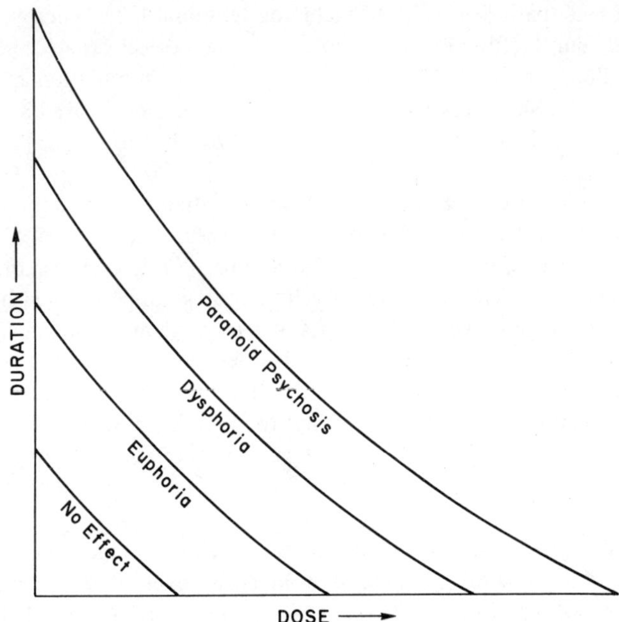

Figure 1 Scheme for interaction of dose and duration in the development of psychomotor stimulant-induced psychopathology.

reviews by Connell, 1958; Ellinwood, 1967; Snyder et al., 1974; Post, 1975; Angrist, 1978; Carlson, 1978). There is also general agreement as to the acute effects of psychomotor stimulants in humans. Many studies have noted the dose-related increases in euphoria, and at high doses, increases in dysphoria in response to the sympathomimetics (Martin et al., 1971; Janowsky et al., 1973; Post et al., 1974; Jimerson et al., 1977; Resnick et al., 1977; Byck et al., 1977; Fischman et al., 1977). In many volunteer and patient populations, acute administration of low to moderate doses appears to produce primarily euphoria, while more chronic and high-dose administration often leads to the emergence of dysphoric, asocial, and bizarre behavior not dissimilar to an evolving paranoid process observed during schizophrenia (Fig. 1).

Although there are differences in relative potencies and selective behavioral and biochemical effects between compounds, the psychomotor stimulants as a class appear to exert many of their activating effects through the catecholamines norepinephrine and dopamine. Dopamine in particular has been implicated in a variety of the activating and stereotypic effects in animals (van Rossum, 1970; Randrup and Munkvad, 1970; Snyder et al., 1974; Creese and Iverson, 1974; Scheel-Kruger et al., 1977). Data implicating dopaminergic mechanisms in some of the psychiatric symptomatology are consistent with the observations that neuroleptics, which relatively specifically block dopamine receptors, are capable not only of blocking and effectively reducing most of the symptoms of psychosis but also of blocking many of the effects of the psychomotor stimulants in animals and humans (Synder et al., 1974; Carlson, 1978).

A particularly intriguing aspect of the progressive nature of the psychomotor stimulant effect in humans has been the issue of behavioral sensitization versus tolerance. Several early studies with cocaine (Tatum and Seevers, 1929; Downs and Eddy, 1932a,b) suggested that repetitive administration of the same dose of cocaine once daily might produce increases in susceptibility to cocaine-induced excitability, convulsions, and lethality. Our work and that of Ellinwood et al. have provided further support for the observations that there may be a progressively increasing response to the behavioral-activating, stereotypic, and convulsive responses to cocaine over time (see Table 1 and Fig. 2). Similar changes have also been reported following chronic amphetamine or methylphenidate administration in a number of animal species. Of particular interest are the reports that directly acting dopamine receptor agonists are also capable of producing behavioral sensitization (Table 1). Borison and collaborators (1977) reported that administration of phenylethylamine (PEA), a naturally occurring substance in the body, also is associated with the sensitization effect on stereotypies in animals.

Several studies have reported that L-dopa similarly sensitizes animals to subsequent activation with other dopaminergic compounds. These studies are thus consistent with those available in the clinical literature that chronic levodopa therapy of parkinsonism leads to an increased freqeuncy of dyskinesias (Klawans et al., 1975) and "on-off" phenomena (Barbeau, 1974) with increasing duration of treatment. The on-off effect refers to a rapid alteration between

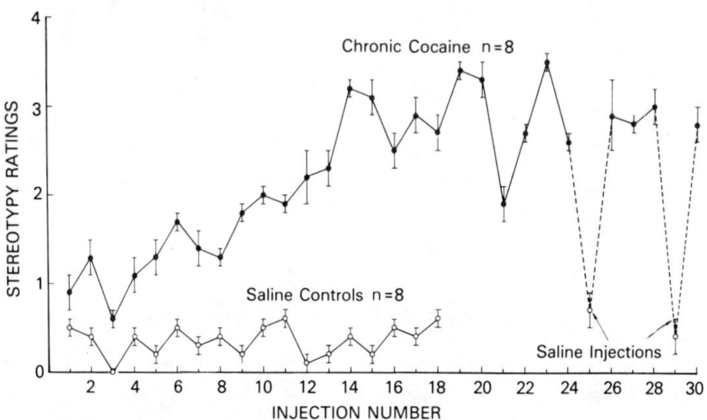

Figure 2 Increasing effect of repetitive cocaine injection on stereotypic behavior.

Table 1 Selected Evidence for Behavioral Sensitization to Dopamine-Active Compounds

Drug	Effects	Selected references
Indirect agonists		
Cocaine	Hyperactivity, stereotypy, catalepsy (In dog and monkey), dyskinesias	Tatum and Selvers, 1929; Downs and Eddy, 1932a,b; Gutierrez-Noriega and Zapata-Ortiz, 1945; Gutierrez-Noriega, 1950; Post and Rose, 1976; Stripling and Ellinwood, 1977a,b; Kilbey and Ellinwood, 1977; Ho et al., 1977; Post et al., 1976; Shuster et al., 1977
Amphetamine	Stereotypy, dyskinesias	Mago, 1969; Tilson and Reich, 1973; Segal and Mandell, 1974; Kilbey and Ellinwood, 1977; Klawans and Margolin, 1975; Short and Shuster, 1976; Ranje and Ungerstadt, 1974; Ellinwood, 1967; Hitzemann et al., 1977; Schiff and Bridger, 1977; Borison et al., 1977; Browne and Segal, 1977; Bailey and Jackson, 1978
Methylphenidate	Stereotypy	Browne and Segal, 1977; Peachey et al., 1977; Schreiber et al., 1976
L-dopa	Stereotypy (in man: dyskinesias, psychosis)	Klawans et al., 1977a,b; Klawans et al., 1975; Moskovitz et al., 1978
Phenylethylamine (PEA)	Stereotypy	Borison et al., 1977, 1978
Direct dopamine agonists		
Apomorphine	Stereotypy and locomotion	Martres et al., 1977; Nausieda et al., 1978; Bailey and Jackson, 1978
Bromocriptine	Stereotypy	Nausieda et al., 1978; Smith et al., 1979
Ergometrine	Motility	Scheel-Kruger et al., 1977; Pijnenburg et al., 1976

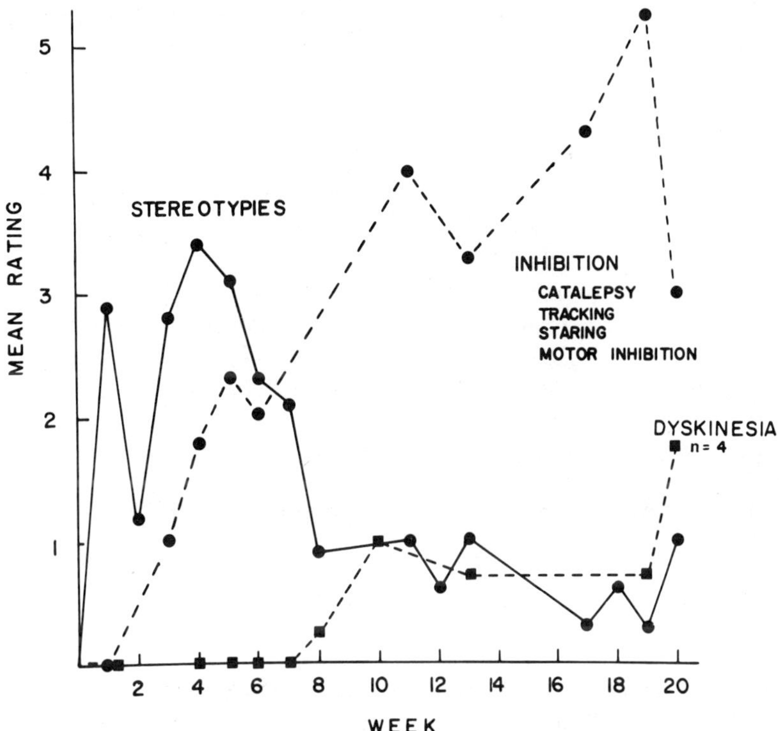

Figure 3 Progressive development of inhibitory behavior in initially stereotypic monkeys, $n = 8$.

dyskinesias and parkinsonian immobility. Most interestingly, the psychiatric side effects also increase with chronic L-dopa treatment. Patients initially report vivid dreams which then spill over into waking life to become hallucinatory phenomena and eventually a paranoid psychosis may emerge (Moskovitz et al., 1978). Increased behavioral pathology and dyskinesias also emerge following chronic, high-dose cocaine in the rhesus monkey (Fig. 3).

Thus, many compounds which directly or indirectly activate dopaminergic receptors have been reported to produce progressive effects on hyperactivity or stereotypy in animals or a psychotic process in humans.

Many of these studies (see Tables 1 and 2 and Kosman and Unna, 1968) report conclusions opposite those traditionally accepted, i.e., that repeated use of psychomotor stimulants leads only to the development of tolerance (Lewander, 1968; Sever et al., 1976; Matsuzaki et al., 1976; Fischman et al., 1977; Wood et al., 1977). Some of the reasons for these apparent discrepancies are discussed below.

Table 2 Characteristics of Kindling-Like Effects on the Development of Seizures

Agent	Interval	References
Cocaine		
Rat	Once daily	Downs and Eddy, 1932b; Post, 1977a; Stripling and Ellinwood, 1977a,b
Monkey[a]	Twice daily	Post et al., 1976
Lidocaine (rat)	Once daily	Post et al., 1975,1979
Flurothyl ether (rat)	Once daily	Prichard et al., 1969
Pentylenetetrazol (Metrazol)	2-day interval	Mason and Cooper, 1972; Pinel and Cheung, 1977
Electroconvulsive therapy (ECT)	3-day interval	Ramer and Pinel, 1976
Carbachol (intra-amygdaloid)	Once daily	Vosu and Wise, 1975
Alcohol withdrawal	2 weeks	Baker and Cannon, 1979

[a]Matsuzaki et al. (1976) report tolerance develops to the convulsive effects of intravenous cocaine.

III. PROPOSED SYNAPTIC AND RECEPTOR MECHANISMS FOR SENSITIZATION (TABLE 3)

Klawans and Margolin (1975) have proposed an "agonist supersensitivity" concept to explain the increased responsivity of their chronic amphetamine pretreated animals to either amphetamine- or apomorphine-induced stereotypy and dyskinesias. Recently, it has been suggested that behavioral sensitization to dopamine-active agonists may be associated with increased numbers of dopamine receptor sites and possibly alterations in [^{3}H] dopamine binding (Klawans, 1977a,b; Borison et al., 1979). Baudry et al. (1977) report that single high-dose injection of amphetamine increases [^{3}H] pimozide binding, indicating an increase in number or affinity of receptors.

McManus et al. (1978) reported that in vitro application of large doses of dopamine or norepinephrine to caudate homogenates led to selective increases in binding to [^{3}H] apomorphine, but not to [^{3}H] WB-4101 or [^{3}H] naloxone. Howlett and Nahorski (1978) reported that chronic amphetamine administration was associated with decreases in dopamine-stimulated adenylate cyclase activity, no change in β-noradrenergic receptor function, but increases in [^{3}H] spiperone binding in limbic system (at 4 but not 20 days) and decreases in striatal tissue. These findings stress the complexity of the agonist-induced receptor changes.

Not only are the receptor changes time- (Banerjee et al., 1977) and dose-dependent (Baudry et al., 1977), but they are also regionally specific (limbic↑, striatum↓), dependent upon pretreatment duration, and not necessarily related to adenylate cyclase generation (Howlett and Nahorski, 1978).

In contrast to the studies reporting direct receptor binding evidence compatible with agonist sensitization, Burt et al. (1977) and Friedhoff et al. (1977) reported that amphetamine did not change radioligand binding. Muller and Seeman (1979) reported that chronic amphetamine and apomorphine significantly decreased apomorphine binding without changing [^{3}H] haloperidol binding. They suggested that these changes were consistent with a presynaptic dopamine receptor subsensitivity accounting for behavioral sensitization.

Schwartz and collaborators (1978) also argue that behavioral facilitation developing even in response to weak dopamine agonists such as piribedil, which in themselves are not sufficient to cause stereotypy, is in accord with the presynaptic desensitization hypothesis. Behavioral sensitization requires the integrity of dopaminergic neurons, they point out, since responsiveness is not further increased by apomorphine pretreatment in 6-OH-dopamine pretreated animals, as is observed in the disuse supersensitivity model. Walters et al. (1975) reported that low doses of dopamine agonists eventually lost their ability to inhibit firing of nigrostriatal neurons, which is consistent with desensitization of presynaptic dopamine receptors. Preliminary data from our laboratory also support a presynaptic receptor desensitization component in cocaine-induced behavioral sensitization. Repeated daily doses of cocaine (10 mg/kg × 13 days) were associated with decreased behavioral suppression to a low dose of apomorphine (0.05 mg/kg) thought to act at presynaptic dopamine receptors. Higher doses of apomorphine (0.5 mg/kg) also produced increased stereotypy in cocaine-pretreated animals compared to controls.

Banerjee et al. (1978) and Chanda et al. (1979) reported increased β-adrenergic receptor binding with [^{3}H] dihydroalprenolol following either chronic amphetamine or cocaine administration. Specific binding of [^{3}H] dihydroalprenolol was greater at 12, 24, and 48 hr (but not at 1 hr or 96 hr) after 10 mg/kg, i.p. d-amphetamine daily for 6 weeks. Preliminary data from our laboratory (A. Pert et al., unpublished data, 1979) suggest that the behavior effects of chronic cocaine administration (10 mg/kg i.p.) may be inhibited by lithium coadministration. Thus it is possible that lithium may block some behavioral and biochemical indices of stimulant-induced sensitization, just as it appears to block the development of neuroleptic withdrawal supersensitivity (Pert et al., 1978; Gallager et al., 1978).

Table 3 Hypothetical Mechanisms for Dopamine Agonist Behavioral Sensitization

Molecular-synaptic
Postsynaptic receptor supersensitivity
Direct increase in receptor number or affinity
Indirect increase secondary to presynaptic transmitter deficit, depletion, or decreased turnover
Presynaptic receptor desensitization
Increased transmitter availability
Increased turnover, release, or decrease reuptake
Pharmacokinetic alteration in drug availability
Neuroanatomical shift in balance:
From *inhibitory* dopamine receptors to *excitatory* dopamine receptors
From one dopaminergic area to another (i.e., *striatal* to *limbic-cortical*)
With *other transmitters or neuromodulators*
Neurophysiological
Post-tetanic potentiation (enhancement)
Kindling
Increased synaptic efficacy
Progressively wider area of effect
Neuropsychological
Neuronal-behavioral *conditioning*

Several presynaptic neurotransmitter mechanisms (including longlasting amine depletion and alterations in enzyme activity, transmitter release, and reuptake) have also been postulated for the behavioral sensitization effect (Segal, 1975; Trendelenberg and Graefe, 1975; Short and Schuster, 1976; Seiden et al., 1977), although these do not appear sufficient to account for the sensitization phenomena in many instances.

Pharmacokinetic explanations do not appear to fully explain the sensitization phenomena. Although alterations in amphetamine uptake into selective areas of brain (Kuhn and Schanberg, 1977) or in cocaine levels with chronic administration have been reported (Ho et al., 1977; Mule and Misra, 1977), other studies have not found substantial acute-chronic differences in peak drug levels (Misra et al., 1974; Post, 1977a). In addition, several studies have demonstrated that the sensitization effect may last for weeks to months following initial pretreatment with the same or even a different dopamine active agent (Table 4). These data would make a differential drug accumulation or metabolism a highly unlikely explanation of the sensitization effect.

IV. KINDLING MODEL FOR BEHAVIORAL SENSITIZATION

We were particularly struck with the parellelism between the development of convulsions to a previously subthreshold dose of cocaine or lidocaine and a variety of temporal characteristics of electrical kindling (Post et al., 1975,1976, 1980a). Similar observations and conclusions were presented by Ellinwood and co-workers (1977,1978). Careful exploration and dissection of a variety of critical variables for the classic electrical kindling process may offer useful avenues of exploration for drug sensitization or apparent "pharmacological

Table 4 Cross-Sensitization: Evidence for Increased Behavioral Response to a Different Drug Following Drug and Electrical Pretreatments

Pretreatment		Test agent	Selected references
Amphetamine	To:	Apomorphine	Klawans and Margolin, 1975 Martres et al., 1977 Kilbey and Ellinwood, 1977 Bailey and Jackson, 1978 Weston and Overstreet, 1976
	Not to:	Morphine or cocaine	Short and Shuster, 1976
Cocaine	To:	Apomorphine	Kilbey and Ellinwood, 1977
	Not to:	Amphetamine	Shuster et al., 1977
Morphine	To:	Cocaine	Shuster et al., 1977
Lidocaine	To:	Cocaine	Squillace et al., 1978
Apomorphine	To:	Amphetamine	Bailey and Jackson, 1978
Bromocriptine	To:	Amphetamine, apomorphine	Nausieda et al., 1978
L-dopa	To:	Amphetamine, apomorphine	Klawans et al., 1977a and b
Piribedil, S584 and L-dopa	To:	Apomorphine	Martres et al., 1977
Electroconvulsive shock	To:	Methamphetamine, apomorphine	Green et al., 1977
	To:	5-methoxy-N,N-dimethyltryptamine	Evans et al., 1976
	To:	Apomorphine and clonidine	Modigh, 1975
	To:	Alcohol withdrawal	Pinel and Van Oot, 1977
Amygdala kindling	To:	Lidocaine seizures	Post et al., 1980a
	To:	Decreased cocaine	Post et al., 1980a
	To:	Alcohol withdrawal	Pinel and Van Oot, 1975

Table 5 Electrical Kindling: Major Characteristics[a]

1. Repeated stimulations
   a. Initially subseizure threshold
   b. Intermittent
2. Local after-discharges and seizure activity
   a. Increase in amplitude
   b. Increase in duration
   c. Increase in complexity of wave form
   d. Increase in anatomical spread
      (1) Limbic → neostriatum → midbrain reticular formation → cortex
3. Replicable sequence of seizure stages
   Behavioral arrest, blinking, and masticatory movements, head nodding, opsithotonis, contralateral then bilateral forelimb clonus, rearing and falling
4. Discharges kindle in quantum jumps
5. Limbic system kindles more readily than cortex
6. In kindled animals the history of convulsion development is recapitulated as seizure builds
7. Transfer effects to secondary sites; kindling facilitated in other sites even after primary site destroyed
8. Interference: A secondary kindled site interferes with primary site rekindling
9. No toxic or neuropathological changes evident; kindling is a transsynaptic process
10. Relatively permanent change in connectivity; a kindled animal will still seize after a 1-year seizure-free interval
11. Seizure may develop spontaneously in chronically kindled animals
12. Interictal spikes and spontaneous epileptiform potentials develop
13. Kindled animals have decreased ability to learn conditioned emotional responses and altered predatory aggression.

[a]See reference for Goddard et al., 1969 regarding 1, 4-10; Wada and Sato, 1974 regarding 2-4, 6; Wada et al., 1974, and Wada, 1978 regarding 10-12; McIntyre, 1976, and Adamec, 1975 regarding 13.

kindling" (Tables 1 and 2). As noted above in the introduction and as reviewed in Table 5, classically described kindling involves repeated, once daily electrical stimulation, particularly of limbic sites such as the amygdala, which eventually produces sequential increases in seizure stage complexity and culminates in bilateral tonic-clonic convulsions to an electrical current which was previously subconvulsive. The electrical kindling process is associated with both an increased duration of after-discharges at the stimulating electrode site (Fig. 4) and an increased spread of after-discharge activity to other neuronal substrates synaptically related to the initial stimulation site. Careful studies by Goddard et al.

(1969), Racine (1972a,b), Wada and co-workers (1974), Goddard and Douglas (1975), and Wada and Osawa (1976) clearly demonstrated that the kindling phenomena is not an artefact of tissue damage and involves an orderly and sequential spread of altered electrical activity from limbic structures into the striatum and brainstem, and finally into the cerebral cortex in association with the appearance of major motor convulsions. This spatiotemporal spread of increased neuronal activity has also been documented by the 2-deoxyglucose technique (Engel et al., 1978).

Racine (1972a,b) documented that kindling may be demonstrated by lowered after-discharge thresholds even in the absence of seizure manifestations.

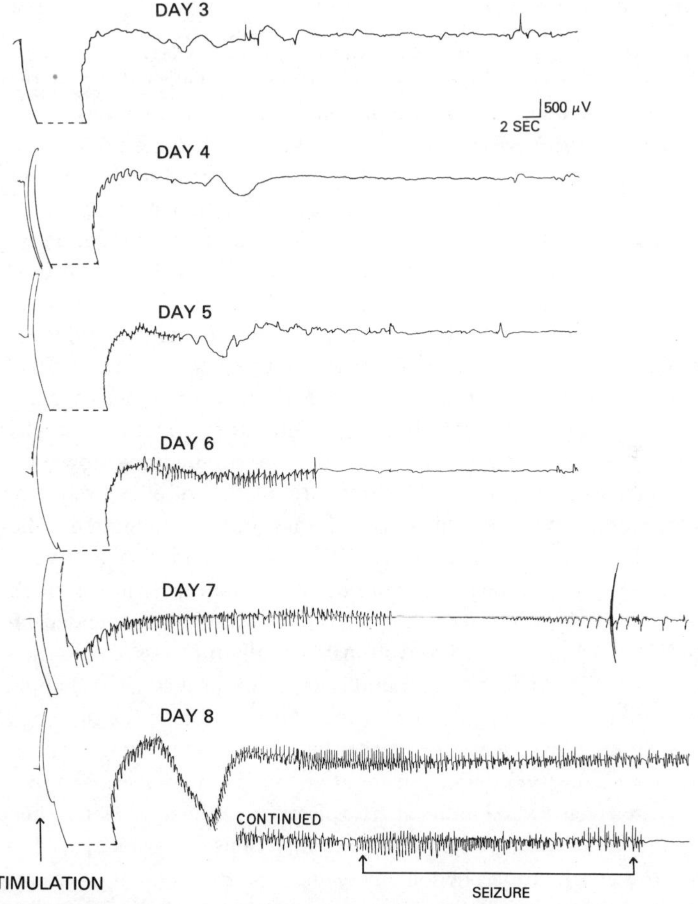

Figure 4 Kindling: development of after-discharge following repetitive stimulation of the amygdala.

Once an animal has been kindled it will remain more sensitive to stimulation for months to years (Goddard et al., 1969). Thus, the kindling model has been used as a model for synaptic plasticity, memory, and learning phenomena, as well as for epileptogenesis (Goddard and Douglas, 1975). We have suggested elsewhere that various characteristics of this model may be particularly applicable to dissection of the development of pathological behavioral phenomena as well (Post and Kopanda, 1976).

V. ASPECTS OF KINDLING RELEVANT TO OTHER SENSITIZATION MODELS

A. Interval Between Stimulation

The time interval between successive kindling stimuli is critical to the rate of development of kindling. For example, continuous electrical stimulation of the amygdala is not associated with kindling and actually retards subsequent kindling (Goddard et al., 1969). Even intermittent stimulation spaced once every 5-10 min leads to adaptation and not kindling. As the interval increases to several hours, or optimally 24 hr, the rapidity of kindling is enhanced. Spaced as far apart as one per week, the number of electrical stimulations required to produce the major motor convulsion is not substantially different from that produced by once a day stimulation (Goddard et al., 1969). Similarly, Mucha and Pinel (1977) have documented that the length of after-discharge in fully kindled seizures decreases following a sequence of stimulations once every hour and a half, but returns toward normal when stimulations are resumed on a once a day basis. Thus, either no kindling effect or an inhibitory effect on after-discharge duration is evident with chronic or short-interval stimulations; however, as the interval increases to a clearly intermittent stimulation of once a day, once every 3 days, or even once a week, the sensitization process is facilitated. These data are consistent with those of Ramer and Pinel (1976) and Pinel and Van Oot (1975), suggesting that longer intervals between electroconvulsive shock therapy may be associated with a decreased seizure threshold and increased intensity (sensitization), while shorter intervals may actually increase seizure threshold.

The time interval between stimulus applications may also be applicable to drug administration paradigms. Behavioral sensitization to the running effect of morphine in mice has been documented in animals administered the drug at intervals of once every 3 days (Shuster et al., 1975). However, when morphine injections are given several hours apart, tolerance to the hyperactivating effects of morphine develops rapidly. When the injections are again spaced at long intervals, the sensitization phenomena reemerges. Few studies of the effects of continuous drug administration versus intermittent drug administration have been conducted with the psychomotor stimulants, although preliminary data from our laboratory and those in the literature (Tables 1 and 2) underline the importance of the length of the interval between drug applications in determining sensitization versus tolerance phenomena.

Nelson and Ellison (1978) did investigate this variable in relation to amphetamine-induced hyperactivity and stereotypy in the rat. Continuous administration of d-amphetamine in pellet form did not lead to behavioral sensitization following one week's treatment, while repeated intermittent injection of amphetamine (3 mg/kg, once daily) for either 7 or 30 days produced significant increases in stereotypy ratings. In addition, when animals were retested 30 days after drug pretreatment, both the 7- and 30-day intermittent injected animals showed significantly enhanced stereotypy ratings compared with continuous pellet drug administrated animals or controls. Most interestingly, pellet-treated animals showed increases in *hyperactivity* compared with saline or intermittent injected animals. Thus, there was an interaction of the endpoint measured and the continuous and intermittent variable. Continuous amphetamine administration was associated with sensitization to running behavior while intermittent injections increased stereotypies both acutely and subsequently on retest 30 days later.

Challenge of the animals with the direct agonist apomorphine was also revealing in relation to continuous versus intermittent pretreatment. Continuous administration of d-amphetamine in pellet form resulted in a decreased stereotypic response to an apomorphine challenge (0.2 mg/kg) immediately following pretreatment but not 30 days later. In contrast, apomorphine-induced stereotypy was significantly enhanced 30 days later in the intermittent pretreated animals. Thus, both amphetamine rechallenge and apomorphine testing demonstrated that intermittent amphetamine pretreatments more significantly sensitized to increases in stereotypy compared with continuous administration.

B. Stimulation Intensity and Drug Dose

Just as the intensity of electrical stimulation is an important factor for the development of kindling, the dose of drug appears to be a critical factor as well. Although behavioral sensitization phenomena have been documented following relatively low or moderate doses of psychomotor stimulants (Segal and Mandell, 1974; Post and Rose, 1976), higher doses of the stimulants (Shuster et al., 1975, 1977; Stripling and Ellinwood, 1977a,b; Ellinwood and Kilbey, 1977,1978) or apomorphine, a direct dopamine receptor agonist (Martres et al., 1977), appear to produce greater effects on several behavioral or convulsive endpoints than lower doses.

These data, taken in conjunction with the importance of the interval between stimulations, may be meaningful from an evolutionary perspective. It might be adaptive for an organism to become tolerant to chronic, low-level stimuli, but an intermittent larger stimulus might signal a more important event and therefore be usefully associated with a facilitated or sensitized response.

C. Sensitization Versus Tolerance: Dependence on Variable and Substrate Studied

It should be reemphasized that under many conditions of drug administration, tolerance phenomena rather than sensitization become evident clinically both in humans and in laboratory animals (Lewander, 1968; Kosman and Unna, 1968; Fischman et al., 1977). The behavioral endpoint or biophysiological variable to be studied appears important in whether tolerance or sensitization appears. For example, many studies demonstrate that repeated administration of a variety of psychomotor stimulants producces tolcrancc to autonomic effects of the drug. It would be interesting to observe whether sensitization were occurring to the hyperactivating or stereotypic effects of the stimulants while tolerance were occurring to the autonomic effects. In our studies of chronic cocaine administration in the rhesus monkey, we observed that eventually oral stereotypies decreased in severity in association with the late emergence of dyskinesias and inhibitory, cataleptic, and visual scanning behavior (Post et al., 1976) (Fig. 3). One way of conceptualizing this observation is that striatal mechanisms subserving oral stereotypies manifest tolerance to the repeated effects of cocaine while the neural substrates (perhaps in the limbic system) (Scheel-Kruger et al., 1977; Costall and Naylor, 1977) which may mediate the inhibitory and cataleptic effects become increasingly affected over time. A differential time course of biochemical and behavioral effects of the neuroleptics have similarly been related to striatal versus mesolimbic or mesocortical mechanisms. For example, there is clinical and laboratory evidence for tolerance to parkinsonian side effects of neuroleptics and to their effect on HVA (presumably related to striatal mechanisms) (Post and Goodwin, 1975). There is little evidence for tolerance to either the antipsychotic effects of the neuroleptics (presumably mediated through mesolimbic or mesocortical systems) or to the increases in prolactin (mediated by the hypothalamic pituitary axis).

D. Conditioning

Tilson and Rech (1973) suggested that conditioning variables might account for some of the sensitization phenomena observed with amphetamine. However, Segal and Mandell (1974) argued that the de novo emergence of new behaviors following chronic amphetamine administration suggests that conditioning factors alone could not account for the sensitization phenomenon. In a recent study, Browne and Segal (1977) manipulated a variety of environmental and conditioning factors and found that they did not contribute to the increased effect of amphetamine over time. However, our work (Post et al., 1980b) and that

that of Scheel-Kruger et al. (1977) suggests that the novelty of the test environment and whether animals repeatedly experience the drug in the test cage markedly alter some components of the cocaine-induced syndrome in rats. For example, animals injected with cocaine (once daily for 9 days) in the test cage show substantial increases in vertical hyperactivity and in rearing behavior compared with animals given the same dose and number of cocaine injections in their home cage. Predrug activity levels were similar in both groups, indicating that there was no conditioned hyperexcitability to the test cage per se, and the differences emerged only in response to a cocaine injection administered in the context of the different test cages. These data are consistent with those of Schiff and Bridger (1977), indicating that some components of amphetamine-induced stereotypy but not others showed sensitization and could be differentially conditioned.

E. Genetics and Individual Differences

Jori and Garratini (1973) reported marked differences in behavioral, biochemical, and physiological responsivity to amphetamine among different genetic strains of mice. Shuster et al. (1977) also observed this effect with cocaine and also reported strain differences in the degree of sensitization effect to repeated cocaine injections. Large differences in individual responsivity to psychomotor stimulants have been observed in rat, monkey, and in humans, suggesting that genetic as well as environmental-experiential variables are importantly related to the sensitization phenomena (Ranje and Ungerstedt, 1974; Post et al., 1976; Weston and Overstreet, 1976; Jimerson et al., 1977).

F. Cross-Sensitization Phenomenon

Another approach to dissection of mechanisms underlying the sensitization phenomenon is to study the interaction between a variety of pretreatments and test agents resulting in cross-sensitization. These data are reviewed in Table 4. For example, Klawans and Margolin (1975) reported that repeated administration of amphetamine is associated with an increased reactivity to challenge with apomorphine, a direct dopamine receptor agonist. Groves and Rebec (1977) demonstrated that repeated administration of amphetamine was associated with increased suppression of unit firing both in the striatum and in the reticular formation following an amphetamine or apomorphine challenge. Chronic administration of lidocaine (60 mg/kg i.p.) for 21 days was associated with an increased response to cocaine-induced hyperactivity (Squillace et al., 1978). Lidocaine produced behavioral sedation and ataxia at these doses and not hyperactivity and stereotypy, yet rechallenge with cocaine (10 mg/kg i.p.) resulted in increased behavioral activation in the lidocaine-pretreated animals compared to saline controls. These data are also highly suggestive that drug conditioning phenomena are not the sole mediators of the sensitization effect.

Martres et al. (1977), in their test of apomorphine-induced vertical climbing behavior, demonstrated sensitization by prior treatment with a variety of drugs acting directly and indirectly on dopamine receptors, including amphetamine, piribedil, apomorphine, and L-dopa. Pinel and Van Oot (1975,1977) demonstrated that either amygdala kindling or prior treatment with electroconvulsive therapy increased the severity of the alcohol withdrawal syndromes in rats. This study demonstrates a possible cross-sensitization or involvement of an amygdala-kindled substrate in alcohol withdrawal symptomatology (as discussed in detail below).

Another strategy for studying cross-sensitization phenomenon has been to pretreat with a sensitizing drug such as cocaine and then study alterations in the rate of electrical kindling. Once daily administration of cocaine (40 mg/kg i.p.) for 10 days was not associated with a facilitation of the rate of amygdala kindling compared to sham-stimulated animals (Post et al., 1978a). Ellinwood and Kilbey (1978) also reported no change in the rate of amygdala kindling, but did observe an increase in the rate of spread of after-discharges to the striatum in animals pretreated with cocaine compared to saline-treated controls. These data are of particular interest since the local anesthetics cocaine and lidocaine produce notable spindling and seizure effects in limbic and particularly amygdala sites (Eidelberg et al., 1963; Wagman et al., 1967; Riblet and Tuttle, 1970; Munson et al., 1972; Stripling and Ellinwood, 1977a,b).

G. Behavioral Effects of Kindling

Another pertinent question is whether amygdala kindling alters relevant spontaneous or drug-induced behavior. Initial studies of McIntyre (1976) suggested that amygdala kindling does alter conditioned emotional responsivity. In collaboration with Squillace and Pert, we have also documented that amygdala kindling decreases spontaneous as well as cocaine-induced vertical hyperactivity. This is particularly interesting since bilateral amygdala lesions appear to facilitate cocaine-induced vertical activity (Squillace et al., 1978). Thus, there appear to be reciprocal effects between amygdala kindling and bilateral lesions of the amygdala on this aspect of the cocaine-induced syndrome (Post et al., 1980a). Amygdala kindling also alters aggressivity in cats and rats (Adamec, 1975; Pinel et al., 1977).

These studies suggest a strategy for producing long-term alterations in neuronal and behavioral excitability by focal electrical stimulation of the brain. This paradigm may become a useful strategy for dissecting the role of specific neural substrates in relation to a particular behavior. While lesion techniques are focused at decreasing the input from a specific system, the kindling paradigm, in contrast, might be viewed as facilitating or at least increasing the excitability of specific neural substrates of behavioral interest.

VI. KINDLING AND THE DEVELOPMENT OF PSYCHOPATHOLOGY WITH CHRONIC TEMPORAL LOBE EPILEPSY

A number of investigators have described the development of significant psychopathology in association with chronic temporal lobe epilepsy (Gibbs, 1951; MacLean, 1973; Slater et al., 1963; Glaser et al., 1963; Stevens et al., 1969; Gloor, 1972; Dalby, 1975; Blumer, 1975; Stevens, 1973,1975; Bear and Fedio, 1977; Stevens and Livermore, 1978; Flor-Henry, 1969,1974,1978). Although Stevens (1975) argued that some of the apparent increase in psychopathology with temporal lobe epilepsy as compared to other types of epilepsy is due in part to sample bias, many investigators agree that psychopathology increases with increased duration of epilepsy. Slater et al. (1963) emphasized the long interval between the onset of epilepsy and the emergence of psychopathology, while Flor-Henry (1969,1977) emphasized the interval between seizures as important for the emergence of psychopathology.

We hypothesize that chronic intermittent convulsive or subconvulsive stimulation by the epileptic focus could be associated with kindling-like phenomena which facilitate spread of abnormal discharges to synaptically related temporal lobe and limbic areas (Post and Kopanda, 1976). Some experimental evidence for the behavioral relevance of this phenomena is available in animal models. Pinel et al. (1977) chronically kindled the amygdala and hippocampus in rats and showed that this is associated with increases in aggressiveness.

In a different species, Adamec (1975) documented that basal levels of predatory aggression in the cat are associated with differences in amygdala afterdischarge threshold; rat-killing cats have a higher threshold for amygdala afterdischarges than nonkillers. Following amygdala kindling, which lowers the afterdischarge threshold, cats which previously were spontaneous rat killers became nonkillers (Adamec, 1975). These and related data cited above suggest that chronic stimulation of a temporal or limbic focus can produce associated changes in exploratory, emotional, and aggressive behavior in animals.

We recently demonstrated that repeated lidocaine-induced seizures in the rat increase glucose consumption in the hippocampus, amygdala, and perirhinal cortex as measured by the $[^{14}C]$2-deoxyglucose method of Sokoloff and Kennedy (Post et al., 1979). Animals experiencing repeated lidocaine seizures develop bizarre eating behaviors and become extremely aggressive. These behavioral data, taken with the specificity of lidocaine's effects on limbic structures, indicate that lidocaine-kindled seizures may be a useful experimental model for human temporal lobe epilepsy.

We suggest that the development of psychopathology in relation to temporal lobe epilepsy may be in part mediated by a kindling mechanism and may represent an important experiment in nature for the elucidation of critical factors necessary for the development of kindling-like phenomena in humans.

Many of the relationships derived from the kindling model could be subjected to specific retro- and prospective tests. For example, does psychopathology emerge with increasing number of psychomotor seizure episodes? Are the behaviors manifested related to the specific neural substrate involved in the seizure focus? Does adequate seizure control alter the underlying electrical abnormality and retard the development of psychiatric sequelae? Is there a role for psychotropic prophylaxis? Bear and Fedio (1977) documented a variety of personality changes associated with left and right temporal lobe epileptics. The personality profile in these patients was substantially different depending on whether the focus was in the left or right hemisphere. On the basis of these and related data, Bear (1979) suggested that many of the personality changes observed in the temporal lobe epileptics are related to a hyperfunctional connectivity of a variety of limbic and cortical systems. He argued that personality traits such as circumstantial concern with detail, increases in religious and philosophical interests, and intense and sober affect are stable characteristics which correlate with the duration of the illness and may be related to increased connectivity between limbic and temporal lobe substrates, a formulation consistent with the kindling paradigm.

VII. THE ALCOHOL WITHDRAWAL SYNDROMES: A KINDLING MODEL

We recently presented data and reviewed the literature consistent with the finding that the severity of the alcohol withdrawal syndromes increases with increasing duration of alcohol abuse (Ballenger and Post, 1978a). Alcohol is a central nervous system depressant and alcohol withdrawal leads to a state of central hyperirritability and heightened seizure susceptibility (McQuarrie and Fingl, 1958; Mendelson, 1972; Begleiter et al., 1973; Hunt, 1973). Recently, several studies employing implanted depth electrodes demonstrated gross electroencephalographic abnormalities during withdrawal (Guerrero-Figueroa et al., 1970; Hunter et al., 1973; Walker and Zornetzer, 1974). These include epileptiform spikes and seizure activity similar to that observed during electrical kindling. In particular, these electroencephalographic abnormalities and the concomitant behavioral symptomatology are cumulative, becoming progressively more severe with each subsequent episode (Baker and Cannon, 1979). We hypothesized that the fall in seizure threshold and the subsequent electrical abnormalities accompanying each alcohol *withdrawal* serve as "kindling stimuli" for subsequent alterations in susceptibility to alcohol withdrawal symptomatology. Implied in the association between total duration of alcohol abuse and severity of alcohol withdrawal symptoms is the presumed direct relationship between the duration of alcohol abuse and the number of *episodes* of alcohol withdrawal. The alcoholic partially withdraws every 24 hours associated with sleep as well as

Table 6 Duration of Alcohol Abuse and Withdrawal Symptomatology (Index Admission)

	Severity of withdrawal				
Years of alcohol abuse	(0) None	(1) Mild tremor	(2) "Shakes," automatic hyperactivity	(3) Seizures, confusion	(4) DTs
½-3 (n=95)	87(91%)	8 (9%)	0	0	0
3-5 (n=36)	15 (42%)	13 (42%)	8 (22%)	0	0
5-10 (n=48)	15 (31%)	12 (25%)	17 (35%)	3 (6%)	1 (3%)
10-15 (n=15)	3 (20%)	2 (14%)	6 (40%)	3 (20%)	1 (6%)
15-20 (n=4)	1 (25%)	0 (0%)	1 (25%)	0	2 (50%)
>20 (n=2)	0	1 (50%)	1 (50%)	0	0

experiencing more full-blown withdrawal effects following cessation of a prolonged period of inebriation. Thus, we would postulate that either the minor nightly episodes of alcohol withdrawal or the major episodes of withdrawal occurring more intermittently with the complete cessation of drinking lead to a kindling-like facilitation of subsequent alcohol withdrawal episodes and symptoms.

As illustrated in Table 6, the majority of alcoholics studied with less than 5 years of alcohol abuse experienced no withdrawal symptoms upon hospitalization for their alcohol problem, and none experienced more than a mild tremor. After 6 years of abuse, withdrawal was associated with increased incidence and severity of withdrawal symptomatology. The more severe symptoms of alcohol withdrawal involving seizures and confusion (stage 3) and delirium tremens (stage 4) began to occur after 6-10 years of abuse. This relationship of severity to duration of abuse (and presumedly to the number of withdrawal episodes) occurs independently of age. The relationship of duration of alcohol abuse to the onset of delirium tremens is also illustrated in Figure 5 in a larger sample of patients.

It is relatively straightforward to conceptualize seizures as an end point of alcohol withdrawal-induced kindling, while the other symptoms of alcohol withdrawal may be more difficult to conceptualize within the context of the kindling model (Fig. 6). While the specific neural substrates showing increased reactivity

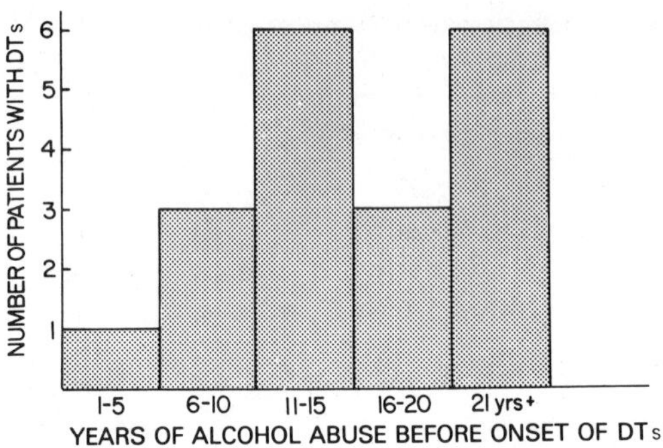

Figure 5 Frequency distribution of delirium tremens in relation to duration of prior alcohol abuse.

with each alcohol withdrawal phenomena have only been preliminarily explored in several animal studies, there is evidence to suggest that a variety of diencephalic and limbic structures do manifest progressively increasing excitability (Branchey et al., 1971; Hunter et al., 1973; Walker and Zornetzer, 1974). The increased activation of these pathways important for the regulation of autonomic, emotional, and cognitive function could facilitate the progressive

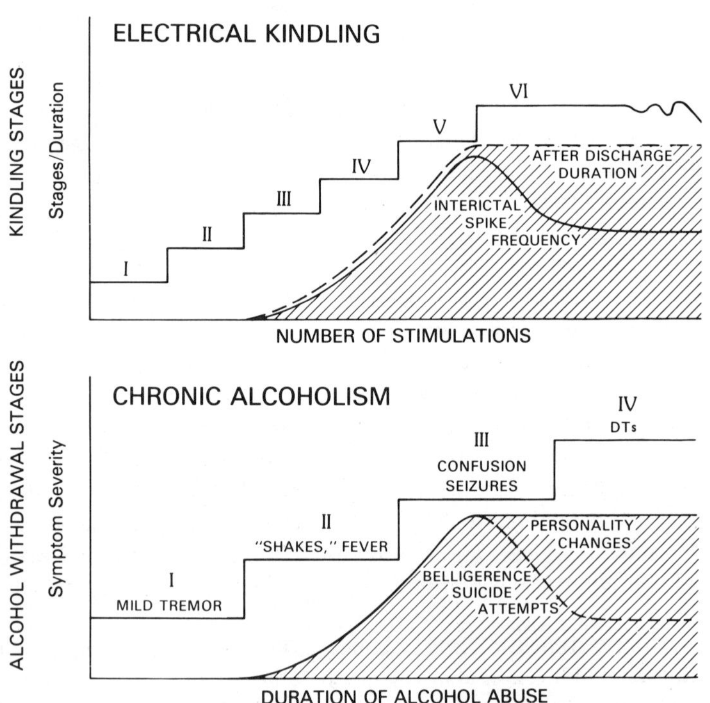

Figure 6 Kindling model for symptomatology of chronic alcoholism.

development of autonomic and psychiatric sequelae observed over time in the alcohol withdrawal syndromes.

Consistent patterns of progressive and serially ordered personality changes also appear to develop in the chronic alcoholic in the interval between episodes of withdrawal. It is of particular interest that many of these personality variables, as described by Jellinek and collaborators (1952), are highly similar to those reported in temporal lobe epileptics (Bear and Fedio, 1977). It is possible that recurrent activation of at least partially similar neural substrates in the temporal-limbic system are related to the overlapping aspects of these clinical syndromes.

VIII. CLINICAL IMPLICATIONS OF KINDLING-LIKE MECHANISMS

A. Alcohol Withdrawal

As cited above, one of the more convincing demonstrations of the possible interaction of kindling and alcohol withdrawal phenomenon are derived from the studies of Pinel and Van Oot (1975,1977). They reported that amygdala-kindled animals had increased severity of alcohol withdrawal syndromes. Our more specific formulation of the alcohol withdrawal syndromes and of the interval-related behavioral pathology as manifestations of kindling after repeated episodes of alcohol withdrawal (Ballenger and Post, 1978a) is subject to further direct experimental and clinical investigative testing. It may open the avenue for new approaches to treatment of the alcohol withdrawal syndromes with a specific focus on prevention of recurrent episodes of alcohol withdrawal. One treatment strategy may involve "covering" each episode of alcohol withdrawal with an appropriate anticonvulsant-tranquilizer such as diazepam or with the anticonvulsant carbamazepine. We suggest these agents both because of their demonstrated efficacy in the acute treatment of the alcohol withdrawal syndromes (Brune, 1966; Brune and Busch, 1971; Bjorkqvist et al., 1976) and also because they are among the most effective agents in retarding a variety of kindling models (Babington and Wedeking, 1973; Wise and Chinerman, 1974; Racine, 1975; Wada et al., 1976). It is worth noting that diphenylhydantoin, which is not particularly effective in the alcohol withdrawal syndromes (Rothstein, 1973), is also not effective in inhibiting the kindling process (Racine, 1975; Wada et al., 1976). As summarized in Table 7, a variety of agents appear to have greater anticonvulsant efficacy at limbic sites compared to more classic cortical sites. This relative selectivity may be relevant to the psychotropic activity of many of the compounds which are more effective at limbic than cortical sites.

Table 7 Pharmacological Effects on Limbic Versus Cortical Kindled Seizures: Evidence for Partial Regional Selectivity[a]

Drug	Effectiveness in retarding amygdala kindling	Suppression of completed kindled seizures		References
		Limbic	Cortical	
Carbamazepine	++	++	+	Babington and Horovitz, 1973; Wada et al., 1976; Wada, 1977
Diazepam	++	++	+	Racine et al., 1975; Babington, 1977; Wise and Chinerman, 1974
Electroconvulsive shock	++	++	+	Babington, 1977
Tricyclic antidepressants		++	+	Babington, 1977
Phenobarbital	++	++	++	Babington and Wedeking, 1973; Wise and Chinerman, 1974; Wada et al., 1976; Turner et al., 1977
Atropine, raphe stimulation, handling stress	++			Arnold et al., 1973; Kovacs and Zoll, 1974
Diphenylhydantoin	0,–	±	++	Wise and Chinerman, 1974; Babington and Wedeking, 1973; Racine et al., 1975; Tanaka, 1972; Wada, 1977; Turner et al., 1977
Procaine	–	–	++	Racine et al., 1975
Reserpine, 6-hydroxydopamine, α-methyl-p-tyrosine	––			Arnold et al., 1973; Sato et al., 1976; Corcoran et al., 1974

[a]Effect on seizures: ++, marked inhibition; +, inhibition; ±, equivocal; 0, no effect; –, potentiation; ––, marked potentiation.

B. Model Psychoses

One experimental approach which also links possible dopaminergic mechanisms with the kindling phenomena derives from the work of Stevens and Livermore (1978). These investigators subjected a small number of cats to kindling by stimulation of the ventral tegmental area (A10), the area of origin of dopaminergic cell bodies projecting to the mesolimbic and mesocortical systems. Following repetitive electrical stimulation, these cats displayed marked asocial behavior, fear reactions, bizarre posturing, and loss of normal social and affectionate behavior. The animals also displayed increased electrical abnormalities following a challenge with the dopamine agonist apomorphine. In two of the cats, reversal of this kindled behavioral syndrome following repetitive stimulation of A10 was produced by prolonged stimulation of the nucleus accumbens, presumably activating an inhibitory feedback pathway to the A10 dopaminergic neurons. This work may also provide a conceptual link between kindling, dopaminergic abnormalities, and bizarre behavioral changes.

Klawans and collaborators (1975,1977a,b) noted the progressive development of L-dopa-induced psychiatric effects (vivid dreams → hallucinations → paranoid psychosis → confusional psychosis) and neurologic sequelae (dyskinesias) in parkinsonian patients.

C. Two Types of Tardive Dyskinesia

It is of interest that similar to the time course of emergence of dyskinesias in parkinsonian patients treated with chronic L-dopa, dyskinesias in animals emerge following long-term indirect dopamine agonist treatment with amphetamine or cocaine (see Fig. 3). Tardive dyskinesias also emerge following long-term treatment with dopamine antagonists (neuroleptics). Recently, Jeste et al. (1978) reported that the emergence and severity of tardive dyskinesia is more specifically associated with the number of times a patient had been withdrawn (for more than 3 months) from chronic neuroleptic treatment, rather than with total duration of neuroleptic treatment. It is possible that repeated episodes of neuroleptic withdrawal, which produce dopamine receptor supersensitivity (Tarsy and Baldessarini, 1973; Snyder et al., 1977), lead to a kindling-like facilitation of receptor sensitivity following each subsequent neuroleptic withdrawal.

D. The Functional Psychoses

We have reviewed several areas of research in which repeated stimulation of the brain, either electrically or chemically, is associated with the development of progressive behavioral, neurologic, or convulsive abnormalities. The broader and more speculative question concerns whether repeated activation of similar neuronal pathways by particular environmental events or severe stresses might also be capable of progressively activating given neural substrates (Meyersburg and Post, 1979). In working with the kindling-like model of post-tetanic potentiation in the hippocampus, Goddard (1978), Racine (1978), and Lynch (1978) demonstrated that repetitive activation of the hippocampus utilizing stimulation characteristics not markedly different from those naturally occurring in the organism are capable of producing increased responses to a subsequent single-stimulus challenge. This "enhancement" effect reported by Douglas and McNaughton (1977) is thought to involve postsynaptic mechanisms and to last for as long as several months.

We would suggest that physiological activation of given neuronal pathways induced by severe environmental stresses or by neurotransmitter alterations associated with a given functional illness, may sensitize that neuronal substrate and facilitate its subsequent activation. In this fashion, it might be conceptualized that repeated stresses during infancy, e.g., the repeated experience of separation and loss, could be a stimulus which sensitizes the subject and predisposes to subsequent depressions on repetition of loss or psychological trauma as an adult. Experimental support for this hypothesis is derived from the work with repetitive primate separations. Young and co-workers (1973) showed that an experience of separation from the mother during infancy is associated with a increased predisposition to a protest and despair reaction following separation again in adulthood. Their data on repeated infant-infant separations also demonstrate that there is no tolerance or accommodation to the separation reaction over time (Suomi et al., 1977).

E. Rapid Cycling Affective Illness

Does each episode of affective illness affect the likelihood of occurrence of the next episode, consistent with a progressive kindling-like model? Grof et al. (1974) reported, with a patient population sample of 594 recurrent unipolar depressives, that on the average each episode of depression tended to occur with shorter intervals between successive episodes (Fig. 7). This apparent sensitization phenomena was more evident in the older age ranges but also occurred following repeated depressive episodes independent of age. Thus, there appears to be a mechanism facilitating the recurrence of depressive episodes, as reflected by the progressively decreasing duration of the asymptomatic interval between episodes. The dopamine agonist behavioral sensitization model and the kindling model may also be relevant for recurrent manic episodes. To the extent that dopaminergic mechanisms are involved in manic illness, repeated exposure to dopamine agonists, either exogenously or endogenously produced, could lead to a sensitization process and an increased frequency of affective episodes (Post, 1977b,c).

It is perhaps noteworthy that electroconvulsive therapy, one of the major treatments for psychotic depression, can alter the kindling process (Babington,

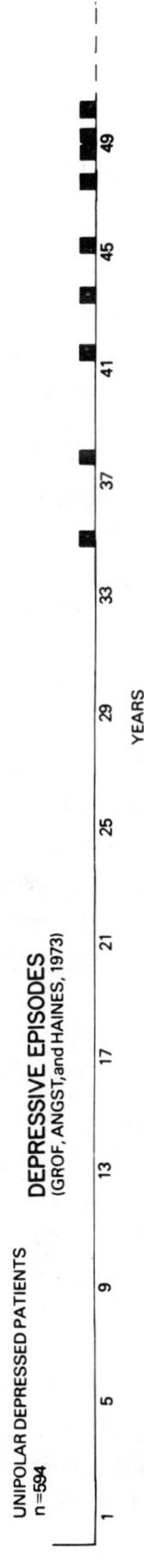

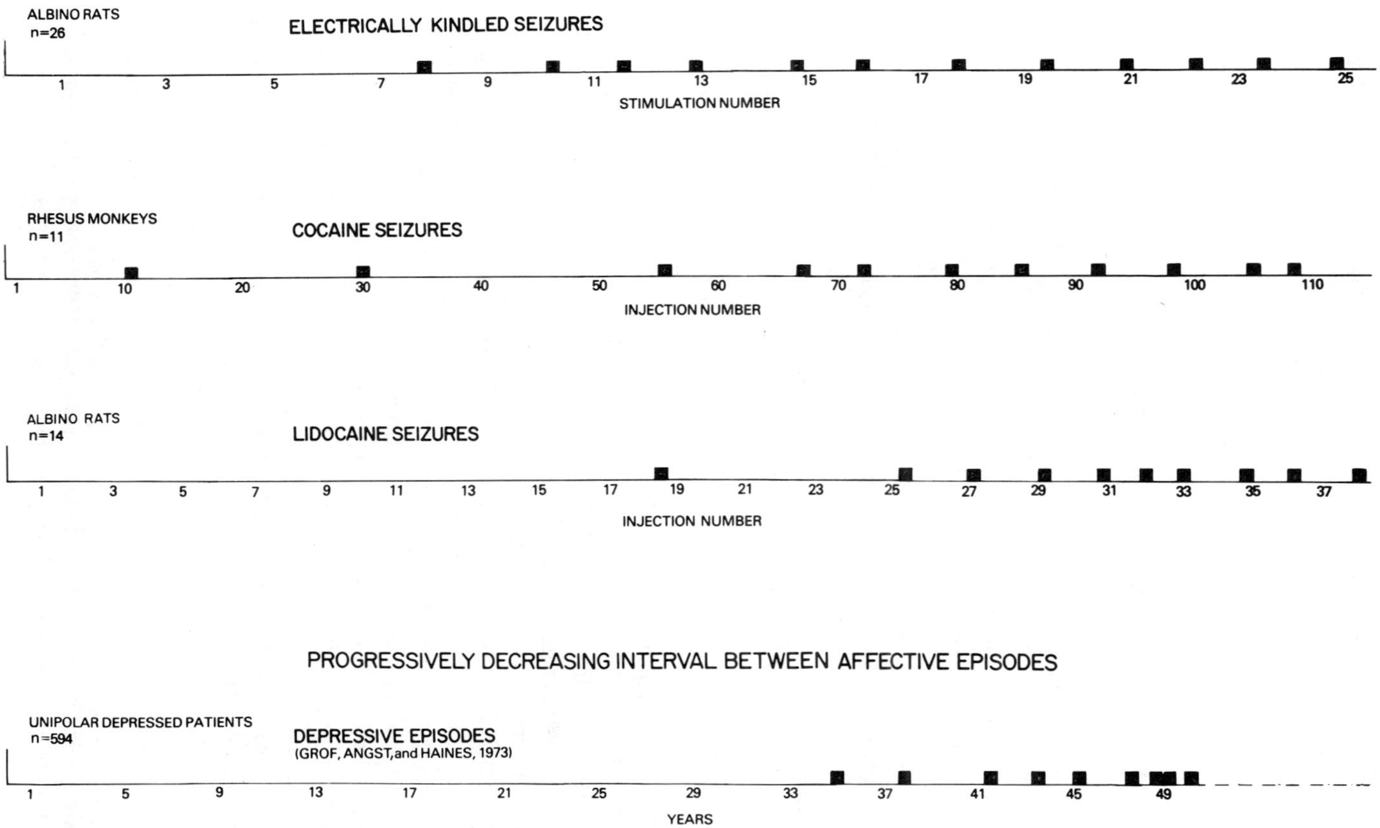

Figure 7 Decreasing interval between episodes of seizures as kindling is established.

1977) and also sensitizes to the activating effects of a variety of agents acting on dopamine, norepinephrine, and serotonin receptors (Modigh, 1975; Evans et al., 1976; Green et al., 1977). The kindling or sensitization formulation may thus lead to new conceptual approaches to the mechanism of action of ECT. Several psychotropic manipulations also have significant effects on the kindling process (Table 7).

F. A Limbic Anticonvulsant in Affective Illness

While the kindling mechanism and neurotransmitter-receptor-mediated changes underlying sensitization are obviously a highly speculative approach to recurrent affective illness, they do emphasize the temporal characteristics and apparent progressive aspects of the clinical course in some patients. In this fashion, this model may also lead to the formulation of new clinical and theoretical approaches to the illness. For example, we recently undertook a preliminary clinical trial of the anticonvulsant carbamazepine in affectively ill patients with no evidence of a convulsive disorder (Ballenger and Post, 1978b, 1980; Post et al., 1978b). The rationale for this clinical trial was based in part on the kindling paradigm with the hypothesis that pathological activation of one or more temporal-limbic substrates may be one of the mechanisms underlying recurrent manic and depressive episodes. It was also based on the empirical observations that many patients with psychomotor epilepsy showed improvement in their psychiatric status when treated with carbamazepine (Dalby, 1975). In addition, preliminary evidence from a nonblind trial by Okuma et al. (1973) in Japan reported therapeutic responses to carbamazepine in both acute and recurrent episodes of affective illness, including positive prophylactic effects in some patients who were lithium nonresponders.

Of our first 14 affectively ill patients tested, 8 appeared to show positive therapeutic effects to carbamazepine. In this double-blind placebo-controlled study, several patients showed acute antimanic responses and then dramatic rebounds in psychotic psychopathology following drug withdrawal (Fig. 8). Two patients showed evidence of a continued and prophylactic effect on recurrent manic episodes. Three patients also showed apparent antidepressive responses and some prophylaxis against recurrent depressive episodes during treatment with carbamazepine. The data from our double-blind clinical trial taken together with the larger open series of Okuma et al. (1973) are suggestive that carbamazepine may be of both acute and longer term therapeutic value when used alone or in combination with other drugs in some patients with affective illness.

At this time, it is not known whether carbamazepine's anticonvulsant properties and its ability to suppress, in a relatively selective fashion, limbic versus cortical excitability are related to the apparent therapeutic effects in patients with affective illness. It may be that carbamazepine (a tricyclic with a

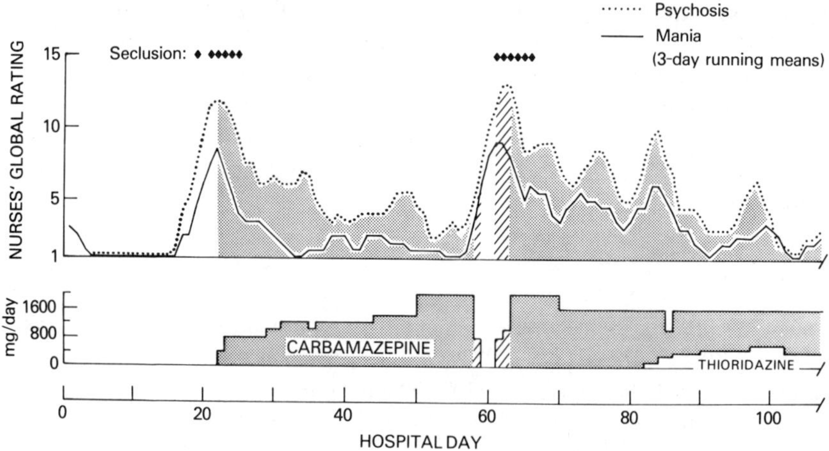

Figure 8 Therapeutic effect of carbamazepine in a manic patient.

structure closely resembling imipramine) is acting via biogenic amine pathways or some other neurochemical system to produce its therapeutic effects. Our preliminary data suggest that it does alter several peripheral and central indices of norepinephrine metabolism in humans (Post et al., 1978b). Exploration of the mechanism of action of carbamazepine in affective illness remains an intriguing problem, which hopefully may shed some light on the neuronal mechanisms underlying the illness. In this regard, it is of particular interest that lithium carbonate, obviously the mainstay of prophylactic treatment of recurrent manic-depressive illness, was shown by Delgado and DeFeudis in 1967 to exert some inhibitory effects on limbic and amygdala excitability. Preliminary data from our laboratory suggest that lithium administration to rats, producing the equivalent of low therapeutic levels in humans (0.4 to 0.8 mEq/liter), did not alter the rate of amygdala electrical kindling, however.

IX. CONCLUSIONS

We have attempted to organize a wide range of clinical and experimental data around the concept of the temporal progression of behavioral pathology. Many drug-induced changes, particularly involving chronic, high-dose dopaminergic stimulation, may be associated with increased disruption of normal behavior in animals and humans. A focus on neurophysiological, transmitter, and receptor changes accompanying this evolving process may help elucidate mechanisms involved in the endogenous psychoses.

The kindling model, in which repeated electrical stimulation of various brain sites eventually evokes major behavioral and convulsive responses to a previously subthreshold stimulation, may also be useful for conceptualizing the development of psychiatric symptoms in temporal lobe epilepsy, the alcohol withdrawal syndromes, and the functional psychoses. The model also directs attention to the biochemical and neurophysiological stimulus characteristics which promote behavioral sensitization. Hopefully, such a formulation may lead to new conceptual approaches to the evaluation of several psychotic syndromes and their treatment.

REFERENCES

Adamec, R. (1975). Behavioral and epileptic determinants of predatory attack behavior in the cat. *Can. J. Neurol. Sci. 2,* 457-466.

Angrist, B. M., and Gershon, S. (1970). The phenomenology of experimentally induced amphetamine psychosis. Preliminary observations. *Biol. Psychiatry 2,* 95-107.

Angrist, B. M., and Sudilovsky, A. (1978). Central nervous system stimulants. Historical aspects and clinical effects. In *Handbook of Psychopharmacology,* Vol. 11, L. Iverson, S. Iverson, and S. Snyder (Eds.). Plenum, New York, pp. 99-165.

Angrist, B. M., Sathananthan, G., Wilk, S., and Gershon, S. (1974). Amphetamine psychosis. Behavioral and biochemical aspects. *J. Psychiatr. Res. 11,* 13-23.

Arnold, P. S., Racine, R. J., and Wise, R. A. (1973). Effects of atropine, reserpine, 6-hydroxydopamine, and handling on seizure development in the rat. *Exp. Neurol. 40,* 457-470.

Babington, R. G. (1977). The pharmacology of kindling. In *Animal Models in Psychiatry and Neurology,* I. Hanin and E. Usdin (Eds.). Pergamon, New York, pp. 141-150.

Babington, R. G., and Horovitz, Z. P. (1973). Neuropharmacology of SQ 10,996, a compound with several therapeutic indications. *Arch. Int. Pharmacodyn. Ther. 202,* 106-118.

Babington, R. G., and Wedeking, P. W. (1973). The pharmacology of seizures induced by sensitization with low intensity brain stimulation. *Pharmacol. Biochem. Behav. 1,* 461-467.

Bailey, R. C., and Jackson, D. M. (1978). A pharmacological study of changes in central nervous system receptor responsiveness after long-term dextroamphetamine and apomorphine administration. *Psychopharmacology 56,* 317-326.

Baker, T. B., and Cannon, D. S. (1979). Potentiation of ethanol withdrawal by prior dependence. *Psychopharmacology 60,* 105-110.

Ballenger, J. C., and Post, R. M. (1978a). Kindling as a model for the alcohol withdrawal syndromes. *Br. J. Psychiatry 133,* 1-14.

Ballenger, J. C., and Post, R. M. (1978b). Therapeutic effects of carbamazepine in affective illness: A preliminary report. *Comm. Psychopharmacol. 2,*159-175.

Ballenger, J. C., Goodwin, F. K., Major, L. F., and Brown, G. L. (1979). Alcohol and central serotonin metabolism in man. *Arch. Gen. Psychiatry 226,* 224-227.

Ballenger, J. C., and Post, R. M. (1980). Carbamazepine in manic-depressive illness: a new treatment. *Am. J. Psychiatry 137,* 782-790.

Banerjee, S. P., Sharma, V. K., Kung, L. S., and Chanda, S. K. (1978). Amphetamine induces β-adrenergic receptor supersensitivity. *Nature 271,* 380-381.

Barbeau, A. (1974). The clinical physiology of side effects of long-term L-DOPA therapy. In *Advances in Neurology,* Vol. 5, F. H. McDowell and A. Barbeau (Eds.). Raven, New York, pp. 347-366.

Baudry, M., Martres, M. P., and Schwartz, J. C. (1977). In vivo binding of ^{3}H-pimozide in mouse striatum. Effects of dopamine agonists and antagonists. *Life Sci. 21,* 1163-1170.

Bear, D. M. (1979). Temporal lobe epilepsy. A syndrome of sensory-limbic hyperconnection. *Cortex 15,* 357-384.

Bear, D. M., and Fedio, P. (1977). Quantitative analysis of interictal behavior in temporal lobe epilepsy. *Arch. Neurol. 34,* 454-467.

Begleiter, H., Gross, M. M., and Porjesz, B. (1973). Recovery function and clinical symptomatology in acute alcoholization and withdrawal. In *Alcohol Intoxication and Withdrawal: Experimental Studies,* M. M. Gross (Ed.). Plenum, New York, pp. 406-413.

Bjorkqvist, S. G., Isohanni, M., Makela, R., and Malinen, L. (1976). Ambulant treatment of alcohol withdrawal symptoms with carbamazepine: A formal multicentre double-blind comparison with placebo. *Acta. Psychiatr. Scand. 53,* 333-342.

Blumer, D. (1975). Temporal lobe epilepsy and its psychiatric significance. In *Psychiatric Aspects of Neurological Disease,* D. F. Benson and D. Blumer (Eds.). Grune and Stratton, New York, pp. 171-198.

Borison, R. L., Havdala, H. S., and Diamond, B. I. (1977). Chronic phenylethylamine stereotypy in rats. A new animal model for schizophrenia? *Life Sci. 21,* 117-122.

Borison, R. L., Diamond, B. I., and Walter, R. (1978). Peptide role in animal models of schizophrenia. In *Proc. 23rd Ann. Meet. Soc. Biol. Psychiatry,* Atlanta, Georgia, 1978, Abstr. 39.

Branchey, M., Rauscher, G., and Kissin, B. (1971). Modifications in the response to alcohol following the establishment of physical dependence. *Psychopharmacologia 22,* 314-322.

Browne, R. G., and Segal, D. S. (1977). Metabolic and experiential factors in the behavioral response to repeated amphetamine. *Pharmacol. Biochem. Behav. 6,* 545-552.

Brune, F. (1966). Anhebung der krampfschwelle als therapeutisches prinzip bei der behandlung von alkolhol-delirien. *Der Nervenarzt 37,* 415-418.

Brune, F., and Busch, H. (1971). Anticonvulsive-sedative treatment of delirium alcoholism. *Q. J. Stud. Alcohol 32,* 334-342.

Burt, D. R., Creese, I., and Snyder, S. H. (1977). Antischizophrenic drugs. Chronic treatment elevates dopamine receptor binding in brain. *Science 197,* 326-328.

Byck, R., Jatlow, P., Barash, P., and van Dyke, C. (1977). Cocaine. Blood concentration and physiological effect after intranasal application in man. In *Advances in Behavioral Biology,* Vol. 21, *Cocaine and Other Stimulants,* E. H. Ellinwood and M. M. Kilbey (Eds.). Plenum, New York, pp. 629-646.

Carlsson, A. (1978). Antipsychotic drugs, neurotransmitters, and schizophrenia. *Am. J. Psychiatry 135,* 164-173.

Chanda, S. K., Sharma, V. K., and Banerjee, S. P. (1979). β-Adrenoceptor (β-AR) sensitivity following psychotropic drug treatment. In *Catecholamines: Basic and Clinical Frontiers,* E. Usdin, I. J. Kopin, and J. Barchas (Eds.). Pergamon, New York, pp. 586-588.

Connell, P. H. (1958). *Amphetamine Psychoses.* Oxford University Press, New York.

Corcoran, M. E., Fibiger, H. C., McCaughran, J. A., Jr., and Wada, J. A. (1974). Potentiation of amygdaloid kindling and metrazol-induced seizures by 6-hydroxydopamine in rats. *Exp. Neurol. 45,* 118-133.

Costall, B., and Naylor, R. (1977). Mesolimbic and extrapyramidal sites for the mediation of stereotyped behavior patterns and hyperactivity by amphetamine and apomorphine in the rat. In *Advances in Behavioral Biology,* Vol. 21, *Cocaine and Other Stimulants,* E. H. Ellinwood and M. M. Kilbey (Eds.). Plenum, New York, pp. 47-76.

Dalby, M. A. (1975). Behavioral effects of carbamazepine. In *Advances in Neurology,* Vol. 11, J. K. Penry and D. D. Daly (Eds.). Raven, New York, pp. 331-343.

Delgado, J. M. R., and DeFeudis, F. V. (1967). Effects of lithium injections into the amygdala and hippocampus of awake monkeys. *Exp. Neurol. 25,* 255-267.

Douglas, R. M., and McNaughton, B. L. (1977). Enhancement of synaptic responses to stimulation of the perforant path is dependent on the number of fibers activated. *Proc. 7th Ann. Meet. Soc. Neurosci.,* Abstract #1640, p. 514.

Downs, A. W., and Eddy, N. B. (1932a). The effect of repeated doses of cocaine on the dog. *J. Pharmacol. Exp. Ther. 46,* 195-198.

Downs, A. W., and Eddy, N. B. (1932b). The effect of repeated doses of cocaine on the rat. *J. Pharmacol. Exp. Ther. 46,* 199-200.

Eidelberg, E., Lesse, H., and Gault, F. P. (1963). An experimental model of temporal lobe epilepsy. Studies of the convulsant properties of cocaine. In *EEG and Behavior,* G. H. Glaser (Ed.). Basic Books, New York, pp. 272-283.

Ellinwood, E. H. (1967). Amphetamine Psychosis. I. Description of the individuals and process. *J. Nerv. Ment. Dis. 144,* 273-283.

Ellinwood, E. H., and Kilbey, M. M. (1977). Chronic stimulant intoxication models of psychosis. In *Animal Models in Psychiatry and Neurology,* I. Hanin and E. Usdin (Eds.). Pergamon, New York, pp. 61-74.

Ellinwood, E. H., and Kilbey, M. M. (1978). Paper presented at the Workshop on The Chronic Use of Cocaine: Tolerance and Dependence? at the 11th Ann. Meet. Winter Conf. Brain Research, Keystone, Colorado, January 1978.

Ellinwood, E. H., Kilbey, M. M., Castellani, S., and Khoury, C. (1977). Amygdala hyperspindling and seizures induced by cocaine. In *Advances in Behavioral Biology,* Vol. 21, *Cocaine and Other Stimulants,* E. H. Ellinwood and M. M. Kilbey (Eds.). Plenum, New York, pp. 303-326.

Engel, J., Jr., Wolfson, L., and Brown, L. (1978). Anatomical correlates of electrical and behavioral events related to amygdaloid kindling. *Ann. Neurol. 3,* 538-544.

Evans, J. P. M., Grahame-Smith, D. G., Green, A. R., and Tordoff, A. F. C. (1976). Electroconvulsive shock increases the behavioral responses of rats to brain 5-hydroxytryptamine accumulation and central nervous system stimulant drugs. *Br. J. Pharmacol. 56,* 193-199.

Fischman, M. W., Schuster, C. R., and Krasnegor, A. (1977). Physiological and behavioral effects of intravenous cocaine in man. In *Advances in Behavioral Biology,* Vol. 21, *Cocaine and Other Stimulants,* E. H. Ellinwood and M. M. Kilbey (Eds.). Plenum, New York, pp. 647-664.

Flor-Henry, P. (1969). Schizophrenic-like reactions and affective psychoses associated with temporal lobe epilepsy. Etiological factors. *Am. J. Psychiatry 126,* 400-403.

Flor-Henry, P. (1974). Psychosis, neurosis, and epilepsy. Developmental and gender-related effects and their aetiological contribution. *Br. J. Psychiatry 124,* 144-150.

Flor-Henry, P. (1978). The endogenous psychoses. A reflection of laterized dysfunction of the anterior limbic system. In *Limbic Mechanisms: The Continuing Evolution of the Limbic System Concept,* K. E. Livingston and O. Hornykiewicz (Eds.). Plenum, New York.

Friedhoff, A. J., Bonnet, K., and Rosengarten, H. (1977). Reversal of two manifestations of dopamine receptor supersensitivity by administration of L-DOPA. *Chem. Path. Pharmacol. (Res. Comm.) 16,* 411-423.

Gallager, D. W., Pert, A., and Bunney, W. E., Jr. (1978). Haloperidol-induced presynaptic dopamine supersensitivity is blocked by chronic lithium. *Nature 273,* 309-312.

Gibbs, F. A. (1951). Ictal and nonictal psychiatric disorders in temporal lobe epilepsy. *J. Nerv. Ment. Dis. 113,* 522-528.

Glaser, G. H., Newman, R. J., and Schafer, R. (1963). Interictal psychosis in psychomotor-temporal lobe epilepsy. An EEG-psychological study. In *EEG and Behavior,* G. H. Glaser (Ed.). Basic Books, New York, pp. 345-365.

Gloor, P. (1972). Temporal lobe epilepsy. Its possible contribution to the understanding of the functional significance of the amygdala and of its interaction with neocortical-temporal mechanisms. In *Advances in Behavioral Biology,* Vol. 2, *The Neurobiology of the Amygdala,* B. E. Eleftheriou (Ed.). Plenum, New York, pp. 423-458.

Goddard, G. V. (1978). Paper presented at the Workshop on Post Activation Potentiation at the 11th Ann. Winter Conf. Brain Research, Keystone, Colorado, January 1978.

Goddard, G. V., and Douglas, R. M. (1975). Does the engram of kindling model the engram of normal long term memory? *Can. J. Neurol. Sci. 2,* 385-394.

Goddard, G. V., McIntyre, D. C., and Leech, C. K. (1969). A permanent change in brain function resulting from daily electrical stimulation. *Exp. Neurol. 25,* 295-330.

Green, A. R., Heal, D. J., and Grahame-Smith, D. G. (1977). Further observations on the effect of repeated electroconvulsive shock on the behavioral responses of rats produced by increases in the functional activity of brain 5-hydroxytryptamine and dopamine. *Psychopharmacology 52,* 195-200.

Griffith, J. D., Cavanaugh, J. H., Held, J., and Oates, J. A. (1970). Experimental psychosis induced by the administration of d-amphetamine. In *Amphetamines and Related Compounds,* E. Costa and S. Garattini (Eds.). Raven, New York, pp. 897-904.

Grof, P., Angst, J., and Haines, T. (1974). The clinical course of depression. Practical issues. In *Symposia Medica Hoest,* Vol. 8, *Classification and Prediction of Outcome of Depression,* F. K. Schattauer (Ed.). Schattauer Verlag, New York, pp. 141-148.

Groves, P. M., and Rebec, G. V. (1977). Changes in neuronal activity in the neostriatum and reticular formation following acute or long-term amphetamine administration. In *Advances in Behavioral Biology,* Vol. 21, *Cocaine and Other Stimulants,* E. H. Ellinwood and M. M. Kilbey (Eds.). Plenum, New York, pp. 269-302.

Guerrero-Figueroa, R., Rye, M. M., Gallant, D. M., and Bishop, M. (1970). Electrographic and behavioral effects of diazepam during alcohol withdrawal stage in cats. *Neuropharmacology 9,* 143-150.

Gunne, L. M., Anggard, E., and Jonsson, L. E. (1972). Clinical trials with amphetamine-blocking drugs. *Psychiatr. Neurol. Neurochir. 75,* 225-226.

Gutierrez-Noriega, C. (1950). Inhibition of central nervous systems produced by chronic cocaine intoxication. *Fed. Proc. 9,* 280.

Gutierrez-Noriega, C., and Zapata-Ortiz, V. (1945). Una neuva accion pharmacologica de la cocaina la accion anticonvulsivante. *Rev. Med. Exp. 4,* 59-100.

Hitzemann, R. J., Tseng, L. F., Hitzemann, B. A., Sampath-Khanna, S., and Loh, H. H. (1977). Effects of withdrawal from chronic amphetamine intoxication on exploratory and stereotyped behaviors in the rat. *Psychopharmacology 54,* 295-302.

Ho, B. T., Taylor, D. L., and Estevez, V. S. (1977). Behavioral effects of cocaine. Metabolic and neurochemical approach. In *Advances in Behavioral Biology,* Vol. 21, *Cocaine and Other Stimulants,* E. H. Ellinwood and M. M. Kilbey (Eds.). Plenum, New York, pp. 229-240.

Howlett, D. R., and Nahorski, S. R. (1978). Effect of acute and chronic amphetamine administration on β-adrenoceptors and dopamine receptors in rat corpus striatum and limbic forebrain. *Br. J. Pharmacol. 64,* 411-412.

Hunt, W. A. (1973). Changes in the neuro-excitability of alcohol dependent rats undergoing withdrawal as measured by the pentylenetetrazole seizure threshold. *Neuropharmacology 12,* 1097-1102.

Hunter, B. E., Boast, C. A., Walker, D. W., and Zornetzer, S. F. (1973). Alcohol withdrawal syndrome in rats. Neural and behavioral correlates. *Pharmacol. Biochem. Behav. 1,* 719-725.

Janowsky, D. S., El-Yousef, M. K., Davis, J. M., and Sekerke, H. J. (1973). Provocation of schizophrenic symptoms by intravenous administration of methylphenidate. *Arch. Gen. Psychiatry 28,* 185-191.

Jellinek, E. M. (1952). Phases of alcohol addiction. *Q. J. Stud. Alcohol 13,* 673-684.

Jeste, D. V., Potkin, S. G., Sinha, S., Feder, S., and Wyatt, R. J. (1978). Tardive dyskinesia. Reversible or persistent. *Arch. Gen. Psychiatry 36,* 585-590.

Jimerson, D. C., Post, R. M., Reus, V. I., van Kammen, D. P., Docherty, J., Gillin, J. C., Buchsbaum, M., Ebert, M., and Bunney, W. E., Jr. (1977). Predictors of amphetamine response on depression. *Sci. Proc. Am. Psychiatr. Ass. 130,* 100-101, Abstr. 170.

Jori, A., and Garratini, S. (1973). Catecholamine metabolism and amphetamine effects on sensitive and insensitive mice. In *Frontiers in Catecholamine*

Research, E. Usdin and S. H. Snyder (Eds.). Pergamon, New York, pp. 939-942.

Kilbey, M. M., and Ellinwood, E. H. (1977). Chronic administration of stimulant drugs. Response modification. In *Advances in Behavioral Biology,* Vol. 21, *Cocaine and Other Stimulants,* E. H. Ellinwood and M. M. Kilbey (Eds.). Plenum, New York, pp. 409-430.

Klawans, H. L., and Margolin, D. I. (1975). Amphetamine-induced dopaminergic sensitivity in guinea pigs. *Arch. Gen. Psychiatry 32,* 725-732.

Klawans, H. L., Crossett, P., and Dana, N. (1975). Effect of chronic amphetamine exposure on stereotyped behavior. Implications for pathogenesis of L-DOPA-induced dyskinesias. In *Advances in Neurology,* Vol. 9, D. B. Calne, T. N. Chase, and A. Barbeau (Eds.). Raven, New York, pp. 105-

Klawans, H. L., Goetz, C., Nausieda, P. A., and Weiner, W. J. (1977a). Levodopa-induced dopamine receptor hypersensitivity. *Ann. Neurol. 2,* 125-129.

Klawans, H. L., Hitri, A., Nausieda, P. A., and Weiner, W. J. (1977b). Animal models of dyskinesia. In *Animal Models in Psychiatry and Neurology,* I. Hanin and E. Usdin (Eds.). Pergamon, New York, pp. 351-364.

Kosman, M. E., and Unna, K. P. (1968). Effects of chronic administration of the amphetamines and other stimulants on behavior. *Clin. Pharmacol. Ther. 9,* 240-254.

Kovacs, D. A., and Zoll, J. G. (1974). Seizure inhibition by median raphe nucleus stimulation in rat. *Brain Res. 70,* 165-169.

Kuhn, C. M., and Schanberg, S. M. (1977). Distribution and metabolism of amphetamine in tolerant animals. In *Advances in Behavioral Biology,* Vol. 21, *Cocaine and Other Stimulants,* E. H. Ellinwood and M. M. Kilbey (Eds.). Plenum, New York, pp. 161-178.

Lewander, T. (1968). Urinary excretion and tissue levels of catecholamines during chronic amphetamine intoxication. *Psychopharmacologia 13,* 394-407.

Lynch, G. S. (1978). Hippocampal potentials and related events. In Symposium III: Physiological Mechanisms Related to Learning and Memory. Presented at the Ann. Meet. Soc. Biol. Psychiatry, Atlanta, May 1978.

MacLean, P. D. (1973). A triune concept of the brain and behavior. In *Clarance M. Hincks Memorial Lectures, 1969,* T. J. Boag and D. Campbell (Eds.). University of Toronto Press, Toronto.

Mago, L. (1969). Persistence of the effect of amphetamine on stereotyped activity in rats. *Eur. J. Pharmacol. 6,* 200-201.

Martin, W. R., Sloan, J. W., Sapira, B. S., and Jasinski, D. R. (1971). Physiologic, subjective, and behavioral effects of amphetamine methamphetamine, ephedrine, phenmetrazine, and methylphenidate in man. *Clin. Pharmacol. Ther. 12,* 245-258.

Martres, M. P., Costentin, J., Baudry, M., Marcais, H., Protais, P., and Schwartz, J. C. (1977). Long-term changes in the sensitivity of pre-and postsynaptic dopamine receptors in mouse striatum evidenced by behavioral and biochemical studies. *Brain Res. 136,* 319-337.

Mason, C. R., and Cooper, R. M. (1972). A permanent change in convulsive threshold in normal and brain damaged rats with small repeated doses of pentylenetetrazol. *Epilepsia 13,* 663-674.

Matsuzaki, M., Spingler, P. J., Misra, A. L., and Mule, S. J. (1976). Cocaine. Tolerance to its convulsant and cardiorespiratory stimulating effects in the monkey. *Life Sci. 19,* 193-204.

McIntyre, D. C. (1976). Kindling and memory. The adrenal system and the bisected brain. In *Limbic Mechanisms: The Continuing Evolution of the Limbic System Concept,* K. E. Livingston and O. Hornykiewicz (Eds.). Plenum, New York, p.p. 495-506.

McManus, C., Hartley, E. J., and Seeman, P. (1978). Increased binding of [^{3}H]-apomorphine in caudate membranes after dopamine pretreatment in vitro. *J. Pharm. Pharmacol. 30,* 444-447.

McQuarrie, D., and Fingl, E. (1958). Effect of single doses and chronic administration of ethanol on experimental seizures in mice. *J. Pharmacol. Exp. Ther. 124,* 264-271.

Mendelson, J. H. (1972). Biochemical mechanisms of alcohol addiction. In *The Biology of Alcoholism,* Vol. 1, B. Kissin and H. Begleiter (Eds.). Plenum, New York, pp. 513-544.

Meyersburg, H. A., and Post, R. M. (1979). An holistic developmental view of neural and psychological processes. *Br. J. Psychiatry 135,* 139-155.

Misra, A. L., Nayak, P. K., Patel, M. N., Vadlamani, N. L., and Mule, S. J. (1974). Identification of norcocaine as a metabolite of [^{3}H]-cocaine in rat brain. *Experientia* (Basel) *30,* 1312-1314.

Modigh, K. (1975). Electroconvulsive shock and postsynaptic catecholamine effects: Increased psychomotor stimulant action of apomorphine and clonidine in reserpine pretreated mice by repeated ECS. *J. Neural Transm. 36,* 19-32.

Moskovitz, C., Moses, H., and Klawans, H. L. (1978). Levodopa-induced psychosis. A kindling phenomenon. *Am. J. Psychiatry 135,* 669-675.

Mucha, R. F., and Pinel, J. P. J. (1977). Postseizure inhibition of kindled seizures. *Exp. Neurol. 54,* 266-282.

Mule, S. J., and Misra, A. L. (1977). Cocaine. Distribution and metabolism in man. In *Advances in Behavioral Biology,* Vol. 21, *Cocaine and Other Stimulants,* E. H. Ellinwood and M. M. Kilbey (Eds.). Plenum, New York, pp. 215-228.

Muller, P., and Seeman, P. (1979). Presynaptic subsensitivity as a possible basis for sensitization by long-term dopamine mimetics. *Eur. J. Pharmacol. 55,* 149-157.

Munson, E. S., Martucci, R. W., and Wagman, I. H. (1972). Bupivacaine and lignocaine induced seizures in rhesus monkeys. *Br. J. Anaesth. 44,* 1025-1029.

Nausieda, P. A., Weiner, W. J., Kanapa, D. L., and Klawans, H. L. (1978). Bromocriptine-induced behavioral hypersensitivity. Implications for the therapy of Parkinsonism. *Ann. Neurol. 20,* 1183-1188.

Nelson, L. R., and Ellison, G. (1978). Enhanced stereotypies after repeated injections but not continuous amphetamines. *Neuropharmacology 17,* 1081-1084.

Okuma, T., Kishimoto, A., Inoue, K., Matsumoto, H., Ogura, A., Matsushita, T., Naklao, T., and Ogura, C. (1973). Antimanic and prophylactic effects of carbamazepine on manic-depressive psychosis. *Folia Psychiatr. Neurol.* Jap. *27,* 283-297.

Peachey, J. E., Rogers, B., and Brien, J. F. (1977). A comparative study of the behavioral responses induced by chronic administration of methamphetamine and amphetamine in mice. *Psychopharmacology 51,* 137-140.

Pert, A., Rosenblatt, J. E., Sivit, C., Pert, C. B., and Bunney, W. E., Jr. (1978). Long term treatment with lithium prevents the development of dopamine receptor supersensitivity. *Science 201,* 171-173.

Pijnenburg, A. J. J., Honig, W. M. M., Struyker-Boudier, H. A. J., Cools, A. R., van der Heyden, J. A. M., and van Rossum, J. M. (1976). Further investigations on the effects of ergometrine and other ergot derivatives following injection into the nucleus accumbens of the rat. *Arch. Int. Pharmacodyn. Ther. 222,* 103-115.

Pinel, J. P. J., and Van Oot, P. H. (1975). Generality of the kindling phenomenon. Some clinical implications. *Can. J. Neurol. Sci. 2,* 467-475.

Pinel, J. P. J., and Van Oot, P. H. (1977). Intensification of the alcohol withdrawal syndrome following periodic electroconvulsive shocks. *Biol. Psychiatry 12,* 479-486.

Pinel, J. P. J., and Cheung, K. F. (1977). Controlled demonstration of metrazol kindling. *Pharmacol. Biochem. Behav. 6,* 599-600.

Pinel, J. P. J., Phillips, A. G., and MacNeill, B. (1973). Blockage of highly stable "kindled" seizures in rats by antecedent footshock. *Epilepsia 14,* 29-37.

Pinel, J. P. J., Van Oot, P. H., and Mucha, R. F. (1975). Intensification of the alcohol withdrawal syndrome by repeated brain stimulation. *Nature 254,* 510-511.

Pinel, J. P. J., Treit, D., and Rovner, L. J. (1977). Temporal lobe aggression in rats. *Science 197,* 1088-1089.

Post, R. M. (1975). Cocaine psychoses. A continuum model. *Am. J. Psychiatry 132,* 627-634.

Post, R. M. (1977a). Progressive changes in behavior and seizures following chronic cocaine administration. Relationship of kindling and psychosis. In *Advances in Behavioral Biology,* Vol. 21, *Cocaine and Other Stimulants,* E. H. Ellinwood and M. M. Kilbey (Eds.). Plenum, New York, pp. 353-372.

Post, R. M. (1977b). Clinical implications of a cocaine-kindling model of psychosis. In *Clinical Neuropharmacology,* Vol. 2, H. L. Klawans (Ed.). Raven, New York, pp. 25-42.

Post, R. M. (1977c). Approaches to rapidly cycling manic-depressive illness. In *Animal Models in Psychiatry and Neurology,* I. Hanin and E. Usdin (Eds.). Pergamon, Oxford, pp. 201-210.

Post, R. M., and Goodwin, F. K. (1975). Time-dependent effect of phenothiazines on dopamine turnover in psychiatric patients. *Science 190,* 488-489.

Post, R. M., and Kopanda, R. T. (1975). Cocaine, kindling, and reverse tolerance. *Lancet 1,* 409-410.

Post, R. M., and Kopanda, R. T. (1976). Cocaine, kindling, and psychosis. *Am. J. Psychiatry 133,* 627-634.

Post, R. M., and Rose, H. (1976). Increasing effects of repetitive cocaine administration in the rat. *Nature 260,* 731-732.

Post, R. M., Kotin, J., and Goodwin, F. K. (1974). The effects of cocaine on depressed patients. *Am. J. Psychiatry 131,* 511-517.

Post, R. M., Kopanda, R. T., and Lee, A. (1975). Progressive behavioral changes during chronic lidocaine administration. Relationship to kindling. *Life Sci. 17,* 943-950.

Post, R. M., Kopanda, R. T., and Black, K. E. (1976). Progressive effects of cocaine on behavior and central amine metabolism in rhesus monkeys. Relationship to kindling and psychosis. *Biol. Psychiatry 11,* 403-419.

Post, R. M., Squillace, K. M., and Pert, A. (1978a). Rhythmic oscillations in amygdala excitability during kindling. *Life Sci. 22,* 717-726.

Post, R. M., Ballenger, J. C., Reus, V. I., Lake, C. R., and Lerner, P. (1978b). Effects of carbamazepine in mania and depression. *Scientific Proc. 131st Ann. Meet. American Psychiatric Association,* Atlanta, May 1978. New Research Abstr. 7.

Post, R. M., Kennedy, C., Shinohara, M., Squillace, K., Miyaoka, M., Suda, S., Ingvar, D. H., and Sokoloff, L. (1979). Local cerebral glucose utilization in lidocaine-kindled seizures. *Soc. Neurosci. Abstr. 5.* Society for Neuroscience, Bethesda, Maryland.

Post, R. M., Squillace, K. M., Pert, A., and Sass, W. (1980a). The effect of amygdala kindling on spontaneous and cocaine induced motor activity and lidocaine seizures. *Psychopharmacology.* In press.

Post, R. M., Lockfield, A., Squillace, K. M., and Contel, N. R. (1980b). Drug-environment interaction: context dependency of cocaine-induced behavioral sensitization. *Commun. Psychopharmacol.* In press.

Prichard, J. W., Gallagher, B. B., and Glaser, G. H. (1969). Experimental seizure-threshold testing with flurothyl. *J. Pharmacol. Exp. Ther. 166,* 170-178.

Racine, R. J. (1972a). Modification of seizure activity by electrical stimulation. I. After-discharge threshold. *Electroencephalogr. Clin. Neurophysiol. 32,* 269-279.

Racine, R. J. (1972b). Modification of seizure activity by electrical stimulation. Motor seizures. *Electroencephalogr. Clin. Neurophysiol. 32,* 281-294.

Racine, R. J. (1975). Modification of seizure activity by electrical stimulation. Cortical areas. *Electroencephalogr. Clin. Neurophysiol. 38,* 1-12.

Racine, R. J. (1978). Paper presented at the Workshop on Post Activation Potentiation at the 11th Ann. Winter Conf. Brain Research, Keystone, Colorado, January 1978.

Racine, R. J., Livingston, K., and Joaquin, A. (1975). Effects of procaine hydrochloride, diazepam, and diphenylhydantoin on seizure development in cortical and subcortical structures in rats. *Electroencephalogr. Clin. Neurophysiol. 38,* 355-365.

Ramer, D., and Pinel, J. P. J. (1976). Progressive intensification of motor seizures produced by periodic electroconvulsive shock. *Exp. Neurol. 51,* 421-433.

Randrup, A., and Munkvad, I. (1970). Biochemical, anatomical, and psychological investigations of stereotyped behavior induced by amphetamines. In *Amphetamines and Related Compounds,* E. Costa and S. Garattini (Eds.). Raven, New York, pp. 695-713.

Ranje, C., and Ungerstedt, U. (1974). Chronic amphetamine treatment. Vast individual differences in performing a learned response. *Eur. J. Pharmacol. 29,* 307-311.

Resnick, R. B., Kestenbaum, R. S., and Schwartz, L. K. (1977). Acute systemic effects of cocaine in man. A controlled study by intranasal and intravenous routes. *Science 197,* 696-698.

Riblet, L. A., and Tuttle, W. W. (1970). Investigation of the amygdaloid and olfactory electrographic response in the cat after toxic dosage of lidocaine. *Electroencephalogr. Clin. Neurophysill. 28,* 601-608.

Rothstein, E. (1973). Prevention of alcohol withdrawal seizures. The roles of diphenylhydantoin and chlordiazepoxide. *Am. J. Psychiatry 130,* 1381-1382.

Sato, M., Nakashima, T., Mitsunobu, K., and Otsuki, S. (1976). Correlation between seizure susceptibility and brain catecholamine level in the kindled cat preparation. *Brain Nerve 28,* 471-477.

Scheel-Kruger, J., Braestrup, C., Nielson, M., Golembrowska, K., and Mogilnicka, E. (1977). Cocaine. Discussion on the role of dopamine in the biochemical mechanism of action. In *Advances in Behavioral Biology,* Vol. 21, *Cocaine and Other Stimulants,* E. H. Ellinwood and M. M. Kilbey (Eds.). Plenum, New York, pp. 373-408.

Schreiber, H. L., Wood, W. G., and Carlson, R. H. (1976). The role of locomotion in conditioning methylphenidate-induced locomotor activity. *Pharmacol. Biochem. Behav. 4,* 393-395.

Schiff, S. R., and Bridger, W. H. (1977). The behavioral effects of chronic administration of d-amphetamine and apomorphine and the development of conditioned stereotypy. *Proc. 7th Ann. Meet. Soc. Neurosci.,* Abstr. 1432, p. 448.

Schwartz, J. C., Costentin, J., Martres, M. P., Protais, P., and Baudry, M. (1978). Modulation of receptor mechanisms in the CNS. Hyper- and hyposensitivity to catecholamines. In *Neuropharmacology,* Vol. 17. Pergamon, Great Britain, pp. 655-685.

Segal, D. S. (1975). Behavioral and neurochemical correlates of repeated d-amphetamine administration. In *Neurobiological Mechanisms of Adaptation and Behavior,* A. J. Mandell (Ed.). Raven, New York, pp. 247-262.

Segal, D. S., and Mandell, A. J. (1974). Long-term administration of d-amphetamine. Progressive augmentation of motor activity and stereotypy. *Pharmacol. Biochem. Behav. 2,* 249-255.

Seiden, L. S., Fischman, M. W., and Shuster, C. R. (1977). Changes in brain catecholamines induced by long-term methamphetamine administration in rhesus monkeys. In *Advances in Behavioral Biology,* Vol. 21, *Cocaine and Other Stimulants,* E. H. Ellinwood and M. M. Kilbey (Eds.). Plenum, New York, pp. 179-186.

Sever, P. S., Caldwell, J., and Williams, R. T. (1976). Tolerance to amphetamine in two species (rat and guinea pig) that metabolize it differently. *Psychol. Med. 6,* 35-42.

Short, P. H., and Shuster, L. (1976). Changes in brain norepinephrine associated with sensitization to d-amphetamine. *Psychopharmacology 48,* 59-67.

Shuster, L., Webster, G. W., and Yu, G. (1975). Perinatal narcotic addiction in mice. Sensitization to morphine stimulation. *Addict. Dis. 2,* 277-292.

Shuster, L., Yu, G., and Bates, A. (1977). Sensitization to cocaine stimulation in mice. *Psychopharmacology 52,* 185-190.

Slater, E., Beard, A. W., and Glithers, E. B. (1963). The schizophrenia-like psychoses of epilepsy. I. Psychiatric aspects. *Br. J. Psychiatry 109,* 95-150.

Smith, R. C., Strong, J. R., Hicks, P. B., and Samorajski, T. (1979). Behavioral evidence for supersensitivity after chronic bromocriptine administration. *Psychopharmacology 60,* 241-246.

Snyder, S. H., Banerjee, S. P., Yamamura, H. I., and Greenberg, D. (1974). Drugs, neurotransmitters, and schizophrenia: Phenothiazines, amphetamines, and enzymes synthesizing psychotomimetic drugs aid schizophrenia research. *Science 184,* 1243-1253.

Squillace, K. M., Pert, A., and Post, R. M. (1978). Effects of amygdala lesions on development of lidocaine and cocaine-induced behaviors. Unpublished manuscript.

Stevens, J. R. (1973). Psychomotor epilepsy and schizophrenia. A common anatomy. In *Epilepsy, Its Phenomena in Man,* M. A. B. Brazier (Ed.). Academic, New York, pp. 189-214.

Stevens, J. R. (1975). Interictal clinical manifestations of complex partial seizures. In *Advances in Neurology,* Vol. 11, *Complex Partial Seizures and*

Their Treatment, J. K. Penry and D. D. Daly (Eds.). Raven, New York, pp. 85-112.

Stevens, J. R., and Livermore, A., Jr. (1978). Kindling of the mesolimbic dopamine system. Animal model of psychosis. *Neurology 28,* 36-46.

Stevens, J. R., Mark, V. H., Erwin, F., Pacheco, P., and Suematsu, K. (1969). Deep temporal stimulation in man. Long latency, long lasting psychological changes. *Arch. Neurol. 21,* 157-167.

Stripling, J. S., and Ellinwood, E. H. (1977a). Potentiation of the behavioral and convulsant effects of cocaine by chronic administration in the rat. *Pharmacol. Biochem. Behav. 6,* 571-579.

Stripling, J. S., and Ellinwood, E. H. (1977b). Sensitization to cocaine following chronic administration in the rat. In *Advances in Behavioral Biology,* Vol. 21, *Cocaine and Other Stimulants,* E. H. Ellinwood and M. M. Kilbey (Eds.). Plenum, New York, pp. 327-352.

Suomi, S. J., Seaman, S. F., Lewis, J. K., DeLizio, R. D., and McKinney, W. T. (1977). Effects of imipramine treatment on separation-induced social disorders in rhesus monkey. *Arch. Gen. Psychiatry 35,* 321-325.

Tanaka, A. (1972). Progressive changes of behavioral and electroencephalographic responses to daily stimulation of the amygdala in rabbit. *Fukuoka Acta Med. 63,* 152-164.

Tarsy, D., and Baldessarini, R. J. (1973). Pharmacologically induced behavioral supersensitivity to apomorphine. *Nature 245,* 262-263.

Tatum, A. L., and Seevers, M. H. (1929). Experimental cocaine addiction. *J. Pharmacol. Exp. Ther. 36,* 401-410.

Tilson, H. A., and Rech, R. H. (1973). Conditioned drug effects and absence of tolerance to d-amphetamine induced motor activity. *Pharmacol. Biochem. Behav. 1,* 149-153.

Trendelenberg, U., and Graefe, K. H. (1975). Supersensitivity to catecholamines after impairment of extraneuronal uptake or catechol-O-methyl transferase. *Fed. Proc. 34,* 1971-1974.

Turner, I. M., Newman, S. M., Louis, S., and Kutt, H. (1977). Pharmacological prophylaxis against the development of kindled amygdaloid seizures. *Ann. Neurol. 2,* 221-224.

van Rossum, J. M. (1970). Mode of action of psychomotor stimulant drugs. *Int. Rev. Neurobiol. 12,* 307-383.

Vosu, H., and Wise, R. A. (1975). Cholinergic seizure kindling in the rat. Comparison of caudate, amygdala and hippocampus. *Behav. Biol. 13,* 491-495.

Wada, J. A. (1977). Pharmacological prophylaxis in the kindling model of epilepsy. *Arch. Neurol. 34,* 389-395.

Wada, J. A. (1978). Spontaneous recurrent seizures. Relevance to human epilepsy. In *Limbic Mechanisms: The Continuing Evolution of the*

Limbic System Concept, K. E. Livingston and O. Hornykiewicz (Eds.). Plenum, New York.

Wada, J. A., and Osawa, T. (1976). Spontaneous recurrent seizure state induced by daily electric amygdaloid stimulation in Senegalese baboons (Papio papio). *Neurology 26,* 273-286.

Wada, J. A., Sato, M., and Corcoran, M. E. (1974). Persistent seizure susceptibility and recurrent spontaneous seizure in kindled cats. *Epilepsia 15,* 465-478.

Wada, J. A., Sato, M., Wake, A., Green, J. R., and Troupin, A. S. (1976). Prophylactic effects of phenytoin, phenobarbital, and carbamazepine examined in kindled cat preparations. *Arch. Neurol. 33,* 426-434.

Wagman, I. H., de Jong, R. H., and Prince, D. A. (1967). Effects of lidocaine on the CNS. *Anesthesiology 28,* 155-172.

Walker, D. W., and Zornetzer, S. F. (1974). Alcohol withdrawal in mice. Electroencephalographic and behavioral correlates. *Electroencephalogr. Clin. Neurophysiol. 36,* 233-243.

Walters, J. R., Bunney, B. S., and Roth, R. H. (1975). Piribedil and apomorphine. Pre- and postsynaptic effects on dopamine synthesis and neuronal activity. In *Advances in Neurology,* D. B. Calne, T. N. Chase, and A. Barbeau (Eds.). Raven, New York, pp. 273-284.

Weston, P. F., and Overstreet, D. H. (1976). Does tolerance develop to low doses of d- and l-amphetamine on locomotor activity in rats? *Pharmacol. Biochem. Behav. 5,* 645-649.

Wise, R. A., and Chinerman, J. (1974). Effects of diazepam and phenobarbital on electrically-induced amygdaloid seizures and seizure development. *Exp. Neurol. 45,* 355-363.

Wood, W. G., Schreiber, H. L., Villescas, R., and Carlson, R. H. (1977). Effects of prior experience and "functional disturbance" on acute and chronic tolerance to methylphenidate. *Psychopharmacology 51,* 165-168.

Young, L. D., Suomi, S. J., Harlow, H. F., and McKinney, W. T. (1973). Early stress and later response to separation in rhesus monkeys. *Am. J. Psychiatry 130,* 400-405.

NUTRITIONAL DISORDERS AND PSYCHIATRIC STATE

19

Nutritional Disorders and the Psychiatric State

Arthur H. Crisp
St. George's Hospital Medical School
London, England

I. NUTRITIONAL ASPECTS OF MENTAL ILLNESS

A. Constitutional Aspects

An association between body shape and mood was first postulated by Hippocrates. Interest was more recently rekindled by Kretschmer (1936), who suggested that individuals with so-called pyknic body build often show cyclothymic personality traits and are also more than normally liable to manic-depressive illness. The term pyknic was given by Kretschmer specifically to individuals with large visceral cavities and a tendency to fat on the trunk, especially its lower part, as well as slightly built shoulder girdle and slender extremities tapering to small hands and feet. The term, however, has generally come to be used in a less specific way as synonymous with obesity. The view that obesity is more frequent in patients suffering from manic-depressive illness than in the general population has had wide support (Mayer Gross et al., 1969) although it has recently been challenged (Beck, 1967; Angst and Perris, 1972; Crisp et al., 1975; Crisp and McGuinness, 1976). Psychoanalytic theory, and especially Kleinian theory, emphasize the strong associations which can develop during the first six months of life between feeding experiences and mood (Winnicot, 1958). Great significance is attached to this phase of development as an important determinant of adult personality and the propensity to experience depression in the face of loss.

B. Phenomenological Aspects

Attention has been devoted to both changes in appetite and weight in psychiatric illness. There are several reasons for this: Changes in appetite and weight are frequent complaints among psychiatric patients and cause for concern by their relatives and they are readily elicited at interview; furthermore, changes in weight during the course of illness have for long been regarded as medically important and they can also be measured easily.

Weight changes may occur throughout the range of psychiatric illness, weight loss most commonly being described during the illness with subsequent weight gain on recovery (Post, 1956). Weight gain during illness is not infrequently encountered (Crisp and Stonehill, 1973), more often in less severe neurotic illness as well as in association with the consumption of some psychotropic drugs. Such weight changes are usually associated with changes in calorie intake (Duquay and Flach, 1964; Pollitt, 1965), but changes in activity and more general energy expenditure also occur in psychiatric illness and a relationship between depression and inactivity which provides a basis for the development of obesity in some individuals has been postulated by Stunkard (1958). Weight change, seemingly independent of calorie intake but probably related to changes in water metabolism, may also occur and has been the subject of investigation in both schizophrenic and affective psychoses (Crammer, 1957).

Weight loss is a common feature of disorders of affect, particularly severe depression and mania, and is also described as an aspect of neurotic disorders, e.g., anxiety phobic states (Mayer Gross et al., 1969). Marked weight loss associated with reduction or cessation of calorie intake is common in stuporous states and is of course present in all conditions in which there is refusal to eat or a marked reduction in calorie intake. Such nonspecific changes led Bliss and Branch (1960) to coin the phrase "nervous malnutrition," within which they also included anorexia nervosa, but many workers have since challenged the latter proposition (Crisp, 1965a; Dally, 1969; Bruch, 1974). Brennan (1945) had found that cases of organic brain disease with mental disturbance showed a statistically significant greater average weight loss than patients in all other diagnostic categories. Among this population are many who are unable to care for themselves and weight loss may be one reflection of the inadequacy of those caring for them to meet such patients' basic needs. Major weight loss during a psychiatric illness is associated with having once been obese (Crisp and Stonehill, 1976).

C. Role of Nutritional Disorder in Psychiatric Symptomatology

An observation (vide infra) that individuals with anorexia nervosa slept very little, waking particularly early in the morning irrespective of their mood, led to the hypothesis (Crisp, 1967a) that sleep disturbance in the second half of the night in patients with psychiatric illness would be more related to their nutritional status than to specific diagnostic syndromes. In a careful study it was found that, among a wide range of such patients, reduced total sleep time, interrupted sleep, and early final waking were associated with weight loss and increased total sleep time, uninterrupted sleep, and later final waking with weight gain, irrespective of diagnosis or mood state. The latter bore a relationship more to sleep in the first half of the night (Crisp and Stonehill, 1973,1976; Stonehill et al., 1976). Restlessness and constipation are also often enhanced by reduced food intake and weight loss. It was suggested that this "nutritional" mechanism might contribute to the "functional shift" observed by Pollitt (1965) in respect of endogenous depression and also operate in other disorders such as narcolepsy (Sours, 1963), the Kleine-Levin syndrome (Green and Cracco, 1970), and the syndrome of hypersomnia and megaphagia (Critchley, 1962).

II. DISORDERS OF WEIGHT AND SHAPE WITH MAJOR PSYCHOBIOLOGICAL DIMENSIONS

A. Introduction

The remainder of this chapter is devoted to the states of obesity and anorexia nervosa. Consonant with the book's overall theme, the content, brief treatment sections apart, will be mainly concerned with the immediate psychobiological aspects, clinical and experimental, of these disorders. Reference is made only in passing to the more experiential psychodynamic and social aspects. The reader is referred elsewhere (Crisp and Stonehill, 1976) for the author's and others' views on the relationship to the above of such disorders as Kleine-Levin syndrome, Pickwickian syndrome, and narcolepsy.

B. Obesity

1. Definition

Obesity is a state of excessive fatness, obvious to the beholder and almost always associated with being overweight. Indeed, lean body mass being a relatively fixed component of body weight (Parisova, 1968), clinicians usually measure obesity and especially changes in it by weighing the individual.

The concepts of "ideal body weight" or "best weight" associated with freedom from illness during life and longevity (Fig. 1) have become established as an actuarial concept (Society of Actuaries, 1959; Metropolitan Life Insurance Co., 1959,1960). Major deviations from them, especially after allowance has been made for the different body builds, mainly reflect variations in the quantity of adipose tissue. Fat is less dense than other components of body mass and estimates of its amount can also be made on this basis (Keys and Brozek, 1953; von Doblen, 1959). Skin fold thicknesses also provide a good measure (Keys and Brozek, 1953; Tanner and Whitehouse, 1962; Steinkamp et al., 1965).

2. Epidemiological Aspects

Obesity is often common in affluent societies and always rare, respected, envied, and often linked to social standing in impoverished societies.

Obesity is already present in 6-15% of children in places like Scandinavia and North America, especially among girls (Quaade, 1955; Johnson et al., 1956; Borjeson, 1962; Dwyer et al., 1967). Fatness is also more common in adolescent females than males (von Doblen, 1959; Tanner and Whitehouse, 1962; Maaser and Droese, 1971). The degree of fatness often characterizes individuals from early life (Eid, 1970; Crisp et al., 1970), but the female puberty further differentiates the sexes in this respect in that the former is associated with further specific deposition of fat.

Among adult populations obesity has usually been found to be increasingly prevelant with increasing age, to remain more common in women than men, and to be less common among professional and managerial classes than among those from working classes (Borjeson, 1962; Moore et al., 1962; Goldblatt et al., 1965; Silverstone, 1968). There are, however, important exceptions to these associations.

3. Biological Functions

Fatness is rare among nondomesticated animals, apart from those that periodically store food in the form of fat in preparation for hibernation or else live actively in cold climates.

The amount of female fatness conferred by puberty probably has an active biological purpose of a sexual kind, albeit only of evolutionary significance for the human. Thus it may provide a food reservoir for the fetus, given the greater

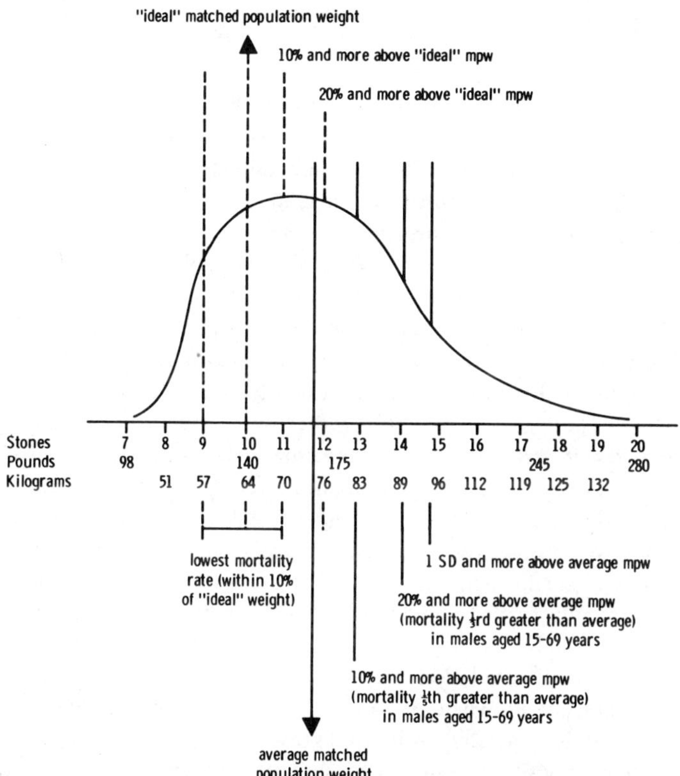

Figure 1 This chart displays some statistical approaches to the definition of obesity. It shows in diagrammatic form the kind of differences that often exist between "ideal" matched population weight (mpw) (10 stones in this instance, e.g., a woman of 5 ft 9 in. and 25 years or older and of medium frame, or a man of 5 ft 7 in. and 25 years or older and of medium frame) and an estimate of the actual present-day average matched population weight. It also shows some related mortality characteristics. It can be seen that the definitions of obesity in these terms are statistical and can offer useful guides, but no more, to the clinical problem of assessment of obesity in an individual.

unpredictability and variability of food supplies in primitive times. Such fatness, in other words, may declare the female's biological readiness for reproduction. Its appearance attracts the male and may, through such social implications as this, reflect an aspect of herself that the individual female who develops anorexia nervosa has needed, defensively, to totally eliminate (vide infra).

Fatness in the male would seem to have little biological significance or value unless one is, say, an Eskimo. For the majority of human males it merely represents, biologically speaking, a useless load to be carried around.

4. Psychological Aspects

a. General

The battle concerning cause and effect in the psychological area has long been joined. Conclusions cannot be drawn from cross-sectional studies of obese populations and especially that minority of obese individuals, often grossly obese and highly self-selected, who appear in the clinic.

The following things can be said:

1. Obesity runs in families and this may have cultural as well as genetic determinants. Such families may eat more than others and "clean their plates more" (Quaade, 1955). Over-feeding and over-eating may reflect family attitudes to well-being and material security and/or compensatory protective devices in relation to children viewed ambivalently (Bruch and Touraine, 1940; Crisp, 1967a). These findings, taken together with the social class finding, invite explanations ranging from the biological to the social. Furthermore, it is noteworthy that the obese adult's over-eating has often been done previously during childhood. If the present adult obese weight is stable, then, in his or her presently relatively inactive state, this reflects a relatively small food intake for much of the time. This is usually achieved through various eating avoidance maneuvers. However, obese adults often remain potentially hyperphagic. Thus they hyper-respond to palatable foods (Wooley et al., 1976), to the presence of available food irrespective of time relationship to previous meal, and they tend not to reduce their food intake when anxious (Abramson and Wunderlich, 1972).

2. Obesity is associated with rapid growth during childhood, with being the later born among siblings, and with subsequent greater assertiveness in adolescence (Crisp et al., 1970). The tendency to a shorter life-span for the obese may to some extent be a function of this overall rapid growth process which is probably a reflection of excessive or optimal infant and childhood nutrition and associated freedom from infection.

3. The majority of obese people (being between 30 and 50% above average population weights) in the general population report themselves as being less anxious and less depressed than others (Crisp and McGuinness, 1976). This finding is consistent with clinical psychiatric experience and again invites various interpretations ranging from the biological to the social (Crisp, 1967a).

4. Massively obese individuals report gross overestimates of their body widths (Kalucy et al., 1975a). They share this propensity with patients with anorexia nervosa and with female adolescents (Crisp and Kalucy, 1974).

5. Massively obese individuals are less sexually active than they were prior to the onset of their present state and less than a matched nonobese population (Crisp, 1967a). It has been argued that this inactivity reflects both a biological process and a factor of self-esteem but that, whatever the basis, it may sometimes be psychologically protective to the individual.

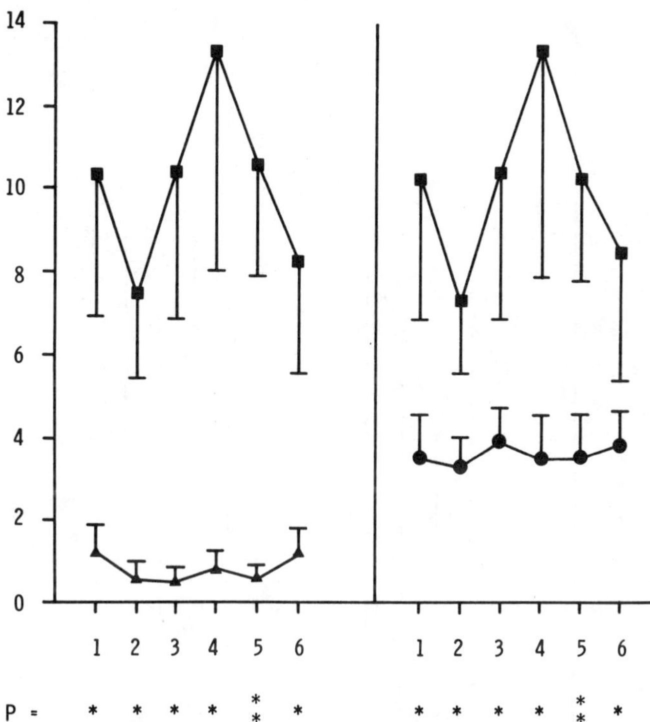

Figure 2 Mean LH levels in mU/ml during six 80-min periods of the night. The left-hand space compares anorexia nervosa subjects (▲) with normal subjects (■); the right-hand space obese subjects (●) with normal subjects (■). The significance of the differences (*P*) between groups is shown below each space; *P* = <.5 (*), *P* = <.01 (**). (Reproduced from Kalucy et al., 1976.)

Certainly the grossly obese state is associated with impairment of reproductive capacity (Crisp, 1967,1978a), reflected in a disturbance of gonadotropic activity. Thus Figures 2 and 3 show nocturnal hormonal profiles (Kalucy et al., 1976) of LH and FSH in 11 severely obese premenopausal females compared with a group of normal females and a group of patients with anorexia nervosa. It can be seen that the obese, while not showing levels so characteristically very low as do the anorectics, nevertheless display significantly low levels of LH at all stages of the night. It was argued that such low levels might reflect these patients' current tendencies to restrict their carbohydrate intake much of the time.

The interplay of psychological and biological factors in the above five areas is probably complex (Crisp, 1967a; Kalucy, 1976). To some extent one

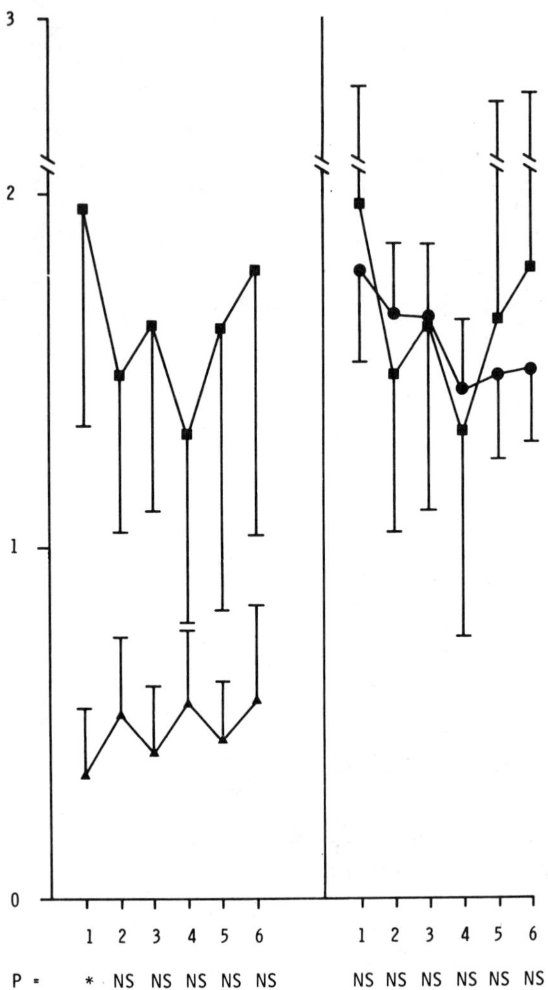

Figure 3 Mean FSH levels in mU/ml during six 80-min periods of the night. The left-hand space compares anorexia nervosa subjects (▲) with normal subjects (■); the right-hand space obese subjects (●) with normal subjects (■). The significance of the difference (P) between groups is shown below each space; $P = < .5$ (*), $P = < .01$ (**). (Reproduced from Kalucy et al., 1976.)

can hope that it will be unraveled by the study of changes that arise during and following treatment which is effective in eliminating the obesity.

b. Treatment

If over-eating and/or obesity have been or become socially meaningful and/or psychologically adaptive for the individual, then they can be seen to be an aspect of personality, the way one deals with and responds to the environment and ones experience of one's self. Any major direct external manipulation of them might lead the individual to social and/or psychological decompensation. So runs the psychodynamic theme. Such views stemming from observations such as those outlined above have derived mainly from cross-sectional studies often of clinic populations and also from the often-stated clinical observation that many people's appetite and ingestion of food is affected by their mood, especially many obese clinic patients who report over-eating in relation to emotional upset. There is a concept of a vicious cycle of insecurity and low self-esteem leading to loneliness leading to over-eating leading to increasing obesity leading to increased sensitivity about shape through projection of one's social difficulties onto it and hence leading to increasing social isolation and so on.

Such theories have unfortunately contributed little to effective treatment. Obese patients (i.e., fat people ostensibly wishing to reduce their obesity) tend to remain or revert to their obese destiny despite everyone's efforts. Psychotherapeutic approaches sometimes tend to enlarge the obese individual's capacity to adjust socially, but seldom succeed in the long term in their initial aim of reducing the patient's fatness.

From a psychological and psychobiological standpoint, two relatively independent factors may have a bearing: (1) the need to eat, which for the obese may have a neurotic component and (2) the consequences of the obese shape and the state of being overweight, which for the obese may have both social and biological components as well as experiential ones.

A number of studies have reported on massively obese individuals who have complied for many months, often as inpatients, with a prescribed rigidly restricted dietary intake and who have lost substantial amounts of body weight, but who have relapsed shortly after reverting to a more liberal and freely chosen diet. Often such individuals became depressed toward the end of the treatment period (Bruch, 1957; Crisp, 1967a; Glucksman and Hirsch, 1968). They also became more socially and sexually active as weight was lost (Kollar and Atkinson, 1966; Crisp, 1967a; Glucksman and Hirsch, 1968; Crisp and Stonehill, 1970). It has been argued that the depression is partly and inevitably a consequence of the food restriction and partly a consequence of the patient's difficulties in coping with a new-found appearance and vigor in the face of what sometimes comes to be more starkly revealed to them as a barren life situation (Crisp, 1967a; Glucksman and Hirsch, 1968; Crisp and Stonehill, 1970). However, as stated previously, such patients are very unlikely to be representative of the larger population of obese or even massively obese individuals.

In recent years, ileojejunal bypass surgery has provided an opportunity for more extensive studies. Initially it seemed that such procedures would allow study of the psychopathological effects of major weight/shape reduction within the context of continued normal food intake. In the event, it has become evident that the major weight loss that usually supervenes during the 6 months following this operation is due to reduced food intake during this period (Pilkington et al., 1976) and that only thereafter and in association with a plateauing of body weight does food intake become normal. Eating patterns often become much more normal and in particular there is less tendency to binge—this change probably having both physiological and psychosocial determinants (Kalucy and Crisp, 1974; Crisp et al., 1977a). A minority, however, seem unable to cope with their newfound state. These tend to be males who had been more ambivalent about major weight loss in the first instance, and females, often with life-long major obesity and socially isolated, who tended in the past to "blame" their obesity for the social inadequacy and now, stripped of the former, are confronted instead by the latter's more widespread origins. Supervening depression is usually followed by determined over-eating and increasing obesity once more, despite the bypass. Among those whose weight remains more normal postoperatively, the hormonal characteristics described earlier and others too, such as insulin, cortisol, and growth hormone, revert to normal (Crisp, 1978a).

In conclusion, psychobiological explanations of obesity need to take account of (1) the presence of age, sex, birth order, and social class factors, (2) the relationship of eating to family attitudes toward welfare, individual children, and mood, especially during childhood, and (3) the relationship of obesity to mood and sexual behavior evident both in the static obese state and also when obesity is being eliminated from the system by reducing food intake or else creating the conditions for malabsorbtion.

C. Anorexia Nervosa

1. Definition

Anorexia nervosa has been accurately described in the English language medical literature for several centuries (Bliss and Branch, 1960). The diagnosis remains an act of considerable clinical skill, mainly because the evident disorder is nevertheless psychologically adaptive for the individual concerned who therefore resists investigation and clarification of her (and sometimes his) condition, deceiving others when necessary.

All the evident pathology stems from (1) the individual's need to achieve and maintain a low and immature body weight and (2) the manifestations of the accompanying starvation.

The former requires sustained control over the impulse to eat. This may become hedged around by ritualistic and/or manipulative behavior as necessary or, when decompensation in this respect has occurred, then by (secret) vomiting, exercise, purging, or ingestion of other relevant drugs following eating.

The individual's secretiveness, hostility, moments of elation and despair, regular weighing of herself, and desperate commitment to school work are other manifestations and psychological devices operating within this need.

Her restlessness by day and by night (especially her early morning waking), her hoarding and stealing and, ironically for her, her preoccupation with food and its acquisition and preparation, together with her impoverished metabolic status, reflect her starved state.

Her fear of examinations, of sexual encounters, and her social isolation reflect her concurrently regressed biological state and provide hints of her premorbid adolescent turmoil and related factors determining the onset of the illness (Crisp, 1965a,b,1967a,b,1970, 1973).

The diagnosis needs to be made at a number of levels of pathology:

1. The manifest syndrome as outlined briefly above.
2. The underlying burgeoning terror of normal body weight and the consequent need to maintain a low "subpubertal" body weight (Fig. 2).
3. The context within which the adolescent fear has arisen: (a) the initial presence of a concern about shape and a determination to "diet" by excluding carbohydrate. This is a commonplace need among female adolescents and has been elaborated on elsewhere (Crisp, 1967b, 1977a). In the anorectic-to-be it becomes "overdetermined" because of its effect through the accompanying biological regression in providing a "solution" to (b) specific adolescent turmoil, i.e., the coexistence with the dieting behavior of major maturational conflict within the adolescent and her family and also the absence of other ways of coping (Crisp, 1967b,1970,1977b).
4. Other background factors not necessarily present but often contributory, such as (a) being female; (b) coming from a family with professional and managerial backgrounds and thus being subject to middle-class value systems, extended adolescence, and an increasing culture clash in our present day society; (c) being obese and with attendant rapid growth; (d) having a family with excessive involvement in nurturing and/or displaying an excess of obesity and/or anorexia nervosa; (e) having been excessively good and compliant as a child or otherwise ill equipped to cope with adolescence; (f) having parents with a propensity for social avoidance patterns or the development of depression.

2. *Natural History*

This has been described in detail elsewhere (see also Fig. 1). The disorder is common (Crisp et al., 1976). The onset is usually in adolescence and otherwise later in life. Approximately 1 in 15 clinic cases is male.

The majority (perhaps 60-70%) of patients are recovered 10 years after first being seen (Crisp et al., 1977b); of the remainder, 3-5% die. Death is usually due to suicide or else inanition; rarely to infection (Crisp, 1965a,b,1970; Seidensticker and Tzagournis, 1968; Morgan and Russell, 1975).

3. *Physical Aspects*

a. Introduction

There is now good evidence that the vast majority of the physical abnormalities found in individuals with anorexia nervosa are a product of the illness and that they revert to normal following restoration of weight to normal and maintenance of normal dietary intake. The same often applies to the perceptual disorders evident within the condition (Crisp and Kalucy, 1974; Lacey et al., 1977). Residual abnormalities following restoration of normal weight, such as delay in return of menses and aspects of carbohydrate and fat metabolism, reflect more constitutional aspects of the disorder such as premorbid obesity (vide infra).

b. Dietary Aspects

The great majority of anorectics enter their illness within the context of dietary avoidance of carbohydrate, though this is often denied by them.

This condition of carbohydrate starvation is unique to them (Crisp, 1965a,b,1967a,1970). It leaves them in a state of relative well-being despite being emaciated. It probably accounts substantially for their early cessation of menstruation. It probably contributes to the disturbances of fat and carbohydrate metabolism that they display, e.g., sustained insulin response to glucose loading (Crisp, 1965a,1967b; Crisp et al., 1967), high resting plasma insulin levels (Fig. 4) (Kalucy et al., 1976), very high plasma levels of cholesterol and other fats, often related directly to high intake in the diet (Crisp, 1965b; Crisp et al., 1968a; Oberdisse et al., 1965; Blendis and Crisp, 1968). Such patients may also sometimes ingest very large quantities of other substances, e.g., carotene, and hence develop hypercarotenemia (Dally, 1959; Crisp and Stonehill, 1967).

However, once vomiting and/or purging emerge as a corrective to weight gain otherwise threatened by the individual having surrendered to the impulse to eat, then the metabolic picture becomes very different. Some such individuals will settle into a pattern of frequent daily bingeing, vomiting, and/or purging, often all or much of this behavior being secretive. They will often protest their great wish to gain weight. Their underlying fear of so doing will only become evident in a strictly controlled situation wherein they will refuse to eat unless they can still secretively dispose of the calories without absorbing them. Such individuals can present a bizarre metabolic picture which can be extremely puzzling if its behavioral and psychological origins remain concealed, when it tends to become construed instead as some primary disorder of metabolism (Crisp, 1977a).

Thus, such patients may now be eating large quantities of all kinds of food, especially of carbohydrate, but retaining hardly any of it. They begin to get hypoproteinemia, major electrolyte depletion (especially if purging with, say 20-50 times the standard dosage per day), and gross disturbances of fluid balance.

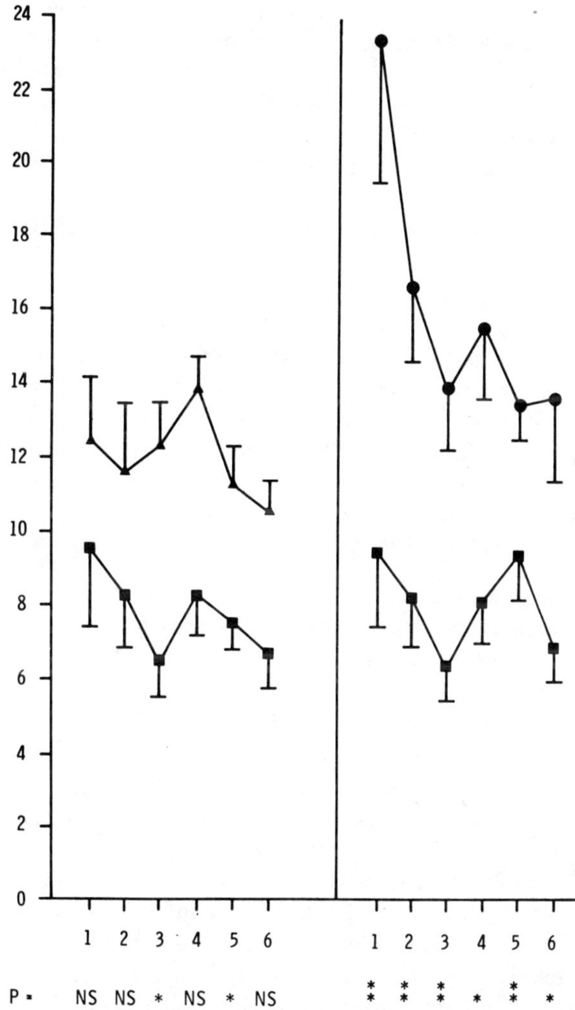

Figure 4 Mean insulin levels in mU/ml during six 80-min periods of the night. The left-hand space compares anorexia nervosa subjects (▲) with normal subjects (■); the right-hand space obese subjects (●) with normal subjects (■). The significance of the differences (P) between groups is shown below each space; $P = < .5$ (*), $P = < .01$ (**). (Reproduced from Kalucy et al., 1976.)

They often look very ill—relatively hot and sweaty and with a bounding peripheral circulation in contrast to the hypometabolic status of the abstaining anorectic. Symptomatic epilepsy can arise and should not be construed as signaling some primary brain damage (Crisp, 1967a, et al., 1968b).

Individuals sometimes alternate between these two patterns of low-weight control but on the whole the latter and more malignant form of bingeing/vomiting/purging is also the more chronic. However, it is adopted at all only by about 50% of all female anorectics but rather more male anorectics. This may reflect the fact that males, who are resistant as a group to developing anorexia nervosa, only do so under more extreme conditions, one of which is a greater tendency to premorbid obesity—a factor itself associated with ultimate bingeing and vomiting as the means of weight control in females as well (Crisp et al., 1977b).

c. Hormonal Aspects

General. The disorder has been construed in psychopathological terms as pivoting around the pubertal process and as having arisen because of the way in which carbohydrate starvation in particular quickly and protectively reverses the endocrine status and hence the entire psychobiological status to that of prepuberty (Crisp, 1967a,b).

In recent years a number of investigators have reported on their studies of the hormonal status of anorectic patients.

Gonadotropins. Luteinizing hormone (LH) and follicle-stimulating hormone (FSH) levels are markedly reduced in the plasma of anorectics, the former more so than the latter (Crisp et al., 1973; Warren and van de Viele, 1973; Palmer et al., 1974,1975; Halmi et al., 1975). This was also found to be true during the sleeping state (Kalucy et al., 1976; Boyar et al., 1974; Hellman et al., 1974; Kalucy et al., 1975b). Low levels have been attributed not only to low body weight but also to chronicity (Garfinkel et al., 1975).

The impact of LH/FSH releasing factors has been investigated (Palmer et al., 1974,1975). It was found that the LH response only occurred above a weight threshold of around 45 kg (Fig. 5). Other workers similarly found only muted responses at low body weight and with a full response only occurring with subjects who had achieved 90% or more of ideal body weight (Halmi et al., 1975). The relationship of puberty to body weight has been investigated at length by Frisch and her collaborators (Frisch and Revelle, 1971; Frisch and McArthur, 1974), and she postulates an intervening factor of change of BMR. It has been pointed out (Crisp, 1967a,1968,1974) that weight for weight, anorectics with the bingeing/vomiting syndrome display much higher levels of metabolic activity consonant with the return of their menstrual bleeding and their fertility at a lower than usual body weight (Crisp, 1977a). Crisp has suggested (1977a) that investigations of the hormonal status of anorectic patients needs to take this sometimes hidden factor into account and, from a research standpoint, are probably best restricted to the abstaining group of anorectics for the time being.

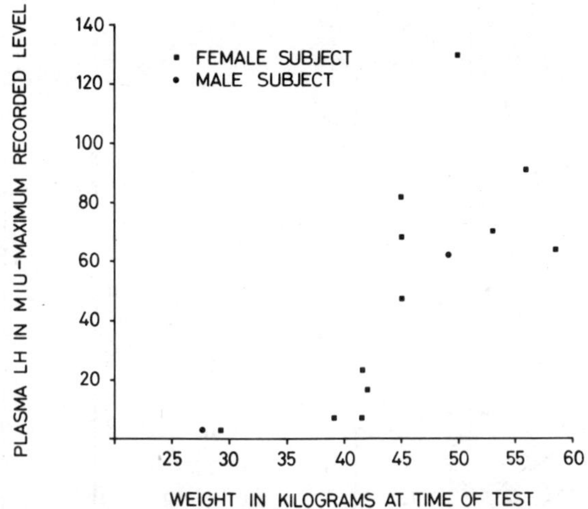

Figure 5 Maximum plasma LH response over basal levels after intravenous injection of 50 μg LH/FSH-RH plotted against body weight of subjects with anorexia nervosa. (From Palmer et al., 1975).

Boyar and his colleagues (1974) found nocturnal LH spikes in some anorectics reminiscent of the very early pubertal state. Unfortunately, in their study they did not discriminate between abstainers and those with the bingeing/vomiting syndrome. It may be that such spikes occur in subjects with the latter means of low-weight control, who thereby generate a higher basal metabolic rate than would otherwise be consistent with their low weight.

Patterns of LH, FSH, estrogen, and progesterone activity have been reported in relation to restoration of patient weight to target level (matched population mean level) in association with a normal diet containing normal amounts of carbohydrate (Crisp et al., 1973). Figures 6-8 illustrate the kinds of outcome found. Figure 6 shows that, despite weight being restored to target level, this patient failed to generate any LH activity. Figures 7 and 8 depict patients in whom such activity was rekindled. The second of these patients (Fig. 8) who underwent a leucotomy procedure (Crisp and Kalucy, 1973) typically, for this group, showed a rapid restoration of menstrual cyclical activity in association with the usual refeeding/psychotherapy treatment program.

These illustrations make the point that the patient displayed in Figure 6 was characterized by premorbid obesity while those displayed in Figures 7 and 8 were not. The other patients in the study, of whom the three described here are illustrative, all divided themselves into these two response groups depending upon their premorbid weight. Moreover, the patient demonstrated in Figure 6 maintained her new target weight for several years, within the context of continued individual and family psychotherapy. She continued to eat normally.

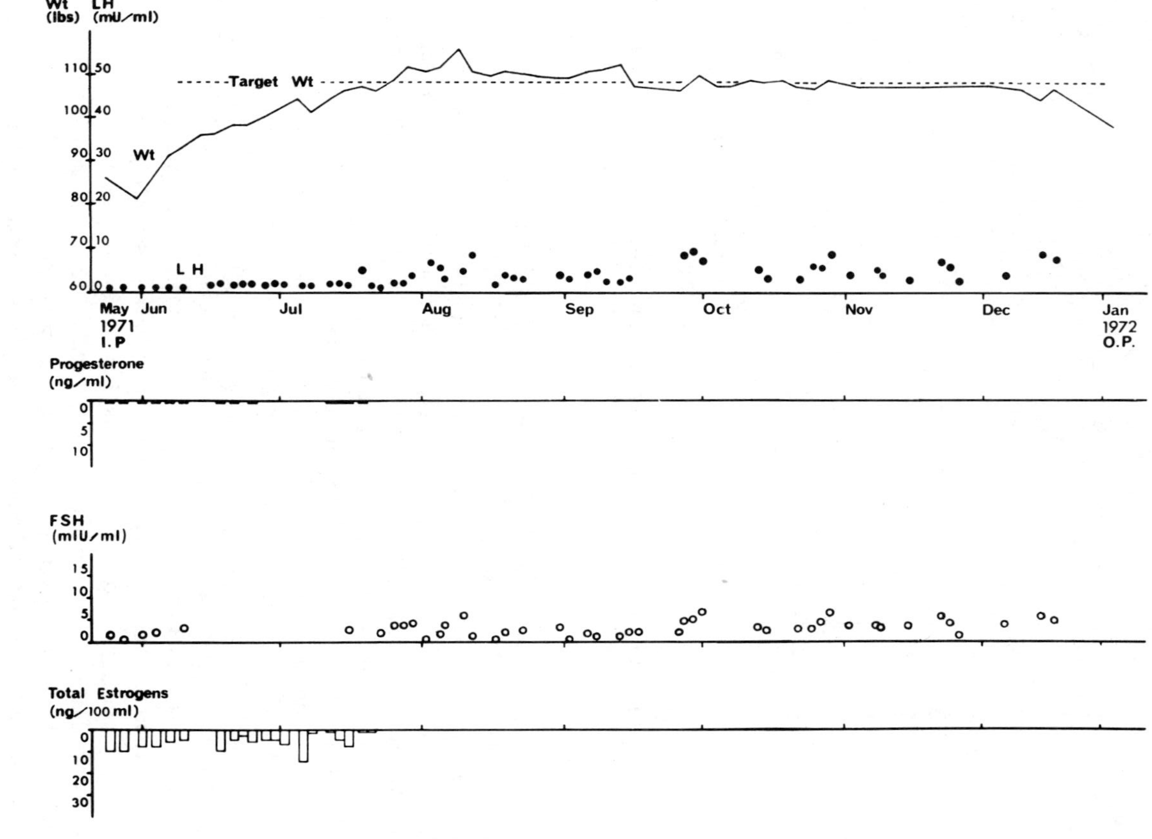

Figure 6 Fifteen-year-old patient, height 5 ft 2 in. (Reproduced from Crisp et al., 1973.)

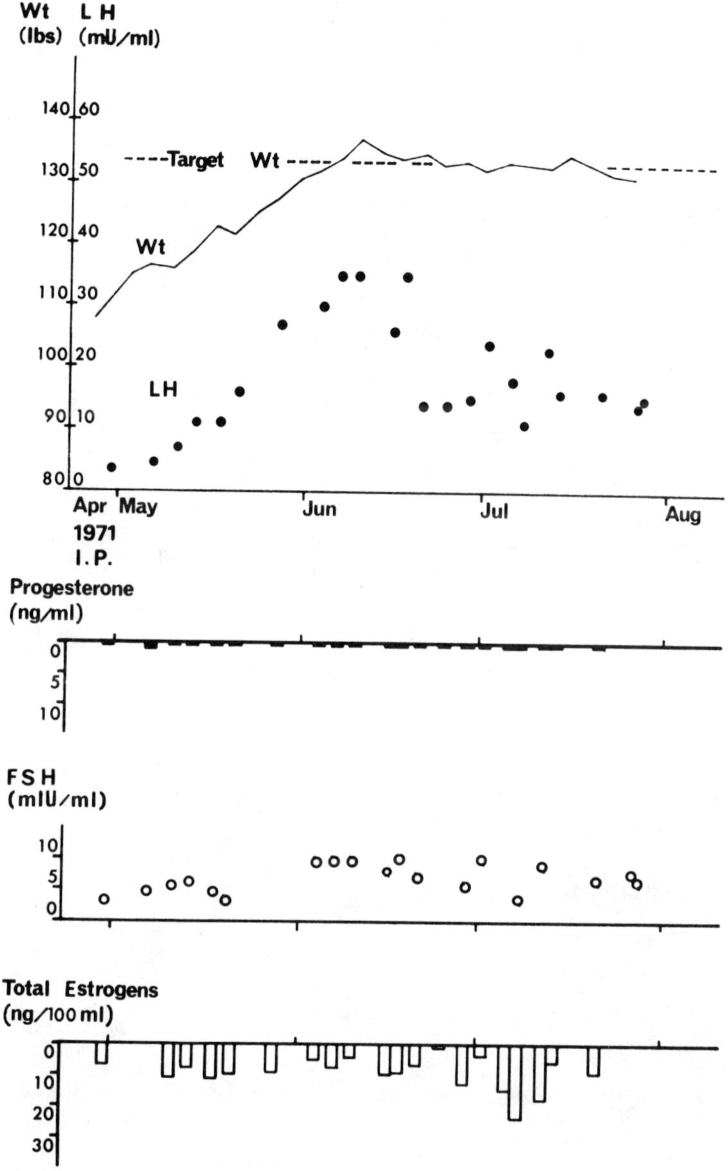

Figure 7 Seventeen-year-old patient, height 5 ft 10 in. (Reproduced from Crisp et al., 1973.)

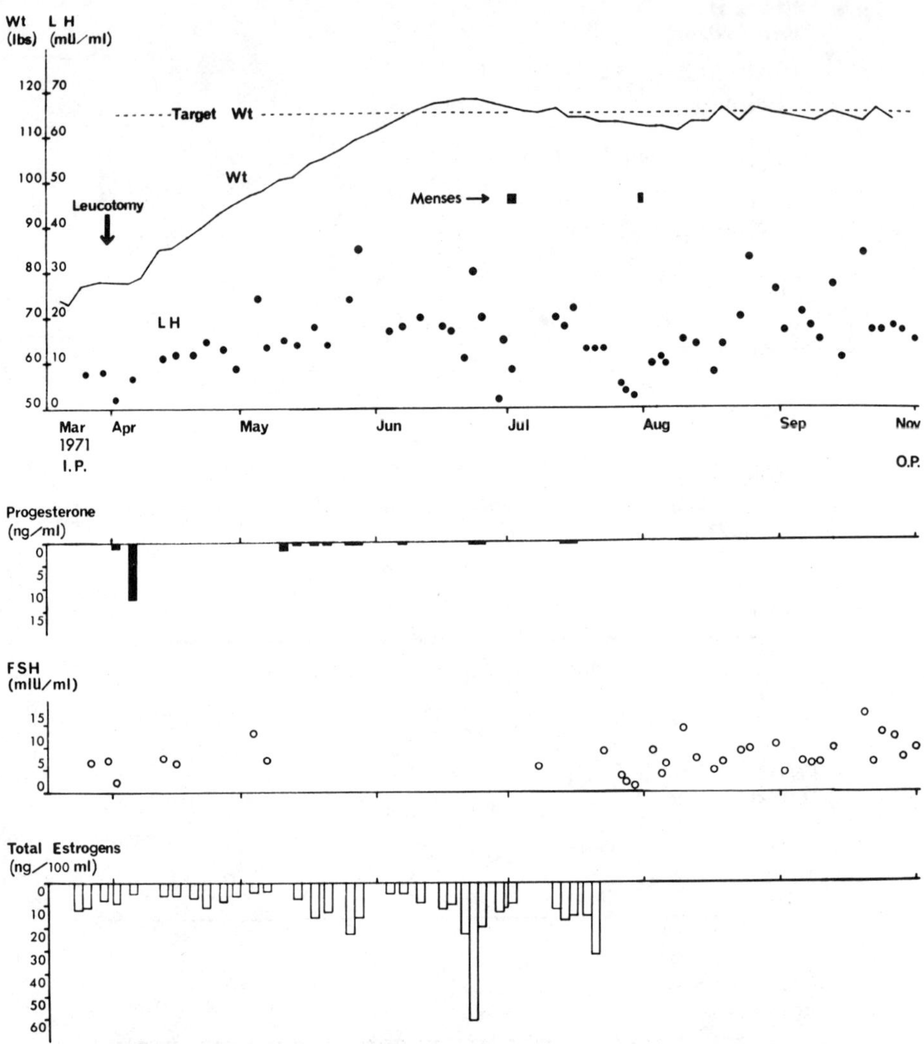

Figure 8 Twenty-year-old patient, height 5 ft 4 in. (Reproduced from Crisp et al., 1973.)

Eventually, her menses restarted at this, for her, new lower weight and fat threshold. Thus such patients have often had a menarchal weight in excess of their present target weight, having grown rapidly throughout childhood and with attendant plumpness. Moreover, they will have lost their menses at the start of the illness at a weight above the present target weight. Nevertheless, given time, they appear able to reset their regulatory mechanisms in the way described above.

Table 1 Relationship of Amenorrhea and Body Weight in Anorexia Nervosa

No.	Patients with anorexia nervosa aged 15 or more	Mean weight s.d. (kg)	Sig. of diff. (*P*)
54	Mean weight at onset of dieting	61.0 ± 11.1	
	Mean matched population mean weight at onset of dieting	55.0 ± 3.7	<.001
	Mean weight at time of LMP	52.1 ± 6.2	<.005
27	Mean weight at time of return of menstruation	53.3 ± 6.2	N.S.
	Mean matched population mean weight at time of return of menses	55.5 ± 3.0	N.S.

Meanwhile, in an earlier study (Crisp and Stonehill, 1971), it had been shown that anorectics as a group were premorbidly obese, although variability in this respect was considerable. Commensurate with this, menstruation ceased at a mean weight of 52 ± 6 kg in those who recovered (Table 1).

Testosterone. Low testosterone levels have been found in male anorectics. Single cases showing levels restored to normal have been described (Palmer et al., 1974,1975; Frankel and Jenkins, 1975). Figure 9 shows data related to four male patients studied as weight was restored to normal (Crisp et al., in press). Levels can be seen to revert to normal once weight is 90% or more of normal.

Growth Hormone. High resting levels which revert to normal with refeeding and substantial weight gain have been described (Garfinkel et al., 1975). Low nocturnal levels (Fig. 10) which have been described (Kalucy et al., 1976a) may reflect the fact that the patients in this study had been eating a normal diet, including normal amounts of carbohydrate, for 1-3 days prior to the study although they were still 30% or more below target weight.

Prolactin. Most investigators have found normal levels in anorectics (Beaumont et al., 1974; Mecklenburg et al., 1974). Low levels (Fig. 11) were found throughout the night (Kalucy et al., 1976). Higher levels were found among anorectics to be associated with premorbid obesity and a failure to resume menstruation following restoration of body weight to matched population mean level (Hafner et al., 1976).

Cortisol. An increased level in the plasma has been found by all workers (Garfinkel et al., 1975; Kalucy et al., 1975b,1976), including during sleep (Fig. 12).

Thyroid Hormone and TSH. Thyroid hormone has generally been found

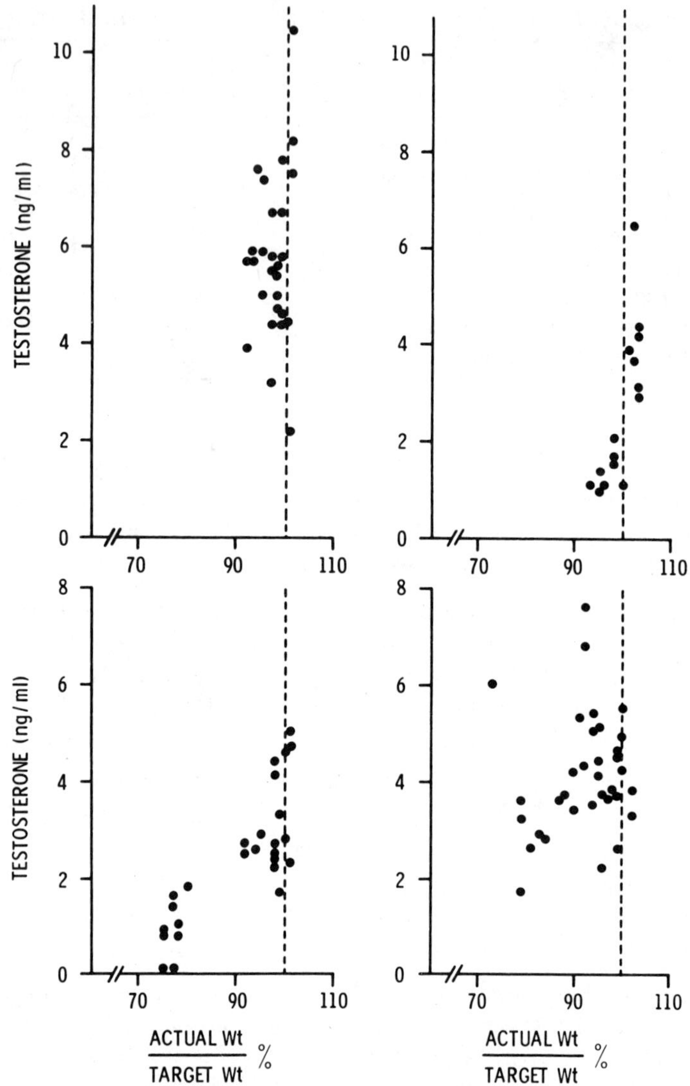

Figure 9 Plasma testosterone levels in four patients with anorexia nervosa during the period that their weight was restored to matched population mean levels (target weights). It can be seen that levels become more normal as weight increases to within 90% of target level.

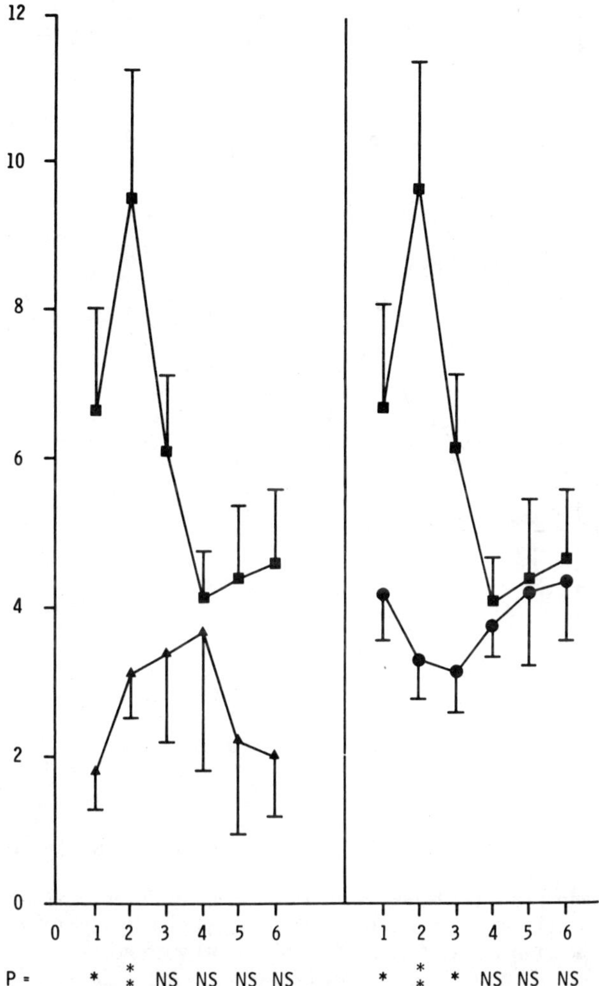

Figure 10 Mean GH levels in mU/ml during six 80-min periods of the night. The left-hand space compares anorexia nervosa subjects (▲) with normal subjects (■); the right-hand space obese subjects (●) with normal subjects (■). The significance of the differences (P) between groups is shown below each space; $P = <.5$ (*), $P = <.01$ (**). (Reproduced from Kalucy et al., 1976.)

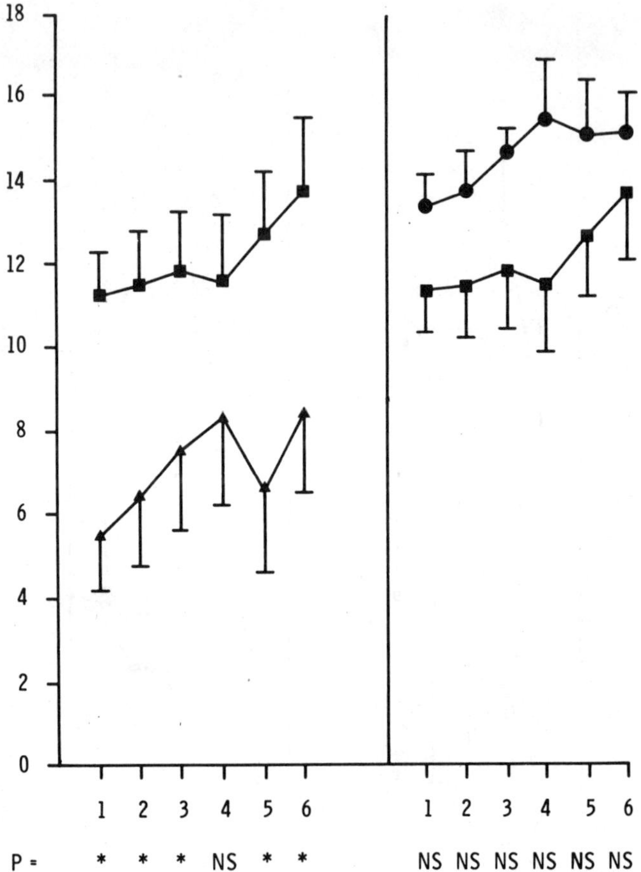

Figure 11 Mean prolactin levels in mU/ml during six 80-min periods of the night. The left-hand space compares anorexia nervosa subjects (▲) with normal subjects (■); the right-hand space obese subjects (●) with normal subjects (■). The significance of the differences (P) between groups is shown below each space; $P = <.5$ (*), $P = <.01$ (⁑). (Reproduced from Kalucy et al., 1976.)

to have a normal or else a slightly low level in the plasma (Werner et al., 1949; Mecklenburg et al., 1974; Kanis et al., 1974; Garfinkel et al., 1975; Frankel and Jenkins, 1975). TSH levels have been found to be near normal (Fig. 13) (Crisp and Roberts, 1962; Lundberg et al., 1972; Frankel and Jenkins, 1975; Kalucy et al., 1975b; Kalucy, 1976).

Metabolic rate is certainly markedly reduced in the abstaining anorectic, whose state of low body temperature, including reversed diurnal temperature rhythm (Crisp and Roberts, 1962; Crisp, 1970; Wakeling and Russell, 1970), poor peripheral circulation, cessation of reproductive function, and reduced

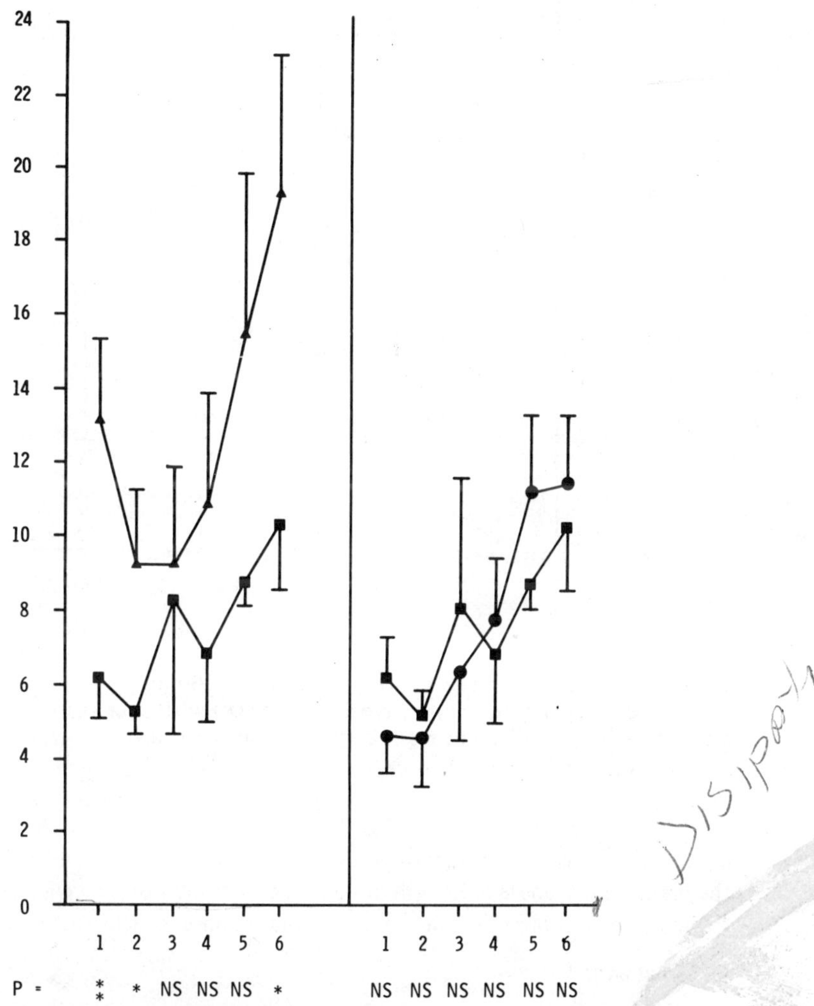

Figure 12 Mean cortisol levels in mU/ml during six 80-min periods of the night. The left-hand space compares anorexia nervosa subjects (▲) with normal subjects (■); the right-hand space obese subjects (●) with normal subjects (■). The significance of the difference (*P*) between groups is shown below each space; $P = <.5$ (*), $P = <.01$ (⁑). (Reproduced from Kalucy et al., 1976.)

cardiac output is consistent with the conservation survival needs of the starved organism. Metabolic rate for a given weight, as previously mentioned, is also related to dietary pattern, abstainers showing a markedly lower rate than bingers/vomiters/purgers (Crisp, 1967b,1974,1978a; Crisp et al., 1968b). The increase in

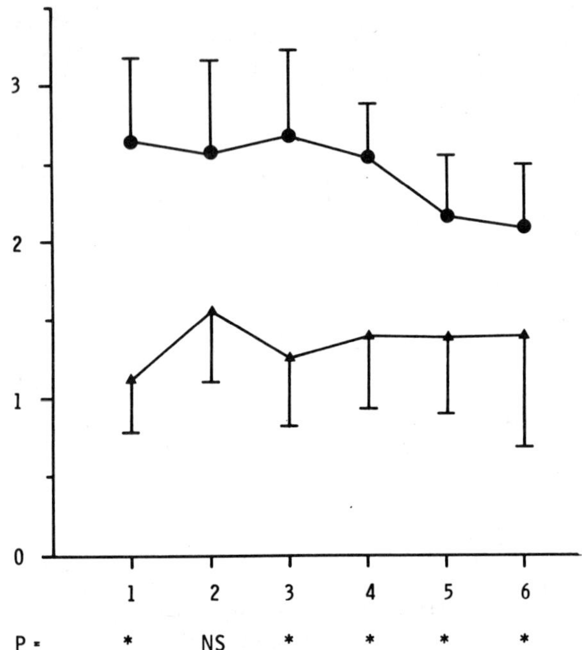

Figure 13 Mean TSH levels in mU/ml during six 80-min periods of the night. The figure compares anorexia nervosa subjects (■) with obese subjects (●). The significance of the differences (P) between groups is shown below; $P = <.5$ (*), $P = <.01$ (⁑). (Reproduced from Kalucy et al., 1976.)

metabolic rate as weight is restored to matched population mean level is less in the premorbidly obese (who will not achieve their premorbid weight under these treatment conditions) than in the premorbidly nonobese (Stordy et al., 1977).

4. *Treatment*

Treatment is a highly complex affair under any circumstances. Some individuals with the condition avoid attention until on the point of collapse. Under these circumstances, acute medical intervention is necessary. The best treatment under these circumstances is to get the individual to ingest either naturally or through a gastric tube. However, it may not be possible to insert the latter under such conditions, due to either resistance by or passivity of the individual concerned. Moreover, the stomach under these conditions may either be contracted down or else distended and unresponsive. Intravenous feeding may be necessary, but despite the other deficiencies, the most important one remains that of calories. Most individuals can be helped to eat even at this stage, providing an appropriate relationship has been established.

More commonly, the individual is thrust into the clinic situation, emaciated but not terminally ill, by increasingly anxious, angry, and embarrassed parents and others who have become involved. The first task in converting such an apparent patient into a real patient (someone wishing to change) involves gaining an understanding of the underlying maturational conflicts within the family. This can only be achieved if some considerable time (2-3 hours) can be spent with the various family members, including the patient in the first instance, seeking and gathering relevant and key information. This is a skilled task, often best undertaken by psychiatrists and others with clinical experience of the maturational problems of adolescence. Such an approach will usually secure the cooperation of the patient and family and lead to treatment such that at least the immediate crisis can be dealt with. However, the longer term requires a carefully planned and often lengthy treatment program which will, nevertheless, not always succeed. For details of various treatment approaches the reader is referred elsewhere (Crisp, 1967b,1970,1974,1978b; Dally, 1969; Russell, 1973; Bruch, 1974; Selvini Palazzoli, 1974; Crisp et al., 1977b,1978).

III. SUMMARY

Nutritional status, including such aspects as body weight and shape, foraging and eating, is interwoven with other important aspects of human experience and behavior. These relationships can be usefully studied when one or other aspect has reached morbid proportions, not least because the related illness model and consequent manipulation by treatment sometimes allows more penetrating examination of the impact upon the other variables of change in the designated morbid variable. In pursuit of clarity, the author polarizes these relationships, in the first instance, into two categories: (1) nutritional characteristics of psychiatric illness and (2) psychological aspects of two major nutritional disorders (obesity and anorexia nervosa). Emphasis is placed on the experimental literature.

REFERENCES

Abramson, E. E., and Wunderlich, R. A. (1972). Anxiety fear and eating. A test of the psychosomatic concept of obesity. *J. of Abnorm. Soc. Psychology 79,* 317-321.

Angst, J., and Perris, C. (1972). The nosology of endogenous depression. *Int. J. Ment. Health 1,* 145-158.

Beaumont, P. J. V., Friesen, H. G., Gelder, M. G., and Kolakowská, T. (1974). Plasma prolactin and luteinising hormone levels in anorexia nervosa. *Psychol. Med. 4,* 219-221.

Beck, A. T. (1967). *Depression.* Staples, London, p. 128.

Blendis, L. M., and Crisp, A. H. (1968). Serum cholesterol levels in anorexia nervosa. *Postgrad. Med. J. 44,* 327-330.

Bliss, E. L., and Branch, C. H. H. (1960). *Anorexia Nervosa.* Hoeber, New York.

Borjeson, M. (1962). Overweight children. *Acta Paed. 51 (supplement 132),* 1-76.

Boyar, R. M., Katz, J., Finkelstein, J. W., Kapen, S., Weiner, H., Weitzman, E. D., and Hellman, L. (1974). Anorexia nervosa. Immaturity of 24 hour L. H. secretory pattern. *N. Engl. J. Med. 291,* 861-865.

Brennan, E. L. (1945). Metabolic facets in psychiatric problems. *Dig. Neurol. Psychiatry 13,* 542-544.

Bruch, H. (1957). *The Importance of Overweight.* Norton, New York.

Bruch, H. (1974). *Eating Disorders.* Routledge and Kegan Paul, London.

Bruch, H., and Touraine, G. (1940). Obesity in childhood. 5. The family frame of obese children. *Psychosom. Med. 2,* 141-206.

Crisp, A. H., Hsu, L. K. G., Chen, C. N., and Wheeler, M. (1981). Reproductive hormone profiles in male anorexia nervosa. *Proc. Carrier Foundation.* In press.

Crammer, J. L. (1957). Rapid weight changes in mental patients. *Lancet 2,* 259-262.

Crisp, A. H. (1965a). Some aspects of the evolution, presentation and follow-up of anorexia nervosa. *Proc. Roy. Soc. Med. 58,* 814-820.

Crisp, A. H. (1965b). Clinical and therapeutic aspects of anorexia nervosa. A study of 30 cases. *J. Psychosom. Res. 9,* 67-68.

Crisp, A. H. (1967a). The possible significance of some behavioural correlates of weight and carbohydrate intake. *J. Psychosom. Res. 11,* 117-131.

Crisp, A. H. (1967b). Anorexia nervosa. *Hosp. Med. (May),* 713-718.

Crisp, A. H. (1970). Anorexia nervosa "feeding disorder," "nervous malnutrition" or "weight phobia." *World Rev. Nutr. Diet. 12,* 452-504.

Crisp, A. H. (1972). The nature of primary anorexia nervosa. In *Symposium: Anorexia Nervosa and Obesity,* R. F. Robertson (Ed.). Royal College of Physicians of Edinburgh, No. 42, 18-30.

Crisp, A. H. (1974). Primary anorexia nervosa or adolescent weight phobia. *Practitioner 212,* 525-535.

Crisp, A. H. (1977a). Some psychobiological aspects of adolescent growth and their relevance for the fat/thin syndrome (anorexia nervosa). *Int. J. Obes. 1,* 231-238.

Crisp, A. H. (1977b). Diagnosis and outcome of anorexia nervosa: the St. George's view. *Proc. Royal Soc. Med. 70,* 464-470.

Crisp, A. H. (1977c). The differential diagnosis of anorexia nervosa. *Proc. Roy. Soc. Med. 70,* 686-694.

Crisp, A. H. (1978a). Some aspects of the relationship between body weight and sexual behaviour with particular reference to massive obesity and anorexia nervosa. *Int. J. Obes. 1.* In press.

Crisp, A. H. (1978b). Some experiential aspects of obesity. Paper read at 2nd Int. Cong. Obesity, Washington, D.C., October.

Crisp, A. H., and Kalucy, R. S. (1973). The effect of leucotomy in intractable adolescent weight phobia (primary anorexia nervosa). *Postgrad. Med. J. 49,* 883-893.

Crisp, A. H., and Kalucy, R. S. (1974). Aspects of the perceptual disorder in anorexia nervosa. *Br. J. Med. Psychology 47,* 349-361.

Crisp, A. H., and McGuinness, B. (1976). Jolly fat. Relation between obesity and psychoneurosis in general population. *Br. Med. J. 1,* 7-9.

Crisp, A. H., and Roberts, F. J. (1962). A case of anorexia nervosa in a male. *Postgrad. Med. J. 38,* 350-353.

Crisp, A. H., and Stonehill, E. (1967). Hypercarotenaemia as a symptom of weight phobia. *Postgrad. Med. J. 43,* 721-725.

Crisp, A. H., and Stonehill, E. (1970). Treatment of obesity with special reference to seven severely obese patients. *J. Psychosom. Res. 14,* 327-345.

Crisp, A. H., and Stonehill, E. (1971). Relationship between aspects of nutritional disturbance and menstrual activity in primary anorexia nervosa. *Br. Med. J. 3,* 149-151.

Crisp, A. H., and Stonehill, E. (1973). Aspects of the relationship between sleep and nutrition. A study of 375 psychiatric out-patients. *Br. J. Psychiatry 122,* 379-394.

Crisp, A. H., and Stonehill, E. (1976). *Sleep, Nutrition and Mood.* Wiley, Chichester.

Crisp, A. H., Ellis, J., and Lowy, C. (1967). Insulin response to a rapid intravenous injection of dextrose in patients with anorexia nervosa and obesity. *Postgrad. Med. J. 43,* 97-102.

Crisp, A. H., Blendis, L. M., and Pawan, G. L. S. (1968a). Aspects of fat metabolism in anorexia nervosa. *Metabolism 17,* 1109-1118.

Crisp, A. H., Fenton, G. W., and Scotton, L. (1968b). A controlled study of the EEG in anorexia nervosa. *Br. J. Psychiatry 114,* No. 514, 1149-1160.

Crisp, A. H., Douglas, J. W. R., Ross, J. M., and Stonehill, E. (1970). Some developmental aspects of disorders of weight. *J. Psychosom. Res. 14,* 313-320.

Crisp, A. H., MacKinnon, P. C. B., Chen, C. N., and Corker, C. S. (1973). Observations of gonadotrophic and ovarian hormone activity during recovery from anorexia nervosa. *Postgrad. Med. J. 49,* No. 547, 584-590.

Crisp, A. H., Stonehill, E., and Koval, J. (1975). The pyknic habitus in psychiatric illness. In *Recent Advances in Obesity Research,* Vol. 1, A. Howard (Ed.). Newman, London, pp. 331-332.

Crisp, A. H., Palmer, R. L., and Kalucy, R. S. (1976). How common is anorexia nervosa? A prevalence study. *Br. J. Psychiatry 128,* 549-554.

Crisp, A. H., Kalucy, R. S., Pilkington, T. R. E., and Gazet, J-C. (1977a). Some psychosocial consequences of ileojejunal bypass surgery. *Am. J. Clin. Nutr. 30,* 109-120.

Crisp, A. H., Kalucy, R. S., Lacey, J. H., and Harding, B. (1977b). The long-term prognosis in anorexia nervosa. Some factors predictive of outcome. In *Anorexia Nervosa,* R. Vigersky (Ed.). Raven, New York, pp. 55-65.

Critchley, M. (1962). Periodic hypersomnia and megaphagia in adolescent males. *Brain 85,* 627-656.

Dally, P. (1959). Carotenaemia occurring in a case of anorexia nervosa. *Br. Med. J. 1,* 1333.

Dally, P. (1969). *Anorexia Nervosa.* Heinemann, London.

Duquay, R., and Flach, F. F. (1964). An experimental study of weight changes in depression. *Acta Psychiatr. Neurol. Scand. 40,* 1-9.

Dwyer, J. T., Feldman, J. J., and Mayer, J. (1967). Adolescent dieters. Who are they? Physical characteristics, attitudes and dieting practices of adolescent girls. *Am. J. Clin. Nutr. 20,* 1045-1056.

Eid, E. E. (1970). Follow-up study of physical growth of children who had excessive weight gain in first six months of life. *Br. Med. J. 2,* 74-76.

Frankel, R. J., and Jenkins, J. S. (1975). Hypothalamic-pituitary function in anorexia nervosa. *Acta Endocrinol. 78,* 209-221.

Frisch, R. E., and McArthur, J. W. (1974). Menstrual cycles. Fatness as a determinant of minimum weight for height necessary for their maintenance or onset. *Science 185,* 949-951.

Frisch, R. E., and Revelle, R. (1971). Height and weight at menarche and a hypothesis of critical body weight and adolescent events. *Arch. Dis. Child. 46,* 695-701.

Garfinkel, P. E., Brown, G. M., Stancer, H. C., and Moldofsky, H. (1975). Hypothalamic pituitary function in anorexia nervosa. *Arch. Gen. Psychiatry 32,* 739-744.

Glucksman, M. L., and Hirsch, J. (1968). The response of obese patients to weight reduction. A clinical evaluation of behaviour. *Psychosom. Med. 30,* 1-11.

Goldblatt, P. B., Moore, M. E., and Stunkard, A. J. (1965). Social factors in obesity. *J. Am. Med. Ass. 192,* 1039-1044.

Green, L. N., and Cracco, R. Q. (1970). Kleine-Levin syndrome. A case with EEG evidence of periodic brain damage. *Arch. Neurol. 22,* 166-175.

Hafner, R. J., Crisp, A. H., and McNeilly, A. S. (1976). Prolactin and gonadotrophin activity in females treated for anorexia nervosa. *Postgrad. Med. J. 52,* 76-79.

Halmi, K. A., Sherman, B. M., and Zamudio, R. (1975). Impaired L.H. response to gonadotrophin-releasing hormone (GnRH) in women with anorexia nervosa. *Psychosom. Med. 37,* 82-83.

Hellman, L., Boyar, R., Weiner, H., Roffwarg, H., Gorzynski, K. G., and Katz, J. (1974). Immaturity of the circadian secretory program for plasma luteinising hormone in anorexia nervosa. *Psychosom. Med. 36,* 457-458.

Johnson, M. L., Burke, B. S., and Mayer, J. (1956). Relative importance of inactivity and overeating in energy balance of obese high school girls. *Am. J. Clin. Nutr. 4,* 37-44.

Kalucy, R. S. (1976). Obesity. An attempt to find a common ground among some of the biological, psychological and sociological phenomena of the obesity/overeating syndromes. In *Modern Trends in Psychosomatic Medicine,* Vol. 3, O. Hill (Ed.). Butterworths, London, pp. 404-429.

Kalucy, R. S., and Crisp, A. H. (1974). Some psychological and social implications of massive obesity. *J. Psychosom. Res. 18,* 465-473.

Kalucy, R. S., Solow, C., Hartmann, M., Crisp, A. H., McGuinness, B., and Kalucy, E. C. (1975a). Self reports of estimated body widths in female obese subjects with major fat loss following ileo-jejunal bypass surgery. In *Recent Advances in Obesity Research,* Vol. 1, A. Howard (Ed.). Newman, London, pp. 331-332.

Kalucy, R. S., Hartmann, M., Chen, C. N., Crisp, A. H., and McNeilly, A. (1975b). A study of some aspects of sleep and nocturnal hormone secretion in a massively obese population. In *Recent Advances in Obesity Research,* A. Howard (Ed.). Newman, London, pp. 111-112.

Kalucy, R. S., Crisp, A. H., Chard, T., McNeilly, A., Chen, C. N., and Lacey, J. H. (1976). Nocturnal hormonal profiles in massive obesity, anorexia nervosa and normal females. *J. Psychosom. Res. 20,* 595-604.

Kalucy, R. S., Crisp, A. H., and Harding, B. (1977). A study of 56 families with anorexia nervosa. *Br. J. Med. Psychology 50,* 381-395.

Kanis, J. A., Brown, P., Fitzpatrick, K., Hibbert, D. J., Horn, D. B., Nairn, I. M., Shirling, D., Strong, J. A., and Walton, H. J. (1974). Anorexia nervosa. A clinical, psychiatric and laboratory study. I. Clinical and laboratory investigation. *Quart. J. Med. (New Series) 43,* No. 170, 321-388.

Keys, A., and Brozek, J. (1953). Body fat in adult man. *Physiol. Rev. 33,* 245-325.

Kollar, E. J., and Atkinson, R. M. (1966). Responses of extremely obese patients to starvation. *Psychosom. Med. 28,* 227-246.

Kretschmer, E. (1936). *Physique and Character,* 2nd Ed. Kegan Paul, London.

Lacey, J. H., Stanley, P. A., Crutchfield, M., and Crisp, A. H. (1977). Sucrose sensitivity in anorexia nervosa. *J. Psychosom. Res. 21,* 17-21.

Lundberg, P. O., Walinder, J., Werner, I., and Wide, L. (1972). Effects of thyrotrophin-releasing hormone on plasma levels of TSH, FSH, LH and GH in anorexia nervosa. *Eur. J. Clin. Invest. 2,* 150-153.

Maaser, R., and Droese, W. (1971). Overnutrition in West German children. *Lancet 2,* 545.

Mayer Gross, W., Slater, E., and Roth, M. (1969). *Clinical Psychiatry.* Bailliere, Tindall and Cassel, London.

Mecklenburg, R. S., Loriaux, D. C., Thompson, R. H., Andersen, A. E., and Lipsett, M. R. (1974). Hypothalamic dysfunction in patients with anorexia nervosa. *Medicine 53,* 147-159.

Metropolitan Life Insurance Co. (1959,1960). Overweight. Its prevention and significance. *Stat. Bull. 40,41.*

Moore, M. E., Stunkard, A., and Srole, L. (1962). Obesity, social class and mental illness. *J. Am. Med. Ass. 181,* 962-966.

Morgan, H. G., and Russell, G. F. M. (1975). The value of family background and clinical features and prediction of long-term outcome in anorexia nervosa. A four-year follow-up study of 41 patients. *Psychol. Med. 5,* 355-371.

Oberdisse, K., Solbach, H. G., and Zimmerman, H. (1965). The endocrinological aspects of anorexia nervosa. In *Symposium on Anorexia Nervosa,* J. Meyer and H. Feldman (Eds.). Thieme Verlag, Stuttgart, pp. 26-43.

Palmer, R. L., Crisp, A. H., MacKinnon, P. C. B., Franklin, M.,Akande, E. O., and Bonnar, J. (1974). Gonodatrophin response to LH/FSH-RH during weight gain in patients with anorexia nervosa. *J. Endocrinol. 63,* No. 2, 32.

Palmer, R. L., Crisp, A. H., MacKinnon, P. C. B., Franklin, M., Bonnar, J., and Wheeler, M. (1975). Pituitary sensitivity to 50 μg LH/FSH-RH in subjects with anorexia nervosa in acute and recovery stages. *Br. Med. J. 1,* 179-182.

Parisova, J. (1968). Nutrition, body fat and physical fitness. In *Borden Review of Nutrition Research,* Vol. 29, 4th Quarter. Borden, New York.

Pilkington, T. R. E., Gazet, J-C., Ang, L., Kalucy, R. S., Crisp, A. H., and Day, S. (1976). Explanations for weight loss after ileojejunal bypass in gross obesity. *Br. Med. J. 1,* 1504-1505.

Pollitt, J. (1965). *Depression and Its Treatment.* Heinemann, London.

Post, F. (1956). Body changes in psychiatric illness. A critical survey of the literature. *J. Psychosom. Res. 1,* 219-226.

Quaade, F. (1955). *Obese Children: Anthropology and Environment.* Danish Science Press, Copenhagen.

Russell, G. F. M. (1973). The management of anorexia nervosa. In *Symposium: Anorexia Nervosa and Obesity,* R. F. Robertson (Ed.). Royal College of Physicians of Edinburgh, No. 42, pp. 44-62.

Seidensticker, J. F., and Tzagournis, M. (1968). Anorexia nervosa. Clinical features and long-term follow-up. *J. Chron. Dis. 21,* 361-367.

Selvini Palazzoli, M. (1974). *Self-Starvation.* Chaucer, London.

Silverstone, J. T. (1968). Psychosocial aspects of obesity. *Proc. Roy. Soc. Med. 61,* 371-375.

Society of Actuaries (1959). *Build and Blood Pressure Study.* Chicago.

Sours, J. A. (1963). Narcolepsy and other disturbances in the sleep-waking rhythm. A study of 115 cases with review of the literature. *J. Nerv. Ment. Dis. 137,* 525-542.

Steinkamp, R. C., Cohen, N. L., Gaffey, W. R., McKay, T., Bron, G., Siri, W. E., Sargent, T. W., and Isaacs, E. (1965). Measures of body fat and related factors in normal adults. II. A simple clinical method to estimate body fat and lean body mass. *J. Chron. Dis. 18,* 1291-1307.

Stonehill, E., Crisp, A. H., and Koval, J. (1976). The relationship of reported sleep characteristics to psychiatric diagnosis and mood. *Br. J. Med. Psychology 49,* 381-391.

Stordy, B. J., Marks, V., Kalucy, R. S., and Crisp, A. H. (1977). Weight gain, thermic effect of glucose and resting metabolic rate during recovery from anorexia nervosa. *Am. J. Clin. Nutr. 30,* 138-146.

Stunkard, A. J. (1958). Physical activity, emotions and human obesity. *Psychosom. Med. 20,* 366-372.

Tanner, J. M., and Whitehouse, R. H. (1962). Standards for subcutaneous fat in British children. *Br. Med. J. 1,* 446-450.

von Doblen, W. (1959). Anthropometric determinations of fat-free body weight. *Acta Med. Scand. 165,* 37-40.

Wakeling, A., and Russell, G. F. M. (1970). Disturbances in the regulation of body temperature in anorexia nervosa. *Psychol. Med. 1,* 30-39.

Warren, M. P., and van de Viele, R. L. (1973). Clinical and metabolic features of anorexia nervosa. *Am. J. Obstet. Gynecol. 117,* 435-449.

Werner, S. C., Quimby, H., and Schmidt, C. (1949). The use of tracer doses of radioactive iodine, I^{131}, in the study of normal and disordered thyroid function in man. *J. Clin. Endocrin. Met. 9,* 342-354.

Winnicot, D. W. (1958). In *Collected Papers.* Tavistock, London, p. 33.

Wooley, S. C., Wooley, O. W., Bartoshuk, L. M., Cabanac, M. J. C., Ferstl, R., Gutezeit, G. W. R., McFarland, D. J., Oetting, M., Pudel, V. E., Rodin, J., and Simmoons, F. J. (1976). Psychological aspects of feeding. Group report. In *Appetite and Food Intake,* T. Silverstone (Ed.). Dahlem Konferenzen, Abakon Verlagsgesellschaft, Berlin, pp. 331-354.

20

Malnutrition and Psychological Development

David V. M. Ashley* **and Alan N. Davison**
Institute of Neurology, The National Hospital
London, England

Marie E. Stewart
Bedford College, University of London
London, England

**Present affiliation:* Nestlé Products Technical Assistance Co., Ltd., La Tour-de-Peilz, Switzerland.

I. INTRODUCTION

Malnutrition has been defined as "an impairment of health and physiological function resulting from failure of an individual to obtain all the essential nutrients in the proper amounts and balance" (Schaefer, 1969). Although overnutrition is a major problem, particularly in the developed world, inadequate nutrition is by far the largest preventable health problem facing the world. The World Health Organization (WHO) estimates that there are at least 100 million children suffering from malnutrition (Bengoa, 1974).

In this chapter we are concerned with the effects of protein energy malnutrition on the morphology and biochemistry of the brain and on behavior. Malnutrition during brain development may have a permanent effect on cerebral morphology which may be of consequence to behavior. Many researchers have been oversimplistic in their interpretation of cause and effect, but the ecology of human malnutrition involves a complex interaction of social and political as well as medical and nutritional factors which preclude any simple explanation.

II. PROTEIN ENERGY MALNUTRITION

Protein energy malnutrition (PEM) is a range of pathological conditions occurring most frequently in infants and young children. The etiology of PEM is complex, and the relative importance of deficiencies of dietary energy and protein in its development is still controversial. In addition, it is difficult to isolate the effect of these deficiencies from deficiencies of other nutrients, infection, and disturbances of metabolism (DeMaeyer, 1976; Alleyne et al., 1977). In many children and in adults, subclinical PEM may be present. Subclinical PEM is difficult to assess, but may be important particularly in women of low socioeconomic status during pregnancy and lactation (DeMaeyer, 1976).

Classification of malnourished children is usually based on the extent of deficits in weight with reference to international standards of expected weight for age (50th percentile, Boston standards; Stuart and Stevenson, 1959). Children with severe malnutrition, or "third degree malnutrition" in the Gomez terminology (Gomez et al., 1956), are grouped as kwashiorkor, marasmus, or marasmic-kwashiorkor by a scoring system based on weight for age and presence or absence of edema (Table 1).

A discussion of prevention and treatment of PEM is beyond the scope of this chapter and has been discussed more fully elsewhere (Bengoa, 1976; DeMaeyer, 1976; Picou et al., 1978). It is sufficient to mention, however, that the basic principle of treatment is to improve the children's nutritional status as quickly as possible by providing sufficient amounts of high energy and high-quality protein foods. Treatment of severe PEM is more complicated than mild-moderate, requiring hospitalization for correction of dehydration, electrolyte imbalances, and infection, after which energy intakes of 840 kJ/kg per day and

Table 1 Classification of Protein Energy Malnutrition

% of expected weight for age	Edema	Type
80-60	0	Mild-moderate
	+	Kwashiorkor
<60	0	Marasmus
	+	Marasmic-kwarshiokor

Source: Adapted from Wellcome Classification, *Lancet,* 1970.

growth rates 20 times faster than normal children can be achieved (Ashworth, 1978).

III. METHODOLOGY

A. Biochemical Indices of Brain Development

The difficulties encountered in identifying various morphological events occurring during development and after nutritional insult have necessitated the use of gross measurements as indices of the anatomical changes. In the earliest studies of undernutrition and brain development, brain size and weight were measured. In later years, quantification of various biochemical constituents of the CNS were used to infer morphological changes. For example, brain lipid or cholesterol, although not wholly characteristic components of myelin, were used to indicate alterations in the extent of myelination. Similarly, determination of DNA, RNA, and protein concentration served as indices of cell number and size. Analysis of DNA for this purpose relies on the assumption that a constant amount of the nucleic acid is present in a stable diploid nucleus. In some respects this does not fully apply, even to predominantly nondividing nervous tissue. Some brain cells are tetraploid, though these are few in number (Lentz and Lapham, 1969, 1970). As well, DNA may not be located entirely within the nucleus (Davison and Dobbing, 1968). In contrast to DNA, RNA may be considered representative of the biosynthetic potential of the cell. When measurements of protein are made as well, indication of cell size and composition may be derived by expressing protein/DNA or RNA/DNA ratio. Although interpretation of these measurements is limited because they do not distinguish between cell types, the more recently used other biochemical correlates, such as gangliosides (e.g., GM_1) for neuronal membranes and nerve endings or glutamine synthetase for glia, are not necessarily more reliable. Nevertheless, these and similar biochemical measures provide a more quantitative assessment of structure change than was possible by histology.

B. Animal Models in the Study of Malnutrition

Ethical and practical considerations limit the nature of definitive research in human populations. For example, it is impossible to intentionally induce malnutrition in humans or to establish adequate controls in populations already affected. Consequently, animal models need to be developed to investigate the sequellae of nutritional insult. The study of the effect of PEM on brain function and intellectual development is made difficult largely because the complex etiology of the disease has not allowed development of completely satisfactory animal models. Moreover, differences in the morphological development in the brain of various species has necessitated the use of a variety of experimental approaches to produce malnutrition at different stages of development, so that the effects of malnutrition at the different stages can be better assessed. Consequently, models for the disease have relied on production of malnutrition in utero during the suckling period and after weaning. Furthermore, many difficulties arise in the development of animal models relevant to human behavior. Extrapolation to humans from the behavior of animals may only be done with extreme caution.

Prenatal malnutrition is usually produced experimentally by restricting intake of food, and therefore energy, of pregnant females. Some paradigms utilize diets deficient in protein, or lacking a single amino acid or other essential nutrient. Warkany (1945) demonstrated that the fetus, although relatively more protected from nutritional insult than the neonate, was not the perfect parasite it was once thought to be.

Severe malnutrition imposed early during pregnancy generally leads to a failure in maintaining the pregnancy. When a protein-free diet was fed for the first 10 days of the 21-day gestation period, 62% of the mated female rats failed to have a live litter (Zamenhof et al., 1971). Later periods of severe protein deficiency had less effect on the maintenance of the pregnancy but resulted in a higher proportion of stillbirths. The critical level of protein in the diet, at or below which significant fetal resorption and stillbirths occur, is approximately 5%. At 10% dietary protein no effects on the offspring were seen. On the other hand, reducing the energy intake by one-third during litter gestation while maintaining an adequate level of protein in the diet resulted in a failure of 30% of the mated females to produce litters. The critical period in the rat during which severe malnutrition can affect the development of the pregnancy appears to be between days 7 and 10 (Zamenhof et al., 1976). This has been related to the failure of the dam to produce the hormones required for implantation of the fetus and for placental development (Zamenhof and van Marthens, 1974). Pregnancy in severely protein-deficient animals has been artificially maintained by hormone administration (Morishige and Leathem, 1972; Niiyama et al., 1973).

The neonate is considerably more susceptible than the developing fetus to severe malnutrition. This is undoubtedly due to the greater nutritional requirement to sustain the rapid growth of the offspring during this early prenatal period. Methods of producing experimental malnutrition during this period rely on limiting the availability of milk to the young offspring. These methods assume that the experimental animal is receiving a well-balanced nutritional intake, but the amount of food received is reduced. Three methods are commonly used to deprive suckling rats. The majority of studies using rodents have employed the method of unequal litter size (Kennedy, 1957). Control litters are most often adjusted to 8-10 animals or less while malnourished litters are increased to up to 20 animals. Other approaches have been to remove the pups from the mother for some part of each day, thus limiting the time available for feeding (Eayrs and Horn, 1955), or to reduce the quantity of milk produced by the lactating dam by feeding protein-deficient diets of restricting intake of a nutritionally adequate diet (Mueller and Cox, 1946). Severe deprivation has been produced by a combination of these approaches (Guthrie and Brown, 1968; Baas et al., 1970a,b). Tube-feeding formula to pups allows the nutritional composition of the diet fed to the suckling animal to be altered, providing a useful technique for assessing the impact of individual nutrients on development (Miller, 1969).

Each of the methods used is associated with unique problems and introduces into the study experimental variables over which adequate control cannot be made. For example, the behavior of nutritionally deprived dams and those nursing large litters toward their young has been noted to be altered (Smart, 1976). In large litters some pups grow well at the expense of the others, and may not therefore be directly compared with each other (Dodge et al., 1975). Removal of pups from dams introduces the problem of temperature control (Perez et al., 1973) and handling (Curzon and Knott, 1975) and their possible effects on the chemistry of the brain and behavior (Fraňková, 1974; Levine and Weiner, 1976).

Postweaning malnutrition in animals results from either restricting intake of protein, or of protein and energy. Many features of kwashiorkor have been successfully produced in the rat (Endozian, 1968; Anthony and Endozian, 1975), guinea pig (Enwonwu, 1973), dog (Platt et al., 1964), pig (Platt et al., 1964), and nonhuman primates (Deo et al., 1965; Coward and Whitehead, 1972).

C. Assessment of Psychological Development in Humans

The subsequent psychological development of nutritionally rehabilitated infants is of increasing importance today as advances in the treatment of malnutrition have resulted in the survival of an increasing proportion of children who have experienced some form of severe nutritional deprivation at an early age. In fact, some centers have reported dramatic decreases in the mortality of severely malnourished infants (Ashworth, 1978). Although it is likely that malnutrition suffered in early infancy will result in stunting of physical growth (Graham and Adrianzen, 1972) any distortion of psychological development has far greater political and social implications. The prevalence of severe and moderate forms of malnutrition in developing countries of the world (Table 2) suggests that the future development of these nations may be greatly affected if malnutrition has serious consequences for psychological development.

Assessment of psychological development in malnourished children is not without its problems. The prime concern in this area has been whether severe malnutrition in infancy results in mental retardation. However, as Vernon (1969) pointed out, mental capacities cannot, like height and weight, be measured on absolute or ratio scales. Results have to be assessed in reference to the distribution of results in a population of comparable individuals, but there are very few tests available which have been developed in the countries in which studies on malnutrition have been conducted. In general, standardized tests from the United States and England, such as the Wechsler Intelligence Scale for children (WISC) and the Griffiths Mental Development Scales, have been utilized. In recognition of the fact that malnutrition has to be viewed as one of a range of variables influencing the functional development of children and that the effects of malnutrition on intellectual performance may not be a direct one, increasingly investigators have included other social and behavioral measures.

The application of tests of mental development in countries in which their validity and reliability have not been established has been questioned repeatedly (Berry and Dasen, 1974; Pollitt and Thompson, 1977). In many studies, including Geber and Dean's classical paper on African children (1957), it has been recognized that the development of children in Africa, Asia, and Latin America follows patterns which make North American and United Kingdom norms inapplicable (Vernon, 1969). However, even where validity of the norms has been established, questions remain as to the interpretation of the results of such tests (Pollitt and Thompson, 1977).

A further issue concerns the nature of tests of infant development and intelligence (IQ). The development of mental abilities in infancy is rapid and difficult to measure (Honzik, 1976). Infant test scores often are not stable over long periods of time (McCall, 1976), and their relationship to previous and concurrent experience is complex and only beginning to be understood (Honzik, 1976). Infant tests, which measure abilities and skills that are regarded as the bases and precursors of later mental development, in fact have poor predictive validity. McCall et al. (1972) report median correlation coefficients of the order of .01 between scores from tests before 6 months and those obtained at 8-18 years and .21 between scores of tests at 13-18 months and scores at 8-18 years. On the other hand, tests of intelligence purport to measure a general intellectual faculty, akin to Spearman's "g" (Butcher, 1968), but there has been considerable debate recently as to the structure of mental abilities and the success of so-called culture fair tests (Block and Dworkin, 1977).

Table 2 Prevalence of Protein Energy Malnutrition in Community Studies (1963-1972)

Region	No. of communities	No. of surveys	No. of children examined	Protein calorie malnutrition (%)		
				Severe	Moderate	Severe and moderate
Latin America	20	29	116,179	0-12.0	3.5-32.0	4.6-36.0
Africa	16	32	34,184	0-9.8	5.6-66.0	7.3-73.0
Asia	10	16	43,326	0-20.0	13.0-73.8	14.8-80.3
Total	46	77	193,689	0-20.0	3.5-73.8	4.6-80.3

Source: Adapted from Bengoa, 1974.

Measured IQ is known to be influenced by social environmental factors (Kamin, 1974; Vernon, 1979). In some circumstances, socioeconomic status in early life is a powerful predictor of IQ levels in middle childhood (Pollitt and Thompson, 1977). As malnutrition occurs mainly in the context of extreme social disadvantage, these factors can be expected to be of considerable importance. In studies of children, therefore, investigators are faced with the task of disentangling the roles of the many influences on psychological development in an attempt to make causal statements on the specific effects of malnutrition. Constraints on experimental manipulation and control in human studies and difficulties arising in the interpretation of data derived from different cultures further complicate the issue.

IV. GROWTH AND DEVELOPMENT OF THE BRAIN

After early embryological development, the central nervous system undergoes a series of interrelated and exceedingly complex morphological and biochemical changes. Cell migration occurs in such a way that different parts of the nervous system undergo development at different times. In all regions, neuroblast multiplication precedes the glial cell precursors (spongioblasts). As a result, the adult number of neurons is achieved early in life. Later, growth of neurons with the formation of dendrites, axons, and synaptic connections overlaps with the synthesis of myelin by the formative glial cell, the oligodendrocyte. Nutritional insults during the development of the central nervous system can therefore affect neuronal and/or glial cell development depending on the time imposed.

The pattern of brain growth relative to birth is different in various species. This is clearly illustrated in Figure 1, where the changes in the rate of increase of wet weight of the brain are plotted on an arbitrary time scale in relation to birth. The period of brain growth occurring when the velocity of brain weight change is maximal is defined as the brain growth spurt. As judged by the rate of increase in brain weight, the sequence of developmental events appears to be common to all species but the timing of the processes varies. The human growth spurt is perinatal, beginning in mid-pregnancy and ending approximately 2 years after birth. Subsequently, brain weight relative to body weight declines exponentially so that in the mature animal brain weight is relatively stable. In contrast to humans, the development of the rat brain is largely postnatal. The brain weight

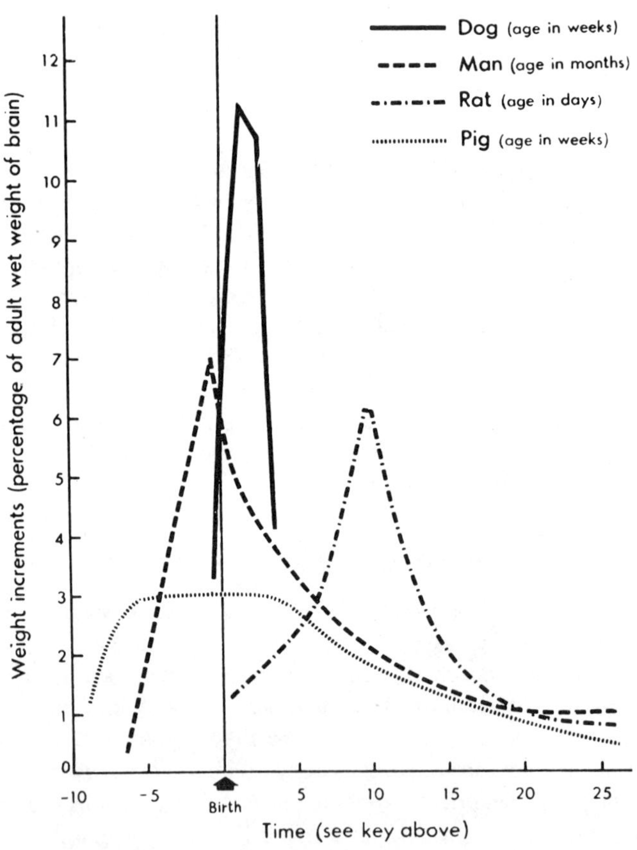

Figure 1 Rate curves of brain growth in relation to birth in different species. Values are calculated at different time intervals in each species. (From Davison and Dobbing, 1963, with kind permission of the British Council.)

increases to a maximum about 10 days after birth, and continues to increase slowly after 6 months. In contrast, the guinea pig brain develops mainly before birth.

These differences among species in the development of the CNS become important in the attempt to relate changes in the brain of experimental animals to those in humans. For example, the newborn rat or rabbit may be regarded as equivalent in brain development terms to that of an 18-week-old human fetus and a newborn guinea pig to that of a 2- to 3-year-old human child. Thus caution must be taken in extrapolating between species, as even the most clear-cut anatomical, biochemical, or behavioral changes in animals resulting from nutritional insult may have little relevance to similar insults in humans.

The rate of change in DNA content of the rat brain (Fig. 2) shows a pattern similar to that of brain weight and indicates that cellular multiplication is maximal at about the 10th postnatal day. This suggests that the increase in

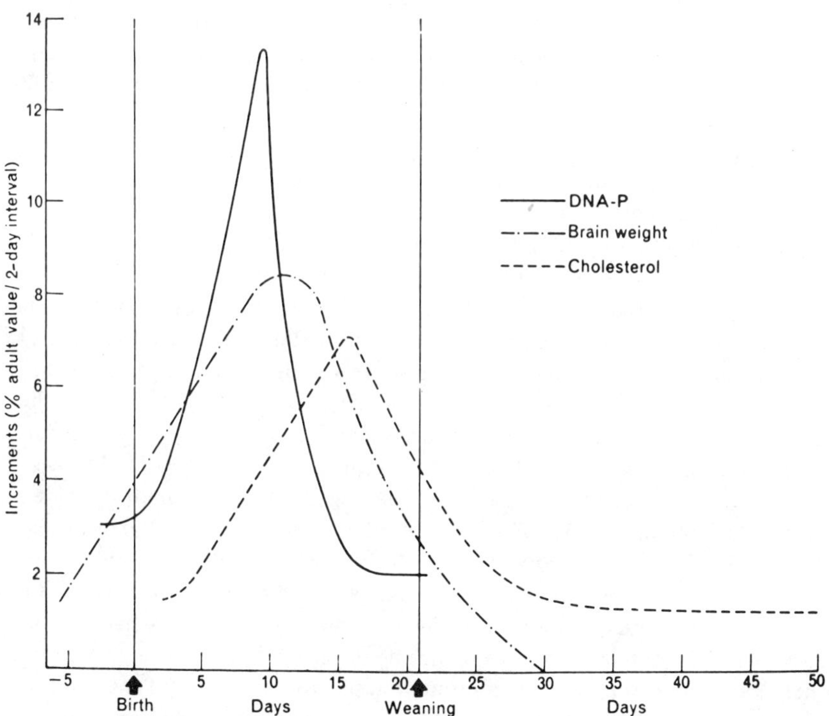

Figure 2 Rate curves for increases in brain weight, DNA, and cholesterol in the rat. (From Davison and Dobbin, 1968, with kind permission of Blackwell's Scientific Publications.)

cell number primarily accounts for the increase in brain weight occurring at about this time. Adult DNA content is essentially achieved by weaning. The rate of increase of DNA falls off sharply long before brain growth or the accumulation of RNA or protein ceases (Davison and Dobbing, 1968), suggesting that the later stages of brain growth result from an increase in cell mass rather than cell number.

In the rat brain, accumulation of DNA after birth represents mainly an accumulation of glial cells, as the neuronal cell population in most regions of the brain (except the cerebellum) is established by that time. Altman (1972a,b) concluded that gliagenesis occurred at the end of and following neurogenesis. These conclusions are in agreement with those of Brizzee and colleagues (1964), who found a progressive rise in glial to neuron cell ratio in the rat cerebral cortex throughout life. The cell counts indicated a continuing increase in the glial cell population while neuronal cell population remained relatively constant after 10 days of age (Fig. 3). However, postnatal neurogenesis appears to take place in at least three areas of the brain. In the cerebellum, 97% of the final number of cells are acquired during the first 3 weeks after birth (Miale and Sidman, 1961; Balázs and Richert, 1973). In addition, postnatal neuronal proliferation has been demonstrated in the hippocampal formation (Altman, 1966a,b) and in the olfactory bulb (Altman and Das, 1966). Thus nutritional insults to rodents after birth are most likely to have their effect on division and migration of neurons in these three regions rather than in other parts of the brain.

Unlike the rat, humans appear to have a temporal separation in the formation of neurons and glia. Accumulation of DNA follows two maxima (Fig. 4), one before birth, presumably due to neuronal acquisition, and the other some 3-6 months after birth, probably due to multiplication of glia.

The likely effect of postnatal nutritional restriction would therefore be on proliferation of glial cells and also on accumulation of lipid and cholesterol and myelin formation, which follow glial cell proliferation (Larroche and Amakawa, 1973). The rate of cholesterol accumulation (Fig. 2) reflects the rate of myelin synthesis, which in the rat is maximal at about 14 days. Different areas of the brain myelinate at different rates. Myelin deposition follows definite temporal and spatial patterns, beginning in the phylogenetically older regions of the brain and proceeding in a caudal-rostral direction. Yakovlev and Lecours (1967) in studying the brains of humans from fetal to adult life found that myelination of sensory, cerebellar, and extrapyramidal tracts were the first to be completed and development of the pyramidal tract began rather late, but advanced rapidly and was completed during the second year of life. Association fibers myelinated very slowly, continuing well into adult life. Thus certain processes, in specific areas, may at any one time appear to be differently susceptible to a retarding stress. Insult to the human infant during 5-11 weeks after birth would be expected to produce marked differences in the myelin

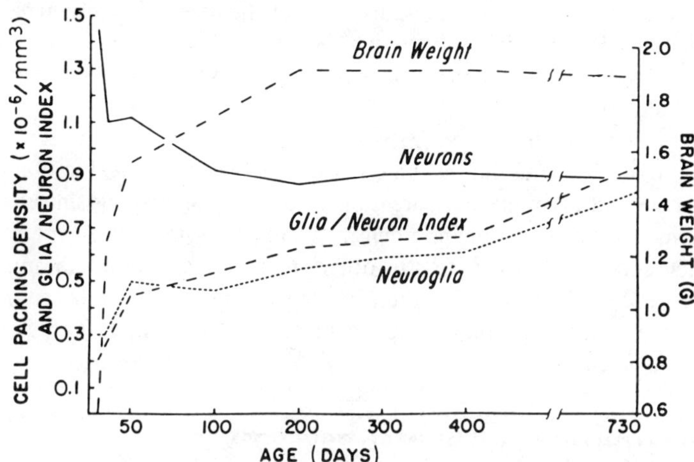

Figure 3 Cell packing densities and glia/neuron index in fixed stained tissues of rat cerebral cortex. (From Brizzee et al., 1964, with kind permission of the authors and publishers.)

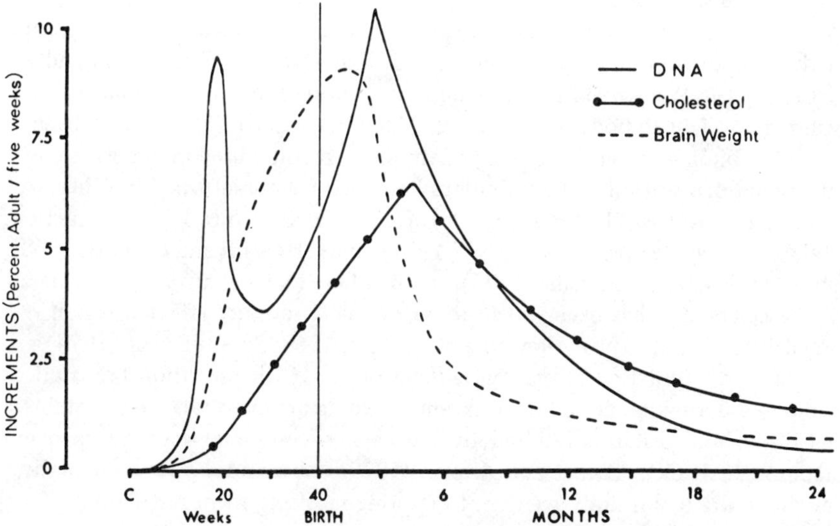

Figure 4 Rate curves for increase in brain weight, DNA, and cholesterol in humans. (From Dobbing and Sands, 1970, with kind permission of the authors and publishers.)

content of the sensory and corticospinal tract of the cerebral hemisphere, but little difference in the motor roots in which myelination is almost complete at this time, or in the frontal association areas, where myelination has barely begun (Dodge et al., 1975).

Increase of dendritic arborization and formation of synaptic contacts occurs at about the same time as the onset of myelination. The duration of synaptogenesis varies in different areas of the brain. For example, in the rat lateral geniculate nucleus synaptic density increases from the fifth postnatal day to the adult level at day 13. In other areas, such as the hippocampus, synaptogenesis extends well after the 20th day (Cragg, 1974). In other areas, synapse formation is apparently dependent on external stimuli (Cragg, 1969; Lund and Lund, 1972).

V. MALNUTRITION AND ANIMAL DEVELOPMENT

A. The Brain

Contemporary investigators have amply corroborated that the brain weight of all species is affected minimally, if at all, when nutritional deprivation begins late in development or after maturity has been attained (Dobbing and Widdowson, 1965; Dickerson and Walmsley, 1967; Platt and Stewart, 1969; Tumbleson et al., 1972). The resistance of the adult brain to nutritional deprivation is evident even when body growth is curtailed severely.

However, nutritional deprivation during pregnancy and the suckling period or throughout both periods severely retards brain growth. Widdowson and McCance (1960) observed that rats underfed during suckling had abnormally high brain weight to body weight ratios. Many investigators have since substantiated the findings of this early study despite the method used in imposing the nutritional deprivation. These findings have also been confirmed in other species, such as pigs (Platt et al., 1964; Dickerson et al., 1966, 1971; Tumbelson et al., 1972), guinea pigs (Chase et al., 1971), mice (Howard and Granoff, 1968), rabbits (Schain and Watanabe, 1973), and monkeys (Kerr et al., 1973). Generally, the cerebellum has been shown to be the most severely affected region (Rajalakshimi et al., 1967; Howard and Granoff, 1968; Sobotka et al., 1974).

Severe retardation of brain growth also occurs if the nutritional restriction is imposed during the period of gestation. Feeding pregnant rats a 6% protein diet throughout gestation resulted, by day 18, in smaller fetal brains (Zeman and Stanbrough, 1969). Barnes and Altman (1973a) observed, however, that the deficits in brain and body weight of offspring resulting from restrictions of maternal food intake during pregnancy were no longer observed 10 days postnatally if they were allowed to suckle from well-nourished mothers. This is not surprising as the brain growth spurt occurs after this period and even a 20% reduction in brain size occurring prior to this time would be obscured by the massive increase in size which later occurs.

The impact of substantial nutritional insult on the cellular development of the brains of adult rats is generally less severe than in young rats. Malnutrition of adult rats had no significant effect on protein and nucleic acid content (Lehr and Gayet, 1963; Mandel and Mark, 1965). Restricting the food intake of rats during weaning caused a reduction in the cell population (DNA) of all organs but did not change their average cell size (protein/DNA). Malnourishing rats by reducing their food intake by 50% between 21 and 42 days of age caused reductions in the cell number, but not the cell size, of most organs, with the exception of the brain and lung. These organs showed reduced cell sizes. Malnutrition imposed after 65 days did not affect the cell number in organs examined except for the spleen and the thymus which continue to divide after this age. A reversal of the effects on cell size but not cell number was obtained when previously deprived rats were refed adequate diets (Winick and Noble, 1966). These data led to the suggestion that the time of most active cell division was the "vulnerable period" during which nutritional insults would lead to permanently reduced cell number and organ size (Dobbing, 1968). Confirmation of these observations has been made in several laboratories (Swaiman et al., 1970; Ahmad and Rahman, 1975). In addition, it has since been shown that severe dietary restriction of pregnant rats also leads to a decrease in the number of brain cells at birth (Winick, 1971). Nutritional deprivation throughout pregnancy and lactation resulted in a 60% reduction in cell number by weaning in contrast to an approximately 15% reduction produced by restricting the diet either during pregnancy or during lactation.

While these general observations have been substantially confirmed, data from Dobbing and Sands (1971) seemed to suggest that the period of DNA accumulation was extended in malnourished rats. In support of this suggestion, Barnes and Altman (1973b) found an increase in cerebellar granule cells between 20 and 30 days in malnourished rats whereas the cerebellum of well-nourished rats showed no increase in cell number during this time. Also, the germinal zone for the cerebral cortex was apparent at 50 days in malnourished rats but disappeared after 20 days in well-nourished animals (Bass et al., 1970a). A more detailed consideration of the effect of undernutrition on cell number and synthesis rate in the developing brain and the possible mechanisms involved in the increased length of the DNA synthesis phase of the cell cycle has been recently given by Balázs et al. (1979).

The brain of newly weaned rats may be more susceptible to a diet deficient in protein rather than in calories. Newly weaned rats fed protein-deficient diets for 8 weeks had severely reduced brain and body weights, while rats fed isocaloric amounts of a protein-adequate diet had brain weights similar to well-fed controls, even though body weights were significantly reduced (Dickerson and Walmsey, 1967).

The suggestion that prenatal malnutrition reduces the number of neurons has been made independently by two groups of investigators utilizing different techniques (Zamenhof et al., 1968; Shrader and Zeman, 1969). In contrast, postnatal malnutrition does not cause a decrease in the number of neurons except in regions like the cerebellum where active neurogenesis is still occurring (Fish and Winick, 1969; Dobbing et al., 1971; Barnes and Altman, 1973a,b). Reduced cell counts in the cerebral cortex of undernourished suckling rats is primarily due to a deficiency of non-neuronal cells (Siassi and Siassi, 1973). However, the density of neurons (i.e., number per microscopic field) may be increased. The density of neuronal cell bodies in the visual and frontal cortical areas was found to be 22-23% higher in rats starved for up to 7 weeks of postnatal life than in well-nourished controls (Cragg, 1972). Although the size of neurons in the lateral vestibular nucleus from the brains of suckling rats, malnourished during the first month after birth, was similar to those from well-nourished control rats, the density of small- and medium-size neurons in that brain region was increased (Johnson and Yoesle, 1975).

More significant perhaps are the effects of early postnatal malnutrition on neuronal events such as dendritic growth and establishment of synaptic connections, which occur during the period of the brain growth spurt (Dobbing and Sands, 1970). Eayrs and Horn (1955) and later Bass (1971) noted that undernutrition in early life resulted in fewer nerve fibers being impregnated by silver. More recent studies have established that early undernutrition of rats reduces the total number of dendritic spines, the density of the basilar dendritic network, and the thickness of the dendritic prolongations of the large pyramidal cells in the frontal and cortical regions (Salas et al, 1974). Escobar (1974) failed to find abnormalities in the dendritic development of large and small pyramidal cells or internucial cells of the cerebral cortex in rats undernourished during the weaning period up to 2 months of age, but found a 20-30% reduction in the number of interneurons in the sixth layer of the cerebral cortex. Similarly, Cragg (1972) noted an absence of abnormalities in synaptic and neuronal structures of rats starved during the first 3-7 weeks of life, but did note that the number of axon terminals associated with one neuron was decreased by 38-41% in the starved rats. In experiments by Gambetti et al. (1974) perinatal malnutrition resulted in a decrease in size and density of presynaptic nerve endings in the somatosensory cortex, although an earlier study had suggested that presynaptic nerve endings were relatively spared (Gambetti et al., 1972). Deficits in the number of synapses per unit area of cerebellum and dentate gyrus of the hippocampus have also been reported (Shoemaker and Bloom, 1977). These results must not yet be taken as unequivocal as other investigations reported similar profiles of synapses in the brains of well and undernourished rats (Burns et al., 1975).

Cravioto et al. (1976) found an increased number of synapses in the brains of perinatally undernourished mice which had been nutritionally rehabilitated from 6 weeks to 6 months of life.

In mature animals, undernutrition affects lipid constituents minimally as the rate of metabolism of most lipids is very slow (Dodge et al., 1975). Rats malnourished after weaning through to adulthood, i.e., during the later stages of myelination, show relatively small deficits in brain lipid content (Dobbing and Widdowson, 1965; Dickerson and Walmsley, 1967) despite severe growth retardation. Similarly, miniature swine, severely malnourished by feeding 4% protein diets between 9 and 41 weeks of age, suffered severe growth retardation, 11% reduction in brain weight, and approximately 10% reduction in the concentration of the lipid fractions examined (Fishman et al., 1972).

In contrast, younger animals malnourished during the period of rapid accumulation of the various myelin constituents are severely affected. Rats undernourished from birth had greatly reduced brain cholesterol concentrations at 12, 21 (Dobbing, 1964), and 35 days of age (Guthrie and Brown, 1968). Phospholipid and proteolipid concentrations were also severely affected by malnutrition imposed from birth to 20 days of age (Culley and Mertz, 1965; Benton et al., 1966). The concentrations of cerebrosides are more severely reduced than any of the other lipids. Of the phospholipids, plasmalogens are most affected (Culley et al., 1966). Regional concentrations of the various lipids are also reduced in the brain of the 20-day-old malnourished rat (Bass et al., 1970b; Ghittoni and Faryna de Raveglia, 1973). Other species, including the pig (Dickerson et al., 1971), the guinea pig (Chase et al., 1971), and the monkey (Kerr and Helmuth, 1973), have been reported to be similarly affected by early malnutrition.

More direct evidence also suggests that myelination is impaired in rats malnourished during the suckling period. In vivo incorporation of [^{35}S] sulfate into sulfatides, specific components of myelin, and the activity of galactocerebroside sulfokinase, the enzyme catalyzing the reaction, was reduced in rats malnourished from birth (Chase et al., 1967). More recently a reduced incorporation of labeled amino acids into myelin protein in the brains of 20-day-old malnourished rats has been observed (Wiggins et al., 1974,1976). Moreover, the total quantity of myelin extracted from the brain of 21- and 53-day-old malnourished rats was respectively 86.5% and 71% less than that recovered from the brain of well-nourished age-matched controls (Fishman et al., 1971; Nakhasi et al., 1975; Wiggins et al., 1976).

Malnutrition appears to exert its major effect by slowing the rate of deposition of the myelin membrane. Consequently, the composition of the myelin membrane is little affected. Fishman et al. (1971) reported that the only qualitative difference in the composition of the myelin membrane of rats undernourished from birth to 53 days of age was a 30% reduction in the content of the plasmalogen phosphatidylethanolamine. Other investigators studying the myelin isolated from the brain of rats have generally supported this observation (Wood, 1973). More recently, however, myelin of malnourished rats was reported to be distorted in its pattern of cerebrosides and sulfatide fatty acids, and to contain 60% less myelin-specific galactolipids (Krigman and Hogan, 1976). Krigman and Hogan (1976) consider these effects to be probably due to a reduction in the number of myelinating glia and to their reduced ability to form myelin. This conclusion is supported by the histological studies of Robain and Ponsot (1978), who found in undernourished animals that glial proliferation was reduced by 50% on the 10th postnatal day in specific tracts of the spinal cord, and that the density of glial cells was 50% that of controls in the corpus callosum at the 19th postnatal day. Such an explanation cannot, however, account for some observations. For example, lipid deficits in the brain of animals malnourished during the suckling period can be reversed to some extent by rehabilitation after weaning, without any increase in glial cell number (Benton et al., 1966; Guthrie and Brown, 1968). In addition, malnutrition imposed after this glial cell population is complete can still affect the process of myelination (Dobbing and Widdowson, 1965; Dickerson and Walmsley, 1967), though not as severely. The recent observation that the specific activity of the myelin constituent 2′,3′-cyclic-nucleotide-3′-phosphohydrolase isolated from the brain of malnourished rats is reduced (Nakhasi et al., 1975) suggests that the effects of myelination may be more subtle than previously recognized.

Interpretation of data arising from studies on the influences of malnutrition on monoaminergic neurotransmitters depends on the manner in which data are expressed (Shoemaker and Bloom, 1977). It is frequently reported that levels of noradrenaline (NA), dopamine (DA), and serotonin (5-HT), expressed as content per brain, are reduced in experimental animals malnourished for varying lengths of time during intrauterine or postnatal life (Sereni et al., 1966; Lee and Dubos, 1972; Shoemaker and Wurtman, 1971, 1973; Sobotka et al., 1974), but concentrations of the neurotransmitters are little altered (Shoemaker and Wurtman, 1971, 1973; Dickerson and Pao, 1975; Ahmad and Rahman, 1975). However, other investigators reported increases in the levels of one or more of the monoamines in the brain of rats subjected to periods of nutritional deprivation (Sobotka et al., 1974; Stern et al., 1975). For example, Stern et al. (1974) found that rats undernourished during the fetal period had higher brain 5-HT and NA concentrations in adulthood than did offspring of control rats fed stock laboratory diet. At weaning, whole-brain content of NA and 5-HT was lower, though in several brain regions concentrations of the amines were elevated (Stern et al., 1975). On the other hand, Ramanamurthy (1977) found that malnutrition during pregnancy had no effect on the concentrations of NA, DA, and 5-HT in utero and up to 7 days of age, but after day 14, the malnourished group had significantly lower levels of all three amines.

Examination of data concerned with other aspects of the metabolism of neurotransmitter amines has not so far allowed a clear picture to emerge with regard to the influence of malnutrition. In general, activities of enzymes involved in the synthesis of monoamines have been reported to be increased in malnourished rats (Shoemaker and Wurtman, 1971, 1973; Nat. Inst. Nutr. Ann. Rep., 1977), except in one instance (Lee and Dubos, 1972), and turnover of catecholamines is decreased (Shoemaker and Wurtman, 1973). However, Tricklebank and Adlard (1974) reported that rats previously malnourished during the fetal or suckling period and then subsequently rehabilitated for 17 weeks had higher turnover rates of 5-HT in the pons medulla, hippocampus, and striatum than did controls. Precise interpretation of these findings within the framework of the vulnerable period hypothesis cannot be made at the present time.

The metabolism of other putative neurotransmitters may also be altered by periods of nutritional deprivation. Acetylcholinesterase was decreased at weaning in rats undernourished prenatally and during suckling (Sereni et al., 1966; Adlard and Dobbing, 1971a). Rehabilitation after weaning resulted in an increased activity of the enzyme (Adlard and Dobbing, 1971b). These observations, however, provide little reliable information on structural alterations in neurons, as the distribution of acetylcholinesterase is not confined to cholinergic nerve terminals (Kasa, 1975; Rossier et al., 1975). Choline acetyltransferase, a more reliable cholinergic marker, is less susceptible to nutritional deprivation than is acetylcholinesterase. The levels of choline acetyltransferase is not altered in malnourished rats or in rats previously malnourished during weaning and then rehabilitated for 4 weeks (Eckhert et al., 1976) or in the cerebral cortex of 24-day-old rats malnourished during the last week of fetal life (Gambetti et al., 1972).

Few studies have focused on effects on other putative neurotransmitters. γ-Aminobutyric acid (GABA) containing neurons are approximately 10,000-fold more numerous in the mammalian brain than any of the catecholamine neurons (Shoemaker and Bloom, 1977) and some work already indicates their vulnerability to undernutrition. For example, the concentrations of glutamate dehydrogenase and glutamate decarboxylase are both reduced in neonatally malnourished rats, although the concentrations are restored to normal after 5 weeks of refeeding (Rajalakashimi et al., 1974). In rats malnourished after the period of weaning, the enzyme activities are affected more by a deficiency of protein than by a deficiency of energy. Feeding low-protein diets to weanling rats resulted in reduced activities of the enzymes whereas feeding restricted amounts of an adequate diet affected enzyme activities only if the rats had been malnourished during suckling (Rajalakshimi et al., 1974). Thus, if the restriction was imposed prior to weaning, some mechanism protecting the neurotransmitter system against nutritional deprivation failed to develop.

The effect of malnourishing rats from birth until weaning on the developmental increases in choline acetyltransferase and glutamate decarboxylase activities in several brain regions was studied recently by Patel et al. (1978). Malnutrition from birth caused a retardation in the normal developmental increases in the activities of the two enzymes in most brain regions (except choline acetyltransferase activity in the cerebellum and glutamate decarboxylase activity in the cerebellum and pons medulla) during the first 2 weeks, but in spite of the continued nutritional deprivation, at weaning the enzyme levels were below control levels only in the hypothalamus and olefactory bulbs. The normal relationship, however, between the regional distribution of the activity of the two enzymes was not established until after rehabilitation for 33 days. Although development of the GABAergic and cholinergic neurotransmitter systems is not irreversibly depressed by early postnatal undernutrition, the retarded development of the two neurotransmitter systems could be important in behavioral development by affecting the chronology of the integrative development of the CNS.

Recent studies have demonstrated that synthesis of neurotransmitters is affected by factors altering the supply of precursor amino acids to the brain (Wurtman and Fernstrom, 1976) and that these alterations may have functional consequences in behavior (Ashley and Anderson, 1975; Anderson, 1977). Change in the brain concentration of amino acids is also important when it is recognized that a number of amino acids and small peptides function as neurotransmitters (Agranoff, 1975; DeFeudis, 1975) and that free amino acids in the brain provide the substrates for synthesis of enzymes and other proteins (Nowark and Munro, 1977) and are probably energy substrates as well (Dodge et al., 1975).

Considerable evidence has accumulated demonstrating that changes in brain amino acids reflect, though not directly, changes in their plasma concentrations (Harper, 1976). Generally, the profile of brain amino acids is less affected in animals malnourished after weaning (Badger and Tumbleson, 1974a,b; Dickerson and Pao, 1975). Even in animals malnourished prior to weaning, feeding of restricted amounts of protein-adequate diets causes fewer significant and parallel changes in the blood and plasma amino acid profiles than does feeding a low-protein diet (Badger and Tumbleson, 1974a,b; Pao and Dickerson, 1975; Kaladhar and Narasinga Rao, 1977).

The effect of deficiencies of protein or energy during pregnancy and the suckling period on amino acid levels in the developing brain has been most systematically investigated in the case of the serotinergic precursor, tryptophan

(Kalyanasundaram, 1976). At birth, tryptophan levels in the brain of pups born to protein- or energy-malnourished rats was several times higher than in pups born to control rats. The level of tryptophan fell progressively after birth so that by the 14th and until the 35th day, tryptophan levels were lower in both the protein- and energy-restricted groups than in the control group. High levels of tryptophan at birth and the progressive decline with age may reflect the immaturity and development of exclusion systems which normally protect the adult brain from severe fluctuation in plasma amino acid concentrations.

Alterations in plasma amino acids may have consequences for the developing brain other than effects on neurotransmitter systems. Experimentally protein synthesis in the brain is affected by administration of large doses of individual amino acids such as phenylalanine (Siegel et al., 1971) and methionine (Wong and Justice, 1972), and deficiencies of leucine, isoleucine, and tryptophan may interfere with the phasing of cell generation time (Balázs et al., 1977).

B. Behavior

1. Learning

An example of the limitations of animal models is nowhere more clearly illustrated than in the attempts to develop models of cognitive development. Many of the early studies, assuming that malnutrition produced brain damage so that learning could not occur (Levitsky, 1975), used stimulus-response (S-R) learning in an effort to investigate the effects of malnutrition on the development of behavior in animals. Deficits in S-R learning were thought to reflect deficits in cognitive development, but this may not necessarily be true. In addition, differences in performance in standard S-R learning tasks which include food reinforcement (Cowley and Griesel, 1959), may not represent differences in learning ability. Levitsky and Barnes (1969) found that the feeding and drinking behavior of rats was affected by earlier periods of malnutrition. These rewards are therefore likely to be inappropriate as they may have different incentive values for groups of malnourished and control animals. In fact, Zimmermann et al. (1976) concede that the superior performance of previously protein-malnourished compared to well-nourished monkeys in learning and memory tasks was probably due to the heightened value of the food reward to the malnourished animals. The conclusion that differences in learning performance may be due to differences in motivation is supported in the experiments of Levitsky and Barnes (1975). These investigators found that when the level of motivation was controlled for, by selecting rats on the basis of rate of bar pressing in a Skinner box during the training period, there were no differences in the ability of malnourished and control rats to learn a visual discrimination problem or a reversal learning problem. The behavioral differences observed were interpreted as a demonstration of increased reactivity of the malnourished animals.

Heightened emotional reactivity has been a consistent finding in malnourished animals. Increased emotionality of rats malnourished during gestation, the suckling and postweaning periods, or postweaning only, has been demonstrated in open-field experiments by decreased horizontal movement with frequent freezing, decreased vertical activity, and increased excretion of urine and feces (Winick and Coombs, 1972; Sobotka et al., 1974). Altered emotionality was also demonstrated in response to aversive stimuli in two ways. Malnourished rats respond to stimuli of lower intensities than normals (Stern et al., 1974; Smart et al., 1975) and give an exaggerated response (Levitsky and Barnes, 1970; Stern et al., 1974). There does not appear to be a direct relationship between emotionality and timing of malnutrition, although there is some evidence for a neurohumoral component in the development of emotionality (Stern et al., 1974; Sobotka et al., 1974). An excessive reaction to stress is likely to interfere with the learning ability of malnourished rats. Reducing the stressfulness of the test situation could improve the learning performance of malnourished rats. By providing a period of familiarization with the test box, thus reducing fear behavior, avoidance learning of previously malnourished rats was equivalent to that of well-nourished controls (Fraňková, 1973). Similarly, Cowley and Griesel (1966) found that performance of malnourished rats in a water maze was improved by raising the temperature of the water, a less stressful situation. Thus it would appear that differences in performance of malnourished and well-nourished animals can be explained by factors other than differences in their capacity to learn.

2. *Behavioral-Environmental Interactions*

Structural changes in the brain induced by perinatal malnutrition are remarkably similar to structural changes in the brain induced by stimulus deprivation in infancy (Rosenzweig, 1966). In addition, many areas of development which are retarded in malnourished animals are enhanced or accelerated in animals reared with increased stimulation. For example, retardation in body growth and development as well as the structural and functional development of the CNS have been reported in malnourished animals while acceleration of somatic growth and enhanced development of motor and sensory functions have resulted in animals reared in enriched environments (Fraňková, 1974). These similarities in brain structure and behavior are shown in Table 3. The many similarities in the behavior of previously malnourished rats and rats reared in experimental isolation suggest that the distortions in the behavior of malnourished animals may be due, at least in part to some kind of stimulus deprivation. It has been proposed that malnutrition may affect the development of an animal by reducing the amount of contact it makes with its environment, i.e., "functionally isolating" the animal (Levitsky and Barnes, 1972). Studies demonstrating that malnourished animals behave in a manner that results in a reduced amount of

Table 3 Some Effects of Early Malnutrition and Stimulation in Animals

Malnutrition	Stimulation
A. Growth and development of tissues and functions	
Marked retardation of growth	Acceleration of growth
Retardation in development of spontaneous motor activity	Enhanced development of motor and sensory functions and their coordination
Delayed appearance of reflexes and maturation of physical features	Earlier eye opening and more rapid development of response to sound
B. Structural and functional development of the CNS	
Lower brain weight, total DNA, RNA, lipid, and protein in brain	Increased brain weight. Increased weight and depth of cortex
Retardation of myelination processes	More rapid myelination
Disturbance in EEG activity	Accelerated development of adult EEG
C. Influence on neurohumoral system	
Smaller pituitaries containing a lower concentration of growth hormone	Earlier maturation of hypothalamo-pituitary system
D. Behavior	
Decreased exploratory behavior	Increased exploratory behavior
Increased emotional reactivity	Lower emotionality, less emotional response to stress situations
E. Resistance to stress and disease	
Disturbance in ability to respond to stress and disease	Better adaptation to different pathogenic agents
	Better survival from starvation and smaller gastrointestinal lesions in conflict situations

Source: Adapted from Fraňková, 1974.

contact with its environment would lend support to this postulate. Functional isolation of the malnourished animal may arise from changes in the behavior of the pup itself or the behavior of the dam toward the malnourished offspring.

Differences in the behavior of malnourished and well-nourished rat pups may be the result of differences in factors such as locomotor development and motivation. Retarded development of spontaneous motor activity has been reported in malnourished rat pups (Smart and Dobbing, 1971a). The appearance of reflexes and maturation of physical features are delayed (Cowley and Griesel,

1966; Simonson et al., 1969; Smart and Dobbing, 1971b). In addition, dispersal of pups throughout the housing area during the first days of life and climbing behavior are delayed in pups born to dams nutritionally deprived during pregnancy (Levitsky et al., 1975) and in pups malnourished from birth (Massaro et al., 1977). Thus, the quantity and the course of the physical contact of the malnourished pup with its environment were altered.

Motivational changes, demonstrated in malnourished monkeys, rats, and pigs, also result in reduced exploration of the animals' environment. Rats malnourished pre- or postweaning have been observed to avoid, or at least not to approach, novel objects in their environment (Levitsky, 1975). This neophobic reaction has been shown also in malnourished monkeys (Zimmermann et al., 1976) and pigs (Levitsky, 1975). Even when malnourished pigs do not show the neophobic reaction, they appear to be indifferent to new objects in their environment (Barnes et al., 1976). Motivational changes are best demonstrated in the studies using protein-malnourished monkeys. Non-food-oriented behaviors of these animals, such as visual curiosity, puzzle solving, and social behavior, are reduced. Malnourished monkeys can solve mechanical puzzles at a level at least equal to that of control animals, but only in the presence of extrinsic motivation. If the reward is manipulation itself (intrinsic motivation) the interest in puzzle-solving activity is uncharacteristically low (Aakre et al., 1973). Zimmermann et al. (1976) reviewed several experiments exploring the motivational and behavioral consequences of protein malnutrition in monkeys. It may be that attentional as well as motivational differences may explain the apparent inability of malnourished rats to profit from information available to them. Levitsky and Barnes (1975), utilizing the latent learning paradigm, demonstrated that rats already malnourished at the time of the original (unrewarded) exposure to a maze performed less well than adequately nourished animals when they were returned to the maze and had to learn to find food.

The behavior of the dam toward the malnourished offspring can also result in functionally isolating the pups from their environment as an altered pattern of interactions between the dam and pup may result in decreased exploration of the environment by the pup. For example, irrespective of the methods used to produce malnourished pups, dams alter their behavior so that they spend an increased amount of time in the nest with their pups (Massaro et al., 1974; Levitsky et al., 1975). This altered pattern of maternal behavior may be stimulated by the pup itself, through changes in their pattern of sucking (Massaro et al., 1974; Galler and Turkewitz, 1977), their retarded physical development (Massaro et al., 1974), or simply by their smaller body size (Wiener et al., 1977). Slob et al.'s (1973) inability to find any differences between previously malnourished and control rats in open-field behavior, tests of motor coordination, and learning when the interactions between dam and pup were experimentally controlled for, implies that maternal behavior is an important factor influencing the functional development of malnourished animals.

Maternal behavior of animals malnourished during pregnancy and lactation has been shown to be altered regardless of the nutritional status of the pups (Smart, 1976). In addition, disturbances in maternal behavior in animals with a familial history of malnutrition remained apparent after two generations of nutritional rehabilitation (Galler and Rosenthal, 1977). These latter studies demonstrate the complexity of the relationship between nutrition and behavioral development, and also the importance of previous nutritional history. Intergenerational malnutrition has been reported to produce greater deficits in physical growth and behavior than postnatal malnutrition alone (Galler, 1979).

3. *Environmental Enrichment*

Observations that malnutrition and environmental enrichment affect similar components of morphological and behavioral development (Table 3) suggest that the effects of malnutrition may be ameliorated by enriching the environment of the malnourished animal. This suggestion gains further support if it is recognized that the functional isolation of the malnourished pup may be the cause of the behavioral deficits in adulthood (Smart, 1974; Whatson et al., 1974). Thus, enriching the environment during the period of nutritional insult would be expected to compensate for the effects of inadequate nutrition.

In animal studies, increased stimulation is often provided by a variety of handling procedures. Handling influences the development of numerous physiological and behavioral functions (Fraňková, 1974; Eckhert et al., 1975). Levitsky and Barnes (1972) studied the effects of handling during the period of early nutritional deprivation on the subsequent behavior of rats. Handling malnourished rats normalized total horizontal locomotor activity, increased their exploratory activity, and decreased their fear responses. Conversely, environmental isolation exacerbated the effects of malnutrition on locomotor activity and other behaviors. The provision of stimulation with a minimum of human contact with the developing malnourished rats, achieved by the introduction of an additional female into the home cage, enhances exploratory behavior (Fraňková, 1974). Pups raised with the "aunt" did as well as normal control animals in behavioral tests.

Evidence reviewed seems to emphasize that the relationship between nutrition and behavior is not a simple one of cause and effect. Of major importance are such nonnutritional variables as environmental conditions. The findings from animal studies have helped to highlight the pertinent issues which need clarification in the study of the effects of malnutrition on the psychological development of human populations.

VI. MALNUTRITION AND HUMAN DEVELOPMENT

A. The Brain

In contrast to the many detailed studies on the development of the CNS in malnourished animals, few investigators have examined the effects of malnutrition on human brain development. Human studies in this area are dependent on the availability of specimens from nonsurvivors, an unpredictable event, and are therefore particularly difficult to control with respect to genetic, nutritional, and environmental influences. As a result, data from these studies must be considered within the framework of the concepts derived from studies with animals.

The general principles derived from animal studies apparently hold for the human brain. Brain weight of infants dying from malnutrition is known to be reduced (Brown, 1965). Attempts to assess brain size in infants suffering from malnutrition have most commonly used head circumference measurements. Although head circumference in healthy children is regarded to be an accurate estimate of brain size, in malnourished infants alterations in brain growth, tissue and fluid content may make these measurements less useful. However, correlations between IQ and head circumference have been made in malnourished children (Stoch and Smythe, 1963,1967) but it is arguable as to whether they reflect the importance of brain size.

Other indices of brain development are also affected by malnutrition. In one study, infants dying during the second year of life from kwashiorkor showed little deficit in DNA but considerable reduction in brain weight/DNA, lipid/DNA, and protein/DNA ratios (Winick et al., 1972). In contrast, infants dying during the first year of life from marasmus had lower brain weights, DNA, RNA, and protein than infants dying from other causes. Cell size was not affected (Winick and Rosso, 1969). Of these infants, three who had particularly low birth weights, perhaps indicative of prenatal malnutrition, had the most severe deficits in all parameters. Thus, it would appear that in humans, as in animals, the severity and nature of the effects of cellular development are related to the time of the nutritional insult.

As well as the effects of malnutrition on whole brain, effects on regional brain development have also been shown. In one study, Chilean and Jamaican infants, severely malnourished and dying during the first year of life, had marked reductions in cell number in the cerebellum, cerebrum, and brainstem (Winick et al., 1970). Chase et al. (1974) did not find a significant reduction in the DNA content of the cerebellum-brainstem and cerebrum-brainstem regions in Guatamalan infants dying of marasmus or marasmic-kwashiorkor in the second year of life. As the children in this study were initially breastfed and most of them had normal birthweights, it can be assumed that the differences between the two studies result from differences in the timing of the malnutrition.

The importance of reduction in the number of brain cells to behavioral development is unknown. It has been suggested that loss of cells in the cerebrum may be more important than loss of cells in other regions (Chase, 1976). Furthermore, loss of neuronal cells may be of greater importance than loss of glial cells.

Although the effect of malnutrition on neuronal and dendritic growth has been little studied in humans, infants dying from malnutrition between 1 and 2 years did not appear to have a deficit in the number of nerve terminals as estimated by total brain gangliosides (Chase et al., 1974). In contrast, deficits in myelin, possibly resulting from failure of glial cell proliferation, have been observed in infants malnourished in early life. As with animals, deficits in total lipids and pronounced reductions in the cerebroside, plasmalogen, and proteolipid fractions (Fishman et al., 1969; Rosso et al., 1970; Chase et al., 1974) and extractable myelin (Fox et al., 1972) have been observed in the brains of infants malnourished during the first 2 years of life. Though the composition of the myelin isolated from these infants' brains was reported to be unchanged, the suggestion from animal studies that the effects on myelin composition may be more subtle than previously recognized remains.

Functional consequences of myelin deficits are unknown, but changes in the myelination of neuronal axons may contribute to altered nerve conductance velocities. In studies of severely malnourished Ethiopian children, reduced motor nerve conduction velocities of the order of half the normal value for age were reported, but these changes cannot be explained solely by deficits in myelination (Engsner, 1974). Electroencephalographic (EEG) investigations have also revealed abnormalities in malnourished children in the acute stage (Coursin, 1974; Montelli et al., 1974) and after recovery. The earliest investigations were largely restricted to the visual inspection of standard resting EEG records, but there has been an increasing use of computers to analyze cortical evoked responses to visual and auditory stimuli. It is still not possible to fully interpret the significance of the EEG changes observed because the field of electrophysiology is still in relatively early development. Also, as standards are derived from American populations, problems of cross-cultural validity arise (Platt and Stewart, 1971). Nevertheless these EEG changes are thought to reflect functional disorders of the CNS and may provide the link between anatomical and biochemical changes and behavior (Coursin, 1975).

The levels of neurotransmitters or amino acids in the brain of malnourished infants have not been measured. However, the levels of these compounds may be altered in malnourished infants as alterations in plasma amino acid levels occur. Human infants with kwashiorkor have depressed levels of most plasma essential amino acids and elevation of the nonessential amino acids (Holt et al., 1963; Endozian, 1966). Moderate forms of malnutrition and marasmus cause similar patterns of change in the plasma amino acid levels but the changes are not as severe (Whitehead, 1964, 1968; Waterlow, 1969). The consequences of some alterations in plasma amino acid levels to brain function are well known in some instances. For example, infants with excessively high blood levels of phenylalanine and branched chain amino and keto acid levels become mentally retarded (Wiltse and Menkes, 1972). In adults neuroendocrine function is sensitive to dihydroxyphenylalanine (DOPA) administered for Parkinson's disease (Mena and Cotzias, 1975). Plasma amino acid pattern in patients with liver cirrhosis may be important in the development of hepatic coma (Munro et al., 1975). Alteration in amino acid supply to the brain limits not only neurotransmitter synthesis but the synthesis of proteins integral to the morphological development of the brain, and may be the factor primarily mediating biochemical and structural effects of malnutrition on the development of the CNS.

B. Behavior

The effects of nutrition on psychological development have been investigated in children with mild-moderate malnutrition or the more severe forms. A rigorous classification and comparison of the human studies is difficult because of the diversity of experimental designs. Some researchers have confined observations to one syndrome while others have included patients with different forms of PEM. In addition, samples of different ages and sexes have been selected on the basis of a variety of criteria (e.g., medical histories or present anthropometry) and assessed at different stages. In general, however, the experimental designs employed in human studies of malnutrition and psychological development fall into four main categories:

1. Cross-sectional.
   a. Comparisons of tall and short children in at-risk populations (e.g., Cravioto et al., 1966; Klein et al., 1972).
   b. Recovered malnourished children compared with children without previous history of clinical malnutrition (e.g., Richardson et al., 1975; Pollitt and Granoff, 1967; Chase and Martin, 1970; Hoorweg and Stanfield, 1976).
2. Follow-up.
   Children studied from admission to hospital, followed for varying lengths of time (e.g., McLaren et al., 1973; Grantham-McGregor et al., 1979).
3. Prospective longitudinal.
   Regular observation of cohort from birth in at-risk community (e.g., Botha-Antoun et al., 1968; Cravioto et al., 1969).
4. Intervention.
   a. Behavioral intervention in hospital (e.g., Yaktin and McLaren, 1970; Cravioto, 1977).

b. Behavioral intervention in hospital plus home visiting after discharge (e.g., Grantham-McGregor et al., unpublished).
c. Nutritional and/or behavioral intervention in at-risk community (e.g., Mora et al., 1979; Irwin et al., 1979; Sinisterra et al., 1979; Chavez and Martinez, 1979).
d. Adoption studies (e.g., Winick, 1979).

Malnourished children have been compared with (usually North American) norms on tests of mental development (e.g., Cravioto and Robles, 1965). This practice is obviously unsatisfactory, so other studies have selected for comparison siblings (Pollitt and Granoff, 1967) or children from similar social backgrounds more or less well matched to the index children (Champakam et al., 1968; Stoch and Smythe, 1976) or both (Richardson et al., 1975). The use of intracommunity comparison groups does not completely eradicate the problems caused by the choice of tests standardized elsewhere (Pollitt and Thompson, 1977), but nevertheless facilitate observations of the psychological development of malnourished children.

In this chapter, severe and mild-moderate malnutrition are discussed separately. More studies have been conducted on children with severe malnutrition than with mild-moderate malnutrition, probably because hospitalization of the former made them more easily accessible for study. The experience of a period of hospitalization in infancy (Stewart and Grantham-McGregor, 1979) may of itself have adverse long-term consequences for psychological development (Douglas, 1975), and this must be considered to be an important difference between the two groups, as the severely malnourished children studied had been hospitalized for periods of up to 1 year.

1. Severe Malnutrition

The effect of severe malnutrition on psychological development is difficult to assess in relation to the critical periods of brain development largely because few prospective studies exist in this area. As a result, the timing of the nutritional insult and the psychological development of the infant prior to hospitalization often cannot be determined with certainty. Attempts to relate age at hospital admission to subsequent development have produced inconsistent results. For example, Cravioto and Robles (1965) found that children admitted to hospital with kwashiorkor before the age of 6 months had a poorer prognosis for development than children admitted after this age. In contrast, Richardson and colleagues (Hertzig et al., 1972) were unable to find a consistent effect of age of admission on children's later performance in tests of psychological development. Other approaches to the study of malnutrition and psychological development have led to modifications in the emphasis placed on relating behavioral deficits to critical periods of brain development.

a. Intellectual Development

IQs, or developmental quotients (DQs) in younger children, have been measured in the acute stage of the illness or after recovery. Gessell DQs of children in hospital recovering from kwashiorkor showed an initial deficit in all spheres of the test when compared with American norms (Cravioto and Robles, 1965). Scores in most areas improved as hospitalization progressed, but large deficits remained in children admitted before 6 months of age. An increase in DQs has also been reported in children in hospital recovering from marasmus and marasmic-kwashiorkor (Yaktin and McLaren, 1970; Grantham-McGregor et al., 1978). However, as children hospitalized for nonnutritional reasons also show increases in scores (Grantham-McGregor et al., 1978), improvement of scores must be attributed to factors other than changing nutritional status, such as changes in behavior during test sessions (Grantham-McGregor et al., 1979). The severely malnourished children failed to reach the mean IQ level of the well-nourished children and were significantly behind at discharge from hospital and 1 month later.

Previously severely malnourished children have also shown IQ deficits when compared with other children in the same community or siblings in studies in many countries including Jamaica (Hertzig et al., 1972), Yugoslavia (Cabak and Najdanvic, 1965), USA (Chase and Martin, 1970), Peru (Pollitt and Granoff, 1967), and Uganda (Hoorweg and Stanfield, 1976). In one study (Hertzig et al., 1972), the mean IQ of school age boys who had been treated for severe malnutrition before the age of 2 was significantly lower than the mean IQs of classmates and siblings. In these children, IQ depression was significantly correlated with the severity of malnutrition as indicated by the degree of growth stunting at time of hospitalization (Richardson, 1979). Pollitt (1973), reviewing eight studies of severely malnourished children, concluded that in marasmus, when malnutrition resulted in severe retardation of weight gain (e.g., 50% weight deficit plus stunting) behavioral deficits were as much as 50% below norms even when compared with equivalent social groups. Children with kwashiorkor tended to show less behavioral retardation than children with marasmus. However, the apparent differences in the effects of kwashiorkor and marasmus may reflect the differences between the children in age at admission to hospital or may be due to differences in the natural histories of the two syndromes. Waterlow and Rutishauser (1974) hypothesize that maramus may be the result of more chronic undernutrition than kwashiorkor (see Fig. 5). If this is the case, then differences in long-term behavioral sequelae could be a reflection of the chronicity of the nutritional deprivation.

In addition to lowered IQ levels, specific deficits in intellectual performance have been reported in survivors of severe PEM. For example, Champakam et al. (1968) found deficits in memory, abstract thinking, and verbal and perceptual ability in Indian children previously treated for kwashiorkor. Previously

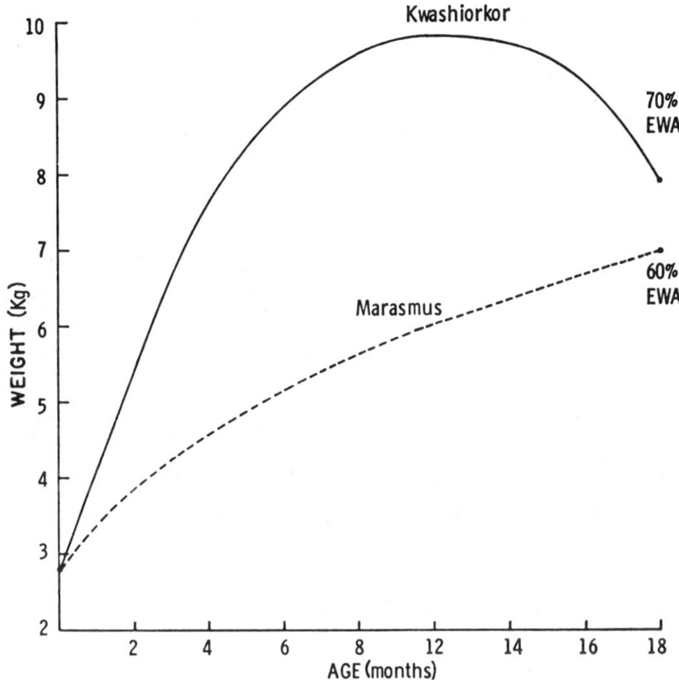

Figure 5 Hypothetical pattern of weight gain, showing the natural histories of kwashiorkor and marasmus. EWA = expected weight for age, Boston standards; 100% EWA ≅ 10.9 kg at 18 months of age. (From Waterlow and Rutishauer, 1974, with kind permission of the authors and publisher.)

severely malnourished children also obtained significantly lower scores on sorting tasks than comparison children (Brockman and Ricciuti, 1971) while others were deficient in intersensory integration when compared with siblings (Cravioto and Delicardie, 1975).

It would seem that severe malnutrition in infancy does affect intellectual development, affecting specific cognitive skills and causing some degree of mental retardation, depending on the severity of the nutritional insult. However, the matter is not that simple. As with animals, there is evidence suggesting that apparent differences in performance may not truly reflect differences in ability. Klein and colleagues (1973) reported that what was initially thought to be a memory deficit in survivors of PEM could also be interpreted as the result of attentional and motivational differences between these children and the comparison group. Children recovered from kwashiorkor did significantly worse than comparison children on a test of intersensory integration (Witkop et al.,

1970), but in addition, response speed was related to number of errors that a child made in the task. Some of the differences between malnourished and well-nourished children on cognitive tasks need to be demonstrated independently of individual differences in response style which may be important predictors of performance on difficult tasks (Klein et al., 1973).

b. Behavioral-Environmental Interactions

Even accepting that impairment of intellectual function has been found in survivors of severe PEM, the task remains to disentangle nutrition from the many environmental influences on the development of these children. The deprived environments in which severely malnourished children live may themselves be sufficient to produce the deficits demonstrated. Alcoholism, marital instability, unemployment, large families, and inadequate finances are common in the family life of recovered malnourished children (Stoch and Smythe, 1963, 1967; Chase and Martin, 1970). Mothers of severely malnourished children assessed at follow-up have been found to have fewer human and material resources and in general to be less capable than mothers of adequately nourished children (Richardson, 1974). Cravioto's prospective study in Mexico offered the unique opportunity of comparing the homes of a cohort of children before some of them became severely malnourished (Cravioto and DeLicardie, 1976). When compared with adequately nourished children matched for birth size and gestational age, children who became severely malnourished had significantly lower scores on the Caldwell Home Inventory* before the diagnosis of severe malnutrition and continued to do so after recovery. The behavioral responses of the mothers of severely malnourished children were also observed to be significantly different from the responses of the other mothers from soon after birth (Cravioto and DeLicardie, 1976). In this cohort of children, examination of microenvironmental factors allowed the identification of families having a child at high risk of developing severe malnutrition. Therefore, the microenvironments of the severely malnourished children could be a sufficient cause of any mental retardation that they may demonstrate. Richardson's (1974) data on school age children suggested than an episode of severe malnutrition in infancy in the context of a lifetime of generally favorable experiences for child development does not appear to cause any intellectual impairment, but when severe malnutrition occurs in an ecology generally unfavorable for intellectual development, the early malnutrition has a clear relation to later intellectual impairment (Hertzig et al., 1972).

A current Jamaican study presents a somewhat different picture. Severely malnourished children had a mean DQ significantly lower than well-nourished

*The Bettye Caldwell Home Observation for Measurement of the Environment Inventory assesses the stimulation available to children in the home through a questionnaire to the caretaker and observation of the adult and child at home (Caldwell et al., 1966).

comparison children 1 month after discharge from hospital (Grantham-McGregor et al., 1979). In contrast to Cravioto's sample, however, these two groups had very similar (low) scores on the Home Inventory, although they differed on other social background variables. Preliminary analysis of the data reveals that, at this stage, nutritional status made the largest independent contribution to the variance in DQ, unlike Richardson's findings with older children that social background factors made the largest independent contribution to IQ variance (Richardson, 1976). Further analysis of Grantham-McGregor's data may clarify the apparent contradiction in these two studies. However, as these relationships were investigated in children of different ages, the differences in these data may merely represent different patterns in the influence of nutritional and non-nutritional variables at different stages in a child's life (Ramos-Galvan et al., 1968). Moreover, little informaton is available on the nutritional history of Richardson's comparison groups. The contradiction may also be explained by the fact that developmental assessment and IQ tests are derived from different theoretical concepts of the nature and organization of mental abilities (Butcher, 1968; Pollitt and Thompson, 1977), with DQs being poor predictors of IQ (McCall et al., 1973).

It may be, however, that the state of severe malnutrition has a major effect on early developmental levels because it reduces the ability of the individual to benefit from the limited opportunities in his impoverished environment. Animal studies have supported the hypothesis of the functional isolation of the malnourished individual. Data from human studies also support this hypothesis. Severely malnourished children have been described as apathetic and unresponsive (Geber and Dean, 1956; Barrera-Moncada, 1963). The absence of changes in heart rate of moderately and severely malnourished infants in response to novel auditory stimuli that elicited this response in well-nourished children is taken as evidence of attentional deficits in the former group (Lester et al., 1975; Lester, 1975, 1976). Moreover, when observed in hospital, severely malnourished children and well-nourished comparisons were found to have different patterns of behavioral responses when alone in their cribs and when presented with a standard set of toys (Stewart et al., 1978). There have also been many anecdotal reports of reduced exploratory behavior in severe malnutrition, but most observational studies have been carried out with moderately malnourished children. In general, however, we have a picture of a severely malnourished infant who is apathetic, depressed, irritable, and lacking in responsiveness to persons and objects (Richardson et al., 1975).

The active role of the child in the evolution of intellectual competence is a recurring principle in genetic psychology. Piaget (1953) stressed the dynamic relationship between the child and his or her environment. Any period of reduced exploration of the environment can therefore be expected to affect the intellectual development of a child. When this period coincides with a stage of rapid development the effects can be expected to be particularly marked, although subsequent events may be able to compensate for early experience (Clarke and Clarke, 1976). The malnourished child's altered behavioral responsiveness in itself, which could be due to CNS dysfunction, but could also be an adaptation to reduced energy intake or to metabolic factors, could possibly explain any mental retardation demonstrated.

The possible ameliorative effects of subsequent environments on the development of children after recovery from severe PEM would be greatly influenced by any persistent abnormalities in the behavior of these children. The social behavior of children of school age has been largely ignored in studies of severe malnutrition, but this was investigated in the study of Jamaican boys (Richardson et al., 1972; Richardson et al., 1975). When assessed on average 6 years after treatment, there were differences in social behavior between these boys and peers who had not experienced an acute episode of PEM. Selecting behaviors which have been emphasized in clinical reports of children thought to have minimal brain dysfunction and those thought to be a result of unfavorable social environments, Richardson and colleagues obtained assessments of the children at home and at school. The index boys were more often described by their parent or guardian as withdrawn, solitary, or unsociable. They more often behaved immaturely, were more clumsy and were either more highly active or lethargic. They were also less liked by siblings. At school, they differed from classmates both in behaviors related to classwork (poor attention and memory, more distractible, contributing less to class discussion) and in social functioning (less popular with peers, less cooperative with teachers, more behavior and conduct problems). Although identification of the causes of the aberrant pattern of social behavior in the survivors of PEM was not possible in this study, it is evident that this behavior would put them at a disadvantage both at home and in the characteristically crowded classrooms of Jamaican primary schools and could have contributed to the significantly lower achievement levels of the previously malnourished schoolboys (Richardson et al., 1973).

The development of children may be influenced not only by nutritional and environmental factors operating within their own lifetimes, but also by the influence of these factors on the development of their parents or even previous generations of the family. For example, a variety of data support a logical chain of consequences starting from malnutrition of the mother when she was a child, to her growth stunting, to her reduced efficiency as a reproducer, to intrauterine and perinatal risk to the child, and to his subsequent retarded development (Birch and Gussow, 1970; Birch, 1972). Moreover, animal models suggest that the effects of several generations of malnutrition may be particularly difficult to reverse (Galler, 1979). The effects of intergenerational malnutrition are difficult to assess in human studies, largely because of the unavailability of relevant information. Nevertheless, intergenerational malnutrition must be recognized as a feature of deprived populations. In the context of a familial history of undernutrition, a child experiencing an acute episode of severe malnutrition may therefore be particularly vulnerable.

c. Environmental Enrichment

Animal studies have shown that increased stimulation can ameliorate some of the effects of malnutrition (Levitsky and Barnes, 1972; Fraňková, 1974). Although stimulation of the animals was often contemporaneous with the nutritional deprivation, it has been hypothesized that extra stimulation from enriched environments combined with nutritional rehabilitation could aid the psychological development of severely malnourished children. Yaktin and McLaren (1970) introduced a program of stimulation for one of two groups of severely malnourished Arab children, which included improved play facilities, increased visual and auditory stimulation, and more social contact between children and nursing staff. The stimulated group showed significantly greater improvement when assessed on the Griffiths Mental Development Scales during recovery in hospital than the unstimulated group, although both groups failed to achieve normal quotients by discharge from hospital. Cravioto (1977) also reports improvements in behavioral recovery resulting from systematic stimulation in hospital.

Differences in the mean DQs of the stimulated and unstimulated groups of Arab children had disappeared 1 year after discharge home (Yaktin et al., 1971) and approximately 3 years afterward both groups had IQs significantly lower than the IQs of a comparison group of adequately nourished children (McLaren et al., 1973). It may be that the program of stimulation was not sufficiently structured or lengthy to bring about long-term IQ gains. American intervention studies have shown the necessity for the involvement of the children's families if IQ gains are to be sustained (Bronfenbrenner, 1974), and it does not appear that families were included in this study. There is some evidence of the cumulative effect of a structured program of behavioral intervention, started in hospital and continued at home after discharge, on the development of a group of severely malnourished children (Grantham-McGregor and Steward, unpublished data). Long-term behavioral intervention programs are also being carried out with moderately malnourished children (Sinisterra et al., 1979).

The effects of adoption, a more radical and permanent kind of environmental change, have also been investigated (Winick et al., 1973; Nguyen et al., 1977; Winick, 1979). IQ levels of Korean children of school age who were either moderately or severely malnourished or well nourished in infancy, adopted into the "enriched environments" of American families, were related to their nutritional history. Age at adoption was an important influence on the magnitude of the differences between the groups. Children adopted before 2 years of age achieved normal IQs. The mean IQs were 102 for previously severely malnourished children, 106 for previously moderately malnourished children, and 116 for well-nourished children. In children adopted after 2, the mean IQs were 95, 101, and 105, respectively. It is not possible from this retrospective study to determine the relative roles of nutrition, duration of malnutrition, and age at adoption, but these data viewed with the results of the behavioral intervention programs support the suggestion that a lifetime of favorable experiences may nullify the effect of severe malnutrition in infancy.

2. *Mild-Moderate Malnutrition*

The estimated prevalence of moderate PEM in Third World countries is greater than for severe malnutrition (see Table 2). Effects of chronic undernutrition on the development of children could therefore be of even greater importance for human populations than the effects of the less prevalent severe forms of malnutrition. Through the observation of groups of mild-moderately malnourished children and their well-nourished peers, and the use of multivariate statistical analysis, further attempts have been made to investigate the relationship between nutritional and nonnutritional variables and child development.

a. Intellectual Development

A history of mild-moderate malnutrition has been inferred from reduced anthropometric measurements in children in cross-sectional studies of socially disadvantaged communities. The validity of such inferences may be questioned (Birch, 1972; Habicht et al., 1974), but significant correlations between physical growth and IQ have been interpreted, at least in part, as evidence of the effects of nutrition on intellectual development (Klein et al., 1972; Mora et al., 1974). Low associations were found between mild-moderate malnutrition and mental and motor development in one study of Guatemalan infants (Klein et al., 1974). On the other hand, Graves (1972) found no systematic relationships between nutritional status and intellectual development in Nepalese children of similar ages. In another study, differences in weight were accompanied by differences in neurointegrative competence in rural Guatemalan children up to the age of 11 (Cravioto et al., 1966). Although the absence of this relationship in well-nourished urban schoolchildren has been interpreted as strengthening the case for the causal role of malnutrition, the possible effects of social differences between the children on neurointegrative performance have not been eliminated.

b. Behavioral-Environmental Interaction

In studies of mild-moderate malnutrition, as in severe malnutrition, differences in microenvironmental characteristics may exist between groups of undernourished children and their well-nourished peers which could account for any developmental differences between the groups. In Columbia, when children up to the age of 66 months were classified as well nourished or moderately malnourished on the basis of anthropometry, well-nourished children obtained higher DQs than malnourished children (Mora et al., 1974), but in the families of malnourished children, more people were sharing less living space, less food, and fewer material goods in comparison with families of well-nourished children in the same neighborhood. Malnourished children were also at a disadvantage in the nature of the attention that they received from their mothers, in their pre- and postnatal medical history and current health status. A significant percentage of DQ variance could be attributed to differences in nutritional status as measured by height and weight even when all the variance explained by the recorded health and social factors was accounted for. As a result, these investigators concluded that the effect of malnutrition on cognitive functioning was significant and can be isolated from effects of social and health factors, while conceding that if other health and social parameters had been measured the results could have been different.

Klein and colleagues (1979) claim that their data on nutritionally supplemented and unsupplemented children suggest more strongly than have those of any previous studies that effects of moderate malnutrition on mental development are causal. When the possible effects of the quality of the home environment were controlled for, there was an association between the amount of supplementation given to mother and child and mental test performance. There was, in addition, an interaction between supplementation and home environment, supplementation having a greater effect where the home environment was most deprived.

As with severe malnutrition, studies of moderately malnourished children have provided data in support of the functional isolation hypothesis. In cross-sectional studies in India and Nepal, Graves (1976, 1978) reported lowered levels of exploratory and play activity in malnourished children when compared with adequately nourished children. There was also more passive physical contact between mothers and children.

Prospective longitudinal investigations of nutritionally supplemented and unsupplemented children in communities where malnutrition is endemic also reveal clear differences in behavior which follow a pattern of decreased interaction with the environment by the undernourished children. These differences are clearly illustrated in a study in rural Mexico (Chavez and Martinez, 1975; Chavez et al., 1975; Chavez and Martinez, 1979). Nutritional supplementation of half of a group of 34 mothers from the sixth week of pregnancy and during lactation and their offspring from 3 months of age resulted in significant differences in anthropometry as well as behavior between the two groups of children. Levels of interaction with people and objects were considerably reduced in malnourished children and this appeared to operate in two ways. First, the malnourished children showed less active exploration of the environment. From

24 weeks of age they were significantly less active and by 18 months the supplemented children were moving six times more than the unsupplemented children. At 56 months, the supplemented children were more talkative, cried less, and were more aggressive and independent. The malnourished children were described as apathetic, withdrawn, passive, timid, and dependent. Second, the malnourished children, apparently by being less demanding than well-nourished children, did not elicit certain kinds of adult attention. Supplemented children were spoken to more often, were cleaned and bathed more often, and received their fathers' attention in a way that was not observed in unsupplemented children.

On the Gesell Scales there were consistent differences in favor of the supplemented children from 2 months of age. The unsupplemented children were described as being limited in cognitive and expressive capacity.

c. Environmental Enrichment

Some studies combined psychoeducational programs with nutritional supplementation. In one such study in Bogota, data are now available on Griffiths Developmental Assessments at 4, 6, and 12 months (Mora et al., 1979). At this stage, it appears that the two types of intervention affected different areas of development. Nutritional supplementation had a significant effect on the locomotor and performance subscales of the test while the effect of behavioral intervention was only significant in language. In another Colombian study, behavioral intervention and/or nutritional supplementation and health care were introduced 9, 18, 27, or 36 months before school entry for seven groups of children (McKay et al., 1974). There were significant gains in cognitive ability in response to intervention, and the magnitude of the gains was positively related to treatment duration. Significant differences between treated and untreated groups were present 2 years after school entry, but all groups fell well below an upper-class comparison group (Sinisterra et al., 1979).

Analysis of data from these important longitudinal studies continues, but reports to date support the view that moderately malnourished children, like severely malnourished children, behave in ways that may themselves be sufficient to cause developmental retardation. Moreover, nutritional and behavioral intervention may to some degree prevent such retardation. These studies, prospective in design, with large numbers of children and combining several of the elements of animal models and human studies with severe malnutrition, offer the opportunity to further disentangle the many factors in this important area of human development.

VII. OTHER NUTRITIONAL INFLUENCES ON BRAIN STRUCTURE AND BEHAVIOR

The emphasis of this chapter has been given to describing the influence of dietary restriction of protein and energy on the structural development of the brain and behavior. However, it must be recognized that deficiencies or excesses of other individual nutrients may also be important in affecting the development of the brain. With regard to the protein-energy-malnourished infant, some nutrients may be more important than others. For example, infants with PEM often have associated deficiencies of vitamin A due to a failure of transport mechanisms in the gut (McLaren, 1970). Deficiencies of vitamins A, E, thiamine, riboflavin, niacin, B_{12}, pyridoxine, and folic acid have been associated with effects on the developing nervous system. Similarly, deficiencies of essential fatty acids may affect the composition of the myelin membrane and impair learning and motor abilities of developing mice (Gozzo and D'Udine, 1977). Dodge et al. (1975) documented in some detail the effects of vitamin deficiencies and excesses on the central nervous system. As well, the authors have considered the effects of minerals and other essential nutrients on the development of the central nervous system.

VIII. CONCLUSIONS

There is undoubtedly compelling evidence that malnourished children are developmentally disadvantaged when compared with their well-nourished peers. However, although both animal and human studies have demonstrated distortion and deficits in brain structure as a consequence of malnutrition and both groups have some aberrant patterns of behavior, factors such as motivation and environmental stimulation have also been shown to influence development. Because of the complexity of the ecology of malnutrition and the inadequacy of some experimental models, it is not yet possible to draw definite conclusions on the relative importance of nutritional and nonnutritional factors in psychological development. It must be recognized, however, that any attempts to understand and find solutions in this area must include consideration of the encompassing conditions of political disadvantage and social deprivation.

REFERENCES

Aakre, B., Strobel, D. A., Zimmermann, R. R., and Geist, C. R. (1973). Reactions to intrinsic and extrinsic rewards in protein-malnourished monkeys. *Percept. Mot. Skills 36*, 787-790.

Adlard, B. P. F., and Dobbing, J. (1971a). Vulnerability of developing brain. III. Development of four enzymes in the brains of normal and undernourished rats. *Brain Res. 28*, 97-107.

Adlard, B. P. F., and Dobbing, J. (1971b). Elevated cholinesterase activity in adult rat brain after undernutrition in early life. *Brain Res. 30*, 198-199.

Agranoff, B. (1975). Neurotransmitters and synaptic transmission. *Fed. Proc. 34*, 1911-1913.

Ahmad, G., and Rahman, M. A. (1975). Effect of undernutrition and protein malnutrition on brain chemistry of rats. *J. Nutr. 105,* 1090-1103.

Alleyne, G. A. O., Hay, R. W., Picou, D., Stanfield, J. P., and Whitehead, R. G. (1977). *Protein-Energy Malnutrition.* Edward Arnold, London.

Altman, J. (1966a). Autoradiographic and histological studies of postnatal neurogenesis. II. A longitudinal investigation on the kinetics, migration and transformation of cells incorporating thymidine in infant rats, with special reference to postnatal neurogenesis of some brain regions. *J. Comp. Neurol. 128,* 431-473.

Altman, J. (1966b). Proliferation and migration of undifferentiated precursor cells in the rats during postnatal gliogenesis. *Exp. Neurol. 16,* 263-278.

Altman, J. (1972a). Postnatal development of the cerebellar cortex in the rat. II. Phases in the maturation of Purkinje cells and of the molecular layer. *J. Comp. Neurol. 145,* 399-463.

Altman, J. (1972b). Postnatal development of the cerebellar cortex in the rat. III. Maturation of the components of the granular layer. *J. Comp. Neurol. 145,* 465-513.

Altman, J., and Das, G. D. (1966). Autoradiographic and histological studies of postnatal neurogenesis. I. A longitudinal investigation of the kinetics, migration and transformation of cells incorporating tritiated thymidine in neonate rats, with special reference to postnatal neurogenesis in some brain regions. *J. Comp. Neurol. 126,* 337-389.

Anderson, G. H. (1977). Regulation of protein intake by plasma amino acids. *Adv. Nutr. Res. 1,* 145-166.

Anthony, L. E., and Endozian, J. C. (1975). Experimental protein and energy deficiencies in the rat. *J. Nutr. 105,* 631-648.

Ashley, D. V. M., and Anderson, G. H. (1975). Correlation between the plasma tryptophan to neutral amino acid ratio and protein intake in the self-selecting weanling rat. *J. Nutr. 105,* 1412-1421.

Ashworth, A. (1978). Progress in the treatment of protein-energy malnutrition. *Proc. Nutr. Soc. 38,* 89-97.

Badger, T. M., and Tumbleson, M. E. (1974a). Protein-calorie malnutrition in young miniature swine. Serum free amino acids. *J. Nutr. 104,* 1339-1347.

Badger, T. M., and Tumbelson, M. E. (1974b). Protein-calorie malnutrition in young miniature swine. Brain free amino acids. *J. Nutr. 104,* 1329-1338.

Balázs, R., and Richter, D. (1973). Effects of hormones on the biochemical maturation of the brain. In *Biochemistry of the Developing Brain,* W. Himwich (Ed.). Dekker, New York, pp. 255-299.

Balázs, R., Patel, A. J., and Lewis, P. D. (1977). Metabolic influences on cell proliferation in the brain. In *Biochemical Correlates of Brain Structure and Function,* A. N. Davison (Ed.). Academic, London, pp. 43-83.

Balázs, R., Lewis, P. D., and Patel, A. J. (1979). Nutritional deficiencies and brain development. In *Human Growth: A Comprehensive Treatise,* Vol. 3. F. Falkner and J. M. Tanner (Eds.). Plenum, New York, pp. 415-480.

Barnes, D., and Altman, J. (1973a). Effects of different schedules of early undernutrition on the preweanling growth of the rat cerebellum. *Exp. Neurol. 38,* 406-419.

Barnes, D., and Altman, J. (1973b). Effects of two levels of gestational-lactational undernutrition on postweaning growth of the rat cerebellum. *Exp. Neurol. 38,* 420-428.

Barnes, R. H., Levitsky, D. A., Pond, W. G., and Moore, V. (1976). Effect of postnatal dietary protein and energy restriction on exploratory behaviour in young pigs. *Dev. Psychobiol. 9,* 425-435.

Barrera-Moncada, G. (1963). *Estudios Sobre Alteraciones del Crecimiento y del Desarrollo Psicológico del Sindrome Pluricarencial (Kwashiorkor.* Editora Grafos, Venezuela.

Bass, N. H. (1971). Influence of neonatal malnutrition on the development of rat cerebral cortex. A microchemical study. *Adv. Exp. Med. Biol. 13,* 413-429.

Bass, N. H., Netsky, M. D., and Young, E. (1970a). Effect of neonatal malnutrition on developing cerebrum. I. Microchemical and histological study of cellular differentiation in the rat. *Arch. Neurol. 23,* 289-302.

Bass, N. H., Netsky, M. G., and Young, E. (1970b). Effect of neonatal malnutrition on developing cerebrum. II. Microchemical and histologic study of myelin formation in the rat. *Arch. Neurol. 23,* 303-313.

Bengoa, J. M. (1974). The problem of malnutrition. *W.H.O. Chron. 28,* 3-7.

Bengoa, J. M. (1976). Nutritional rehabilitation. In *Nutrition in Preventive Medicine,* G. H. Beaton and J. M. Bengoa (Eds.). WHO Monograph Series No. 62, Geneva, pp. 321-334.

Benton, J. W., Moser, H. W., Dodge, P. R., and Carr, S. (1966). Modification of the schedule of myelination by early nutritional deprivation. *Pediatrics 38,* 801-807.

Berry, J. W., and Dasen, P. (Eds.) (1974). *Culture and Cognition: Readings in Cross-Cultural Psychology.* Methuen, London.

Birch, H. G. (1972). Issues of design and method in studying the effects of malnutrition on mental development. In *Nutrition, the Nervous System and Behaviour.* Scientific Publication No. 251, PAHO, pp. 115-128.

Birch, H., and Gussow, J. D. (1970). *Disadvantaged Children. Health, Nutrition and School Failure.* Harcourt, Brace and World, New York.

Block, N., and Dworkin, G. (Eds.) (1977). *The IQ Controversy,* Quartet, London.

Botha-Antoun, E., Babayan, S., and Harfouche, J. K. (1968). Intellectual development related to nutritional status. *J. Trop. Ped. 14,* 112-115.

Brizzee, K. R., Vogt, J., and Kharetchko, X. (1964). Postnatal changes in glia/neuron index with a comparison of methods of cell enumeration in the white rat. *Progr. Brain Res. 4,* 136-149.

Brockman, L. M., and Ricciuti, H. N. (1971). Severe protein-calorie malnutrition and cognitive development in infancy and early childhood. *Dev. Psychology 4,* 312-319.

Bronfenbrenner, U. (1974). *A Report on Longitudinal Evaluations of Pre-School Programs.* Vol. 2. *Is Early Intervention Effective?* DHEW Publication No. (NIH) 74-25, Washington, D.C.

Brown, R. E. (1965). Decreased brain weight in malnutrition and its implications. *East Afr. Med. J. 42,* 584-595.

Burns, E. M., Richards, J. G., and Kuhn, H. (1975). An ultrastructural investigation of the effects of perinatal malnutrition on E-PTA stained synaptic junctions. *Experientia 32,* 1451-1453.

Butcher, H. (1968). *Human Intelligence: Its Nature and Assessment.* Methuen, London.

Cabak, V., and Najdanvic, R. (1965). Effect of undernutrition in early life on physical and mental development. *Arch. Dis. Child. 40,* 532-534.

Caldwell, B., Heider, J., and Kaplan, B. (1966). The inventory of home stimulation. Paper presented at the meeting of the Am. Psychological Assoc., New York.

Champakam, S., Srikantia, S. G., and Gopalan, G. (1968). Kwashiorkor and mental development. *Am. J. Clin. Nutr. 21,* 844-852.

Chase, H. P. (1976). Undernutrition and growth and development of the human brain. In *Malnutrition and Intellectual Development,* J. D. Lloyd-Still (Ed.). MTP Press, Lancaster, England, pp. 13-38.

Chase, H. P., and Martin, H. P. (1970). Undernutrition and childhood development. *N. Engl. J. Med. 282,* 933-939.

Chase, H. P., Corsey, J., and McKhann, G. M. (1967). The effect of malnutrition on the synthesis of a myelin lipid. *Pediatrics 46,* 551-559.

Chase, H. P., Dabiere, C. S., Welch, N. N., and O'Brien, D. (1971). Intrauterine undernutrition and brain development. *Pediatrics 47,* 491-500.

Chase, H. P., Canosa, C. A., Dabiere, C. S., Welch, N. N., and O'Brien, D. (1974). Postnatal undernutrition and human brain development. *J. Ment. Def. Res. 18,* 355-366.

Chavez, A., and Martinez, C. (1975). Nutrition and development of children from poor rural areas. V. Nutrition and behavioral development. *Nutr. Rep. Int. 11,* 477-489.

Chavez, A., and Martinez, C. (1979). Effects of nutrition on child behaviour. In *Proceedings of International Conference on Behavioural Effects of Energy and Protein Deficits,* J. Brožek (Ed.). DHEW Publication No. (NIH) 79-1906. Washington, D.C., pp. 216-228.

Chavez, A., Martinez, C., and Yaschine, T. (1975). Nutrition, behavioural development, and mother-child interaction in young rural children. *Fed. Proc. 34,* 1574-1582.

Clarke, A. M., and Clarke, A. D. B. (1976). The formative years? In *Early Experience: Myth and Evidence,* A. M. Clarke and A. D. B. Clarke (Eds.). Open Books, London, pp. 3-24.

Coursin, D. B. (1974). Electrophysiological studies in malnutrition. In *Early Malnutrition and Mental Development,* J. Cravioto, L. Hambraeus, and B. Vahlquist (Eds.). Symposia of the Swedish Nutrition Foundation. XII. Uppsala, Almquist and Wiksell: Stockholm, pp. 72-84.

Coursin, D. B. (1975). Malnutrition, brain development and behavior: anatomical, biochemical and electrophysiologic constructs. In *Growth and Development of the Brain, Nutritional, Genetic and Environmental Factors,* M. Brazier (Ed.). IBRO Monograph Series, Vol. 1. Raven, New York, pp. 289-305.

Coward, D. G., and Whitehead, R. G. (1972). Experimental protein-energy malnutrition in baby baboons: Attempts to reproduce the pathological features of kwashiorkor as seen in Uganda. *Br. J. Nutr. 28,* 223-237.

Cowley, J. J., and Griesel, R. D. (1959). Some effects of a low protein diet on a first filial generation of white rats. *J. Gen. Psychol. 95,* 187-201.

Cowley, J. J., and Griesel, R. D. (1966). The effect on growth and behavior of rehabilitating first and second generation low-protein rats. *Anim. Behav. 14,* 506-517.

Cragg, B. G. (1969). The effects of vision and dark-rearing on the size and density of synapses in the lateral geniculate nucleus measured by electron microscopy. *Brain Res. 13,* 53-67.

Cragg, B. G. (1972). The development of cortical synapses during starvation in the rat. *Brain 95,* 143-150.

Cragg, B. G. (1974). Plasticity of synapses. *Br. Med. Bull. 30,* 141-144.

Cravioto, J. (1977). Not by bread alone. Effects of early malnutrition and stimuli deprivation on mental development. In *Perspectives in Pediatrics,* O. P. Ghai (Ed.). Interprint, New Delhi, pp. 87-104.

Cravioto, J., and Delicardie, E. R. (1975). Neurointegrative development and intelligence in children rehabilitated from severe malnutrition. In *Brain Function and Malnutrition: Neuropsychological Methods of Assessment,* J. W. Prescott, M. S. Read, and D. B. Coursin (Eds.). Wiley, New York, pp. 53-72.

Cravioto, J., and Delicardie, E. R. (1976). Microenvironmental factors in severe protein-calorie malnutrition. In *Nutrition and Agricultural Development,* N. S. Scrimshaw and M. Béhar (Eds.). Plenum, New York, pp. 25-35.

Cravioto, J., and Robles, B. (1965). Evolution of adaptive and motor behavior during rehabilitation from kwashiorkor. *Am. J. Orthopsychiatry 35,* 449-464.

Cravioto, J., Delicardie, E. R., and Birch, H. G. (1966). Nutrition, growth and neurointegrative development. An experimental and ecologic study. *Pediatrics 38,* 319-372.

Cravioto, J., Birch, H. G., Delicardie, E., Rosales, L., and Vega, L. (1969). The Ecology of Growth and Development in a Mexican Preindustrial Community. *Monographs of the Society for Research in Child Development* No. 129, *34.*

Cravioto, J., Randt, C. T., Derby, B. M., and Diaz, A. (1976). A quantitative ultrastructural study of synapses in the brains of mice following early life undernutrition. *Brain Res. 118,* 304-306.

Culley, W. J., and Mertz, E. T. (1965). Effect of restricted food intakes on growth and composition of preweanling rat brain. *Proc. Soc. Exp. Biol. Med. 118,* 233-235.

Culley, W., Yuan, L., and Mertz, E. (1966). Effect of food restriction and age on rat brain phospholipid levels. *Fed. Proc. 25,* 674.

Curzon, G., and Knott, P. J. (1975). Rapid effects of environmental disturbance on rat plasma unesterified fatty acid and tryptophan concentrations and their prevention by antilipolytic drugs. *Br. J. Pharmacol. 54,* 389-396.

Davison, A. N., and Dobbing, J. (1963). Myelination as a vulnerable period in brain development. *Br. Med. Bull. 22,* No. 1, 40-44.

Davison, A. N., and Dobbing, J. (1968). The developing brain. In *Applied Neurochemistry,* A. N. Davison and J. Dobbing (Eds.). Blackwell, Oxford, pp. 253-286.

DeFeudis, F. V. (1975). Amino acids as central neurotransmitters. *Ann. Rev. Pharmacol. 15,* 105-130.

DeMaeyer, E. M. (1976). Protein-energy malnutrition. In *Nutrition in Preventive Medicine,* G. H. Beaton and J. M. Bengoa (Eds.). WHO Monograph Series, No. 62, Geneva, pp. 23-53.

Deo, M. G., Sood, S. K., and Ramalingaswami, V. (1965). Experimental protein deficiency: Pathological features in the rhesus monkey. *Arch. Pathol. 80,* 14-23.

Dickerson, J. W. T., and Pao, S. K. (1975). Effect of pre- and post-natal maternal protein deficiency on free amino acids and amines of rat brain. *Biol. Neonate 25,* 114-124.

Dickerson, J. W. T., and Walmsley, A. L. (1967). The effect of undernutrition and subsequent rehabilitation on the growth and composition of the central nervous system of the rat. *Brain 90*, 897-906.

Dickerson, J. W. T., Dobbing, J., and McCance, R. A. (1966). The effect of undernutrition on the postnatal development of the brain and cord in pigs. *Proc. Roy. Soc. London (Biology) 166*, 396-407.

Dickerson, J. W. T., Merat, A., and Widdowson, E. M. (1971). Intrauterine growth retardation in the pig. III. The chemical structure of the brain. *Biol. Neonate 19*, 354-362.

Dobbing, J. (1964). The influence of early nutrition on the development and myelination of the brain. *Proc. Roy. Soc. Lond. (Biology) 159*, 503-509.

Dobbing, J. (1968). Vulnerable periods in developing brain. In *Applied Neurochemistry*, A. N. Davison and J. Dobbing (Eds.). Blackwell, Oxford, pp. 287-316.

Dobbing, J., and Sands, J. (1970). Timing of neuroblast multiplication in developing human brain. *Nature* (London) *226*, 639-640.

Dobbing, J., and Sands, J. (1971). Vulnerability of developing brain. IX. The effect of nutritional growth retardation on the timing of the brain growth spurt. *Biol. Neonate 19*, 363-378.

Dobbing, J., and Widdowson, E. M. (1965). The effect of undernutrition and subsequent rehabilitation on myelination of rat brain as measured by its composition. *Brain 85*, 357-366.

Dobbing, J., Hopewell, J. W., and Lynch, A. (1971). Vulnerability of developing brain. VII. Permanent deficits of neurons in cerebral and cerebellar cortex following early mild undernutrition. *Exp. Neurol. 32*, 439-447.

Dodge, P. R., Prensky, A. L., and Feigin, R. D. (1975). *Nutrition and the Developing Nervous System*. Mosby, St. Louis.

Douglas, J. W. B. (1975). Early hospital admissions and later disturbances of behaviour and learning. *Dev. Med. Child Neurol. 17*, 456-480.

Eayrs, J. T., and Horn, G. (1955). The development of cerebral cortex in hypothyroid and starved rats. *Anatom. Rec. 121*, 53-61.

Eckhert, C. D., Levitsky, D. A., and Barnes, R. H. (1975). Postnatal stimulation: The effects on cholinergic enzyme activity in undernourished rats. *Proc. Soc. Exp. Biol. Med. 149*, 860-863.

Eckhert, C. D., Barnes, R. H., and Levitsky, D. A. (1976). Regional changes in rat brain choline acetyltransferase and acetylcholinesterase activity resulting from undernutrition imposed during different periods of development. *J. Neurochemistry 27*, 227-283.

Endozian, J. C. (1966). The free amino acids of plasma and urine in kwashiorkor. *Clin. Sci. 31*, 153-166.

Endozian, J. C. (1968). Experimental kwashiorkor and marasmus. *Nature 220,* 917-919.

Engsner, G. (1974). Brain growth and motor nerve conduction velocities in children with marasmus and kwashiorkor. In *Early Malnutrition and Mental Development,* J. Cravioto, L. Hambraeus, and B. Vahlquist (Eds.). Symposia of the Swedish Nutrition Foundation. XII. Uppsala, Almquist and Wiksell, Stockholm, pp. 85-89.

Enwonwu, C. O. (1973). Experimental protein-calorie malnutrition in the guinea pig and evaluation of the role of ascorbic acid status. *Lab. Invest. 29,* 17-26.

Escobar, A. (1974). Cytoarchitectonic derangement in the cerebral cortex of the undernourished rat. In *Early Malnutrition and Mental Development,* J. Cravioto, L. Hambraeus, and B. Vahlquist (Eds.). Symposia of the Swedish Nutrition Foundation. XII. Uppsala, Almquist and Wiksell, Stockholm, pp. 55-60.

Fish, I., and Winick, M. (1969). Effect of malnutrition and regional growth of the developing rat brain. *Exp. Neurol. 25,* 534-540.

Fishman, M. A., Prensky, A. L., and Dodge, P. R. (1969). Low content of cerebral lipids in infants suffering from malnutrition. *Nature 221,* 552-553.

Fishman, M. A., Madyastha, P., and Prensky, A. L. (1971). The effect of undernutrition on the development of myelin in the rat central nervous system. *Lipids 6,* 458-465.

Fishman, M. A., Prensky, A. L., Tumbleson, M. E., and Daftari, B. (1972). Relative resistance of the later phase of myelination to severe undernutrition in miniature swine. *Am. J. Clin. Nutr. 25,* 7-10.

Fox, J. H., Fishman, M. A., Dodge, P. R., and Prensky, A. L. (1972). The effect of malnutrition on human central nervous system myelin. *Neurology* (Minneapolis) *22,* 1213-1216.

Fraňková, S. (1973). Influence on the familiarity with the environment and early malnutrition on the avoidance learning and behavior in rats. *Activitas Nervosa Superior 15,* 207-216.

Fraňková, S. (1974). Interaction between early malnutrition and stimulation in animals. In *Early Malnutrition and Mental Development,* J. Cravioto, L. Hambraeus, and B. Vahlquist (Eds.). Symposia of the Swedish Nutrition Foundation. XII. Uppsala, Almquist and Wiksell, Stockholm, pp. 202-209.

Galler, J. R. (1979). Intergenerational malnutrition and behaviour. In *Proc. Int. Conf. Behavioural Effects of Energy and Protein Deficits,* J. Brožek (Ed.). DHEW Publication No. (NIH) 79-1906. Washington, D.C., pp. 22-38.

Galler, J., and Rosenthal, M. (1977). Maternal behavior in the rat following intergenerational malnutrition. (Personal Communication to M. E. S.).

Galler, J., and Turkewitz, G. (1977). The use of partial mammectomy to produce undernutrition in the rat. *Biol. Neonate 31,* 260-265.

Gambetti, P., Autillio-Gambetti, L., Gonatas, N., Shafer, B., and Stieber, A. (1972). Synapses and malnutrition. Morphological and biochemical study of synaptosomal fractions from rat cerebral cortex. *Brain Res. 47,* 477-484.

Gambetti, P., Autillio-Gambetti, L., Rizzuto, N., Shafer, B., and Pfaff, L. (1974). Synapses and malnutrition. Quantitative ultrastructural study of rat cerebral cortex. *Exp. Neurol. 43,* 464-473.

Geber, M., and Dean, R. F. A. (1956). The psychological changes accompanying kwashiorkor. *Courrier 6,* 3-14.

Geber, M., and Dean, R. F. A. (1957). The state of development of newborn African children. *Lancet 1,* 1216-1219.

Ghittoni, N. E., and Faryna de Raveglia, J. (1973). Effects of malnutrition and subsequent rehabilitation on the lipid composition of cerebral cortex and cerebellum of the rat. *J. Neurochem. 21,* 983-987.

Gomez, F., Ramos-Galvan, R., Frenk, S., Cravioto, J. M., Chavez, R., and Vazquez, J. (1956). Mortality in second and third degree malnutrition. *J. Trop. Ped. 2,* 77-83.

Gozzo, S., and D'Udine, B. (1977). Diet deprived in essential fatty acids affect brain myelination. *Neurosci. Lett. 7,* 267-275.

Graham, G. G., and Adrianzen, B. (1972). Late "catch up" growth after severe infantile malnutrition. *Johns Hopkins Med. J. 131,* 204-211.

Grantham-McGregor, S. M., Stewart, M. E., and Desai, P. (1978). A new look at the assessment of mental development in young children recovering from severe malnutrition. *Dev. Med. Child Neurol. 20,* 773-778.

Grantham-McGregor, S., Stewart, M., and Desai, P. (1979). Mental development of young children recovering from severe protein-energy malnutrition. In *Proceedings of International Conference on Behavioural Effects of Energy and Protein Deficits,* J. Brožek (Ed.). DHEW Publication No. (NIH) 79-1906. Washington, D.C., pp. 131-141.

Graves, P. L. (1972). Malnutrition and behaviour. In *Annual Report of the Johns Hopkins Center for Medical Research and Training.* Baltimore, cited in Klein et al., 1974.

Graves, P. L. (1976). Nutrition, infant behaviour and maternal characteristics: a pilot study in West Bengal, India. *Am. J. Clin. Nutr. 29,* 305-319.

Graves, P. L. (1978). Nutrition and infant behavior. A replication study in the Katmandu Valley, Nepal. *Am. J. Clin. Nutr. 31,* 541-551.

Guthrie, H. A., and Brown, M. L. (1968). Effect of severe undernutrition in early life on growth, brain size and composition in adult rats. *J. Nutr. 94,* 419-426.

Habicht, J. P., Yarbrough, C., and Klein, R. E. (1974). Assessing nutritional status in a field study of malnutrition and mental development. Specificity, sensitivity and congruity of indices of nutritional status. In *Methodology in Studies of Early Malnutrition and Mental Development,* J. Cravioto, L. Hambraeus, and B. Vahlquist (Eds.). Symposia of the Swedish Nutrition Foundation. XII. Uppsala, Almquist and Wiksell, Stockholm, pp. 35-42.

Harper, A. E. (1976). Protein and amino acids in the regulation of food intake. In *Hunger: Basic Mechanisms and Clinical Implications,* D. Novin, W. Wyrwicka, and G. Bray (Eds.). Raven, New York, pp. 103-113.

Hertzig, M. E., Birch, H., Richardson, S., and Tizard, J. (1972). Intellectual levels of school children severely malnourished during the first two years of life. *Pediatrics 49,* 814-824.

Holt, L. E., Jr., Snyderman, S. E., Norton, P. M., Roitman, E., and Finch, J. (1963). The plasma aminogram in kwashiorkor. *Lancet 2,* 1343-1348.

Honzik, P. (1976). Value and limitations of infant tests. An overview. In *Origins of Intelligence,* M. Lewis (Ed.). Plenum, New York, pp. 59-95.

Hoorweg, J., and Stanfield, J. P. (1976). The effects of protein energy malnutrition in early childhood on intellectual and motor abilities in later childhood and adolescence. *Dev. Med. Child Neurol. 18,* 330-350.

Howard, E., and Granoff, D. M. (1968). Effect of neonatal food restriction in mice on brain growth, DNA, cholesterol and on adult delayed response learning. *J. Nutr. 95,* 111-121.

Irwin, M., Klein, R. E., Townshend, J. W., Owens, W., Lechtig, A., Martorell, R., Yarbrough, C., and Delgado, H. L. (1979). The effects of food supplementation on cognitive development and behaviour among rural Guatemalan children. In *Proceedings of International Conference on Behavioural Effects of Energy and Protein Deficits,* J. Brožek (Ed.). DHEW Publication No. (NIH) 79-1906. Washington, D.C., pp. 239-254.

Johnson, J. E., Jr., and Yoesle, R. A. (1975). The effects of malnutrition on the developing brain stem of the rat. A preliminary experiment using the lateral vestibular nucleus. *Brain Res. 89,* 170-174.

Kaladhar, M., and Narasinga Rao, B. S. (1977). Experimental protein and energy deficiencies: effects on brain free amino acid composition in rats. *Br. J. Nutr. 38,* 141-144.

Kalyanasundaram, S. (1976). Effect of dietary protein and calorie deficiency on tryptophan levels in developing rat brain. *J. Neurochem. 27,* 1245-1247.

Kamin, L. J. (1974). *The Science and Politics of IQ.* Erlbaum, Potomac.

Kasa, D. (1975). Histochemistry of choline acetyltransferase. In *Cholinergic Mechanisms,* P. G. Waser (Ed.). Raven, New York, pp. 271-281.

Kennedy, G. C. (1957). The development with age of hypothalamic restraint upon the appetite of the rat. *J. Endocrinol. 16,* 9-17.

Kerr, G. R., and Helmuth, A. C. (1973). Malnutrition studies on Macaca mulatta. III. Effect on cerebral lipids. *Am. J. Clin. Nutr. 26,* 1053-1059.

Kerr, G. R., Waisman, H. A., Allen, J. R., Wallace, J., and Scheffler, G. (1973). Malnutrition studies in Macaca mulatta. II. The effect on organ size and skeletal growth. *Am. J. Clin. Nutr. 26,* 620-630.

Klein, R. E., Freeman, H. E., Kagan, J., Yarbrough, C., and Habicht, J. P. (1972). Is big smart? The relation of growth to cognition. *J. Health Soc. Behav. 13,* 219-225.

Klein, R. E., Habicht, J. P., and Yarbrough, C. (1973). Some methodological problems in field studies on nutrition and intelligence. In *Nutrition, Development and Social Behavior,* D. Kallen (Ed.). DHEW Publication No. (NIH) 73-242, Washington, D.C., pp. 61-75.

Klein, R. E., Yarbrough, C., Lasky, R. E., and Habicht, J. P. (1974). Correlations of mild-moderate protein-calorie malnutrition among rural Gautemalan infants and preschool children. In *Early Malnutrition and Mental Development,* J. Cravioto, L. Hambraeus, and B. Vahlquist (Eds.). Symposia of the Swedish Nutrition Foundation. XII. Uppsala, Almquist and Wiksell, Stockholm, pp. 168-181.

Krigman, M. R., and Hogan, E. L. (1976). Undernutrition in the developing rat. Effect upon myelination. *Brain Res. 107,* 239-255.

Lancet (1970). Classification of infantile malnutrition. *Leader 2,* 302.

Larroche, J. C., and Amakawa, H. (1973). Glia of myelination and fat deposit during early mylogenesis. *Biol. Neonate 22,* 421-435.

Lee, C. J., and Dubos, R. (1972). Lasting biological effects of early environmental influences. VIII. Effects of neonatal injection, perinatal malnutrition, and crowding on catecholamine metabolism of brain. *J. Exp. Med. 136,* 1031-1042.

Lehr, P., and Gayet, J. (163). Response of the cerebral cortex of the rat to prolonged protein depletion. *J. Neurochem. 10,* 169-176.

Lentz, R. D., and Lapham, L. W. (1969). A quantitative cytochemical study of the DNA content of neurons of rat cerebellar cortex. *J. Neurochem. 16,* 379-384.

Lentz, R. D., and Lapham, L. W. (1970). Postnatal development of tetraploid DNA content in rat Purkinje cells. A quantitative cytochemical study. *J. Neuropathol. Exp. Neurol. 29,* 43-56.

Lester, B. M. (1975). Cardiac habituation of the orienting response to an auditory signal in infants of varying nutritional status. *Dev. Psychology 11,* 432-442.

Lester, B. M. (1976). Spectrum analysis of the cry sounds of well-nourished and malnourished infants. *Child Dev. 47,* 237-241.

Lester, B. M., Klein, R. E., and Martinez, S. J. (1975). The use of habituation in the study of the effects of infantile malnutrition. *Dev. Psychobiology 8,* 541-546.

Levine, S., and Wiener, S. (1976). A critical analysis of data on malnutrition and behavioral deficits. *Adv. Ped. 22,* 113-130.

Levitsky, D. A. (1975). Malnutrition and animal models of cognitive development. In *Nutrition and Mental Functions,* G. Serban (Ed.). Plenum, New York, pp. 75-89.

Levitsky, D. A., and Barnes, R. H. (1969). *Effects of Early Malnutrition on Animal Behavior.* American Association for the Advancement of Science Publication, Washington, D.C.

Levitsky, D. A., and Barnes, R. H. (1970). Effects of early malnutrition on the reaction of adult rats in aversive stimulation. *Nature 225,* 468-469.

Levitsky, D. A., and Barnes, R. H. (1972). Nutritional and environmental interactions in the behavioural development of the rat: Long term effects. *Science 176,* 68-71.

Levitsky, D. A., and Barnes, R. H. (1975). Malnutrition and the biology of experience. In *Proceedings of the IXth Int. Cong. Nutrition, Mexico City, 1972.* Karger, Basel, pp. 330-334.

Levitsky, D. A., Massaro, T. F., and Barnes, R. H. (1975). Maternal malnutrition and the neonatal environment. *Fed. Proc. 34,* 1583-1586.

Lund, J. S., and Lund, R. D. (1972). The effects of varying periods of visual deprivation on synaptogenesis in the superior colliculus of the rat. *Brain Res. 42,* 21-32.

McCall, R. B. (1976). Toward an epigenetic conception of mental development in the first three years of life. In *Origins of Intelligence,* M. Lewis (Ed.). Plenum, New York, pp. 97-122.

McCall, R. B., Hogarty, P. S., and Hurlburt, N. (1972). Transitions in infant sensorimotor development and the prediction of childhood IQ. *Am. Psychol. 27,* 728-748.

McCall, R. B., Appelbaum, M., and Hogarty, P. S. (1973). Developmental changes in mental performance. *Monographs of the Society for Research in Child Development 38,* Serial No. 150.

McKay, H. E., McKay, A., and Sinisterra, L. (1974). Intellectual development of malnourished preschool children in programmes of stimulation and nutritional supplementation. In *Early Malnutrition and Mental Development,* J. Cravioto, L. Hambraeus, and B. Vahlquist (Eds.). Symposia of the Swedish Nutrition Foundation. XII. Uppsala, Almquist, and Wiksell, Stockholm, pp. 226-232.

McKean, C. M., Boggs, D. E., and Peterson, N. A. (1968). The influence of high phenylalanine and tyrosine on the concentrations of essential amino acids in brain. *J. Neurochem. 15,* 235-241.

McLaren, D. S. (1970). Effects of vitamin A deficiency in man. In *'Vitamins', Chemistry, Physiology, Pathology, Methods,* Vol. 1. W. H. Sebrell and R. S. Harris (Eds.). Academic, New York, pp. 267-280.

McLaren, D. S., Yaktin, U. S., Kanawati, A. A., Sabbagh, S., and Kadi, Z. (1973). The subsequent mental and physical development of rehabilitated marasmic infants. *J. Ment. Defic. Res. 17,* 273-281.

Mandel, P., and Mark, J. (1965). The influence of nitrogen deprivation on free amino acids in rat brain. *J. Neurochem. 12,* 987-992.

Massaro, T. F., Levitsky, D. A., and Barnes, R. H. (1974). Protein malnutrition in the rat. Its effects on maternal behaviour and pup development. *Dev. Psychobiol. 7,* 551-561.

Massaro, T. F., Levitsky, D. A., and Barnes, R. H. (1977). Protein malnutrition induced during gestation. Its effect on pup development and maternal behavior. *Dev. Psychobiol. 10,* 339-345.

Mena, I., and Cotzias, G. C. (1975). Protein intake and treatment of Parkinson's disease with levodopa. *N. Engl. J. Med. 292,* 181-184.

Miale, I. L., and Sidman, R. L. (1961). An autoradiographic analysis of histogenesis in the mouse cerebellum. *Exp. Neurol. 4,* 227-296.

Miller, S. A. (1969). Protein metabolism during growth and development. In *Mammalian Protein Metabolism,* Vol. 3. H. N. Munro (Ed.). Academic, New York, pp. 183-233.

Montelli, T. B., Moura Ribeiro, V., Moura Ribeiro, R., and Ribeiro, M. A. C. (1974). Electroencephalographic changes and mental development in malnourished children. *J. Trop. Ped. Environ. Child Health 20,* 201-204.

Mora, J. O., Amezquita, A., Castro, L., Christiansen, N., Clement-Murphy, J., Cobos, L. F., Cremer, H. D., Dragastin, S., Elias, M. F., Franklin, D., Herrera, M. G., Ortiz, N., Pardo, F., DeParedes, B., Ramos, C., Riley, R., Rodriguez, H., Vuori-Christiansen, L., Wagner, M., and Stare, F. J. (1974). Nutrition, health and social factors related to intellectual performance. *World Rev. Nutr. Diet. 19,* 205-236.

Mora, J. O., Clement, J., Christiansen, N., Ortiz, N., Vuori, L., Wagner, M., and Herrera, M. G. (1979). Nutritional supplementation, early home stimulation and child development. In *Proceedings of International Conference on Behavioural Effects of Energy and Protein Deficits,* J. Brožek (Ed.). DHEW Publication No. (NIH) 79-1906. Washington, D.C., pp. 255-269.

Morishige, W. K., and Leathem, J. H. (1972). Pregnancy maintenance with corticosterone in protein-depleted rats. A study on fetal protein composition. *Endocrinology 90,* 318-322.

Mueller, A. J., and Cox, W. M. (1946). The effect of changes in diet on the volume and composition of rat milk. *J. Nutr. 31,* 249-259.

Munro, H. N., Fernstrom, J. D., and Wurtman, R. J. (1975). Insulin, plasma amino acid imbalance, and hepatic coma. *Lancet 1,* 722-724.

Nakhasi, H. L., Toews, A. D., and Horrocks, L. A. (1975). Effects of a postnatal protein deficiency on the content and composition of myelin from the brains of weanling rats. *Brain Res. 83*, 176-179.

National Institute of Nutrition Annual Report. (1977). Hyderabad, India. Nutrition and mental development. 126-137.

Nguyen, M. L., Meyer, K. K., and Winick, M. (1977). Early malnutrition and "late" adoption. A study of their effects on the development of Korean orphans adopted into American families. *Am. J. Clin. Nutr. 30*, 1734-1739.

Niiyama, Y., Kishi, K., Endo, S., and Inoue, G. (1973). Effect of diets devoid of one essential amino acid on pregnancy of rats maintained by ovarian steroids. *J. Nutr. 103*, 207-212.

Noward, T. S., and Munro, H. N. (1977). Effects of protein-caloric malnutrition on biochemical aspects of brain development. In *Nutrition and the Brain*, Vol. 2. R. J. Wurtman and J. J. Wurtman (Eds.). Raven, New York, pp. 193-260.

Pao, S.-K., and Dickerson, J. W. T. (1975). Effect of a low protein diet and isoenergetic amounts of high protein diet in the weanling rat on the free amino acids of the brain. *Nutr. Metab. 18*, 204-216.

Patel, A., del Vecchio, M., and Atkinson, D. J. (1978). Effect of undernutrition on the regional development of transmitter enzymes. Glutamate decarboxylase and choline acetyltransferase. *Dev. Neurosci. 1*, 41-53.

Perez, V. J., Olney, J. W., and Robin, S. J. (1973). Glutamate accumulation in infant mouse hypothalamus. Influence of temperature. *Brain Res. 59*, 181-189.

Piaget, J. (1953). *The Origin of Intelligence in the Child.* Routledge and Kegan Paul, London.

Picou, D., Alleyne, G. A. O., Brooke, O., Kerr, D. S., Miller, C., Jackson, A., Hill, A., Bogues, J., and Patrick, J. (1978). *Malnutrition and Gastroenteritis in Children: A Manual for Hospital Treatment and Management.* Revised ed. Caribbean Food and Nutrition Institute/PAHO, Jamaica.

Platt, B. S., and Stewart, R. J. C. (1969). Effects of protein-calorie deficiency on dogs. II. Morphological changes in the nervous system. *Dev. Med. Child Neurol. 11*, 174-192.

Platt, B. S., and Stewart, R. J. C. (1971). Reversible and irreversible effects of protein-calorie deficiency on the central nervous system of animals and man. *World Rev. Nutr. Diet. 13*, 43-85.

Platt, B. S., Heard, C. R. C., and Stewart, R. J. C. (1964). Experimental protein-calorie deficiency. In *Mammalian Protein Metabolism*, Vol. 2. H. N. Munro and J. B. Allison (Eds.). Academic, New York, pp. 451-521.

Pollitt, E. (1973). Behavioural correlates of severe malnutrition in man. In *Nutrition, Growth and Development of North American Indian Children,*

W. M. Moore, M. M. Silverberg, and M. S. Read (Eds.). DHEW Publication No. (NIH) 72-76, Washington, D.C., pp. 151-156.

Pollitt, E., and Granoff, D. M. (1967). Mental and motor development of Peruvian children treated for severe malnutrition. *Rev. Interamerican Psychology 1,* 93-102.

Pollitt, E., and Thompson, C. (1977). Protein-calorie malnutrition and behavior. A view from psychology. In *Nutrition and the Brain,* Vol. 2. R. J. Wurtman and J. J. Wurtman (Eds.). Raven, New York, pp. 261-302.

Rajalakshimi, R., Ali, S. Z., and Ramakrishnan, C. V. (1967). Effect of inanition during the neonatal period on discrimination learning and brain biochemistry in the albino rat. *J. Neurochem. 14,* 29-34.

Rajalakshimi, R., Parameswaran, M., Telang, S. D., and Ramakrishnan, C. V. (1974). Effect of undernutrition and protein deficiency on glutamate dehydrogenase and decarboxylase in rat brain. *J. Neurochem. 23,* 129-133.

Ramanamurthy, P. S. V. (1977). Maternal and early postnatal malnutrition and transmitter amines in rat brain. *J. Neurochem. 28,* 253-254.

Ramos-Galvan, R., Viniegra-C., A., and Mariscal-A, C. (1968). Aspectos sociales y epidemiologicos. In *Humanismo y Pediatria.* Nestle Editorial Fund of the Mexican Academy of Pediatrics, Mexico City, pp. 415-433.

Richardson, S. A. (1974). The background histories of school children severely malnourished in infancy. *Adv. Ped. 21,* 167-195.

Richardson, S. A. (1976). The relation of severe malnutrition in infancy to the intelligence of school children with differing life histories. *Ped. Res. 10,* 57-61.

Richardson, S. (1979). The relationship between different degrees of early malnutrition and intelligence at school age. In *Proceedings of International Conference on Behavioural Effects of Energy and Protein Deficits,* J. Brožek (Ed.). DHEW Publication No. (NIH) 79-1906. Washington, D.C., pp. 172-184.

Richardson, S. A., Birch, H. G., Grabie, E., and Yoder, K. (1972). Behavior of children in school who were severely malnourished in the first two years of life. *J. Health Soc. Behav. 12,* 276-284.

Richardson, S. A., Birch, H. G., and Hertzig, M. (1973). School performance of children who were severely malnourished in infancy. *Am. J. Ment. Defic. 77,* 623-632.

Richardson, S. A., Birch, H. G., and Ragbeer, C. (1975). The behaviour of children at home who were severely malnourished in the first two years of life. *J. Biosoc. Sci. 7,* 255-267.

Robain, O., and Ponsot, G. (1978). Effects of undernutrition on glial maturation. *Brain Res. 149,* 379-397.

Rosenzweig, M. R. (1966). Environmental complexity, cerebral change and behavior. *Am. Psychol. 21*, 321-332.

Rossier, J., Bauman, A., Reiger, F., and Benda, P. (1975). Immunological studies on the enzymes of the cholinergic system. In *Cholinergic Mechanisms,* P. G. Waser (Ed.). Raven, New York, pp. 283-293.

Rosso, P., Hormazabel, J., and Winick, M. (1970). Changes in brain weight, cholesterol phospholipid and DNA content in marasmic children. *Am. J. Clin. Nutr. 23,* 1275-1279.

Salas, M., Diaz, S., and Nieto, A. (1974). Effects of neonatal food deprivation on cortical spines and dendritic development of the rat. *Brain Res. 73,* 139-144.

Schaefer, A. E. (1969). Statement read before the Senate Select Committee on Nutrition and Related Human Needs, January 22, 1969. Quoted in Dodge, P. R., Prensky, A. L., and Feigin, R. D. (1975). *Nutrition and the Developing Nervous System.* Mosby, St. Louis, p. 183.

Schain, R. J., and Watanabe, K. S. (1973). Effects of undernutrition on early brain growth in the rabbit. *Exp. Neurol. 41,* 366-370.

Seigel, F. L., Aoki, K., and Colwell, R. E. (1971). Polyribosome disaggregation and cell free protein synthesis in preparations from cerebral cortex of hyperphenylalaninemic rats. *J. Neurochem. 18,* 537-547.

Sereni, F., Principi, N., Perletti, L., and Piceni-Sereni, L. (1966). Undernutrition and developing rat brain. I. Influence on acetylcholinesterase and succinic acid dehydrogenase activities and on norepinephrine and 5-OH-tryptamine tissue concentrations. *Biol. Neonate 10,* 254-265.

Shoemaker, W. J., and Bloom, F. E. (1977). Effect of undernutrition on brain morphology. In *Nutrition and the Brain,* Vol. 2. R. J. Wurtman and J. J. Wurtman (Eds.). Raven, New York, pp. 147-192.

Shoemaker, W. J., and Wurtman, R. J. (1971). Perinatal undernutrition. Accumulation of catecholamines in rat brain. *Science 171,* 1017-1019.

Shoemaker, W. J., and Wurtman, R. J. (1973). Effect of perinatal undernutrition on the metabolism of catecholamines in the rat brain. *J. Nutr. 103,* 1537-1547.

Shrader, R. E., and Zeman, F. J. (1969). Effect of maternal protein deprivation on morphological and enzymatic development of neonatal rat tissue. *J. Nutr. 99,* 401-421.

Siassi, F., and Siassi, B. (1973). Differential effects of protein-calorie restriction and subsequent repletion on neuronal and nonneuronal components of cerebral cortex in newborn rats. *J. Nutr. 103,* 1625-1633.

Simonson, M., Sherwin, R. W., Anilane, J. K., Yu, W. Y., and Chow, B. F. (1969). Neuromotor development in progeny of underfed mother rats. *J. Nutr. 98,* 18-24.

Sinisterra, L., McKay, H., McKay, A., Gómez, H., and Korgi, J. (1979). Response of malnourished pre-school children to multidisciplinary intervention. In *Proceedings of International Conference on Behavioural Effects of Energy and Protein Deficits,* J. Brožek (Ed.). DHEW Publication No. (NIH) 79-1906. Washington, D.C., pp. 229-238.

Slob, A. K., Snow, C. E., and de Natris-Mathot, E. (1973). Absence of behavioral deficits following neonatal undernutriton in the rat. *Dev. Psychobiol. 6,* 177-186.

Smart, J. L. (1974). Activity and exploratory behaviour of adult offspring of undernourished mother rats. *Dev. Psychobiol. 7,* 315-321.

Smart, J. L. (1976). Maternal behaviour of undernourished mother rats towards well fed and underfed young. *Physiol. Behav. 16,* 147-149.

Smart, J. L., and Dobbing, J. (1971a). Vulnerability of developing brain. *Brain Res. 28,* 85-95.

Smart, J. L., and Dobbing, J. (1971b). Vulnerability of developing brain. VI. Relative effects of foetal and early postnatal undernutrition on reflex ontogeny and development of behaviour in the rat. *Brain Res. 33,* 303-314.

Smart, J. L., Whatson, T. S., and Dobbing, J. (1975). Thresholds of response to electric shock in previously undernourished rats. *Br. J. Nutr. 34,* 511-516.

Sobotka, T. J., Cook, M. P., and Brodie, R. E. (1974). Neonatal malnutrition, neurochemical, hormonal and behavioral manifestations. *Brain Res. 65,* 443-457.

Stern, W. C., Forbes, W. B., Resnick, O., and Morgane, P. J. (1974). Seizure susceptibility and brain amine levels following protein malnutrition during development in the rat. *Brain Res. 79,* 375-384.

Stern, W. C., Miller, M., Forbes, W. B., Morgane, P. J., and Resnick, O. (1975). Ontogeny of the levels of biogenic amines in various parts of the brain and in peripheral tissues in normal and protein malnourished rats. *Exp. Neurol. 49,* 314-326.

Stewart, M. E., and Grantham-McGregor, S. M. (1979). The experiences of young children in a Kingston hospital. *W. Ind. Med. J. 27,* 30-35.

Stewart, M. E., Schofield, W. N., and McGregor, S. M. (1978). The behaviour of severely malnourished Jamaican children during recovery. Paper presented at 23rd Scientific Meeting, Commonwealth Caribbean Medical Research Council, Barbados.

Stoch, M. B., and Smythe, P. M. (1963). Does undernutrition during infancy inhibit brain growth and subsequent intellectual development? *Arch. Dis. Child. 38,* 546-552.

Stoch, M. B., and Smythe, P. M. (1967). The effect of undernutrition during infancy on subsequent brain growth and intellectual development. *S. Afr. Med. J. 41*, 1027-1030.

Stoch, M. B., and Smythe, P. M. (1976). Fifteen year developmental study on effects of severe undernutrition during infancy on subsequent physical growth and intellectual functioning. *Arch. Dis. Child. 51*, 327-335.

Stuart, H. C., and Stevenson, S. S. (1959). Physical growth and development. In *Textbook of Pediatrics*, 7th Ed. W. E. Nelson (Ed.). Saunders, Philadelphia, pp. 12-61.

Swaiman, K. F., Daleiden, J. M., and Wolfe, R. N. (1970). The effect of food deprivation on enzyme activity in the developing brain. *J. Neurochem. 17*, 1387-1391.

Tricklebank, M. D., and Adlard, B. P. F. (1974). Regional brain 5-hydroxytryptamine turnover in adult rats growth retarded in early life. *Biochem. Soc. Trans. 2*, 127-129.

Tumbleson, M. E., Tinsley, O. W., Hicklin, K. W., and Mulder, J. B. (1972). Fetal and neonatal development of Sinclair (S-1) miniature piglets effected by maternal dietary protein deprivation. *Growth 36*, 373-387.

Vernon, P. (1969). *Intelligence and Cultural Environment*. Methuen, London.

Vernon, P. E. (1979). *Intelligence: Heredity and Environment*. Freeman, San Francisco.

Warkany, J. (1945). Manifestations of prenatal nutritional deficiency. *Vitam. Horm. 3*, 73-103.

Waterlow, J. C. (1969). The assessment of protein nutrition and metabolism in the whole animal with special reference to man. In *Mammalian Protein Metabolism*, Vol. 3. H. N. Munro (Ed.). Academic, New York, pp. 325-390.

Waterlow, J. C., and Rutishauser, I. H. E. (1974). Malnutrition in man. In *Early Malnutrition and Mental Development*, J. Cravioto, L. Hambraeus, and B. Vahlquist (Eds.). Symposia of the Swedish National Foundation. XII. Uppsala, Almquist and Wiksell, Stockholm, pp. 13-26.

Whatson, T. S., Smart, J. L., and Dobbing, J. (1974). Social interactions among adult male rats after early undernutrition. *Br. J. Nutr. 32*, 413-419.

Whitehead, R. G. (1964). Rapid determination of some plasma amino acids in subclinical kwashiorkor. *Lancet 1*, 250-252.

Whitehead, R. G. (1968). Biochemical changes in kwashiorkor and nutritional marasmus. In *Calorie Deficiencies and Protein Deficiencies*, R. A. McCance and E. M. Widdowson (Eds.). Churchill, London, pp. 109-118.

Widdowson, E. M., and McCance, R. A. (1960). Some effects of accelerating growth. 1. General somatic development. *Proc. Roy. Soc. London (Biology) 152*, 188-206.

Wiener, S. G., Fitzpatrick, K. M., Levin, R., Smotherman, W. P., and Levine, S. (1977). Alterations in the maternal behaviour of rats rearing malnourished offspring. *Dev. Psychobiol. 10,* 243-254.

Wiggins, R. L., Miller, S. L., Benjamins, J. A., Krigman, M. R., and Morell, P. Synthesis of myelin proteins during starvation. *Brain Res. 80,* 345-349.

Wiggins, R. C., Miller, S. L., Benjamins, J. A., Krigman, M. R., and Morell, P. (1976). Myelin synthesis during postnatal nutritional deprivation and subsequent rehabilitation. *Brain Res. 107,* 257-273.

Wiltse, H. E., and Menkes, J. H. (1972). Brain damage in the aminoacidurias. In *Handbook of Neurochemistry,* Vol. 7. A. Lajtha (Ed.). Plenum, New York, pp. 143-167.

Winick, M. (1971). Cellular changes during placental and fetal growth. *Am. J. Obstet. Gynecol. 109,* 166-176.

Winick, M. (1979). Malnutrition and behaviour: Data from adoption studies of Korean children. In *Proceedings of International Conference on Behavioural Effects of Energy and Protein Deficits,* J. Brožek (Ed.). DHEW Publication No. (NIH) 79-1906. Washington, D.C., pp. 195-198.

Winick, M., and Coombs, J. (1972). Nutrition, environment and behavioural development. *Ann. Rev. Med. 23,* 149-160.

Winick, M., and Noble, A. (1966). Cellular response in rats during malnutrition at various ages. *J. Nutr. 89,* 300-306.

Winick, M., and Rosso, P. (1969). The effect of severe early malnutrition on cellular growth of human brain. *Ped. Res. 31,* 181-184.

Winick, M., Rosso, P., and Waterlow, J. (1970). Cellular growth of cerebrum, cerebellum, and brain stem in normal and marasmic children. *Exp. Neurol. 26,* 393-400.

Winick, M., Rosso, P., and Brasel, J. H. (1972). Malnutrition and cellular growth in the brain. *Bibl. Nutr. Diet. 17,* 60-68.

Winick, M., Katchadurian Meyer, K., and Harris, R. C. (1975). Malnutrition and environmental enrichment by early adoption. *Science 190,* 1173-1175.

Witkop, C. J., Baldizon, G. C., Castro, O. R. P., and Umana, R. (1970). Auditory memory span and oral stereognosis in children recovered from kwashiorkor. In *Second Symposium on Oral Sensation and Perception,* J. S. Bosma (Ed.). Thomas, Springfield, Illinois, pp. 444-465.

Wong, P. W. K., and Justice, P. (1972). Effect of amino acid imbalance on polyribosome profiles and protein synthesis in fetal cerebral cortex. In *Sphingolipids, Sphingolipidoses and Allied Disorders,* B. W. Volk and S. M. Aronson (Eds.). Plenum, New York, pp. 163-174.

Wood, J. G. (1973). The effect of undernutrition on the proteins of optic and sciatic nerves during development. *J. Neurochem. 20,* 423-429.

Wurtman, R. J., and Fernstrom, J. D. (1976). Control of brain monoamine synthesis by precursor availability and nutritional state. *Biochem. Pharmacol. 25,* 1691-1696.

Yakovlev, P. I., and Lecours, A. R. (1967). The myelogenetic cycles of regional maturation of the brain. In *Regional Development of the Brain in Early Life,* A. Minkowski (Ed.). Blackwell, Oxford, pp. 3-70.

Yaktin, U. S., and McLaren, D. S. (1970). The behavioural development of infants recovering from severe malnutrition. *J. Ment. Def. Res. 14,* 25-31.

Yaktin, U. S., McLaren, D. S., Kanawati, A. A., and Sabbagh, S. (1971). Effect of undernutrition in early life on subsequent behavioural development. *Proc. 13th Int. Congr. Ped. 2,* 71-75.

Zamenhof, S., and van Marthens, E. (1974). Study of factors influencing prenatal brain development. *Mol. Cell Biochem. 4,* 157-168.

Zamenhof, S., van Marthens, E., and Margolis, F. (1968). DNA (cell number) and protein in neonatal brain. Alteration by maternal dietary protein restriction. *Science 160,* 322-323.

Zamenhof, S., van Marthens, E.,and Grauel, L. (1971). DNA (cell number) in neonatal brain. Alteration by maternal dietary caloric restriction. *Nutr. Rep. Int. 4,* 269-274.

Zamenhof, S., van Marthens, E., and Shimomaye, S. Y. (1976). The effects of early maternal protein deprivation on fetal development. *Fed. Proc. 35,* 422.

Zeman, F. J., and Stanbrough, E. C. (1969). Effect of maternal protein deficiency on cellular development in the fetal rat. *J. Nutr. 99,* 274-282.

Zimmermann, R. R., Strobel, D. A., Maguire, D., Steere, R. R., and Hom, H. L. (1976). The effects of protein and deficiency on activity, learning, manipulative tasks, curiosity, and social behaviour of monkeys. In *Play,* J. S. Bruner, A. Jolly, and K. Sylva (Eds.). Penguin, England, pp. 496-511.

MODE OF ACTION OF PSYCHOTROPIC DRUGS

21

Mode of Action of Antidepressants and Central Stimulants

Irwin J. Kopin
National Institute of Mental Health
Bethesda, Maryland

I. INTRODUCTION

Although it has been recognized for centuries that a variety of substances can alter mood and behavior, only within the last 20 years have drugs come into wide use for the treatment of psychiatric disorders. The appearance of effective psychopharmacological agents for the treatment of mental disturbances and the demonstrable genetic basis for the susceptibility to schizophrenia and depression (Kallmann, 1953) have led to the prevalent conviction that there exist biological bases for mental disorders. Hypotheses that specific functional abnormalities in neuronal activity and neurotransmission may be involved in human psychiatric states have been based largely on indirect evidence from pharmacological studies in animals. These hypotheses have generated studies which seek to explain, on a molecular basis, how drugs act to alter the processes controlling brain neurotransmission. Three important classes of drugs have played an extremely important role in the development of hypotheses regarding the biology of affective disorders.

About 20 years ago the first of each of two distinct groups of antidepressant drugs were discovered. Iproniazid (see Fig. 1), a monoamine oxidase (MAO) inhibitor, was described as a "psychic energizer" which was useful in the treatment of depression (Crane, 1957; Loomer et al., 1957). At about the same time, Kuhn (1958) found that imipramine, a dibenzazepine compound (see Fig. 2) in which the sulfur atom of promazine (the parent compound of chlorpromazine) had been replaced by two carbons (an ethylene link), was useful in alleviating the symptoms of retarded depressed patients (although the drug exacerbated the symptoms of agitated depression). In 1952, a third drug, reserpine, isolated from the *Rauwolfia* preparations which had been in medical use in India for treatment of psychoses and hypertension, was introduced to Western medicine (see Bein, 1956) and provided an important contrast to the antidepressants. In animals, reserpine produces a calming effect, a decline in aggressiveness, sleep which can be interrupted by external stimuli (the term "tranquilizer" was used to distinguish this type of sedation from that of barbiturates), and a moderate decrease in blood pressure. When the drug was introduced into clinical use for treatment of hypertension, the incidence of mental depression in patients treated with *Rauwolfia* was found to be much higher than in untreated hypertensive patients (Anchor et al., 1955; Muller et al., 1955; Lemieux et al., 1956; Quetsch et al., 1959). The behavioral effects produced in animals by administration of reserpine then came to be regarded as an experimental model for depression. Reversal of the reserpine-induced behavioral effects in animals was then used as a method to detect potential antidepressant activity of new drugs. Considerable overlap in antireserpine activity was found between central stimulants, such as amphetamine and cocaine, which are euphoriants but not particularly useful in treatment of depression, and antidepressants (monoamine oxidase inhibitors and tricyclic antidepressants). This

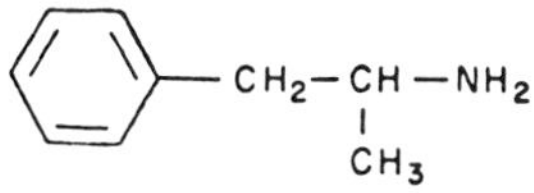

AMPHETAMINE

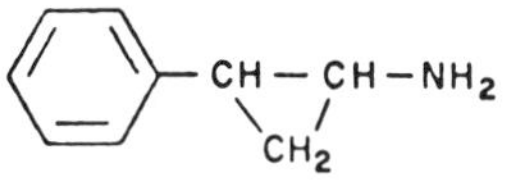

TRANYLCYPROMINE

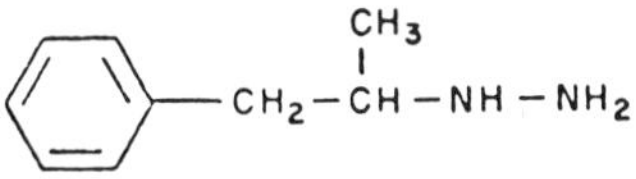

PHENIPRAZINE

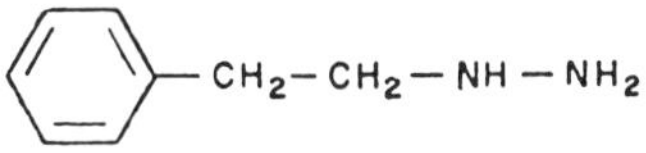

PHENELZINE

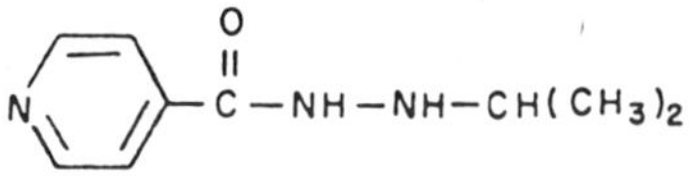

IPRONIAZID

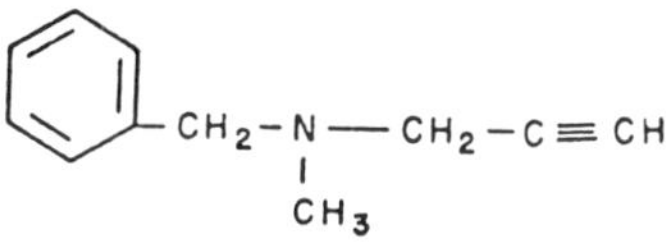

PARGYLINE

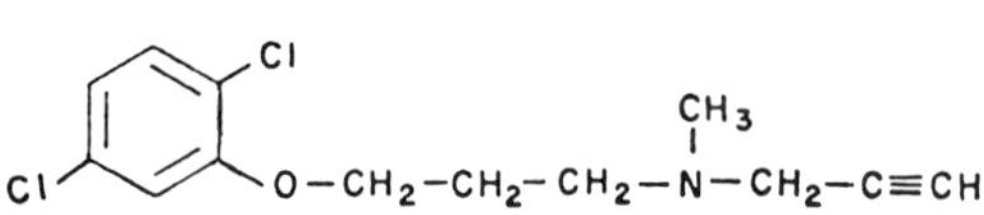

CLORGYLINE

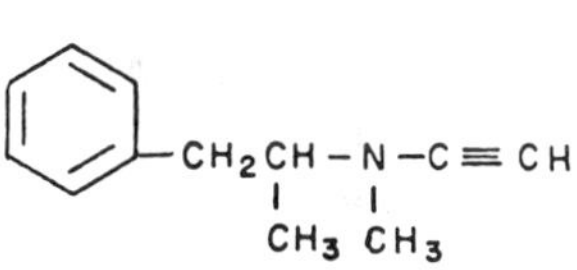

DEPRENYL

Figure 1 Chemical structures of amphetamine and monoamine oxidase inhibitors.

suggested that these compounds might share common actions and thus in considering modes of drug action it appears appropriate to discuss central stimulants along with clinically useful antidepressants.

The development of specific and sensitive methods for assay of many compounds which normally occur in brain and nerves throughout the body and the introduction of isotopic techniques for study of the metabolism and disposition of putative transmitters provided the techniques needed to explore the possible modes of action of drugs. It soon became apparent that monoamines

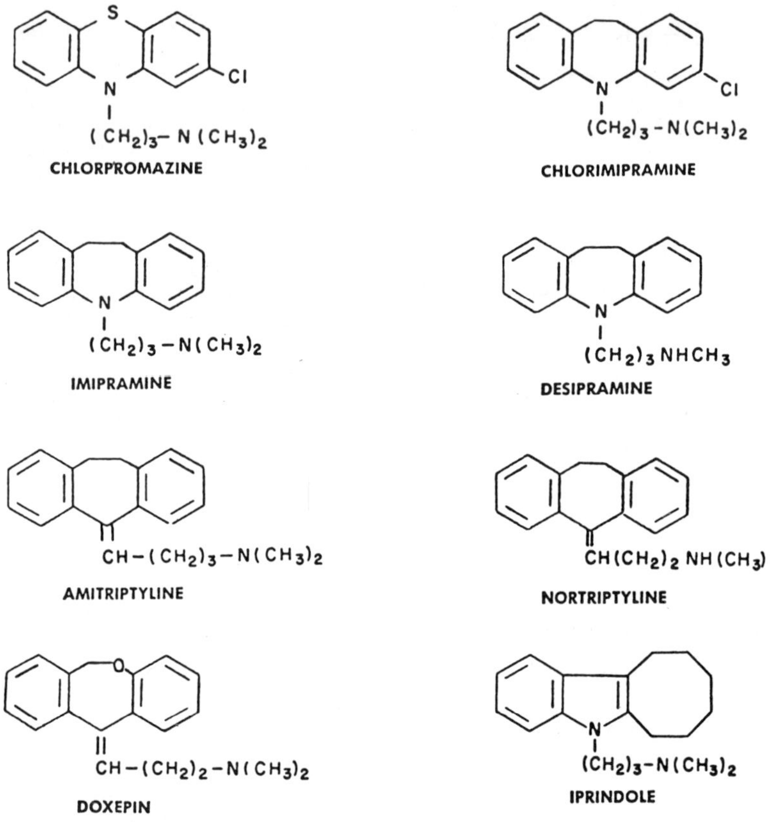

$(CH_2)_3-N(CH_3)_2$
CHLORPROMAZINE

$(CH_2)_3-N(CH_3)_2$
CHLORIMIPRAMINE

$(CH_2)_3-N(CH_3)_2$
IMIPRAMINE

$(CH_2)_3NHCH_3$
DESIPRAMINE

$CH-(CH_2)_3-N(CH_3)_2$
AMITRIPTYLINE

$CH(CH_2)_2NH(CH_3)$
NORTRIPTYLINE

$CH-(CH_2)_2-N(CH_3)_2$
DOXEPIN

$(CH_2)_3-N(CH_3)_2$
IPRINDOLE

Figure 2 Chemical structures of chlorpromazine and tricyclic antidepressants.

provided a focus on which the various biochemical and behavioral observations converged. Norepinephrine was identified as the neurotransmitter released from peripheral sympathetic nerves (von Euler, 1948) and its regional localization in brain suggested it is also a neurotransmitter in brain (Vogt, 1954). Similarly, serotonin (Bogdanski et al., 1957) and dopamine (Carlsson, 1959) were implicated as central neurotransmitters. Reserpine was found to deplete tissue stores of norepinephrine, dopamine, and serotonin (see Shore, 1962) while monoamine oxidase inhibitors elevated tissue levels of these amines and partially prevented their decrease after administration of reserpine (see Spector et al., 1963). Imipramine, cocaine, and amphetamine were found to prevent uptake (and presumably inactivation) of norepinephrine (see Axelrod, 1965). Thus monoamines were implicated as being intimately involved in the mode of action of antidepressants and central stimulants. It is the purpose of this chapter to provide an overview of the evidence implicating each of the monoamines (or other putative central neurotransmitters) in the mode of action of these various drugs and to indicate briefly how these actions have provided the bases for provocative hypotheses to explain on a biochemical level how drugs may act to alter mood or induce alterations of behavior in animals.

II. FUNDAMENTAL PROCESSES AT AMINERGIC SYNAPSES

Communication among neurons in the central nervous system, in peripheral ganglia, and at axon terminals of neuroaffector junctions is usually mediated by release of a specific chemical substance into the synaptic cleft. The neurotransmitter substance released from the axon terminal interacts with a receptor on the postsynaptic membrane to trigger a series of events which result in alteration of activity of the postjunctional cell. Several mechanisms involved in the process of neurochemical transmission are probably common to different types of neurons, regardless of the chemical nature of the transmitter. These mechanisms are particularly susceptible to the actions of drugs, so that before considering the possible modes of action of antidepressants or central excitants it will be useful to describe briefly the current concepts of the processes involved in chemical, particularly aminergic, neurotransmission. These concepts have been developed largely as a result of studies of catecholamines at peripheral sympathetic nerve endings (see Kopin, 1967), but there is considerable evidence that these concepts may be extended validly to the central nervous system (see Glowinski and Baldessarini, 1966).

A diagrammatic representation of an aminergic synapse is presented in Figure 3. Amine neurotransmitters are synthesized mainly in the axon terminals. The enzymes required for their synthesis are formed in the cell bodies and transported along the axon to the nerve terminals. The neurotransmitter formed at the nerve ending is sequestered in an inactive form by being bound to a protein confined to synaptic vesicles. Amines which are free in the cytosol are destroyed by the action of monoamine oxidase. Elevation of cytosol levels of the amine produces feedback inhibition of neurotransmitter synthesis. Arrival of nerve impulse at the nerve endings results in a change in ion permeability and entry of calcium ions appears to trigger a process which results in a fusion of the membranes of the storage vesicles with the axonal ending in the region of the synapse and discharge exocytosis of the contents of the vesicles into the synaptic cleft. Receptors which are activated by the released neurotransmitter substance appear to be present on both the presynaptic and postsynaptic membrane. The effect of stimulation of presynaptic receptors is to diminish the rate of transmitter release so that the burst of release of the substance is short-lived. The action of amine neurotransmitters on intrasynaptic receptors appears to be terminated

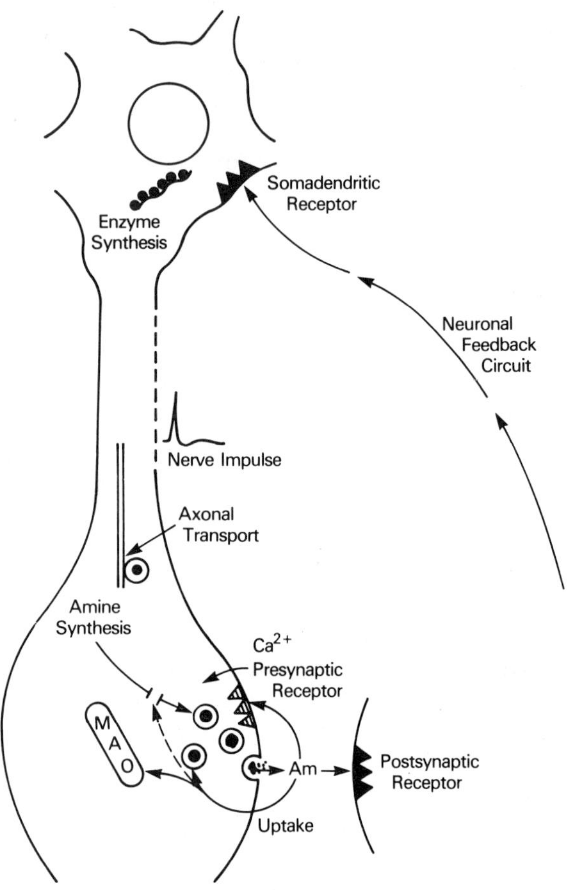

Figure 3 Diagrammatic representation of aminergic neuron and the mechanism controlling release of its neurotransmitter (Am).

mainly by physical removal of the transmitter substance, usually by reuptake of the amine into the presynaptic neuron where it may be destroyed by monoamine oxidase. The actions of amines on the receptors of postsynaptic cells are frequently mediated by activation of adenylcyclase and consequent formation of cyclic AMP or by alterations in ion permeability. There are, of course, variations in this general scheme. For example, termination of the action of acetylcholine is the result of enzymatic hydrolysis of the transmitter by acetylcholinesterase, but the presynaptic terminal has an active transport system to recapture the liberated choline. Inactivation of γ-aminobutyric acid (GABA), an inhibitory neurotransmitter, appears to be largely by uptake into glia. The mode of presynaptic storage of acetylcholine, however, does appear to involve synaptic vesicles and it was at cholinergic nerve endings that Katz and his co-workers first provided evidence that packets of neurotransmitters are released in quantal amounts (see Katz and Miledi, 1965). Receptors for other transmitters (acetylcholine, GABA, or peptides) may also be present on presynaptic membranes and activation of these receptors may modulate amine transmitter release.

III. APPROACHES TO DEFINING MODES OF DRUG ACTION

Drugs may influence the efficacy of neurochemical transmission by alteration, directly or indirectly, of the biosynthesis, storage and availability, release, action on receptor or inactivation of the neurotransmitters. One drug may alter one or more of these processes and may act in different neurons containing different transmitters. Discussion of possible modes of action of drugs in producing behavioral effects, in altering mood, or in alleviating depression must include some consideration of the neuronal basis for the psychological effect as well as the biochemical alterations produced by the drugs. Since hypotheses regarding particular transmitters systems involved in control of the behavioral of psychological state are often based on the known pharmacological effects of the drugs, there is a danger that some of the reasoning may become circular. Support for the hypotheses is generated by use of drugs with different biochemical actions or by use of precursors for specific neurotransmitters.

A large body of evidence has been generated to support the notion that abnormalities of one or more of the biogenic amine neurotransmitter systems is involved in disorders of mood and that these systems mediate the effects of central excitants. As indicated above, the triad of reserpine (which depletes amines and causes depression), iproniazid (which inhibits monoamine oxidase and reverses the effects of reserpine as well as acting as an antidepressant), and imipramine (which interferes with uptake of amines at nerve endings and is an antidepressant) provide the foundation for the aminergic hypotheses for control of mood and behavior. While suitable methods to evaluate unequivocally and directly the effects of drugs on aminergic neurons in human brain are not available, there are a host of techniques which have been used in animals to assess behavioral changes and to determine alterations in aminergic neuronal activity. Activation of neurons, which may be monitored directly by cellular recordings, is attended by accelerated release and formation of the neurotransmitter and appearance of its metabolites, which may be measured biochemically. Alterations in neuronal activity, however, may be mediated by direct action of the drug on the neuron or indirectly by alteration of activity of a neuronal system which controls the activity of the aminergic neuron. Thus, a drug which stimulates the aminergic receptors may, by stimulating an inhibitory neuronal feedback loop, diminish activity of the aminergic neuron while producing the effects which would be the result of release of the transmitter. From examination of the behavioral, physiological, and biochemical effects of a series of drugs, preferably with different modes of action, it is hoped that there will emerge a clearer picture of the relevant drug actions and biochemical events important in control of mood and behavior.

In attempting to define the mode of action of drugs it is important to realize that our knowledge is continually expanding. Drugs have multiple sites at which they can act with varying degrees of potency. Consideration of newly discovered transmitters, of new roles for known transmitters, or demonstration of alterations in the organism in response to the drug after continued exposure to the agent (changes in drug metabolism, enzyme levels, receptor sensitivity, etc.) result in an evolution of concepts of drug action with modification or discarding of hypotheses. Thus descriptions of the mode of action of drugs must be tempered with some skepticism as to our knowledge of the drug. It is for these reasons that there has been, and will continue to be, changes in our views of the modes of action of the different classes of antidepressants.

IV. MONOAMINE OXIDASE INHIBITORS

The discovery by Zeller and Barsky (1952) that iproniazid is a potent inhibitor of MAO and the subsequent clinical descriptions of its antidepressant activity (Crane, 1957; Loomer et al., 1957) stimulated thousands of investigations to seek other drugs of this type, to utilize those chemical agents as pharmacological tools to study amine metabolism, effects on other drugs, behavioral changes, etc., as well as to determine their therapeutic usefulness. The structures of some MAO inhibitors are shown in Figure 1. As indicated above, MAO inhibitors increase levels of amines in the tissues, partially prevent the depletion of amines produced by reserpine, and reverse the pharmacological effects of this drug.

A. Multiple Types of MAO

When these enzyme inhibitors were first described, MAO was generally assumed to be a single enzyme. Examination of inhibition by drugs and inactivation by temperature elevation of deamination of different substrates for MAO led to the discovery that there are at least two forms, A and B, of the enzyme (see reviews by Youdim, 1973; Tipton, 1975). Johnston (1968) found that clorgyline (Fig. 1) more effectively inhibited deamination of serotonin by type A MAO than deamination of benzylamine by type B MAO. Deprenyl (Fig. 1), introduced by Knoll et al. (1965), has been found to inhibit selectively type B MAO. The relative amounts of types A and B MAO varies in different tissues (see Knoll and Magyar, 1972; Neff and Goridis, 1973; Squires, 1972). Both clorgyline and deprenyl are irreversible inhibitors of MAO and are not absolutely specific for types A and B. Their selectivity for types A and B MAO, respectively, are based on different rates of inhibition of the enzymes (Tipton, 1971).

The existence of multiple forms of MAO appears to result from the effects of neighboring lipid molecules in the mitochondrial membrane. Houslay and Tipton (1973) claim to have abolished selective sensitivity to enzyme inhibitors of rat liver mitochondrial MAO by solubilization of the enzyme. Furthermore, they found that substrates for one species (A or B) may act as inhibitors for the other type (B or A) of MAO (Houslay and Tipton, 1975). The latter observations suggest that even if one type of MAO were specifically inhibited in vivo, accumulation of its substrates could lead to reversible inhibition of the other type of MAO. This phenomenon does not appear to be important in acute experiments, however, since inhibition of both A and B forms of MAO are required for behavioral changes seen in rats after tryptophan loading (Squires and Lassen, 1975). Under in vivo conditions, however, where drug distribution, affinity for the enzymes, and rates of formation of new active enzyme may vary, the rules of specificity are far less rigid than under in vitro conditions.

B. Molecular Basis for Inhibition of MAO

The molecular mechanisms for inhibition of MAO have recently been the subject of intensive investigation. Hellerman and Erwin (1968) showed that $[^{14}C]$pargyline combines stoichiometrically with bovine kidney MAO when inhibition of the enzyme is complete. Initially inhibition is competitive, but irreversible inhibition develops as a first-order reaction between substrate and enzyme; the enzyme undergoes chemical reduction. The adduct was later found to involve the flavin moiety in MAO (Chuang et al., 1974) and recently the chemical nature of acetylenic adducts to the flavin of MAO have been identified (Gärtner and Hemmerich, 1975; Maycock et al., 1976). Irreversible inhibition of MAO by hydrazine derivatives (e.g., iproniazid) also appears to involve formation of a highly reactive intermediate which reacts with the enzyme to produce a chemical change which results in inactivation of the enzyme (see Bloom, 1963), but the nature of this reaction has not been described. The site of the reaction with the reactive products formed from oxidation of hydrazines or N-cyclopropylamines is not necessarily the same as that of the products from acetylenic inhibitors.

C. Biochemical Consequences of MAO Inhibitors

MAO is present in high concentrations in liver, kidney, and many other tissues as well as in aminergic nerves. Amines generated by bacteria in the intestine or ingested with food are readily destroyed before they reach the circulation. After inhibition of MAO, however, this enzyme barrier is eliminated and the amines may reach the circulation. Thus, in patients being treated with MAO inhibitors, ingestion of a variety of amine drugs or fermented foods containing tyramine may produce acute hypertensive reactions (Blackwell et al., 1967), presumably as a result of the release by the amine of norepinephrine from sympathetic nerve endings.

Postural hypotension frequently develops in patients being treated with inhibitors of MAO, as do other symptoms of impairment of sympathetic responsivity. The mechanism of interference with sympathetic neuronal activation appears to involve the accumulation of amines. The accumulation of norepinephrine in sympathetic ganglia has been suggested as the basis for diminution of ganglionic transmission (Goldberg and DaCosta, 1960; Gessa et al., 1963) since Marrazzi (1939) had shown that norepinephrine counteracts the excitatory effects of acetylcholine at sympathetic ganglia. More recently, Puig et al., (1972) showed that after chronic treatment of cats with an MAO inhibitor (pargyline), preganglionic-stimulation-induced release of norepinephrine from the spleen is diminished to a greater extent than is postganglionic stimulation. There was also a decrease in norepinephrine content of the spleen and less norepinephrine was released with postganglionic stimulation as well, suggesting that the accumulation of octopamine may have partially replaced norepinephrine at the nerve endings (Kopin et al., 1965). Accumulation of dopamine in the ganglia after MAO inhibition may result in activation of adenylcyclase (Kebabian and Greengard, 1971) and thereby diminish sympathetic ganglion cell responsivity by increasing the negative after-potential interval (Kebabian et al., 1975). Thus both decreased responsivity of ganglion cells and decreased release of norepinephrine at the nerve endings may contribute to the diminished sympathetic reactivity seen after treatment with MAO inhibitors.

Although MAO inhibitors also affect the activity of other enzymes (e.g., drug-metabolizing enzymes, dopamine-β-hydroxylase) their effects on the central nervous system are almost certainly the result of blockade of metabolism of amines. Since metabolism of norepinephrine, dopamine, serotonin, and of several other trace amines (phenylethylamine, tryptamine, octopamine, etc.) is blocked, levels of all of these amines increase in the brain and each has been considered a possible mediator of the effects of MAO inhibitors. Administration of amine precursors to selectively increase the levels of a particular amine has been tried in efforts to determine which amine is responsible for the behavioral effects seen with drugs which interfere with amine storage or metabolism. In animals, administration of the catecholamine precursor, dihydroxyphenylalamine (dopa), or the serotonin precursor, 5-hydroxytryptophan (5-HTP), results in dramatic reversal of the effects of reserpine (Carlsson et al., 1957) and striking hyperactivity after MAO inhibition (e.g., Spector et al., 1963; Grahame-Smith, 1971). Aminergic nerve terminals appear to be dispersed widely in brain and to be involved in control of a myriad of functions (endocrine, cardiovascular, temperature, appetite, motor activity, etc.). No group of neurons operates in isolation and there is interdependency of the various neurotransmitter systems. Alterations in activity of one system are probably reflected in alterations in the activity of others. Thus drugs have multiple secondary effects as well as several primary actions.

The mode of action of MAO inhibitors in alleviating depression in patients probably varies between individuals, depending on the extent of involvement of each of the amine neurotransmitters. There is ample evidence that tryptophan administration may potentiate, at least in some patients, the antidepressant effects of MAO inhibitors (Coppen et al., 1963; Pare, 1963; Glassman and Platman, 1969). The suggestion that serotonin is lacking in some depressed patients has received further support from the observations of van Praag et al. (1973) that the rate of probenecid-induced accumulation in cerebrospinal fluid of 5-hydroxyindole acetic acid (5-HIAA), the major metabolite of serotonin, is diminished in depressed patients. Other investigators have emphasized the importance of catecholamines, particularly of norepinephrine in the pathogenesis of depression (e.g., Schildkraut, 1965; Bunney and Davis, 1965). More recently, however, attempts have been made to distinguish subgroups of depressive patients, based on biochemical criteria, clinical course, and/or pharmacological responses (see e.g., van Praag and Korf, 1971a,b; Maas et al., 1973; Schildkraut, 1973; Bowers and Cohen, 1974; Asberg et al., 1976). Thus, depending on the population studied, the clinical criteria for inclusion in the study, and previous pharmacological therapy, support can be obtained for involvement in depression of catecholamines or of serotonin as the amine which is functionally insufficient. Hypotheses involving either of these amines or implicating other trace amines explain the efficacy of MAO inhibitors in depression by their actions in preventing amine destruction and the consequent overflow of amines onto receptors which are inadequately stimulated in the absence of the enzyme inhibitor. There are other secondary effects of MAO-inhibitor-induced amine accumulation. Thus, diminished synthesis due to feedback inhibition of the rate-limiting enzyme and alterations in responsivity of receptors in the presence of excessive amines have been described (Vetulani et al., 1976), but the role of these effects in antidepressant actions of MAO inhibitors is unknown.

V. TRICYCLIC ANTIDEPRESSANTS

The discovery by Kuhn (1958) that imipramine is useful in alleviating endogenous depressions and the subsequent finding that its metabolite, desmethylimipramine (desipramine), is also a potent antidepressant led to a search for related compounds which might be even more useful clinically. The importance of developing antidepressant drugs led to a search for rapid methods for screening of compounds for antidepressant activity. For this purpose attempts were made to relate the effects of drugs in untreated animals (Irwin, 1962), the antagonism of the behavioral effects of reserpine or tetrabenazine (Costa et al., 1960; Askew, 1963), or the potentiation of the effects of amphetamine (Carlton, 1961) to antidepressant activity.

In such tests, only analogs of antidepressant compounds were usually studied and unrelated substances not tested, so that new entities were not discovered. The tests have, however, resulted in clinical testing of many chemically related compounds and several of these have proven clinically useful. Among these, protryptaline, doxipin, amitryptaline, noritryptaline, and chlorimipramine as well as imipramine and desipramine have been used to treat depression. The chemical structures of these compounds are shown in Figure 2.

A. Effects of Tricyclic Antidepressants on Amine Uptake

At the time that imipramine was introduced by Kuhn (1958) as an antidepressant, pharmacologists had no explanation for its action. Although Sigg (1959) soon demonstrated that imipramine potentiated the effects of sympathetic nerve stimulation, it was not until it was found that termination of the activity of norepinephrine at sympathetic nerve endings depended on reuptake of the released transmitter (Hertting et al., 1961), and until Axelrod et al. (1961) showed that imipramine inhibits this reuptake process, that an explanation of the effects of imipramine could be offered. Tricyclic antidepressants also inhibit uptake of norepinephrine in brain (Glowinski and Axelrod, 1964) but not of dopamine (Carlsson et al., 1966), suggesting that norepinephrine is the more important catecholamine in reversing depressive states. Most antidepressants have some effect in blocking uptake of serotonin as well as that of norepinephrine. The relative efficacy in blocking uptake of the indoleamine appears to be greater for tertiary amines, while the secondary amines seem to be more selective blockers of norepinephrine uptake (Carlsson, 1970; Shashkan and Snyder, 1970). Treatment with drugs which prevent reuptake should enhance effectiveness of released amines by increasing synaptic levels of the neurotransmitter. Norepinephrine regulates its own release by activation of presynaptic α-adrenoreceptors which inhibit further release of the amine (Langer, 1977). There may also be neuronal inhibitory feedback loops which limit adrenergic neuronal activity when excess neurotransmitter is available. The resultant activation of presynaptic α-receptors and postsynaptic receptors may thereby result in compensatory decreases in the rates of neuronal firing and of amine turnover. After acute administration of tricyclic antidepressants, neuronal firing rates and amine turnover are reduced in both adrenergic and serotonergic neurons (see Sheard et al., 1972). This compensatory diminution in aminergic activity may explain why these drugs do not greatly alter behavior in animals or in normal subjects and are excitants only when there is a rapid, pharmacologically-induced release of amines (Sulser et al., 1964). The onset of antidepressant actions in patients is delayed, so that acute effects may not entirely explain the antidepressant efficacy of the drugs. Schildkraut et al. (1971) showed that chronic administration of imipramine increases, rather than reduces, turnover of norepinephrine, although inhibition of norepinephrine uptake persists.

Pharmacological bases for these observations have been provided recently by the demonstration that chronic treatment with antidepressants is attended by changes in receptor sensitivity. Crews and Smith (1978) demonstrated that subsensitivity of autoregulation of presynaptic α receptors diminishes after rats are treated with desmethylimipramine for 3 weeks and suggested that the increase in norepinephrine release caused by this deficit in autoregulation is important in the action of tricyclic antidepressants. Wolfe et al. (1978) and Sarai et al. (1978) showed that chronic treatment with desmethylimipramine resulted in a diminution of β-receptor density and decrease isoproterenol activation of adenylcyclase. If β receptors mediate the neuronal circuits which may exert a negative feedback on adrenergic neurons, decreased β-receptor sensitivity might also play a role in enhancing release of norepeinephrine. The increase in availability of norepinephrine as a result of these chronic effects of tricyclic antidepressants may account for the delay in onset of therapeutic effects.

On the basis of the selective effects of chlorimipramine on serotonin uptake and the potentiation of antidepressant effects of drugs by tryptophan, Carlsson (1976) made a strong case for the role of serotonin, as well as norepinephrine, in depressive illnesses. As indicated above, different subgroups of patients may respond differently, depending on a number of factors. Furthermore, it is becoming increasingly clear that antidepressant effects may also be mediated by actions not involving alterations in amine metabolism or uptake.

B. Other Actions of Tricyclic Antidepressants

In addition to their effects on catecholamine uptake, the tricyclic antidepressants diminish parasympathetic activity by a central action (Sulser et al., 1964). Neither atropine nor serotonin antagonists reverse the effects of reserpine (Sigg et al., 1965), and it appears unlikely that the central antimuscarinic actions of these antidepressants can be related to their behavioral effects in reserpine-pretreated animals (Valliant, 1969) or in patients (Blackwell et al., 1972).

Until relatively recently it was believed that "all drugs or treatments that modify depression or mania have significant effects on the metabolism of norepinephrine" (Byck, 1975a). This rule appears to have been broken by iprindole (Fig. 1). Iprindole is an effective antidepressant (Hicks, 1965; Johnson and Maden, 1967; Ayd, 1969) but does not inhibit uptake of [^{3}H]NE in the heart or brain (Gluckman and Baum, 1969; Lahti and Maickel, 1971; Freeman and Sulser, 1972) and does not alter norepinephrine turnover or uptake, even when given chronically (Rosloff and Davis, 1974). Furthermore, iprindole could not be shown to alter serotonin metabolism in mouse brain (Sanghri and Gershon, 1975). Clearly inhibition of amine uptake is not a necessary feature of antidepressant activity.

Until relatively recently attention had been directed toward presynaptic events, but during the last few years methods for assessing biochemically the activity and density of adrenergic receptors have been developed. In brain, as well as in peripheral organs, activation of adenyl cyclase often attends activation of receptors (Robison et al., 1969) and cyclic AMP has been implicated in aminergic transmission in brain (see Siggins et al., 1973). Recently Vetulani et al. (1976) reported that chronic (but not short-term) treatment with iprindole, as well as with desmethylimipramine, reduced the sensitivity to norepinephrine of the cyclic AMP generating system in rat limbic forebrain. The effects were unrelated to levels of the drug in brain at the time of assay, suggesting there were adaptive changes in the receptor. While it would be convenient to attempt to explain this apparent change in receptor sensitivity by suggesting that chronic exposure to excess catecholamines was responsible, as in the case for the pineal gland (Deguchi and Axelrod, 1973), the fact that iprindole also had this affect makes this explanation untenable since this drug does not influence amine disposition or metabolism. Furthermore, this explanation of the antidepressant activity of drugs would be valid only if depression were associated with increased sensitivity of receptors or a relative excess of norepinephrine, which is the opposite of the usual amine hypothesis of depression (see Schildkraut, 1965, 1973).

VI. AMPHETAMINE

Sympathomimetic drugs, such as amphetamine (Fig. 1), methamphetamine, and ephedrine, which are able to pass the blood-brain barrier, act as powerful central stimulants. Amphetamine is the prototype of these drugs and has been studied most intensely. It produces a wide variety of effects which depend on the route and dose administered, the state of the patient, and the time after administration. In moderate doses (10-20 mg) the more active D isomer has a euphoriant effect, diminishes fatigue, and enhances motor activity (Weiss and Laties, 1962). Higher doses have deleterious effects on mood and may produce extremes of hyperactivity (see below), while chronic use may result in a state clinically indistinguishable from schizophrenia. In animals, the characteristic changes in behavior produced by amphetamine are easily quantified. In rats, doses in the range of 1.5 mg/kg produce persistent increases in motor activity while somewhat higher doses (5 mg/kg) results in a syndrome of sniffing, rearing, licking, biting, and gnawing which has been termed stereotypy (Randrup and Munkvad, 1966). Repetitive motor activity seen in patients who have taken large doses of amphetamine over prolonged periods have been described as "punding" by Rylander (1969).

Explanations for the molecular pharmacological basis of the effects of amphetamine have centered on the interactios of the drug with biogenic amines in brain. The obvious chemical structural resemblance of amphetamine and phenylethylamine at first led to the suggestion by Gaddum and Kwiatkowski (1938) that amphetamine acted by competing with epinephrine and monoamine oxidase and for receptors. After norepinephrine was discovered to be the neurotransmitter at peripheral sympathetic nerve endings, evidence accumulated that it was also a neurotransmitter in brain. Amphetamine was found to stimulate release of both dopamine and norepinephrine and to inhibit termination of their action by blocking uptake into the presynaptic neurons (see review by Glowinski and Baldessarini, 1966). The involvement of norepinephrine in the actions of amphetamine has been supported by observations that drugs which selectively deplete or antagonize norepinephrine inhibit the motility stimulated by amphetamine. During the last decade, however, dopamine has received increasing attention in explaining the effects of amphetamine (Scheel-Krüger and Randrup, 1967; Taylor and Snyder, 1970; Creese and Iversen, 1972). There appears to be some regional specificity in brain for the responses to amphetamine. Pijnenburg and van Rossum (1973) found that injection of dopamine into the nucleus accumbens stimulates locomotor activity. Injection of haloperidol into this nucleus blocked amphetamine-induced locomotor activity (Pijnenburg et al., 1975). Kelly et al. (1975) reported that in rats, 6-OH-dopamine-induced lesions in the nucleus accumbens septi prevent the locomotor, rearing, and sniffing responses to 1.5 mg/kg of amphetamine while enhancing these responses to apomorphine. These observations suggest that dopaminergic neurons in the nucleus accumbens mediate the locomotor and exploratory responses to amphetamine and that destruction of these neurons is followed by the development of supersensitivity of the dopaminergic receptors. Kelly et al. (1975) also found that lesions in the caudate nucleus blocked the stereotopic responses to 5 mg/kg amphetamine, while lesions of the dorsal or ventral noradrenergic pathways had no effect. These are typical of a number of studies in which brain lesions have altered selectively amphetamine-induced behavioral changes. Many of these responses share the property of being attentuated by drugs, such as haloperidol, which block dopaminergic receptors and are produced by apomorphine which stimulates dopaminergic receptors. Thus dopaminergic neurons in different areas of brain are involved in the diverse effects of amphetamine.

The possible role of norepinephrine in mediating some of the amphetamine-induced behavioral changes which were suggested in early studies (see review by Glowinski and Baldessarini, 1966) have not been excluded. Stein and Wise (1973) summarized the evidence that norepinephrine is involved in mediating the enhanced "reward" responses in self-stimulating rats. Lal and Sourkes

(1972) reported that lithium did not alter amphetamine-induced stereotypy or excitation in rats, but in humans the euphoriant and antidepressant effects of amphetamine are attenuated by lithium treatment (Flemenbaum, 1974; van Kammen and Murphy, 1975). These results are compatible with the notion that the euphoriant, and perhaps alerting, effects of amphetamine are mediated by noradrenergic neurons, while the motor system effects involve dopaminergic neurons.

Amphetamine also releases serotonin from some areas of brain (Azzaro and Rutledge, 1973; Moore et al., 1977) and depletion of serotonin produced by blockade of tryptophan hydroxylase (with p-chlorophenylalanine) potentiates markedly the locomotor activity produced by the drug (Breese et al., 1974). This potentiation of the locomotor effects of amphetamine is reversed by administration of 5-hydroxytryptophan.

Stein and Wise (1975) have attempted to relate this action to the punishment-enhancing effects of amphetamine. The hyperthermia seen after amphetamine may also be related to release of serotonin. These observations are consistent with the accumulating evidence (see Cools, 1975) that dopamine-mediated and serotonin-mediated behavioral states may be interdependent.

Changes in responses after repeated doses of amphetamine may be related to alterations in levels of enzymes concerned with biosynthesis of the amines or with alterations in the receptor sensitivity. Clearly, the relatively nonspecific nature of the interaction of amphetamine with various enzymes, amine binding and transport sites, and aminergic receptors lead to a myriad of effects which are mediated by both direct and indirect acctions.

VII. COCAINE

Cocaine has been known as a central stimulant and local anesthetic for over a century. Its early history has been reviewed by Byck (1975b) and the available information on the effects of cocaine have been summarized by Woods and Downs (1974). Cocaine produces an intense euphoria and has been tried as an antidepressant, first by Freud (see Byck, 1975b) and more recently by Post et al. (1974). Cocaine has multiple actions in the peripheral as well as central nervous systems. It inhibits the uptake of amines into peripheral sympathetic nerves (Hertting et al., 1961) and this action has been used to explain its actions in potentiating the actions of norepinephrine in the synapse while preventing the action of indirectly acting sympathomimetics, such as tyramine. The central actions of cocaine result in stimulation of the sympathoadrenal medullary system, particularly of the adrenal medulla, so that it causes levels of epinephrine to increase in plasma while other blockers of uptake, such as desmethylimipramine, do not have this effect (Chiueh and Kopin, unpublished observations). Although cocaine inhibits uptake of norepinephrine in brain slices, this effect could not be demonstrated when [^{3}H]norepinephrine was injected intraventricularly (see Glowinski and Baldessarini, 1966).

The resemblance of the effects of large doses of cocaine to those of amphetamine supported the view that dopaminergic mechanisms are important in cocaine-induced hypermotility (van Rossum and Hurkman, 1964). Confirmation of this hypothesis has been obtained in several studies in which cocaine has been studied along with amphetamine. Pijnenburg et al. (1975) found that administration into the nucleus accumbens of haloperidol blocked the locomotor effects of cocaine as well as of amphetamine, and Kelly et al. (1975) showed that lesions of the substantia nigra block the locomotor response to both drugs.

Cocaine is less effective than amphetamine in releasing newly formed [^{3}H]dopamine into perfusates from the cat cerebral ventricle (Moore et al., 1977), suggesting that differences in potency at particular sites may account for differences in the effects of cocaine and amphetamine. The mode of action of cocaine in promoting release may inolve its local anesthetic action as well as its ability to inhibit amine uptake. Blockade of inhibitory neurons could have the same effects as direct stimualtion of dopamine release, particularly if the mechanisms for reuptake of the released transmitter were also blocked. Thus, although cocaine-induced hypermotility involves dopaminergic neurons, its effect could be indirectly mediated by an action at a neuronal system which normally inhibits dopaminergic neurons. The euphoriant and other effects of cocaine could be mediated by norepinephrine or other (? peptide) neurotransmitters.

VIII. OTHER CENTRAL STIMULANTS

There is an enormous literature devoted to the pharmacology of drugs which in high doses produce central excitation, tremors, and other abnormal movements, and convulsions. Some, such as methylphenidate, appear to act by mechanisms similar to those of cocaine and amphetamine and produce similar stereotypic effects. Apomorphine acts directly on dopamine receptors to produce these effects and inhibition of the chewing and hyperactivity produced by this drug and amphetamine were used by Janssen et al. (1965) to identify haloperidol and other compounds with possible neuroleptic activity. In addition to drugs which act directly on dopaminergic mechanisms, there are a host of agents which at certain doses act as central stimulants. Local anesthetics, particularly those, such as lidocaine, which are not rapidly metabolized, may produce central excitation, presumably by blockade of inhibitor neurons. Excitation is seen in stage 2 of anesthesia. Anticholinesterases which can penetrate into brain (eserine and organophosphorus compounds) cause stimulation followed by depression. Moderate overdoses of cholinolytic compounds (scopolamine, atropine) may also produce central stimulation resulting in restlessness, tremor, and incoordinations. Little is known of the mechanisms by which these diverse agents produce excitation, but the types of central stimulation seen are not suggestive of the more specific syndromes produced by amphetamine, cocaine, and apomorphine, and it is clearly beyond the scope of this review to do more than make mention of them and to contrast them with the central stimulants which appear to interact more directly and specifically with the biogenic amines.

IX. CONCLUSIONS

Antidepressant drugs include two major groups: inhibitors of monoamine oxidase and tricyclics. While there is a considerable body of evidence that the mode of action of these drugs involves their effects of biogenic amine metabolism on disposition, more recently it has become apparent that receptor mechanisms may also be important. The delay in therapeutic efficacy of these drugs suggests that adaptive changes are involved in their mode of action and in normal subjects these drugs have only minimal effects.

The central stimulants amphetamine, cocaine, and related compounds have striking effects on behavior, produce euphoria, and are subject to abuse. The mechanisms of action of these drugs appear to involve dopamine, but other biogenic amines are also affected. There are differences in the effects of even closely related compounds which may be attributed to differences in their distribution and affinities for specific molecular sites and efficacy in altering processes of neurotransmission at multiple sites in brain. Clearly a great deal more information about the actions of these drugs on specific neurons in different regions of brain is needed before all of their effects can be explained at molecular, neurophysiological, and behavioral levels.

REFERENCES

Anchor, R. W. P., Hanson, N. O., and Gifford, R. W., Jr. (1955). Hypertension treated with *Rauwolfia serpentina* (whole root) and with reserpine. *J. Am. Med. Assoc. 159,* 841-845.

Asberg, M., Thoren, P., Traskman, L., Bertilsson, L., and Ringberger, V. (1976). Serotonin depression. A biochemical subgroup within the affective disorders? *Science 191,* 478-480.

Askew, B. M. (1963). A simple screening procedure for imipramine-like antidepressant agents. *Life Sci. 10,* 725-730.

Axelrod, J. (1975). Metabolism and inactivation of noradrenaline and adrenaline and the effect of drugs. In *Pharmacology of Cholinergic and Adrenergic Transmission,* G. B. Koelle, W. W. Douglas, and A. Carlsson (Eds.). Pergamon, Oxford, pp. 205-220.

Axelrod, J., Whitby, L. G., and Hertting, G. (1961). Effect of psychotropic drugs on the uptake of H^3-norepinephrine by tissues. *Science 133,* 383-384.

Ayd, F. J., Jr. (1969). Clinical evaluation of a new tricyclic antidepressant iprinodole. *Dis. Nerv. Sys. 30,* 818-823.

Azzaro, A. J., and Rutledge, C. O. (1973). Selectivity of release of norepinephrine, dompamine, and 5-hydroxy tryptamine in various regions of rat brain. *Biochem. Pharmacol. 22,* 2801-2813.

Bein, H. J. (1956). The pharmacology of *Rauwolfia. Pharmacol. Rev. 8,* 435-483.

Blackwell, B., Marley, E., Price, J., and Taylor, D. (1967). Hypertensive interactions between monoamine oxidase inhibitors and foodstuffs. *Br. J. Psychiatry 113,* 349-365.

Blackwell, B., Lipkin, J. O., Meyer, J. H., Kuzma, R., and Boulter, W. V. (1972). Dose responses and relationships between anticholinergic activity and mood with tricyclic antidepressants. *Psychopharmacologia* (Berlin) *25,* 205-217.

Bloom, B. M. (1963). Some structural considerations regarding compounds that influence monoamine metabolism. *Ann. N.Y. Acad. Sci. 107,* 878-890.

Bogdanski, D. F., Weissbach, H., and Udenfriend, S. (1957). The distribution of serotonin, 5-hydroxytryptophan decarboxylase and monamine oxidase in brain. *J. Neurochem. 1,* 272-278.

Bowers, M. B.,and Cohen, A. (1974). (Cited in Bowers, M. B.) Lumbar CSF 5-hydroxyindoleacetic acid and homovanillic acid in affective syndromes. *J. Nerv. Ment. Dis. 158,* 325-330.

Breese, G. R., Cooper, B. R., and Mueller, R. A. (1974). Evidence for involvement of 5-hydroxytryptamine in the actions of amphetamine. *Br. J. Pharmacol. 52,* 307-314.

Bunney, W. E., Jr., and Davis, J. M. (1965). Norepinephrine in depressive reactions. A review. *Arch. Gen. Psychiatry 13,* 483-494.

Byck, R. (1975a). Drugs and the treatment of psychiatric disorders. In *The Pharmacological Basis of Therapeutics,* L. S. Goodman and A. Gilman (Eds.). MacMillan, New York.

Byck, R. (1975b). *Cocaine Papers: Sigmund Freud.* Stonehill, New York.

Carlsson, A. (1959). The occurrence, distribution, and phsyiological role of catecholamines in the nervous system. *Pharmacol. Rev. 11,* 490-493.

Carlsson, A. (1970). Structural specificity for inhibition of ^{14}C-5-hydroxytryptamine uptake by cerebral slices. *J. Pharm. Pharmacol. 22,* 729-732.

Carlsson, A. (1976). The contribution of drug research to investigating the nature of endogenous depression. *Pharmakopsychiatrie 9,* 2-10.

Carlsson, A., Lindqvist, M., and Magnusson, T. (1957). 3,4-Dihydroxyphenylalanine and 5-hydroxytryptophan as reserpine antagonists. *Nature* (London) *180,* 1200.

Carlsson, A., Fuxe, K., Hamberger, B., and Lindqvist, M. (1966). Biochemical and histochemical studies on the effects of imipramine-like drugs and (+)-amphetamine on central and peripheral catecholamine neurons. *Acta Physiol. Scand. 67,* 481-497.

Carlton, P. L. (1961). Potentiation of the behavioral effects of amphetamine by imipramine. *Psychopharmacologia 2,* 364-367.

Chuang, H. Y. K., Patek, D. R., and Hellerman, L. (1974). Mitochondrial monoamine oxidase. Inactivation by pargyline. Adduct formation. *J. Biol. Chem. 249,* 2381-2384.

Cools, A. R. (1975). An integrated theory of the etiology of schizophrenia. Impairment of the balance between certain in series connected, dopaminergic, serotonergic, and noradrenergic pathways within the brain. In *Symposium on Schizophrenia, Biological and Behavioral Aspects.* International Society of Biological Psychiatry, Amsterdam.

Coppen, A., Shaw, D. M., and Farrell, J. P. (1963). Potentiation of antidepressive effect of a monoamine-oxidase inhibitor by tryptophan. *Lancet 1,* 79-81.

Costa, E., Garattini, S., and Valzelli, L. (1960). Interactions between reserpine, chlorpromazine, and imipramine. *Experientia 16,* 461-463.

Crane, G. E. (1957). Iproniazid (Marsilid) phosphate. A therapeutic agent for mental disorders and debilitating diseases. Psychiatry research. *Rep. Am. Psychiatry Assoc. 8,* 142-152.

Creese, I., and Iversen, S. D. (1972). Amphetamine response after dopamine neurone destruction. *Nature (New Biology) 238,* 247-248.

Crews, F. T., and Smith, C. B. (1978). Presynaptic alpha-receptor subsensitivity after long term antidepressant treatment. *Science 202,* 322-324.

Deguchi, T., and Axelrod, J. (1973). Supersensitivity and subsensitivity of β-adrenergic receptor in pineal gland regulated by catecholamine transmitter. *Proc. Natl. Acad. Sci.* (USA) *70,* 2411-2414.

Flemenbaum, A. (1974). Does lithium block the effects of amphetamine? A report of three cases. *Am. J. Psychiatry 131,* 7.

Freeman, J. J., and Sulser, F. (1972). Iprindole-amphetamine interactions in the rat. The role of aromatic hydroxylation of amphetamine in its mode of action. *J. Pharmacol. Exp. Ther. 183,* 307-315.

Gaddum, J. N., and Kwiatkowski, H. (1938). The action of ephedrine. *J. Physiol. 94,* 87-100.

Gärtner, B., and Hemmerich, P. (1975). Inhibition of monoamine oxidase by propargylamine. Structure of the inhibitor complex. *Angewandte Chem. Int.* English Ed. *14,* 110-111.

Gessa, G. L., Cuenca, E., and Costa, E. (1963). On the mechanism of hypotensive effects of MAO inhibitors. *Ann. N.Y. Acad. Sci. 107*, 935-944.

Glassman, A. M., and Platman, S. R. (1969). Potentiation of a monoamine oxidase inhibitor by tryptophan. *J. Psychiatr. Res. 7*, 83-88.

Glowinski, J., and Axelrod, J. (1964). Inhibition of uptake of tritiated noradrenaline in the intact rat brain by imipramine and structurally related compounds. *Nature 204*, 1318-1319.

Glowinski, J., and Baldessarini, R. J. (1966). Metabolism of norepinephrine in the central nervous system. *Pharmacol. Rev. 18*, 1201-1238.

Gluckman, M. I., and Baum, T. (1969). The pharmacology of iprindole, a new antidepressant. *Psychopharmacology 15*, 169-185.

Goldberg, L. L., and DaCosta, I. M. (1960). Selective depression of sympathetic transmission by intravenous administration of iproniazid and harmine. *Proc. Soc. Exp. Biol. Med. 105*, 223-227.

Grahme-Smith, D. G. (1971). Studies in vivo on the relationship between brain tryptophan brain 5-HT synthesis and hyperactivity in rats treated with a monoamine oxidase inhibitor and L-tryptophan. *J. Neurochem. 18*, 1953-1066.

Hellerman, L., and Erwin, V. G. (1968). Mitochondrial monoamine oxidase. II. Action of various inhibitors for the bovine kidney enzyme. Catalytic mechanism. *J. Biol. Chem. 243*, 5234-5243.

Hertting, G., Axelrod, J., Kopin, I. J., and Whitby, L. G. (1961). Lack of uptake of catecholamines after chronic denervation of sympathetic nerves. *Nature* (London) *169*, 66.

Hertting, G., Axelrod, J., and Patrick, R. W. (1961). Actions of cocaine and tyramine on the uptake and release of H^3-norepinephrine in the heart. *Biochem. Pharmacol. 8*, 246-247.

Hicks, J. T. (1965). Iprindole, a new antidepressant for use in general office practice. A double-blind, placebo-controlled study. *Ill. Med. J. 128*, 622-626.

Houslay, M. D., and Tipton, K. F. (1973). The nature of the electrophoretically separable multiple forms of rat liver monoamine oxidase. *Biochem. J. 135*, 173-186.

Houslay, M. D., and Tipton, K. F. (1975). Amine competition for oxidation by rat liver mitochondrial monoamine oxidase. *Biochem. Pharmacol. 24*, 627-631.

Irwin, S. (1962). Drug screening and evaluation procedures. *Science 136*, 123-128.

Janssen, P. A., Niemegeers, C. J. E., Schellekens, K. H. L., and Leanaerts, F. M. (1965). Is it possible to predict the clinical effects of neuroleptic drugs (major tranquillizers) from animal data? *Arz. Forsch. 15*, 841-854.

Johnson, J., and Maden, J. G. (1967). A new antidepressant pramindole (WY-3263). A double-blind controlled trial. *J. Clin. Trials 4,* 787-791.

Johnston, J. P. (1968). Some observations upon a new inhibitor of monoamine oxidase in brain tissue. *Biochem. Pharmacol. 17,* 1285-1297.

Kallmann, F.J. (1953). *Heredity in health and mental disorders: Principles of psychiatric genetics in the light of comparative twin studies.* W. W. Norton, New York.

Katz, B., and Miledi, R. (1965). The quantal release of transmitter substances. In *Studies in Physiology,* D. R. Curtis and A. K. McIntyre (Eds.). Springer, New York, pp. 118-125.

Kebabian, J. W., and Greengard, P. (1971). Dopamine-sensitive adenyl cyclase. Possible role in synaptic transmission. *Science 174,* 1346-1349.

Kebabian, J. W., Steiner, A. L., and Greengard, P. (1975). Muscarinic cholinergic regulation of cyclic guanosine 3′,5′ monophosphate in autonomic ganglia. Possible role in synaptic transmission. *J. Pharmacol. 193,* 474-488.

Kelly, P. H., Seviour, P. W., and Iversen, S. D. (1975). Amphetamine and apomorphine responses in the rat following 6-OHDA lesions of the nucleus accumbens septi and corpus striatum. *Brain Res. 94,* 507-522.

Knoll, J., and Magyar, K. (1972). Some puzzling pharmacological effects of monoamine oxidase inhibitors. In *Monoamine Oxidases: New Vistas,* E. Costa and M. Sandler (Eds.). Advances in Biochemical Psychopharmacology, 5, Raven, New York and North-Holland, Amsterdam, pp. 393-408.

Knoll, J., Ecseri, Z., Kelemen, K., Nievel, J. G., and Knoll, B. (1965). Phenylisopropylmethylpropinylamine (E-250). A new spectrum psychic energizer. *Arch. Int. Pharmacodyn. Ther. 155,* 154-164.

Kopin, I. J. (1967). The adrenergic synapse. In *The Neurosciences: A Study Program,* G. C. Quarton, T. Melnechuk, and F. O. Schmitt (Eds.). Rockefeller University Press, New York.

Kopin, I. J., Fischer, J. E., Musacchio, J. M., Horst, W. D., and Weise, V. K. (1965). False neurochemical transmitters and the mechanism of sympathetic blockade by monoamine oxidase inhibitors. *J. Pharmacol. Exp. Ther. 147,* 186-193.

Kuhn, R. (1958). The treatment of depressive states with G22355 (imipramine hydrochloride). *Am. J. Psychiatry 115,* 459-464.

Lahti, R. A., and Maickel, R. P. (1971). The tricyclic antidepressants. Inhibition of norepinephrine uptake as related to potentiation of norepinephrine and clinical efficacy. *Biochem. Pharmacol. 20,* 482-486.

Lal, S., and Sourkes, T. L. (1972). Potentiation and inhibition of the amphetamine stereotypy in rats by neuroleptics and other agents. *Arch. Int. Pharmacodyn. Ther. 199,* 289-301.

Langer, Z. (1977). Presynaptic receptors and their role in the regulation of transmitter release. *Br. J. Pharmacol. 60,* 481-497.

Lemieux, G., Davignon, A., and Genest, J. (1956). Depressive states during *Rauwolfia* therapy for arterial hypertension. A report of 30 cases. *Can. Med. Assoc. J. 74,* 522-526.

Loomer, H. P., Saunders, J. C., and Kline, N. S. (1957). A clinical and pharmacodynamic evaluation of iproniazid as a psychic energizer. *Psychiatr. Res. Rep., Am. Psychiatr. Assoc. 8,* 129-141.

Maas, J. W., Kekirmenkian, H., and Jones, F. (1973). The identification of depressed patients who have a disorder of NE metabolism and/or disposition. In *Frontiers in Catecholamine Research,* E. Usdin and S. Snyder (Eds.). Pergamon, New York, pp. 1091-1096.

Marrazzi, A. S. (1939). Adrenergic inhibition at sympathetic synapses. *Am. J. Physiol. 127,* 738-744.

Maycock, A., Abeles, R. H., Salach, J. I., and Singer, T. P. (1976). Structure of the flavin-inhibitor adduct from monoamine oxidase. *Biochemistry 15,* 114-125.

Moore, K. E., Chiueh, C. C., and Zeldes, G. (1977). Release of neurotransmitters from the brain in vivo by amphetamine, methylphenidate, and cocaine. In *Cocaine and Other Stimulants. Advances in Behavioral Biology,* Vol. 21, E. H. Ellinwood and M. M. Kilbey (Eds.). Plenum, New York, pp. 143-160.

Muller, J. C., Pryer, W. W., Gibbons, J. E., and Orgain, E. S. (19955). Depression and anxiety occurring during *Rauwolfia* therapy. *J. Am. Med. Assoc. 159,* 836-839.

Neff, N. H., and Goridis, C. (1972). Neuronal monoamine oxidase. Specific enzyme types and their rates of formation. In *Monoamine Oxidases: New Vistas,* E. Costa and M. Sandler (Eds.). Advances in Biochemical Psychopharmacology. Raven, New York, and North-Holland, Amsterdam.

Pare, C. M. B. (1963). Potentiation of monoamine-xoidase inhibitors by tryptophan. *Lancet 2,* 527-528.

Pijnenburg, A. J. J., and van Rossum, J. M. (1973). Stimulation of locomotor activity following injection of dopamine into the nucleus accumbens. *J. Pharm. Pharmacol. 25,* 1003-1105.

Pijenburg, A. J. J., Honig, W. M. H., and van Rossum, J. M. (1975). Inhibition of D-amphetamine-induced locomotor activity by injection of haloperidol into the nucleus accumbens of rats. *Psychopharmacologia* (Berlin) *41,* 87-95.

Post, R. M., Kotin, J., and Goodwin, F. K. (1974). The effects of cocaine on depressed patients. *Am. J. Psychiatry 131,* 511-517.

Puig, M., Wakade, A. R., and Kirpekar, S. M. (1972). Effect on the sympathetic nervous system of chronic treatment with pargyline and L-dopa. *J. Pharmacol. Exp. Ther. 182*, 130-134.

Quetsch, R. M., Anchor, R. W. P., Litin, E. M., and Faucett, R. L. (1959). Depressive reactions in hypertensive patients. A comparison of those treated with *Rauwolfia* and those receiving no specific antihypertensive treatment. *Circulation 19*, 366-375.

Randrup, A. and Munkvad, J. (1966). Role of catecholamines in the amphetamine excitatory response. *Nature 211*, 540-541.

Robison, G. A., Butcher, R. W., and Sutherland, E. W. (1969). On the relation of hormone receptors to adenyl cyclase. In *Fundamental Concepts in Drug-Receptor Interactions,* J. F. Danielli, J. F. Moran, and D. J. Triggle (Eds.). Academic, New York, pp. 59-91.

Rosloff, B. N., and Davis, J. M. (1974). Effect of iprindole on norepinephrine turnover and transport. *Psychopharmacologia* (Berlin) *40*, 53-64.

Rylander, G. (1969). Clinical and medico-criminological aspects of addictions to central stimulant drugs. In *Abuse of Central Stimulants,* F. Sjoqvist and M. Totler (Eds.). Raven, New York, pp. 251-253.

Sanghri, I., and Gershon, S. (1975). Effect of acute and chronic iprindole on serotonin turnover in mouse brain. *Biochem. Pharmacol. 24*, 2103-2104.

Sarai, K., Frazer, A., Brunswick, D., and Mendels, J. (1978). Desmethylimipramine-induced decrease in β-adrenergic receptor binding in rat cerebral cortex. *Biochem. Pharmacol. 27*, 2179-2181.

Scheel-Krüger, J., and Randrup, A. (1967). Stereotype hyperactive behavior produced by dopamine in the absence of norepinephrine. *Life Sci. 6*, 1389-1394.

Schildkraut, J. J. (1965). The catecholamine hypothesis of affective disorders. A review of supporting evidence. *Am. J. Psychiatry 122*, 509-522.

Schildkraut, J. J. (1973). Catecholamine metabolism and affective disorders. Studies of MHPG excretion. In *Frontiers in Catecholamine Research,* E. Usdin and S. Snyder (Eds.). Pergamon, New York, pp. 1165-1171.

Schildkraut, J. J., Winokur, A., Drasóczy, P. R., and Hensle, J. H. (1971). Changes in norepinephrine turnover in rat brain during chronic administration of imipramine and protryptaline: A possible explanation for the delay in onset of clinical antidepressant effects. *Am. J. Psychiatry 12*, 1032-1039.

Shashkan, E. G., and Snyder, S. H. (1970). Kinetics of serotonin accumulation into slices from rat brain, relation to catecholamine uptake. *J. Pharmacol. Exp. Ther. 175*, 404-418.

Sheard, M. H., Zolovick, A., and Aghajanian, G. K. (1972). Raphe neurons. Effect of tricyclic antidepressant drugs. *Brain Res. 43*, 690-694.

Shore, P. A. (1962). Release of serotonin and catecholamines by drugs. *Pharmacol. Rev. 14*, 531-550.

Sigg, E. B. (1959). Pharmacological studies with Tofranil. *Can. Psychiatr. Assoc. J. 45,* 75-85.

Sigg, E. B., Gyermek, L., and Hill, R. T. (1965). Antagonism to reserpine induced depression by imipramine, related psychoactive drugs, and some autonomic agents. *Psychopharmacologia 7,* 144-149.

Siggins, G. R., Battenberg, E. F., Hoffer, B. J., Bloom, F. E., and Steiner, A. L. (1973). Noradrenergic stimulation of cyclic adenosine monophosphate in rat Purkinje neurons. An immunocytochemical study. *Science 179,* 585-588.

Spector, S. (1953). Monoamine oxidase in control of brain serotonin and norepinephrine content. *Ann. N.Y. Acad. Sci. 107,* 856-864.

Spector, S., Hirsch, C. W., and Brodie, B. B. (1963). Association of behavioral effects of pargyline, a non-hydrazine MAO inhibitor with increase in brain norepinephrine, *Int. J. Neuropharmacol. 2,* 81-93.

Squires, R. F. (1972). Multiple forms of monoamine oxidase in intact mitochondria as characterized by selective inhibitors and thermal stability. A comparison of eight mammalian species. In *Monoamine Oxidases: New Vistas,* Vol. 5, E. Costa and M. Sandler (Eds.). Advances in Biochemical Psychopharmacology, Raven, New York, and North-Holland, Amsterdam, pp. 355-370.

Squires, R. F., and Lassen, J. B. (1975). Inhibition of both A and B forms of MAO required for production of characteristic behavioural syndrome in rats after tryptophan loading. *Psychopharmacologia 41,* 145-151.

Stein, L., and Wise, C. I. (1973). Amphetamine and noradrenergic reward pathways. In *Frontiers in Catecholamine Research,* E. Usdin and S. H. Snyder (Eds.). Pergamon, New York, pp. 963-968.

Sulser, F., Bickel, M. H., and Brodie, B. B. (1964). The actions of desmethylimipramine in counteracting sedation and cholinergic effects of reserpine-like drugs. *J. Pharmacol. Exp. Ther. 144,* 321-329.

Taylor, K. M., and Snyder, S. H. (1970). Amphetamine. Differentiation by d- and l-isomers of behavior involving brain norepinephrine or dopamine. *Science 168,* 1487-1489.

Tipton, K. F. (1971). Monoamine oxidases and their inhibitors. In *Mechanisms of Toxicity,* W. N. Aldridge (Ed.). MacMillan, London, pp. 13-27.

Tipton, K. F. (1975). Monoamine oxidase. In *Handbook of Physiology,* Sec. 7: *Endocrinology,* Vol. 6: *Adrenal Gland.* H. K. F. Blaschko and A. D. Smith (Eds.). American Physiological Society, Washington, D.C., pp. 667-691.

Valiant, G. E. (1969). Clinical significance of anticholinergic effects of imipramine-like drugs. *Am. J. Psychology 125,* 1600-1602.

van Kammen, D. P., and Murphy, D. L. (1975). Attenuation of the euphoriant and activating effects of d- and l-amphetamine by lithium carbonate. *Psychopharmacologia, 44,* 215-224.

van Praag, H. M., and Korf, J. (1971a). Retarded depression and the dopamine metabolism. *Psychopharmacologia 19,* 199-203.

van Praag, H. M., and Korf, J. (1971b). Endogenous depressions with and without disturbances in the 5-hydroxytryptamine metabolism: a biochemical classification? *Psychopharmacologia 19,* 148-152.

van Praag, H. M., Korf, J., and Schut, T. (1973). Cerebral monoamines and depression. An investigation with the probenecid technique. *Arch. Gen. Psychiatry 28,* 827-831.

van Rossum, J. M., and Hurkman, J. A. T. M. (1964). The mechanism of action of psychomotor stimulant drugs. *Int. J. Neuropharmacol. 3,* 227-239.

Vetulani, J., Stawartz, R. J., and Sulser, F. (1976). Adaptive mechanisms in the noradrenergic cyclic AMP generating system in limbic forebrain of the rat. Adaptation to persistent changes in the availability of norepinephrine. *J. Neurochem. 27,* 661-666.

Vogt, M. (1954). Concentration of sympathin in different parts of central nervous system under normal conditions and after administration of drugs. *J. Physiol. 123,* 451-481.

von Euler, U. S. (1948). Identification of the sympathomimetic ergone in adrenergic nerves of cattle (sympathin N) with laeva-noradrenaline. *Acta Physiol. Scand. 16,* 63-74.

Weiss, B., and Laties, V. G. (1962). Enhancement of human performance by caffeine and the amphetamines. *Pharmacol. Rev. 14,* 1-36.

Wolfe, B. B., Harden, T. K., Sporn, J. R., and Molinoff, P. B. (1978). Presynaptic modulation of β-adrenergic receptor in rat cerebral cortex after treatment with antidepressants. *J. Pharmacol. Exp. Ther. 207,* 446-457.

Woods, J. H., and Downs, D. A. (1974). The Psychopharmacology of Cocaine. Prepared for the National Commission on Marihuana and Drug Abuse.

Youdim, M. B. H. (1973). Multiple forms of mitochondrial monoamine oxidase. *Br. Med. Bull. 29,* 120-122.

Zeller, E. A., and Barsky, J. (1952) In vivo inhibition of liver and brain monoamine oxidase by 1-isonicotinyl-2-isopropylhydrazine. *Proc. Soc. Exp. Biol. Med. 81,* 459-461.

22

Mode of Action of Neuroleptic Drugs

Giuseppe Bartholini
Synthélabo–L.E.R.S.
Paris, France

I. INTRODUCTION

Compounds utilized in the treatment of schizophrenia are referred to as neuroleptic drugs. "Neuroleptic," however, often refers to the neurologic syndromes evoked by these agents rather than to their therapeutic action. "Antipsychotic" is also utilized but does not distinguish between drugs effective in schizophrenia and those acting in psychotic depression (antidepressants). The term "antischizophrenic" is also incorrect because it might improperly suggest that these compounds have a curative action. In the following, the three terms will be used synonymously, referring to those drugs which (1) contain the moiety of phenylethylamine and (2) impair dopaminergic transmission. The latter is considered to be the action mechanism closely involved in the amelioration, by these agents, of some schizophrenic symptoms as well as in extrapyramidal and endocrinological side effects.

II. CHEMISTRY

All of the neuroleptic agents of the various chemical classes (tricyclics, butyrophenones, pentacyclics, diarylbutylamines, indoles, benzamides) (Janssen, 1974; Pletscher and Kyburz, 1976) share structural and steric features with dopamine (DA), and with (R)-apomorphine, a DA receptor agonist which contains the DA moiety in a fixed conformation (Corrodi and Hardegger, 1955). The basic feature appears to be the presence of a tertiary amino group, the nitrogen of which is at a distance of 5-6 Å from the center of a (substituted) aromatic ring (see Fig. 1). This is thought to be the absolute requirement of a compound to fit to the DA receptor. However, other features determine whether such a compound is a DA receptor agonist or antagonist: substituents in the aromatic ring; orientation of the bulky part of the molecule with respect to the aromatic ring and the nitrogen; relative steric position of the N atom and the aromatic ring,

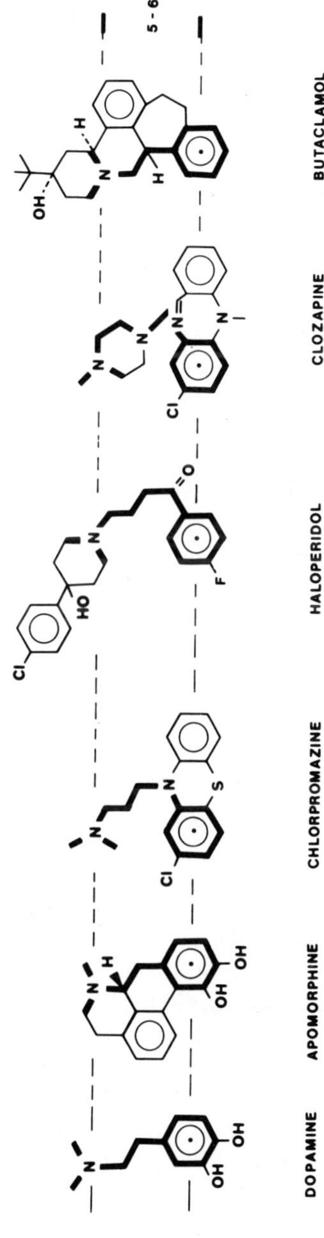

Figure 1 Structural similarity of dopamine, apomorphine, and some neuroleptic drugs.

which is determined by the orientation of a connecting side chain, either free (e.g., chlorpromazine, haloperidol) or incorporated into a semifixed cyclic (e.g., clozapine) or a fixed polycyclic structure (e.g., butaclamol). Figure 1 shows, as examples, the structural similarity of DA, apomorphine, and some neuroleptic compounds.

III. DOPAMINE THEORY

The chemical structure of neuroleptic drugs closely related to that of DA suggests an interaction between these drugs and the receptor(s) for this transmitter. Indeed, neuroleptic agents block the DA receptors, and thus impair dopaminergic transmission. Evidence for the blockade of DA receptors is provided by two orders of data: (1) Electrophysiological results show that neuroleptic compounds antagonize the action of DA administered microiontophoretically onto postsynaptic target cells of dopaminergic neurons (York, 1971; Bunney and Aghajanian, 1974, 1976). (2) Biochemical results indicate that for in vitro preparation (slices or homogenates of DA-rich brain areas), DA activates an adenylate cyclase which transforms ATP into cyclic AMP, considered to be the second messenger of dopaminergic transmission in target cells of DA neurons: The DA action on adenylate cyclase is blocked by neuroleptic agents (Greengard, 1974). These findings support the view that DA and neuroleptic compounds act at the same site and that adenylate cyclase is closely connected with DA receptors.

The impairment of dopaminergic transmission by neuroleptic drugs is thought to be connected with both the extrapyramidal side effects and the antipsychotic action of these agents. Indeed, no antipsychotic compound is known which is devoid of DA receptor-blocking properties. Moreover, dopaminergic agents such as amphetamine (which liberates DA from the neurons), apomorphine (which stimulates DA receptors), L-dopa (which forms DA in the brain), or LSD (which stimulates serotonin but also DA receptors) (Da Prada et al., 1975) cause schizophrenic-like symptoms; particularly in the case of amphetamine, the psychotic syndrome is almost indistinguishable from that of the acute paranoid psychosis (Snyder et al., 1974). Finally, administration of α-methyl-*p*-tyrosine to psychotic patients—which blocks the synthesis of catecholamine—in combination with neuroleptic drugs, allows the reduction of the daily dose of the latter, the antipsychotic action remaining unaltered (Carlsson, 1976). All of these data suggest the involvement of DA in the pathogenesis of schizophrenia and that the antipsychotic action of neuroleptics is connected with the blockade of DA receptors. Although postsynaptic receptor blockade is a well, directly established property of all neuroleptics, alternative or additive mechanisms have been proposed to explain the reduction in dopaminergic transmission, e.g., an action on presynaptic DA receptors (Seeman and Lee, 1974) and/or the anaesthetic action of the compounds (Seeman and Lee, 1975).

IV. NEURONAL EFFECTS OF NEUROLEPTIC AGENTS: GENERALITIES

The blockade of DA receptors by neuroleptic drugs has two distinct effects: the activation of the dopaminergic neurons and the changes in the activity of their target cells.

A. Feedback Activation of Dopaminergic Neurons

The administration of neuroleptic drugs results in an increased firing rate of dopaminergic cells, as shown electrophysiologically (Bunney and Aghajanian, 1974), and in an enhanced liberation of DA. The latter has been demonstrated indirectly by the accumulation in brain tissue of DA metabolites such as 3-methoxytyramine (Carlsson and Lindqvist, 1963), homovanillic acid, and dihydroxyphenylacetic acid (see below); by the accelerated disappearance of DA following tyrosine hydroxylase inhibition by α-methyl-*p*-tyrosine (Andén et al., 1970); by the accumulation of labeled DA following administration of radioactive precursors (Nybäck and Sedvall, 1970); and, directly, by collecting the neurotransmitter released in discrete brain areas by means of the push-pull cannula (see below). The increased liberation of DA is accompanied by an activation of tyrosine hydroxylase which enhances the synthesis of the neurotransmitter. In this condition, the tissue concentration of DA is not changed and the enhanced transmitter liberation reflects an increased turnover (Carlsson, 1976).

The mechanism by which the dopaminergic neurons are activated is still debated: It is generally attributed to a positive feedback triggered by alterations of DA receptors. Thus, the changes in the activity of the postsynaptic cells due to the blockade of the postsynaptic DA receptors may trigger—via a (poly- or multi-) neuronal loop—modifications of excitatory or inhibitory inputs to the DA neurons resulting in their activation (see Section V.A). A second possibility is that neuroleptics block an "autoreceptor" localized on the DA cell through which the neurotransmitter physiologically regulates its own release: Blockade of this receptor results in an enhanced liberation of DA (Carlsson, 1976). Evidence for the occurrence of either mechanism is mainly indirect and it is difficult to assess which component has the main bearing in vivo.

Teleologically, the activation of dopaminergic neurons by neuroleptic drugs is considered a compensatory mechanism which, in some situations (see below), might overcome the blockade of postsynaptic receptors and restore dopaminergic transmission.

B. Changes in DA Target Cell Activity

The changes in the activity of postsynaptic target cells of the DA pathways—due to the removal of the dopaminergic input—must result in an alteration in the release of their transmitters. The knowledge of these changes is of paramount importance for understanding (1) the chain of events which leads to the amelioration of psychotic symptoms and, therefore, the possible pathogenetic alterations of psychoses, and (2) the mechanisms involved in the side effects of neuroleptics.

In the following, the changes due to antipsychotic compounds, both in DA neurons and in the postsynaptic cells, will be discussed in relation to the clinical effects of these drugs in extrapyramidal and limbic systems. Thus, recent data suggest that the blockade of dopaminergic transmission in the basal ganglia is related to the extrapyramidal side effects and in the limbic system to the antipsychotic action of the neuroleptic compounds.

V. EFFECTS OF NEUROLEPTIC DRUGS IN EXTRAPYRAMIDAL SYSTEM

A. Effects on Acetylcholine (ACh) and γ-Aminobutyric Acid (GABA) Neurons: Feedback Mechanisms

Several neuroleptic drugs of different chemical classes (e.g., chlorpromazine, haloperidol, clozapine) increase the release of DA in the cat caudate nucleus perfused by means of the push-pull cannula* (Bartholini et al., 1974a). The DA liberation is dose-dependent (Fig. 2), and is not accompanied by changes of the tissue levels of the transmitter (Lloyd et al.,1973), indicating increased turnover. Neuroleptic drugs cause also an enhanced liberation of ACh in the cat caudate nucleus (Fig. 2) (Stadler et al., 1973; Bartholini et al., 1974a), which is not paralleled by changes of the ACh esterase activity or of the transmitter concentration in the perfused regions (Bartholini et al., 1975b). This indicates that the turnover of ACh is accelerated. The neuroleptic-induced increase in ACh liberation is not connected with the ACh receptor-blocking properties of some of these compounds, which might enhance the ACh release via a positive feedback mechanism. In fact, haloperidol, which is devoid of anticholinergic properties, is one of the most potent neuroleptics in enhancing ACh liberation. The enhanced ACh release by antipsychotic drugs is blocked by apomorphine

*The push-pull cannula consists of two parallel or concentric cannulae (0.2 mm) which are stereotaxically implanted into the brain regions of the cat. Ringer's solution is pushed through the inflow cannula, perfuses the tissue at its tip, and is pulled through the outflow cannula. The minute amounts of transmitters released during the perfusion of brain regions of gallamine-immobilized or freely moving animals can be measured in perfusate by means of radioenzymatic methods.

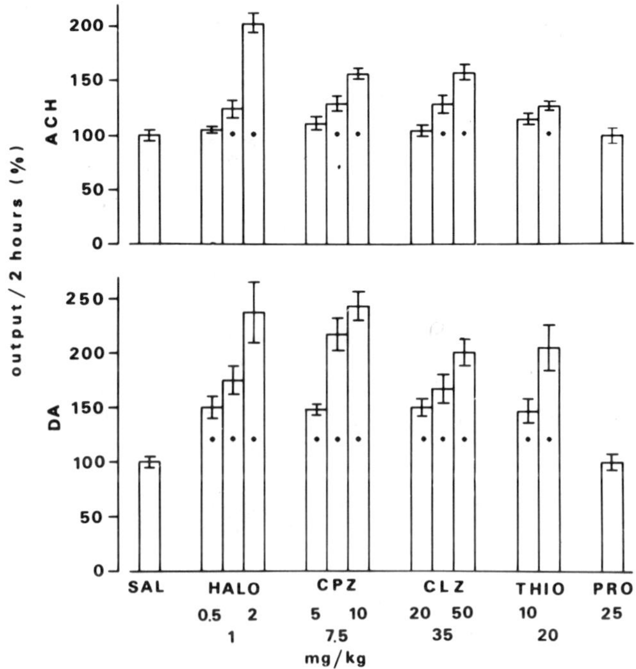

Figure 2 Neuroleptic-induced enhancement of DA and ACh release in the cat caudate nucleus, perfused by means of the push-pull cannula. Saline and neuroleptics were injected i.v. Each bar represents the neurotransmitter liberation for 2 hr following injection. Values are averages (with SEM) of results from 4-8 cats and are represented as percent of those obtained during the control period (= 100). Abbreviations: SAL = saline; HALO = haloperidol; CPZ = chlorpromazine; CLZ = clozapine; THIO = thioridazine; PRO = promethazine. $P < .01$ versus control periods. [From G. Bartholini, H. Stadler, M. Gadea Ciria, and K. G. Lloyd (1976b). Interaction of dopaminergic and cholinergic neurons in extrapyramidal and limbic system. In *Advances in Biochemical Psychopharmacology*, Vol. 16, E. Costa and G. L. Gessa (Eds.). Raven Press, New York.]

(Table 1) and by L-dopa. Apomorphine, administered alone, also diminishes the spontaneous liberation of the transmitter. This antagonism between DA receptor blocking and activating agents suggests that the neuroleptic-induced increase in the ACh output is the result of the blockade of DA receptors. Indeed, promethazine, a phenothiazine derivative devoid of DA receptor-blocking properties, is ineffective on ACh release (Fig. 2). In addition, the electrical stimulation of the DA cell bodies in the pars compacta of the substantia nigra—which releases DA in the striatum—decreases the ACh liberation in the ipsilateral,

Table 1 Reversal by Apomorphine of Chlorpromazine-Induced Increase in Striatal ACh Output[a]

Treatment	Perfusion period (min)		
	0-60	70-120	130-180
Chlorpromazine	100 ± 5.5	157.4 ± 3.1[b]	162.3 ± 4.5[b]
Chlorpromazine plus apomorphine	100 ± 2.6	149.0 ± 2.6[b]	105.8 ± 6.2

[a] In gallamine-immobilized cats, the ACh released from striatal neurons was collected by means of the push-pull cannula. Chlorpromazine (10 mg/kg i.v.) was injected at 60 min, apomorphine (10 mg/kg i.v.) at 120 min. In each cat, the release of ACh was determined in the 5-6 ten-minute samples throughout the perfusion period. For each perfusion period, the values represent averages (with SEM) of results from 4-5 cats per group and are expressed in percent of the average ACh release during the control period (0-60 min = 15.7 ± 0.5 ng/10 min = 100).

[b] $P < .01$ vs. control period.

Note: For further details see Stadler et al., 1973.

but not in the contralateral, caudate nucleus (Bartholini et al., 1974a). These data indicate that cholinergic neurons (or interneurons) in the caudate nucleus are inhibited by a dopaminergic input, which is impaired by neuroleptic agents. This input is possibly tonic in nature, as a section of the nigro striatal DA pathway increases the utilization of ACh in the striatum (Guyenet et al., 1975).

There is also evidence for the opposite regulation, namely, that of the nigro striatal DA pathway by cholinergic neurons. In fact, systemically administered anticholinergic compounds diminish the neuroleptic-induced activation of striatal DA turnover (O'Keeffe et al., 1970) and cholinomimetic agents enhance DA release (Bartholini et al., 1976a). It appears, therefore, that an excitatory cholinergic input activates the dopaminergic cells in the extrapyramidal system. This regulation might occur at different levels, e.g., in the striatum and the substantia nigra, both of which are rich in choline acetylase activity and in ACh. However, it is unlikely that the nigral cholinergic terminals belong to a strionigral pathway as previously postulated (Corrodi et al., 1972); thus, hemitransection of the brain between striatum and substantia nigra fails to change both ACh concentration and choline acetylase activity in the latter structure (Kataoka et al., 1974). In contrast, a striatal mechanism has to be considered, because perfusion of the caudate nucleus with Ringer's solution containing ACh, physostigmine (Fig. 3), or oxotremorine results in an enhanced release of DA (Bartholini and Stadler, 1975a).

From these data, it is reasonable to assume that one of the possible neuronal loops involved in the neuroleptic-induced feedback activation of

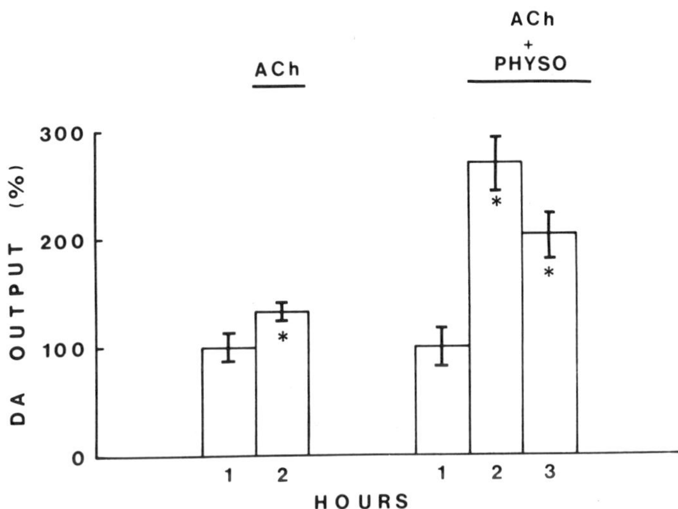

Figure 3 Release of DA in the cat caudate nucleus by ACh. The caudate nucleus of gallamine-immobilized cat was perfused with Ringer's solution by means of the push-pull cannula. ACh (10^{-3} M) or ACh + physostigmine (10^{-3} M) was added to the Ringer's 1 hr after the beginning of the perfusion. The values represent the averages (with SEM) of results obtained from three cats per group and are expressed in percent of those obtained during the 1-hr control period (= 100).

dopaminergic neurons triggered by blockade of DA receptors is of a cholinergic nature. Thus, the increased liberation of striatal ACh due to the impairment of dopaminergic transmission might increase the firing of DA cells and the liberation of the transmitter. Indeed, electrophysiological experiments show that microiontophoretically administered ACh enhances the firing of dopaminergic neurons (Bunney and Adhajanian, 1974).

Another loop involved in the feedback activation of dopaminergic neurons may be the strionigral GABA pathway. GABA neurons exert an inhibitor influence on DA cell bodies in the substantia nigra as shown by electrophysiological experiments (Yoshida and Precht, 1971). In addition, GABA or aminooxyacetic acid—which may increase the GABA concentration in the synaptic cleft—injected into the substantia nigra of the rat reduces the striatal DA turnover; a similar effect is observed with γ-hydroxybutyric acid (Andén and Stock, 1973; Andén, 1974a). In contrast, enhancement of striatal DA liberation is caused by bicuculline—a GABA receptor blocker—when perfused in the substantia nigra of the cat (Bartholini and Stadler, 1975b). Moreover, systematically administered aminooxyacetic acid diminishes the neuroleptic-induced enhancement of DA turnover

(Lahti and Losey, 1974). The inhibitory GABA action on DA neurons is likely to be exerted also in the striatum. Thus, bicuculline or picrotoxin added to Ringer's solution perfusing the caudate nucleus of the cat enhances the DA output. This effect is blocked by the addition of GABA into the perfusion fluid. GABA alone reduces the spontaneous DA liberation (Fig. 4) (Bartholini and Stadler, 1977).

The possible involvement of GABA in the neuroleptic-induced activation of DA neurons is suggested by data showing that neuroleptics such as haloperidol or clozapine enhance the GABA turnover in extrapyramidal centers (Marco et al., 1976). The mechanism which leads to this effect is not known. It could be speculated that neuroleptics block GABA receptors inducing, on the one hand, a feedback activation of GABAergic neurons and, on the other hand, suppression of the GABA inhibitory input on DA cells. However, the increase in GABA turnover could result from the activation of GABA neurons caused by

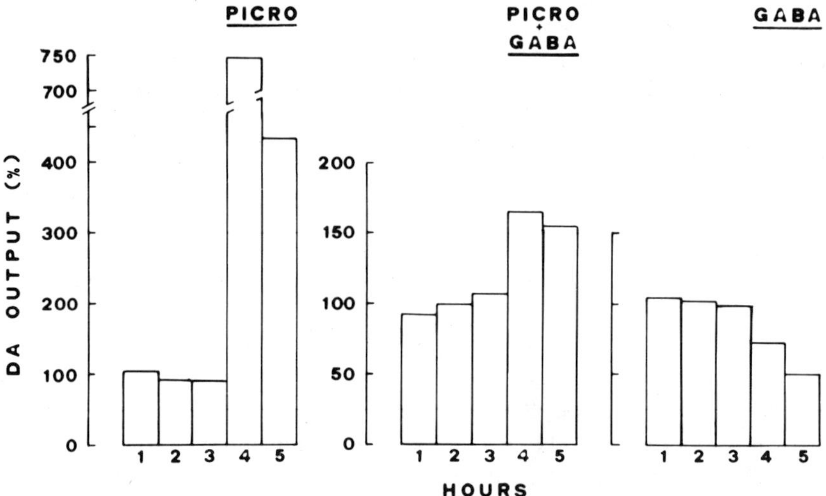

Figure 4 Relase of DA in the cat caudate nucleus: effect of picrotoxin, picrotoxin plus GABA, and GABA. In the gallamine-immobilized cat, the caudate nucleus was perfused with Ringer's solution by means of the push-pull cannula. Compounds (10^{-3} M) were added to the Ringer's during the last 2 hr of perfusion. Values are the averages (with SEM) of results from three to five cats per group. The release of DA (per hour) is expressed as a percentage of the average release during the corresponding 3-hr control period. *P* versus control period (Kruskal-Wallis test): picrotoxin (PICRO) $< .001$; PICRO + GABA $> .05$; GABA $< .05$. (From Bartholini and Stadler, 1977).

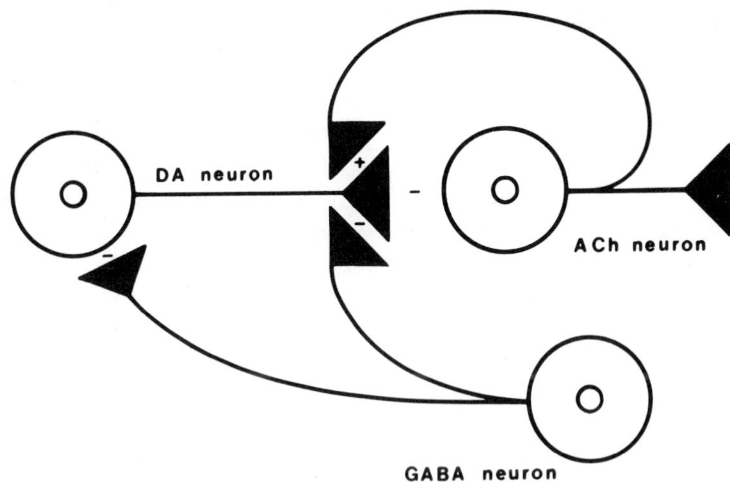

Figure 5 Possible interconnection of DA, ACh, and GABA neurons in extrapyramidal centers. The + and the − refer to excitatory and inhibitory inputs, respectively.

mechanisms other than the blockade of GABA receptors (for instance, it may be secondary to the blockade of DA receptors).

In conclusion, it appears that in extrapyramidal centers, neuroleptics cause changes in activity and in transmitter liberation of various neuronal systems; blockade of DA receptors impairs the dopaminergic inhibitory input on striatal cholinergic (inter)neurons leading to increased ACh liberation. The enhanced cholinergic activity might in turn excite the DA cells, resulting in acceleration of DA turnover. The latter could also be triggered by blockade of the inhibitory GABA input on DA neurons, in both striatum and substantia nigra. A schematic representation of the known interconnection of DA, ACh, and GABA neurons in the extrapyramidal centers is shown in Figure 5 (see also Section XII).

B. Functional Implications

1. Compensatory Role of DA Neuron Activation

The view that the activation of dopaminergic neurons caused by neuroleptic agents may partially compensate the blockade of postsynaptic DA receptors finds support in the different responses of the striatal DA and ACh neurons to these drugs. The dose of neuroleptics which enhances the DA liberation is lower than that which affects ACh (Fig. 2), suggesting that the relative concentration of DA and of the neuroleptic at the receptor site is critical for the changes in activity of the cholinergic target cell. Thus, it could be assumed that a low dose of neuroleptic causes only a partial blockade of the receptors, which is overcome by the increased amount of DA liberated by feedback activation. Under these conditions, no changes in the activity of the target cells is observed, nor are functional alterations perceived. However, if the dose of the neuroleptic reaches a critical threshold, the feedback activation of DA neurons is insufficient to overcome the receptor blockade; consequently, both changes in the activity of the target cells and functional alterations would appear.

This hypothesis is supported by the results of the experiments with γ-butyrolactone, a precursor of γ-hydroxybutyric acid, which possibly acts as a GABA agonist (Section V.A); this compound reduces the activity of dopaminergic neurons and, therefore, the DA liberation. Thus, it has been shown that 20 mg/kg i.v. of clozapine increases the liberation of DA but not that of ACh into the perfusate of the cat caudate nucleus (Table 2); however, in animals pretreated with γ-butyrolactone, the same dose of clozapine causes a marked increase in the liberation of ACh (similar to that induced by 35 or 50 mg/kg of the neuroleptic; see Fig. 2), paralleled by a reduced release of DA (Stadler et al., 1974; Bartholini et al., 1974a). It appears, therefore, that when the activation of DA neurons is impaired by γ-butyrolactone, relatively low doses of neuroleptics cause a disinhibition of cholinergic target cells similar to that provoked by higher doses of these drugs. Moreover, in the rat, γ-butyrolactone (or its main metabolite, γ-hydroxybutyrate) decreases the neuroleptic-induced

Table 2 Release of Striatal ACh and DA by Clozapine: Effect of γ-Butyrolactone[a]

Treatment (mg/kg i.v.)	ACh	DA
Saline	100 ± 8	100 ± 9
γ-Butyrolactone (500)	78 ± 13	99 ± 7
Clozapine (20)	105 ± 5	148 ± 15[b]
γ-Butyrolactone (500) followed by clozapine (20)	150 ± 7[c]	91 ± 8[c]

[a]In gallamine-immobilized cats, the head of the caudate nucleus was perfused by means of the push-pull cannula. When given alone, γ-butyrolactone and clozapine were administered 1 hr after saline; otherwise, clozapine was injected 1 hr after γ-butyrolactone. The average values (with SEM) indicate ACh and DA released during the 1-hr perfusion period following γ-butyrolactone or clozapine administration, and are expressed as a percent of those in saline-injected animals (= 100).

[b]$P < .01$ vs. saline.

[c]$P < .001$ vs. clozapine.

Source: Data from Bartholini et al., 1974a, 1976.

enhancement of cerebral homovanillic acid (Roth, 1971), as well as the firing rate of DA neurons (Walters et al., 1972). γ-Butyrolactone lowers the ED_{50} of neuroleptics for catalepsy (unpublished), an effect which probably originates via a cholinergic hyperactivity (see below).

These data strongly support the idea that the increased liberation of DA by a low dose of neuroleptics overcomes the receptor blockade and maintains the critical degree of inhibition of the cholinergic target cells.

The antagonism at the receptor site of DA and neuroleptic agents is probably essential for understanding the pathogenesis of extrapyramidal side effects as well as the possible mechanism of the antipsychotic action of these compounds.

2. *Extrapyramidal Side Effects*

The finding that dopaminergic cells inhibit striatal cholinergic (inter)neurons might explain the genesis of extrapyramidal side effects during neuroleptic medication.

a. Parkinsonian Syndrome

The parkinsonian syndrome, a frequent neuroleptic side effect, is probably the result of a blockade of DA receptors which cannot be overcome by the feedback activation of the dopaminergic neurons. Apart from hypokinesia, the pathogenesis of which does not seem to have a cholinergic component, some symptoms such as rigidity and possibly tremor have been proposed to originate from a cholinergic hyperactivity as a consequence of the reduction of the inhibitory dopaminergic input on striatal cholinergic neurons (Fig. 6) (Stadler et al., 1973; Bartholini et al., 1974). These symptoms, in fact, are ameliorated by anticholinergic drugs (Munkvad et al., 1976). The involvement of hyperactive cholinergic neurons in the pathogenesis of these symptoms is also supported by the inverse correlation between the incidence of extrapyramidal reactions by neuroleptic drugs in humans and the threshold dose of these agents which increases the liberation of striatal ACh in the cat (Table 3). The less potent a compound is in causing striopallidal reactions, the higher its threshold dose affecting ACh release.

Blockade of DA receptors → Hypokinesia

↓

Disinhibition of striatal
cholinergic neurons

↓

Enhanced release of ACh

↓

Rigidity (tremor)

Figure 6 Possible pathogenesis of neuroleptic-induced parkinsonian symptoms.

Table 3 Tentative Correlation of Neuroleptic-Induced Changes in Humans and Cats

	Humans		Cats	
Drug	Daily average dose (mg/kg p.o.)[a]	Incidence of extrapyramidal reactions	Threshold dose[b]	ACh output[c]
Clozapine	10	Low	35	142 ± 10[d]
Chlorpormazine	5	High	10	153 ± 4[d]
Haloperidol	0.1	Very high	0.5	144 ± 10[d]

[a]See Snyder et al., 1974.
[b]For enhancing the striatal output of ACh in experiments of perfusion of the caudate nucleus by means of the push-pull cannula in the gallamine-immobilized cat.
[c]Average 1-hr release (with SEM) as percent of the corresponding 1-hr preinjection (control) period (= 100).
[d]$P < .01$ vs. control period.
Source: Data from Bartholini and Stadler, 1975b.

Parkinsonian symptoms in humans, however, tend to ameliorate spontaneously in the course of the neuroleptic medication (Ayd, 1976). Similarly, repeated administration of neuroleptic drugs to the rat leads to a tolerance to the cataleptogenic action (Asper et al., 1973; Ezrin-Waters and Seeman, 1977). Biochemically, in both humans and animals, there is a concomitant progressive decrease in the neuroleptic-induced enhancement of DA turnover as determined by measuring the transmitter synthesis in the rat brain (Scatton et al., 1975), as well as the changes in the accumulation of homovanillic acid in human cerebrospinal fluid (Post and Goodwin, 1975) and in the rat striatum (Bower and Rozitis, 1974; Waldeimer and Maître, 1976a,b). In addition, experiments in the cat have shown that after repeated administration of haloperidol or chlorpromazine, the enhancement in the release of striatal ACh is reduced as compared to that observed following a single administration of these drugs (Bartholini et al., 1974b). It appears, therefore, that the biochemical effects of neuroleptic drugs on both dopaminergic neurons and their target cells, as well as the functional effects such as parkinsonian symptoms, are reduced during prolonged medication. This tolerance is thought to be connected with the development of supersensitivity to DA of the postsynaptic cells. Indeed, the threshold dose of dopaminergic agents (apomorphine, L-dopa) for inducing stereotypies is reduced in the course of prolonged treatment of rat with neuroleptics (Asper et al., 1973; Gianutsos et al., 1974).

The mechanisms underlying supersensitivity to DA are not known (cf. Moore and Thornburg, 1975; Ungerstedt et al., 1975). The effect is, however, similar to the "denervation supersensitivity" occurring in the peripheral autonomic system (Langer and Trendelenburg, 1966). It is therefore reasonable to assume that, due to supersensitivity, the blockade of postsynaptic receptors by neuroleptic drugs is partly overcome by DA, resulting in a reduction of both feedback activation of dopaminergic neurons and disinhibition of their target cells. Furthermore, a higher degree of supersensitivity may lead to functional consequences such as tardive dyskinesias.

b. Tardive Dyskinesias

In the course of the treatment with neuroleptics, another type of extrapyramidal disturbance appears, the tardive dyskinesias. This syndrome is reminiscent of chorea, of choreiform movements induced in parkinsonian patients by L-dopa, and of stereotyped behavior elicited by DA-mimetic compounds. As a working hypothesis (Fig. 7), it is assumed that tardive dyskinesias originate from such a supersensitivity to DA of target cells that the transmitter does not only overcome the neuroleptic-induced blockade of the receptors but also leads to an enhanced transmission to the postsynaptic neurons and possibly to a decreased striatal cholinergic activity. In fact, the apomorphine-induced decrease in ACh utilization is more marked in the denervated than in the intact caudate nucleus (Fibiger and Grewaal, 1974). Although more experimental work is needed, this hypothesis seems likely as tardive dyskinesias are ameliorated either by switching to a more potent neuroleptic drug (which restores the blockade of the receptors) or by administering reserpine or tetrabenazine (which deplete DA stores and impair dopaminergic transmission); moreover, anticholinergic compounds aggravate and physostigmine ameliorates the clinical picture (Klawans, 1973; Fann et al., 1974; Munkvad et al., 1976). This supports the hypothesis of a reduced cholinergic transmission in the pathogenesis of tardive dyskinesias.

While there is some knowledge of the link between DA and ACh neurons and of their role in the extrapyramidal function in connection with the action mechanism of neuroleptic drugs, the involvement of GABA is still obscure.

Supersensitivity of DA target cells
↓
Increased response to DA
↓
Inhibition of striatal cholinergic neurons
↓
Decreased release of ACh
↓
Tardive dyskinesias

Figure 7 Possible pathogenesis of neuroleptic-induced tardive dyskinesias.

As previously stated, one can assume that GABA is involved in the regulation of the activity of DA neurons. On the other hand, DA neurons probably exert an influence on striatal GABA cells. Thus, the activity of glutamic acid decarboxylase is low in the caudate nucleus of parkinsonian patients not treated with L-dopa, whereas after medication with the amino acid, it tends to be restored; in addition, glutamic acid decarboxylase activity is enhanced in the striatum of rat chronically treated with L-dopa (Lloyd and Hornykiewicz, 1973). The possible link between DA and GABA neurons leads to the speculation that changes in striatal GABAergic activity are involved in the genesis of symptoms connected with altered dopaminergic transmission. For instance, during long-term medication with neuroleptics, the tardive dyskinesias may result, in part, from decreased GABA function. A similar imbalance between GABA and DA has been postulated in Huntington's chorea, which is ameliorated by neuroleptic drugs and in which a decrease of striatal glutamic acid decarboxylase activity has been established (McGeer and McGeer, 1976). Thus, for both neuroleptic-induced tardive dyskinesias and Huntington's chorea, a medication with GABA-mimetic compounds can be envisaged (see Section XII).

In conclusion (compare Figures 6 and 7), during treatment with neuroleptic drugs, two kinds of extrapyramidal disturbances appear, which may be considered mirror images: (1) the parkinsonian syndrome, which originates from a decreased dopaminergic activity leading to a cholinergic preponderance (indeed, anticholinergic compounds are the drugs of choice) and (2) the tardive dyskinesias attributed to a supersensitivity of DA target cells, and thus to a relatively excessive dopaminergic transmission, possibly leading to a decreased cholinergic activity (GABAergic drugs might ameliorate this syndrome) (see Section XII).

VI. LIMBIC SYSTEM

As in the extrapyramidal system, neuroleptic drugs block the dopaminergic transmission in the limbic system. Thus, the turnover of DA is increased in limbic regions as indicated by the accumulation of homovanillic acid and by the increased liberation of DA in perfusion experiments utilizing the push-pull cannula (Bartholini et al., 1974a).

A. Effect on ACh and GABA Neurons

The fact that in the striatum cholinergic neurons represent target cells of the DA pathway and probably mediate some extrapyramidal effects of neuroleptic drugs leads to the following questions: Does a similar link between DA and ACh neurons exist in the limbic system? If so, is the possible alteration of the activity of limbic cholinergic neurons—due to the blockade of dopaminergic transmission—implicated in the antipsychotic action of neuroleptic compounds?

Results of perfusion experiments in the nucleus accumbens septi—one of the limbic regions with the most dense dopaminergic input—do not confirm these hypotheses. In fact, following administration of neuroleptic agents, although the liberation of DA (and of noradrenaline, Section IX) is markedly enhanced—indicating blockade of receptors—no changes in the ACh output occur (Table 4) (Lloyd et al., 1973; Stadler et al., 1975). This indicates that the activity of cholinergic neurons afferent to, or of interneurons in, the nucleus accumbens septi is not affected by the impairment of the dopaminergic transmission. Neither does the septal dopaminergic input influence the activity of cholinergic projections from the septum such as the septohippocampal pathways. These neurons have been demonstrated histochemically (Shute and Lewis, 1967) and biochemically (Sethy et al., 1973). In addition, the electrical stimulation of the nucleus accumbens septi evokes, in the ventral hippocampus, potentials which are highly dependent on cholinergic transmission (Schaffner et al., 1974). Accordingly, the electrical stimulation of septal nuclei releases ACh in both the ipsilateral ventral and dorsal hippocampal formation. However, neuroleptic compounds do not alter the liberation of ACh in the latter structures (Table 4) (Stadler et al., 1975).

The mesocortical DA pathway which terminates in the limbic prefrontal cortex of animals (Thierry et al., 1973) and humans (Olson et al., 1973) is also affected by neuroleptic compounds which increase DA turnover in this region. Whether or not the mesocortical DA neurons modify cholinergic activity is still an open question. Some authors claim that cortical cholinergic neurons are activated by DA, but the data are contradictory. Thus, amphetamine (which liberates both DA and noradrenaline) increases the liberation of ACh collected from the frontal cortex of rat, rabbit, and cat by means of epidural perfusion

Table 4 Liberation of DA and ACh in Cat Limbic Regions Perfused by Means of the Push-Pull Cannula: Effect of Chlorpromazine[a]

	Nucleus accumbens		ACh	
Minutes	DA	ACh	Hippocampal ventral	Formation dorsal
0-60	100 ± 29	100 ± 11	100 ± 7	100 ± 9
60-120	197 ± 15[b]	96 ± 9	119 ± 8	105 ± 9
120-180	201 ± 16[b]	104 ± 10	–	–

[a]Chlorpromazine (10 mg/kg i.v.) was injected at 60 min. Average values (with SEM) from 4-6 cats per group are expressed in percent of those of the control period (0-60 min, = 100).
[b]$P < .01$ vs. corresponding control period.
Note: For further details see Stadler et al., 1975.

cups. This effect is prevented by chlorpromazine and haloperidol, but at doses which also block the noradrenergic transmission; similarly, propanolol, but not other β blockers or phenoxybenzamine, antagonizes the amphetamine effect. In addition, the release of cortical ACh is increased by DL-dopa (and this effect is not antagonized by propanolol) as well as by DA-β-hydroxylase inhibitors. In contrast, dl-threo-3,4-dihydroxyphenylserine (a noradrenaline precursor) decreases the cortical ACh output (for references, see Pepeu, 1974).

Although these data are not completely coherent, they suggest that cortical cholinergic neurons may be influenced, directly or indirectly, by a noradrenergic input. However, an excitatory DA action is not excluded with certainty.

Some evidence exists in animals for the regulation of limbic DA pathways by a cholinergic input. In fact, experiments in the rabbit (Andén, 1974b) and the rat (Bartholini et al., 1975) show that the turnover of DA is accelerated by muscarinic agents such as oxotremorine; anticholinergic drugs counteract this effect as well as the increase in DA turnover caused by neuroleptic agents. In the cat, anticholinergic compounds diminish the release of DA from the nucleus accumbens septi perfused by means of the push-pull cannula (Bartholini, unpublished data). Therefore, an excitatory cholinergic input, as in the striatum, may modulate the activity of DA cells in the limbic system and may be altered by neuroleptic agents, leading to functional modifications (see Section VI.B).

Limbic GABA neurons also, may be involved in the action mechanism of neuroleptic drugs. Thus, compounds supposed to increase GABAergic transmission (e.g., aminooxyacetic acid) diminish the DA turnover in the limbic system (Andén, 1974a). This is also suggested by histofluorimetric experiments (Fuxe et al., 1975). It is likely, therefore, that, as in the striatum, DA neurons in the limbic system receive an inhibitory GABA input.

B. Functional Implications

From the previously discussed data, it appears that a fundamental difference exists between striatal and limbic cholinergic neurons. In the striatum, a cholinergic activity is under the inhibitory control of the nigrostriatal DA pathway and mediates some effects of the DA receptor blockade by neuroleptics (extrapyramidal syndromes); in contrast, the dopaminergic transmission in the limbic system does not seem to affect the activity of cholinergic neurons. This allows the speculation that, although the limbic system is purportedly the anatomical substrate for the antipsychotic action of neuroleptic drugs (see Section VII), limbic cholinergic activity is not involved. Neither is the cholinergic involvement suggested by the few contradictory clinical data; thus, schizophrenic symptoms do not seem to be affected by anti-ACh drugs or by physostigmine. In contrast, the latter compound has been claimed to antagonize the methylphenidate-induced exacerbation of the acute paranoid syndrome (Davis, 1974). The involvement of striatal, and the lack of involvement of limbic, cholinergic neurons in the action mechanism of neuroleptic drugs might explain why anti-ACh compounds ameliorate the parkinsonian syndrome induced by these agents, apparently without altering their antipsychotic action.

Several of the above-discussed results suggest that the limbic DA neurons are controlled by an excitatory ACh and by an inhibitory GABA input, as schematically represented in Figure 8. On the basis of these results in animals and because a great deal of data suggest that schizophrenia is improved by the impairment of the limbic dopaminergic transmission (see Section VII), inhibition of the cholinergic, or activation of the GABAergic, influence on limbic DA neurons should result in a reduced dopaminergic activity and, therefore, in amelioration of the psychosis. Thus, it could be speculated that the anticholinergic properties of some neuroleptics (see Section VII) contribute to the reduction of limbic dopaminergic transmission by blocking the excitatory

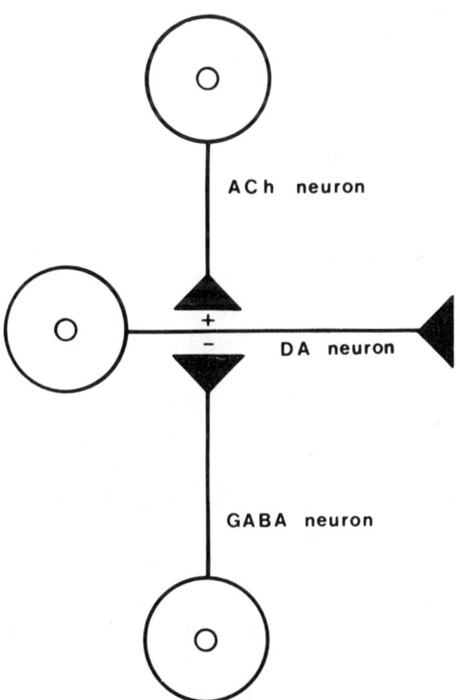

Figure 8 Possible interconnection of DA, ACh, and GABA neurons in the limbic system. The + and the – refer to excitatory and inhibitory inputs, respectively.

cholinergic input on DA neurons. However, the few available clinical data (see above) do not support this hypothesis. Neuroleptics may also alter the GABA input on limbic DA neurons since some of these agents (e.g., haloperidol) increase GABA turnover in the limbic system (Marco et al., 1976). The activation of GABA neurons may originate either from the direct blockade of GABA receptors or from the primary blockade of DA receptors. The action of neuroleptics on GABA neurons remains to be investigated; however, as a working hypothesis, an interaction of haloperidol with GABA receptors can be assumed, because of the presence of the GABA moiety in its structure (Janssen, 1976).

Recently, β-(*p*-chlorophenyl)GABA (baclofen) has been shown to reduce limbic dopaminergic transmission, and since it contains the GABA moiety, it has been hypothesized to act as a GABA receptor stimulant (Fuxe et al., 1975). However, several experiments do not confirm this hypothesis. In fact, this compound does not antagonize convulsions induced by picrotoxin (Fehr and Bein, 1974) or by bicuculline (unpublished) and does not mimic GABA on mammalian neurons (Curtis et al., 1974). In addition, the depressant action of baclofen on cortical neurons is not antagonized by bicuculline (Davis and Watkins, 1974). Finally, baclofen does not potentiate the neuroleptic-induced catalepsy in the rat (Worms, personal communication), in contrast to the action of muscimol, a known GABA-mimetic compound (Johnston, 1976). Nevertheless, bacoflen has been claimed to exert an antipsychotic action (Fredericksen, 1975) which, however, could not be confirmed by others (Beckmann et al., 1977; Bigelow et al., 1977; Simpson et al., 1978). Whether or not the decreased limbic dopaminergic transmission by baclofen in animals (see above) results from an interference with GABAergic mechanisms, remains to be investigated. However, these data may lead to the development of GABA receptor stimulant drugs, which will possibly represent a new approach in the therapy of schizophrenia (see Section XII).

In conclusion, neuroleptic drugs block the dopaminergic transmission in the limbic system and this effect is thought to be connected with the antipsychotic action of these agents (see Section VII). This action, however, does not seem to be mediated by changes of cholinergic activity since the latter is not apparently altered by the blockade of dopaminergic transmission. The involvement of changes in ACh and GABA input on DA neurons in the action mechanism of neuroleptic drugs remains an open problem; there is no clear evidence as yet that, in humans, GABA and ACh neurons influence limbic dopaminergic transmission and, therefore, that compounds acting on these neurons have an effect on schizophrenia (see Section XII).

VII. "ATYPICAL" NEUROLEPTICS

A. Preferential Effect on Limbic Dopaminergic Transmission

Since the advent of neuroleptic medication, it has appeared clear that some patients do improve without showing striopallidal disturbances while others, in the absence of a significant amelioration, develop severe extrapyramidal reactions. Nevertheless, the erroneous view often persists that the blockade of extrapyramidal dopaminergic transmission is connected with the therapeutic action of neuroleptic drugs.

However, various compounds, i.e., clozapine, sulpiride, and thioridazine, have been recently claimed to display an antipsychotic action being virtually devoid of extrapyramidal side effects both in humans and in animals (for references, see Bartholini, 1976). The pattern of such compounds—referred to in the following as "atypical" neuroleptics, as compared to the classical agents of chlorpromazine and haloperidol type—clearly indicates that the therapeutic action and the extrapyramidal side effects of neuroleptics are dissociable.

Moreover, due to the low incidence of extrapyramidal side effects, it is reasonable to assume that atypical neuroleptic drugs block less effectively the striatal than the limbic dopaminergic transmission. Evidence for a preferential impairment of limbic dopaminergic transmission by atypical neuroleptics is provided by the fact (Table 5) that, in contrast to chlorpromazine and haloperidol, which enhance DA turnover similarly in extrapyramidal and limbic areas, clozapine, sulpiride, and thioridazine cause a more marked accumulation of homovanillic acid in the limbic system than in the striatum. This effect of neuroleptics clearly occurs after blockade of the acid clearance by probenecid (Bartholini, 1976). In fact, in the absence of probenecid, several authors (for references, see Scatton et al., 1977) did not find a difference in the accumulation of acidic DA metabolites by neuroleptic drugs (with the exception of sulpiride at low doses; Scatton et al., 1977) in the two cerebral regions. It appears likely, therefore, that the transport mechanism of homovanillic acid is more efficient in the limbic system than in the striatum and that only after blockade of the acid transport does the preferential effect of the drugs clearly appear. However, utilizing other methods, the preferential effect of sulpiride, clozapine, and thioridazine on limbic dopaminergic structures has been confirmed (Zivkovic et al., 1975; Scatton et al., 1977; Westerink et al., 1977). Finally, the preferential activation of limbic DA neurons is directly demonstrated in experiments of perfusion of the caudate nucleus and the nucleus accumbens by means of the push-pull cannula. Thus, clozapine causes a more marked liberation of DA in the limbic than in the extrapyramidal region, in contrast to chlorpromazine, which leads to a similar effect in both areas (Table 6) (Bartholini, 1976).

Table 5 Effect of Neuroleptic Drugs on the Accumulation of Homovanillic Acid in Limbic System and Striatum of Probenecid-Pretreated Rats

Drug	Homovanillic acid increase (%)[a]	
	Limbic system	Striatum
Sulpiride	81.0 ± 8.4[b]	31.0 ± 7.4
Clozapine	87.0 ± 8.2[b]	56.0 ± 9.1
Thioridazine	61.5 ± 3.9[b]	47.5 ± 2.1
Haloperidol	134.5 ± 13.5[c]	139.3 ± 15.9
Chloropromazine	85.3 ± 23.4[c]	104.3 ± 12.1

[a] Average values (with SEM) represent the net effect of neuroleptics, namely, the difference between the homovanillic acid increase in rat administered neuroleptic plus probenecid and probenecid alone. The increase is expressed in percent of values in untreated control animals (= 100).
[b] $P < .001$ vs. striatum.
[c] $P > .05$ vs. striatum.
Note: For further details see Bartholini, 1976.

The mechanisms of atypical neuroleptics for inducing a preferential activation of limbic DA neurons is still obscure. It might be connected with a selective accumulation of these drugs in the limbic system as compared to the striatum resulting from a difference in the blood-brain barrier of the two regions. Alternatively, these compounds might have a higher affinity for limbic than for striatal DA receptors. In vitro experiments, however, show that atypical neuroleptics, as the classical compounds, block the DA-sensitive adenylate

Table 6 Chloropromazine and Clozapine-Induced Release of DA into the Push-Pull Cannula Perfusate of Nucleus Caudatus and Nucleus Accumbens of the Gallamine-Immobized Cat

Drug	DA output/3 hr[a]	
	Nucleus caudatus	Nucleus accumbens
Chlorpromazine	257 ± 13.0[b]	220 ± 10.6
Clozapine	143 ± 6.3[c]	350 ± 12.0

[a] Average values (with SEM) represent the DA liberated into the 3 hr perfusate following i.v. injection of chlorpromazine (10 mg/kg) or clozapine (20 mg/kg) and are expressed in percent of those obtained in saline-injected animals (controls = 100).
[b] $P > .05$ vs. nucleus accumbens.
[c] $P < .01$ vs. nucleus accumbens.
Note: For further details see Bartholini, 1976.

cyclase to a similar extent in limbic and extrapyramidal structures (Scatton et al., 1977). The less marked activation of striatal than of limbic DA neurons by atypical neuroleptics could be explained by the anticholinergic properties of some of these compounds (e.g., clozapine and thioridazine). Thus, antimuscarinic properties may diminish the feedback activation of DA cells. This assumption is, however, unlikely, since (1) clozapine enhances the striatal ACh output only at doses of 35 mg/kg i.v. (see Section V.B.1), in contrast to the low doses of anti-ACh drugs (e.g., 2 mg/kg atropine) which activate cholinergic neurons, probably via a feedback mechanism; (2) clozapine causes intense salivation in humans; (3) clozapine and thioridazine do not antagonize (in contrast to low doses of anti-ACh compounds) the sinistrotorsion in the guinea pig (Bartholini et al., 1972) and the increase in rat brain ACh caused by physostigmine (Sethy and Van Woert, 1974); (4) sulpiride is devoid of anticholinergic properties since it does not antagonize the arecoline-induced activation of the rabbit electrocorticogram (Depoortere, personal communication) or the behavioral effects of oxotremorine (Worms, personal communication), yet sulpiride is one of the less active atypical neuroleptics on striatal DA turnover.

Therefore, as previously postulated (Bartholini et al., 1972), the less marked activation of the nigrostriatal DA pathway by atypical neuroleptics rather than from their anti-ACh properties likely results from a weak blockade of DA receptors as compared to that caused by classical antipsychotic agents. This conclusion is also supported by (1) the fact that clozapine and thioridazine are less potent than chlorpromazine in enhancing the striatal ACh release in the cat, an effect which is the consequence of the DA receptor blockade (see Section V.A); (2) the electrophysiological observation that administration of clozapine results in a more marked blockade in nucleus accumbens than in striatum of the depression of cells postsynaptic to dopaminergic neurons elicited by micro-iontophoretically applied DA (Bunney and Aghajanian, 1976).

Many other nonneuroleptic drugs affect preferentially limbic, as compared to striatal, DA neurons, putting some doubt on the view that this effect is related to the antipsychotic action of atypical compounds (see Westerink et al., 1977). However, none of these non-neuroleptic drugs has been shown to block DA receptors, in contrast to sulpiride, clozapine, and thioridazine. Therefore, the increase in DA turnover caused by non-neuroleptics occurs via different mechanisms (for instance, physostigmine and oxotremorine are known to activate cholinergic receptors on DA neurons; see Section VI.A) which, not being related to the DA receptor blockade, explain the lack of antipsychotic properties of these compounds.

B. Functional Implications

The above discussed data support the assumption that atypical neuroleptics are weak DA receptor blocking agents in the striatum, and preferentially affect

Table 7 "Atypical" and Classical Neuroleptics: Degree of Limbic vs. Striatal DA Receptor Blockade as Compared to Incidence of Extrapyramidal Reactions

Drug	Limbic system striatum[a]	Incidence of extrapyramidal reactions
Sulpiride	2.1	Low
Clozapine	1.6	Low
Thioridazine	1.3	Medium
Haloperidol	0.97	High
Chlorpromazine	0.82	High

[a]The data, calculated from those of Table 5, indicate for each drug the ratio between the limbic and the striatal increase in homovanillic acid levels.

the limbic dopaminergic transmission. This leads to two main conclusions concerning the functional implications of this differential effect:

(1) The less marked effect in striatum explains the lower incidence of extrapyramidal side effects during medication with these drugs as compared to that occurring with classical compounds such as haloperidol and chlorpromazine, which influence, to a similar extent, limbic and striatal dopaminergic transmission. Thus, the lower the striatal DA receptor blockade by neuroleptics as compared to that in the limbic system, the lower the incidence of their striopallidal reactions. Table 7 shows a tentative correlation.

The low incidence of extrapyramidal side effects associated with clozapine and thioridazine has been alternatively claimed to be connected with the anticholinergic properties of these compounds, which may block the cholinergic hyperactivity triggered by the blockade of striatal DA receptors (see Section V). This hypothesis is based on the apparent inverse correlation between the affinity of these drugs for cholinergic binding sites in brain homogenates and the frequency of extrapyramidal disturbances (Snyder et al., 1974; Miller and Hiley, 1974). However, the data discussed in Section VII.A indicate that the anticholinergic properties of atypical neuroleptics may contribute to, but cannot play a major role for, the virtual absence of parkinsonian symptoms during medication with these drugs.

(2) The preferential impairment of limbic dopaminergic transmission by sulpiride, clozapine, and thioridazine also reinforces the hypothesis that the limbic system is the anatomical substrate for the antipsychotic action of neuroleptic drugs.

VIII. DIFFERENTIAL DEVELOPMENT OF NEUROLEPTIC-INDUCED TOLERANCE IN EXTRAPYRAMIDAL AND LIMBIC STRUCTURES: FUNCTIONAL EFFECTS

The data discussed in the previous sections indicate that the blockade of dopaminergic transmission by neuroleptic agents in the limbic system is responsible for the antipsychotic action of, and in the striatum, for the parkinsonian syndrome induced by, these drugs. It appears, however, that during neuroleptic medication, supersensitivity of DA target cells develops in the striatum, explaining the spontaneous reduction of parkinsonian symptoms and the development of tardive dyskinesias (see Section V.B.2). Thus, the question arises as to why supersensitivity does not develop in the target cells of limbic DA pathway, leading to a gradual disappearance of the antipsychotic action of neuroleptic drugs. Recent results in animals have shown that during repeated administration of both classical and atypical neuroleptic agents, the doses required to induce tolerance to the increase in the striatal DA turnover are lower than those needed to affect the limbic system (nucleus accumbens, tuberculum olfactorium, and cortex); and for a given dose, tolerance develops earlier in striatum than in the other regions (Scatton, 1977). These data suggest, therefore, that the target cells of limbic DA neurons are less sensitive to the induction of tolerance than those in striatum. Thus, if the antipsychotic action of neuroleptic drugs is connected with the blockade of DA receptors in limbic system, it may be assumed that the concentration of the drugs required to induce tolerance in this structure may seldom be reached in humans, explaining the persistence of the antipsychotic action.

IX. NEUROLEPTIC DRUGS AND NORADRENERGIC TRANSMISSION

Several neuroleptic drugs block cerebral noradrenaline receptors: their relative potency, however, differs greatly (Keller et al., 1973). In addition, other neuroleptics are pure DA receptor antagonists. Therefore, the blockade of noradrenaline receptors by neuroleptics does not seem to be related to the antipsychotic action of the drugs but rather may be connected to a sedative effect of some of these compounds. In fact, the noradrenergic system is involved in alertness and impairment of noradrenergic transmission may contribute unspecifically to the amelioration of psychotic symptoms.

X. NEUROLEPTIC DRUGS, PROLACTIN, AND GONADOTROPIN SECRETION

All of the DA receptor blocking agents suppress the inhibitory influence of hypothalamic DA on the secretion of prolactin and gonadotropin, leading to increased release of these hormones and to side effects such as gynecomasty, galactorrhea, and blockade of ovulation. For further details, see McLeod and Login, 1976; Agnati et al., 1976.

XI. SUMMARY

Neuroleptic drugs block postsynaptic DA receptors. Evidence for this blockade is provided by the chemical structure of these drugs, which is closely related to that of DA (Section II), the antagonism of neuroleptics toward the electrophysiological changes induced by microiontophoretically administered DA, the blockade of a DA-sensitive adenylate cyclase, which is supposed to be connected with DA receptors (Section III).

Blockade of DA receptors impairs dopaminergic transmission in extrapyramidal and limbic structures. In the striatum, this blockade suppresses the inhibitory dopaminergic input on cholinergic interneurons (Section V.A), leading to cholinergic hyperactivity and to the appearance of parkinsonian symptoms (Section V.B.2.a). The increased activity of striatal cholinergic neurons may also repesent a feedback mechanism of activation of DA neurons since an excitatory cholinergic influence on the DA cells has been demonstrated (Section V.A). An inhibitory GABA input also may intervene in the neuroleptic-induced feedback activation of the DA neurons as neuroleptic drugs enhance the turnover of GABA in the striatum (Section V.A). The enhanced DA release may overcome the postsynaptic receptor blockade by neuroleptic agents. In fact, some experiments suggest that the relative concentration of DA and neuroleptics in the synaptic cleft is critical for the inhibition of the DA target cells (Section V.B.1). The compensatory activation of DA neurons may lead, in the presence of supersensitivity of DA postsynaptic cells, to reduction of parkinsonian syndrome (Section V.B.2.a) and to the development of tardive dyskinesias (Section V.B.2.b).

In the limbic system, dopaminergic neurons do not apparently influence cholinergic cells. Thus, the blockade of DA receptors by neuroleptics does not lead to alterations of limbic cholinergic activity, which therefore appears not to be involved in the antipsychotic action of these drugs (Section VI.A). However, a dopaminergic influence on cortical cholinergic neurons is not excluded with certainty.

Limbic dopaminergic neurons seem to be modulated by an excitatory cholinergic, and an inhibitory GABAergic, input. Thus, the anticholinergic properties of some neuroleptics may contribute to the impairment of dopaminergic transmission, although no clear evidence is provided by clinical data. The involvement of GABA in the action of these drugs is still obscure (Section VI.B). The impairment of limbic dopaminergic transmission is probably connected with the antipsychotic action of neuroleptics. Evidence for this view is provided by the preferential activation of limbic DA turnover by atypical neuroleptics (e.g., clozapine, sulpiride, and thioridazine), suggesting a preferential blockade of limbic DA receptors. The mechanism of this preferential blockade is still obscure. It may be connected with a difference in brain distribution of the drugs and/or in the affinity for receptors; or, less probably, with the anticholinergic properties of neuroleptics (Section VII.A). However, the pattern of atypical neuroleptics suggests that the limbic system is the anatomical substrate of the antipsychotic action of DA receptor blockers and explains why atypical compounds display fewer extrapyramidal side effects than classical neuroleptics (Section VII.A).

Finally, recent data indicate that supersensitivity of the postsynaptic target cells of DA neurons during neuroleptic medication develops in striatum after low doses of the drugs and earlier than in the limbic system. This difference might explain why tolerance does not apparently develop to the antipsychotic action of neuroleptics (Section VIII).

XII. RECENT DEVELOPMENTS

Since this chapter was written, new data have appeared which are relevant to (1) the mode of action of neuroleptics and (2) the GABA involvement in the regulation of DA neurons and its relation to the treatment of tardive dyskinesias and schizophrenia.

A. Substituted Benzamides and Adenylate Cyclase Activity

The pharmacological pattern of sulpiride, a benzamide derivative, is briefly described in Section VII; the compound differs from classical neuroleptics in as much as it preferentially affects limbic dopaminergic transmission and does not cause catalepsy in animals. In addition, it was recently reported that sulpiride does not block DA-sensitive adenylate cyclase (Elliot et al., 1977). However, other benzamide derivatives which have a pharmacological and biochemical pattern similar to that of "classical" neuroleptics (increase of striatal ACh turnover, induction of catalepsy) also do not affect the enzyme; this indicates that biochemical and behavioral effects of DA receptor blockade can occur in the absence of alterations of adenylate cyclase stimulated by DA (Scatton et al., 1979). As a consequence, it cannot be generally stated anymore that this enzyme is the second messenger of DA neurons (see Section III); probably, two types of DA receptors (or two conformational states of the receptor) exist, one connected with adenylate cyclase and affected by classical neuroleptics and one independent from the enzyme and affected by substituted benzamides.

All of the neuroleptics, however, share the common property of displacing labeled ligands from binding sites of brain membrane preparations (Creese et al.,

1976; Jenner et al., 1978); this property can be considered, to date, the biochemical evidence for the action of neuroleptics on DA receptors.

B. GABA and DA Neurons: Relation to the Treatment of Tardive Dyskinesias and Schizophrenia

The recent synthesis of the first, nontoxic GABA-mimetic compound, SL 76 002,* has given new light on the relation between GABA and DA systems in both animals and humans. SL 76 002 [{α(chloro-4-pehnyl)fluoro-5-hydroxy-2-benzilideneamino}-4-butyramide] (Fig. 9) (Kaplan et al., 1980) is a GABA derivative (gabamide) attached by an imine link to a lipophilic, substituted benzophenone allowing penetration into the brain. In the mammalian organism, SL 76 002 is converted to its acidic derivative SL 75 102 by deamination of the amide moiety; it releases gabamide by hydrolysis of the imine bond; both SL 75 102 and gabamide form GABA.

SL 76 002 and its metabolites displace labeled GABA from binding sites of brain membrane preparations; the soluble compound SL 75 102 has been shown to cause changes in membrane conductance and depolarization in the rat dorsal sensory root ganglia similar to those produced by GABA; SL 76 002 decreases the firing of the cat Deiter's nucleus cells (which are densely innervated by cerebellar GABAergic neurons) and antagonizes the increase in their activity caused by picrotoxin; SL 76 002 antagonizes bicuculline-induced

*Synthesized by Dr. J. P. Kaplan, Chemistry Department, Synthélabo (L.E.R.S.), Paris.

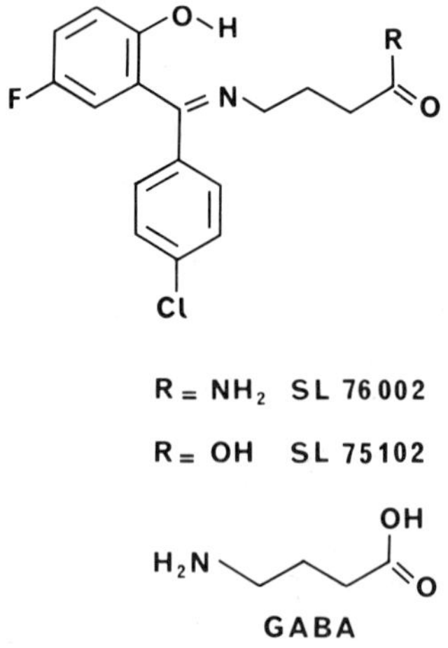

R = NH_2 SL 76002

R = OH SL 75102

GABA

Figure 9 Chemical structure of SL 76 002, SL 75 102, and GABA.

convulsion in the cat; no changes in GABA transaminase or glutamic acid transaminase activity or in GABA uptake are observed with SL 76 002 and its metabolites. These data indicate SL 76 002 as GABA receptor agonist and precursor of GABA receptor stimulants, including GABA (Bartholini et al., 1979a; Lloyd et al., 1979; Desarmenien et al., 1980).

SL 76 002, systemically administered, decreases synthesis and release of DA. Thus, the compound diminishes the accumulation of striatial dopa in vivo and formation of $[1\text{-}^{14}C]O_2$ in vitro from labeled tyrosine, this effect being blocked by picrotoxin; also, SL 76 002 reduces the rate of disappearance of DA due to α-methyl-p-tyrosine and decreases the amount of DA liberated into the perfusate of the cat caudate nucleus implanted with the push-pull cannula.

These results clearly support the view that GABA reduces the activity of DA neurons (see Sections V.A and VI.A). This GABAergic influence is more marked on striatal than on limbic DA pathway as SL 76 002 only slightly affects the activity of the latter. However, it appears that the GABA input on DA neurons is more pronounced when these neurons are activated as, for instance, after neuroleptics (Bartholini et al., 1979a).

As discussed in Section V.A, the GABA influence on DA neurons is probably exerted on both cell bodies and terminals. GABA, however, does not only affect the dopaminergic function by a presynaptic input (on DA neurons) but also influences the postsynaptic system(s) involved in behavioral responses to changes of dopaminergic transmission; thus, SL 76 002 administered chronically with neuroleptics prevents the development of tolerance to their cataleptogenic action as well as the increased sensitivity to DA receptor stimulants (e.g., apomorphine). In contrast, SL 76 002 does not prevent the tolerance of the striatal cholinergic system to neuroleptics, indicating that (1) behavioral effects resulting from alteration of dopaminergic transmission are not exclusively mediated by changes of cholinergic activity (see Section V) and (2) GABA may affect behavioral responses independently from the changes in activity of striatal cholinergic neurons. These results suggest a therapeutic action of SL 76 002 in tardive dyskinesias. In this syndrome, some symptoms are probably related to development of DA target cell supersensitivity (see Section V.B.2.b); thus, GABA-mimetic drugs by acting beyond both dopaminergic and cholinergic systems may damp the effect of an exaggerated response to DA (Bartholini et al., 1979b). This may be of beneficial effect not only in tardive dyskinesias but also in L-dopa-induced involuntary movements in parkinsonian patients as well as in Huntington's chorea. Indeed, preliminary open pilot studies with SL 76 002 in these disorders support this view (Bartholini et al., 1979a,c,d).

In section VI, the possible involvement of GABA in the regulation of limbic DA neurons has been discussed in relation to the therapy of schizophrenia. Thus, compounds such as GABA receptor agonists, which decrease the firing of the mesolimbic DA pathway, may be useful in the treatment of this psychosis, which is thought to be connected with a relative exaggeration of limbic DA transmission. In this light, SL 76 002 has been administered to schizophrenic (hebephrenic and paranoid) subjects, alone or associated with neuroleptic drugs. No effect has been observed on the clinical status. The lack of effect on SL 76 002 may be related to the possibility that the compound does not sufficiently affect limbic DA transmission which, in animals, has been shown to be less sensitive to the drug than in striatum (see above). Alternatively, GABA transmission does not play a major role in humans for the regulation of limbic dopaminergic activity (Bartholini et al., 1979c).

In summary, the availability of the first, nontoxic GABA receptor agonist, SL 76 002, has confirmed that DA pathways are inhibited by a GABA input. In addition, it appears that GABA inhibits the mesolimbic less than the extrapyramidal DA neurons. The inhibitory influence of GABA on dopaminergic activity is more marked when DA neurons are activated (e.g., after neuroleptics). GABA also affects striatal function beyond DA and ACh neurons; thus, during chronic treatment with neuroleptics, SL 76 002 antagonizes the tolerance to their cataleptogenic action as well as the increased sensitivity to apomorphine but not the tolerance of the cholinergic system. This suggests a beneficial action of GABA-mimetic compounds in disorders such as neuroleptic-induced tardive dyskinesias, Huntington's chorea, and involuntary movement caused by L-dopa in parkinsonian patients. Results of preliminary open pilot studies appear to confirm this view. In contrast, SL 76 002 alone or associated with neuroleptic medication is not effective in schizophrenia.

REFERENCES

Agnati, L., Fuxe, K., Löfström, A., and Hökfelt, T. (1976) Dopaminergic drugs and ovulation. Studies on PMS-induced ovulation and changes in median eminence DA and NE turnover in immature female rats. In *Advances in Biochemical Psychopharmacology*, Vol. 16. E. Costa and G. L. Gessa. Symposium on nonstriatal dopaminergic neurons. Raven, New York, pp. 159-168.

Andén, N.-E. (1974a). Inhibition of the turnover of brain dopamine after treatment with the gammaaminobutyrate: 2-oxyglutarate transaminase inhibitor aminooxyacetic acid. *Nauyn Schmiedeberg's Arch. Pharmacol. 283*, 419-428.

Andén, N.-E. (1974b). Effect of oxotremorine and physostigmine on the turnover of dopamine in the corpus striatum and the limbic system. *J. Pharm. Pharmacol. 26*, 738-740.

Andén, N.-E., and Stock, G. (1973). Inhibitory effect of γ-hydroxybutyric acid and γ-aminobutyric acid on the dopamine cells in the substantia nigra. *Nauyn Schmiedeberg's Arch. Pharmacol. 289*, 89-92.

Andén, N.-E., Butcher, S. G., Corrodi, H., Fuxe, K., and Ungerstedt, U. (1970). Receptor activity and turnover of dopamine and noradrenaline after neuroleptics. *Eur. J. Pharmacol. 11*, 303-314.

Asper, H. M., Baggiolini, H. R., Burki, H., Lauener, W., Ruch, H., and Stille, G. 1973). Tolerance phenomena with neuroleptics, catalepsy, apomorphine stereotypies and striatal dopamine metabolism in the rat after simple and repeated administration of loxapine and haloperidol. *Eur. J. Pharmacol. 22*, 287-294.

Ayd, F. J. (1976). Haloperidol update. In Haloperidol. A new profile. *Proc. Roy. Soc. Med. 69*, No. 1, 14-18.

Bartholini, G. (1976). Differential effect of neuroleptic drugs on dopamine turnover in the extrapyramidal and limbic system. *J. Pharm. Pharmacol. 28*, 429-433.

Bartholini, G., and Stadler, H. (1975a). Cholinergic and GABA-ergic influence on the dopamine release in extrapyramidal centers. In *Chemical Tools in Catecholamine Research. II. Regulation of Catecholamine Turnover,* O. Almgren, A. Carlsson, and J. Engel (Eds.). North-Holland, Amsterdam, pp. 235-241.

Bartholini, G., and Stadler, H. (1975b). Neurotransmitter interaction in the basal ganglia. Relation to extrapyramidal disorders. In *Advances in Parkinsonism,* W. Birkmayer (Ed.). Editiones Roche, pp. 115-123.

Bartholini, G., and Stadler, H. (1977). Evidence for an intrastriatal GABA-ergic influence on dopamine neurons of the cat. *Neuropharmacology 16*, 343-347.

Bartholini, G., Haefely, W., Jalfre, M., Keller, H. H., and Pletscher, A. (1972). Effect of clozapine on cerebral catecholaminergic neurone systems. *Br. J. Pharmacol. 46*, 736-740.

Bartholini, G., Stadler, H., Gadea Ciria, M., and Lloyd, K. G. (1974a). The effect of antipsychotic drugs on the release of neurotransmitters in various brain areas. In *Antipsychotic Drugs: Pharamcodynamics and Pharmacokinetics,* G. Sedvall, B. Uvnäs, and Y. Zotterman (Eds.). Pergamon, New York, pp. 105-116.

Bartholini, G., Stadler, H., and Lloyd, K. G. (1974b). *The Effect of Drugs on the Release of Striatal Neurotransmitters.* CINP Meeting, Paris, 1974. Excepta Medica International Congress Series No. 359, pp. 487-492.

Bartholini, G., Keller, H. H., and Pletscher, A. (1975a). Drug-induced changes of dopamine turnover in striatum and limbic system of the rat. *J. Pharm. Pharmacol. 27*, 439-442.

Bartholini, G., Stadler, H., and Lloyd, K. G. (1975b). Cholinergic-dopaminergic inter-regulations within the extrapyramidal system. In *Cholinergic Mechanims,* P. G. Waser (Eds.). Raven, New York, pp. 411-418.

Bartholini, G., Stadler, H., Gadea Ciria, M., and Lloyd, K. G. (1976a). The use of the push-pull cannula to estimate the dynamics of acetylcholine and catecholamines within various brain areas. *Neuropharmacology 15,* 515-519.

Bartholini, G., Stadler, H., Gadea Ciria, M., and Lloyd, K. G. (1976b). Interaction of dopaminergic and cholinergic neurons in extrapyramidal and limbic system. In *Symposium on Extrastriatal Dopamine Neurons, Advances in Biochemical Pharmacology,* Vol. 16, E. Costa and G. L. Gessa (Eds.). Raven, New York, pp. 391-395.

Bartholini, G., Scatton, B., Zivkovic, B., and Lloyd, K. G. (1979a). On the mode of action of SL 76 002, a new GABA receptor agaonis. In *GABA-Neurotransmitters,* H. Kofod, P. Krogsgaard-Larsen, and Scheel-Krüger (Eds.). Munksgaard, Copenhagen, pp. 326-339.

Bartholini, G., Scatton, B., and Zivkovic, B. (1979b). Effect of the new GABA agonist SL 76 002 on striatial acetycholine. Relation to neuroleptic-induced extrapyramidal alterations. In *Long-Term Effects of Neuroleptics,* F. Cattabeni, S. Gorini, G. Racagni, and P. F. Spano (Eds.). Raven, New York, pp. 207-213.

Bartholini, G., Cuche, H., Zarifian, E., and Morselli, P. L. (1979c). Involvement of cholinergic and GABAergic systems in schizophrenia. In *Biological Psychiatry Today,* J. Obiols, C. Ballús, E. Gonzales Monclus, and J. Pujol (Eds.). Elsevier/North-Holland Biomedical Press, Amsterdam, pp. 439-444.

Bartholini, G., Lloyd, K. G., Worms, P., Constantinidis, J., and Tissot, R. (1979d). GABA and GABAergic medication. Relation to striatal DA function and Parkinsonism. In *Parkinson's Disease,* L. J. Poirier, T. Sourkes, and P. J. Bedard (Eds.). Raven, New York. pp. 253-257.

Beckmann, H., Frische, M., Rüther, E., and Zimmer, R. (1977). Baclofen (para-chlorophenyl-GABA) in schizophrenia. *Pharmakopsychiat. 10,* 26-31.

Bigelow, L. B., Nasrallah, H., Carman, J., Gillin, J. C., and Wyatt, R. J. (1977). Baclofen treatment in chronic schizophrenia. A clinical trial. *Am. J. Psychiatry 134,* No. 3, pp. 318-320.

Bower, M. B., and Rozitis, A. (1974). Regional differences in homovanillic acid concentrations after acute and chronic administration of antipsychotic drugs. *J. Pharm. Pharamcol. 26,* 743-745.

Bunney, B. S., and Aghajanian, G. K. (1974). The effect of antipsychotic drugs on the firing of dopaminergic neurons. A reappraisal. In *Antipsychotic Drugs: Pharmacodynamics and Pharmacokinetics,* G. Sedvall, B. Uvnäs, and Y. Zotterman (Eds.). Pergamon, New York, pp. 305-318.

Bunney, B. S., and Aghajanian, G. K. (1976). Incidence of neuroleptic extrapyramidal side-effects. An alternative explanation to the "antimuscarinic hypothesis" for variations between drugs. In Biochemical Basis of Drug

Side-Effects in Psychiatry. Ann. Meet. Soc. Biological Psychiatry, San Francisco, June 1976 (Abstr.).

Carlson, A. (1976). The impact of pharmacology on the problem of schizophrenia. In *Schizophrenia Today*, D. Kemali, G. Bartholini, and D. Richter (Eds.). Pergamon, New York, pp. 89-103.

Carlsson, A., and Lindqvist, M. (1963). Effect of chlorpromazine and haloperidol on formation of 3-methoxytyramine and normetanephrine in mouse brain. *Acta Pharmacol. Toxicol. 20,* 104-144.

Corrodi, H., and Hardegger, E. (1955). Die Konfiguration des Apomorphins und verwander verbindugnen. *Helv. Chim. Acta 32,* 2038.

Corrodi, H., Fuxe, K., and Lidbrink, P. (1972). Interaction between cholinergic and catecholaminergic neurons in rat brain. *Brain Res. 43,* 397-416.

Creese, I., Burt, D., and Snyder, S. H. (1976). Dopamine receptor binding predicts clinical and pharmacological potencies of antischizophrenic drugs. *Science 192,* 481-483.

Curtis, D. R., Game, C. J. A., Johnston, G. A. R., and McCulloch, R. M. (1974). Central effect of β-(p-cholophenyl)-γ-aminobutyric acid. *Brain Res. 70,* 493-499.

Da Prada, M., Saner, A., Burkard, W. P., Bartholini, G., and Pletscher, A. (1975). Lysergic acid diethylamide. Evidence for stimulation of cerebral dopamine receptors. *Brain Res. 94,* 67-73.

Davis, J. M. (1974). A two factor theory of schizophrenia. *J. Psychiatr. Res. 11,* 25-29.

Davis, J. M., and Watkins, J. C. (1974). The action of β-phenyl-GABA derivatives in neurons of the rat cerebral cortex. *Brain Res. 70,* 501-505.

Desarmenien, M., Feltz, P., Haedley, P. M., and Santangelo, F. (1980). SL 75 102 as a GABA agonist. Experiments on dorsal root ganglion neurons in vitro. *Br. J. Pharmacol.* In press.

Elliot, P. N. C., Jenner, P., Huizing, G., Marsden, C. D., and Miller, R. (1977). Substituted benzamides as cerebral dopamine antagonists in rodents. *Neuropharmacology 16,* 333-342.

Ezrin-Waters, C., and Seeman, P. (1977). Tolerance to haloperidol catalepsy. *Eur. J. Pharmacol. 41,* 321-327.

Fann, W. E., Lake, C. R., Gerber, C. J., and McKenzie, G. M. (1974). Cholinergic suppression of tardive dyskinesia. *Psychopharmacology 37,* 101-107.

Fehr, H V., and Bein, H. J. (1974). Site of action of a new muscle relaxant (baclofen, Lioresal^{R}, Ciba 34.647 Ba). *J. Int. Med. Res. 2,* 36-47.

Fibiger, H. C., and Grewaal, D. S. (1974). Neurochemical evidence for denervation supersensitivity. The effect of unilateral substantia nigra lesions on apomorphine-induced increase in neostriatal acetylcholine levels. *Life Sci. 15,* 57-63.

Frederiksen, P. K. (1975). Baclofen in the treatment of schizophrenia. *Lancet 1,* 702-703.

Fuxe, K., Hökfelt, T., Ljungdahl, A., Agnati, L., Johansson, O., and Perez Ia, Mora M. (1975). Evidence for an inhibitory GABA-ergic control of the mesolimbic dopamine neurons. Possibility of improving treatment of schizophrenia by combined-treatment with neuroleptics and GABA-ergic drugs. *Med. Biol. 53,* 177-183.

Gianutsos, G., Drawbangh, R. R., Hynes, M. D., and Lal, H. (1974). Behavioral evidence for dopaminergic supersensitivity after chronic haloperidol. *Life Sci. 14,* 887-898.

Greengard, P. (1974). In *Molecular Studies on the Nature of Dopamine Receptor in the Caudate Nucleus of the Mammalian Brain,* P. Seeman and G. M. Brown (Eds.). The University of Toronto Press, Toronto, 12-15.

Guyenet, P., Agid, Y., Yavoy, F., Beaujouan, J., Rossier, J., and Glowinski, J. (1975). Effects of dopaminergic receptor agonists and antagonists on the activity of the neo-striatal cholinergic system. *Brain Res. 84,* 227-236.

Janssen, P. A. J. (1967). The pharmacology of haloperidol. *Int. J. Neuropsychiatry 3,* 10-18.

Janssen, P. A. J. (1974). Structure-activity relations (SAR) and drug design as illustrated with neuroleptic agents. In *Antipsychotic Drugs: Pharmacodynamics and Pharmacokinetics,* G. Sedvall, B. Unväs, and Y. Zotterman (Eds.)., Pergamon, New York, pp. 5-31.

Jenner, P., Elliot, P. N. C., Clow, A., Reavill, C., and Marsden, C. D. (1978). A comparison of "in vitro" and "in vivo" dopamine receptor antagonism produced by substituted benzamide drugs. *J. Pharm. Pharmacol. 30,* 46-48.

Johnston, G. A. R. (1976). Physiologic pharmacology of GABA and its antagonists in vertebrate nervous system. In *GABA in Nervous System Function,* E. Roberts, T. N. Chase, and D. B. Tower (Eds.). Raven, New York, pp. 395-411.

Kaplan, J. P., Worms, P., Raison, B., Feltz, P., Lloyd, K. G., and Bartholini, G. (1980). New anticonvulsants. Schiff's bases of GABA and GABAMIDE. *J. Med. Chem. 23,* 702-704.

Kataoka, K., Bak, I. J., Hassler, R., Kim, J. S., and Wagner, A. (1974). L-Glutamate decarboxylase and choline acetyltransferase activity in the substantia nigra and the striatum after surgical interruption of the strio-nigral fibres of the baboon. *Exp. Brain Res. 19,* 217-222.

Keller, H. H., Bartholini, G., and Pletscher, A. (1973). Increase in 3-methoxy-4-hydroxyphenylethylene glycol in rat brain by neuroleptic drugs. *Eur. J. Pharmacol. 23,* 183-186.

Kalwans, H. L. (1973). Some observations on the pharmacology of striatum. *Psychiatr. Forum,* 16-26.

Lahti, R. A., and Losey, E. G. (1974). Antagonism of the effect of chlorpromazine and morphine on dopamine metabolism by GABA. *Res. Comm. Chem. Pathol. Pharmacol. 1,* 31-40.

Langer, S. Z., and Trendelenburg, N. (1966). The onset of denervation supersensitivity. *J. Pharmacol. Exp. Ther. 151,* 76-86.

Lloyd, K. G., and Hornykiewicz, O. (1973). L-glutamic acid decarboxylase in Parkinson's disease. Effect of L-DOPA therapy. *Nature 243,* 521-522.

Lloyd, K. G., Stadler, H., and Bartholini, G. (1973). Dopamine and acetylcholine neurons in striatal and limbic structures. Effect of neuroleptic drugs. In *Frontiers in Catecholamine Research,* E. Usdin and S. Snyder (Eds.). Pergamon, New York, pp. 777-779.

Lloyd, K. G., Worms, P., Depoortere, H., and Bartholini, G. (1979). Pharmacological profile of SL 76 002, a new GABA-mimetic drug. In *GABA-Neurotransmitters,* H. Kofod, P. Krogsgaard-Larsen, and J. Scheel-Krüger (Eds.). Munksgaard, Copenhagen, pp. 308-325.

Marco, E., Mao, C. C., Cheney, D. L., Rivuelta, A., and Costa, E. (1976). The effect of antipsychotics on the turnover rate of GABA and acetylcholine in rat brain nuclei. *Nature 264,* 363-365.

McGeer, P. L., and McGeer, E. G. (1976). The GABA system and function of the basal ganglia: Huntington's disease. In *GABA in Nervous System Function,* E. Roberts, T. N. Chase, and D. B. Tower (Eds.). Raven, New York, pp. 487-495.

McLeod, R. M., and Login, I. S. (1976). Regulation of prolactin secretion through dopamine, serotonin and cerebro-spinal fluid. In *Symposium on Nonstriatal Dopaminergic Neurons, Advances in Biochemical Psycho-Psychopharmacology,* Vol. 16, E. Costa and G. L. Gessa (Eds.). Raven, New York, pp. 147-157.

Miller, R. J., and Hiley, C. R. (1974). Antimuscarinic properties of neuroleptics and drug-induced parkinsonism. *Nature 284,* 596-597.

Moore, K. E., and Thornberg, J. E. (1975). Drug-induced dopaminergic supersensitivity. *Adv. Neurol. 9,* 93-104.

Munkvad, I., Fog, R., and Kristjansen, P. (1976). The drug approach to therapy. Long-term treatment of schizophrenia. In *Schizophrenia Today,* D. Kemali, G. Bartholini, and D. Richter (Eds.). Pergamon, New York, pp. 173-182.

Nybäck, H., and Sedvall, G. (1970). Further studies on the accumulation and disappearance of catecholamines formed from tyrosine-^{14}C in mouse brain. Effect of some phenothiazine analogues. *Eur. J. Pharmacol. 10,* 193-205.

O'Keeffe, R., Sharman, D. F., and Vogt, M. (1970). Effect of drugs used in psychoses on cerebral dopamine metabolism. *Br. J. Pharmacol. 38,* 287-304.

Olson, L., Nyström, B., and Seiger, Å. (1973). Monoamine fluorescence histochemistry of human postmortem brain. *Brain Res. 63,* 231-247.

Pepeu, G. (1974). The release of acetylcholine from the brain: an approach to the study of central mechanisms. *Progr. Neurobiol. 2,* 257-288.

Pletscher, A., and Kyburz, E. (1976). Neuroleptic drugs. Chemical versus biochemical classification. In *Schizophrenia Today,* D. Kemali, G. Bartholini, and D. Richter (Eds.). Pergamon, New York, pp. 183-200.

Post, R. M., and Goodwin, F. K. (1975). Time dependent effects of phenothiazines on dopamine turnover in psychiatric patients. *Science 190,* 488-489.

Roth, R. H. (1971). Effect of anesthetic doses of γ-hydroxybutyrate on subcortical concentrations of homovanillic acid. *Eur. J. Pharmacol. 15,* 52-59.

Scatton, B. (1977). Differential regional development of tolerance to increase in dopamine turnover upon repeated neuroleptic administration. *Eur. J. Pharmacol. 46,* 363-369.

Scatton, B., Glowinski, J., and Jolou, L. (1975). Neuroleptics. Effects on dopamine synthesis in the nigro-neostriatal, mesolimbic and meso-cortical dopaminergic systems. In *Antipsychotic Drugs: Pharmacodynamics and Pharmacokinetics,* G. Sedvall, B. Unväs, and Y. Zotterman (Eds.). Pergamon, New York, pp. 243-260.

Scatton, B., Bischoff, S., Dedek, J., and Korf, J. (1977). Regional effects of neuroleptics on dopamine metabolism and dopamine sensitive adenylate cyclase activity. *Eur. J. Pharmacol. 44,* 287-292.

Scatton, B., Worms, B., Zivkovic, B., Depoortere, H., Dedek, J., and Bartholini, G. (1979). On the neuropharmacological spectra of "classical" (Haloperiodol) and "atypical" (Benzamide derivatives) neuroleptics. In *International Workshop on Sulpiride and Other Benzamides,* G. L. Gessa, G. U. Corsini, P. F. Spano, and M. Trabucchi (Eds.). Italian Brain Research Foundation Press. Raven, New York, pp. 53-66.

Schaffner, R., Jalfre, M., and Haefely, W. (1974). Effect of different pharamcological agents on the septo-hippocampal evoked potentials. CINP Congress, Paris 1974 (Abstr. CJ4).

Seeman, P., and Lee, T. (1974). The dopamine releasing actions of neuroleptics and ethanol. *J. Pharmacol. Exp. Ther. 190,* 131-140.

Seeman, P., and Lee, T. (1975). Antipsychotic drugs. Direct correlation between clinical potency and presynaptic action on dopamine neurons. *Science 188,* 1217-1219.

Sethy, V. H., and Van Woert, M. H. (1974). Modifications of striatal acetylcholine concentration by dopamine receptor agonists and antagonists. *Res. Comm. Chem. Pathol. Pharmacol. 8,* 13-28.

Sethy, V. H., Roth, R. H., Kuhar, M. J., and Van Woert, M. H. (1973). Choline and acetylcholine. Regional distribution and effect of degeneration of cholinergic nerve terminal in rat hippocampus. *Neuropharmacology 12,* 819-823.

Shute, C. C. D., and Lewis, P. R. (1967). The ascending reticular system. Neocortical, olfactory and subcortical projections. *Brain Res. 90,* 497-520.

Simpson, G. M., Hillary Lee, J., Shrivastava, R. K., and Branchey, M. H. (1978). Baclofen in the treatment of tardive dyskinesia and schizophrenia. *Psychopharmacol. Bull. 14,* No. 2, pp. 16-18.

Snyder, S. H., Banerjee, S. P., Yamamura, H. I., and Greenberg, A. (1974). Drugs, neurotransmitters and schizophrenia. *Science,* 1243-1253.

Stadler, H., Lloyd, K. G., Gadea Ciria, M., and Bartholini, G. (1973). Enhanced striatal acetylcholine release by chlorpromazine and its reversal by apomorphine. *Brain Res. 55,* 476-480.

Stadler, H., Lloyd, K. G., and Bartholini, G. (1974). Dopaminergic inhibition of striatal cholinergic neurons. Synergistic blocking action of γ-butyrolactone and neuroleptic drugs. *Naunyn Schmiedeberg's Arch. Pharmacol. 283,* 129-134.

Stadler, H., Gadea Ciria, M., and Bartholini, G. (1975). In vivo release of endogenous neurotransmitters in cat limbic regions. Effect of chloropromazine and of electrical stimulation. *Naunyn Schmiedeberg's Arch. Pharmacol. 288,* 1-6.

Thierry, A. M., Blanc, G., Sobel, A., Stinus, L., and Glowinski, J. (1973). Dopaminergic terminals in the rat cortex. *Science 182,* 499-501.

Ungerstedt, U., Ljungberg, T., Hopper, B., and Siggins, G. (1975). Dopaminergic supersensitivity in the striatum. *Adv. Neurol. 9,* 57-65.

Waldeimer, P. C., and Maître, L. (1976a). Clozapine. Reduction of the initial dopamine turnover increase by repeated treatment. *Eur. J. Pharmacol. 38,* 197-203.

Waldeimer, P. C., and Maître, L. (1976b). On the relevance of the preferential increase of mesolimbic versus striatal dopamine turnover for the prediction of the antipsychotic action of psychotropic drugs. *J. Neurochem. 27,* 589-597.

Walters, J. R., Aghajanian, G. K., and Roth, R. H. (1972). Dopaminergic neurons. Inhibition of firing by γ-hydroxybutyrate. *Proc. 5th Congr. Pharmacol.,* San Francisco, p. 242.

Westerink, B. H. C., Lejeune, B., Korf, J., and van Praag, H. M. (1977). On the significance of regional dopamine metabolism in the rat brain for the classification of centrally active drugs. *Eur. J. Pharmacol. 42,* 179-190.

York, D. H. (1971). Dopamine receptor blockade. A central action of chlorpromazine on striatal neurons. *Brain Res. 37,* 91-101.

Yoshida, M., and Precht, W. (1971). Monosynaptic inhibition of neurons of the substantia nigra by caudato-nigral fibres. *Brain Res. 32,* 225-231.

Zivkovic, B., Guidotti, A., Rivuelta, A., and Costa, E. (1975). Effect of thioridazine, clozapine and other antipsychotics on the kinetic state of tyrosine hydroxylase and on the turnover rate of dopamine in striatum and nucleus accumbens. *J. Pharmacol. Exp. Ther. 194,* 37-46.

23

Mode of Action of Lithium

Mogens Schou
Aarhus University Institute of Psychiatry,
The Psychiatric Hospital, Risskov, Denmark

Erling T. Mellerup and Ole J. Rafaelsen
Psychochemistry Institute, Rigshospitalet
Copenhagen, Denmark

All psychotropic drugs are enigmas as regards their mode of action. Lithium (lithium salts, Li^+) is more enigmatic than most because it has such special properties with respect to psychotropic effects, to adverse reactions, and to physical and chemical nature.

I. SPECIAL FEATURES OF LITHIUM

A. Double Action in Manic-Depressive Disorder

Lithium differs from the conventional antimanic and antidepressive drugs in being active against both manifestations of manic-depressive disorder (Baastrup and Schou, 1967; Schou, 1976a). It exerts a clear therapeutic action in mania; it has a weak therapeutic action in depression; and it has a pronounced prophylactic action against both manias and depressions. By prophylactic action is meant the ability to attenuate or prevent further manic and depressive recurrences.

This peculiar double action of lithium is worth keeping in mind. There has been a tendency to disregard the action of lithium against depressive recurrences because doing so meant that it was easier to formulate coherent amine hypotheses. But it cannot be proper to consider only data that fit one's favorite hypothesis. The clinical facts indicate that one must look for biochemical models in which lithium does not simply stimulate or suppress, but in which it exerts a stabilizing action on cerebral processes that are out of balance, stabilizing through attentuation of a positive feedback mechanism or stimulation of a negative one.

B. Special Side Effects

Side effects observed during lithium treatment are different from those produced by conventional antimanic and antidepressive drugs (Vacaflor, 1975; Brown 1976; Schou, 1977). Lithium has for example no distinct autonomic side effects, and in therapeutic doses it very rarely, if ever, produces extrapyramidal symptoms. During lithium treatment one may, on the other hand, encounter specific adverse reactions such as development of goiter or myxedema, aggravation of physiological hand tremor, renal concentrating defect, polyuria, polydipsia, and interstitial nephropathy, and in some instances it has been possible to demonstrate the biochemical effects underlying these functional defects (Geisler et al., 1972; Wraae et al., 1972; Berens and Wolff, 1975; MacNeil and Jenner, 1975; Singer, 1976; Wolff, 1976). It seems reasonable to expect that information obtained through the study of such side effects may provide clues to what lithium does in the central nervous system.

C. Physicochemical Properties

While the conventional psychotropic drugs are large organic molecules, lithium is a monovalent cation. It is not metabolized, its quantitative determination is rapid and accurate, and its pharmacokinetics have been studied in considerable detail. Table 1 shows some of the special features of lithium. It belongs to the group I alkali metals together with sodium and potassium, and it is adjacent to the group II alkaline earth metals, among which magnesium and calcium are

Table 1 Special Features of Lithium

Element	Group	Charge	Atomic no.	Ionic radius (Å)	Charge density (Coul/$Å^2$)
Lithium		1+	3	0.8	0.22
Sodium	I	1+	11	1.0	0.09
Potassium		1+	19	1.3	0.05
Magnesium	II	2+	12	0.7	0.38
Calcium		2+	20	1.0	0.16

biologically important. It appears from Table 1 that lithium has the same charge as sodium and potassium, but is closer to the former than to the latter; this is found to be the case also in most biological systems. Lithium has approximately the same radius as magnesium and about the same charge density as calcium. These similarities are reflected in chemical and biological relationships betweeen lithium on one hand and magnesium and calcium on the other (Mellerup and Jørgensen, 1975; Lehn, 1976; Williams, 1976). Lithium and magnesium both bind nitrogen-containing ligands. Like calcium lithium is characterized by poorly defined coordination number and site geometry; this may explain why lithium competes effectively for calcium binding sites in systems using carboxyl groups as chelators.

On the basis of the physicochemical properties of the lithium ion biophysicists have deduced certain characteristics of the acceptor or binding sites to which lithium must be attached in order to exert biological actions (Eigen, 1976; Eisenman, 1976; Lehn, 1976; Winkler, 1976). (The word *binding* does not denote firm locking together such as that between a heavy metal and a protein; the binding sites discussed here are locations to which the lithium ion is attached transiently and reversibly.) Lithium binding sites must be of appropriate size to fit the ion. Since the unhydrated radius of the lithium ion is 0.8 Å, the lower limit of the binding site cavity is 1.6 Å. The upper limit would be only slightly larger because the ligands at the binding site could not favorably compete with the water molecules, and if water molecules are not substituted, the interaction will not be sufficiently specific. If the binding site is not specific, lithium cannot be attracted in the presence of the other cations in the biological system. The binding site must possess such properties that it can strip the hydrated lithium ion of several of its water molecules in order to hold it. The cavity must be flexible so that it can contract as the water molecules are gradually replaced by receptor ligands. It is likely that the binding sites are of the chelate type, since only in this way can they gain sufficient specificity.

Lithium binding sites and carrier systems are at present being studied in artificial systems such as macropolycyclic polyethers, cyclic peptides, antibiotic ionophores, and peptide-like ion carriers (Blout, 1976; Eisenman, 1976; Lehn, 1976; Winkler, 1976). The properties of these systems are altered step by step to produce lithium acceptors with varying degrees of specificity, stability, interaction with other ions, etc. The studies may eventually yield information of relevance to the binding and mode of action of lithium in the brain.

Attachment of lithium to a binding site alters the geometry of the latter and thereby produces functional changes in the system (Blout, 1976). The influence may be exerted through a direct action of the lithium ion, or it may be due to displacement of or interaction with one or more of the biologically active cations. Interaction with ammonium groups, including those of the biogenic amines, is also a possibility.

Physicochemical considerations concerning the properties of biological lithium receptors led Eigen (1976) to speculate on various ways in which lithium might work: (1) As the effector ion in an unperturbed (normal) receptor system. Unlikely. (2) As the effector in an unperturbed (normal) transport system. Unlikely. (3) Through repairing a biological defect specific to manic-depressive illness: (a) a substrate lack or (b) a genetically determined alteration of a central nervous system receptor or carrier. Eigen favored this last hypothesis and pointed out that a lithium-correctable "receptor" would need to be studied in manic-depressive patients, since in normal subjects and animals there would be nothing to correct.

II. TARGET SYSTEMS

The number of known biological effects of lithium is very large, and a complete list cannot be presented. Such a catalog would also be boring. We have chosen instead to list five fairly general target systems which are known to be affected by lithium and through which conceivably lithium might exert its therapeutic and prophylactic action in patients suffering from manic-depressive disorder. There are of course innumerable other systems, and they are not mutually exclusive. On the contrary, they are strongly interdependent, and interference with one usually means affection also of others.

A. Membranes

Membrane permeability may take several forms. In addition to unspecific permeability, where diffusion alone determines the passage of compounds, there are specific permeability devices. One of these consists of the so-called channels, which are seen as pores extending through the cell membrane (Hille, 1972, 1973, 1976; Campbell, 1976). There are specific sodium channels, specific potassium channels, and specific calcium channels. The movement of ions through the channels is determined by the dimensions and the charge of the channel and the degree to which ions have to be stripped of their hydrating water molecules to pass. Lithium ions have been found able to substitute for extracellular sodium ions at certain sodium channels, e.g., in the neuronal membrane during impulse conduction. Intracellular lithium ions may in sufficient concentration block certain potassium channels. They are sucked down the channel by electrostatic forces and once inside will prevent potassium ions from passing by electrostatic repulsion.

Another specific transport mechanism involves the so-called ion pumps, now more often referred to as ionophore carriers, which are substances that can move through or across the cell membrane carrying one or more cations (Baker et al., 1969; Baker and Crawford, 1971, 1972; Blaustein and Ector, 1976).

The lithium ion is transported into and out of the cell, but not simply like sodium and not simply like potassium. The mechanisms involved differ from one tissue to another, and the erythrocyte is the best-studied system. There seem to be at least four different mechanisms for lithium transport across the red cell membrane. One is outward transport with the ouabain-sensitive sodium-potassium-ATPase system (Duhm and Becker, 1977c). A second is inward transport in ion pair formation with chloride or bicarbonate via the anion exchange pathway; this lithium transport can be inhibited by various inhibitors of anion transfer (Funder et al., 1978; Becker and Duhm, 1978). A third mechanism is outward transport with lithium substituting for sodium in the saturable sodium-sodium exchange system which is driven by the sodium gradient across the cell wall (Haas et al., 1975; Duhm et al., 1976; Greil et al., 1977c; Pandey et al., 1976). This transport system may be inhibited with phloretin. Even when all these transport systems are inhibited, there still seems to be a fourth transport mechanism, namely simple leaking resulting from the lithium concentration gradient across the cell wall (Funder et al., 1978).

At therapeutic plasma lithium levels and in the presence of normal plasma concentrations of sodium, potassium, chloride, and bicarbonate one-third of the lithium *influx* seems to take place through the last mentioned leakage and two thirds via the anion exchange pathway (Funder et al., 1978). Lithium *efflux* takes place mainly via the lithium-sodium exchange system, whereas extrusion via the sodium-potassium-activated ATPase system plays a minor role (Duhm et al., 1976; Fewil et al., 1977; Frazer et al., 1978).

Whereas the lithium erythrocyte/plasma ratio is fairly stable in the individual patient, there is considerable interindividual variation. It seems to be due solely to variation of the activity of the lithium-sodium exchange mechanism (Greil et al., 1977; Frazer et al., 1978). The activity of this system is genetically determined (Mendlewicz et al., 1978; Ostrow et al., 1978), and variation of the activity may reflect differences in the number of transport sites per cell (Duhm and Becker, 1977c).

In vitro determinations of the lithium-sodium exchange mechanism shows lower activity with erythrocytes drawn from the patients during periods of lithium treatment than during periods when no lithium is given (Meltzer et al., 1977).

Many studies have aimed at using the erythrocyte lithium concentration or the lithium erythrocyte/plasma ratio as predictors of response to lithium treatment or of lithium toxicity, but findings are controversial.

B. Enzymes

Enzymes involved in transport are not the only ones that may be affected by lithium (Schou, 1973; Blout, 1976). Many enzymes which take part in the general metabolism are activated by cations, most often magnesium but sometimes also potassium or sodium. When potassium is the activator, lithium usually inhibits enzyme activity. When sodium is the activator, lithium stimulates. There are even some enzymes which prefer lithium to sodium. In these studies on tissue preparations lithium concentrations have often been high, and it is difficult to draw functional conclusions about the intact organism.

Also in vivo studies with animals and studies with patients have shown lithium interference with intermediary metabolism. It has been found, for example, that lithium treatment of patients leads to a rise in the urinary excretion of α-ketoglutaric acid and other tricarboxylic acid cycle metabolites (Bond and Jenner, 1975). It has further been shown that lithium affects lipid metabolism, liver hexokinase, activation of liver adenyl cyclase and protein kinase, glycogen synthesis, and pyruvate kinase (Mellerup and Rafaelsen, 1975). These effects may or may not be related to the therapeutic and prophylactic actions of lithium in manic-depressive patients. They may have to do with the lithium-induced weight gain seen in some patients during treatment (Vendsborg et al., 1976).

Lithium also exerts an action on ATPases, interfering with their transport function and with their effect on general cellular metabolism. Lithium effects on ATPase activity cannot, however, be brought on a simple formula, for they vary from one tissue preparation to another, they depend on the lithium concentration, and they are influenced by the presence of other ions. Three examples: In the classical sodium-potassium-ATPase system from crab nerve lithium exerts in the presence of magnesium and sodium a stimulating action on the enzyme, similar to but weaker than that exerted by potassium (Skou, 1957). In mucosa tissue from colon lithium lowers the activity of sodium-potassium-ATPase, but stimulates the activity of magnesium-dependent ATPase (Gutman et al., 1973). And in salivary gland preparations lithium elevates sodium-potassium-ATPase activity (Gutman et al., 1973).

It may be of more clinical relevance that lithium treatment of patients produces a significant increase of ouabain-sensitive ATPase activity in the erythrocytes with a resultant increase in erythrocyte sodium pump activity

(Hokin-Neaverson et al., 1974; Naylor et al., 1974). There is even a study which indicates that patients with low erythrocyte sodium-potassium-ATPase activity before treatment tend to respond clinically better to lithium than patients with a high enzyme activity (Naylor et al., 1976). A comprehensive hypothesis has been proposed (Glen and Reading, 1973), according to which lithium may prevent recurrent attacks of mania and depression by regulating cell membrane ATPases through potassium-like stimulation of the sodium pump, through intracellular competition with sodium, and through stimulation of the magnesium-activated ATPase.

Adenyl cyclase, not the least interesting of the enzymes affected by lithium, will be dealt with later.

C. Electrolytes

It has often been suggested that derangement of electrolyte balance and metabolism might be the cause of manic-depressive disorder, and although this has never been proved, the advent of lithium as an active psychotropic agent has given new life to such speculations.

Observations concerning lithium effects on electrolyte concentrations and balance are often conflicting, and experimental conditions play an important role. Among the more consistent findings in patients may be mentioned an excess excretion of sodium and potassium during the first days of lithium treatment (Hullin, 1975). This is followed by a retention, and still later equilibrium is restored. During long-term lithium treatment there is an increase of plasma magnesium and plasma calcium and a decrease in the urinary excretion of calcium (Nielsen, 1964; Mellerup et al., 1976).

Lithium treatment is accompanied by a slight, but statistically significant, decrease of bone density (Christiansen et al., 1975; Hullin, 1975). One does not know whether these changes are secondary or coincident to the therapeutic and prophylactic actions of lithium, or whether they reflect cellular changes which are part of its mode of action.

The peculiar way in which lithium both resembles and differs from the biological cations is well illustrated by the way it is handled by the kidney (Fyrö and Sedvall, 1975; Thomsen, 1976, 1977a,b). Lithium is filtered freely through the glomerular membrane and is reabsorbed together with, and to the same extent as, sodium in the proximal tubules. In the distal parts of the nephron very little or no lithium is reabsorbed, and there is no secretion of the ion. Nevertheless, potassium has a preventive action against fatal lithium intoxication in rats (Olesen and Thomsen, 1976).

D. Neurotransmitters

Lithium exerts a large number of actions on neurotransmitters (Schou, 1973; Berl and Clarke, 1975; Shaw, 1975; Murphy, 1976). One may at random mention stimulation of serotonin turnover; alteration of norepinephrine breakdown; inhibition of stimulus-induced norepinephrine and serotonin release; stimulation or inhibition of amine reuptake; changes in brain and spinal fluid concentrations of amine precursors, amines, and amine metabolites; inhibition of platelet serotonin uptake; and increase of platelet MAO activity. Lithium may also influence other established or putative neurotransmitters, e.g., acetylcholine and GABA.

Calcium ions are essential for the secretion or release of neurotransmitters, presumably by crosslinking vesicle membranes to the plasma membrane. Lithium inhibits stimulation-induced release of norepinephrine (Bogdanski et al., 1968; Katz et al., 1968), and presumably it does so by being attached to the calcium binding sites, thereby interfering with the crosslinking, stabilizing the vesicle membrane, and inhibiting release of the vesicle contents. If the calcium concentration is raised, lithium inhibition is overcome (Katz and Kopin, 1969). This emphasizes the competitive nature of the interaction between the two ions.

Earlier transmitter hypotheses concentrated on lithium effects on release and uptake of norepinephrine and serotonin at the nerve ending. With these hypotheses the authors succeeded in accounting for the antimanic action of lithium, but not very easily for its ability to prevent depressions. More recent studies have focused on precursor uptake and amine synthesis (Mandell, 1976; Mandell and Knapp, 1976). Tryptophan is taken up through the neuronal membrane and in the cell converted to serotonin, which is released from the nerve ending. After short-term lithium treatment tryptophan uptake is augmented, and since intraneuronal tryptophan hydroxylase is not saturated with regard to substrate, synthesis and release of serotonin are increased. Initial experiments indicated that long-term lithium treatment led to reduction of the enzyme activity as a compensation for the initial augmentation of serotonin release, thus providing a metabolic feedback system. However, later experiments (Mandell, personal communication, 1978; Samuel Gershon, personal communication, 1978) have failed to confirm the late fall of hydroxylase activity, and the hypothesis is in need of revision.

There are observations in patients which may support the notion that lithium interacts with serotonin through lowering of the probenecid-induced accumulation of 5-hydroxyindoleacetic acid in the spinal fluid (Goodwin et al., 1976). This seems to be an acute rather than a chronic effect of lithium, and it may not be relevant to the clinical action of the drug.

Animal experiments have shown that neuronal synthesis and content of acetylcholine are decreased by lithium administration, and that the stimulation induced release of acetylcholine is decreased and the resting release increased in lithium treated animals (Vizi, 1975). During lithium administration the influx of choline into rat brain is reduced, but since efflux is reduced still more, the choline in the brain is higher after administration of lithium plus choline than after administration of choline alone (Millington et al., 1979).

E. Receptors

Lithium binding sites may be identical with or closely bound to receptor sites for messenger substances such as hormones and neurotransmitters. In fact, several instances of lithium interference with hormone response are known; some are responsible for well-known side effects of lithium.

First, lithium lowers the ability of the kidneys to conserve sodium (Thomsen et al., 1976); the treatment produces a lowered response of the kidney to the sodium-retaining adrenocortical hormone aldosterone. Second, during lithium treatment some patients develop nephrogenic diabetes insipidus with polyuria and polydipsia (MacNeil and Jenner, 1975; Singer, 1976). The reason, or part of the reason, is that the kidneys have lost their ability to respond to ADH, the antidiuretic hormone. Third, thyroid function is affected in a number of ways by lithium treatment (Wolff, 1976). One effect is a lowering of the response to TSH, the thyroid-stimulating hormone.

We know that adenyl cyclase and cyclic AMP are involved in the two latter systems, and it has been demonstrated that lithium treatment lowers the hormone-induced stimulation of adenyl cyclase activity in kidneys and thyroid so that less cyclic AMP is produced (Wolff et al., 1970; Williams et al., 1971; Geisler et al., 1972; Wraae et al., 1972). Kidney and thyroid are not the only tissues in which lithium inhibits hormone-stimulated adenyl cyclase activity. Inhibition has been demonstrated also in fat cells (Birnbaumer et al., 1969), in ovary (Smith et al., 1972), in toad bladder (Rotenberg et al., 1971), in lymphocytes (Gelfand et al., 1979), and in brain (Dousa and Hechter, 1970; Forn and Valdecasas, 1971). Some of the brain experiments were done in vitro with lithium in as high concentrations as 25-50 mmol/liter. It is probably of more relevance that administration of nontoxic lithium doses to rats lowers the cyclic AMP content of the brain (Berndt, 1975) and that lithium administration may prevent the dopamine receptor supersensitivity which is induced in both presynaptic and postsynaptic neurons by haloperidol (Gallager et al., 1978).

III. EXPERIMENTAL CONDITIONS

In any discussion of the mode of action of lithium it seems necessary to stress the importance of the experimental conditions used in the studies, because these determine the possible relevance of the data (Schou, 1976b). We select for illustration two significant variables: the lithium concentration and the duration of the exposure to lithium.

Table 2 shows the extracellular and intracellular concentrations of the four biologically important cations. Table 2 also shows the approximate extracellular and intracellular lithium concentrations encountered during lithium treatment of manic-depressive patients. The serum lithium concentration is maintained at about 1 mmol/liter or slightly lower; steady-state tissue concen-

Table 2 Extra- and Intracellular Concentrations of Biologically Important Cations

Ion	Conc. outside cells (mmol/liter)	Conc. inside cells (mmol/kg wet wt)
Lithium	1	0.5-5
Sodium	150	5-10
Potassium	5	100
Magnesium	1	5-10
Calcium	2.5	<1

trations range from 0.5 mmol/kg wet weight in a tissue such as liver to about 5 mmol/kg wet weight in the thyroid. Extracellular sodium and intracellular potassium concentrations are much higher, but the other concentrations are at least of the same order of magnitude, so interaction with lithium is not at all unlikely.

Due to the partial similarity of lithium with sodium, physiologists have for many years carried out experiments in which sodium in the incubation medium was partly or totally replaced by lithium. It cannot be entirely excluded that some of these observations may be of relevance in this connection, but lithium concentrations have usually been 50-150 mmol/liter, and caution in the use of the data is on the whole advisable.

When lithium is used therapeutically, full antimanic action develops in the course of 6-10 days. When it is used prophylactically, achievement of full protection against relapses may take weeks or months. It is therefore unlikely that one can obtain relevant data by doing experiments with a single or a few injections of lithium to an animal. Studies with lithium administration for a prolonged period are much more likely to yield interesting information. Acute and chronic lithium administration may have entirely different effects; this has been seen with for example brain amine concentration and turnover (Corrodi et al., 1967, 1969; Genefke, 1972), thyroid iodine transport and metabolism (Berens and Wolff, 1975), and the development of polyuria and polydipsia (Thomsen, 1970).

It is also prudent to remember that certain biological effects of lithium may persist not only after lithium administration has been stopped but also after complete disappearance of lithium from the organism. Such independence of the actual presence and concentration of the lithium ion has been observed in studies on lithium-induced polyuria, renal adenyl cyclase activity, synaptosome transport systems, and choline transport in red blood cells (Baldessarini and

Yorke, 1970; Thomsen, 1970; Geisler et al., 1972; Harris and Jenner, 1972; Wraae et al., 1972; Lee et al., 1974). These observations indicate that some lithium effects may be indirect, produced by changes that persist after disappearance of the ion.

IV. HYPOTHESES

Numerous hypotheses have been proposed about the mode of action of lithium in manic-depressive illness. Some have been elaborate and incorporated many sets of clinical and experimental data, others have been extrapolations from a few data with a single system. We do not know whether any of the hypotheses is relevant to the point at issue.

In this section we shall refer to a few hypotheses that have been advanced during recent years. We shall also describe in some detail an integrative hypothesis of our own, based primarily on our personal data. We realize that it does not conform in all respects to the criteria for experimental conditions and data assessment set out above. The hypothesis is presented merely to illustrate a way of reasoning; it does not pretend to be of higher veracity than other working models.

Bunney and Murphy (1976) proposed two hypotheses, one according to which lithium acts mainly on the presynaptic membrane regulating or correcting transmitter amine release, and one according to which lithium acts on postsynaptic neuronal receptors by stabilizing pathologically labile receptor site transitional processes. Frausto da Silva and Williams (1976) suggested that lithium competes with magnesium for particular ligands and so affects important regulatory processes in the central nervous system. Lehmann (1975) hypothesized that lithium influences membrane ATPase and hereby regulates transmitter release, electrolyte changes, and postsynaptic cyclic AMP. According to Tissot (1977) lithium may exert its action by influencing the ionic balance in the cells (increased sodium gradient across the cell wall) and affecting monoamine metabolism (activated serotonin metabolism without stimulation of cerebral serotoninergic activity). Sen et al. (1976) presented evidence indicating the existence of a sodium pump deficiency in both manic and depressed phases of manic-depressive illness and suggested that lithium therapy might correct this deficiency. This assumption is related to the hypothesis by Glen and Reading (1973) which was mentioned above. Byck (1976) proposed that enkephalin is a neurotransmitter which controls mood through its binding to opiate receptors; he suggested that lithium may act through modifiction of receptor affinity for the endogenous morphine-like substance. Green and Grahame-Smith (1976) felt that lithium administration might cause an initial increase of the serotonin available for release at the nerve ending, followed during further treatment by an increase in the rate of serotonin synthesis.

All of the above-mentioned hypotheses have in common that the site of the direct lithium action is assumed to be a site which also is directly involved in processes postulated to be of etiological importance for affective disorder. This is true whether it is competition with magnesium at particular ligands in the central nervous systems, effects on ATPases, adenyl cyclase, presynaptic membranes, neurotransmitter metabolism, or opiate receptors.

We should like to emphasize another possibility, namely that indirect and eventually peripheral effects of lithium may lead to the antimanic and/or prophylactic effect of lithium.

An example of this general idea is the previously mentioned changes in magnesium and calcium metabolism in lithium-treated organisms. The chemical similarity between sodium, potassium, magnesium, and calcium on the one side, and lithium on the other, has been emphasized in this chapter because it is one way to encompass the molecular basis for all direct lithium effects. However, this chemical similarity also indicates that the number of possible lithium effects may be very large and in every single case it should be studied, whether the function of lithium was similar to an increase, respectively a decrease in concentration of one of the other cations.

The importance of constancy in the serum concentration of calcium and magnesium is well known, and it is also known that many different symptoms (including mental symptoms) are associated with even slight deviations from normal levels of calcium and magnesium concentration. These symptoms are not generally observed during lithium treatment, indicating that lithium in the organism only to moderate degree may function like or compete with calcium and magnesium.

Thus the functional change due to substitution or competition between lithium and magnesium or calcium may in several systems be quantitatively less important than changes produced by increases in magnesium or calcium concentrations.

Accordingly, in a number of hypotheses where a direct lithium effect on some system is the central concept, it can be postulated that it might as well be the increase in magnesium and/or calcium concentration in the very same system, which indirectly produces the lithium effects.

The value of a hypothesis depends largely upon its testability, and in some respects it may be an easier (although difficult) task to test a hypothesis stressing the indirect effects.

To test whether a given biochemical and physiological effect of lithium has anything to do with the psychotropic effect is very difficult (a fact which is best illustrated by the lack of progress in this field, especially compared with the increasing accumulation of knowledge of lithium effects on the biochemical level). This is partly due to the problems in producing the same effect as a direct lithium effect by some other means, e.g., if it is suggested that the proplylactic effect of lithium specifically is based on the lithium produced inhibition of adenyl cyclase, then a quantitatively similar inhibition by some other drug should also have a prophylactic effect. Normally such kind of test cannot be performed regarding direct lithium effects due to the specificity of lithium. Indirect effects on the other hand might eventually be produced by some other treatment.

The changes in serum magnesium and calcium during lithium treatment are obviously indirect effects, which may be produced by a number of possible lithium effects on other systems, e.g., intestinal uptake, renal excretion, parathyroid hormone and calcitonin secretion, bone metabolism, phosphate metabolism, etc.

Similar changes may possibly be produced by some means other than lithium treatment, hereby offering possibilities for falsification of the hypothesis that changes in calcium and magnesium metabolism are involved in the psychotropic effect of lithium.

V. CONCLUSION

Our conclusion is brief. Lithium is of value to many patients with recurrent affective disorders. Its molecule is simple, but its biology is not. As could have been expected with a cation related to sodium, potassium, magnesium, and calcium, lithium exerts a multitude of effects in a variety of biological systems. Lithium is a challenge to our ingenuity; in the end it may give us deeper insight.

REFERENCES

Baastrup, P. C., and Schou, M. (1967). Lithium as a prophylactic agent. Its effect against recurrent depressions and manic-depressive psychosis. *Arch. Gen. Psychiatry 16*, 162-172.

Baker, P. F., and Crawford, A. C. (1971). Sodium-dependent transport of magnesium ions in giant axons of *Loligo forbesi*. *J. Physiol.* (London) *216*, 38P-40P.

Baker, P. F., and Crawford, A. C. (1972). Mobility and transport of magnesium in squid giant axons. *J. Physiol.* (London) *227*, 855-874.

Baker, P. F., Blaustein, M. P., Keynes, R. D., Manil, J., Shaw, T. I., and Steinhardt, R. A. (1969). The ouabain-sensitive fluxes of sodium and potassium in squid giant axons. *J. Physiol.* (London) *200*, 459-496.

Baldessarini, R. J., and Yorke, C. (1970). Effects of lithium and of pH on synaptosomal metabolism of noradrenaline. *Nature 228*, 1301-1303.

Becker, B. F., and Duhm, J. (1978). Evidence for anionic cation transport of lithium, sodium and potassium ions across the human erythrocyte membrane induced by divalent anions. *J. Physiol.* (London) *282*, 149-168.

Berens, S. C., and Wolff, J. (1975). The endocrine effects of lithium. In *Lithium Research and Therapy*, F. N. Johnson (Ed.). Academic, London, pp. 443-472.

Berl, S., and Clarke, D. D. (1975). Lithium and amino acid metabolism. In *Lithium Research and Therapy*, F. N. Johnson (Ed.). Academic, London, pp. 425-441.

Berndt, S. F. (1975). Inhibition by lithium of cyclic AMP metabolism in rat brain. In *Neuropsychopharmacology*, J. R. Boissier, H. Hippius, and P. Pichot (Eds.). Excerpta Med., Amsterdam, pp. 970-978.

Birnbaumer, L., Pohl, S. L., and Rodbell, M. (1969). Adenyl cyclase in fat cells. I. Properties and the effects of adrenocorticotropin and fluoride. *J. Biol. Chem. 244*, 3468-3476.

Blaustein, M. P., and Ector, A. C. (1976). Carrier-mediated sodium-dependent and calcium-dependent calcium efflux from pinched-off presynaptic nerve terminals (synaptosomes) in vitro. *Biochim. Biophys. Acta* (Amsterdam) *419*, 295-308.

Blout, E. R. (1976). Ion complexing with natural and synthetic peptides. In *The Neurobiology of Lithium*, W. E. Bunney and D. L. Murphy (Eds.). Neurosciences Research Program Bulletin (Boston), Vol. 14, No. 2, pp. 137-139.

Bogdanski, D. F., Tissari, A., and Brodie, B. B. (1968). The effects of inorganic ions on uptake, storage and metabolism of biogenic amines in nerve endings. In *Psychopharmacology: A Review of Progress 1957-1967*, D. H. Efron, J. O. Cole, J. Levine, and J. R. Wittenborn (Eds.). PHS Publication No. 1836, U.S. Government Printing Office, Washington, D.C., pp. 17-26.

Bond, P. A., and Jenner, F. A. (1975). The effects of lithium on organic acid excretion. In *Lithium Research and Therapy*, F. N. Johnson (Ed.). Academic, London, pp. 499-506.

Brown, W. T. (1976). Side effects of lithium therapy and their treatment. *Can. Psychiatr. Assn. J. 21*, 13-21.

Bunney, W. E., and Murphy, D. L. (1976). Neurobiological considerations on the mode of action of lithium carbonate in the treatment of affective disorders. *Pharmakopsychiat. 9*, 142-147.

Byck, R. (1976). Peptide transmitters. A unifying hypothesis for euphoria, respiration, sleep, and the action of lithium. *Lancet 2*, 72-73.

Campbell, D. T. (1976). Ionic selectivity of the sodium channel of frog skeletal muscle. *J. Gen. Physiol. 67*, 295-307.

Christiansen, C., Baastrup, P. C., and Transbøl, I. (1975). Osteopenia and dysregulation of divalent cations in lithium-treated patients. *Neuropsychobiology 1*, 344-354.

Corrodi, H., Fuxe, K., Hökfelt, T., and Schou, M. (1967). The effect of lithium on cerebral monoamine neurons. *Psychopharmacologia* (Berlin) *11*, 345-353.

Corrodi, H., Fuxe, K., and Schou, M. (1969). The effect of prolonged lithium administration on cerebral monoamine neurons in the rat. *Life Sci. 8*, 643-652.

Dousa, T., and Hechter, O. (1970). Lithium and brain adenyl cyclase. *Lancet 1*, 834-835.

Duhm, J., Eisenried, F., Becker, B. F., and Greil, W. (1976). Studies on the lithium transport across the red cell membrane. I. Li^+ uphill transport by the Na^+-dependent Li^+ counter-transport system of human erythrocytes. *Pflügers Arch. 364*, 147-155.

Duhm, J., and Becker, B. F. (1977a). Studies on the lithium transport across the red cell membrane. II. Characterization of ouabain-sensitive and ouabain-insensitive Li^+ transport. Effects of bicarbonate and dipyridamole. *Pflügers Arch. 367*, 211-219.

Duhm, J., and Becker, B. F. (1977b). Studies on the lithium transport across the red cell membrane. III. Factors contributing to the intraindividual variability of the in vitro Li^+ distribution across the human red cell membrane. *Pflügers Arch. 368*, 203-208.

Duhm, J., and Becker, B. F. (1977c). Studies on the lithium transport across the red cell membrane. *Pflügers Arch. 370*, 211-219.

Eigen, M. (1976). Possible mechanisms of action of lithium from the perspective of "receptor"-Li^+ interaction. In *The Neurobiology of Lithium*, W. E. Bunney and D. L. Murphy (Eds.). Neurosciences Research Program Bulletin (Boston), Vol. 14, No. 2, pp. 142-144.

Eisenman, G. (1976). The molecular basis for ion selectivity and its possible bearing on the neurobiology of lithium. In *The Neurobiology of Lithium*, W. E. Bunney and D. L. Murphy (Eds.). Neurosciences Research Program Bulletin (Boston), Vol. 14, No. 2, pp. 154-161.

Forn, J., and Valdecasas, F. G. (1971). Effects of lithium on brain adenyl cyclase activity. *Biochem. Pharmacol. 20*, 2773-2779.

Frausto da Silva, J. J. R., and Williams, R. J. P. (1976). Possible mechanism for the biological action of lithium. *Nature 263*, 237-239.

Frazer, A., Mendels, J., Brunswick, D., London, J., Pring, M., Ramsey, T. A., and Rybakowski, J. (1978). Erythrocyte concentrations of the lithium ion. Clinical correlates and mechanisms of action. *Am. J. Psychiatry 135*, 1065-1069.

Funder, J., Tosteson, D. C., and Wieth, J. O. (1978). Effects of bicarbonate on lithium transport in human red cells. *J. Gen. Physiol. 71*, 721-746.

Fyrö, B., and Sedvall, G. (1975). The excretion of lithium. In *Lithium Research and Therapy*, F. N. Johnson (Ed.). Academic, London, pp. 287-312.

Gallager, D. W., Pert, A., and Bunney, W. E., Jr. (1978). Haloperidol-induced presynaptic dopamine supersensitivity is blocked by chronic Lithium. *Nature 273*, 309-312.

Geisler, A. Wraae, O., and Olesen, O. V. (1972). Adenyl cyclase activity in kidneys of rats with lithium-induced polyuria. *Acta Pharmacol.* (Kbh.) *31*, 203-208.

Gelfand, E. W., Dosch, H.-M., Hastings, D., and Shore, A. (1979). Lithium. A modulator of cyclic AMP-dependent events in lymphocytes? *Science 203*, 365-404.

Genefke, I. K. (1972). The concentration of 5-hydroxytryptamine (5-HT) in hypothalamus, grey and white brain substance in the rat after prolonged oral lithium administration. *Acta Psychiatr. Scand. 48*, 400-404.

Glen, A. I. M., and Reading, H. W. (1973). Regulatory action of lithium in manic-depressive illness. *Lancet 2*, 1239-1241.

Goodwin, F. K., Wehr, T., and Sack, R. L. (1976). Studies on the mechanism of action of lithium in man. A contribution to neurobiological theories of affective illness. In *Lithium in Psychiatry: A Synopsis*, A. Villeneuve (Ed.). Presses Univ. Laval, Québec, pp. 23-48.

Green, A. R., and Grahame-Smith, G. (1976). Effects of drugs on the processes regulating the functional activity of brain 5-hydroxytryptamine. *Nature 260*, 478-491.

Greil, W., Eisenried, F., and Duhm, J. (1976). Ueber die Verteilung von Lithium zwischen Erythrozyten und Plasma. In-vitro-Untersuchung zum Transport von Lithium an menschlichen Erythrozyten. *Arz. Forsch. 26*, 1147-1149.

Greil, W., Eisenried, F., Becker, B. F., and Duhm, J. (1977). Interindividual differences in the Na^+-dependent Li^+ countertransport system and in the Li^+ distribution ratio across the red cell membrane among Li^+-treated patients. *Psychopharmacology 53*, 19-26.

Gutman, Y., Hochman, S., and Strachman, D. (1973). Effect of lithium treatment on microsomal ATPase activity in several tissues. *Int. J. Biochem. 4*, 315-318.

Haas, M., Schooler, J., and Tosteson, D. C. (1975). Coupling of lithium to sodium in human red cells. *Nature 258*, 425-427.

Harris, C. A., and Jenner, F. A. (1972). Some aspects of the inhibition of antidiuretic hormone by lithium ions in the rat kidney and bladder of the toad *Bufo marinus*. *Br. J. Pharmacol. 44*, 223-232.

Hille, B. (1972). The permeability of the sodium channel to metal cations in myelinated nerve. *J. Gen. Physiol. 59*, 637-658.

Hille, B. (1973). Potassium channels in myelinated nerve. Selective permeability to small cations. *J. Gen. Physiol. 61*, 669-686.

Hille, B. (1976). Channels and ion transport in axons and synapses. In *The Neurobiology of Lithium*, W. E. Bunney and D. L. Murphy (Eds.). Neurosciences Research Program Bulletin (Boston), Vol. 14, No. 2, pp. 161-164.

Hokin-Neaverson, M., Spiegel, D. A., and Lewis, W. C. (1974). Deficiency of erythrocyte sodium pump activity in bipolar manic-depressive psychosis. *Life Sci. 15,* 1739-1748.

Hullin, R. P. (1975). The effect of lithium on electrolyte balance and body fluids. In *Lithium Research and Therapy,* F. N. Johnson (Ed.). Academic, London, pp. 359-379.

Katz, R. I., and Kopin, I. J. (1969). Release of norepinephrine-^{3}H evoked from brain slices by electricalfield stimulation-calcium dependency and the effects of lithium, ouabain and tetrodotoxin. *Biochem. Pharmacol. 18,* 1935-1939.

Katz, R. I., Chase, T. N., and Kopin, I. J. (1968). Evoked release of norepinephrine and serotonin from brain slices. Inhibition by lithium. *Science 162,* 466-467.

Lee, G., Lingsch, C., Lyle, P. T., and Martin, K. (1974). Lithium treatment strongly inhibits choline transport in human erythrocytes. *Br. J. Clin. Pharmacol. 1,* 365-370.

Lehmann, K. (1975). Zur Wirkungsmechanismus und zur Kinetik von Lithium. I. Biochemische und experimentell-pharmakologische Befunde nach Lithiumapplikation. Schlussfolgerungen zum Mechanismus des therapeutischen Lithiumeffektes. *Psychiatr. Neurol. Med. Psychol.* (Lpz.) *27,* 705-719.

Lehn, J.-M. (1976). Design of synthetic receptor and carrier molecules for the Li^+ cation. In *The Neurobiology of Lithium,* W. E. Bunney and D. L. Murphy (Eds.). Neurosciences Research Program Bulletin (Boston), Vol. 14, No. 2, pp.133-139.

MacNeil, S., and Jenner, F. A. (1975). Lithium and polyuria. In *Lithium Research and Therapy,* F. N. Johnson (Ed.). Academic, London, pp. 473-484.

Mandell, A. J. (1976). Effects of lithium on serotonin synthesis. In *The Neurobiology of Lithium,* W. E. Bunney and D. L. Murphy (Eds.). Neurosciences Research Program Bulletin (Boston), Vol. 14, No. 2, pp. 169-173.

Mandell, A. J., and Knapp, S. (1976). A neurobiological model for the symmetrical prophylactic action of lithium in bipolar affective disorder. *Pharmakopsychiat. 9,* 116-126.

Mellerup, E. T., and Jørgensen, O. S. (1975). Basic chemistry and biological effects of lithium. In *Lithium Research and Therapy,* F. N. Johnson (Ed.). Academic, London, pp. 353-358.

Mellerup, E. T., and Rafaelsen, O. J. (1975). Lithium and carbohydrate metabolism. In *Lithium Research and Therapy,* F. N. Johnson (Ed.). Academic, London, pp. 381-389.

Mellerup, E. T., Lauritsen, B., Dam, H., and Rafaelsen, O. J. (1976). Lithium effects on diurnal rhythm of calcium, magnesium, and phosphate metabolism in manic-melancholic disorder. *Acta Psychiatr. Scand. 53,* 360-370.

Meltzer, H., Kassir, S., Dunner, D. L., and Fieve, R. R. (1977). Represssion of a lithium pump as a consequence of lithium ingestion by manic-depressive subjects. *Psychopharmacology 54,* 113-118.

Mendlewicz, J., Verbanck, P., Linkowski, P., and Wilmotte, J. (1978). Lithium accumulation in erythrocytes of manic-depressive patients. An in vivo twin study. *Br. J. Psychiatry 133,* 436-444.

Millington, W. R., McCall, A. L., and Wurtman, R. J. (1979). Lithium and brain choline levels. *N. Engl. J. Med. 300,* 196-197.

Murphy, D. L. (1976). Effects of lithium on catecholamines and other brain neurotransmitters. In *The Neurobiology of Lithium,* W. E. Bunney and D. L. Murphy (Eds.). Neurosciences Research Program Bulletin (Boston), Vol. 14, No. 2, pp. 165-169.

Naylor, G. J., Dick, D. A. T., and Dick, E. G. (1976). Erythrocyte membrane cation carrier, relapse rate of manic-depressive illness and prediction of response to lithium. *Psychol. Med. 6,* 257-263.

Naylor, G. J., Dick, D. A. T., Dick, E. G., and Moody, J. P. (1974). Lithium therapy and erythrocyte membrane cation carrier. *Psychopharmacologia* (Berlin) *37,* 81-86.

Nielsen, J. (1964). Magnesium-lithium studies. *Acta Psychiatr. Scand. 40,* 190-196.

Olesen, O. V., and Thomsen, K. (1976). A preventive effect of potassium against fatal lithium intoxication in rats. *Neuropsychobiology 2,* 112-117.

Ostrow, D. G., Pandey, G., Davis, J. M., Hurt, S. W., and Tosteson, D. C. (1978). A heritable disorder of lithium transport in erythrocytes of a subpopulation of manic-depressive patients. *Am. J. Psychiatry 135,* 1070-1078.

Pandey, G. N., Javaid, J. I., Davis, J. M., and Tosteson, D. C. (1976). Mechanism of lithium transport in red blood cells. *Physiologist 19,* 321.

Rotenberg, D., Puschett, J. B., Ramsey, P., Stokes, J., Mendels, J., and Singer, I. (1971). Effects of lithium on vasopressin responsiveness in vivo and in vitro. *Clin. Res. 19,* 546.

Schou, M. (1973). Possible mechanisms of action of lithium: Approaches and perspectives. *Biochem. Soc. Trans. 1,* 81-87.

Schou, M. (1976a). Current status of lithium therapy in affective disorders and other diseases. In *Lithium in Psychiatry: A Synopsis,* A. Villeneuve (Ed.). Presses Univ. Laval, Québec, pp. 49-77.

Schou, M. (1976b). Pharmacology and toxicology of lithium. *Ann. Rev. Pharmacol. 16*, 231-243.

Schou, M. (1977). Effects secondaires et intoxication provoqués par les sels de lithium. Mécanisme, traitement et prévention. *Actualités pharmacol. 29*, 7-24.

Sen, A. K., Murthy, R., Stancer, H. C., Awad, A. G., Godse, D. D., and Grof, P. (1976). The mechanism of action of lithium ion in affective disorders. A new hypothesis. In *Membranes and Disease*, L. Bolis, J. G. Hoffman, and A. Leaf (Eds.). Raven, New York, pp. 109-122.

Shaw, D. M. (1975). Lithium and amine metabolism. In *Lithium Research and Therapy*, F. N. Johnson (Ed.). Academic, London, pp. 411-423.

Singer, I. (1976). Lithium effects on water metabolism. In *The Neurobiology of Lithium*, W. E. Bunney and D. L. Murphy (Eds.). Neurosciences Research Program Bulletin (Boston), Vol. 14, No. 2, pp. 175-177.

Skou, J. C. (1957). The influence of some cations on an adenosine triphosphatase from peripheral nerves. *Biochim. Biophys. Acta* (Amsterdam) *23*, 394-401.

Smith, B. M., Harris, C. A., and Major, P. W. (1972). The effect of lithium ions on the activation of ovarian adenyl cyclase. In *Physiology and Pharmacology of Cyclic AMP*, P. Greengard, J. D. Robinson and M. Paoletti (Eds.). Raven, New York, p. 588, abstr.

Thomsen, K. (1970). Lithium-induced polyuria in rats. *Int. Pharmacopsychiat. 5*, 233-241.

Thomsen, K. (1976). Renal elimination of lithium in rats with lithium intoxication. *J. Pharmacol. Exp. Ther. 199*, 483-489.

Thomsen, K. (1977a). The renal handling of lithium: Relation between lithium clearance, sodium clearance and urine flow in rats with diabetes insipidus. *Acta Pharmacol.* (Kbh.) *40*, 491-496.

Thomsen, K. (1977b). Renal handling of lithium at non-toxic and toxic serum lithium levels. *Dan. Med. Bull. 25*, 106-115 .

Thomsen, K., Jensen, J., and Olesen, O. V. (1976). Effect of prolonged lithium ingestion on the response to mineralocorticoids in rats. *J. Pharmacol. Exp. Ther. 196*, 463-468.

Tissot, R. (1977). Hypothéses sur les mécanismes d'action de lithium. *Rev. Méd.* (Paris) *18*, 159-162.

Vacaflor, L. (1975). Lithium side effects and toxicity. The clinical picture. In *Lithium Research and Therapy*, F. N. Johnson (Ed.). Academic, London, pp. 211-225.

Vendsborg, P. B., Bech, P., and Rafaelsen, O. J. (1976). Lithium treatment and weight gain. *Acta Psychiatr. Scand. 53*, 139-147.

Vizi, E. S. (1975). Lithium and acetylcholine metabolism. In *Lithium Research and Therapy*, F. N. Johnson (Ed.). Academic, London, pp. 391-410.

Williams, J. A., Berens, S. C., and Wolff, J. (1971). Thyroid secretion in vitro. Inhibition of TSH and dibutyryl cyclic-AMP stimulated ^{131}I release by Li^+. *Endocrinology 88*, 1385-1388.

Williams, R. J. P. (1976). Ion complexing with proteins and other macromolecules. In *The Neurobiology of Lithium*, W. E. Bunney and D. L. Murphy (Eds.). Neurosciences Research Program Bulletin (Boston), Vol. 14, No. 2, pp. 145-154.

Winkler, R. (1976). Kinetics of "receptor"-Li^+ interaction. In *The Neurobiology of Lithium*, W. E. Bunney and D. L. Murphy (Eds.). Neurosciences Research Program Bulletin (Boston), Vol. 14, No. 2, pp. 139-142.

Wolff, J. (1976). Effects of lithium on thyroid gland function. In *The Neurobiology of Lithium*, W. E. Bunney and D. L. Murphy (Eds.). Neurosciences Research Program Bulletin (Boston), Vol. 14, No. 2, pp. 178-180.

Wolff, J., Berens, S. C., and Jones, A. B. (1970). Inhibition of thyrotropin-stimulated adenyl cyclase activity of beef thyroid membranes by low concentration of lithium ion. *Biochem. Biophys. Res. Commun. 39*, 77-82.

Wraae, O., Geisler, A., and Olesen, O. V. (1972). The relation between vasopressin stimulation of renal adenyl cyclase and lithium-induced polyuria in rats. *Acta Pharmacol.* (Kbh.) *31*, 314-317.

24

Interaction of Benzodiazepines with Known and Putative Neurotransmitters in the Brain

Herbert Ladinsky, Silvana Consolo, Cesario Bellantuono,* and Silvio Garattini
Mario Negri Pharmacology Research Institute
Milan, Italy

**Additional affiliation:* University of Bari, Bari, Italy

I. INTRODUCTION

Which central sites the 1,4-benzodiazepines act at and which neurotransmitters they affect in specific situations is still virtually unknown despite wide clinical use and extensive laboratory study. Independent investigations have yielded evidence to sustain several neurotransmitter hypotheses for the powerful anticonvulsant, antianxiety, and muscle relaxant actions of the benzodiazepines. Emphasis has recently been laid on GABAergic, serotoninergic, catecholaminergic, cholinergic, and glycinergic mechanisms.

The different amine actions are not mutually exclusive for two reasons: (1) Recent findings show coupling between various neurons, e.g., the GABA-mimetic action of the benzodiazepines may be a common feature primary to their influence on other putative neurotransmitter mechanisms and (2) the benzodiazepines may have a generalized action on synaptic mechanisms shared by all the central monoaminergic neurons and perhaps by other neurons too.

II. PHARMACOLOGICAL ASPECTS

In animals diazepam is effective in a variety of neuropharmacological and psychopharmacological tests in doses ranging from 0.14 to 88 μmol/kg (0.04 to 25 mg/kg) and greater. Some of the most powerful effects of diazepam in rats are listed in Table 1. At doses up to 1 μmol/kg, the drug prevents isoniazid, picrotoxin, and pentylenetetrazol convulsions; suppresses the tetrabenazine-stimulated avoidance rate in iproniazid-treated rats; depresses Purkinje cell-firing rate; and blocks the isoniazid-induced increase in cerebellar cyclic 3′,5′-guanosine monophosphate (cGMP). At around 2 μmol/kg, diazepam decreases cerebellar cGMP content, increases deprivation-induced water consumption, and releases punished behavior from suppression.

The potency of antagonistic effects of diazepam versus some actions of three convulsants, isoniazid, picrotoxin, and pentylenetetrazol, are shown in Table 2. Diazepam prevents pentylenetetrazol seizures in rats at doses from 8 μmol/kg (ED_{80}) to 42 μmol/kg (ED_{50}). This wide range most likely depends upon differences in the interval selected between diazepam pentylenetetrazol administrations. The importance of the time factor in the antipentylenetetrazol action of some benzodiazepines in rats and mice has recently been demonstrated in a careful study by Banerjee and Yeoh (1977). These authors found that the doses of diazepam, nitrazepam, and clonazepam required to prevent pentylenetetrazol seizures in 50% of the animals increased several fold relative to the time (in hr) between the benzodiazepine and pentylenetetrazol administrations. The impact of the interval on the ED_{50} value is further illustrated in Figure 1. The ED_{50} of lorazepam for the antipentylenetetrazol action in rats differed by a factor of 30 depending on whether lorazepam was administered 5 or 180 min before the convulsant. Qualitatively similar data were described for oxazepam

Table 1 Some Potent Effects of Diazepam in Rats

Action of diazepam	Dose (μmol/kg)	Ref.
Prevents isoniazid convulsions (ED_{50})	0.14 i.p.	Mao et al., 1975
Attenuates tetrabenazine-stimulated avoidance rate of iproniazid-treated rats (MED)[a]	0.18 i.p.	Zbinden and Randall, 1967
Depresses Purkinje-cell-firing rate (MED)	0.35 i.v.	Haefely et al., 1975
Blocks isoniazid-induced increase in cerebellar cGMP content (MED)	0.52 i.p.	Costa et al., 1975b
Prevents pentylenetetrazol convulsions (MED)	0.61 i.p.	Consolo and Ladinsky, 1978
Prevents picrotoxin convulsions (ED_{50})	1.0 i.p.	Mao et al., 1975
Decreases cerebellar cGMP (MED)	1.75-2.4 i.p.	Mao et al., 1975; Govoni et al., 1976
Increases deprivation-induced water consumption (MED)	1.8 i.p.	Maickel and Maloney, 1973
Disinhibits punishment-suppressed behavior (conflict test MED)	2.2 p.o.	Cook and Sepinwall, 1975

[a]MED = minimum effective dose.

Table 2 Potency Comparisons of Antagonistic Effects of Diazepam vs. Some Actions of Three Convulsants in Rats

	Convulsant and dose (μmol/kg)					
	Isoniazid		Picrotoxin		Pentylenetetrazol	
Action of diazepam	2200[a]	3300	3.3-4.2	7.5	289	579
Anticonvulsant (ED_{50})	–	0.14[b]	–	1.0[b]	3.5[b]	3.0[c] 42[d] 5.5[e]
(ED_{80})					8.0[f]	–
(MED)					–	0.61[g]
Inhibits convulsant-stimulated increase in cerebellar cGMP (MED)	0.52[h]	–	1.7[h]	–	–	–
Interacts with convulsant on striatal ACh (MED)	–	–	17.6[i]	–	–	0.61[g]
Inhibits convulsant-stimulated increase in ant. pituitary cAMP (MED)	5.0[j]	–	–	–	–	–

The doses of diazepam are expressed in μmol/kg

[a]Subconvulsant dose.

[b]Mao et al., 1975.

[c]Garattini et al., 1973.

[d]Banziger, 1965.

[e]Banerjee and Yeoh, 1977 vs. 470 μmol/kg of pentylenetetrazol.

[f]Doteuchi and Costa, 1973.

[g]Consolo and Ladinsky, 1978.

[h]Costa et al., 1975b

[i]Javoy et al., 1977.

[j]Guidotti et al., 1978a

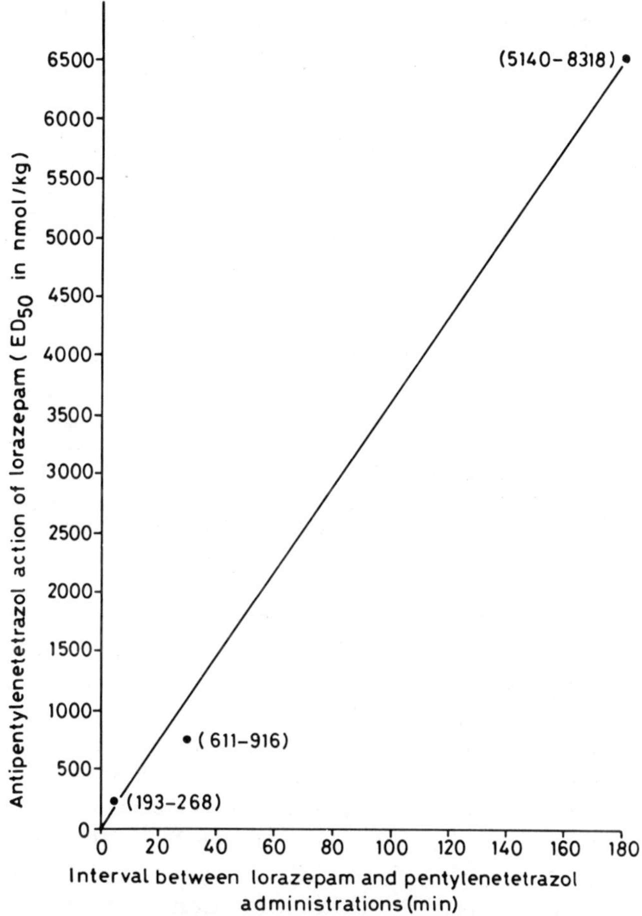

Figure 1 The ED_{50} of lorazepam vs. pentylenetetrazol convulsions with time in rats. Lorazepam was injected intravenously into male rats 5, 30, and 180 min before intraperitoneal administration of pentylenetetrazol, 868 μmol/kg. The onset of convulsions was followed for up to 6 hr after pentylenetetrazol administration. The ED_{50} increased 30-fold over the 175-min difference in the interval between lorazepam and pentetrazole. Numbers in brackets indicate the confidence limits (95%) for 40 animals per group. The ED_{50} of lorazepam (in nmol/kg) is shown on the ordinate. The time (in min) between lorazepam and pentylenetetrazol administrations is shown on the abscissa. (From A. Guaiatani, personal communication, by permission.)

(Garattini et al., 1973). It was found in our laboratory that 100% of the rats were protected against pentylenetetrazol convulsions by 0.61 μmol/kg of diazepam (Tables 2 and 3) given 12 min before pentetrazole and measuring the protective effect 15 min. later.

Table 3 Dose-Response Relationship of Diazepam's Interaction with Pentylenetetrazol on Striatal ACh and Convulsions

Dose of diazepam (μmol/kg i.v.)	No. of rats convulsed / No. of rats treated	Striatal acetylcholine level (nmol/g wet wt)[a]
Solvent-treated	17/17	26.9 ± 0.8 (17)
0.35	5/5	29.3 ± 1.2 (5)
0.61	0/7	18.7 ± 1.4 (7)[b]
0.875	0/9	19.7 ± 0.6 (9)[b]
1.75	0/9	18.7 ± 0.7 (9)[b]
3.5	0/10	19.5 ± 1.5 (10)[b]
8.75	0/9	15.5 ± 1.3 (9)[b]
17.5	0/14	18.0 ± 1.1 (14)[b]

[a]Striatal acetylcholine level in untreated rats: 29.2 ± 0.8 (20). The animals were killed 15 min after diazepam and 12 min after pentylenetetrazol, 579 μmol/kg i.p. Diazepam alone, at 8.75 and 17.5 μmol/kg, significantly increased ACh content. Data are mean ± s.e. (*n*).
[b]$P < .01$ Dunnett's test.

Because of the rapid metabolism and elimination of diazepam in rats (Garattini et al., 1977), the time within which measurements are made also determines the potency of the drug. The half-lives of diazepam and some other benzodiazepines in rat brain are short, of the order of 15-40 min (Table 4). In contrast, pentylenetetrazol persists in rat brain for a long period, its half-life being 160 min (Dal Bo et al., 1979). This is reflected in the drug's longlasting convulsant effect in rats. The time courses of the elimination of diazepam and pentylenetetrazol from rat brain are shown in Figure 2. By 60 min after its administration, the brain level of diazepam had fallen 10-fold, and from this time onward pentylenetetrazol convulsions may appear.

Table 4 Half-Lives ($t_{1/2}$) of Some Benzodiazepines in Rat Brain and Plasma

Benzodiazepines	$t_{1/2}$ (min)[a] Brain	Plasma
N-Demethyldiazepam	16.8	–
N-Methyloxazepam	14.7	–
Camazepam	30.8	24.1
Diazepam	13.9	22.4
Oxazepam	39.1	–

[a]The $t_{1/2}$ values were calculated from data reported by Garattini et al. (1973, 1977) and Marcucci and Mussini (1968).

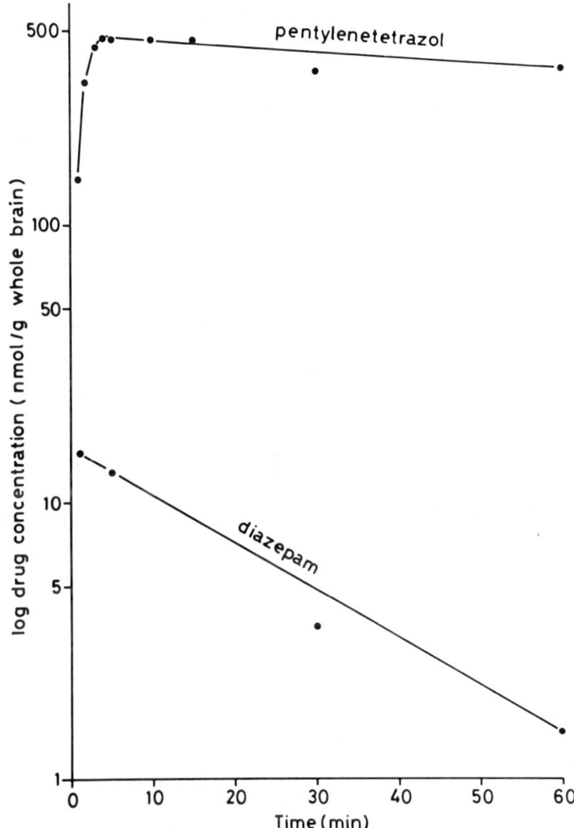

Figure 2 Levels of diazepam and pentylenetetrazol in rat whole brain at different times after administration. Diazepam was injected i.v. at a dose of 17.6 μmol/kg and pentylenetetrazol was given i.p. at a dose of 543 μmol/kg to male rats. The drug concentrations in the brain (in nmol/g) are given on the ordinate in log units. The time (in min) after drug administration is shown on the abscissa. Pentylenetetrazol reached a peak after about 4 min and then slowly declined with a half-life ($t_{1/2}$) of 160 min. Pentylenetetrazol convulsions are long-lasting in rats. The whole-brain concentration of diazepam fell 10-fold over the 60-min period with a $t_{1/2}$ of 13.9 min. Metabolites of diazepam are not found in whole rat brain except for a trace amount of N-desmethyldiazepam which is eliminated rapidly. The antipentylenetetrazol action of diazepam lasts about 120 min in these conditions (Marucci et al., 1968), the shortfall possibly being due to diazepam rapidly falling to below effective levels while pentylenetetrazol remains high enough to maintain the convulsive state. Each point represents the mean of at least 4 determinations. The data for diazepam were taken from Marcucci et al. (1970) and the data for pentylenetetrazol were taken from Marcucci et al. (1971). Pentylenetetrazol does not interfere with diazepam's metabolism and diazepam does not interfere with pentylenetetrazol's metabolism (Marcucci, personal communication).

The antipentylenetetrazol action of the benzodiazepines lasts much longer in mice and guinea pigs (Marcucci et al., 1968; Banerjee and Yeoh, 1977; Garattini, 1978) because of species differences in their metabolism and pharmacokinetics. In these two animals, oxazepam, the metabolite of diazepam, accumulates in the brain because of reabsorption of oxazepam glucuronide via the enterohepatic circulation (Bertagni et al., 1972; Garattini, 1978).

III. CATECHOLAMINES

The benzodiazepines affect the levels and turnovers of brain catecholamines in rats (Table 5) and mice (Fennessy and Lee, 1972). At a moderate dose (35 μmol/kg) diazepam reduced norepinephrine (NE) turnover in some regions of the rat brain (Taylor and Laverty, 1969,1973) while at a dose as low as 3.5 μmol/kg it decreased dopamine (DA) turnover in limbic and caudate areas (Fuxe et al., 1975). It has been suggested that these drugs impede the release of NE and DA, leading to an increase in their levels. Support for this view is provided by the finding that diazepam significantly lowered HVA, the metabolite of physiologically released DA, but raised the level of DOPAC, the metabolite of nonfunctional intraneuronal DA in the striatum (Rastogi et al., 1977). The authors suggested that the drug either acts directly at the nerve terminals or decreases nerve impulse flow. Consistent with these results are recent findings by Biswas and Carlsson (1978) showing that diazepam significantly decreased dopa formation only in the DA-rich limbic forebrain at a dose of 3.5 μmol/kg while higher doses (10 and 35 μmol/kg) were required to decrease dopa formation in the NE-dominated hemisphere portion and in the DA-rich striatum. These authors found that diazepam affected DA synthesis even after acute transection of ascending dopaminergic axons, suggesting an action at the synaptic level.

Several reports proposed that benzodiazepines reduce the turnover of brain DA by facilitating the inhibitory action of the GABAergic striatonigral pathway on dopaminergic neurons of the substantia nigra (Fuxe et al., 1975; Costa et al., 1975a; Keller et al., 1976; Cheramy et al., 1977) (see Table 6). However, Biswas and Carlsson (1978) were unable to relate the inhibitory action of diazepam on DA synthesis to enhanced GABAergic transmission. In fact, unlike diazepam, GABA, and the presumed GABA-like drugs, γ-butyrolactone (GBL) and γ-hydroxybutyric acid, are capable of stimulating DA synthesis in the brain probably by inhibiting the firing of dopaminergic neurons. Diazepam inhibited DA synthesis even in the absence of firing by these neurons in GBL-anesthetized rats. Biswas and Carlsson concluded that GABA and diazepam differ not only in the direction of their effects on DA synthesis but also in the site of their action. GABA acts on the dopaminergic cell bodies and diazepam on the nerve terminals.

In a different type of study, Weiner et al. (1977) concluded that clonazepam influences the central dopaminergic system through a direct effect on

Table 5 Compendium of Diazepam's Effects on the Activity of Aminergic Systems in Rat Brain Areas

Biochemical parameter	Effect and MED (μmol/kg)		Ref.
GABA level in cerebellar cortex	No effect up to	16	Costa et al., 1975a,b
n. caudatus	No effect up to	35	Peričić et al., 1977
pyriform cortex	No effect up to	35	Peričić et al., 1977
cingulate cortex	No effect up to	35	Peričić et al., 1977
s. nigra	Increase at	17.5	Peričić et al., 1977
GABA turnover in cerebellar cortex	No effect at	35	Peričić et al., 1977
pyriform cortex	No effect at	35	Peričić et al., 1977
globus pallidus	No effect at	3.5	Mao et al., 1977
enterhinal cortex	Decrease at	35	Peričić et al., 1977
parietal cortex	Decrease at	35	Peričić et al., 1977
n. caudatus	Decrease at	3.5	Mao et al., 1977
n. accumbens	Decrease at	3.5	Mao et al., 1977
DA level in whole brain	No effect at	17.5	Consolo et al., 1975
striatum	Increase at	35	Rastogi et al., 1977
hypothalamus	Increase at	35	Rastogi et al., 1977
pons medulla	Increase at	35	Rastogi et al., 1977
hippocampus	Decrease at	35	Rastogi et al., 1977
midbrain	Decrease at	35	Rastogi et al., 1977
striatum	No effect up to	35	Taylor and Laverty, 1969; Doteuchi and Costa, 1973
HVA level in striatum	Decrease at	35	Rastogi et al., 1977
striatum	No effect at	17.5	Consolo et al., 1975
whole brain	Decrease at	35	Bartholini et al., 1973

Table 5 (Continued)

Biochemical parameter	Effect and MED (μmol/kg)		Ref.
DOPAC level in striatum	Increase at	35	Rastogi et al., 1977
DOPA formation in striatum	Decrease at	10	Biswas and Carlsson, 1978
hemisphere	Decrease at	10	Biswas and Carlsson, 1978
limbic region	Decrease at	3.5	Biswas and Carlsson, 1978
DA turnover in n. caudatus	Decrease at	3.5	Fuxe et al., 1975
n. accumbens	Decrease at	3.5	Fuxe et al., 1975
tuberculum olf.	Decrease at	3.5	Fuxe et al., 1975
striatum	No effect at	18	Doteuchi and Costa, 1973
ACh level in striatum	No effect at	10	Zsilla et al., 1976
striatum	No effect at	35	Javoy et al., 1977
striatum	Increase at	8.8	Consolo et al., 1975; Consolo et al., 1977
striatum	Increase at	350	Sethy, 1978
hippocampus	No affect at	10	Zsilla et al., 1976
hippocampus	Increase at	17.6	Consolo et al., 1975
hippocampus	No effect at	350	Sethy, 1978
cerebral hemispheres	Increase at	17.6	Consolo et al., 1975
n. accumbens	Increase at	17.6	Consolo et al., 1977
brainstem	No effect at	10	Zsilla et al., 1976
brainstem	No effect at	350	Sethy, 1978
cortex	No effect at	10	Zsilla et al., 1976
cortex	Increase at 350		Sethy, 1978
ACh turnover in brainstem	Decrease at	7	Zsilla et al., 1976

striatum	No effect at	7	Zsilla et al., 1976
hippocampus	No effect at	7	Zsilla et al., 1976
cortex	Decrease at	7	Zsilla et al., 1976
NE level in striatum	No effect up to	35	Taylor and Laverty, 1969; Doteuchi and Costa, 1973
midbrain	No effect up to	35	Taylor and Laverty, 1969; Doteuchi and Costa, 1973
cerebellum	No effect up to	35	Taylor and Laverty, 1969; Doteuchi and Costa, 1973
cortex	No effect up to	35	Taylor and Laverty, 1969; Doteuchi and Costa, 1973
cortex	Decrease at	35	Rastogi et al., 1977
medulla pons	No effect up to	35	Taylor and Laverty, 1969; Doteuchi and Costa, 1973
medulla pons	Increase at	35	Rastogi et al., 1977
hypothalamus	No effect up to	35	Taylor and Laverty, 1969; Doteuchi and Costa, 1973
hypothalamus	Increase at	35	Rastogi et al., 1977
hippocampus	Increase at	35	Rastogi et al., 1977
cortex cerebri	No effect at	35	Corrodi et al., 1971
MOPEG-SO_4 level in whole brain	No effect at	17.5	Consolo et al., 1975
Tyrosine level in striatum	No effect at	35	Rastogi et al., 1977
pons medulla	No effect at	35	Rastogi et al., 1977
NE turnover in median eminence	Increase at	35	Fuxe et al., 1975
cerebellum	No effect at	18	Doteuchi and Costa, 1973
cerebellum	Decrease at	35	Taylor and Laverty, 1969
cortex	Decrease at	35	Taylor and Laverty, 1969
midbrain	Decrease at	35	Taylor and Laverty, 1969
cortex cerebri	No effect at	35	Corrodi et al., 1971
5-HT level in hippocampus	Increase at	35	Rastogi et al., 1977
hypothalamus	Increase at	35	Rastogi et al., 1977

Table 5 (Continued)

Biochemical parameter	Effect and MED (μmol/kg)		Ref.
midbrain	Increase at	35	Rastogi et al., 1977
pons medulla	No effect at	35	Rastogi et al., 1977
whole brain	No effect at	17.5	Consolo et al., 1975
whole brain	Increase at	20	Bourgoin et al., 1975
5-HIAA level in whole brain	No effect at	17.5	Consolo et al., 1975
hippocampus	No effect at	35	Rastogi et al., 1977
hypothalamus	Increase at	35	Rastogi et al., 1977
midbrain	Increase at	35	Rastogi et al., 1977
pons medulla	Increase at	35	Rastogi et al., 1977
whole brain	Increase at	70	Bourgoin et al., 1975
Tryptophan level in midbrain	Decrease at	35	Rastogi et al., 1977
whole brain	Increase at	70	Bourgoin et al., 1975
5-HTP formation in limbic areas	Decrease at	10	Biswas and Carlsson, 1978
striatum	No effect up to	35	Biswas and Carlsson, 1978
hemispheres	Decrease at	3.5	Biswas and Carlsson, 1978
5-HT turnover in cortex	Decrease at	88	Lidbrink et al., 1974
whole brain	Decrease at	70	Chase et al., 1970
whole brain less cortex	No effect at	88	Lidbrink et al., 1974
Histamine level in hypothalamus	No effect at	35	Taylor and Laverty, 1973

dopaminergic presynaptic mechanisms. These authors found that clonazepam blocked L-dopa- and amphetamine-induced stereotypy (presynaptic DA agonists) but not lergotrile- or apomorphine-induced stereotypy (postsynaptic DA agonists).

Fuxe et al. (1975) found that diazepam reduced apomorphine-induced contraversive turning in rats with unilateral lesions of the ascending dopaminergic pathway. It is unlikely that the drug prevented turning by blocking DA receptors. This was also shown by Tarsy and Baldessarini (1974), i.e., chronic treatment with diazepam did not induce a supersensitive stereotypy response to apomorphine and thus did not produce pharmacological "denervation" by blockade of dopamine receptors. Fuxe et al. (1975) proposed that diazepam may act on nonmonoaminergic pathways beyond the DA receptors to interfere with the behavioral consequences of increased DA receptor activity.

Extremely low doses of diazepam (0.175 μmol/kg) and chlordiazepoxide (1.5 μmol/kg) attenuated the stimulation of continuous avoidance response elicited by an acute dose of tetrabenazine in rats pretreated with the monoamine oxidase inhibitor iproniazid (Boff and Heise, 1963; Zbinden and Randall, 1967). Probably tetrabenazine stimulation is due to central release of NE since the drug induced no stimulation when brain NE was reduced by blockade of tyrosine hydroxylase or dopamine-β-hydroxylase (Zbinden and Randall, 1967). This interesting action of the two benzodiazepines appears to involve inhibition of impulse flow in noradrenergic neurons and hence a decrease in NE release. The potency of diazepam in this test is even more striking in the light of the duration of its action. The rats were pretreated with diazepam 2 hr before tetrabenazine administration, an interval amounting to almost 9 half-lives of diazepam or its metabolites in rat brain (see Fig. 2).

The benzodiazepines have other effects on catecholamines under stressful conditions (see Table 6). Chlordiazepoxide, diazepam, and nitrazepam prevented the depletion of NE in selective areas of the brain caused by electrofootshock stress (Taylor and Laverty, 1969) and by immobilization (Corrodi et al., 1971; Keim and Sigg, 1977). Pretreatment with diazepam, but not with pentobarbital, prevented electrofootshock-stress-induced increase in DOPAC levels in the rat frontal cortex and n. accumbens (Fadda et al., 1978). Diazepam reduced the turnover rate of striatal DA and cerebellar and hypothalamic NE in rats exposed to cold (Doteuchi and Costa, 1973). Impairment of the DA system by reserpine or haloperidol facilitates the cataleptic action of small doses of nitrazepam (Matsui and Deguchi, 1977) or diazepam, respectively. Diazepam is potent in preventing seizures in rats and cats induced by cocaine (Eidelberg et al., 1965), which blocks NE uptake, but also is potent in preventing seizures in cats induced by procaine (Feinstein et al., 1970), which is a less effective blocker in this regard.

Table 6 Compendium of Diazepam's Effects on the Actions of Drugs or Stress Designed to Affect Behavior and/or Monoaminergic Activity in Rats

Action of drug or stress	Effect of diazepam and MED (μmol/kg)		Ref.
Haloperidol-stimulated increase in HVA in striatum and limbic forebrain	Attenuates	35	Keller et al., 1976
Pimozide-induced DA disappearance in striatum	No effect at	17.6	Keller et al., 1976
Picrotoxin-stimulated release of DA from striatum (cats)	Blocks	35	Cheramy et al., 1977
γ-Butyrolactone-increased DA synthesis	Counteracts	10	Biswas and Carlsson, 1978
γ-Butyrolactone-increased 5-HT synthesis	Counteracts	10	Biswas and Carlsson, 1978
Cold-stress-induced increase in brain area catecholamine turnover	Slows	18	Doteuchi and Costa, 1973
Electrofootshock-induced increase in brain area NE turnover	Prevents	35+35	Taylor and Laverty, 1973 Taylor and Laverty, 1969
Electrofootshock-induced increase in DOPAC in frontal cortex and n. accumbens	Prevents	7	Fadda et al., 1978
Restraint-induced reduction in hypothalamic NE	Prevents	17.5	Keim and Sigg, 1977

Immobilization-induced increase in cortical NE turnover	Counteracts	35	Corrodi et al., 1971
Haloperidol-induced prolactinemia	Reduces	35	Chieli et al., 1978
Cold-stress-induced reduction in hypothalamic histamine	Prevents	35	Taylor and Laverty, 1973
Audiogenic increase in plasma corticoids	Lowers	17.5	Lahti and Barsuhn, 1974
Restraint-induced increase in plasma corticoids	Lowers	17.5	Keim and Sigg, 1977
Haloperidol-induced catalepsy	Potentiates	35	Haefely et al., 1975; Keller et al., 1976
Apomorphine-induced turning in unilateral-nigral-lesioned rats	Blocks	8.8	Fuxe et al., 1975
Methamphetamine-induced locomotor activity	Inhibits	22	Babbini et al., 1971
Methamphetamine-induced stereotypy	Enhances	22	Babbini et al., 1971
Cocaine seizures	Protects 100%	8.8	Eidelberg et al., 1965
L-dopa-induced increase in flexor reflex activity in spinal cats	Reduces	17.5	Fuxe et al., 1975
Water immersion despair immobility	No effect up to	14	Porsolt et al., 1978
Strychnine seizures	Protects 33%	28	Soubrie and Simon, 1978
Bemegride seizures	Protects 75%	7	Soubrie and Simon, 1978

IV. SEROTONIN (5-HT)

A number of biochemical studies have suggested that benzodiazepines affect central serotoninergic mechanisms (see Table 5). After intracerebroventricular (i.c.v.) or intracisternal injections of [^{14}C] serotonin ([^{14}C]-5-HT), the brain counts attributable to [^{14}C]-5-HT or [^{14}C]-5-HIAA increased after a single large dose of diazepam (Chase et al., 1970) or oxazepam (Stein et al., 1975). The latter workers found that benzodiazepines reduce 5-HT turnover and, in agreement with Chase et al. (1970), concluded that the increase in [^{14}C]-5-HIAA was due to interference with its egress from brain. Such a mechanism is reminiscent of probenecid's action. In line with these data are the findings of Rastogi et al. (1977) and Jenner et al. (1975), who showed that the benzodiazepines increased brain 5-HT and 5-HIAA of the rat and mouse, respectively.

Diazepam, 35 μmol/kg, reduced tryptophan content in the midbrain (Rastogi et al., 1977). Several benzodiazepines can compete with tryptophan binding for serum albumin (Bourgoin et al., 1975). These workers suggested that the increase in both 5-HIAA and tryptophan found in brains of rats after high doses (about 70 μmol/kg) of chlordiazepoxide, diazepam, and oxazepam may, at least partially, be the consequence of its effect on tryptophan binding in blood.

Studies have demonstrated that pharmacological agents which reduce 5-HT turnover and in turn raise its level elevate seizure threshold, whereas those which lower 5-HT content increase seizure susceptibility (Kilian and Frey, 1973). Diaz (1970) acknowledged the important role of 5-HT in pentylenetetrazol convulsions although he found essentially opposite results, i.e., pentylenetetrazol reduced 5-HT turnover at a subconvulsant dose. The possibility remains, however, that benzodiazepines may exert anticonvulsive effects by lowering 5-HT turnover.

Whether these serotoninergic neurons are affected directly or convey the effects of another neuronal system, e.g., GABAergic neurons (Stein et al., 1975), is still to be ascertained. Biswas and Carlsson (1978) observed, for example, that a moderate dose of diazepam counteracted the increase in rat forebrain 5-HT synthesis induced by the putative GABA-mimetic agent γ-butyrolactone. These authors proposed that the benzodiazepines generally inhibit transmitter synthesis and utilization at the synaptic level, an action not necessarily bearing any direct relationship to GABA.

V. ACETYLCHOLINE

Several benzodiazepines and their metabolites at moderate doses (10-35 μmol/kg) increased the level of acetylcholine (ACh) in rat and mouse brain (Domino and Wilson, 1972; Gatti et al., 1973; Ladinsky et al., 1973; Consolo et al., 1972, 1974, 1975, 1977; Garattini, 1978). The increase was limited to hemispheric structures (striatum, hippocampus, n. accumbens, and cortex) and the most pronounced effect was in the striatum (Consolo et al., 1975). Sethy (1978), however, required a much larger dose of diazepam (350 μmol/kg) to increase striatal ACh (Table 5).

Diazepam did not affect either the choline level or the activities of choline acetyltransferase and cholinesterase (Ladinsky et al., 1973; Consolo et al., 1974, 1975), the enzymes responsible for ACh synthesis and hydrolysis. The high-affinity uptake of choline by rat synaptosomal fraction of hippocampus was also not affected by in vivo administration of diazepam (unpublished results from this laboratory). The hypothesis that diazepam prevents the release of ACh from presynaptic nerve terminals (Consolo et al., 1974) is compatible with these data and with reports that diazepam decreased the turnover of ACh in mouse brain (Cheney et al., 1973) and rat cortex and brainstem (Zsilla et al., 1976).

It is conceivable that the cholinergic effect of diazepam is indirect, mediated by an action on other central monoaminergic neurons or other neurons. Mediation through dopaminergic neurons can probably be ruled out because pimozide cannot prevent diazepam's increase in striatal ACh (Consolo et al., 1975). Zsilla et al. (1976) proposed that the effect was due to blockade of impulse flow secondarily to an action of diazepam at GABA sites since its effect is similar to that of muscimol, a putative GABA mimetic, on ACh turnover in various rat brain areas.

If diazepam acts as a GABA agonist to increase ACh, then GABA antagonists, such as picrotoxin, can be expected to decrease it. On the contrary, it was found that mouse whole-brain ACh content (Svenneby and Roberts, 1974) and rat striatal ACh content (Ladinsky et al., 1976; Javoy et al., 1977) were increased by picrotoxin and that the effect in striatum was summated with that of diazepam when supramaximal doses of each drug were administered in combination (Consolo and Ladinsky, 1978).

The action of picrotoxin, unlike diazepam, was blocked by both pimozide and α-methyl-p-tyrosine, suggesting mediation by dopaminergic neurons (Ladinsky et al., 1976). Furthermore, whereas diazepam was able to increase the ACh content equally in the hippocampus and n. accumbens (Consolo et al., 1975,1977), picrotoxin was ineffective in both these areas (Ladinsky et al., 1976; Consolo et al., 1977). These data support the hypothesis that GABA does not mediate the action of diazepam as far as the cholinergic system is concerned and it is more likely that they act at different sites in affecting cholinergic activity.

VI. BENZODIAZEPINES AND CHOLINERGIC MECHANISMS IN CONVULSIONS

A number of studies have implicated the central cholinergic system in the anticonvulsant effect of benzodiazepines. The benzodiazepines can antagonize the stimulatory effects of anticholinesterases (Gatti et al., 1973; Lipp, 1973; Rump et al., 1973; Johnson and Lowndes, 1974). The LD_{50} of diisopropylfluorophosphate was increased by diazepam in mice (Gatti et al., 1973). Intravenous administration of clonazepam or nitrazepam effectively terminated the convulsions and suppressed the seizure activity induced by soman (Lipp, 1973). Diazepam also abolished soman-induced repetitive electrical activity at the motor end plate in rats (Johnson and Lowndes, 1974). In rabbits diazepam, at a dose of 4.4 μmol/kg, can both block and prevent fluostigmine-induced epileptiform patterns (Rump et al., 1973). Diazepam also blocked seizures in cats produced by the application of acetylcholine crystals to the amygdala, midbrain, or n. habenularis (Hernández-Peón et al., 1964), although benzodiazepines probably do not directly block cholinergic receptors (Madan et al., 1963).

The benzodiazepines are by far the most powerful antipentylenetetrazol drugs known (Zbinden and Randall, 1967). Pentylenetetrazol may induce convulsions partly through its action on cholinergic neurons. The drug, in fact, decreases the level of ACh in rat whole brain (Giarman and Pepeu, 1962), striatum (Longoni et al., 1974), and hippocampus but not striatum (Consolo et al., 1975). Pentylenetetrazol can induce massive release of ACh from rat and cat cortex (Mitchell, 1963; Beleslin et al., 1965; Hemsworth and Neal, 1968; Gardner and Webster, 1973). Furthermore, its convulsive activity can be potentiated by cholinesterase inhibitors in the rat (Green, 1964).

The increase in hemispheric ACh induced by the benzodiazepines may be a contributing factor to their antipentylenetetrazol action. In both rats and mice the cholinergic and antipentylenetetrazol effects of oxazepam (Garattini, 1979) and diazepam (Ladinsky et al., 1973; Consolo et al., 1974,1975) were related in time (Table 7).

In rats, an unusual interaction between diazepam and pentylenetetrazol was observed on the striatal cholinergic system (Consolo et al., 1975). Pentylenetetrazol, at a convulsive dose of 579 μmol/kg, had no effect on the level of ACh but significantly reduced ACh to below the control value when administered to diazepam-pretreated rats (Table 3).

Diazepam's antagonism of pentylenetetrazol-induced convulsions and the decrease in striatal ACh produced by combined administration of the two drugs were clearly related both with the diazepam dose and in time (Tables 3 and 7). The decrease in striatal ACh was constant for all doses of diazepam down to 0.61 μmol/kg, the dose which still protected all the animals from convulsions. Both the biochemical action and the antipentylenetetrazol effect of diazepam disappeared in rats at the dose of 0.35 μmol/kg. Similarly, in time, these effects persisted up to 60 min after diazepam administration (Table 7); the ACh content had almost returned to the control level by 120 min when less than 50% of the animals were protected against convulsions.

This type of interaction between the two drugs cannot be considered simply a blockade of diazepam's action by pentylenetetrazol. The data can at

Table 7 Time Course of the Relationship of Diazepam's Interaction with Pentylenetetrazol on Striatal ACh and Convulsions

Time (min) after diazepam	No. of rats convulsed / No. of rats treated	Striatal acetylcholine level (nmol/g wet wt)[a]
Solvent-treated	24/24	25.3 ± 0.9 (24)
15	0/10	14.0 ± 1.2 (10)[b]
60	0/7	14.9 ± 2.2 (6)[b]
120	8/13	22.3 ± 1.2 (13)
240	9/10	21.6 ± 1.9 (10)
360	10/10	27.0 ± 0.9 (10)

[a]Striatal acetylcholine level in untreated rats: 27.9 ± 0.6 (27). The rats were killed 12 min after pentylenetetrazol, 579 μmol/kg i.p.; diazepam was injected i.v. at a dose of 17.5 μmol/kg. Diazepam alone increased ACh content at 15 and 60 min. Data are means ± s.e. (*n*).
[b]$P < .01$ Dunnett's test.

present be best interpreted as indicating two different sites of attack of the drugs. This is borne out by pentylenetetrazol's inability to block the increase in ACh produced by diazepam in the hippocampus (Consolo et al., 1975). It is thus significant that Braestrup and Squires (1978) did not detect displacement of [^{3}H] diazepam binding by pentylenetetrazol, suggesting that the two drugs act not at a common site but possibly in series at different sites within a common polysynaptic circuit.

VII. BENZODIAZEPINES AND CHOLINERGIC MECHANISMS IN THE RAT CONFLICT TEST

Restoration of suppressed response in rats was obtained not only with chlordiazepoxide, but also with scopolamine and atropine (Heise et al., 1970), perhaps indicating a common site of action, or possibly different sites within a common neuronal circuit. This conjecture would fit in with the elaborate study by Ruch-Monachon et al. (1976), indicating that in cats the benzodiazepines initiate a reaction in the limbic system that eventually affects norepinephrine release in the locus coeruleus. A cholinergic synapse was identified within this circuit by pharmacological means.

VIII. GABA

A. Electrophysiology

γ-Aminobutyric acid (GABA) is the putative inhibitory neurotransmitter at several synapses where the benzodiazepines cause presynaptic inhibition: superior cervical ganglion (Suria and Costa, 1975), spinal cord (Polc et al., 1974), and cuneate nucleus (Polc and Haefely, 1976); or postsynaptic inhibition: cuneate nucleus (Polc and Haefely, 1976) and substantia nigra (Haefely et al., 1975). The benzodiazepines may also potentiate the inhibitory action of GABA on Purkinje cells (Haefely et al., 1975), although their primary site in depressing Purkinje-cell-firing rates could not be deduced.

These electrophysiological data contributed to the contention first put forward by Haefely et al. (1975) and Costa et al. (1975b) that GABA mediates several of the benzodiazepines' effects.

Other electrophysiological studies have revealed actions of the benzodiazepines which are not GABA-like (Steiner and Felix, 1976; Gähwiler, 1976; Curtis et al., 1976; Lippa and Critchett, 1981). The former two studies presented evidence that these drugs antagonize GABA in Deiter's nucleus and cerebellum, sites at which there is irrefutable evidence for GABA-mediated inhibition. Curtis et al. (1976) noted that benzodiazepines neither mimic nor antagonize the action of GABA or glycine on spinal or cerebellar neurons in pentobarbitone-anaesthetized cats.

Lippa and Critchett (1981) observed that the depression of rat Purkinje-cell-firing rate by flurazepam was not mediated through direct action on the GABA recognition site since bicuculline, probably the most selective GABA antagonist, was ineffective versus flurazepam in this test. On the other hand, picrotoxin, believed to antagonize GABA by interfering with a chloride ionophore distinct from the GABA recognition site, antagonized flurazepam in 56% of the cells. The authors made the interesting speculation that this picrotoxin-sensitive site may denote a type B benzodiazepine receptor (not the GABA recognition site), responsible for the benzodiazepines' sedative and ataxic properties. The type A receptor mediates the benzodiazepines' anticonflict and antipentylenetetrazol properties.

B. Psychopharmacology

Benzodiazepines are effective against chemical seizures induced by a variety of drugs believed to act as GABA antagonists at receptor sites, e.g., picrotoxin, bicuculline, and perhaps bemegride (Soubrie and Simon, 1978) and naloxone (Dingledine et al., 1978), or as GABA synthesis inhibitors (thiosemicarbazide and isoniazid).

Restoration of conditioned suppression of drinking by diazepam in rats was blocked by prior treatment with bicuculline or thiosemicarbazide (Zakusov et al., 1977). The authors inferred that the action of diazepam was mediated by GABA and suggested that the benzodiazepines increase the sensitivity of postsynaptic GABAergic receptors. Naloxone, too, reverses chlordiazepoxide's action, perhaps via GABA receptor blockade (Billingsley and Kubena, 1978).

Both picrotoxin and strychnine were effective against oxazepam-induced release of punished behavior from suppression (Stein et al., 1975).

C. Neuropharmacology

The ED_{50} of diazepam for preventing isoniazid-induced convulsions in rats is 0.14 μmol/kg (Mao et al., 1975). It is widely assumed that diazepam, as a GABA mimetic, counteracts the convulsions once isoniazid has inhibited GABA synthesis and lowered GABA levels. It remains to be established whether isoniazid interferes with the metabolism or elimination of benzodiazepines in rats, thus increasing their bioavailability and contributing to their potency. This is suggested because isoniazid is known to inhibit metabolism of phenytoin in rats (Kutt et al., 1968). Other presumed GABA-mimetic actions of the benzodiazepines have not revealed such a high potency (see Table 2). For example, the ED_{50} of diazepam for picrotoxin convulsions was seven times higher (Mao et al., 1975). In mice, the ED_{50} of diazepam in preventing convulsions produced by thiosemicarbazide, which also impairs GABA synthesis, was 12 μmol/kg p.o. (Schallek et al., 1972).

The benzodiazepines do not affect GABA content or turnover in the cerebellum and only minimally alter these parameters in other brain regions (Table 5). Biochemical studies in cerebellum, however, provide general support for the GABA-like action of benzodiazepines based most notably on the finding that the drugs are potent in decreasing the level of cGMP and in antagonizing isoniazid- and picrotoxin-induced increases in cGMP (Mao et al., 1975; Tables 1 and 2). The cGMP content of Purkinje cells is considered a marker for GABA activity and is taken as a second messenger response to the activation of GABA receptors (Guidotti et al., 1978a). The cGMP level may thus inversely reflect GABA release from stellate cells or basket cells during their inhibitory effect on Purkinje cell activity.

The action of GABA receptor agonists and antagonists on the cAMP content of anterior pituitary probably depends on an action at hypothalamic GABAergic synapses (Guidotti et al., 1978a). It is seen in Table 2 that there are 10-fold differences in the potency of diazepam in antagonizing isoniazid's and picrotoxin's effects on cerebellar cGMP as compared with their other GABA-related effects on pituitary cAMP or striatal ACh contents, respectively.

The benzodiazepines do not affect cerebellar cGMP content in newborn rats (Govoni et al., 1976), where Purkinje cells and dendrites lack synaptic contacts (Woodward et al., 1971). However, GABA receptors may already be present since i.c.v. administration of GABA lowered cGMP content (Govoni et al., 1976).

The benzodiazepines do not appear to act directly on GABA receptors as they do not displace labeled GABA from its specific binding sites (Snyder and

Enna, 1975); conversely, GABA and the presumed GABA receptor agonist muscimol do not displace tritiated diazepam from its specific binding sites (Braestrup and Squires, 1978). The evidence thus points to an indirect GABA-mimetic action of the benzodiazepines. It is unlikely that they augment the synaptic concentration of GABA since at reasonable concentrations they apparently neither inhibit GABA uptake (Harris et al., 1973) nor affect GABA transaminase (Sawaya et al., 1975) and do not enhance the action of GABA applied electrophoretically to the synapse (Curtis et al., 1976).

It has been proposed by Costa et al. (1975a) that the benzodiazepines sensitize GABA receptors possibly by "modifying allosterically the affinity of GABA for its own postsynaptic receptors. Thus, GABA receptors are seen as a multimolecular entity in which the affinity of the natural agonist for the recognition site can be modified by changes in the tertiary structure of a protein which is part of the multimolecular complex." The specific benzodiazepine binding sites (Braestrup et al., 1977; Squires and Braestrup, 1977; Braestrup and Squires, 1977,1978) might provide a means by which benzodiazepines alter the sensitivity of GABA receptors. It has been reported that the benzodiazepines do increase the affinity of [^{3}H]GABA for rat brain GABA receptors (Guidotti et al., 1978b), perhaps by removing a protein inhibitor.

The benzodiazepines (and their endogenous ligand) thus appear more likely to act as postsynaptic neuromodulators than as neurotransmitters. If such were the case, then the distribution of benzodiazepine receptors and GABA receptors throughout the brain might be expected to be parallel. However, as noted by Braestrup and Squires (1977), "marked regional variations in specific [^{3}H] diazepam binding existed and failed to parallel the regional distribution of γ-aminobutyric acid, glycine, substance P, endorphins or opiate receptors, neurotensin or dopamine, norepinephrine and acetylcholine." The rank orders of binding of diazepam and some other ligands in rat brain areas are shown in Table 8. GABA binding is highest in the cerebellum. Diazepam binding ranks second lowest in this area where many biochemical studies have been done to sustain the GABA hypothesis of the benzodiazepines' actions. In the hypothalamus, GABA binding is considered intermediate whereas benzodiazepine binding is weak. In some regions, such as the pons medulla, hippocampus, corpus striatum, and cortex, there is better parallelism. The most marked benzodiazepine receptor binding was found in cortical and limbic forebrain structures.

The lack of parallelism in the regional distribution of diazepam and quinuclidinyl benzilate (QNB), α-bungarotoxin, strychnine, spiroperidol, and fentanyl binding, shown in Table 8, illustrates the conclusion of Braestrup and Squires (1977) quoted above.

Biswas and Carlsson (1978) stated, "In view of the actions of diazepam on the synthesis of DA, NA and 5-HT, it may be suggested that we are dealing with a generalized action of benzodiazepines on a synaptic mechanism shared by all

Table 8 Rank Order of Distribution of Specific Receptor Binding of Diazepam and Several Ligands in Rat Brain Areas[a]

Area	diazepam[b]	QNB[c]	α-bungarotoxin[d]	strychnine[e]	spiroperidol[f]	GABA[g]	fentanyl[h]
Cortex	1	1	2	4^i	2	2	2
Limbic forebrain	1						1
Hippocampus	2	2	1	4^i	3	2	
Hypothalamus	3	3	1	3	3	2	2
Corpus striatum	3	1	4	4^i	1	3	1
Cerebellum	3	4	4^i	4^i	4^i	1	4
Midbrain and pons		3		3	3	2	
Pons medulla	4		2	2		4	
Medulla-cervical spinal cord		4		1	3	4	3
Thalamus		3	3	3		2	1
Superior and inferior colliculi		2					

[a]Numbers represent the rank order of specific receptor binding with respect to brain area. The rank was assigned by us based on the data tabulated and discussed in the references. Values close together, but not necessarily identical, were assigned the same rank. In general, 1 = highest binding; 2 and 3 = high and intermediate binding; 4 and 4^i = low and no detectable binding.
[b]Braestrup and Squires, 1977.
[c]Yamamura and Snyder, 1974 (muscarinic sites).
[d]Segal et al., 1978 (nicotinic sites).
[e]Young and Snyder, 1973 (glycinergic sites).
[f]Fields et al., 1977 (dopaminergic sites).
[g]Zukin et al., 1974 (Na^+-independent binding).
[h]Leyson and Laduron, 1977 (opiate sites).

the central monoaminergic neurons and perhaps by other neurons as well. If this is indeed a general inhibitory action located at synapses, it is not surprising that in many instances it may bear a close resemblance to the action of GABA, even though the action at the molecular level may be different."

IX. TOLERANCE TO SOME NEUROPHARMACOLOGICAL AND PSYCHOPHARMACOLOGICAL ACTIONS OF THE BENZODIAZEPINES

Tolerance arises to some of the benzodiazepines' properties after chronic treatment, but not to others. This characteristic is useful in relating neuropharmacological to psychopharmacological actions. Chronic treatment with some benzodiazepine derivatives stimulates hepatic autoinduction (Valerino et al., 1973), which may contribute to the tolerance in select cases. But since autoinduction occurs only at very high doses and tolerance does not develop uniformly to all the benzodiazepines' effects in the same species, so hepatic enzyme induction can be ruled out as a major factor. Some examples of tolerance and nontolerance to various effects of benzodiazepines are listed in Table 9. Tolerance does not develop to the drug's anticonflict effect (Stein et al., 1975) while in contrast it arises within a few days to the depression by oxazepam in rats (Stein et al., 1975) and chlordiazepoxide in humans (Goldberg et al., 1967).

Lippa and Regan (1977) determined the effect of chronic treatment with diazepam on the antagonism of pentylenetetrazol-, strychnine-, and bicuculline-induced convulsions. Tolerance to the antistrychnine and antibicuculline (see also Juhasz and Dairman, 1977) activities of diazepam developed while there was no tolerance to the pentylenetetrazol antagonism (Table 9). These data minimize the importance of any glycinergic and GABAergic actions of diazepam in mediation of the anticonflict and anticonvulsant effects. It would be of interest to know whether tolerance develops to diazepam's isoniazid antagonism. On the other hand, this drug's antipentylenetetrazol action, which might be a correlate of its antianxiety activity (Cook and Sepinwall, 1975), does not appear to be GABA-mediated.

The decrease in NE turnover, but not the decrease in 5-HT turnover, in the midbrain-hindbrain region induced by oxazepam rapidly undergoes tolerance (Stein et al., 1975). Behavioral tolerance to the depressant action and an apparent enhancement of antianxiety activity followed repeated doses (Margules and Stein, 1968). Primarily based on these studies, Stein et al. (1975), Margules and Stein (1968), and others (Rastogi et al., 1977) suggested that the benzodiazepines exert their anxiolytic effects by reducing the synthesis and turnover of 5-HT. On the other hand, in mice tolerance does develop to the diazepam- and clonazepam-induced increase in whole-brain 5-HT and 5-HIAA contents (Table 9; Jenner et al., 1975; Chadwick et al., 1978).

Table 9 Tolerance and Nontolerance to Effects of the Benzodiazepines in Rat and Mouse

Benzodiazepine, dose (μmol/kg), species and reference	Neuropharmacological parameter		Psychopharmacological parameter	
	Tolerant	Nontolerant	Tolerant	Nontolerant
Oxazepam 35 μmol/kg p.o.; 1/d × 6d; rats (Stein et al., 1975)	NE turnover in midbrain-hindbrain	5-HT turnover in midbrain-hindbrain	Depression of non-punished lever pressing	Release of suppressed behavior
Diazepam 17.6 μmol/kg i.p.; 3/d × 7d; rats (Consolo and Ladinsky, 1978 and unpublished results)	ACh increase in striatum	ACh decrease in striatum induced by diazepam-pentetrazol combination		Antagonism of pentetrazol convulsions muscle relaxation hypothermia
Diazepam 7 μmol/kg p.o.; 1/d × 7d; mice (Lippa and Regan, 1977)			Antagonism of strychnine and bicuculline convulsions	Antagonism of pentetrazol convulsions
Diazepam 7 μmol/kg p.o., 1/d × 4d; mice (Juhasz and Dairman, 1977)			Antagonism of bicuculline convulsions	Antagonism of pentetrazol convulsions
Chlordiazepoxide 167 μmol/kg 1/d × 14d; rats (Goldberg et al., 1967)			Protection against maximal electroshock	
Diazepam 113 μmol/kg i.p. 1/d × 8d; mice (Chadwick et al., 1978)	5-HT and 5-HIAA increase in whole brain			
Clonazepam 12.7 μmol/kg 1/d × 8d; mice (Jenner et al., 1975)	5-HT and 5-HIAA increase in whole brain			

The increase in the striatal ACh level produced by an acute dose of diazepan shows tolerance after repeated doses (Table 9). In contrast, the decrease in the striatal ACh content to below the normal level produced by the combination of diazepam and pentylenetetrazol does not show tolerance to repeated treatment with diazepam.

It may be safely assumed that psychopharmacological actions which do not succumb to tolerance are probably not related to neuropharmacological effects which do. The converse should also hold true. Thus, any possible cause-effect relationships may be ruled out. However, a "nontolerant" psychopharmacological action may be attributable to any one or any combination of nontolerant neuropharmacological actions or even to none of them. A similar reasoning holds for the tolerant psychopharmacological and neuropharmacological actions of the benzodiazepines.

REFERENCES

Babbini, M., Montanaro, N., Strocchi, P., and Gaiardi, M. (1971). Enhancement of amphetamine-induced stereotyped behavior by benzodiazepines. *Eur. J. Pharmacol. 13,* 330-340.

Banerjee, U. and Yeoh, P. N. (1977). The temporal dimensions of anticonvulsant action of some newer benzodiazepines against metrazol induced seizures in mice and rats. *Med. Biol. 55,* 310-316.

Banziger, R. F. (1965). Anticonvulsant properties of chlordiazepoxide, diazepam, and certain other 1,4 benzodiazepines. *Arch. Int. Pharmacodyn. Ther. 154,* 131-136.

Bartholini, G., Keller, H., Pieri, L., and Pletscher, A. (1973). The effect of diazepam on the turnover of cerebral dopamine. In *The Benzodiazepines,* S. Garattini, E. Mussini, and L. O. Randall (Eds.). Raven, New York, pp. 235-240.

Beleslin, D., Polak, R. L., and Sproull, D. H. (1965). The effect of leptazol and strychnine on the acetylcholine release from the cat brain. *J. Physiol. 181,* 308-316.

Bertagni, P., Marcucci, F., Mussini, E., and Garattini, S. (1972). Biliary excretion of conjugated hydroxylbenzodiazepines after administration of several benzodiazepines to rats, guinea pigs, and mice. *J. Pharmaceut. Sci. 61,* 965-966.

Billingsley, M. L. and Kubena, R. K. (1978). The effects of naloxone and picrotoxin on the sedative and anticonflict effects of benzodiazepines. *Life Sci. 22,* 897-906.

Biswas, B. and Carlsson, A. (1978). On the mode of action of diazepam on brain catecholamine metabolism. *Naunyn Schmiedeberg's Arch. Pharmacol. 303,* 73-78.

Boff, E. and Heise, G. A. (1963). Attenuation of tetrabenazine "reversal" by chlordiazepoxide hydrochloride. *Fed. Proc. 22,* 510.

Bourgoin, S., Héry, F., Ternaux, J. P., and Hamon, M. (1975). Effects of benzodiazepines on the binding of tryptophan in serum. Consequences on 5-hydroxyindoles concentrations in the rat brain. *Psychopharmacol. Comm. 1,* 209-216.

Braestrup, C., Albrechtsen, R., and Squires, R. F. (1977). High densities of benzodiazepine receptors in human cortical areas. *Nature* (London) *269,* 702-704.

Braestrup, C., and Squires, R. F. (1977). Specific benzodiazepine receptors in rat brain characterized by high-affinity [^{3}H] diazepam binding. *Proc. Nat. Acad. Sci. USA 74,* 3805-3809.

Braestrup, C., and Squires, R. F. (1978). Pharmacological characterization of benzodiazepine receptors in the brain. *Eur. J. Pharmacol. 48,* 263-270.

Chadwick, D., Gorrod, J. W., Jenner, P., Marsden, C. D., and Reynolds, E. H. (1978). Functional changes in cerebral 5-hydroxytryptamine metabolism in the mouse induced by anticonvulsant drugs. *Br. J. Pharmacol. 62,* 115-124.

Chase, T. N., Katz, R. I., and Kopin, I. J. (1970). Effect of diazepam on fate of intracisternally injected serotonin-C^{14}. *Neuropharmacology 9,* 103-108.

Cheney, D. L., Trabucchi, M., Hanin, I., and Costa, E. (1973). Effect of several benzodiazepines on concentrations and specific activities of choline and acetylcholine in mouse brain. *Pharmacologist 15,* 162.

Chéramy, A., Nieoullon, A., and Glowinski, J. (1977). Blockade of the picrotoxin-induced in vivo release of dopamine in the cat caudate nucleus by diazepam. *Life Sci. 20,* 811-816.

Chieli, T., Cocchi, D., Fregnan, G. B., and Muller, E. E. (1978). Interaction between different neuronal systems and the prolactin rise-induced by blockade of dopamine receptors. In Università degli Studi di Ancona *Giornate Nazionali e Internazionali di Farmacologia, XIX Congresso della Società Italiana di Farmacologia,* Ancona, Italy, 24-27 Sept. 1978, Abstracts, 438 (Abstr. 115).

Consolo, S., and Ladinsky, H. (1978). Interaction of diazepam (DZ) with other drugs on rat brain area acetylcholine (ACh) Abstract presented to 11th C.I.N.P. Congress, Wien, July 1978.

Consolo, S., Ladinsky, H., Peri, G., and Garattini, S. (1972). Effect of central stimulants and depressants on mouse brain acetylcholine and choline levels. *Eur. J. Pharmacol. 18,* 251-255.

Consolo, S., Ladinsky, H., Peri, G., and Garattini, S. (1974). Effect of diazepam on mouse whole brain and brain area acetylcholine and choline levels. *Eur. J. Pharmacol. 27,* 266-268.

Consolo, S., Garattini, S., and Ladinsky, H. (1975). Action of the benzodiazepines on the cholinergic system. In *Mechanism of Action of Benzodiazepines,* E. Costa and P. Greengard (Eds.). Raven, New York, pp. 45-61.

Consolo, S., Ladinsky, H., Bianchi, S., and Ghezzi, D. (1977). Apparent lack of a dopaminergic-cholinergic link in the rat nucleus accumbens septi-tuberculum olfactorium. *Brain Res. 135,* 255-263.

Cook, L., and Sepinwall, J. (1975). Behavioral analysis of the effects and mechanisms of action of benzodiazepines. In *Mechanism of Action of Benzodiazepines,* E. Costa and P. Greengard (Eds.). Raven, New York, pp. 1-28.

Corrodi, H., Fuxe, K., Lidbrink, P., and Olson, L. (1971). Minor tranquillizers, stress and central catecholamine neurons. *Brain Res. 29,* 1–16 .

Costa, E., Guidotti, A., Mao, C. C., and Suria, A. (1975a). New concepts on the mechanism of action of benzodiazepines. *Life Sci. 17,* 167-186.

Costa, E., Guidotti, A., and Mao, C. C. (1975b). Evidence for the involvement of GABA in the action of benzodiazepines. Studies on rat cerebellum. In *Mechanism of Action of Benzodiazepines,* E. Costa and P. Greengard (Eds.). Raven, New York, pp. 113-130.

Curtis, D. R., Lodge, D., Johnston, G. A. R., and Brand, S. J. (1976). Central actions of benzodiazepines. *Brain Res. 118,* 344-347.

Dal Bo, L., Marcucci, F., and Mussini, E. (1979). Gas chromatographic determination of pentetrazole in blood and brain of rats and blood of humans. *J. Pharmacol. Meth. 2,* 29-33.

Díaz, P. M. (1970). Pentylentetrazol and ethamivan effects on brain serotonin metabolism. *Life Sci. 9,* part 1, 831-840.

Dingledine, R., Iversen, L. L., and Breuker, E. (1978). Naloxone as a GABA antagonist. Evidence from iontophoretic, receptor binding and convulsant studies. *Eur. J. Pharmacol. 47,* 19-27.

Domino, E. F., and Wilson, A. E. (1972). Psychotropic drug influences on brain acetylcholine utilization. *Psychopharmacology 25,* 291-298.

Doteuchi, M., and Costa, E. (1973). Pentylenetetrazol convulsions and brain catecholamine turnover rate in rats and mice receiving diphenylhydantoin or benzodiazepines. *Neuropharmacology 12,* 1059-1072.

Eidelberg, E., Neer, H. M., and Miller, M. K. (1965). Anticonvulsant properties of some benzodiazepine derivatives. *Neurology* (Minneapolis) *15,* 223-230.

Fadda, F., Argiolas, A., Melis, M. R., Tissari, A. H., Onali, P. L., and Gessa, G. L. (1978). Stress-induced increase in 3,4-dihydroxyphenylacetic acid (DOPAC) levels in the cerebral cortex and n. accumbens. Reversal by diazepam. *Life Sci. 23,* 2219-2224.

Feinstein, M. B., Lenard, W., and Mathias, J. (1970). The antagonism of local anesthetic induced convulsions by the benzodiazepine derivate diazepam. *Arch. Int. Pharmacodyn. Ther. 187,* 144-154.

Fennessy, M. R., and Lee, J. R. (1972). The effect of benzodiazepines on brain amines of the mouse. *Arch. Int. Pharmacodyn. Ther. 197,* 37-44.

Fields, J. Z., Reisine, T. D., and Yamamura, H. I. (1977). Biochemical demonstration of dopaminergic receptors in rat and human brain using [^{3}H] spiroperidol. *Brain Res. 136,* 578-584.

Fuxe, K., Agnati, L. F., Bolme, P., Hökfelt, T., Lidbrink, P., Ljungdahl, A., Pérez de la Mora, M., and Ögren, S.-C. (1975). The possible involvement of GABA mechanisms in the action of benzodiazepines on central catecholamine neurons. In *Mechanism of Action of Benzodiazepines,* E. Costa and P. Greengard (Eds.). Raven, New York, pp. 45-61.

Gähwiler, B. H. (1976). Diazepam and chlordiazepoxide: powerful GABA antagonists in explants of rat cerebellum. *Brain Res. 107,* 176-179.

Garattini, S. (1978). Biochemical and pharmacological properties of oxazepam. *Acta Psychiatr. Scand. (suppl. 274),* 9-18.

Garattini, S., Marcucci, F., and Mussini, E. (1977). The metabolism and pharmacokinetics of selected benzodiazepines. In *Psychotherapeutic Drugs.* Part 2. *Applications,* Dekker, New York, pp. 1039–1087.

Garattini, S., Mussini, E., Marcucci, F., and Guaitani, A. (1973). Metabolic studies on benzodiazepines in various animal species. In *The Benzodiazepines,* S. Garattini, E. Mussini, and L. O. Randall (Eds.). Raven, New York, pp. 75-97.

Gardner, C. R., and Webster, R. A. (1973). The effect of some antidepressant drugs on leptazol and bicuculline induced acetylcholine efflux from rat cerebral cortex. *Br. J. Pharmacology 47,* 652P.

Gatti, G. L., Bonavoglia, F., and Michalek, H. (1973). Brain acetylcholine levels in diazepam attenuation of DFP toxicity in mice. In *Abstracts 4th. Int. Meet. Int. Soc. Neurochemistry,* Tokyo, Aug. 26-31, 1973, 492.

Giarman, N. J., and Pepeu, G. (1962). Drug-induced changes in brain acetylcholine. *Br. J. Pharmacol. 19,* 226-234.

Goldberg, M. E., Manian, A. A., and Efron, D. H. (1967). A comparative study of certain pharmacologic responses following acute and chronic administrations of chlordiazepoxide. *Life Sci. 6,* 481-491.

Govoni, S., Fresia, P., Spano, P. F., and Trabucchi, M. (1976). Effect of desmethyldiazepam and chlordesmethyldiazepam on 3′,5′-cyclic guanosine monophosphate levels in rat cerebellum. *Psychopharmacology* (Berlin) *50,* 241-244.

Green, V. A. (1964). Alterations in the activity of pentothal, phenobarbital, pentylenetetrazol and strychnine by cholinesterase inhibitors. *J. Pharmaceut. Sci. 53,* 762-766.

Guidotti, A., Toffano, G., Grandison, L., and Costa, E. (1978a). Second messenger responses and regulation of high affinity receptor binding to study pharmacological modifications of gabergic transmission. In *Amino Acids As Chemical Transmitters,* F. Fonnum (Ed.). Plenum, New York.

Guidotti, A., Toffano, G., and Costa, E. (1978b). An endogenous protein modulates the affinity of GABA and benzodiazepine receptors in rat brain. *Nature* (London) *275,* 553-555.

Haefely, W., Kulcsár, A., Möhler, H., Pieri, L., Polc, P., and Schaffner, R. (1975). Possible involvement of GABA in the central actions of benzodiazepines. In *Mechanism of Action of Benzodiazepines,* E. Costa and P. Greengard (Eds.). Raven, New York, pp. 131-151.

Harris, M., Hopkin, J. M., and Neal, M. J. (1973). Effect of centrally acting drugs on the uptake of γ-aminobutyric acid (GABA) by slices of rat cerebral cortex. *Br. J. Pharmacol. 47,* 229-239.

Heise, G. A., Laughlin, N., and Keller, C. (1970). A behavioral and pharmacological analysis of reinforcement withdrawal. *Psychopharmacologia* (Berlin) *16,* 345-368.

Hemsworth, B. A., and Neal, M. J. (1968). The effect of central stimulant drugs on acetylcholine release from the rat cerebral cortex. *Br. J. Pharmacol. 34,* 543-550.

Hernández-Peón, R., Rojas-Ramirez, J. A., O'Flaherty, J. J., and Mazzuchelli-O'Flaherty, A. L. (1964). An experimental study of the anticonvulsive and relaxant actions of Valium. *Int. J. Neuropharmacol. 3,* 405-412.

Javoy, F., Euvrard, C., Herbet, A., and Glowinski, J. (1977). Involvement of the dopamine nigrostriatal system in the picrotoxin effect on striatal acetylcholine levels. *Brain Res. 126,* 382-386.

Jenner, P., Chadwick, D., Reynolds, E. H., and Marsden, C. D. (1975). Altered 5-HT metabolism with clonazepam, diazepam and diphenylhydantoin. *J. Pharm. Pharmacol. 27,* 707-710.

Johnson, D. D., and Lowndes, H. E. (1974). Reduction by diazepam of repetitive electrical activity and toxicity resulting from soman. *Eur. J. Pharmacol. 28,* 245-250.

Juhasz, L., and Dairman, W. (1977). Effect of sub-acute diazepam administration in mice on the subsequent ability of diazepam to protect against metrazol and bicuculline induced convulsions. *Fed. Proc. 36,* 377.

Keim, K. L., and Sigg, E. B. (1977). Plasma corticosterone and brain, catecholamines in stress. Effect of psychotropic drugs. *Pharmacol. Biochem. Behav. 6,* 79-86.

Keller, H. H., Schaffner, R., and Haefely, W. (1976). Interaction of benzodiazepines with neuroleptics at central dopamine neurons. *Naunyn Schmiedeberg's Arch. Pharmacol. 294,* 1-7.

Kilian, M., and Frey, H.-H. (1973). Central monoamines and convulsive thresholds in mice and rats. *Neuropharmacology 12,* 681-692.

Kutt, H., Verebely, K., and McDowell, F. (1968). Inhibition of diphenylhydantoin metabolism in rats and in rat liver microsomes by antitubercular drugs. *Neurology* (Minneapolis) *18,* 706-710.

Ladinsky, H., Consolo, S., Peri, G., and Garattini, S. (1973). Increase in mouse and rat brain acetylcholine levels by diazepam. In *The Benzodiazepines,* S. Garattini, E. Mussini, and L. O. Randall (Eds.). Raven, New York, pp. 241-242.

Ladinsky, H., Consolo, S., Bianchi, S., and Jori, A. (1976). Increase in striatal acetylcholine by picrotoxin in the rat: Evidence for a gabergic-dopaminergic-cholinergic link. *Brain Res. 108,* 351-361.

Lahti, R. A., and Barsuhn, C. (1974). The effect of minor tranquilizers on stress-induced increases in rat plasma corticosteroids. *Psychopharmacologia* (Berlin) *35,* 215-220.

Leysen, J., and Laduron, P. (1977). Differential distribution of opiate and neuroleptic receptors and dopamine-sensitive adenylate cyclase in rat brain. *Life Sci. 20,* 281-288.

Lidbrink, P., Corrodi, H., and Fuxe, K. (1974). Benzodiazepines and barbiturates. Turnover changes in central 5-hydroxytryptamine pathways. *Eur. J. Pharmacol. 26,* 35-40.

Lipp, J. A. (1973). Effect of benzodiazepine derivatives on soman-induced seizures activity and convulsions in the monkey. *Arch. Int. Pharmacodyn. Ther. 202,* 244-251.

Lippa, A. S., and Critchett, D. J. (1981). Benzodiazepines, GABA and chloride conductance. *Nature* (London). Submitted.

Lippa, A. S., and Regan, B. (1977). Additional studies on the importance of glycine and GABA in mediating the actions of benzodiazepines. *Life Sci. 21,* 1779-1783.

Longoni, R., Mulas, A., and Pepeu, G. (1974). Drug effect on acetylcholine level in discrete brain regions of rats killed by microwave irradiation. *Br. J. Pharmacol. 52,* 429P-430P.

Madan, B. R., Sharma, J. D., and Vyas, D. S. (1963). Actions of methaminodiazepoxide on cardiac, smooth and skeletal muscles. *Arch. Int. Pharmacodyn. Ther. 143,* 127-137.

Maickel, R. P., and Maloney, G. J. (1973). Effects of various depressant drugs on deprivation-induced water consumption. *Neuropharmacology 12,* 777-782.

Mao, C. C., Guidotti, A., and Costa, E. (1975). Evidence for an involvement of GABA in the mediation of the cerebellar cGMP decrease and the anticonvulsant action of diazepam. *Naunyn Schmiedeberg's Arch. Pharmacol. 289,* 369-378.

Mao, C. C., Marco, E., Revuelta, A., Bertilsson, L., and Costa, E. (1977). The turnover rate of γ-aminobutyric acid in the nuclei of telencephalon. Implications in the pharmacology of antipsychotics and of a minor tranquilizer. *Biol. Psychiatry 12,* 359-371.

Marcucci, F., and Mussini, E. (1968). A metabolic explanation for differences between species of the anticonvulsant activity of diazepam. *Br. J. Pharmacol. 34,* 667P-668P.

Marcucci, F., Guaitani, A., Kvetina, J., Mussini, E., and Garattini, S. (1968). Species difference in diazepam metabolism and anticonvulsant effect. *Eur. J. Pharmacol. 4,* 467-470.

Marcucci, F., Fanelli, R., Mussini, E., and Garattini, S. (1970). Further studies on species difference in diazepam metabolism. *Eur. J. Pharmacol. 9,* 253-256.

Marcucci, F., Airoldi, M. L., Mussini, E., and Garattini, S. (1971). Brain levels of metrazol determined with a new gas chromatographic procedure. *Eur. J. Pharmacol. 16,* 219-221.

Margules, D. L., and Stein, L. (1968). Increase of "antianxiety" activity and tolerance of behavioral depression during chronic administration of oxazepam. *Psychopharmacologia* (Berlin) *13,* 74-80.

Matsui, Y., and Deguchi, T. (1977). Cataleptic action of nitrazepam and brain dopamine function in mice. *Neuropharmacology 16,* 253-258.

Mitchell, J. F. (1963). The spontaneous and evoked release of acetylcholine from the cerebral cortex. *J. Physiol. 165,* 98-116.

Peričić, D., Walters, J. R., and Chase, T. N. (1977). Effect of diazepam and pentobarbital on aminooxyacetic acid-induced accumulation of GABA. *J. Neurochem. 29,* 839-846.

Polc, P., and Haefely, W. (1976). Effects of the benzodiazepines, phenobarbitone, and baclofen on synaptic transmission in the cat cuneate nucleus. *Naunyn Schmiedeberg's Arch. Pharmacol. 294,* 121-131.

Polc, P., Möhler, H., and Haefely, W. (1974). The effect of diazepam on spinal cord activities. Possible sites and mechanisms of action. *Naunyn Schmiedeberg's Arch. Pharmacol. 284,* 319-337.

Porsolt, R. D., Anton, G., Blavet, N., and Jalfre, M. (1978). Behavioural despair in rats. A new model sensitive to antidepressant treatments. *Eur. J. Pharmacol. 47,* 379-391.

Rastogi, R. B., Agarwal, R. A., Lapierre, Y. D., and Singhal, R. L. (1977). Effects of acute diazepam and clobazam on spontaneous locomotor activity and central amine metabolism in rats. *Eur. J. Pharmacol. 43,* 91-98.

Ruch-Monachon, M. A., Jalfre, M., and Haefely, W. (1976). Drugs and PGO waves in the lateral geniculate body of the curarized cat. IV. The effects of acetylcholine, GABA and benzodiazepines on PGO wave activity. *Arch. Int. Pharmacodyn. Ther. 219,* 308-325.

Rump, S., Grudzinska, E., and Edelwejn, Z. (1973). Effects of diazepam on epileptiform patterns of bioelectrical activity of the rabbit's brain induced by fluostigmine. *Neuropharmacology 12,* 813-817.

Sawaya, M. C. B., Horton, R. W., and Meldrum, B. S. (1975). Effects of anticonvulsant drugs on the cerebral enzymes metabolizing GABA. *Epilepsia 16,* 649-655.

Schallek, W., Schlosser, W., and Randall, L. O. (1972). Recent developments in the pharmacology of the benzodiazepines. *Adv. Pharmacol. Chemother. 10,* 119-183.

Segal, M., Dudai, Y., and Amsterdam, A. (1978). Distribution of an α-bungarotoxin-binding cholinergic nicotinic receptor in rat brain. *Brain Res. 148,* 105-119.

Sethy, V. H. (1978). Effect of hypnotic and anxiolytic agents on regional concentration of acetylcholine in rat brain. *Naunyn Schmiedeberg's Arch. Pharmacol. 301,* 157-161.

Snyder, S. H., and Enna, S. J. (1975). The role of central glycine receptors in the pharmacologic actions of benzodiazepines. In *Mechanism of Action of Benzodiazepines,* E. Costa and P. Greengard (Eds.). Raven, New York, pp. 81-91.

Soubrie, P., and Simon, P. (1978). Comparative study of the antagonism of bemegride and picrotoxin on behavioural depressant effects of diazepam in rats and mice. *Neuropharmacology 17,* 121-125.

Squires, R. F., and Braestrup, C. (1977). Benzodiazepine receptors in rats. *Nature* (London) *266,* 732-734.

Stein, L., Wise, C. D., and Belluzzi, J. D. (1975). Effects of benzodiazepines on central serotoninergic mechanisms. In *Mechanism of Action of Benzodiazepines,* E. Costa and P. Greengard (Eds.). Raven, New York, pp. 29-44.

Steiner, F. A., and Felix, D. (1976). Antagonistic effects of GABA and benzodiazepines on vestibular and cerebellar neurones. *Nature* (London) *260,* 346-347.

Suria, A., and Costa, E. (1975). Action of diazepam, dibutyryl cGMP and GABA on presynaptic nerve terminals in bullfrog sympathetic ganglia. *Brain Res. 87,* 102-106.

Svenneby, G., and Roberts, E. (1974). Elevated acetylcholine contents in mouse brain after treatment with bicuculline and picrotoxin. *J. Neurochem. 23,* 275-277.

Tarsy, D., and Baldessarini, R. J. (1974). Behavioural supersensitivity to apomorphine following chronic treatment with drugs which interfare with the synaptic function of catecholamines. *Neuropharmacology 13,* 927-940.

Taylor, K. M., and Laverty, R. (1969). The effect of chlordiazepoxide, diazepam and nitrazepam on catecholamine metabolism in regions of the rat brain. *Eur. J. Pharmacol. 8,* 296-301.

Taylor, K. M., and Laverty, R. (1973). The interaction of chlordiazepoxide, diazepam, and nitrazepam with catecholamines and histamine in regions of the rat brain. In *The Benzodiazepines,* S. Garattini, E. Mussini, and L. O. Randall (Eds.). Raven, New York, pp. 191-202.

Valerino, D. M., Vesel, E. S., Johnson, A. O., and Aurori, K. C. (1973). Effects of various centrally active drugs on hepatic microsomal enzymes. A comparative study. *Drug. Met. Dispos. 1,* 669-678.

Weiner, W. J., Goetz, C., Nausieda, P. A., and Klawans, H. L. (1977). Clonazepam and dopamine-related stereotyped behavior. *Life Sci. 21,* 901-906.

Woodward, D. J., Hoffer, B. J., Siggins, G. R., and Bloom, F. E. (1971). The ontogenetic development of synaptic junctions, synaptic activation and responsiveness to neurotransmitter substances in rat cerebellar purkinje cells. *Brain Res. 34,* 73-97.

Yamamura, H. I., and Snyder, S. H. (1974). Muscarinic cholinergic binding in rat brain. *Proc. Nat. Acad. Sci. USA 71,* 1725-1729.

Young, A. B., and Snyder, S. H. (1973). Strychnine binding associated with glycine receptors of the central nervous system. *Proc. Nat. Acad. Sci. USA 70,* 2832-2836.

Zakusov, V. V., Ostrovskaya, R. U., Kozhechkin, S. N., Markovich, V. V., Molodavkin, G. M., and Voronina, T. A. (1977). Further incidence for GABA-ergic mechanisms in the action of benzodiazepines. *Arch. Int. Pharmacodyn. Ther. 229,* 313-326.

Zbinden, G., and Randall, L. O. (1967). Pharmacology of benzodiazepines: Laboratory and clinical correlations. *Adv. Pharmacol. Chemother. 5,* 213-291.

Zsilla, G., Cheney, D. L., and Costa, E. (1976). Regional change in the rate of turnover of acetylcholine in rat brain following diazepam or muscimol. *Naunyn Schmiedeberg's Arch. Pharmacol. 294,* 251-255.

Zukin, S. R., Young, A. B., and Snyder, S. H. (1974). Gamma-aminobutyric acid binding to receptor sites in the rat central nervous system. *Proc. Nat. Acad. Sci. USA 71,* 4802-4807.

25

Mode of Action of Hallucinogenic Drugs

Daniel X. Freedman
The University of Chicago
Chicago, Illinois

To understand mediating mechanisms in disease and in therapies, and to design rational interventions, we must grasp and delineate the underlying neurobiological organizations, the mechanisms by which chemical and neuronal feedbacks are organized and regulated, and by which neurochemical equilibria are maintained and shift. These are of abiding concern for clinical psychiatry, and all psychotropic drugs have been a tool in the growing science base. The measures of substrates and metabolites and clinical descriptive distinctions that we can undertake in humans become meaningful the more we understand of intrinsic physiological organizations and controls. In general, neuropsychopharmacology has been discovering the "alphabet" (e.g., brain receptor systems and their specific neuronal organizations) and a few of the rules of syntactical transformations: the logic of nature as it involves the link of brain chemistry, neuronal transmission, and behavior. Although experiments with none of the available psychotropic drugs have as yet established any unequivocal and primary etiological link to clinical disorder, many useful leads are in hand. The fact that in humans we can now glimpse events inside of a nerve ending through relatively noninvasive measures of CNS amine metabolites and logically deduce how a drug may have affected amine synthesis, reuptake, or release provides psychiatry with an astonishing grasp of processes and an array of measures which 30 years ago would have been hard to predict. There is now a reason for the clinician to note whether Parkinson's disease has ever occurred in a previously schizophrenic patient or to search for subgroup differences in clinical response to antidepressants with primary effects on one or another neurotransmitter. The interplay of animal and clinical research is, then, of increasing importance, and this is as true for hallucinogenic drugs as for other major psychotropics.

This chapter focuses, as has the attention of the field over the past 30 years, on d-lysergic acid diethylamide (d-LSD) as the prototypical agent thought to be an hallucinogen. There is a similarity in the fundamental pattern of mental and perceptual changes produced by LSD and its proven psychoactive indoleamine congeners (psilocin and psilocybin, N,N-dimethyltryptamine or DMT) and the phenylethylamine mescaline (Freedman and Aghajanian, 1959; Isbell et al., 1959,1961; Wolbach et al., 1962; Appel and Freedman, 1968; Winters, 1971). These represent a group of hallucinogens with which cross-tolerance has been clearly noted in humans and animals, as have similar mental and behavioral effects. Without doubt, the astonishingly high potency of LSD (less than a billionth of a gram per gram of brain is required in a human being for reliable effects); the specificity and reliability with which it produces a time-limited period of altered perceptual, emotional, and mental functioning; and its striking structural and functional links with physiologically active indoles elicited both the experimental and clinical attention. These features stimulated the hope that the drug would provide a salient lead by which behaviorally relevant biobehavioral substrates could be defined.

The reliability with which *single* doses of LSD and the far less potent related drugs produce a specific mental state (Freedman, 1968) contrasts with the uncertain psychotomimetic effects of single doses of amphetamine or with the variability of mental response produced by amine precursors (such as L-dopa) and enzyme inhibitors. The mental effects of this family of indole and phenylethylamines differs from the cholinolytic deliriants with their atropine-like amnestic and confusional effects. Rather, they produce psychedelic, mysticomimetic, or psychotomimetic perceptions and thought which occur in the presence of clear consciousness and without significant impairment of neurological or neurosensory function (thus differing from phencyclidine, or PCP). From this specificity of pharmacological activation of a fluid and multipotential mental state (Bowers and Freedman, 1966) any number of theoretical or clinical hypotheses of concern to clinical psychiatry and experimental psychopathology were suggested and tested. Thus LSD motivated a search for its therapeutic uses or for an endogenous indole or methylated indole or phenylethylamine psychotoxin, or for common molecular or neural mechanisms of hallucinogenesis.

Both literature review (Siegal and West, 1975) and reflection, however, would make the likelihood of a common biological trigger or mechanism underlying all illusory and hallucinatory phenomena highly unlikely. For the many clinical states, from the epilepsies to delirium tremens, from the various hallucinoses to the functional psychoses, common mediating mechanisms are not evident and, in perspective, not probable. Indeed, for *all* drugs or ionic and metabolic shifts that lead to altered mental states accompanied by illusions or hallucinatory activity, there is as yet no known common mechanism. Even among the related indole and phenylethylamines, we now know that for similar *biological* effects, similar chemical structure–e.g., an indole ring–is more important than common behavioral effects (Freedman et al., 1970). Among all drugs with which any hallucinatory phenomena are associated, there are phenomenological similarities and differences which descriptive psychiatry can note and which biology must yet explain. Thus there are the toxic states or deliria that can be observed with febrile response to disease and with a very wide range of medications in which dosage regimen is critical. There are also the toxic states more closely resembling paranoid psychoses that occur only with chronic high-dose regimens of drugs such as Atabrine (Newell and Lidz, 1946); there are the inconstant effects of prolonged or high dosage with steroids, as well as the hallucinatory phenomena observed in drug withdrawal states with the sedative antianxiety agents including alcohol. It currently appears more fruitful to study each of these phenomena in its own right rather than at the outset to require of them a common mechanism which, in any event, remains undiscerned.

Among those drugs which are now commonly abused, and which in sufficient dosage lead to altered perceptual states, marijuana preparations, in which Δ^9-THC is the active ingredient, and phencyclidine–abused as PCP or "angel dust"–are receiving increasing study, but have not had the extensive multisystems testing and multidisciplinary study which has attended the indole and phenylethylamine hallucinogens. Phencyclidine, an anesthetic in sufficient dosage, produces a number of neurologic symptoms–notably numbness. As yet, the drug has produced no clear trail to central neural or biochemical systems that might provide a basis for deducing its mode of action; presynaptic dopaminergic actions are currently under study. Early studies of PCP emphasized its effects on proprioception (Luby et al., 1962) and described a kind of chemically induced sensory isolation with the induction of confusional states, perceptual distortion, and affective perturbation when the subject was provoked into coping with people or the environment. Hallucinatory and paranoid states with Δ^9-THC are well known, but the marijuana derivatives show no cross-tolerance with drugs such as LSD, psilocybin, DMT, or mescaline, or even the substituted phenylpropylamines such as DOM (known as STP), even though the drug has effects (albeit highly variable) on brain biogenic amines (Braude and Szara, 1976). Nor has study of Δ^9-THC as yet yielded electrophysiological and biochemical changes that trace a meaningful or correlatable pattern of relatively specific brain changes that might lead to the cogent formulation of hallucinogenic mechanisms.

In highlighting LSD and related drugs, we will emphasize those mechanisms which are in clearest focus, emphasizing among the veritable myriad of often confusing and questionably reliable biochemical and behavioral test systems (ranging from invertebrates to rodents, cattle, goats, cats, dogs, primates, and humans), those for which the vast bulk of congruent evidence would warrant both clinical and experimental attention. Thus it is clear that the solid and compelling leads have been the study of LSD and related drugs on neural and chemical mechanisms regulating 5-HT and to a lesser extent catecholamines. The drug has indeed been a primary tool in identifying and elucidating the raphe system: cell assemblies morphologically, biochemically, and functionally specific for serotonin (5-HT, or 5-hydroxytryptamine) (Aghajanian et al., 1975). The extent to which these midline systems explain LSD effects will require focus since this appears to be a key, yet certainly not sufficient and a questionably necessary system to explain the array of LSD effects. While effects on norepinephrine (NE) and dopamine (DA) are noted, as well as effects in NE- or DA-sensitive adenylate cyclase in mammals, their significance is less certain and requires some perspective. Similarly, there has recently been extensive study of stereospecific, high-affinity "receptors"–binding or acceptor sites for LSD; these are likely in the coming few years to receive enhanced experimental and clinical study. There are also long- and short-term effects on the regulation of the turnover of 5-HT and catechols, which may be related to tolerance and possibly to long-term behavioral effects of clinical interest. Finally, subcellular work with LSD appears to be leading to the identification of nerve ending mechanisms and endogenous carrier systems (Halaris and Freedman, 1977; Freedman and Halaris, 1978) or substances (Tamir and Rapport, 1978) regulating the binding and release of monoamines which may have increasing clinical relevance.

I. A HISTORICAL NOTE

LSD and congeners were the third of the major classes of psychotropics to be linked to the chemistry of brain, following detection of the effects of reserpine and MAO inhibitors. By 1963, Axelrod had shown that serotonin, like the catecholamines, could be conserved by reuptake mechanisms in tissues, and through his work and that of Axelrod and Carlson and Lindquist (1963) it was established that blockade at a receptor would alter amine metabolites and thus rates of synthesis and turnover. Impulse flow and the synthetic and releasing properties of the presynaptic neuron could be viewed as controlled by the degree of receptor activation of the transmitter or agonistic drugs (through neural loop or chemical feedback signals). An agonist should slow turnover and decrease impulse flow ("There is too much of me") and an antagonist enhance it ("There is not enough of me. Make more"). Actual electrophysiological measurements at cell bodies and nerve endings between 1967 and the present, for both norepinephrine and serotonin, have demonstrated instances of what originally was a biochemically inferred link—increase discharge rates with antagonists and the reverse with agonists. No doubt the startling visualization in 1964 by Dahlstrom and Fuxe (1965) with fluorescence histochemistry of monoaminergic-containing perikaria and terminals led to the definitions of the specificity of each of the known monoaminergic neural systems.

Thus the alphabet of measurable substrates and enzymes and some of the syntax began to be in place by the late sixties and the explanation of drug action has required combinations of behavioral, electrophysiological, and biochemical studies. The effect of receptor blockade by phenothiazines and reuptake blockade by tricyclics on dopamine and norepinephrine and their metabolites have (in part because of the ease with which peripheral mechanisms could be studied in sympathetically innervated systems) been far more extensively characterized than have the actions of hallucinogens. But any who follow the field can note similar experimental paradigms. With the experimental systems and measures now available, there has recently been a vast increase in the pace of research into hallucinogens (Freedman and Halaris, 1978), different animal systems to evaluate their behavioral effects (Trulson et al., 1977), operant (Appel and Freedman, 1965) and state-dependent learning designs (Cameron and Appel, 1973; Hirschorn et al., 1975; Winters, 1978) (capable of detecting very low doses of different or similar drugs). Inferences and deductions from many of these leave much to be desired, e.g., the lack of systematic criteria for assessing "low" and "high" doses in animal behavior, electrophysiological, biochemical, and human test systems, and the frequent unavailability of "coupled" behavioral, electrophysiological, and biochemical measures in the same organism. Such cautionary concern, while not stipulated in this review, guides the discussion.

For perspective, it is interesting that the first published clinical description of LSD appeared in 1947, 4 years after Hoffman's bicycle trip from his laboratory where he noted the odd effects of the ergot derivative he had synthesized in 1938. It is startling that we then did not know whether we could understand more than the fact that the limits of consciousness and coma were dependent on oxygen and glucose. A functional brain chemistry—as Sir Henry Dale envisioned it—to account for the dissociations and shifts in behavior which descriptive psychiatry delineated (and which pellagra, and hormonal and metabolic disorders suggested ought to occur) was simply not in hand. The exciting leads were coming from the brain's "wires" rather than the "juices"; from studies of the aggressive, regressive, compulsive, and stereotyped automatisms linked to the limbic brain and the loss of pathological drive, the indifference to anticipatory anxiety, noted after frontal lobe surgery. Yet in the next 2 or 3 years, appreciation of reticular systems, and electrophysiological studies at the synaptic level showing graded inhibitory or excitatory potentials, provided a picture of a nervous system in which graded changes in consciousness rather than simple off or on switching mechanisms could be accommodated.

Serotonin was but 6 years old when it was identified in brain by Twarog and Page (1953). At that time, Gaddum (1953) and Woolley and Shaw (1954), noting that competitive antagonism by LSD of serotonin at smooth muscle receptors, proposed in effect that serotonin might be necessary for sanity and that excesses or deficiencies of the amine in brain could be important to altered mental states. The key hypothesis was that binding and release of endogenous amines were key to mental function. It is interesting that there was then no evidence that endogenous monoamines were themselves directly psychotomimetic—and there are still no such data; rather, methylated tryptamines (DMT) or phenylethylamines (dimethoxyphenylethylamine, DMPEA) have been linked, albeit unsuccessfully (Cohen et al., 1974; Gillin et al., 1976; Friedhoff et al., 1977), with clinical disorder. On the other hand, insufficient or excess amine at different receptor sites, perhaps contingent on different rates of neural transmission (which are in turn regulated by different balances among the transmitters), continues to be a viable hypothesis. In brief, we might in retrospect note that the question has been what regulates excesses or deficiencies in the binding and release of amines and their availability at different receptors and what order of magnitude of change is necessary for behavior change.

In spite of fruitful hypotheses, a direct link of LSD to brain serotonin was apparently not even sought until, in 1955, reserpine was found to deplete granular stores of amines and simultaneously to produce striking associated behavioral shifts (Brodie et al., 1956). This finding marks a distinct impetus to attempt to link behavior change with brain amine change. Since full repletion of storage sites in humans requires several weeks at the least to achieve (Freedman and Benton, 1961), reserpine provided the opportunity to study amine behavior interactions as well as drug behavior interactions. Thus the germinal notion that the binding and release of amine might affect neural function and behavior had a tangible demonstration. Indeed, it was the detection of an increase in brain 5-HT *after* reserpine depletion that made possible the initial detection of an LSD effect on brain levels of serotonin (Freedman, 1960).

By 1957, the behavioral effects of MAO inhibitors had been correlated with an increase in brain amine and a decrease in urinary 5-hydroxyindoleacetic acid (5-HIAA), the catabolite of serotonin (measurement of which in brain was not technically feasible until the sixties). 5-Hydroxytryptophan (5-HTP), the precursor of 5-HT, was soon noted to elevate brain 5-HT and to produce central excitatory effects in part similar to LSD [recently elevated mood was reported (Pühringer et al., 1976)]. But since measures of brain 5-HT taken 4 hr after LSD showed no effect, and since LSD failed when given before reserpine to inhibit release of amine, and since powerful 5-HT antagonists such as 2-brom-LSD (BOL) had no mental effects, there was little to be said for the link of LSD to 5-HT by the end of 1957.

By that time, studies on the "wires" of the brain had shown that 5-HT and catecholamines when tested directly at corticodendritic synapses in both animals (Marrazzi and Hart, 1955) and humans (Purpura et al., 1957) were inhibitory, as was LSD; the drug changed transmission at the geniculate synapse in the optic system (Evarts et al., 1955); LSD even in doses as low as 5 μg/kg in the cat had selective action on optical and auditory cortex and relays. Thus low doses of LSD could enhance sensory systems and simultaneously inhibit the response of cortical systems (Purpura, 1956a,b). It was thought that the drug by enhancing reticular transmission increased sensitivity to input but diminished control and led to dehabituation to familiar inputs which would now appear "novel." Yet after this initial thrust such work subsided and few of these early definitions and test systems have been systematically pursued.

By 1957, then, biochemical pharmacology was turning to catecholamines, to the discovery of other mechanisms controlling the equilibria of amines, such as synthetic enzymes and uptake. LSD was indeed beginning to be rediscovered but mainly by overwrought (if not addled) clinicians and seekers of transcendent truth, laying the groundwork for the psychedelic decade of the sixties and a period of lay experimentation which posed new problems to biological psychiatry. It is striking that in the present decade we are generally unable to undertake systematic studies with LSD in humans, which would yield a crisper picture of the psychopharmacology of this drug and remove many ambiguities about drug effects in humans which still (as later noted) persist. Nevertheless by 1957 after-effects (flashbacks) had been noted, as had the therapeutic potential of hallucinogens and the potential for adverse effects (Elkes et al., 1955; Cooper, 1955) later known as bad trips.

In 1960, when periods of acute behavioral change in rat were precisely coupled with biochemical measures, the direct effect of LSD on elevating brain 5-HT was found (Freedman, 1960,1961a). At the same time, small decreases in brain norepinephrine were measured (Freedman, 1961b) and a similar pattern of effects was noted for acute physiological stress (Barchas and Freedman, 1963). Seven years later the major effect of LSD on 5-HT metabolism—a slowed turnover—was measurable in brain: an initial 45 min decrease in 5-HIAA (differently mediated than that in the subsequent 90 min).

II. LSD AND 5-HT METABOLISM

There is a characteristic pattern of initial brain biochemical effects in species studied: increased brain 5-HT (a small change of 15-20% in whole brain) and a decrease in the catabolite 5-HIAA (Rosecrans et al., 1967). This is a stereospecific effect and neither 1-LSD nor nonpsychoactive congeners, such as BOL or methysergide, produce it. This slowed-down turnover of brain amine was originally ascribed to an LSD-induced "binding" of serotonin in nerve-ending particles, sparing 5-HT from catabolism without any direct action on MAO (Freedman, 1961a; Collins et al., 1970). Similar effects were adduced for psilocybin, psilocin, and DMT but *not* mescaline or DOM (Freedman et al., 1970). While mescaline (and physiological stress) elevated brain levels of 5-HT (Freedman, 1963), the drug effect is probably, as with stress, due to increased turnover. Thus we could not replicate studies which indicated the LSD pattern on 5-HT-5-HIAA for *all* psychotomimetics (Freedman and Halaris, 1978). The hope for a uniform explanation even for psychotomimetic drugs related by mental effect and cross-tolerance in terms of biogenic amine metabolism has not been fulfilled. Rather, indole psychotomimetic amines appear to be linked, and all, including the short-acting DMT, show tolerance and cross-tolerance (Kovacic and Domino, 1976). The basis for cross-tolerance with mescaline [there is none with amphetamines (Vaupel et al., 1978)] remains obscure.

Biochemical changes induced by LSD are not mediated by intermediate metabolites. Brain concentrations of drug peak early and they are always about a 1000-fold less than the plasma; clearance faithfully follows the plasma half-life of LSD which marks the termination of acute behavioral effects (about 45 min to a behavioral threshold dose of 130 μg/kg in rat) (Rosecrans et al., 1967; Freedman and Boggan, 1974). There is a preferential drug concentration in optical and limbic areas, and drug binding in various cells of interest. This has little precise explanatory value, apart from the fact that radioactive LSD in minute amounts can be identified in brain 12 hr or more after injection.

Thus the peak retention of serotonin [normally occurring almost entirely in synaptic vesicles (Halaris and Freedman, 1977; Freedman and Halaris, 1978)] occurs as drug has cleared the brain and as the termination of acute behavioral effects is observed. The conversion of the amino acid precursor tryptophan, through 5-hydroxytryptophan to serotonin, is slowed for about 2 hr after LSD (Lin et al., 1969); without evidence of direct effect on the enzyme, this is due either to indirect feedback signals or the LSD-induced inhibition of raphe soma firing. Synthesis, nevertheless, still occurs and it is the newly synthesized serotonin which we have concluded is retained in vesicular storage sites (Freedman and Halaris, 1973; 1978).

What, however, is most salient to the effect of LSD are actions which render nerve-ending 5-HT—whether it is bound in vesicles or in a newly characterized, soluble "juxtavesicular" fraction (Freedman and Halaris, 1978)—*inaccessible to the adjacent mitochondrial MAO.* Diminished catabolism of 5-HT is evident even when huge increases of 5-HIAA are produced by the intracellular amine release induced by reserpine. With various drugs (PCPA, PCA, RO4-460, or during chlorimipramine-feedback-induced inhibition) inhibiting the conversion of precursor to 5-HT, no 5-HT increment is evident, but 5-HIAA decreases occur. Thus the 5-HT increase and 5-HIAA decrease can be dissociated. In brief, there are nerve-ending events which indicate a failure of the normal conversion of nerve-ending serotonin to 5-HIAA, whether or not an increment in 5-HT can be measured after LSD.

The nerve-ending membrane and the intracellular, presynaptic effects of LSD compose a unit for intensive study. There appear to be biophysical or biochemical effects of LSD which are independent or semi-independent of the transmission of the nerve impulse and events at the raphe soma. Thus in incubated brain slices, after a brief inhibition of [^{3}H] 5-HT uptake, there is a subsequent retention of labeled amine (Ziegler et al., 1973). There is an inhibition of 5-HT release in electrically stimulated brain slices (Chase et al., 1967), since studies of the efflux of labeled 5-HT and metabolites into ventricular fluid also show a retention of 5-HT after LSD, but not after reuptake blockaders (Gallager and Aghajanian, 1975). Inhibition of 5-HT reuptake at the nerve membrane by LSD does not appear to be involved as once noted (Marchbanks, 1967), and there is no effect of LSD on high-affinity, synaptosomal uptake of 5-HT when studied at 37°C rather than 0°C (Lovell and Freedman, 1974; Freedman and Halaris, 1978).

That retention of 5-HT and protection from MAO after LSD may be an effect of the drug on soluble macromolecules, which normally have a carrier function, is one favored hypothesis. The normal picture of a serotonin nerve ending—a large proportion of amine in vesicles and various presynaptic compartments with low concentrations of 5-HT to be readily released across the nerve membrane into the synaptic cleft and to the postsynaptic receptors—may not be the case. Rather, approximately 80% of the 5-HT in the nerve-ending fraction is held in a soluble compartment, and only 20-30% in the vesicular subfractions. Crude 100,000 g spins, which showed "particulate" increases after LSD and a ratio of 75:25 of particulate to supernatant amine (Freedman, 1961a), are in fact now explained by the fact that the soluble juxtavesicular materials are within that crude particulate fraction, which on subfractionation reveals a strikingly different picture of possible nerve-ending events. After reserpine, this juxtavesicular fraction binds serotonin and, while reserpine-sensitive, has a many times greater concentration of serotonin than the impaired vesicles. Thus one can conceive of carrier materials which normally deliver an increment of the newly synthesized serotonin to vesicles, to the terminal nerve-ending membrane for release, and to the nerve-ending MAO for catabolism. Interference by LSD with this normal traffic leads to less amine available at postsynaptic elements, leaving LSD free to bind to postsynaptic receptors and to exert its characteristic combined agonistic and antagonistic postsynaptic effects at sites normally "expecting" 5-HT and perhaps at other acceptor sites as well.

Tamir (1978) has recently characterized a soluble substance capable of binding serotonin; probably an actin-like molecule, it is found in serotonin neurons in the myenteric plexus as well as in the CNS, and while its characteristics do not accord with those required from biochemical studies with LSD, such a substance or other related materials should be a current focus of study. After all, if soluble binding or carrier substances were abnormal in human disease, the measurable changes produced might be of small magnitude, but of great consequence. This would be a "model" deduced from these studies of LSD in rat brain nerve endings.

Other carrier functions are implicated in a peculiar effect of LSD in increasing brain tryptophan at a time when serotonin synthesis is slowed down (Freedman and Boggan, 1974). This disappears after a daily dosage tolerance regimen. Corticosterone in rat also shows large increases and, similarly, a decrement on the tolerance dosage regimen. With adrenalectomy the corticosterone effect is of course abolished, but so too is the increased brain tryptophan, while the LSD effects on 5-HT and 5-HIAA continue (Halaris et al., 1975). Since the ratio of plasma free to bound tryptophan does not change with LSD, it is possible that there is a common carrier for steroids and indole compounds, and this represents yet another avenue for both animal and, subsequently, clinical study.

III. TOLERANCE DOSAGE SCHEDULES

Tolerance to LSD is a dose-dependent phenomenon, and a progressive decrement of behavioral and autonomic LSD effects in rats are not easily observed in rat with doses higher than 260 μg/kg. Effects of behavioral tolerance can be summed up as a diminished duration and magnitude (or intensity) of effects. Parasympathomimetic effects of LSD do not show tolerance, whereas sympathomimetic and mental and behavioral effects do. The changes, both of endogenous indoles and catecholamines, observed *in the first 45 min* after LSD (during the period of acute behavioral effects in rat) are speeded up after 7 daily doses. While the basis of tolerance is not evident, studies of low daily dosage (20 μg/kg) over 14-30 days, with measures of catechol and indoleamine turnover made at 18-24 hr *after* the last dose, clearly indicate dose-dependent alterations in the long-term regulation of 5-HT and NE; in general, 5-HT and NE turnover appear to be *increased* (Diaz and Huttunen, 1971; Peters, 1974a,b). We may assume, with tolerance, that the initial 60 min effect is speeded up (Freedman and Boggan, 1974), but 18-24 hr later there is also a change. Thus there appear to be compensatory events in the regulation of 5-HT turnover occurring in all probability at least over a 24-hr period, perhaps after single, but certainly after multiple, daily doses. Basic studies must now map events consequent to the 45 min effect over a 24-hr period and longer following a single dose and multiple doses. Peters and Tang (1977) find effects (elevated 5-HT) 2 weeks after daily LSD dosages.

The possibility that these compensatory changes in turnover may account for some of the after effects of LSD in humans has been raised. Bowers (1972, 1975) reported lowering of CSF 5-HIAA in a group of patients who suffered for schizophreniform reactions following LSD, as well as in good premorbid acute schizophrenia as compared to chronic schizophrenia. A negative correlation of 5-HIAA with agitation ratings and telemetered movement counts was noted in schizophrenic patients, but not in the depressive group. He notes that animal studies using raphe lesions or administration of PCPA would lend support to the idea that the central 5-HT systems play a significant inhibitory role in modulating arousal. Whether or not acute schizophrenics and the post-LSD schizophreniform states have a central 5-HT system which is defective remains to be determined. With respect to hallucinogens, the question is whether LSD induces a specific neurochemical insult, perhaps at the raphe, which then would lead to less ability to inhibit and modulate stimuli leading to overarousal (Bowers, 1975).

IV. EFFECTS OF LSD ON CATECHOLAMINES

Various studies replicate the 5-HT increase and concomitant slight decrease in NE originally observed with LSD in the rat. An increase in brain DA and tyrosine [and changes with tolerance dosage schedule (Smith et al., 1975)] has been observed. In the rabbit, the excitatory effects of LSD are diminished when synthesis of NE is inhibited; the effects can be restored with L-dopa (Horita et al., 1973), although the drug-induced pyrexia is not affected. In other species, 5-HT- and NE-mediated responses have not been as clearly differentiated.

What is clear in rat is that an enhanced sensitivity to the effects of LSD—a fourfold lowering of the requisite dosage of the drug—occurs after reserpine or tetrabenazine pretreatment (Appel and Freedman, 1964). Enhanced vulnerability to LSD so induced does not discriminate 5-HT or NE as mediating the intensity of the LSD response. Drug levels, we find, do not account for pretreatment-induced sensitivity. However, lesions of the raphe (Appel et al., 1970a), which indeed do selectively reduce serotonin, or PCPA inhibiting serotonin synthesis (Appel et al., 1970b), produce similar sensitizing effects, thus indicating a critical role for serotonin in modulating the intensity (and perhaps the duration) of the LSD behavioral and autonomic response.

Among psychotomimetics in rats, LSD has a weak and secondary effect on NE (Stolk et al., 1974). During the acute phase, slight shifts occur in NE metabolites, NE levels decrease, the synthesis of NE is minimally increased; the specific activity of NE, but not DA, is increased; however, these effects are not always observed (Persson, 1970). The pattern of altered metabolites after psychotomimetics shows no common mechanism among or across the indole and phenylethylamine groups of drugs. Mescaline initially enhances intracellular catabolism of NE, but in subsequent hours increases O-methylated metabolites, as does amphetamine and, to a marked degree, psilocybin, which shows potent and long-term effects. In summary, those psychotomimetics that are milder or less potent than LSD may have a greater and more direct effect on the synthesis and utilization of NE. Perhaps the intensity of the LSD response is linked to a *lack* of a sufficient compensatory catecholamine synthesis or to an imbalance in catechol and indole neural systems (Stolk et al., 1970).

In studies of adenylate cyclase, theoretically, one seeks nanomolar concentrations for molecularly significant effects. Thus in the thoracic ganglia of the cockroach, a cyclase is specifically activated by 5-HT and selectively inhibited by extremely low—physiological—concentrations of 5-HT, LSD, and BOL, with drug interactions in accord with observed effects in humans (Nathanson and Greengard, 1974). But in cell-free preparations from mammalian rat brain, we deal with micromolar concentrations in studies of NE- or DA-stimulated cyclase (Von Hungen et al., 1974,1975). In general, these studies indicate that LSD acts stereospecifically as both a DA agonist and antagonist, while BOL is only a DA antagonist. Yet against the cyclase story for a unified view of hallucinogenesis is the fact that mescaline, DMT, and psilocin had no parallel effects. Adenylate cyclase interactions in the striatum thus differentiate LSD from its antagonists and nonpsychoactive congeners and conform to the requirement of an antagonistic effect of BOL and LSD; however, they leave the phenomenon of cross-tolerance with psilocin and mescaline unexplained.

The finding that LSD can potently displace in vitro DA receptor binding (Burt et al., 1976) (although the reverse is not true) and findings of DA agonistic circling behavior induced by LSD (Pieri et al., 1974; Kelly and Iversen, 1975) along with the biochemical measures of changes in tyrosine NE, and DA levels after LSD clearly show the drug to have some action on catechols, the relevance of which remains to be clarified. Persson (1977a) summarized extensive studies (Persson, 1977b; Kehr and Speckenbach, 1978) of the effect of LSD on a variety of catechol systems, indicating that LSD can act as both DA agonist and antagonist, whioe BOL appears only to be an antagonist. Persson notes that only with manipulations which damage the normal function of DA systems can one demonstrate behavioral and some of the biochemical effects of LSD linked to DA. No behavioral study in the intact rat has yet been presented which convincingly demonstrates that LSD has a pure DA agonistic effect. Indeed DA antagonists, even at high doses, can fail to completely block the effects of LSD in animal studies (Menon et al., 1977); DA antagonists such as chlorpromazine were effective in startlingly low doses, 30 μg/kg, in blocking 130 μg/kg LSD, but at higher doses produced effects of their own compounding the LSD impairment in bar-pressing behavior (Ray and Marrazzi, 1961; Appel and Freedman, 1964). Electrophysiological studies of dopamine cells are conflicting (Svensson et al., 1975; Christoph et al., 1977), and unsubstantiated claims of psychotomimetic activity in humans of bufotenin and of "potent" DA effects of LSD are to be cautiously interpreted.

Pituitary DA receptors perhaps show the most potent pure agonistic effect of LSD on a mammalian DA system (Meltzer et al., 1977). LSD lowers prolactin levels while other psychotomimetic indoles increase it by 5-HT agonist effects—again illustrating the range of different 5-HT and DA receptor systems and different effects of drugs with a common behavioral effect. Persson demonstrated that LSD and BOL act at presynaptic DA autoreceptors and uniquely stimulate tyrosine hydroxylase without changing the nigroneostriatal impulse flow (Persson, 1977b). He suggests two autoreceptors sensitive to LSD: one a DA receptor and the other, stimulated by LSD and blocked by BOL, possibly a 5-HT receptor. The effect of LSD in increasing tyrosine hydroxylation may depend on the median, but *not* the dorsal raphe, and perhaps this is a link of LSD with the mescaline-stimulated median nuclei.

The effects of LSD on DA-mediated systems are obscure and difficult to clarify, and far less uniform with respect to hallucinogenics than are the 5-HT effects. The only possible implication of DA involvement and the effects of LSD in humans was found 48 hr after reserpine, where 3 of 10 female subjects not only developed a prolonged and intense LSD effect, but displayed oculogyric crises for the first time (Freedman, 1961b); this implies DA antagonism by LSD. Further, the effects of DA receptor blockade on LSD in humans are not at all clear (Schwarz et al., 1955; Isbell and Logan, 1957; Clark and Bliss, 1957). We simply do not have sufficiently compelling and replicated data that DA blocking agents are effective in specifically blocking rather than masking LSD effects; given clinically during LSD bad trips, the effects are mixed and complete blockade not at all evident.

V. STEREOSPECIFIC RECEPTORS

Whether receptor interactions are studied in the cockroach, snail, mollusk, or smooth muscle, there is a close and potent interaction between LSD and 5-HT acceptor sites. A high affinity binding of d-LSD to synaptic membrane fractions was first found with equilibrium dialysis (Farrow and Von Vunakis, 1973). Several groups have since reported on high affinity binding of [^{3}H] LSD (Bennett and Aghajanian, 1974; Bennett and Snyder, 1975, 1976; Lovell and Freedman, 1976). The most potent displacer of [^{3}H] LSD is d-LSD, followed by the 5-HT antagonist methiothepin and BOL. Among the transmitters, the most potent displacer is 5-HT; whereas 5-HT acts physiologically in concentrations as high as 100 nM, the IC_{50} values (the concentration displacing 50% of the labeled ligand) range from 200 to 1900 nM. Neither psychotomimetic potency of a drug (psilocybin and mescaline are very weak displacers) nor antagonism of 5-HT, LSD, or DA correlates directly with the [^{3}H] LSD site. A molecule does not have to act like or antagonize LSD to block stereospecific binding. In brief, the physiological significance of the range of binding studies is obscure.

At issue is whether the acceptor sites for LSD are postsynaptic or presynaptic—or both—and whether they are all identical with 5-HT acceptor sites, or whether there are several such acceptor sites. Snyder's group argue that all [^{3}H] LSD sites are postsynaptic, implying their identity with 5-HT receptors, and, analogous to his elegant findings with the opiate receptor, appear to favor interconvertibility of a single receptor as explaining binding and displacement. Yet LSD and tryptamines are potent in displacing [^{3}H] 5-HT, but 5-HT is 100-fold less potent in displacing [^{3}H] LSD (Bennett and Snyder, 1976). Our own view (from a subcellular study which systematically differentiated l from d-LSD acceptor sites) is that there are closely related acceptor sites for 5-HT and LSD, but they are all not identical; both pre- and postsynaptic and other neuronal elements bind LSD; thus there is a high binding in myelin fractions. Consideration of the enormous number of LSD acceptor sites throughout brain, and the fact that manipulation of endogenous levels of 5-HT have not been shown to affect LSD binding, along with structural characteristics of the molecule, indicates an overlap but lack of identity of 5-HT and LSD sites. LSD is also strikingly capable of acting at H_2 receptors for histamine (Green et al., 1977). Direct leads to specific serotonin receptor sites activating psychotomimetic effects have not yet appeared.

Nevertheless, a compelling physiological hypothesis is that any drug affecting brain function should have activity because of a link to endogenous ligands. We may expect that these tools may be used with increasing precision to help decode various interactions, but it is the better part of wisdom to recall that not all that binds can be viewed as a physiological receptor. With these precautions, there are 5-HT and LSD displacement studies in human CSF (Mehl et al., 1977) and in autopsied brain of schizophrenics, the latter showing a marked reduction in [^{3}H] LSD binding sites, although not in [^{3}H] 5-HT sites (Bennett et al., 1979). Studies in animals of biological changes which would reduce LSD acceptor sites would enhance interpretability of such intriguing findings.

VI. RAPHE SYSTEMS AND HALLUCINOGENS

The clarity and precision of electrophysiological data at the dorsal raphe in linking 5-HT to LSD and congeners are in sharp contrast to attempts to deduce DA or NA activity. The effects of LSD on 5-HT metabolism; the fourfold lower dose of LSD required for behavioral effects after reduction of 5-HT levels; the fact that cyclic AMP interactions in invertebrates are the most sensitive, specific, and physiologically relevant with respect to 5-HT at the molecular level (Nathanson and Greengard, 1974); and the myriad of receptor studies on transmission in the clam heart and the like, coupled with the raphe data, provide the overwhelming basis for 5-HT-LSD interactions as crucial to the mode of action of LSD.

The serotoninergic raphe system may be viewed as a pacemaker to a range of postsynaptic target areas which are variably coupled to the raphe nerve endings. Increases or decreases in the availability of 5-HT will influence electrophysiological events *both* at the raphe *and* at the postsynaptic target cells. On the soma, 5-HT inhibits firing. With release of 5-HT from terminals, the amine inhibits postsynaptic cellular assemblies. The firing of the raphe neurons at a regular rhythm keeps postsynaptic systems under tonic inhibition (Aghajanian et al., 1975). Perhaps only 15 or 20% of 5-HT in nerve endings conform to the model of a classical neuron with specialized subsynaptic thickening; the more typical are unmyelinated fibers with varicosities containing vesicles, mitochondria, and the synthetic enzyme. These occur throughout the brain and cerebral cortex and may in fact shift in physical space. Physiologically, this means that events at the raphe are "noted" in a very wide variety of different neuronal operations and brain areas. Caution should be exercised in globally generalizing the impact of both raphe and drugs on this very wide variety of postsynaptic assemblies, and given the range of inhibitory and excitatory electrical events at postsynaptic areas and the varied parameters required to assess postsynaptic response (Ruch-Monachon et al., 1976; Segal, 1976) and presynaptic events as well (Couch, 1976), global inferences should be guarded.

There is no substance much more potent in inhibiting the dorsal raphe than LSD. The drug acts as a 5-HT agonist, inhibiting neuronal firing probably by direct action on the soma and at a 5-HT receptor. All *psychoactive* indole congeners of LSD inhibit dorsal raphe firing with a potency in accord with their behavioral potency. Aghajanian characterizes the indole psychotomimetics by their differential potency: high potency at the raphe soma, but diminished potency (which does *not* mean impotency!) on postsynaptic cells. There is a mixture of inhibitory and agonistic effects on postsynaptic brainstem and limbic areas (Tebecis and DiMaria, 1972; Horn and McKay, 1973; Conrad et al., 1974). It is probable that the drug acts postsynaptically on both 5-HT and LSD acceptor sites. The data not only emphasize the sensitivity and relevance of the raphe to indole psychotomimetic drug action, but indicate that in the future, analysis of differing postsynaptic systems are key.

Unfortunately the antagonisms, attenuations, and enhancements observed with LSD in humans do not occur at the raphe soma. There is no tolerance (Trulson et al., 1977) or cross-tolerance (Aghajanian et al., 1975) with psychotomimetics, and mescaline differs. BOL does not antagonize the electrophysiological effects of LSD *either* at the raphe *or* at postsynaptic areas; potent displacers of LSD in stereospecific binding do not inhibit the raphe LSD effect. As a unit, the raphe soma, its axons, and its nerve terminals are "postsynaptic" to other nerve terminals with cell bodies originating in various brainstem NE, 5-HT, and GABA systems.

Since the raphe may respond to doses as low as 12 μg/kg of intravenous LSD, the selectivity and sensitivity for LSD of this membrane is the most potent one found in mammals. LSD acts on individual units throughout the brainstem (Couch, 1976) and in the median raphe stimulates as well as depresses cells. Mescaline has mixed actions mostly stimulating the median raphe, but with a few dorsal raphe neurons turning off. Certain state-dependent learning paradigms in rat can detect even lower doses of LSD than the raphe, but neither system detects tolerance.

Release of raphe inhibition on postsynaptic areas consequent to cessation of firing should be produced by lesioning the soma or by LSD, or by a 5-HT excess at the soma. Are *low* dose LSD effects identical to lesion effects and due solely to "disinhibition?" Or does LSD produce postsynaptic effects *in addition* to those contingent on the absence of 5-HT release? Such questions arise in the literature.

Since the array of behaviorally and clinically relevant LSD effects are impossible to obtain without LSD (which probably is acting simultaneously in a variety of cortical and subcortical brain areas), one might best search for components of the LSD response for which raphe nonfiring is accountable. The raphe-lesioned animal indeed shows a shift in sensitivity and reactivity to sensory input, as does the LSD animal. Yet when low-dose LSD is given to a lesioned animal, the characteristic LSD response occurs; the unique pattern of disruption of fixed-ratio bar pressing is evident and is *not* evident with the lesion alone (Appel et al., 1970a). The supersensitivity to LSD is also noted with the 5-HT precursor. In studies of pontine-geniculate-occipital (PGO) spiking at the lateral geniculate, LSD *or* 5-HTP *or* raphe stimulation *inhibit* the spiking; a raphe lesion *releases* spiking, thus differentiating the *postsynaptic effects* of soma nonfiring due to lesions and LSD inhibition of the soma, when LSD is *also* postsynaptically acting as a 5-HT agonist at relatively low dosage. Raphe stimulation (which *increases* 5-HT turnover)—or a raphe lesion—induces dehabituation, but failure to habituate to repeated stimuli was long noted (Key and Bradley, 1958) as a low- *or* high-dose effect of LSD—and LSD *decreases* turnover. The point is that too much or too little 5-HT (or LSD) at postsynaptic sites has not explained some of the general effects on dehabituation. Mechanisms and definitions of habituation and sensitization are relevant, and there may be component aspects that are raphe-specific (Davis and Sheard, 1974). Thus components of the LSD response may or may not be evoked with very low-dose LSD acting solely to release tonic inhibition, but it is clear that postsynaptic actions of LSD are necessary to hallucinogenesis; in humans, dosages 4-5 times the threshold dose enhance the psychotomimetic effects. Depression of raphe firing, then, may (or may not) be necessary, but certainly is *not* a sufficient explanation for the LSD psychotomimetic effects.

While there is a fair correlation between the first 45-min period of biochemical change and lack of raphe firing, events at the nerve terminal—where biochemical effects are measured—are probably semi-independent of transmission from the raphe soma. Our preliminary studies on biochemical effects after raphe lesions indicate that for the first 3 days the characteristic LSD decrement in 5-HIAA and increment in 5-HT occur; and several weeks later, as sprouting and regeneration occur, LSD biochemical effects are evident (Freedman and Halaris, 1978). Thus raphe-lesioned animals will show an LSD response, *both* behaviorally and biochemically, and while the "release" of postsynaptic areas may enhance some characteristics of sensitization to input and dehabituation, these are not events solely contingent on the activity or inactivity of the LSD-sensitive neuronal element in the dorsal raphe.

VII. CLINICAL-ANIMAL CORRELATIONS

To construct a comprehensive picture of hallucinogenic drug action, the absence of replicated and well-designed clinical definitions is complicating. In humans there is a threshold dose (20-50 μg) for the characteristic sequence of fundamental changes upon which set and setting provide variability. Subthreshold doses have not been sufficiently studied (Greiner et al., 1958). There have been attempts with substituted phenylethylamines or low-dose LSD to produce a fluidity of associations without the attendant florid psychedelic state and illusory and hallucinatory phenomena. In smooth muscle, low doses are often agonistic rather than antagonistic. In view of the proposition of a "pure" disinhibited serotonin system with low LSD doses, such study is critical. With these clinical distinctions in mind, a focus in animals on components of response within the human LSD state is relevant, e.g., the dehabituation to familiar stimuli, the breakdown of perceptual constancies, failure to suppress a previous perceptual input (leading to an experiential coexistence of what is being seen and what has just been seen), the persistence of perceptions and memories evoked in the drug state, etc., all require study (Freedman, 1968).

Dose effects relevant to humans require testing in animals. In humans, it is *not* possible to have the sequence of psychedelic events without a concomitant mydriasis (which is dose-dependent in magnitude and duration) (Freedman, 1968). This centrally mediated sympathomimetic effect has not been sufficiently investigated in terms of dose thresholds in animals.

In humans, tolerance to both the mental effects and mydriasis occur in 3 or 4 days, and full sensitivity is restored within 4 or 5 days, and this can be seen for certain behavioral and sympathomimetic effects in rat (Freedman and Boggan, 1974). But the effect of BOL in humans requires further study. Because of limited research design, we do not know if BOL truly blocks or if, as is likely, daily doses of BOL are initially needed to produce what would then be a cross-tolerance rather than a blockade (Clark and Bliss, 1957; Murphree et al., 1958; Abramson et al., 1958; Isbell et al., 1959; Balestrieri and Fontanari, 1959). The same is true for the question of NE and DA blocking agents. It is fairly easy to block amphetamine in humans, but this has not been demonstrated in a truly satisfactory way for LSD. Today a variety of interesting agonists and antagonists, if cogently tested clinically, could clarify underlying mediating mechanisms, including the question of NE-5-HT imbalance with LSD.

Further, early studies showed that reserpine could enhance the intensity of effects in humans (Isbell and Logan, 1957). In an amine behavior paradigm—48-72 hr *after* reserpine when the acute drug effects were over—the experience was enhanced and prolonged with elements of clouded consciousness (Freedman, 1961b). Since in animals this postdepletion sensitivity can occur even when amine levels have reached 85-90% repletion, a very *small* change in amine levels may indeed influence the *intensity* of some of the *component* events within an LSD response. This has not been tested in humans, but if disease affects the previous state of amines, and this is what leads to variable response to amine precursors and drugs, there is a logic that could be fruitfully pursued here as it has with 5-HT synthesis inhibition in the depressions (Shopsin et al., 1976).

There is dubiety that bufotenin or the biologically interesting harmaline analogs yohimbine or methysergide are indeed psychotomimetic, and no data on how they compare to LSD. A conservative view is warranted. Shulgin et al., using substituted amphetamines, have attempted some comparative studies in humans (Shulgin, 1969), but current ethical constraints make future study unlikely. Thus many, like Bowers (1975), undertake biochemical and clinical studies in patients who have misused drugs.

Finally, in all discussions of model psychoses, researchers have ignored the second phase of the LSD response (Freedman, 1968). Most of the electrophysiological and biochemical work in rats and humans has focused on the first phase: the "TV show in the head." Yet the second 4 hours post-LSD in humans are accompanied by ideas of reference in which Schneiderian symptoms generally dissipate about the time at which pupil size has returned to normal. If we are interested in compensatory neuroregulatory response after the LSD effect—which occurs in animals—this is another area for fruitful study.

Thus to achieve a comprehensive picture of the psychedelic state, a number of combined biochemical, neurophysiological, and neurobehavioral studies in animals and humans lie ahead. There is no reason to anticipate that a biochemical or electrophysiological change in itself must necessarily be directly coupled to the phenomena under review. Nevertheless, there are electrophysiological studies in animals which are congruent with what we know to occur in humans; some (the enhancement of sensory systems and simultaneous inhibition of cortical systems) have been noted. More recently noted are EEG signs in animals of a general shift in attentiveness and valuation of positive reinforcement (Winters and Wallach, 1970; Brooks, 1975), which is coupled behaviorally with enhanced sensitivity to stimuli and noxious input. In animals, sensitivity to noxious input (as in all conditioned avoidance paradigms) is quite evident. Indeed, tolerance to LSD does not occur to behaviors dependent on noxious input. This, however, approximates the effects in humans in which lay experimenters note a vulnerability to unpleasant events to which they appear sensitized. The drug produces an ambivalent pleasure-pain evaluation of the experience in which demands of reality are disregarded, if possible, in favor of attending to a private experience in which ordinary stimuli become novel and vivid, and noxious stimuli highly aversive and disruptive. Yet a lag of neurobehavioral and electrophysiological study of these events still persists. Thus some speculate that LSD might indicate a state of "dreaming while awake." LSD does not induce a release of PGO spiking (which might accompany such a dreaming state) but rather, like the 5-HT precursor (Jouvet, 1967), delays the onset of REM sleep and diminishes both REM percent and REM PGO spiking (Brooks, 1975). Nevertheless, raphe do stop firing prior to this spiking. Thus new brainstem studies of input to the raphe are likely, and electrophysiological measures in humans correlating with these brain events are feasible and may guide neurobiologists.

In brief, the search for biobehavioral mechanisms by which altered states are accommodated can be advanced with various such hypotheses tested between animals and humans. This is the challenge to investigators utilizing the ever-widening array of research techniques which may someday relevantly delineate the mode of hallucinogenic drug action.

REFERENCES

Abramson, H. A., Sklarofsky, B., Baron, M. O., and Fremont-Smith, N. (1958). Lysergic acid diethylamide (LSD-25) antagonists. II. Development of tolerance in man to LSD-25 by prior administration of MLD-41 (l-methyl-d-lysergic acid diethylamide). *Arch. Neurol. Psychiatry 79,* 201.

Aghajanian, G. K., Haigler, H. J., and Bennett, J. L. (1975). Amine receptors in CNS. III. 5-hydroxytryptamine in brain. In *Handbook of Psychopharmacology,* Vol. 6. L. L. Iversen, S. D. Iversen, and S. H. Snyder (Eds.). Plenum, New York, pp. 63-69.

Appel, J. B., and Freedman, D. X. (1964). Chemically-induced alterations in the behavioral effects of LSD-25. *Biochem. Pharmacol. 13,* 861-869.

Appel, J. B., and Freedman, D. X. (1965). The relative potencies of psychomimetic drugs. *Life Sci. 4,* 2181-2186.

Appel, J. B., and Freedman, D. X. (1968). Tolerance and cross-tolerance among psychotomimetic drugs. *Psychopharmacologia* (Berlin) *13,* 267-274.

Appel, J. B., Sheard, M. H., and Freedman, D. X. (1970a). Alterations in the behavioral effects of LSD by mid-brain raphe lesions. *Comm. Behav. Biol., Part A, 5,* 237-241.

Appel, J. B., Lovell, R. A., and Freedman, D. X. (1970b). Alterations in the behavioral effects of LSD by pretreatment with p-chlorophenylalanine and a-methyl-p-tyrosine. *Psychopharmacologia* (Berlin) *18,* 387-406.

Balestrieri, A., and Fontanari, D. (1959). Acquired and crossed tolerance to mescaline, LSD-25, and BOL-148. *Arch. Gen. Psychiatry 1,* 279.

Barchas, J. D., and Freedman, D. X. (1963). Brain amines. Response to physiological stress. *Biochem. Pharmacol. 12,* 1225.

Bennett, J. L., and Aghajanian, G. K. (1974). D-LSD binding to brain homogenates: possible relationship to serotonin receptors. *Life Sci. 15,* 1935.

Bennett, J. P., and Snyder, S. H. (1975). Stereospecific binding of d-lysergic acid diethylamide (LSD) to brain membranes. Relationship to serotonin receptors. *Brain Res. 94,* 523-544.

Bennett, J. P., Jr., and Snyder, S. H. (1976). Serotonin receptor binding in rat brain membranes. *Mol. Pharmacol. 12,* 373-389.

Bennett, J. P., Jr., Salvatore, J. E., Bylund, D. B., Gillin, J. C., Wyatt, R. J., and Snyder, S. H. (1979). Neurotransmitter receptor binding alterations in schizophrenic brain. *Arch. Gen. Psychiatry.* In press.

Bowers, M. B., Jr. (1972). Acute psychosis induced by psychotomimetic drug abuse. I. Clinical findings. *Arch. Gen. Psychiatry 27,* 437-439.

Bowers, M. B., Jr. (1975). Serotonin (5HT) systems in psychotic states. *Psychopharmacol. Comm. 1,* 655-662.

Bowers, M. B., and Freedman, D. X. (1966). "Psychedelic" experiences in acute psychoses. *Arch. Gen. Psychiatry 15,* 240.

Braude, M. C., and Szara, S. (Eds.) (1976). *Pharmacology of Marihuana* (2 vols.). Raven, New York.

Brodie, B. B., Shore, P. A., and Pletscher, A. (1956). Serotonin-releasing activity limited to rauwolfia alkaloids with tranquilizing action. *Science 123,* 992-993.

Brooks, D. C. (1975). The effect of LSD upon spontaneous PGO wave activity and REM sleep in the cat. *Neuropharmacology 14,* 847-857.

Burt, D. R., Creese, I., and Snyder, S. H. (1976). Binding interactions of lysergic acid diethylamide and related agents with dopamine receptors in the brain. *Mol. Pharmacol. 12,* 631-638.

Cameron, O. G., and Appel, J. B. (1973). A behavioral and pharmacological analysis of some discriminable properties of d-LSD in rats. *Psychopharmacologia 33,* 117-134.

Carlsson, A., and Lindqvist, M. (1963). Effect of chlorpromazine or haloperidol on formation of 3-methoxytyramine and normetanephrine in mouse brain. *Acta Pharmacol. Toxicol.* (Kbh.) *20,* 140-144.

Christoph, G. R., Kuhn, D. M., and Jacobs, B. L. (1977). Electrophysiological evidence for a dopaminergic action of LSD. Depression of unit activity in the substantia nigra of the rat. *Life Sci. 21,* 1585-1596.

Clark, L. D., and Bliss, E. L. (1957). Psychopharmacological studies of lysergic acid diethylamide (LSD-25) intoxication. Effects of premedication with BOL-148 (2-bromo-d-lysergic acid diethylamide), mescaline, atropine, amobarbital, and chlorpromazine. *Arch. Neurol. Psychiatry 78,* 653.

Cohen, S. M., Nichols, A., Wyatt, R., and Pollin, W. (1974). The administration of methionine to chronic schizophrenia patients. A review of ten studies. *Biol. Psychiatry 8,* 209-225.

Collins, B. J., Lovell, R. A., Boggan, W. O., and Freedman, D. X. (1970). Effects of hallucinogens on rat brain monoamine oxidase activity. *Pharmacologist 12,* 256.

Conrad, L. C. A., Leonard, C. M., and Pfaff, D. W. (1974). Connections of the median and dorsal raphe nuclei in the rat. An autoradiographic and degeneration study. *J. Comp. Neurol. 156,* 179-205.

Cooper, H. A. (1955). Hallucinogenic drugs. *Lancet 268,* 1078.

Couch, J. R. (1976). Action of LSD on raphe neurons and effect on presumed serotonergic raphe synapses. *Brain Res. 110,* 417-424.

Dahlstrom, A., and Fuxe, K. (1965). Evidence for the existence of monoamine-containing neurons in the central nervous system. I. Demonstration of monoamines in the cell bodies of brain stem neurons. *Acta Physiol. Scand. 62 (supplement 232),* 1-55.

Davis, M., and Sheard, M. H. (1974). Habituation and sensitization of the rat startle response. Effects of raphe lesions. *Physiol. Behav. 12,* 425-431.

Diaz, J. L., and Huttunen, M. O. (1971). Persistent increase in brain serotonin turnover after chronic administration of LSD in the rat. *Science 174,* 62-64.

Elkes, C., Elkes, J., and Mayer-Gross, W. (1955). Hallucinogenic drugs. *Lancet 268,* 719.

Evarts, E. V., Landau, W., Freygang, E., and Marshall, W. H. (1955). Some effects of lysergic acid diethylamide and bufotenine on electrical activity in the cat's visual system. *J. Physiol. 182,* 594.

Farrow, J. T., and Von Vunakis, H. (1973). Characteristics of D-lysergic acid diethylamide to subcellular fractions derived from rat brain. *Biochem. Pharmacol. 22,* 1103-1113.

Freedman, D. X. (1960). LSD-25 and brain serotonin in reserpinized rat. *Fed. Proc. 19,* 266.

Freedman, D. X. (1961a). Effects of LSD-25 on brain serotonin. *J. Pharmacol. Exp. Ther. 134,* 160.

Freedman, D. X. (1961b). Studies of LSD-25 and serotonin in the brain. *Proc. 3rd World Cong. Psychiatry 1,* 653.

Freedman, D. X. (1963). Psychotomimetic drugs and brain biogenic amines. *Am. J. Psychiatry 119,* 843.

Freedman, D. X. (1968). On the use and abuse of LSD. *Arch. Gen.Psychiatry 18,* 330-331.

Freedman, D. X., and Aghajanian, G. K. (1959). Time parameters in acute tolerance, cross tolerance, and antagonism to psychotogens. *Fed. Proc. 18,* 390.

Freedman, D. X., and Benton, A. J. (1961). Persisting effects of reserpine in man. *N. Engl. J. Med. 264,* 529.

Freedman, D. X., and Boggan, W. O. (1974). Brain serotonin metabolism after tolerance dosage of LSD. In *Advances in Biochemical Psychopharmacology,* Vol. 10, Raven, New York.

Freedman, D. X., and Halaris, A. E. (1973). The role of serotonin in the action of psychotomimetic drugs. (Abs.) Presented at 3rd Ann. Meet. Soc. Neurosci.

Freedman, D. X., and Halaris, A. E. (1978). Monoamines and the biochemical mode of action of LSD at synapses. In *Psychopharmacology,* M. A. Lipton, A. L. DiMascio, and K. F. Killam (Eds.). Raven, New York.

Freedman, D. X., Gottlieb, R., and Lovell, R. A. (1970). Psychotomimetic drugs and brain 5-hydroxytryptamine metabolism. *Biochem. Pharmacol. 19,* 1181-1188.

Friedhoff, A. J., Park, S., and Schweitzer, J. W. (1977). Excretion of 3,4-dimethoxyphenethylamide (DMPEA) by acute schizophrenics and controls. *Biol. Psychiatry 12,* 643-654.

Gaddum, J. H. (1953). Antagonism between lysergic acid diethylamide and 5-hydroxytryptamine. *J. Physiol. 121,* 15.

Gallager, D. W., and Aghajanian, G. K. (1975). Effects of chlorimipramine and lysergic acid diethylamide on efflux of precursor-formed ^{3}H-serotonin. Correlations with serotonergic impulse flow. *J. Pharmacol. Exp. Ther. 193,* 785-795.

Gillin, J. C., Kaplan, J., Stillman, R., and Wyatt, R. J. (1976). The psychedelic model of schizophrenia. The case of N-N-dimethyltryptamine. *Am. J. Psychiatry 133,* 203-207.

Green, J. P., Johnson, C. L., Weinstein, H., and Maayani, S. (1977). Antagonism of histamine-activated adenylate cyclase in brain by D-lysergic acid diethylamide. *Proc. Nat. Acad. Sci. USA 74,* 5697-5701.

Halaris, A. E., and Freedman, D. X. (1977). Vesicular and juxtavesicular serotonin. Effects of lysergic acid diethylamide and reserpine. *J. Pharmacol. Exp. Ther. 203,* 575-586.

Halaris, A. E., Freedman, D. X., and Fang, V. S. (1975). Plasma corticoids and brain tryptophan after acute and tolerance dosage of LSD. *Life Sci. 17,* 1467-1472.

Hirschhorn, I. D., Hayes, R. L., and Rosecrans, J. A. (1975). Discriminitive control of behavior by electrical stimulation of the dorsal raphe nucleus. Generalization of lysergic acid diethylamide (LSD). *Brain Res. 86,* 134-138.

Horita, A., and Hamilton, A. E. (1973). The effects of DL-x-Methyltyrosine and L-dopa on the hyperthermic and behavioral actions of LSD in rabbits. *Neuropharmacology 12,* 471-476.

Horn, G., and McKay, J. M. (1973). Effects of lysergic acid diethylamide on the spontaneous activity and visual reseptive fields of cells in the lateral geniculate nucleus of the cat. *Exp. Brain Res. 17,* 271-284.

Isbell, H., and Logan, C. R. (1957). Studies on the diethylamide of lysergic acid (LSD-25). II. Effects of chlorpromazine, azacyclonol, and reserpine on the intensity of the LSD-reaction. *Arch. Neurol. Psychiatry 77,* 350.

Isbell, H., Logan, C. R., and Miner, E. J. (1959). Relationships of psychotomimetic to anti-serotonin potencies of congeners of lysergic acid diethylamide (LSD-25). *Psychopharmacologia* (Berlin) *1,* 20-28.

Isbell, H., Wolbach, A. B., Wikler, A., and Miner, E. J. (1961). Cross tolerance between LSD and psilocybin. *Psychopharmacologia 2,* 147-159.

Jouvet, M. (1967). In *Sleep and Altered States of Consciousness,* S. S. Kety, E. V. Evarts, and H. Williams (Eds.). Williams & Wilkins, Baltimore.

Kehr, W., and Speckenbach, W. (1978). Effect of lisuride and LSD on monoamine synthesis after axotomy or reserpine treatment in rat brain. *Arch. Pharmacol. 301,* 163-169.

Kelly, P. H., and Iversen, L. L. (1975). LSD as an agonist at mesolimbic dopamine receptors. *Psychopharmacologia* (Berlin) *45,* 221-224.

Key, B. J., and Bradley, P. B. (1958). Effect on drugs on conditioning and habituation to arousal stimuli in animals. *Nature 182,* 1517.

Kovacic, B., and Domino, E. F. (1976). Tolerance and limited cross tolerance to the effects of N,N-dimethyltryptamine lysergic acid diethylamide (LSD-25) on food rewarded bar pressing in the rat. *J. Pharmacol. Exp. Ther. 197,* 495-502.

Lin, R. C., Ngai, S. H., and Costa, E. (1969). Lysergic acid diethylamide: Role in conversion of plasma tryptophan to brain serotonin (5-hydroxytryptamine). *Science 166,* 237-239.

Lovell, R. A., and Freedman, D. X. (1974). Compartmental analysis of the LSD-serotonin interaction in the rat brain. *Trans. Am. Soc. Neurochem. 5,* 155.

Lovell, R. A., and Freedman, D. X. (1976). Stereospecific receptor sites for d-lysergic acid diethylamide in rat brain. Effects of neurotransmitters, amine antagonists and other psychotropic drugs. *Mol. Pharmacol. 12,* 620-630.

Luby, E. D., Gottlieb, J. S., Cohen, B. D., Rosenbaum, G., and Domino, E. G. (1962). Model psychoses and schizophrenia. *Am. J. Psychiatry 19,* 61.

Marchbanks, R. M. (1967). Inhibitory effects of lysergic acid derivatives and reserpine on 5-HT binding to nerve ending particles. *Biochem. Pharmacol. 16,* 1971-1979.

Marrazzi, A. S., and Hart, E. R. (1955). Evoked cortical responses under the influence of hallucinogens and related drugs. *Electroenceph. Cl. Neurophysiol. 7,* 146.

Mehl, E., Ruther, E., and Redemann, J. (1977). Endogenous ligands of a putative LSD-serotonin receptor in the cerebrospinal fluid. Higher level of LSD-displacing factors (LDF) in unmedicated psychotic patients. *Psychopharmacology 54,* 9-16.

Meltzer, H. Y., Fessler, R. G., Simonovic, M., Doherty, J., and Fang, V. S. (1977). Lysergic acid diethylamide. Evidence for stimulation of pituitary dopamine receptors. *Psychopharmacology 54,* 39-44.

Menon, M. K., Clark, W. G., and Masuoka, D. T. (1977). Possible involvement of the central dopaminergic system in the antireserpine effect of LSD. *Psychopharmacology 52,* 291-297.

Murphree, H. B., DeMaar, E. W. J., Williams, H. L., and Bryan, L. L. (1958). Effects of lysergic acid derivatives on man; antagonism between d-lysergic acid diethylamide and its 2-brom congener. *J. Pharmacol. Exp. Ther. 122,* 55A.

Nathanson, J. A., and Greengard, P. (1974). Serotonin-sensitive adenylate cyclase in neural tissue and its similarity to the serotonin receptor. A possible site of action of lysergic acid diethylamide. *Proc. Nat. Acad. Sci. USA 71,* 797-801.

Newell, H. W., and Lidz, T. (1946). The toxicity of Atabrine to the central nervous system. *Am. J. Psychiatry 102,* 805.

Persson, T. (1970). Drug induced changes in ^{3}H-catecholamine accumulation after ^{3}H-tyrosine. *Acta. Pharmacol. Toxicol. 28,* 378-390.

Persson, S-A. (1977a). Effects of lysergic acid diethylamide (LSD) and 2-bromo lysergic acid diethylamide (BOL) on central cathecholaminergic pathways—A biochemical study. *UMEA University Medical Dissertations No. 32,* University of Umea, Sweden.

Persson, S-A. (1977b). The effect of LSD and 2-bromo LSD on the striatal dopa accumulation after decarboxylase inhibition in rats. *Eur. J. Pharmacol. 43,* 73-83.

Peters, D. A. V. (1974a). Comparison of the chronic and acute effects of d-Lysergic acid diethylamide (LSD) treatment on rat brain serotonin and norepinephrine. *Biochem. Pharmacol. 23,* 231-237.

Peters, D. A. V. (1974b). Chronic lysergic acid diethylamide administration and serotonin turnover in various regions of rat brain. *J. Neurochem. 23,* 625-627.

Peters, D. A. V., and Tang, S. (1977). Persistent effects of repeated injections of D-lysergic acid diethylamide on rat brain 5-hydroxytryptamine and 5-hydroxyindoleacetic acid levels. *Biochem. Pharmacol. 26,* 1085-1086.

Pieri, L., Pieri, M., and Haefely, W. (1974). LSD as an agonist of dopamine receptors in the striatum. *Nature 252,* 586-588.

Puhringer, W., Wirz-Justice, A., and Lancranjan, I. (1976). Mood elevation and pituitary stimulation after i.v. 1-5-HTP in normal subjects. Evidence for a common serotoninergic mechanism. *Neurosci. Lett. 2,* 349-354.

Purpura, D. P. (1956a). Electrophysiological analysis of psychotogenic drug action. II. General nature of lysergic acid diethylamide (LSD) action on central synapses. *Arch. Neurol. Psychiatry 75,* 132.

Purpura, D. P. (1956b). Electrophysiological analysis of psychotogenic drug action. I. Effect of LSD on specific afferent systems in the cat. *Arch. Neurol. Psychiatry 75,* 122.

Purpura, D. P., Pool, J. L., Ransohoff, J., Frumin, M. J., and Housepian, E. M. (1957). Observations on evoked dendritic potentials of human cortex. *EEG Cl. Neurophysiol. 9,* 453.

Ray. O. S., and Marrazzi, A. S. (1961). A quantifiable behavioral correlate of psychotogen and tranquilizer actions. *Science 133,* 1705-1706.

Rosecrans, J. A., Lovell, R. A., and Freedman, D. X. (1967). Effects on lysergic acid diethylamide on the metabolism of brain 5-hydroxytryptamine. *Biochem. Pharmacol. 16,* 2011-2021.

Ruch-Monachon, M. A., Jalfre, M., and Haefely, W. (1976). Drugs and PGO waves in the lateral geniculate body of the curarized cat. *Arch. Int. Pharmacodyn. Ther. 219,* 269-286.

Schwarz, B. E., Bickford, R. G., and Rome, H. P. (1955). Reversibility of induced psychosis with chlorpromazine. *Proc. Staff Meet. Mayo Clinic 30,* 407.

Segal, M. (1976). 5-HT antagonists in rat hippocampus. *Brain Res. 103,* 161-166.

Shopsin, B., Friedman, E., and Gershon, S. (1976). Parachlorophenylalanine reversal of tranylcypromine effects in depressed patients. *Arch. Gen. Psychiatry 33,* 811-819.

Shulgin, A. T., Sargent, T., and Naranjo, C. (1969). Structure-activity relationships of one-ring psychotomimetics. *Nature 221,* 537-541.

Siegel, R. K., and West, L. J. (Eds.) (1975). *Hallucinations: Behavior, Experience and Theory.* Wiley, New York.

Smith, R. C., Boggan, W. O., and Freedman, D. X. (1975). Effects of single and multiple dose LSD on endogenous levels of brain tyrosine and catecholamines. *Psychopharmacologia* (Berlin) *42,* 271-276.

Stolk, J. M., Barchas, J. D., Goldstein, M., Boggan, W. O., and Freedman, D. X. (1974). A comparison of psychotomimetic drug effects on rat brain norepinephrine metabolism. *J. Pharmacol. Exp. Ther. 189,* 42-50.

Svensson, T. H., Bunney, B. S., and Aghajanian, G. K. (1975). Inhibition of both noradrenergic and serotonergic neurons in brain by the a-Adrenergic agonist clonidine. *Brain Res. 92,* 291-306.

Tamir, H., and Rapport, M. M. (1978). Effects of neurotoxins in vitro on the binding of serotonin to serotonin-binding protein. In *Serotonin Neurotoxins,* J. H. Jacoby and L. D. Lytle (Eds.). N. Y. Acad. Sci., New York.

Tebecis, A. K., and DiMaria, A. (1972). A re-evaluation of the mode of action of 5-hydroxytryptamine on lateral geniculate neurons: comparison with catecholamines and LSD. *Exp. Brain Res. 14,* 480-493.

Trulson, M. E., and Jacobs, B. L. (1977). Usefulness of an animal behavioral model in studying the duration of action of LSD and the onset and duration of tolerance of LSD in the cat. *Brain Res. 132,* 315-326.

Trulson, M. E., Ross, C. A., and Jacobs, B. L. (1977). Lack of tolerance of the depression of raphe unit activity by l sergic acid diethylamide. *Neuropharmacology 16,* 771-774.

Twarog, B. M., and Page, I. H. (1953). Serotonin content of some mammalian tissues and urine and a method for its determinations. *Am. J. Physiol. 175,* 157-161.

Vaupel, D. B., Nozaki, M., Martin, W. R., and Bright, L. D. (1978). Single dose and cross tolerance studies of B-phenethylamine, d-amphetamine and LSD in the chronic spinal dog. *Eur. J. Pharmacol. 48,* 431-437.

von Hungen, K., Roberts, S., and Hill, D. F. (1974). LSD as an agonist and antagonist at central dopamine receptors. *Nature 252,* 588-589.

von Hungen, K., Roberts, S., and Hill, D. F. (1975). Interactions between lysergic acid diethylamide and dopamine-sensitive adenylate cyclase systems in rat brain. *Brain Res. 94,* 57-66.

Winters, W., and Wallach, M. (1970). Drug induced states of CNS excitation. A theory of hallucinosis. In *Psychotomimetic Drugs,* D. H. Efron (Ed.). Raven, New York, pp. 193-214.

Winters, J. C. (1971). Tolerance to a behavioral effect of lysergic acid diethylamide and cross-tolerance to mescaline in the rat. Absence of a metabolic component. *J. Pharmacol. Exp. Ther. 178,* 625-630.

Winters, J. C. (1978). Stimulus properties of phenethylamine hallucinogens and lysergic acid diethylamide. The role of 5-hydroxytryptamine. *J. Pharmacol. Exp. Ther. 204,* 416-423.

Wolbach, A. B., Jr., Miner, E. J., and Isbell, H. (1962). Comparison of psilocin with psilocybin, mesacline and LSD-25. *Psychopharmacologia 3,* 219-223.

Woolley, D. W., and Shaw, E. (1954). A biochemical and pharmacological suggestion about certain mental disorders. *Proc. Nat. Acad. Sci. USA 40,* 228-231.

Ziegler, M. G., Lovell, R. A., and Freedman, D. X. (1973). Effects of lysergic acid diethylamide on the uptake and retention of brain 5-hydroxytryptamine in vivo and in vitro. *Biochem. Pharmacol. 22,* 2183-2193.

Author Index

Numbers indicate that an author's work is referred to. Italic numbers give the page on which the complete reference is listed.

A

C

D

F

G

H

N

O

P

T

Subject Index

D

L

M

N

O

P

T

U

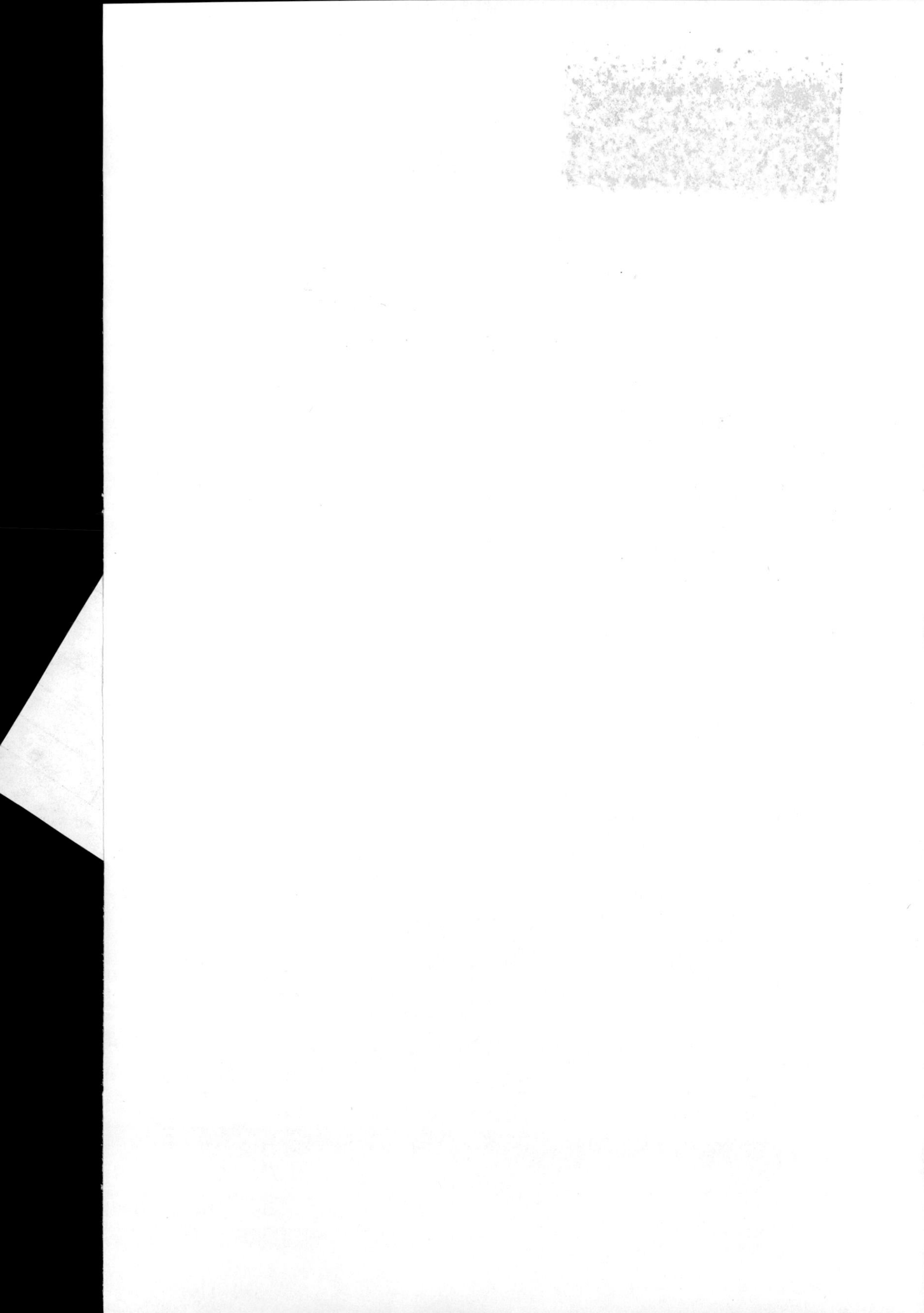

Northern Michigan University
3 1854 003 296 954
EZNO
RC455.4 B5 H35 pt. 4
Brain mechanisms and abnormal behavior-c